Current Chemotherapy and Infectious Disease

Proceedings of the 11th International
Congress of Chemotherapy and the
19th Interscience Conference on
Antimicrobial Agents and Chemotherapy

Volume I

Current Chemotherapy
and
Infectious Disease

Proceedings of the 11th International Congress of Chemotherapy and the 19th Interscience Conference on Antimicrobial Agents and Chemotherapy

Boston, Massachusetts • 1–5 October 1979

Editors:

John D. Nelson
The University of Texas
Southwestern Medical School, Dallas
Dallas, Texas, U.S.A.

Carlo Grassi
Institute of Carlo Forlanini
Pavia, Italy

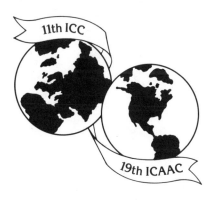

Volume I

Published by
The American Society for Microbiology
Washington, DC
1980

Library of Congress Cataloging in Publication Data

International Congress of Chemotherapy, 11th, Boston, 1979.
    Current chemotherapy and infectious disease.

    Includes indexes.
    1. Communicable diseases—Chemotherapy—Congresses. 2. Cancer—Chemotherapy—Congresses. 3. Anti-infective agents—Congresses. 4. Antineoplastic agents—Congresses. I. Nelson, John D. II. Grassi, Carlo. III. American Society for Microbiology. IV. Interscience Conference on Antimicrobial Agents and Chemotherapy, 19th, Boston, 1979. V. Title. [DNLM: 1. Anti-infective agents—Congresses. 2. Antineoplastic agents—Congresses. 3. Communicable diseases—Drug therapy—Congresses. W3 IN351 11th 1979/QV250 I61 1979c]
RC110.I58 1979   616.9'0461   79-28826

ISBN 0-914826-22-0 (set)

CONTENTS

VOLUME I

Preface

The skies of Boston were gray and gloomy and the streets were damp and empty. Vehicular traffic had been banned because of the visit of Pope John Paul II. The crowds who had watched and cheered the Pope had moved to the Commons to celebrate mass in the rain. Around the Sheraton-Prudential Center, Boston appeared like a deserted city as the opening session of the Congress got underway. Even the walls of the Hynes Auditorium were gray and gloomy. But, as soon as the New England Conservatory Ragtime Ensemble began to play their captivating and infectiously jolly tunes, the mood changed and spirits lifted. The Congress was off to a happy start and the many months of work by the organizational committees and by the staff of the American Society for Microbiology was in the crucible.

In October 1965 the 4th International Congress of Chemotherapy and the 5th Interscience Conference on Antimicrobial Agents and Chemotherapy met jointly at the Shoreham Hotel in Washington, D.C. There were 286 papers presented and approximately 1,000 registrants. During the intervening 14 years both meetings flourished. For the 1979 meeting, the Scientific Program Committee was overwhelmed by 1,776 submitted abstracts (the number of 1,776 was a particularly appropriate one for a meeting held in the historic city of Boston), and there were over 5,600 registrants. Size is an easily measurable factor. Quality is a more elusive one, but those of us who have attended these meetings over the years recognize the immense—perhaps geometric—rise in the scientific quality of our meetings. This makes the selection process by the Scientific Program Committee ever more difficult, but assures excellence in the program.

The Congress was the largest meeting of its kind ever held. That might be considered our salute to the fiftieth anniversary of the discovery of penicillin by Fleming in 1929. The unexpectedly large attendance created some problems, with distant hotels and overcrowded session rooms, but it also created an aura of excitement with the knowledge that virtually all of the major international figures in chemotherapy and infectious diseases were together in one spot. This is a major function that an international congress serves: the opportunity to meet person-to-person with people who may have been only names on journal articles. The social and cultural events stimulate this interpersonal contact.

The format used in this book was devised for the published proceedings of the International Congress of Chemotherapy held in Zurich in 1977. It was widely acclaimed as an excellent means of rapid publication and dissemination of all the essential data from papers and the major points of symposia. The extended abstract concept stresses results and minimizes methodology and references. Publication of a complete summation of a meeting within five months is not unprecedented—it was done after the Zurich Congress—but it is an extraordinary feat! The conciseness and easy accessibility of a massive amount of information means that these two volumes should serve as useful references for many years.

Throughout the three and one-half days of the Congress the air of enthusiasm and excitement was maintained. The scientific level of presentations exceeded that of previous years, and we cannot recall a year when so many unique and potentially useful drugs were introduced. The affiliation of the American Society for Microbiology and the International Society of Chemotherapy seems to have been a synergistic one.

The Editors

John D. Nelson
Dallas, Texas, U.S.A.

Carlo Grassi
Pavia, Italy

11th International Congress of Chemotherapy
19th Interscience Conference on Antimicrobial Agents and
Chemotherapy

1–5 October 1979   Boston, Massachusetts

ORGANIZATION

Officers of the Congress

President: John D. Nelson, University of Texas Southwestern Medical School, Dallas, Texas, U.S.A.
Co-President: Carlo Grassi, Institute of Carlo Forlanini, Pavia, Italy
Secretary-General: Raymond W. Sarber, American Society for Microbiology, 1913 I St., N.W., Washington, D.C. 20006, U.S.A.

Executive Committee
John D. Nelson, *Chairman*
Roy Cleeland
Gladys L. Hobby
George H. Warren
George B. Whitfield, Jr.
Raymond W. Sarber

Scientific Program Committee
John D. Nelson, *Chairman*
Roy Cleeland, *Vice-Chairman*
George H. Warren, *Vice-Chairman*
George Arcieri
William E. Brown
Theodore C. Eickhoff
Francis A. Ennis
Martin Forbes
Thomas C. Hall
George A. Jacoby
Janusz Jeljaszewicz
Karl Karrer
Helmut P. Kuemmerle
Harold P. Lambert
Georges Mathé
Robert C. Moellering, Jr.
Harold C. Neu
Paul G. Quie
George B. Whitfield
Yukimasa Yagisawa

Officers of the American Society for Microbiology

Willis A. Wood, *President*
Albert Balows, *President-Elect*
Joseph M. Joseph, *Secretary*
Brinton M. Miller, *Treasurer*

Finance Committee
George B. Whitfield, Jr., *Chairman*

Special Events Committee
Gladys L. Hobby, *Chairman*
Ann E. Coghlan
Arnold L. Demain
George A. Jacoby
Jerome O. Klein
John E. Lynch
Robert C. Moellering, Jr.
Larry Nathanson

Advisory Committee
Ruedi Lüthy
Walter Siegenthaler
C. G. Schmidt

ISC Correspondent to the Secretary-General
Helmut P. Kuemmerle

Public Affairs Committee
George H. Warren, *Chairman*
Robert L. Vann, *Associate Chairman*
Robert D. Watkins, *ex officio*

Officers of the International Society of Chemotherapy

Carlo Grassi, *President*
Gladys L. Hobby, *Vice-President*
Zdenek Modr, *Vice-President*
Peter Naumann, *Vice-President*
George N. Rolinson, *Vice-President*
Alois Stacher, *Vice-President*
Yukimasa Yagisawa, *Vice-President*
Helmut P. Kuemmerle, *Secretary-General*
Georges Werner, *Treasurer*

The Impact of Antimicrobial Agents on the Natural History of Infectious Disease: Beneficial, Harmful, and Indifferent Effects

LOUIS WEINSTEIN

Infectious Disease Division, Department of Medicine, Peter Bent Brigham Division of the Affiliated Hospitals Center, and the Department of Medicine, Harvard Medical School, Boston, Massachusetts

Before I undertake the discussion of the positive, negative, and indifferent effects of antimicrobial therapy on the natural history of infectious disease, I want to express my deep appreciation to Dr. Nelson, the President, and to the members of the Executive Committee of the 11th International Congress of Chemotherapy for the singular honor you have paid me by your invitation to deliver this lecture. I am particularly pleased to have been asked to present a discourse to a group of American investigators and to our colleagues from abroad whose interests encompass the fields of microbiology, infectious disease, and chemotherapy, because this underscores the total interrelation of these disciplines and, from a personal standpoint, reflects my own experiences first as a microbiologist and later as a physician whose primary interest over more than 30 years has been in infectious diseases and their management. Should you wonder why I have chosen to review as broad an area as is implied by the title of my talk, I want to quote a comment made by Sir William Osler in the late 1890s that points out the need to do what I shall be talking about. "It is of use from time to time to take stock, so to speak, of our knowledge of a particular disease—substitute words *therapeutic modality*—to see where we stand in regard to it, to inquire to what conclusions the accumulated facts seem to point, and to ascertain in what direction we may look for fruitful investigations in the future."

I shall concentrate the first part of my discussion on the positive aspects, that is, all the benefits that have accrued from the use of the antimicrobial agents. I will then turn my attention to the negative effects of these drugs which include not only the situations in which they may be harmful but also those in which they may be partially or totally ineffective or indifferent in their influence on the natural history of infectious disease.

BENEFICIAL EFFECTS OF ANTIMICROBIAL THERAPY

There is no question that the antimicrobial agents have had a tremendous effect on the ability of physicians to cure the vast majority of infectious diseases caused by susceptible organisms. Not only have the fatality rates of these disorders been markedly reduced, in many instances to zero, but, just as important, complications that have often been responsible not only for protracted illness but also for death have decreased in incidence strikingly or have been completely eliminated. A few examples serve to underscore the tremendous impact of these drugs on the clinical behavior of a few selected infections. The effect of penicillin G on streptococcal pharyngitis has been very striking. Suppurative complications such as purulent otitis media, mastoiditis, cellulitis, acute vulvovaginitis (young girls), and peritonsillar abscess have been virtually eliminated when therapy is started early in the course of the disease. When these are already present in untreated patients, they are usually cured readily by administration of an appropriate antimicrobial agent. An outstanding case in point is acute mastoiditis which, when detected early, is eradicated with antibiotics and does not require surgical intervention. Available data indicate that the incidence of rheumatic fever is strikingly reduced when penicillin G is administered in the early stage of streptococcal pharyngitis; however, this is still somewhat controversial. Although it was thought initially that the development of acute proliferative glomerulonephritis was prevented by treatment of the initiating streptococcal infection, later studies have indicated that this is not true.

Treatment with antimicrobial agents has dramatically altered the clinical courses of all types of gonorrhea and syphilis. Gonococcal urethritis, an infection that, in the pre-antibiotic era, required weeks to months of uncomfortable urethral irrigations that often failed to prevent complications such as posterior urethritis and prostatitis, is now readily eradicated with one or two doses of an appropriate antibiotic. Even the more potentially lethal complications of the disease—bacteremia, endocarditis, and meningitis—respond favorably to chemotherapy. In the past, untreated acute gonococcal arthritis often led to early and rapid destruction of cartilage followed later by ankylosis. Now, when treated shortly after onset, it is rapidly cured and leaves little or no residual damage in joints. The change in the behavior of all types of syphilis treated with penicillin are truly most remarkable. From a situation when a year or more of therapy, first with bismuth and then with neoarsphenamine, was required when antibiotics were not available, the disease is now cured by 10 days of exposure to penicillin if the nervous system is not affected, and 15 days if it is. Even long-term involvement of the cardiovascular and/or central nervous system can be arrested, but established damage not reversed, by treatment with adequate doses of penicillin or tetracycline. Acute hematogenous osteomyelitis, often fatal, especially when associated with high-grade bacteremia, is now curable in the vast majority of cases when the diagnosis is established early and appropriate antimicrobial therapy is instituted promptly.

The most striking impact of antibiotics in sharply reducing the risk of complications in and death from an infectious disease is exemplified by the potentially lethal types of staphylococcal infections such as pneumonia, bacteremia, and acute endocarditis. While death still occurs in patients with these disorders, its incidence has been appreciably reduced. The fatality rate of staphylococcal endocarditis was 100% in the pre-antibiotic era. It has now decreased to 40 to 50% or less, even when "late" cases or those involving abusers of the intravenous use of drugs are included. The effect of antimicrobial therapy on the outcome of subacute bacterial endocarditis has been most dramatic. Prior to the availability of antibiotics, about 90% of patients with this disease died. At present, the rate of recovery from the infectious process approaches 100%; when death occurs, it is usually due to noninfectious complications such as embolization to vital areas such as the brain or coronary artery bed or rupture of a mycotic aneurysm. Similar reductions in the risk of a fatal outcome have occurred when other life-threatening infections such as meningitis caused by *Neisseria meningitidis*, *Haemophilus influenzae*, or *Streptococcus pneumoniae*, pneumococcal pneumonia, and typhoid fever have been treated with appropriate antimicrobial drugs (Table 1).

When the effects of treatment with antibiotics of bacterial infections that are, for the most part, not potentially lethal are examined, it is clear that not only has the small risk of death been eliminated, but there has also been a sharp decrease in morbidity related to the development of complications (Table 2). Between 1945

and 1950, a period when penicillin became available and was used in relatively limited quantities, 15 of 37,398 patients in Massachusetts with scarlet fever died. In the next 5 years, when antimicrobial agents of several types were in use, only 2 of 21,819 patients expired. Between 1962 and 1972, when these drugs were used most extensively, there were no fatalities among 28,622 individuals with this disease. Not shown in the table, but very important, has been the almost total elimination of suppurative complications by treatment of the initiating streptococcal infection with an effective antibiotic. Although all of the statistically valid data have indicated that therapy with any antimicrobial agent, even when it has been active in vitro, has exerted no beneficial effect on the clinical course of pertussis, such treatment has nevertheless reduced the fatality rate associated with this disease. The number of babies in Massachusetts dying from complications of whooping cough, most commonly bacterial pneumonia, fell from 183 of 30,045 patients between 1945 to 1950 to only 8 of 10,313 children observed between 1951 and 1955 (Table 2). The effect of the availability of newer drugs active against many of the organisms involved in pneumonia, especially *H. influenzae* and other gram-negative bacteria, is evident in the sharp reduction in the periods 1951 to 1955 and 1962 to 1972.

Tuberculosis is an outstanding example of the beneficial effects of antimicrobial therapy on the course of an infection. Very striking, however, is

TABLE 1. *Effects of antibiotics on death rates of several common infections*

Diseases	% Deaths	
	No antibiotics	Antibiotic therapy
Pneumonia (pneumococcal)	(20–85) 30	About 5
Subacute bacterial endocarditis	99+	5
Meningitis (*H. influenzae*)	100	2–3
Meningitis (pneumococcus)	100	8–10
Meningitis (meningococcal)	20–90	1–5
Typhoid fever	8–10	1–2

TABLE 2. *Bacterial infections (Massachusetts 1945–1972)*

Years	Scarlet fever		Pertussis	
	No. of cases	No. of deaths	No. of cases	No. of deaths
1945–1950	37,398	15	30,045	183
1951–1955	21,819	2	10,313	8
1962–1972	28,622	0	1,715	0

the apparent failure of treatment with strepto-mycin to reduce the fatality rate of this disease in patients in Massachusetts between 1945 and 1950, from about 50% noted in the years before effective tuberculostatic agents became availa-ble. This did not change in the period 1945 to 1950, despite the wide use of streptomycin (Ta-ble 3). The first important reduction in the risk of death to about 26% became apparent only after isoniazid became available in 1951. As more drugs active against the tubercle bacillus have appeared on the scene and prophylaxis of con-tacts has been put into practice, not only has the fatality rate fallen even further, but the inci-dence and prevalence of the disease has also declined.

With the possible exception of encephalitis caused by *Herpesvirus hominis* and the prophy-laxis of influenza with amantadine, there are presently no effective agents for the treatment or prevention of viral infections. However, anti-microbial drugs have been highly effective in reducing the number of deaths from some of the common viral diseases, in an indirect way, by controlling and/or eliminating complications in-duced by secondary bacterial invasion (Table 4). The fatality rate of varicella, most of which is related to secondary bacterial infection, fell sharply from the period 1945 to 1955 to the period 1962 to 1972, despite only a moderate decline in the incidence of the disease. A similar effect of treatment with antibiotics is apparent in the risk of death in cases of measles, usually due to secondary bacterial pneumonia, when the intervals 1945 to 1955 and 1962 to 1972 are compared. Although the frequency of the disease was much lower in the later period, the reduction in the number of deaths is still striking. It must be emphasized that the prophylactic exhibition of antibiotics for the purpose of preventing bac-terial complications of viral infections is not only

TABLE 3. *Tuberculosis (Massachusetts 1945–1970)*

Years	Total no. of cases	% Deaths
1945–1950	15,492	51
1951–1955	10,711	26
1962–1970	7,935	17

TABLE 4. *Comparison of cases and deaths from viral infections in Massachusetts*

Disease	1945–1955		1962–1972	
	Total cases	Total deaths	Total cases	Total deaths
Varicella	177,761	3,535	107,846	19
Measles	270,675	116	62,231	6

without beneficial effect but is, in fact, poten-tially dangerous. This is discussed in detail be-low.

Chemoprophylaxis

The striking effectiveness of antimicrobial agents in eradicating established infections led to what appeared to be the obvious conclusion that, when appropriately selected, these drugs should prevent bacterial implantation and in-vasion and the development of infection. Like many concepts that appear reasonable, this one was quickly found to be only partially true and dependent on the purpose of the prophylaxis. As studies were carried out, it became apparent that attempts to prevent infection in situations in which patients were, for one reason or an-other, predisposed to infection by a variety of microorganisms, prophylaxis not only failed to protect but led to an increased incidence of infections, some of which were caused by uncom-mon bacteria, yeasts, and fungi that were not susceptible to many of the available antimicro-bial compounds. Thus, comatose individuals given antibiotics to prevent pneumonia experi-enced no decrease in incidence of this disease but, in fact, developed it more often than those who were not treated. Controlled studies of the value of chemoprophylaxis in patients with mea-sles, pertussis, poliomyelitis, and varicella have indicated that it is ineffective. The frequency of infections was higher than in untreated patients, and the organisms involved were unusual and resistant to the antibiotic being administered. In sharp contrast to this is the success of prophy-laxis when its purpose is the prevention of in-vasion by a single organism sensitive to the drug used. So, streptococcal pharyngitis, gonorrhea, incubating syphilis, shigellosis, and recurrent in-fection of the urinary tract are prevented when a single active antimicrobial agent is given. These experiences have led to the establishment of two "rules" for chemoprophylaxis that permit prediction of its effectiveness. *First, if the pur-pose of the prophylaxis is to prevent invasion by a single organism highly sensitive to the drug being administered, the chance for success is 100%. Second, if the intent of the chemopro-phylaxis is to inhibit implantation of and in-vasion by all organisms in a patient's internal and external environment,* for example coma, elective surgery, viral infections, and an immu-nosuppressed state, *the chance of failure is 100%.*

Chemoprophylaxis, as it was practiced until relatively recently, was fraught with the same dangers as are associated with the therapeutic application of antimicrobial agents. Untoward effects such as hypersensitization, toxicity, and suprainfection were common. These were related, in good part, to the prolonged periods over which the prophylaxis was carried out. A new approach is now employed that has reduced the risk of these complications. This involves the use of antibiotics prophylactically for much shorter periods of time than in the past. It is now common practice to administer a pre-, intra-, and postoperative dose of a drug in surgical cases and to continue this, at an appropriate interval, for no longer than 2 days after the procedure has been completed. This has led to a sharp reduction in the incidence of toxic reactions and suprainfection. Whether or not the development of hypersensitivity has been decreased is not clear. Although there is still some controversy concerning the effectiveness of "short course" prophylaxis, a striking benefit has been increased safety, as evidenced by a decrease in the frequency of untoward effects.

Identification of "New" Infections

One of the important beneficial effects of the use of antimicrobial agents has been the recognition of previously undescribed infectious disorders. This has come about because of failure of these drugs to cure an infectious process assumed to be caused by an organism susceptible to the agent being administered. An outstanding example of this has been the discovery of the disease presently recognized to be due to *Mycoplasma pneumoniae*. Failure of sulfonamides to alter the course of an outbreak of pneumonia, thought to be bacterial in origin, in a private school in the mid-1940s led to the conclusion that a virus was the etiologic agent, and the disease was labeled "primary atypical pneumonia." As is now well known, studies over a period of years have identified the cause of this disease to be *M. pneumoniae*, an organism not susceptible to the sulfonamides but sensitive to the tetracyclines and erythromycin, drugs that were not available when the syndrome was first observed. It is very likely that attention was drawn to the possibility of a "new" disease when the pulmonary lesion of Legionnaires disease was noted to be unaffected by treatment with antibiotics known to cure most other types of bacterial pneumonia. This has also probably been the reason behind the discovery of the recently described "Pittsburgh pneumonia," the etiologic agent of which appears to be a gram-negative, acid-fast bacillus. It has probably also been the case in instances in which, because the clinical behavior of an infectious process has not been altered by intensive antimicrobial therapy, the question of a nonbacterial cause has been raised and has led eventually to the discovery of a "new" viral disease.

Antimicrobial Agents and Virology

Although, as pointed out above, antimicrobial drugs are, with very few exceptions, of no value in the management of viral infections, the availability of these agents has played a major role in the isolation and identification of viruses and in the development of vaccines for the prophylaxis of disease caused by these organisms. Without incorporation of various antibiotics into the media used in cultures of tissue, it is highly probable that recovery of viruses from sources such as sputum and feces would be impossible because of destruction of the cells by the large number and variety of organisms present in these substances. It is patently clear, therefore, that most of the progress that has been made over the past 20 or more years in the isolation and identification of viruses, definition of their biological, chemical, and genetic features, the diseases they produce, and the development of effective viral vaccines rests solidly on the ability of antimicrobial agents to prevent destruction of tissue cultures by organisms that may be present in the materials being studied.

Impact of Antimicrobial Agents on Public Health

A very important by-product of the treatment of bacterial infections is its impact on public health with respect to the spread of disease and control of epidemics. Two processes are involved in this effect. The first is the prophylaxis of single contacts of patients with specific infections by the administration of an effective drug. This is chemoprophylaxis, as described above. The other, which is less apparent, is a reduction in the incidence and prevalence of a particular infection without administration of a prophylactic antibiotic to a large population in which the infected persons live. Thus, the eradication of streptococcal pharyngitis in several children in a school may sharply decrease or eliminate secondary cases without exposing all the contacts to penicillin G, a procedure often impossible logistically because of the very large number of uninfected individuals involved. This may also apply to other communicable infections such as enteritis caused by salmonella and shigella. In outbreaks of illness caused by these bacteria, it is very likely that much can be accomplished to curb the spread of disease, if the source of the organism is infected patients or asymptomatic carriers, by treating only these individuals with an effective agent, without resorting to prophylaxis of a very large number of contacts. The recent decrease in the incidence of syphilis is probably related to increased detection and treatment of persons with the communicable stages of the disease. It is entirely possible that, until an effective vaccine is developed, a marked reduction in the frequency of gonorrhea could be accomplished were it possible to detect and treat all active cases, asymptomatic carriers, and contacts. In essence, the impact of antimicrobial agents on the public health rests on the principle that elimination of the source of an infecting agent reduces or eliminates its transmission to susceptible individuals and, in this way, controls the spread of disease and prevents the development of an epidemic.

Socioeconomic Impact of Antimicrobial Therapy

A critical evaluation of the overall beneficial effects of antimicrobial agents requires more than mere consideration of their activity in specific infections, because this omits evaluation of their impact on other aspects of illness. Infectious diseases often involve serious and distressing socioeconomic upheaval for patients and important public health problems for their families and friends. Because of the availability and effectiveness of antibiotics, many persons with readily curable infections can now be treated at home and are spared the extended periods of hospitalization required not too long ago. The financial savings, in terms of the present costs of hospital care for the millions of people who suffer this kind of disease in the United States each year, is huge. In addition, rapid cure permits early return to work and reduces, often strikingly, the burden of lack of income associated with prolonged illness. Taken together, the economic impact of these "ripple" effects of antibiotic therapy, although not accurately calculable, are undoubtedly tremendous. Among the other essentially nonmedical benefits of antimicrobial therapy is the reduction of the social disruption that often follows removal of patients from their homes to the hospital, and the avoidance of the associated psychologic trauma, especially in young children but also in many adults.

One of the very important accomplishments of modern medicine has been a significant increase in life expectancy. However, this is mostly related to a sharp reduction in deaths among young children. Improved obstetrical practice, better management of premature babies, repair of correctable, life-threatening congenital defects, treatment of chemical disturbances, and appropriate immunization have contributed greatly to survival in this age group. However, it must be emphasized that the successful treatment of a variety of infectious diseases, especially meningitis, pneumonia, bacteremia, otitis media, and purulent sinusitis and diarrhea caused by bacteria, has played a major role in increasing life expectancy in children. Only a relatively small increment of years has been added to the life of adults. Recent progress in the management of solid tumors and hematologic malignancies, strokes, coronary artery disease, and immunological disorders has contributed only in a small way to an increase in the duration of life in adults. It would appear, however, that the impact of the antimicrobial drugs in increasing longevity has been as important, or even more important, than improvement in the control of noninfectious disorders in this age group. An outstanding example is pneumonia, "the old man's friend," a disease that carried off many of the elderly in great numbers and with dispatch and which is now readily cured if detected early and treated promptly with appropriate antimicrobial agents.

HARMFUL EFFECTS OF ANTIMICROBIAL AGENTS

Reactions to the Drugs

The antimicrobial agents have had a tremendous negative impact on the natural history of the infectious diseases because of the large number and variety of untoward effects associated with their use. These have been responsible for a number of noninfectious and infectious complications that have altered the history of treated infections and that have, in some instances, been more life-threatening than the primary disease. In some cases, the drugs may produce the paradox of death in the course of an infection that, appropriately treated, is associated with a very high rate of survival. The reactions induced by antimicrobial agents fall into three categories on the basis of the mechanisms involved in their pathogenesis: (a) those that result from the development of hypersensitivity; (b) those that are related to the innate toxicity of the drugs, and (c) those that represent biological effects induced by neither hypersensitivity nor toxicity.

Hypersensitization. This is the commonest reaction produced by the antimicrobial drugs. Some of the syndromes that develop are clinically unimportant and represent an inconvenience rather than a potential threat in terms of severity or risk to life. Among the very mild and often evanescent untoward effects of the development of hypersensitivity are all types of dermal eruptions, low- to high-grade fever without eosinophilia, and eosinophilia without elevation of temperature. Among those that may be severe but only uncommonly life-threatening are exfoliative dermatitis, exudative erythema multiforme, especially the Stevens-Johnson Syndrome (sulfonamides, penicillin), generalized weakness and paralysis (nitrofurantoin), acute or chronic pulmonary reactions (nitrofurantoin), serum sickness (penicillins, most often), Arthus reactions, and interstitial nephritis (penicillins and cephalosporins). Anaphylaxis is uncommon but imposes a high risk of death. This occurs most often in patients sensitized to the penicillins; it has been suggested that it is responsible for 300 to 500 deaths per year in the United States. Another uncommon but potentially life-threatening reaction to penicillin, probably resulting from hypersensitization, is vasculitis.

Toxicity. Although the frequency and organ or tissue involved in toxic reactions to the antimicrobial agents are variable, almost all of these drugs have the potential for producing this type of untoward effect. The disorders that develop may be as minor as irritation and pain at sites of injection or as major as loss of function of an organ or even death. The different types of toxic effects associated with specific antimicrobial drugs will not be discussed. Rather, the organs involved and the types of disease that occur are described to emphasize the fact that practically no system is spared the effects of the innate toxicity of these agents. This has added a new dimension to the natural history of infection that may pose, at times, a greater threat to life than that imposed by the infectious process alone. The kidney and inner ear are common sites of the toxic activity of these drugs. Renal problems, ranging in severity from proteinuria to tubular necrosis, are associated with the use of all the aminoglycosides, with the exception of streptomycin. Deafness, represented by loss of perception of high frequency sounds, is also caused by this group of agents. The toxicity of these agents for the ear may be expressed only as vestibular dysfunction in patients treated with gentamicin, tobramycin, or streptomycin. Erythromycin may produce varying degrees of deafness when given intravenously in a dose of 4 g/day; this usually clears within a short time after administration of the drug is stopped. The liver may be the site of the toxic activity of some of the antimicrobial agents. Among the drugs that are known to injure this organ are the sulfonamides, isoniazid, rifampin, and the tetracyclines (when a dose larger than 2 g/day is given). A dose of most tetracyclines greater than 2 g/day has been noted to produce hepatocellular injury in normal persons. This is especially a problem in pregnant

individuals with severe pyelonephritis, even when they are given only 2 g/day of one of these drugs. Doxycycline is an exception because it is excreted primarily via the intestinal tract. All the other members of this class of drugs are both excreted in unchanged form by the kidney and inactivated in the liver, differing only in the degree to which they are metabolized or excreted. The pregnant woman with severe pyelonephritis, because of a varying level of renal failure and because of the well-known increase in fat in the liver associated with the gravid state, is unable to adequately excrete or metabolize a conventional dose of the drug. This leads to the development of blood levels that may be as high or even higher than those produced by the administration of 3 to 4, or more, g and results in hepatocellular necrosis. Deaths have been reported in such cases. Treatment of newborn infants, especially those who are premature, with conventional doses of chloramphenicol (50 mg/kg) may produce the so-called gray syndrome in which the major pathological disturbance is a toxic myocarditis; death is common. This is due to the inability of the infant liver to produce enough glucuronyl transferase, the enzyme involved in inactivation of the antibiotic by conjugation with glucuronic acid, to degrade the usual dose of the drug. Because of this, circulating levels of the antibiotic reach a height associated with injury to the heart. Transient myocardial injury, as indicated by electrocardiographic abnormalities, may occur in patients who develop severe serum sickness as a consequence of sensitization to penicillin. The brain may be the site of maximal impact of the toxic activity of some antibiotics. Seizures due to cortical irritation may be produced by the intrathecal injection of excessive doses of penicillin G or may follow the intravenous infusion of large quantities of the antibiotic, especially in patients with compromised renal function or localized or diffuse cerebral disease. One of the very important toxic effects of chloramphenicol involves the bone marrow. All patients who receive this drug develop anemia; this results from failure of iron to be incorporated into heme. Leucopenia may develop in about 5% and thrombopenia in less than 1% of patients treated with this drug. Both of these are dose-related and return to normal within a week or less after administration of chloramphenicol is discontinued. The sulfonamides have been well known to induce the same types of hematologic abnormalities as have been associated with the use of chloramphenicol. It has recently been noted that oxacillin may also be responsible for the appearance of a striking leucopenia in some individuals. Manifestations of dysfunction of the intestinal tract is common following oral administration of a number of the frequently used antibiotics. This is usually expressed as nausea, vomiting and/or diarrhea, and probably is the result of the irritative effect of the drugs; the mechanism involved differs from that responsible for suprainfection. The toxic, irritative effects of some of the antimicrobial agents on blood vessels is very well illustrated by the moderate to very severe thrombophlebitis associated with the intravenous injection of the penicillins, cephalosporins, and especially erythromycin. Peripheral nerves may be involved in toxic reactions to anti-infective drugs, as emphasized by the paresthesias in the circumoral area, hands, and feet that occur in some persons treated with streptomycin, gentamicin, or tobramycin. The damage produced in teeth (yellow-brown discoloration and hypoplasia of enamel) and inhibition of growth of bone when tetracycline compounds are administered to young children is well known. Optic neuritis develops in about 2 to 3% of patients given chloramphenicol. This agent has also been noted to be responsible for breaks in chromosomes.

Biological effects. Many untoward effects associated with the use of antibiotics, but not induced by the development of hypersensitivity or the toxic activity of the drugs, have been described. While the mechanisms involved in some of these phenomena are well known, they are obscure in some and have been attributed to idiosyncratic reactions. A few examples serve to illustrate this type of untoward effect. Normal individuals treated with standard doses of tetracycline compounds develop negative nitrogen and riboflavin balance that cannot be restored to positive, despite the administration of these substances, as long as these drugs are being given. The oral administration of antibiotics, by suppressing the bacteria in the intestinal flora that convert bilirubin to urobilinogen, may confuse the differential diagnosis of obstructive and hepatocellular jaundice. In this instance, failure to demonstrate an elevated level of urobilinogen does not eliminate the possibility of hepatocellular disease. Orally administered drugs may produce deficiency of vitamin K by the same mechanism; this may lead to bleeding because of decrease in circulating levels of prothrombin, in some cases. Hemolytic anemia may supervene in individuals with the glucose-6-phosphate dehydrogenase defect who are treated with sulfonamides, chloramphenicol, nitrofurantoin, dapsone, and possibly isoniazid; this is more common in black than in white persons. Bleeding may occur in patients receiving carbenicillin because of its propensity to cause aggregation of platelets. Hemolysis is an uncommon complica-

tion of therapy with cephalothin. Neonates are exposed to the risk of developing kernicterus when given a sulfonamide during the period of so-called physiological jaundice. This is related to the greater avidity of the sulfonamide than of bilirubin for binding to albumin. As a result, bilirubin is detached from albumin and reaches high concentrations, as the free compound, in the circulation. This leads to injury to the basal ganglia in the brain and the subsequent development of kernicterus. Aplasia of the bone marrow is a rare complication of therapy with chloramphenicol. This reaction is not dose-related and is not a manifestation of hypersensitivity; its precise mechanism is unknown. Hypokalemia is a well-known but poorly understood complication of therapy with amphotericin. One of the very interesting and possibly clinically important untoward effects of antimicrobial therapy is the suppression of immune responses. This has been demonstrated in patients with streptococcal pharyngitis treated with penicillin G parenterally. Eighty-five percent of untreated cases but only 15% of those who received the antibiotic developed significant elevations of antistreptolysin. Even more striking was the difference in the frequency with which bactericidal activity specific for the serotype of streptococcus responsible for the disease was detected 5 to 7 weeks after the onset of infection. Of those who were not treated, 100% developed this antibody. Bactericidal activity was not detectable in any of those who had received penicillin G. There is also some evidence that exhibition of amphotericin B may lead to immunosuppression.

A relatively common, very important, and potentially lethal biological untoward effect of antimicrobial agents is suprainfection. Although all persons treated, either orally or parenterally, with these drugs undergo changes in the microflora of the intestinal and upper respiratory tracts, only about 2.5%, on average, develop this phenomenon. Overgrowth of one or more organisms in the indigenous microbial population of individuals following antimicrobial therapy occurs in all persons. In the absence of manifestations of active infection, this represents colonization. Suprainfection is defined as the appearance of microbiological and clinical features consistent with a new infectious process that occurs during treatment of another infection. This may lead to death, if it is overlooked or it is caused by highly drug-resistant organisms. Suprainfection is a problem, especially in immunosuppressed patients in whom nonpathogenic organisms such as *Pseudomonas, Serratia, Candida,* and *Aspergillus* overgrow, invade, and cause life-threatening disease; these organisms are also occasionally involved in immunocompetent individuals. In some instances, multiplication of a particular microorganism does not lead to suprainfection but results, nevertheless, in the development of disease. An example of this is pseudomembranous colitis, a disorder that occasionally complicates treatment with clindamycin, ampicillin, and other antibiotics. In this case, *Clostridium difficile*, present in the intestinal tract of some but not all persons, multiplies, as other bacteria are suppressed, to numbers large enough to produce the concentration of toxin required for injury of the bowel to occur.

The following factors are important in the pathogenesis of suprainfection:

(i) *Duration of treatment.* Suprainfection is relatively infrequent in the first 48 hours of exposure to an antibiotic. After this, the incidence increases, reaches a peak between 6 and 8 days of therapy, and then reaches a plateau, the height of which is related to the type of drug given.

(ii) *Age of patients.* Suprainfection is commonest in children 2 years of age and younger; a second peak occurs in adults over 50 years of age, especially when an underlying disease that increases susceptibility to infection is present.

(iii) *Underlying pulmonary disease.* This may be acute, chronic, infectious, or noninfectious in character; pulmonary tuberculosis appears to be an exception.

(iv) *Nature of the antibiotic.* The broader the spectrum of activity of an antibiotic, the greater its tendency to produce suprainfection. While this appears, at first glance, to be paradoxical, it is reasonable because the broader the range of organisms suppressed or killed by an antimicrobial agent, the more likely a single microorganism is to overgrow, as inhibitory factors elaborated by the heterogenous collection of genera and species of bacteria and other living agents susceptible to the drug being given are inhibited or eliminated.

Diagnostic Confusion Produced by Antimicrobial Agents

Administration of an antibiotic before or even after the etiologic agent of an infection has been identified may lead to serious diagnostic confusion. A few examples serve to underscore the clinical importance of this problem. Pharyngeal cultures of patients treated with penicillin often grow large numbers of *E. coli* and other gram-negative bacilli. This is occasionally assumed to represent a suprainfection, especially if fever has not disappeared during treatment, despite the fact that it is usually only an indication of colonization. *Staphylococcus aureus* is a relatively common member of the indigenous microflora of the upper respiratory tract. In untreated in-

dividuals, its numbers in this area are small. However, when an antibiotic to which the staphylococcus is resistant is administered, it overgrows and tends to crowd out many other organisms. When this occurs, a sore throat that may be caused by a virus is attributed to invasion by *S. aureus*, when in fact it has merely colonized the pharynx. The demonstration of *Candida* in the urine and feces of patients treated with antibiotics has led, in some cases, to a diagnosis of infection and to institution of unnecessary antifungal therapy when this has represented only colonization. Of greater clinical importance are the situations in which an infectious process is treated with an antimicrobial drug before the results of cultures are available and the etiology has been defined. For example, the microbiological diagnosis of diphtheria may be difficult or impossible to establish if as few as two or three doses of penicillin G have been administered before the membrane is cultured. As long as 5 days, instead of the usual 24 to 48 hours, may be required for the organism to grow out, even when only a single dose of this antibiotic has been administered. This is also true in some cases of purulent meningitis caused by *N. meningitidis, H. influenzae,* and *S. pneumoniae.* In these, a single dose of a drug active against these organisms often makes it impossible to demonstrate them in Gram stains of cerebrospinal fluid; it may also be difficult to grow them. The treatment of subacute bacterial endocarditis with antibiotics prior to establishing the etiologic diagnosis is an outstanding example of the diagnostic confusion produced by antimicrobial agents. In this instance, defervescence induced by the drug often leads physicians to a diagnosis of some other disease and, most important, makes it difficult or impossible to establish the microbiological diagnosis. Discontinuation of treatment for a short time may not increase the possibility of recovering the organisms from the blood. Until recently, it was thought that the optimal time to begin culturing the blood of patients with this disease was 48 hours after the antibiotic was stopped. However, it is now clear that cultures of blood may not become "positive" until a week or longer after therapy has been stopped. Treatment of so-called fever of unknown origin often produces etiologic confusion and may delay the diagnosis of noninfectious disorders such as some types of lymphoma in which defervescence may be spontaneous.

Infections in Which Antibiotics Alone Are Not Definitive Therapy

It has become very clear, after many years of experience with the management of infections, that, in some instances, the use of therapeutic modalities in addition to or at times in place of antimicrobial agents may be the critical determinant of the clinical outcome of some infectious processes. Among the adjunct measures that have been employed is the use of corticosteroids, transfer factor, antitoxin, and surgery.

Corticosteroids are contraindicated in most infections because of their capacity to impair chemotaxis and phagocytosis and to stabilize lysosomal membranes so that intracellular killing of organisms is inhibited. However, in some situations treatment with these agents in addition to antibiotics is life-saving. The need for these drugs in patients with hypoadrenalism or frank Addison's disease who develop severe infections is obvious. It is now established that the administration of dexamethasone, at 3 mg/kg, together with appropriate antimicrobial drugs has a salutory effect on the course of septic shock. Although not indicated in the average of even advanced cases of pulmonary tuberculosis, individuals with the fulminant type of disease, tuberculous pneumonia or so-called "galloping consumption," benefit from treatment with a corticosteroid for a short period while they are being given three tuberculostatic drugs. Whether steroid compounds are necessary for the successful management of tuberculous meningitis is controversial; most authorities agree that they are of little or no value. The use of corticosteroids in patients with abscess of the brain is without effect on the primary process. It should be restricted to cases in which a threatening degree of increased intracranial pressure is present. Interstitial pneumonia caused by S. aureus is an uncommon complication of viral infection of the respiratory tract, especially when caused by the influenza virus. Experience with this disease has indicated that therapy with antibiotics alone is ineffective and does not reduce significantly the fatality rate of close to 100%. The administration of 100 mg of hydrocortisone intravenously, and titration of the need for additional doses on the basis of the pO_2 arterial blood, has been found to lead to recovery in almost all cases. The corticosteroid is usually not required for longer than 24 to 36 hours, at which time the infection has usually been brought under control by the antibiotic. An outstanding example of the importance of corticosteroids in controlling a life-threatening complication of an infection for which antimicrobial agents are of no value is the thrombopenia that occurs in the course of some of the common viral infections—measles, rubella, varicella. Treatment with these agents usually produces a relatively rapid return of the thrombocyte count to normal levels.

A moderate number of infections may fail to respond to even prolonged administration of antimicrobial agents because of inadequate function of delayed hypersensitivity. Among these is a small number of reported cases of mucocutaneous candidiasis, disseminated tuberculosis, histoplasmosis, or coccidioidomycosis, and the prophylaxis of staphylococcal infection in patients with the Wiskott-Aldrich syndrome. Treatment with transfer factor, together with an appropriate antibiotic, has been helpful in bringing the problem under control in some but not all of these diseases.

The clinical features of some infectious disorders are not due primarily to bacterial invasion but are caused almost completely by exotoxins elaborated by the causative organisms. Diphtheria and tetanus are outstanding examples of this phenomenon. Studies of the treatment of diphtheria with antitoxin plus penicillin and with antitoxin alone (patients matched for age, sex, severity and duration of disease before diagnosis) have shown no difference in the incidence of death or complications. The only benefit produced by antibiotics in this infection is rapid eradication of the carrier state. Antimicrobial agents are without value in the management of tetanus. When given, they eliminate the orgaisms from the site in which they are multiplying and elaborating toxins. However, there is no detectable beneficial effect on the course of the disease for which optimal therapy is the administration of antitoxin plus surgical removal of the area in which Clostridium tetani is growing.

Many localized infectious processes respond either partially or not at all to the most intensive antimicrobial therapy when treated initially or, if they do, relapse within a short time after treatment has been stopped. These are the disorders in which experience has demonstrated the need for appropriate surgical intervention. They fall into three groups: (i) those that respond well to adequate drainage, (ii) those that fail to improve unless they are completely removed, and (iii) those that obstruct the airway and need to be by-passed surgically. Abscesses at various sites may be cured by treatment with antibiotics alone in some cases. However, surgical drainage in addition to chemotherapy is often required. Chronic bronchiectasis, chronic osteomyelitis, infected intravascular and intracranial shunts, arterial or arteriovenous fistulas, chronic otitis media and mastoiditis, and tuberculous lymphadenitis require treatment with antibiotics followed by removal of the infected site. Anaerobic myositis (gas gangrene) is very difficult to cure unless the area of infection is completely removed; when the blood supply of an infected extremity is badly compromised, the administration of antibiotics alone is of no avail unless the limb is amputated. Rapid, recurrent reaccumulation of pericardial fluid in patients with tuberculous pericarditis is influenced little, if at all, by even the most intensive treatment with tuberculostatic drugs, in some instances. This requires total pericardiectomy if death from progressive cardiac tamponade is to be prevented. The fatality rate in patients with the syndrome of salmonella bacteremia who have an atherosclerotic aneurysm (not infected in some cases and present in any area of the aorta and its main branches) approaches 100%, even when the most intensive antimicrobial therapy is applied. However, if the vascular lesion is removed during treatment with an appropriate antibiotic, almost all patients are cured. Another outstanding example of the therapeutic importance of surgery is infection of a natural or prosthetic cardiac valve. Recent reports have indicated that, when endocarditis involving natural tricuspid valves is not benefitted by the administration of antibiotics alone, removal of the valve, continuation of antimicrobial therapy, and implantation of a prosthesis months later is feasible. In patients with valvular infections of the left side of the heart in whom treatment with antibiotics fails to control the disease, it may become necessary to remove the affected valve and, at the same time, replace it with a prosthesis. While infections of prosthetic valves respond to the administration of antibiotics alone in some cases, replacement of the prosthesis during antimicrobial therapy may be the only approach to cure of the disease. Three disorders associated with obstruction of the airway—acute epiglottitis, diphtheria with involvement of the larynx, or obstructing bilateral peritonsillar abscess—exemplify the need for a surgical procedure, tracheostomy, in addition to antimicrobial therapy.

Changes in the Natural History of Infectious Diseases in Which Antimicrobial Therapy Has Played No Role

The infection that most strikingly illustrates a dramatic change in its natural history, unrelated to antimicrobial agents, is syphilis, a disease that, when first described, was acute in nature (the "great pox") and progressed rapidly to death in some instances and became one of the most chronic disorders of man long before antibiotics were known. More modern examples of this phenomenon include subacute bacterial endocarditis, pneumonia caused by *M. pneumoniae,* and scarlet fever. When mycoplasmal pneumonia was first described in the mid-1940s, its commonest features were noted to be severe headache, low- to high-grade fever, nonproduc-

tive cough, frequent involvement of the middle lobe of the right lung, absence of pleural effusion, and spontaneous recovery; relapses or other complications did not occur, young people were most often involved, and treatment was thought to be unnecessary. The disease has changed its character in many ways over the past 30-odd years without any apparent impact attributed to the antimicrobial drugs. Today, this disease produces a variety of infiltrates in different areas in the lungs, and the middle lobe syndrome has become uncommon. An increasing number of older individuals are involved, and pleural effusion develops in about 25% of cases. Recurrent episodes have been documented. Neurological complications, including transverse myelitis and encephalitis, may supervene. Antimicrobial therapy is recommended for all cases; in a rare instance the infection may be fatal. Even more striking have been the changes in the natural history of subacute bacterial endocarditis that have occurred over the last 30 years and which, except for a remarkable reduction in the risk of death, are unrelated to the use of antimicrobial agents. Older people are presently involved much more frequently than in the past; the type of underlying cardiac disease is less often congenital or rheumatic in nature; murmurs are absent in a small number of cases; the types of organisms involved have changed both qualitatively and quantitatively; cultures of blood are sterile in about 20% of patients (the longer the duration of symptoms before cultures are carried out, the higher the incidence of sterile blood); and the classical peripheral manifestations of the disease—Osler's nodes, Janeway lesions, Roth spots, petechiae and subungual hemorrhages—have become relatively uncommon. Scarlet fever is now often featured by rapid disappearance of the diagnostic rash in 24 hours or less in patients who have not been treated with an antibiotic. Even the natural history of tuberculosis has undergone a number of changes unrelated, except for a reduction in the risk of death, to treatment with tuberculostatic agents. An increasing number of patients presently have disease involving the lower lobes of the lungs (the majority do not have diabetes mellitus). In addition, extrapulmonary disease, common in the preantibiotic era and then virtually disappearing, has increased in frequency in the past 15 years. Another example of a change in the behavior of an infectious disease has been the sharp increase in the incidence of gonococcal arthritis in women over the past 15 years. Prior to this, involvement of the joints in this disease was much more common in males than in females.

CONCLUDING COMMENTS

As I have looked back over more than 30 years of experience with antimicrobial agents, it has become clear to me that considerable time is required before a new drug can be adequately evaluated. The development of our knowledge of the usefulness of all of these agents usually progresses through three well-defined stages. The first might be called the *Stage of Hyperenthusiasm*. This encompasses the first 2 or 3 years after a compound has become available. During this period, the medical literature is usually devoted to recitation of a catalog of all of its benefits, with only an occasional reference to reactions or to failure of response. The next 3 to 5 years cover a period that might be labeled the *Stage of Critical Evaluation*. During this, sufficiently large numbers and varieties of infections are treated, careful clinical and microbiological studies are carried out, and the results are critically analyzed. These two stages are required for accumulation of a large enough experience to permit determination of the degree of effectiveness and the types and frequency of reactions that may be associated with the use of a drug. The final stage is usually reached only after a compound has been used widely for 5 to 6 or more years; after this time, enough has usually been learned about it to allow it to be applied effectively and with the least danger. This I have called the *Stage of Established Value*.

That the development of the antimicrobial agents has been one of the very important, if not the most important, advances in medicine in this century cannot be questioned. However, as suggested by Osler, when we "take stock" at this time, it is evident that, while the benefits that have accrued from the use of antimicrobial agents have been tremendous, it is just as clear that they are not the single panacea for the management of all infections and that, in fact, their administration may be harmful. This should be no surprise because it is well known that the solution of any problem in medicine or any other human effort is usually followed by the creation of a new set of problems. In this regard, it is well to be cognizant always of the well-established fact that all therapeutically effective drugs, regardless of their nature and the uses to which they are put, are potentially dangerous. As I have pointed out, the antimicrobial agents exert strongly positive effects as well as negative and indifferent ones that include not only a growing catalog of reactions but also a number of situations in which they are ineffective or serve only as adjunct therapy. It is the custom today, when various therapeutic or prophylactic measures are evaluated, to "cost-benefit" them. As this measure is applied to the antimicrobial agents in relation to benefit in terms of cure and cost with respect to risk, it is clear that the benefits far outweigh the dangers. Although I have spent a good part of my discussion on the null and untoward effects of these drugs, examination of their use from a qualitative and quantitative standpoint underscores the preponderance of their benefit.

Finally, to heed Osler's admonition "to ascertain in what direction we may look for fruitful investigations in the future," it is evident that many new antimicrobial agents are being and will continue to be developed over the coming years. It is also clear that, as the age of the population increases, as more and more people with potentially lethal diseases such as leukemia have their lives prolonged by the use of compounds that are variably immunosuppressive, and as drug resistance becomes an increasing phenomenon, problems with the management of infectious diseases will probably become even more difficult than they are today. The "fruitful investigations" that Osler called for appear to lie primarily in the areas of the discovery of effective antiviral drugs, the development of prophylactic measures, drugs or immunizing agents, that will protect immunosuppressed persons from microbial invasion, the search for clinically applicable methods of curing organisms of resistance, and the production of new chemical classes of antimicrobial agents that will minimize or eliminate the growing problems of cross-resistance and cross-sensitization associated with the availability of more and more congeners of the antimicrobial agents already in use.

Section I. Antimicrobial Agents and Infectious Disease

Symposia

New Developments in Viral Hepatitis

R. J. GERETY
Chairman

Bureau of Biologics
Food and Drug Administration
Bethesda, Maryland 20205, U.S.A.

F. DEINHARDT
Co-Chairman

Max von Pettenkofer-Institut for Hygiene and Medical Microbiology
Munich, Federal Republic of Germany

P. J. PROVOST

Merck Institute for Therapeutic Research
West Point, Pennsylvania 19486, U.S.A.

D. TRICHOPOULOS

Department of Hygiene and Epidemiology
University of Athens School of Medicine
Athens, Greece

W. ROBINSON

Department of Internal Medicine
Stanford University Hospital
Stanford, California 94305, U.S.A.

S. N. HUANG

Department of Pathology
McGill University
Montreal, Canada

L. B. SEEFF

Department of Internal Medicine
Veterans Administration Medical Center
Washington, DC 20422, U.S.A.

J. L. GERIN

National Institute of Allergy and Infectious Diseases
Rockville, Maryland 20205, U.S.A.
and
Georgetown University School of Medicine
Washington, DC 20007, U.S.A.

Many serological methods for the detection of antigens and antibodies associated with hepatitis B virus (HBV) and hepatitis A virus (HAV) have been developed. More recently, candidate serological tests have been described which appear to identify antigens specifically associated with non-A, non-B hepatitis. Rapid progress in the refinement and application of serological techniques and the development of reliable animal models have greatly enhanced our understanding of clinical, virological, and epidemiological aspects of viral hepatitis types A, B, and non-A, non-B. It is now possible to identify high-risk populations for hepatitis B, investigate the role of HBV in hepatocellular cancer, and to commence research and development directed at better control of viral hepatitis by passive and active immunization. Preliminary data suggest that the hepatitis A virus has finally yielded to the persistent effort of virologists to culture it in vitro. With current serological tests, a third form of hepatitis in which there is no serological evidence of infection with either HAV or HBV has been identified; it is presumed to be of viral origin and is termed non-A, non-B hepatitis. The symposium reviewed the clinical and histological characterization of viral hepatitis, serological methods for the detection of hepatitis antigens and antibodies, the current state of the art with respect to the recognition and control of hepatitis via active and passive immunization, our increased knowledge of the biochemistry of HBV, chronic hepatitis produced by HBV and by non-A, non-B agent(s), and finally our current understanding of non-A, non-B hepatitis.

Hepatitis A Virus: a Review of Recent Studies
(P. J. Provost)

A strain of HAV was used to infect *Saguinus mystax* marmosets by intravenous inoculation with blood from a 9-year-old Costa Rican patient with hepatitis A (strain CR326). Using infectious marmoset plasma, a total of five serial passages of the agent were made in this marmoset species. The disease was characterized by serum enzyme elevations, liver damage detectable by histological examination, and incubation periods similar to the human disease, confirming previous studies on the transmission of hepatitis A to certain

3

species of marmoset monkeys. Extensive neutralization experiments were carried out in which the agent in marmoset serum was reacted with human preillness and postillness hepatitis A and hepatitis B sera prior to marmoset inoculation. The CR326 agent was specifically neutralized by the postillness sera of 11 human patients with hepatitis A and by neither of two postillness sera from those with hepatitis B, providing conclusive evidence that the CR326 agent was human hepatitis A virus.

In further studies, it was shown that the CR326 agent was also neutralized by commercial preparations of human immune serum globulin, that the viral infectivity was stable to heat (60°C), ether, and acid pH treatments, and that its size was between 25 and 50 nm by filtration, properties wholly consistent with those seen in patients with HAV carried out earlier by U.S. and British investigators. Viral infectivity was destroyed by formalin, UV irradiation, and 100°C. Infectivity was partially destroyed at 60°C, more so in the presence of ribonuclease. The CR326 agent in marmoset serum was applied to cesium chloride gradients; the greatest infectivity for marmosets was recovered at a buoyant density of 1.34 g/cm^3. This material when concentrated 100× and examined by the electron microscope revealed typical 27-nm virus particles resembling picornaviruses. Similar 27-nm virus particles were revealed in stool extracts of human hepatitis A patients, with application of the technique of immune electron microscopy documenting the immunological relatedness of the 27-nm particles to hepatitis A.

Extracts of liver were examined for virus by inoculation into other marmosets and revealed levels of infectivity far greater than in infectious serum from as early as 3 and 7 days postinoculation. Using a 1% liver extract to transmit HAV in marmosets, enzyme elevations were seen as early as 7 to 14 days postinoculation. When examined by immune electron microscopy, infected liver extracts revealed typical 27-nm virus particles. Further, thin sections of infected livers revealed for the first time the cytoplasmic localization of the 27-nm particles in the hepatocytes.

HAV appeared to be a picornavirus, more specifically an enterovirus, based on size, buoyant density in CsCl, RNA content, cytoplasmic localization in hepatocytes, and stability to heat, ether, and acid pH. That HAV is a picornavirus and most likely an enterovirus has now been proven by several investigators. HAV purified from human stools by the sodium dodecyl sulfate-polyacrylamide gel method demonstrated four major polypeptide components similar in size to the major polypeptides of poliovirus. Additionally, treatment of HAV with urea and formamide released linear single-stranded nucleic acid which, like genomes from other RNA-containing viruses, was hydrolyzed at pH 12.9. Crude extracts of infected liver, heated to 60°C for 2 h and clarified, were used as antigen to detect anti-HAV in standard complement fixation assays. Liver extracts, further purified on CsCl gradients, were used as antigen in immune adherence hemagglutination (IAHA) assays. These practical serological assays for anti-HAV, especially IAHA, made possible the first specific epidemiological studies of hepatitis A, and even more sensitive and specific radioimmunoassays and enzyme immunoassays have now been developed for use in routine diagnostic and research laboratories. The rufiventer marmoset (S. labiatus) also appears susceptible to hepatitis A. The Cr326 strain of HAV was serially passed a total of 26 times in the rufiventer marmoset, providing highly potent liver-derived HAV preparations.

The HAV preparations from liver were used to demonstrate that an inactivated vaccine could be prepared in spite of our inability at the time to propagate HAV in cell culture. HAV, partially purified from infected liver, was inactivated by Formalin and injected subcutaneously into marmosets. In a control study it was shown that anti-HAV was induced and that the vaccinated animals were protected against live HAV challenge. Nevertheless, the absolute prerequisite to practical vaccine development remained the in vitro growth of HAV in cell culture. Within the last 2 years Provost and co-workers have successfully propagated HAV in cell cultures which had been passed many times from marmoset to marmoset by using a highly sensitive direct immunofluorescence assay that made possible detection of the minute fluorescent granules characteristic of HAV infection in cell cultures. The HAV was serially transmissible and could be measured by radioimmunoassay.

Monkey kidney cells, especially a low passage line of normal cells developed from a fetal rhesus monkey (FRhK6), have proven to be excellent and practical substrates for the growth of HAV. HAV was serially transmissible in FRhK6 cells with virus yields higher than obtained in previous liver cell cultures. The virus has now been extensively passed in FRhK6 cells and the ultimate goal of vaccine development appears within grasp.

Additional Remarks on the Propagation of HAV in Cell Cultures
(F. Deinhardt)

HAV recovered directly from human stool (without passage in marmosets), recently was grown in my laboratories in collaboration with

G. Frösner, V. Gaus-Müller, N. Holmes, V. Messelberger, R. Scheid, and G. Siegl in a hepatoma cell line originally isolated by J. J. Alexander. This cell line carries the full genome of HBV but expresses only hepatitis B surface antigen (HBsAg). Cultures of this cell line inoculated with acute phase human hepatitis A stool extracts were positive for intracellular hepatitis A antigen (HAAg) by radioimmune and fluorescent antibody assays beginning 4 to 6 weeks after inoculation. HAAg could not be demonstrated in supernatant culture fluids, but the infection could be passed serially from cell culture to cell culture by cell extracts. The latter reached infectivity titers of 10^4 to 10^5 $TCID_{50}$ from approximately 10^5 infected cells. The virus was identified as HAV by specific blocking with convalescent but not by preinfection human and marmoset hepatitis A sera in radioimmunoassays and by specific staining of the infected but not the control cultures with the same sera in indirect fluorescent antibody tests. It is so far not known whether the hepatitis A infection has any influence on the persistent hepatitis B infection of the hepatoma cells; current studies may answer this question.

Newer Serological Tests for Hepatitis B
(F. Deinhardt)

HBV has a structure more complex than the picornavirus hepatitis A, and determination of the presence of several viral components is important in diagnosing hepatitis B. HBsAg, an antigen located at the surface of the HBV particle, hepatitis B core antigen (HBcAg), located in the core of the HBV particle, and HBe antigen (HBeAg), which only recently has been identified definitively as an additional core protein of HBV, can be distinguished. Previously HBeAg was thought possibly not to be a structural component of HBV but a virus-induced nonstructural or altered host protein. Sensitive radioimmunoassays or enzyme immunoassays, or both, have been developed for these three antigens and their corresponding antibodies (anti-HBs, anti-HBc, and anti-HBe). Tests have also been designed to distinguish between anti-HBc of the IgG and IgM classes. HBsAg can appear in the blood as early as 14 days after infection, and with rare exceptions it is always present during the acute stage of the disease. HBeAg appears somewhat later, is practically always present during the acute disease, and usually disappears before the disappearance of HBsAg. Anti-HBe becomes measurable usually shortly after HBeAg has become no longer detectable.

Persistence of high titers of HBsAg, particularly if associated with persistence of HBeAg, statistically but not in every case indicates a

likely development of chronic active hepatitis. Persistence of HBsAg alone at lower titers is not always associated with significant liver pathology. IgM anti-HBc is the first antibody to appear and is almost always present at the onset of disease. In uncomplicated cases, IgM anti-HBc titers decline after the acute disease and are no longer detectable 6 to 12 months later. IgG anti-HBc appears somewhat later during the acute disease but persists for many years and possibly for life. Persistence of IgM anti-HBc probably indicates a continuing and significant viral activity with liver damage, whereas IgG anti-HBc is the most reliable marker for a past infection with HBV. Anti-HBs is formed weeks to several months after the acute disease; it persists for many years, but possibly not for the lifetime of the individual, and indicates immunity. During the acute disease or periods of continuing or recurrent significant virus production, HBV (Dane particles) can be demonstrated in the circulation by electron microscopy, and HBV DNA polymerase can be detected by appropriate biochemical tests.

In summary, an acute case of hepatitis B can be diagnosed best by evaluating HBsAg, HBeAg, IgM anti-HBc, and IgG anti-HBc. Follow-up examinations should also determine anti-HBs and anti-HBe. For evaluation of the infectivity of human blood or serum HBsAg, HBeAg, anti-HBs, anti-HBe, and anti-HBc should be determined. Blood containing only HBsAg and IgG anti-HBc probably has only a very low if any infectivity, whereas presence of HBsAg together with HBeAg indicates a high infectivity. These latter bloods often also contain IgM anti-HBc. Bloods containing anti-HBs are generally considered to be noninfectious. Of interest are recent observations that bloods containing only anti-HBc may also be infectious. This theory must be evaluated further, particularly whether infectivity is associated with anti-HBc of the IgM class.

Hepatitis B Virus and Hepatocellular Carcinoma
(D. Trichopoulos)

Primary hepatocellular carcinoma (PHC) is among the most common cancers in sub-Saharan Africa and the Far East. Since these areas are heavily populated, it has been postulated that PHC is among the most common cancers worldwide.

The association between hepatitis B and PHC was suspected in the late 1940s by French workers in Africa who observed an association of PHC with the "post-hepatitic" type of cirrhosis. The discovery of HBsAg allowed a more direct evaluation of this hypothesis. Population and case control studies have shown an association between chronic HBV infection and PHC, an association present not only in Africa but also in the United States and Europe. In contrast, there is no association between hepatitis A and PHC.

A causal nature of the association between HBV and PHC has been proposed but has not been proven. It was said that "There is no evidence to support any alternative explanations for this association, i.e., that a third factor relates to both HBV persistence and PHC, or that PHC increases susceptibility to chronic HBV infections," but this, of course, does not prove that third factors do not exist. The potential magnitude of HBV as one factor in the pathogenesis of PHC is indicated by the presence of 200 million HBsAg carriers worldwide.

The pathogenesis of HBV-related PHC is obscure. Integration of viral DNA into the cellular DNA has not been demonstrated unequivocally, although there is some evidence to support this hypothesis. The theory that PHC develops in the regenerative nodules of HBV-related cirrhosis does not explain the occurrences of many cases of HBV-related PHC in an otherwise normal liver. It has also been suggested that persistent, low-grade liver damage may introduce selective pressure on HBV-resistant, dysplastic cells which undergo continuous replication and eventually malignant transformation, or that HBV-related liver damage or liver regeneration, or both, potentiate the carcinogenic effects of other factors. The existing evidence, however, remains inconclusive, and one cannot overlook the fact that HBV infection is not an absolute prerequisite for the development of PHC, as cases also occur in individuals without any indication of a previous HBV infection by currently available serological tests.

Biochemical Studies of HBV
(W. Robinson)

The hepatitis B virion is spherical, approximately 42 nm in diameter, and has a complex structure. The outer layer or viral envelope containing HBsAg and the spherical inner core or nucleocapsid can be seen. HBV forms found in blood include the 22-nm spherical and filamentous forms of HBsAg, the virion or Dane particle, and the nucleocapsid or core which contains HBcAg and the viral DNA. The third antigen associated with HBV infection, HBeAg, now appears to be a part of the nucleocapsid or core of HBV.

Studies of the polypeptide structure of hepatitis B virion cores have established that the major component is a 19,000-dalton polypeptide; minor polypeptides that are larger in size can

also be detected. An interesting recent finding is that the 19,000-dalton core polypeptide recovered from sodium dodecyl sulfate-containing gels after electrophoresis appears to react with anti-HBe and not with anti-HBc. If this finding is confirmed, it establishes the nature of HBeAg and provides a rational basis for the established association between HBeAg and Dane particles or infectious HBV.

Two enzyme activities have been found in core particles isolated from hepatitis virions. One is a DNA polymerase that can be used to assay the relative level of DNA containing hepatitis B virions in serum. This viral marker in the blood has been shown to correlate with relative numbers of Dane particles, HBcAg titers, and HBeAg and with transmission of infection from mothers to newborns and via accidental needle-sticks. It is perhaps the most useful and practical assay for assessing relative levels of Dane particles in the blood.

The second enzyme activity found in core particles is protein kinase. The 19,000-dalton polypeptide is phosphorylated by this protein kinase present in the core particles. This protein phosphorylation reaction provides a gentle and specific method of radiolabeling the polypeptides of core particles. Highly purified 22-nm HBsAg particles contain very little or no protein kinase activity, although high levels of such activity are present in serum.

The HBcAg-antibody (anti-HBc) system is interesting and has potential clinical relevance. After infection with HBV, there is a brisk anti-HBc response just before or at the onset of clinical illness. Anti-HBc titers remain high in virtually all persistently infected patients. Some blood with high anti-HBc titers in the absence of HBsAg or antibody to surface antigen (anti-HBs) may transmit hepatitis B. IgM anti-HBc has been shown to appear early after acute infection and to persist in a high percentage of persistently infected patients. After becoming HBsAg negative, 60% of patients become IgM anti-HBc negative by 3 months and 100% by 1 year. Further studies are needed, however, to establish the clinical usefulness of this serological marker.

The cores of hepatitis B virions contain a circular DNA molecule which has a unique structure among DNAs of known viruses. It is partially double stranded, and the single-stranded portion varies in length from approximately 15 to 50% of the circle length in different molecules; there is a long strand, *a*, of constant length (3,200 nucleotides) and a short strand, *b*, which varies in length from approximately 1,700 to 2,800 nucleotides in different molecules. A

DNA polymerase activity in the virion closes the single-stranded gap in each molecule to make fully double-stranded circular DNA with a uniform length of approximately 3,200 base pairs. DNA synthesis is initiated for this reaction at the 3' end of the short strand that occurs at different sites in different molecules within a specific region consisting of approximately 50% of the DNA.

DNA with a single-stranded region, made double stranded by a virion DNA polymerase activity as found in HBV, has not been found in other viruses. The role of these features in virus infection and replication is not yet clear.

Recently cloning of the hepatitis B viral DNA-plasmid DNA hybrid molecules in procaryotic cells has been reported from four different laboratories. This has provided quantities of DNA sufficient for nucleotide sequence analysis. The surface antigen gene appears to be near the *Eco*RI site within the single-stranded region of the molecule. A second finding concerning the genetic potential of this DNA is the expression of HBcAg in *E. coli* HB 101 transformed by a hepatitis B viral DNA-pRB 322 plasmid DNA hybrid. These findings are the most direct evidence that the DNA described here is hepatitis B viral DNA and that Dane particles are hepatitis B virions.

Ultrastructural Changes in Liver During Viral Hepatitis
(S. N. Huang)

Electron and immunoelectron microscopic studies were carried out on liver tissues from marmosets experimentally infected with HAV and sacrificed during the acute phase of illness. Ultrastructurally, the liver cells demonstrated marked cisternal dilation of endoplasmic reticulum and vesicular transformation and contortion of endoplasmic reticulum profiles. Clusters of viruslike particles of 24 to 27 nm in diameter, both "solid" and "empty," were found in membrane-bound cytoplasmic vesicles. In one marmoset, the viruslike particles were significantly smaller, measuring 17 to 22 nm in size; almost all were "solid" embedded in an amorphous matrix. Clusters of viruslike particles were found in the bile canaliculi of liver cell cords and in lysosomal structures of monocytes or Kupffer cells in the hepatic sinusoids; the latter correlated with the immunofluorescent localization of hepatitis A antigen.

Indirect immunoferritin staining was carried out on fresh and Formalin-fixed liver tissues, using convalescent-phase serum from patients recovered from HAV infection as the primary antibody, and the ferritin-labeled rabbit anti-human IgG or ferritin-labeled staphylococcal protein A as the secondary antibody or identifying agent. Specific staining of the viruslike particles was observed, indicating that they were at least antigenically related to hepatitis A antigen. These findings support the premise that HAV is produced in the liver. The infection seems to produce cytopathic effects especially involving the endoplasmic reticulum organelle of hepatocytes.

Dane particles (HBV) appear to be formed in the cisternae of endoplasmic reticulum as shown by immunoferritin electron microscopy. HBcAg is seen as 22- to 25-nm particles in liver cell nuclei and to a lesser extent in the protoplasmic processes of hepatocytes. The tubular forms of HBsAg are seen in proliferating degranulated endoplasmic reticulum often in association with Dane particles. Core particles resist digestion with protease, DNase, RNase, phospholipase C, lipase, lysozyme, diastase, neuraminidase, or hyaluronidase.

Chronic Viral Hepatitis
(L. B. Seeff)

Chronic viral hepatitis is a disorder characterized by continuing inflammation of the liver for at least 3 months, but generally for 6 months or longer. This entity may occur as chronic persistent hepatitis (CPH) or chronic active hepatitis (CAH). Studies by a number of investigators have shown that the ultimate outcome depends on the initial histological finding in the liver biopsy at the time of diagnosis. Of particular importance was the observation made in some studies of a poor outcome if portal-to-portal bridging necrosis was present in the initial biopsy, whereas bridging necrosis between the central vein and portal area, or between central veins, appeared less important. CPH may progress to CAH; a study by Chadwick and co-workers showed that 9 of 26 patients with CPH ultimately developed CAH when followed for 1 to 17 years. Factors which are associated with the development of CAH of viral etiology include infection in the neonatal period, immunosuppression, renal dialysis, frequent exposure to sources of infection (such as illicit parenteral drug use and therapy for hemophilia), persistence of HBeAg, anicteric infection, and subacute hepatic necrosis during the acute phase of the disease. A comparison between HBsAg-positive and HBsAg-negative hepatitis shows significant differences in the HBsAg-negative CAH cases, including a tendency to occur in younger persons and in females, frequent presence of symptoms, particularly multisystem involvement, autoantibodies, hyperglobulinemia, association with

HLA-A1, HLA-B8, and HLA-DRw4, a poor prognosis, and some benefit from immunosuppressive therapy. Liver biopsies during chronic non-A, non-B hepatitis in 12 patients reported by Berman et al. revealed CPH in 2, CAH in 5, and CAH with early cirrhosis in 1. Treatment of chronic hepatitis with corticosteroids has been shown in several controlled trials to result in improvement primarily in "lupoid" hepatitis. While benefit from corticosteroid therapy of lupoid hepatitis has been established, the response in chronic viral hepatitis has not been sufficiently proven. Corticosteroids, therefore, should not be given in HBsAg-positive CAH, or only in cases with a progressive course and if no improvement occurs after 1 year of observation. Of several experimental forms of treatment, interferon in combination with adenine arabinoside seems to be the most promising, and further studies are in progress.

Hepatitis B Vaccine
(J. L. Gerin)

In the absence of successful propagation of the HBV in vitro, plasma from asymptomatic humans chronically infected with HBV and circulating large amounts of HBsAg have been used by several groups of investigators to prepare subviral vaccines. In collaboration with the National Institutes of Health, National Institute of Allergy and Infectious Diseases, Dr. Gerin's group prepared such vaccines by separating 20-nm HBsAg particles from the plasma of three donors containing high titers of HBsAg by ultracentrifugation. One vaccine contained HBsAg subtype **adw**, one subtype **ayw**, and one a combination of both subtypes. A total of 10,000 40- to 50-µg doses each were prepared and the vaccines were treated with Formalin.

To date each preparation has been safety tested in chimpanzees with no indication of residual infectivity after the Formalin inactivation step. Similarly, they have been shown efficacious; no hepatitis B infections were seen after challenge with infectious HBV. The monovalent vaccines when administered without adjuvant appeared to be less immunogenic in man than would be required, although each was very effective in inducing specific antibodies (anti-HBs) in both guinea pigs and chimpanzees. Clinical trials using sublots of the **adw** vaccine, either aqueous, alum precipitated, ether-Tween 80 aqueous, or ether-Tween 80 alum precipitated are currently under way.

Non-A, Non-B Viral Hepatitis
(R. J. Gerety)

A series of discoveries led to the identification of what is known as non-A, non-B hepatitis. Dr. Prince in 1974, following development of serological tests for markers of hepatitis B virus, described post-transfusion hepatitis cases that were not caused by the hepatitis B virus (HBV). Redeker and Mosely described multiple episodes of acute viral hepatitis, some clearly unrelated to HBV. Finally, serological testing confirmed that few cases of posttransfusion hepatitis were caused by the hepatitis A virus (HAV). Currently, between 80 and 90% of posttransfusion cases in the United States are non-A, non-B hepatitis. More recently Craske, Zuckerman and Tabor have described two sequential episodes of non-B hepatitis associated with the transfusion of clotting factor concentrates to treat hemophilia in humans and in experimentally infected chimpanzees. In the early 1950s, sera from three asymptomatic blood donors were inoculated into 10 to 20 human volunteers. Retrospectively, these sera which caused icteric hepatitis in 10 to 47% of recipients revealed no serological evidence of infection in donors or recipients by other viruses known to cause hepatitis. Homologous immunity was documented by reinoculation of the identical infectious sera.

Most recently, non-A, non-B hepatitis was transmitted to chimpanzees at the Bureau of Biologics by the inoculation of human sera. Aminotransferases in four chimpanzees became elevated at weeks 2 to 4 (peak ALT 210 to 328 IU/liter between weeks 10 and 15). Liver biopsies from all four confirmed acute hepatitis. Additional chimpanzees were inoculated with sera obtained during acute non-A, non-B hepatitis from one of the initially infected chimpanzees. Sera from weeks 4 through 13 transmitted non-A, non-B hepatitis to the additional chimpanzees. The incubation periods in these recipient chimpanzees were 3 to 4 weeks. Peak ALT values were 142 to 386 IU/liter between weeks 9 and 12. Liver biopsies again confirmed acute hepatitis during the period of elevated ALT levels. Thus, the agent of non-A, non-B hepatitis was present during acute disease in a chimpanzee at the time of first ALT elevation (week 4) at least through week 13 while the ALT remained elevated. These data and subsequent data from other laboratories have confirmed that the chimpanzee is an adequate animal model for at least some human non-A, non-B hepatitis agents. The agent is in the blood early during clinical disease and persists for weeks. The agent or agents of the non-A, non-B hepatitis transmitted at the Bureau of Biologics is serologically unrelated to herpes simplex types 1 and 2, varicella-zoster, HAV, HBV, cytomegalovirus, or Epstein-Barr virus based on either the absence of convalescent antibodies to these agents in chimpanzees recovered from non-A, non-B hepatitis or on similar antibody titers before and after experimental infection. In additional studies conducted at the Bureau of Biologics, sera taken over a 6-year period from a chronically infected human have been shown to transmit non-A, non-B hepatitis to chimpanzees which exhibited similar serological and histological alterations. Sera from this human continued to transmit non-A, non-B hepatitis when his ALT level had returned to normal.

Three chimpanzees which had recovered from non-A, non-B hepatitis were challenged by a second of three infectious human sera maintained at the Bureau of Biologics. None had recognizable hepatitis after challenge, suggesting that one agent or several agents with at least one common or similar antigen had caused the non-A, non-B hepatitis. Since the three infectious human sera were obtained from individuals in different geographic areas of the United States, one agent or related agents may cause much of the non-A, non-B hepatitis in this country. These three sera used to infect chimpanzees, however, were selected from chronically infected humans with elevated ALT levels for more than 1½ years. Clearly these studies do not rule out the possibility of there being more than one agent of non-A, non-B hepatitis. Data suggest that two episodes of non-A, non-B hepatitis can be produced in chimpanzees. One cannot, however, rule out the possibility of reinfection in these instances in the absence of specific serological tests. Specific ultrastructural changes characteristic of non-A, non-B infections have recently been described at the Bureau of Biologics and by others. Some have suggested that two different ultrastructural alterations, one cytoplasmic and one nuclear, may define different non-A, non-B agents. This needs to be confirmed.

In vitro studies using sera and liver biopsies from 10 chimpanzees infected with human non-A, non-B hepatitis revealed nuclear fluorescence in hepatocyte nuclei in liver biopsies during acute disease when tested with convalescent sera of chimpanzee or human origin. No fluorescence was seen in liver biopsies obtained prior to inoculation or with sera obtained prior to inoculation. Similarly, no fluorescence was seen in liver biopsies during hepatitis A or B or when antibodies to hepatitis A or B antigens were used. This fluorescence was not due to antinuclear, anti-SM or anti-RNP antibodies.

An antigen has also been detected by agar gel diffusion and counterelectrophoresis associated with non-A, non-B hepatitis after transfusion in humans and in experimentally inoculated chimpanzees. Sera from six of seven chimpanzees with acute human non-A, non-B hepatitis circulated this antigen during acute disease. It was not detected in 35 sera taken prior to inoculation or in sera from chimpanzees during experimental hepatitis A or B. Antibody to this antigen was detected in the convalescent sera from all seven chimpanzees studied. This antigen appears identical to the serum antigen described by others during human posttransfusion hepatitis. The exact relationship between this antigen and the agent or agents of non-A, non-B hepatitis remains unclear at this time. The specificity of these antigen-antibody systems has to be confirmed. Specific tests could permit the identification of those who transmit non-A, non-B hepatitis and determine whether one or more agents is responsible for what we know as non-A, non-B hepatitis.

New Developments in Malaria Chemotherapy Using In Vitro Cultures

W. H. G. RICHARDS
Co-moderator

The Wellcome Foundation, Ltd.
Berkhamstead, England

J. D. HAYNES
Co-moderator

Department of Immunology
Walter Reed Army Institute
of Research
Washington, D.C. 20012, U.S.A.

L. W. SCHEIBEL

Department of Parasitology
The Rockefeller University
New York, New York 10021, U.S.A.

R. SINDEN

Imperial College Field Station
University of London
Ascot, Bearks, SL5 7DE England

R. E. DESJARDINS

Division of Experimental Therapeutics
Walter Reed Army Institute
of Research
Washington, D.C. 20012, U.S.A.

W. H. WERNSDORFER

Malaria Action Programme
World Health Organization
1211 Geneva 27, Switzerland

The control of malaria by chemotherapy has been curtailed by the increasing spread of drug resistance of the parasite, especially *Plasmodium falciparum*, while the global malaria problem has been exacerbated by the return of infection to areas recently freed from the disease. The search for new chemotherapeutic agents and investigations aimed at a better understanding of existing antimalarials is an expensive and time-consuming task, undertaken usually only in the more sophisticated laboratories. The continuous culture of the human malaria parasite, first described by Trager and Jensen in 1976, has now provided the means to examine compounds against the target species quickly and easily; it also allows the biochemistry of the parasite to the investigated, and by exploiting this knowledge it may be possible to develop new antimalarials based on a more rational approach.

Dr. Haynes described a study of the purine metabolism of the parasite, which utilizes preformed purines provided by the host. Examination of five purine salvage enzymes in *P. falciparum* obtained from in vitro cultures revealed high levels of a parasite-specific adenosine deaminase (ADA). The partially purified enzyme from *P. falciparum* was distinguished from erythrocyte ADA by its greater electrophoretic mobility in starch gel and its lack of sensitivity to erythro-9-(2-hydroxy-3-nonyl) adenine

(EHNA), an inhibitor of erythrocyte ADA. When both ADAs were inhibited by deoxycoformycin, low concentrations of adenosine or deoxyadenosine (such as might be found in vivo) inhibited growth of the parasite. Similarly, the toxicity of an adenosine analog with antimalarial activity (cordycepin) was increased 1,000-fold when ADA was inhibited. Thus, in addition to participation in the purine salvage pathways, parasite ADA detoxifies adenine nucleosides and analogs. The results show that there are major differences between the host and parasite enzymes, which might be exploited in the development of adenosine analogs with selective toxicity for the parasite.

Dr. Scheibel presented information on carbohydrate and energy metabolism. *P. falciparum* in culture grows optimally at 3% O_2. Oxygen levels as low as 0.5% still support growth, but anaerobic conditions do not. These findings, plus the absence of the Krebs cycle or a classical Pasteur effect in *Plasmodia*, suggest that the malaria parasite does not rely on oxygen for energy metabolism to the same degree as does aerobic mammalian tissue. It may act to a large extent through metalloprotein biosynthetic oxygenases rather than in electron transport. In theory, therefore, a potent chelating agent with proven activity against metalloproteins might result in selective toxicity to the parasite and little effect on the host tissue. Tetraethylthiu-

10

ram disulfide (Antabuse) and its physiological reduction product diethyldithiocarbamate inhibit many purified metalloprotein oxygenases and have a lipid/water partition coefficient and high binding constant for metal ions, favoring selective toxicity to the intracellular malaria parasite. Antabuse has been used for years in clinical medicine. It is useful in aversion therapy for alcoholism, presumably through inhibition of liver aldehyde dehydrogenase which allows toxic metabolites of alcohol to accumulate. Even though it is highly inhibitory to metalloprotein oxidases, pharmacological doses do not inhibit the terminal electron transport enzyme, cytochrome oxidase, which is present in both *Plasmodium* and mammalian tissue.

In studies reported here, Antabuse and diethyldithiocarbamate exhibited active antimalarial effects in vitro in concentrations as low as 0.1 μg/ml, the lowest level tested. This is 1/100 the concentration reported to circulate in alcoholic patients on this drug. This effect occurred 72 h after addition of the drug to the in vitro system. Higher doses completely inhibited growth within 24 h of contact with the compound. In addition, tetraethylthiuram disulfide at a level as low as 1 μg/ml inhibited parasite glycolysis with no effect on glycolysis in normal erythrocytes.

Two methods were described in which can be studied the direct effect of drugs against the parasite. The first is a semiautomated microtitration technique; the second is a 4-day test in 3.5-cm petri dishes. The work in the latter system, described by Dr. Richards, is uncomplicated yet offers the ability to assess intrinsic drug activity quickly and cheaply. The malaria-infected cells can be exposed to controlled concentrations of drug, often higher than those which can be attained in vivo; this allows less active compounds to be assessed more fully and is important in drug design studies. Only small amounts of a drug or its metabolite are required.

Starting with an initial parasitemia where approximately 1% of the erythrocytes are infected, cultures with known concentrations of drug are incubated for 2 days, the supernatant containing the drugs is then removed and replaced with fresh medium, and the whole is incubated for a further 2 days. Films made daily from the cultures are stained and examined; the parasitemia is then estimated and compared with that of the untreated controls. The effect on the parasite is easily observed and can be measured not only as a decrease in parasite density but also in monitoring the viability of the remaining parasites after drug pressure. The standard antima-

larials chloroquine, primaquine, quinine, pyrimethamine, proguanil, and cycloguanil were all examined, and the inhibitory drug concentrations were evaluated at 10^{-6} M for the first three compounds, 10^{-9} M for pyrimethamine, 10^{-5} M for proguanil, and less than 10^{-10} M for cycloguanil. These levels approximate those obtained in plasma in vivo following routine antimalarial therapy.

The bioassay of human plasma after dosing with antimalarials has also been demonstrated. Samples taken at various periods after dosing and incubated with *P. falciparum*-infected erythrocytes demonstrate the rate at which the drug is absorbed and a blood level reached that is inhibitory to the growth of the parasite. The length of the protective inhibition level can also be measured. The concentration levels with pyrimethamine, for which a maximum concentration is achieved in 2 h and a protective level maintained for 7 days, have been corroborated using gas-liquid chromatographic methods. These techniques will undoubtedly feature prominently in future clinical trials, where initially it will be possible to establish inhibitory drug concentrations without the need to challenge the volunteers with the parasite.

Using a microtitration plate culture technique, Dr. Sinden found five morphologically distinguishable stages of gametocyte development over a period of 10 days. Using specific antimetabolites, the basic organization of the sexual cell cycle was investigated, the inhibitory activity being compared with that against the asexual parasites. Inhibitors used were directed against DNA synthesis, e.g., mitomycin C; RNA synthesis, e.g., actinomycin D, rifampin, and 8-azaguanine; and protein synthesis, e.g., puromycin, cyclohexamide, and emetine. It was possible to demonstrate four phases of gametocyte development: a G_1 period which lasts only a few hours; the S phase in which DNA synthesis occurs, which occupies the remainder of the first 2 days. G_1 and S are confined to stage I and II gametocytes. G_2 is divided into two sections: G_{2A}, characterized by stage II and III gametocytes in which significant RNA and protein synthesis continue to occur; and G_{2B}, in which there is a progressive increase in control (probably at a transcription level) resulting in the depression of both RNA and protein synthesis. Continued morphological differentiation occurs in the latter section, transforming the parasites to stage IV and the mature stage V. The mitotic phase is marked by the brief and explosive events of gametogenesis during which further protein synthesis occurs de novo. Using these criteria for gametocytogenesis, the activity of four antimalarial compounds was investigated. Results suggest that activity against gametocytes during S phase (stages I and II) is at the same level as that against the asexual parasites, and that the antigametocyte activity in vitro of chloroquine and cycloguanil is largely confined to this period. In contrast, while pyrimethamine is highly active during the S phase, its lethal effects continue into G_{2A}. Proguanil has a prolonged antigametocyte activity at least until day 8 of culture. It is well known that proguanil is converted in vivo to the triazine cycloguanil; it may be, however, that some of the parent compound is unchanged and continues to act on the older gametocytes.

Dr. Desjardins described a rapid, semiautomated microdilution method which was developed for measuring the activity of potential antimalarial drugs against cultured intraerythrocytic asexual forms of the human malaria parasite *P. falciparum*. Microtitration plates were used to prepare serial dilutions of the compounds to be tested. Parasites obtained from stock cultures were subcultured in these plates for 42 h. Inhibition of uptake of [^{3}H]hypoxanthine, a nucleic acid precursor capable of crossing the parasite membrane, served as the indicator of antimalarial activity. The data were analyzed by nonlinear curve-fitting techniques using a form of the logistic-logarithmic function which yields direct estimates of the ID_{50}, i.e., the concentration of drug causing a 50% reduction in the uptake of [^{3}H]hypoxanthine. This method of analysis allows precise comparisons among active compounds based on their respective ID_{50} and associated 95% confidence limits.

Results of repeated measurements of activity with chloroquine, quinine, and the investigational new drug mefloquine demonstrated that the method is sensitive and precise. Several additional antimalarial drugs and compounds of interest, including four new amodiaquine analogs, were tested in vitro and the results were consistent with available in vivo data. The use of *P. falciparum* isolates with known susceptibility to antimalarial drugs also permitted evaluation of the cross-resistance potential of each drug tested. Mefloquine was not cross-resistant with chloroquine or quinine, and a dihydrofolate reductase inhibitor (an oxo-triazine, WR 99,210) was not cross-resistant with pyrimethamine. Both are compounds of considerable interest as potential new antimalarial drugs.

In addition to screening large numbers of compounds rapidly and inexpensively, this automated system offers a potential bioassay for antimalarial activity in blood specimens obtained during early clinical studies with potential new drugs. This would greatly facilitate the process of drug development and provide a credible predictor of efficacy in therapeutic trials.

Dr. Wernsdorfer discussed the value of the in vitro culture in determining the level of drug sensitivity in the field. The in vitro test described by Rieckmann in 1968 provided for the first time the opportunity to objectively measure the sensitivity of *P. falciparum* to chloroquine in the field. This method used the measurement of schizont maturation, in short term, noncontinuous culture. In 1978, the principles of continuous culture of *P. falciparum* were applied to a microculture technique and successfully used to assess the sensitivity of the parasite to chloroquine and mefloquine under field conditions. The method starts essentially from synchronized parasite material usually available from patients with *P. falciparum* infections. The technique has been successfully used in Thailand, Brazil, Colombia, and the Sudan. The test is performed in flat-bottomed microtitration plates prepared with appropriate additions of drug, usually chloroquine and mefloquine. A small amount of patient's blood from a fingertip or earlobe is drawn into an anticoagulant capillary tube and ejected into a vial of growth medium and gently mixed. Each well is seeded with 50 μl of blood in medium, and the plate is incubated for 24 h, at which time films are made, stained, and counted. Schizonts, that is, parasites with more than two nuclei, are enumerated, and the values of the respective drug concentrations are compared with the untreated controls. Generally, total inhibition of growth at 4.00 pmol of chloroquine per well indicates a drug-susceptible strain, whereas growth at 5 to 7 pmol or more indicates resistance to chloroquine. Although at an early stage, similar findings are expected with mefloquine. The in vitro microtest is not meant to replace the in vivo assessment of the response to treatment with chloroquine; however, it provides a useful means for monitoring parasite susceptibility to drugs and is a convenient method for detecting the emergence of drug resistance under natural conditions in the field. The phenomenon of the selective uptake of chloroquine by the parasitized erythrocyte seems to be quite marked in the microtest system. However, the interaction of parasite density with drug response merits further investigation with isolates of defined susceptibility, preferably from continuous in vitro culture. Experiences with the in vitro microtest in South America demonstrated that local chloroquine-resistant strains were up to seven times more susceptible to me-floquine than to chloroquine. The 24-h test period makes the system unsuitable for the assessment of growth inhibition by the dihydrofolate reductase inhibitors, but by extending the incubation period this may prove possible.

During the discussion period, Dr. C. Camp-bell, from the Center for Disease Control, mentioned that reference strains of parasites sometimes develop increased or decreased susceptibility to drugs during serial subpassage in vitro, and that the microtest method for drug evaluation in the field continues to be refined.

Biochemistry and Mechanisms of Action of Antiprotozoan Agents

J. JOSEPH MARR
  Co-Chairman

Division of Infectious Diseases
St. Louis University School of Medicine
St. Louis, Missouri 63104, U.S.A.

FERNANDO STEELE DA CRUZ
  Co-Chairman

Institute of Microbiology
Department of General Microbiology
Federal University of Rio de Janeiro
Rio de Janeiro, Brazil

W. E. GUTTERIDGE

Biological Laboratory
University of Kent, Canterbury
Kent, England

MIKLÓS MÜLLER

Rockefeller University
New York, New York 10021, U.S.A.

ROBERT FERONE

Wellcome Research Laboratories
Research Triangle Park
North Carolina 27709, U.S.A.

I. B. R. BOWMAN

Department of Biochemistry
University of Edinburgh Medical School
Edinburgh, EH8 9AG, Scotland

The hemoflagellates that infect man have, to a considerable degree, defied chemotherapy. The specificity of antimicrobial therapy, so useful in the treatment of diseases caused by bacteria, is lacking in these protozoan diseases. The problem is compounded by the fact that these afflictions are of a global magnitude and the organisms which cause them are, at best, poorly understood. This symposium was an attempt to summarize our current knowledge of the biochemistry of these hemoflagellates as it relates to chemotherapy.

The first paper, by Dr. Gutteridge, presented a survey of those agents which have been shown to be active against *Trypanosoma cruzi* in vivo and relates them to their mechanisms of action insofar as is possible. Dr. Müller described in detail the activation of nitroimidazole compounds by protozoans which renders them effective as chemotherapeutic agents. Dr. Marr discussed a new class of antiprotozoan agents, the pyrazolopyrimidines, which enjoy a unique metabolism in *Leishmania* and *Trypanosoma*. The use of antifolate drugs in malaria and the biochemistry of their action were discussed by Dr. Ferone. The action of four antitrypanosomal agents was described by Dr. Bowman. These agents are diverse in their antimetabolic functions and illustrate the importance of understanding the biochemistry of the hemoflagellates

if we are to develop effective chemotherapeutic agents.

Mechanisms of Action of Drugs Active In Vivo in Experimental Chagas' Disease
(*W. E. Gutteridge*)

Extensive study of the modes of action of antibacterial drugs over many years has led to the identification of six key areas of metabolism as targets for drug action: energy metabolism, membrane function, cofactor synthesis, nucleic acid synthesis, protein synthesis, and cell wall synthesis. In parasitic protozoa, there is no real equivalent to the bacterial cell wall. With this exception it appears, though from far less extensive study, that the same key areas are also targets for antiprotozoan drugs.

Compounds active in vivo in experimental Chagas' disease have been described, but unfortunately there is little information available regarding their mechanisms of action. Where there is information, it has rarely been obtained using *T. cruzi* as test organism and only in a few instances have the investigations been carried out systematically.

The likely mechanisms of action of compounds active in vivo in experimental Chagas' disease are summarized in Table 1. Note that, with the exception of protein synthesis, there is at least one group of drugs in each category,

TABLE 1. *Possible modes of action of compounds active in vivo in experimental Chagas' disease*

Energy metabolism	Membrane function	Cofactor synthesis	Nucleic acid synthesis	Protein synthesis	Unknown
Arsenobenzenes 8-Aminoquinolines	Polyenes	Quinazolines	Purine analogs Phenanthridines Bisquinaldines 5-Nitrofurans 2-Nitroimidazoles 5-Nitroimidazoles 5-Nitrothiazoles	None	Naphthoquinones Piperazines Thioisonicotinic acid amides Thiosemicarbazones

though there are four groups where it is impossible so far to make even tentative suggestions. Nucleic acid synthesis appears to be the metabolic area in *T. cruzi* affected by the largest number of compounds. Included here are nifurtimox (a 5-nitrofuran) and benznidazole (a 2-nitroimidazole), the only two compounds so far on general release in Latin America for the treatment of Chagas' disease.

Mode of Action of Nitroimidazoles on Protozoa
(*Miklós Müller*)

Nitroimidazole derivatives were used as antiparasitic drugs for many years and more recently also as drugs against procaryotic microorganisms. Metronidazole (1-hydroxyethyl-2-methyl-5-nitroimidazole), introduced in 1960 for the treatment of human trichomoniasis, is extensively used today also in amoebiasis, giardiasis, and in certain bacterial infections. This successful drug served as a parent compound for the synthesis of a large number of nitroimidazole derivatives which differ greatly in their chemotherapeutic selectivity. Metronidazole and a number of similar drugs represent a group of compounds whose selectivity is defined by the anaerobic nature of the susceptible organisms. These compounds are effective not only against trichomonads and other anaerobic protozoa but also against strictly anaerobic bacteria. In addition, however, a number of nitroimidazoles with activity on strict anaerobes were found to act also on protozoa and bacteria which are not strict anaerobes, e.g., benznidazole on *T. cruzi* or SC 28538 on *Neisseria gonorrhoeae*.

The antimicrobial properties of these compounds depend on the presence of a nitro group on the imidazole ring. Evidence obtained on anaerobic protozoa and bacteria shows that these organisms activate the drug by reducing the nitro group. Neither the unreduced original compound nor the final products of reduction exhibit marked biological activity, but certain intermediate products of the reduction with

short half-lives are highly cytotoxic. The nature of these products and their action on the target cells are not clarified yet, although interaction with DNA has been demonstrated.

The reduction of the nitro group is performed by biological electron donors of the cell. The nitro group competes with other electron acceptors present. Under aerobic conditions, i.e., in the presence of O_2 which is a good electron acceptor, the antimicrobial activity of nitroimidazoles is markedly diminished, but not eliminated completely. Some *Trichomonas vaginalis* strains isolated from patients who were unsuccessfully treated with metronidazole were suspected of having decreased susceptibility to the drug. Such lowered susceptibility could indeed be detected but only if the assay was performed under aerobic conditions, suggesting that the relative resistance of these strains is due to an altered competition between metronidazole and O_2.

The spectrum of antimicrobial action of various nitroimidazoles is correlated with the relative electron affinity, i.e., reducibility of the nitro group. Nitroimidazoles with very low electron affinity (e.g., the 4-nitro analog of metronidazole) are not reduced by microorganisms and have no antimicrobial activity. Metronidazole and closely related drugs have a somewhat higher electron affinity, and their effective reduction requires electrons donated by low redox potential electron donors, e.g., ferredoxin- or flavodoxin-type electron transport proteins. The major metabolic role of such proteins in susceptible anaerobic protozoa and bacteria has been demonstrated or strongly implicated. At the same time, it is known that such compounds are absent from, or play only a subordinate role in, nonsusceptible facultative anaerobes or aerobes. Derivatives with still higher electron affinity often show a broader spectrum of action, including organisms which are not anaerobic. Although the interactions of these compounds with nonanaerobic target cells have been insufficiently studied, it is likely that the nitro group of such compounds can be reduced by a greater variety of cellular electron donors, explaining their broader action.

Antileishmanial and Antitrypanosomal Effects of Pyrazolopyrimidines
(*J. Joseph Marr*)

Pyrazolopyrimidines are purine analogs in which the carbon and nitrogen atoms of the imidazole ring are inverted. These compounds will not serve as purines in mammalian cells to any significant degree. Allopurinol [4-hydroxy-pyrazolo(3,4-d)pyrimidine; HPP], widely used in the treatment of hyperuricemic conditions, undergoes a unique metabolism in members of the genera *Leishmania* and *Trypanosoma*. In these organisms the pyrazolopyrimidine ring is converted to a ribonucleotide and then aminated to produce an analog of adenosine monophosphate (AMP) which is toxic.

This metabolic sequence was described first in three members of the genus *Leishmania*: *L. donovani*, *L. braziliensis,* and *L. mexicana*. These organisms concentrate allopurinol approximately 1,000-fold to produce intracellular concentrations of 1 to 2 mM. At these concentrations, HPP serves as a substrate for the hypoxanthine-guanine phosphoribosyltransferase (HGPRTase) and is activated in a single-step reaction to the ribonucleotide (HPPR-MP). The large concentration of HPPR-MP in the cell competes effectively with inosinic acid for the adenylosuccinate synthase. This enzyme aminates the nucleotide to 4-aminopyrazolopyrimidine monophosphate (APPR-MP). Since the V_{max} of the reaction with the analog is substantially slower than the V_{max} with the normal substrate, this becomes a rate-limiting step and decreases the amount of AMP synthesized by the cell. The APPR-MP is subsequently phosphorylated to its di- and triphosphate analogs and incorporated into the RNA of the cell. Investigations currently in progress have shown that HPP can inhibit RNA and protein synthesis in *L. donovani*, although it has not been demonstrated that this is the lethal event in the cell.

A similar metabolic sequence has been described for *T. cruzi*. The enzymology is not yet complete, but the metabolic transformations of HPP appear in the same sequence, that is, conversion to the ribonucleotide and subsequent conversion to APPR-MP and incorporation of the amino analogs into RNA. Investigations in progress have shown that HPP also inhibits RNA and protein synthesis in *T. cruzi*.

An analog of HPP, allopurinol ribonucleoside (HPPR), has been shown to be 100-fold more effective than its parent. The ribonucleoside undergoes a single-step activation by a phosphotransferase in *L. donovani* and, after conversion to the ribonucleotide, follows the metabolic sequence described above. A significant difference exists between the leishmania and *T. cruzi*: HPPR is ineffective against the latter. Studies with radiolabeled HPPR have shown that this compound does penetrate the cell but is neither hydrolyzed to the base nor phosphorylated to the ribonucleotide in any significant amounts. The chemotherapeutic usefulness of this relative inability to hydrolyze ribonucleosides remains to be explored.

The intracellular forms of *L. donovani* and *T. cruzi* have been shown to metabolize HPP in the same manner as do their extracellular forms. *L. donovani*, growing in P388D₁ macrophage tissue culture, converts HPP to the metabolic products given above and, apparently, in the same sequence. In addition, these parasites can be eliminated from macrophage tissue culture by the addition of HPP or HPPR. *T. cruzi*, growing in L929 fibroblasts, converts radiolabeled HPP to the same metabolic products as the epimastigote form.

Recently, several species of African trypanosomes, *T. rhodisiense*, and *T. brucei* (4 strains), all have been shown to convert HPP to HPPR-MP and APPR-mono, di-, and triphosphates. This latter compound is incorporated into the RNA of all of the African strains. The metabolism of allopurinol in these forms appears to be identical to that described in *T. cruzi* and the leishmaniae.

Folic Acid Antagonists as Antimalarial Agents
(*Robert Ferone*)

Many compounds that interfere with the biosynthesis or utilization of folate cofactors inhibit the growth of malarial parasites. These include: sulfa drugs, whose antimalarial activity and *p*-aminobenzoate (pAB) antagonism have been known for approximately four decades; diaminopyrimidines and -triazines, which have been studied and used clinically for almost three decades; and the more recent diaminoquinazolines and related compounds, whose place in antimalarial chemotherapy is yet undecided. In the case of the established compounds, the loci of action have been well established, but little is known about most of the recent ones.

The sulfonamides and sulfones inhibit the biosynthesis of folate by competing with pAB for the enzyme dihydropteroate synthase. Recent work with *Escherichia coli* has established that the sulfonamides are good alternate substrates for this enzyme, forming dihydropterinsulfonamide products. If this occurs in plasmodia, these products also should be tested for additional inhibitory action. Analogs of the pterins used in folate biosynthesis also can be antiplasmodial agents, since tetrahydrohomopteroate inhibits the growth of *Plasmodium cynomolgi* and is a potent inhibitor of plasmodial dihydropteroate synthase.

In the late 1940s, Hitchings and co-workers at Burroughs Wellcome developed a series of "nonclassical" folic acid antagonists that inhibited the growth of certain bacteria, protozoa, and tumor cells. The antifolate action was determined by the metabolite-reversal pattern of inhibition of *Lactobacillus casei*, but these compounds were termed nonclassical antagonists because they do not contain the complete pteridine structure of a classical analog such as aminopterin. The most active member of the series, pyrimethamine (2,4-diamino-5-*p*-chlorophenyl-6-ethyl pyrimidine), has been widely used in antimalarial chemotherapy; its selective toxicity is due to the approximately 1,000-fold tighter binding to the parasite dihydrofolate (FH_2) reductase than to the host enzyme. This locus of action has been demonstrated for most of the important antifolate antimalarials. The consequences of the resultant depletion of tetrahydrofolate cofactor pools in the parasite are still in question, because, contrary to expectations, the growth of the inhibited cells is arrested at a stage after that in which the bulk of the DNA is synthesized.

Trimethoprim, an FH_2 reductase inhibitor in clinical use as an antibacterial, also has useful antimalarial activity. Certain close analogs which are more potent inhibitors of malarial dihydrofolate reductase than trimethoprim are better against *P. berghei*, in vivo. The relative ability of a compound to inhibit the parasite dihydrofolate reductase compared to that of the host can be predictive in determining in vivo activity and/or toxicity; a lack of correlation among a series of compounds indicates differences in absorption, metabolism, excretion, etc.

After it was discovered that the biguanide, proguanil, is active as an antimalarial agent only after metabolism to a dihydrotriazine, many triazines were tested. The high activity but rapid excretion of cycloguanil led workers at Parke, Davis & Co. to try less soluble salts as repository forms of the compound, resulting in the extensive testing of the long-acting salt, cycloguanil pamoate. Cross-resistance to antifolate-resistant strains proved to be a major drawback, which is not surprising since cycloguanil and related dihydrotriazines share the same locus of action as pyrimethamine, that is, inhibition of plasmodial dihydrofolate reductase. Several newer dihydrotriazines, with 1-(substituted) benzyloxy group in place of the usual 1-(substituted) phenyl group, are still being investigated since they do not show cross-resistance to existing antifolate-resistant laboratory strains of malaria. Studies on the mode of action of these compounds should prove interesting.

2,4-Diamino-pteridines similar to "classical" folic acid antagonists are usually not effective antimalarials, possibly because they are not taken up by the parasite. Deaza-pteridine analogs such as pyrido[2,3-d] pyrimidines and quinazolines are, in general, more potent than pteridines, and several 2,4-diamino-substituted quinazolines have been widely studied. The most active, 2,4-diamino-6-(2-naphthyl)-sulfonylquinazoline, was less active in antifolate-resistant laboratory strains than in susceptible strains and does not have as favorable a ratio of parasite/host FH_2 reductase inhibition as does pyrimethamine.

All of the FH_2 reductase inhibitors of interest have also been used in combination with sulfa drugs, since the configuration of this metabolic pathway leads to a synergistic interaction between the two types of inhibitors. Synergistic combinations are inhibitory to most malaria strains resistant to either component alone and are currently in use for the prophylaxis and treatment of *P. falciparum*.

Chemotherapy of African Trypanosomiasis (*I. B. R. Bowman*)

Four drugs are available for the treatment of human trypanosomiasis caused by *Trypanosoma rhodesiense* and *T. gambiense*. They are melarsoprol (MelB), suramin, and nitrofurazone, which are curative, and pentamidine which is also prophylactic. MelB penetrates the CSF so that only it is effective in the terminal stages of sleeping sickness. No new drugs have been introduced for the last 20 years, and all suffer from the disadvantages of toxic side effects and from emerging resistance in the causative organism. An understanding of the action of these drugs and related model compounds at the molecular level could lead to improvements in treatment. To this end a knowledge of the basic biochemistry and of the function of organelles in the trypanosomes is essential.

The diamidine drugs and nitrofurazone act on nuclear DNA and kinetoplast DNA (kDNA), of which kDNA is probably the main target for selective action. MelB and suramin affect various enzymes of aerobic glycolysis. For trypanosomes in the mammalian bloodstream, this is the principal system for ATP generation and is distributed in three compartments. The first six enzymes of glycolysis, together with L-glycerol-3-phosphate dehydrogenase and glycerokinase, are found in microbodies; the remaining glycolytic enzymes exist in the cytoplasm and the cytochrome-independent glycerophosphate oxidase in the promitochondrion.

Pentamidine and related aromatic diamidines such as berenil, used in animal trypanosomiasis, bind to kDNA and selectively inhibit kinetoplast replication. The spacing between the amidino groups is critical. Removal of a nitrogen atom from the triazine bridge of berenil decreases the spacing from 1.3 to 0.5 nm, causing loss of growth inhibitory activity in *T. mega*. Replacement of this diazo bridge with an imino link gives a spacing of 1.1 nm restoring activity. Phenanthridinium drugs such as ethidium and related compounds which are used in the treatment of animal trypanosomiasis act by intercalation with nuclear DNA and kDNA.

Suramin inhibits the promitochondrial glycerophosphate oxidase. Analogs of suramin are, in order of their decreasing therapeutic effectiveness, correspondingly less active inhibitors of this oxidase. However, this cannot be the only site of action of this drug, as the organism survives anaerobically or under specific inhibition of the oxidase by salicylhydroxamate (SHAM). When a second reaction is inhibited by glycerol in the presence of SHAM, the trypanosomes are killed. Such treatment cures infections of *T. brucei* and of *T. vivax* in rats but only at near-lethal doses of SHAM. In conditions where the oxidase is inactive, glycerokinase is the only enzyme so far demonstrated which catalyzes a reaction leading to a net gain in ATP. This is synthesized from glycerophosphate and ADP when their concentrations in the microbody are elevated, as occurs when the oxidase is inactive. Thus the trypanocidal action is due to inhibition of the oxidase by SHAM and concurrent inhibition of ATP synthesis by a mass action effect of glycerol. Recent evidence shows that suramin satisfies this need for multisite action by inhibiting not only the oxidase but also glycerophosphate dehydrogenase.

Melarsen oxide, the active form of MelB, is a trivalent arsenical; it inhibits hexokinase, glycerokinase, and pyruvate kinase in solubilized extracts of trypanosomes. Pyruvate kinase is considered to be the primary target in vivo. Because of melarsen oxide's action on glycerokinase, a prime target, it might be predicted from the reasoning above that SHAM should potentiate the action of the arsenical and permit less toxic doses to be used. However, the action of malarsen oxide in *T. brucei* infections in rats is not potentiated by SHAM. It can be shown that the microbody membrane is impermeable to melarsen oxide, making glycerokinase inaccessible to the drug.

Other trivalent arsenicals, such as a dimerized melarsen oxide of the arsenobenzene type, should be tested for ability to penetrate the microbody. Such a molecule should then show a synergistic effect with SHAM.

Beta-Lactamase: a Major Form of Bacterial Resistance

HAROLD C. NEU
   Chairman

Columbia University
New York, New York 10032, U.S.A.

MARK RICHMOND
   Co-Chairman

University of Bristol
Bristol, England

SUSUMU MITSUHASHI

Gunma University
Maebashi, Japan

CARL-ERIK NORD

Karolinska Institute
Stockholm, Sweden

GORDON W. ROSS

Glaxo-Allenburys Research
Greenford, England

JEREMY R. KNOWLES

Harvard University
Cambridge, Massachusetts 02138, U.S.A.

ROBERT SUTHERLAND

Beecham Pharmaceuticals
Surrey, England

The importance of β-lactamases as a bacterial defense mechanism against β-lactam antibiotics has been appreciated since the 1940s. However, the increasing problem of infections due to gram-negative species resistant to many of the older β-lactam compounds has prompted intense research into the distribution, characterization, and activity of β-lactamases as well as research into ways by which these enzymes can be inhibited. This symposium attempted to clarify some of the aspects of what we know of β-lactamases and their role in bacterial resistance.

Distribution of β-Lactamases in Nature
(Susumu Mitsuhashi)

In studies of drug resistance in bacteria, we discovered that there were two types of resistance plasmids. One is conjugally transmissible (R) and the other is nontransmissible (r) by conjugation. About 60 to 80% of resistances to tetracycline, chloramphenicol, streptomycin, sulfonamide, kanamycin, ampicillin, and gentamicin are conjugally transferable in clinical isolates.

Most R plasmids confer multiple resistance on their host bacteria and are isolated only from gram-negative bacteria. Nonconjugative (r) plasmids are demonstrated at a high frequency from both gram-positive and gram-negative bacteria carrying nontransferable resistance, and they are also isolated from gram-negative bacteria carrying R plasmids. Most r plasmids confer single resistance on their host and exist as multiple copies in a cell. Epidemiological studies have disclosed the presence of chromosome-mediated and plasmid-mediated resistance in clinical iso-

lates. There are five types of plasmid-mediated resistance. Resistance due to the presence of both R and r in a cell (group 3) is most common in gram-negative bacteria. Resistance due to the presence of various r plasmids in a cell is often seen in *S. aureus*. Chromosome-mediated resistance to cephalosporins is most common in gram-negative bacteria with the production of cephalosporinase (CSase). Chromosome-mediated resistance to penicillins is seen in *Proteus mirabilis* and *Klebsiella pneumoniae* due to the production of penicillinase (PCase).

Sixty to 80% of ampicillin resistance in gram-negative bacteria is due to the presence of R plasmids, and most R plasmids showing ampicillin resistance are capable of conferring multiple resistance. Most penicillin resistance in *Staphylococcus aureus*, *Neisseria gonorrhoeae*, and *Haemophilus influenzae* is due to the presence of r plasmids. In gram-positive bacteria, penicillin-resistant and penicillin-susceptible groups with 75% of *S. aureus* strains are penicillin resistant. *Streptococcus pneumoniae* and *S. pyogenes* are still penicillin susceptible. In gram-negative bacteria, *Escherichia coli*, *Salmonella*, indole-negative *Proteus*, and *H. influenzae* mostly are susceptible to ampicillin. By contrast, most *Enterobacter cloacae*, *Citrobacter freundii*, *Klebsiella*, *Pseudomonas aeruginosa*, and *Serratia marcescens* are resistant to ampicillin.

β-Lactamases mediated by R plasmids are of PCase type and can be classified into four types according to their substrate profiles, inhibition profiles, molecular weight, isoelectric points, and immunological properties. The type I PCase is most often seen in gram-negative bacteria and is capable of hydrolyzing both ampicillin and cephaloridine at a high rate. The type II and type III are cloxacillin- and dicloxacillin-hydrolyzing enzymes, but are different in their molecular weight, immunological properties, and inhibition profiles. The type IV is a carbenicillin-hydrolyzing enzyme often seen in *P. aeruginosa*.

Gram-negative bacteria produce chromosomally mediated CSases, although some bacteria produce two types of β-lactamase: chromosome-mediated CSase and R-mediated PCase.

The properties of the β-lactamases produced by bacteria are summarized in Table 1. In general, *K. pneumoniae* and *P. mirabilis* produce the chromosomally mediated PCases and the production is noninducible. By contrast, the β-lactamases produced by other gram-negative bacteria are of CSase type and the production is enhanced by the prior treatment with β-lactam antibiotics, indicating the inducible production. The chromosomally mediated β-lactamases in *Proteus vulgaris*, *Pseudomonas cepacia*, and *Bacteroides fragilis* have broad substrate profiles and different inhibition profiles from other β-lactamases.

Genetic Organization Underlying Expression of β-Lactamase by Bacteria
(Mark Richmond)

Despite the fact that studies on the substrate profiles of bacterial β-lactamases suggest that a wide range of different types of enzyme are to be found in penicillin-resistant organisms, detailed examination of the amino acid sequences

TABLE 1. *β-Lactamase produced by bacteria*

Organisms	PCase	CSase	Inducibility
Gram-positive			
S. aureus	+	−	+
E. coli	−	+	−
K. pneumoniae	+	−	−
E. aerogenes	−	+	+
E. cloacae	−	+	+
S. marcescens	−	+	+
Gram-negative (chromosomally mediated)			
C. freundii	−	+	+
P. morganii	−	+	+
P. mirabilis	+	−	−
P. vulgaris	−	+	+
P. rettgeri	−	+	+
P. inconstans	−	+	+
P. aeruginosa	−	+	+
H. influenzae	+	−	−
P. cepacia	−	+	+
R-mediated PCase	+	−	−

of the enzymes reveals that some of those most different in properties are considerably alike in structure. Thus there is accumulating evidence that the β-lactamases which give rise to resistance in many strains of clinical significance are actually variants of the same evolutionary invention.

It is likely that there has been a stepwise modification of the primary sequence of the enzymes through point mutations in the gene concerned giving rise to a series of single amino acid changes, and this in turn is likely to have given rise to a gradual alteration of the substrate profiles of the enzymes in a number of directions. The second process is the transfer of the β-lactamase gene from one bacterial strain or species to another, and a given sensitive strain will receive the full apparatus needed to express resistance or not. The first type of process primarily has strategic consequences, whereas the second may give rise to changes of much more tactical import.

There is an additional genetic process which facilitates the spread of antibiotic resistance genes. This is transposition, a process whereby a gene moves from one bacterial replication unit to another but not by genetic recombination. No sequence homology between the interacting pieces of DNA is necessary for the process to occur.

The gene must be part of a highly specialized organizational DNA unit known as a transposon, an element characterized by specialized DNA sequences. In β-lactamase transposons—generically known as Tn*A*'s—the flanking sequences are 38 nucleotide pairs in length which are arranged as "inverted repeats": the 38-base-pair sequence at one end of the transposon is the same as the equivalent sequence at the other end of the transposon when that sequence is read in the opposite direction.

Transposons have evolved so that not all Tn*A*'s are identical and some bacteria carry fragments of transposons. For example, a strain of *N. gonorrhoeae* carrying the plasmid pMR0360 has a portion of a typical Tn*A* transposon with one of the inverted repeats as well as the genetic material for the β-lactamase gene. But the other end of the transposon is totally missing. Such a structure cannot transpose, so it appears that the evolutionary sequence has been to establish the β-lactamase gene in the strain concerned and to lock it there by elimination of its transpositional potential. An analogous situation also is to be found in some strains of *H. parainfluenzae*.

Although β-lactamase synthesis commonly is mediated by bacterial plasmids, one must not conclude that this is always so. The genes can be located on the bacterial chromosome and there is speculation whether a plasmid or a chromosomal location for a β-lactamase gene is the primitive state. There is a fluid situation where β-lactamase genes in some species are usually plasmid located, whereas in others they are carried as part of the chromosome.

Role of β-Lactamase in the Resistance of *Bacteroides fragilis* to β-Lactam Compounds
(Carl-Erik Nord)

Among the anaerobic gram-negative rods, *B. fragilis*, *B. melaninogenicus*, *B. bivius*, *B. oralis*, and *B. disiens* have been shown to possess β-lactamases, but the role of these enzymes in the antibiotic resistance to different β-lactam antibiotics is not completely understood. The most studied β-lactamase in anaerobic bacteria is that of *B. fragilis*. The enzymes from *B. fragilis* strains have mainly CSase activity, with some cephalosporins more rapidly hydrolyzed than others. The β-lactamases do not seem to be inducible with β-lactam antibiotics.

The enzymes have lower isoelectric points than those of aerobic gram-negative rods. The isoelectric points of *B. fragilis* β-lactamases are found between pI 4.3 and 5.2.

Anaerobic β-lactamases are inhibited by both cloxacillin and *p*-chloromercuribenzoate, and this is in contrast to most β-lactamases with CSase activities.

Observations on the cellular location of the enzymes have not yet resolved whether they are cell bound or periplasmically located. The release of the enzyme into the growth medium during cultivation suggests a loose association with the cell envelope, which is supported by the fact that β-lactamase activity is found in the osmotic shock fluid. The molecular weights of the β-lactamases have been reported to be about 29,000 to 31,000 as determined by gel filtration and 40,000 to 43,000 as determined by gel electrophoresis.

B. fragilis strains can be divided into three resistance categories: group 1, highly resistant (MIC > 128 μg/ml); group II, relatively resistant (MIC, 4 to 64 μg/ml); group III, relatively sensitive (MIC $\leq$ 4 μg/ml). Group 1 strains produced about 10 times as much β-lactamase as that produced by group II strains, whereas group III strains produced only minute amounts of β-lactamase or no β-lactamase at all. The most active β-lactam antibiotic compounds against *B. fragilis* β-lactamase are the cephamycins. Three new cephalosporins, cefamandole, cefuroxime, and cefotaxime, are resistant to most β-lactam-

ases from facultative anaerobic bacteria but they are hydrolyzed by *B. fragilis* β-lactamase.

Clavulanic acid and penicillanic acid sulfone reduce the MICs of cephaloridine for β-lactamase-producing strains of *B. fragilis* but do not influence the MICs for strains showing low or no enzyme production.

The genetic control of *B. fragilis* β-lactamases has not yet been clarified. There is no correlation between β-lactamase production and the presence of plasmids in *B. fragilis*.

Characterization of β-Lactamases
(Gordon W. Ross)

The widespread occurrence of β-lactamases in all species of bacteria together with their key role in the resistance of certain bacteria to β-lactam antibiotics has led to the characterization of these enzymes.

Early characterization was achieved by determination of substrate and inhibitor profiles, measurements of molecular weights, and use of antisera.

Such methods have proved most useful when, for example, the substrate profiles of a number of β-lactamases have been compared by one investigator using enzyme preparations of similar purity under carefully controlled conditions and with the use of one well-tried assay procedure. It is possible to obtain similar substrate profiles for an enzyme by the careful use of several different assay methods, but problems have arisen when substrate profiles of the same enzyme have been obtained by different workers using enzyme preparations of different degrees of purity and employing different assay methods. Confusion may also occur when a β-lactamase has been labeled as resistant or sensitive to an inhibitor without the precise conditions used to assess the inhibition being emphasized.

Isoelectric focusing has simplified some aspects of β-lactamase classification by demonstrating that enzymes isolated in different parts of the world are identical; for example, the plasmid-mediated β-lactamases R1, RGN 14, and TEM, which were first isolated in England, Japan, and Greece, respectively, are clearly identical. Conversely, other β-lactamases thought to be identical on the basis of biochemical and immunological properties have clearly distinguishable isoelectric focusing patterns; for example, until recently the only way of distinguishing the common TEM-1 and TEM-2 types of enzyme was by isoelectric focusing. It is now known there is probably only one amino acid difference.

The technique has proved especially useful for monitoring the spread of antibiotic resistance due to transfer of plasmid-mediated β-lactamases, because the β-lactamase specified by a plasmid gives an identical isoelectric focusing pattern even when located in different hosts. Antibiotic resistance due to transfer of known plasmids mediating β-lactamase has been identified by this technique in *Haemophilus*, *Neisseria*, and *Pseudomonas* spp.

New β-lactamases continue to be found. The properties of β-lactamases determined by plasmids in over 350 strains of gram-negative bacteria have been classified into 11 types on the basis of clear differences in key properties. TEM-type β-lactamases occurred most frequently and were the most widespread; they constituted over 77% of plasmid-determined β-lactamases examined, and the TEM-1 type alone has been found in 19 different species from 8 countries. The oxacillin-hydrolyzing β-lactamases make up over 15% of the total and have been located in 8 species from 10 countries while the interesting SHV-1 type, which is inhibited by p-chloromercuribenzoate when cephaloridine is the substrate but not when benzylpenicillin is the substrate, makes up over 4% of the total and has been found with increasing frequency. The four PSE types of plasmid-determined β-lactamase have been found only in *P. aeruginosa*.

The enzymes from *S. aureus* PC1, *Bacillus licheniformis* 749/C, *B. cereus* 569H (β-lactamase 1), and *E. coli* R TEM (TEM-2) clearly belong to the same homology group. Work on the secondary and tertiary structure of the TEM-2 enzyme is well advanced and studies on other sequenced enzymes are in progress. The major β-lactamases are now well characterized, and new β-lactamases that undoubtedly have yet to be discovered can be compared with those already characterized.

Inactivation of β-Lactamases
(Jeremy R. Knowles)

There are two approaches that can be taken to overcome the defensive production of β-lactamase by β-lactam-resistant bacteria. The first approach is to develop new β-lactam antibiotics poorly hydrolyzed by β-lactamases. Yet the promiscuous transfer of genetic information amongst bacteria in the form both of plasmids and of transposons carrying the β-lactamase gene has resulted in a continuing struggle to maintain the efficacy of β-lactam antibiotics and has encouraged the search for β-lactamase inactivators that could be used in synergy with existing β-lactam antibiotics. This second approach met with early failure, as it was found that a variety of classical "affinity reagents" were quite ineffective in the inactivation of β-lactamase. The discovery in a *Streptomyces* strain of the first β-lactamase inactivator, clavulanic acid, was followed by the discovery of other materials that were effective in synergy with β-lactam antibiotics against β-lactamase-producing organisms. Consideration of the possible modes of action of these compounds has led, in the past year or so, to the synthesis of several new reagents, such as the penicillanic acid sulfone and 6-β-bromopenicillanic acid, that have clearly demonstrated that β-lactamases are susceptible to inactivation by the more subtle pathways of so-called suicide reagents.

Studies of the mechanistic pathway followed by the TEM β-lactamase from *E. coli* during the hydrolysis of the poor substrate cefoxitin has shown that the reaction proceeds via the formation of an acyl-enzyme intermediate. This intermediate derives from the acylation of an enzymic hydroxyl group by the β-lactam and then hydrolyzes to produce the product cephalosporoic acid.

Consider the simplest of the group inactivators, the 6-desamino-penicillanic acid sulfone. This molecule is a substrate for the TEM β-lactamase having a k_{cat} of 60 min^{-1} and a k_m of 0.9 M. These values may be compared with those for the excellent substrate benzylpenicillin, which has a k_{cat} of 10^5 min^{-1} and a k_m of 20 μM. The sulfone also is an inactivator of the enzyme, and the kinetic and spectroscopic characteristics of its interaction with the β-lactamase are consistent with the partition of the acyl-enzyme between hydrolysis and a β-elimination process that produces a relatively more stable acyl-enzyme. The inactive enzyme is either α,β-unsaturated ester itself or is derived from it by the attack of an enzyme nucleophile at what was C-5 of the original β-lactam. This simple mechanistic postulate accommodates, with minor variations, all the kinetic, chemical, and spectroscopic behavior of the five major β-lactamase inactivators.

Consideration of this scheme led us to propose that effective inactivators of β-lactamase must fulfill three criteria: (i) the inactivator must contain a β-lactam ring that is susceptible to at least the first steps of the normal hydrolytic reaction catalyzed by the β-lactamase, up to and including the formation of the acyl-enzyme intermediate; (ii) the inactivator must possess an α-proton at C-6 that can participate in a β-elimination to an α,β-unsaturated ester; (iii) the inactivator must possess a good leaving group for the β-elimination reaction to occur either across C-6 and C-5 or (as in the case of II) from C-6 out into the C-6 side chain.

These features are not prerequisites for any

effective inhibitor of β-lactamase action, and a competitive inhibitor of extremely low K_i might well fulfill none of the above criteria. The conditions can be met by selecting β-lactams that are poor substrates for the enzyme. This maximizes the chances of producing a long-lived acyl-enzyme that may survive long enough for the putative β-elimination to occur and oxidizing the sulfur to a sulfone, thus simultaneously providing lability of the 6-α proton and a good leaving group from C-5. For the sulfones of cloxacillin, methicillin, and quinacillin, the k_{cat} values for the parent penams were 24, 10, and 7 s^{-1}, respectively. In vitro, each of these molecules is a more effective inactivator of the TEM β-lactamase than is the 6-desamino-penicillanic acid sulfone (k_{cat} 40 s^{-1}), which supports the validity of the mechanistic analysis proposed above.

Inhibition of β-Lactamases by Clavulanic Acid and Similar Compounds
(Robert Sutherland)

Semisynthetic penicillins such as methicillin and cloxacillin have been shown to act as competitive inhibitors of β-lactamases, but the level of activity is low and the breadth of spectrum of inhibition limited. Following the discovery of β-lactamase inhibitory activity in cultures of *Streptomyces olivaceus*, a series of bicyclic β-lactam compounds, the olivanic acids, were isolated. The olivanic acids, chemically related to the antibiotic thienamycin, have been shown to be active broad-spectrum bactericidal antibiotics as well as β-lactamase inhibitors. Further investigations of microbial metabolites led to the isolation of another bicyclic β-lactam compound, clavulanic acid, in culture filtrates of *S. clavuligeris* ATCC 27064, also known to produce cephalosporins and cephamycin C. Clavulanic acid was found to be a potent progressive inhibitor of β-lactamases from a broad spectrum of gram-positive and gram-negative bacteria. More recently, the β-lactamase-inhibitory properties of two semisynthetic compounds, penicillanic acid sulfone (CP 45899) and β-bromopenicillanic acid, have been reported, and the sulfone has been shown to potentiate the activity of ampicillin and other β-lactam antibiotics.

Clavulanic acid is a potent progressive inhibitor, and β-lactamases susceptible to the compound include plasmid-mediated enzymes (TEM, OXA) and the chromosomally mediated β-lactamases produced by *Klebsiella* spp., *B. fragilis*, *Proteus* spp., and *S. aureus*. The CSase's found in many gram-negative bacilli are inhibited to a much lesser extent. When combined with penicillin or cephalosporins, marked enhancement of antibiotic activity against many β-lactamase-producing bacteria has been demonstrated.

Clavulanic acid is well absorbed by the oral route in animals and man, and pharmacokinetic studies have shown that the compound is compatible with amoxicillin. Accordingly, the properties of a formulation comprising amoxicillin (two parts) and clavulanic acid (one part) (BRL 25000, Augmentin) have been studied in detail. The association of the broad-spectrum penicillin and the β-lactamase inhibition has been shown to demonstrate significant activity against a high proportion of β-lactamase-producing gram-negative bacteria, including amoxicillin-resistant strains of *H. influenzae* and *N. gonorrhoeae*, and against penicillin-resistant *S. aureus*. The results of in vitro tests are reflected in experimental chemotherapy, and amoxicillin plus clavulanic acid was efficacious against a variety of experimental infections refractory to amoxicillin. Bioavailability studies in man have shown that clavulanic acid is rapidly absorbed after oral administration to human volunteer subjects and produces peak serum levels similar to those obtained with amoxicillin. When the amoxicillin/clavulanic acid formulation was administered to volunteers, peak serum concentrations of both compounds were attained at 1 h, and the ratio of amoxicillin:clavulanic acid in the serum ranged from 1.0 to 2.0 during the 6-h period after dosing. Both compounds were excreted in high concentrations in the urine.

Comparative Activity of New Cephalosporins Against β-Lactamase-Producing Bacteria
(Harold C. Neu)

Over the past few years we have evaluated the efficacy of a number of novel cephalosporins (Fig. 1) in inhibiting bacteria containing β-lactamases (Table 2), as well as the relative stability of these compounds to β-lactamases of diverse origins.

The first compound of the third-generation agents that has been extensively studied is cefotaxime. It is as resistant to hydrolysis by the most common β-lactamases as are cefoxitin and cefuroxime. Thus the most commonly encountered β-lactamase, the so-called TEM-1, Richmond type III, or more properly plasmid-mediated β-lactamase active against both penicillins and cephalosporins does not hydrolyze this agent. Presence of this enzyme in *E. coli*, *H. influenzae*, *N. gonorrhoeae*, *S. sonnei*, *S. typhimurium*, and *P. aeruginosa* does not make these species resistant to cefotaxime. This compound is active against organisms which possess β-lactamases which primarily act as CSase's, such as

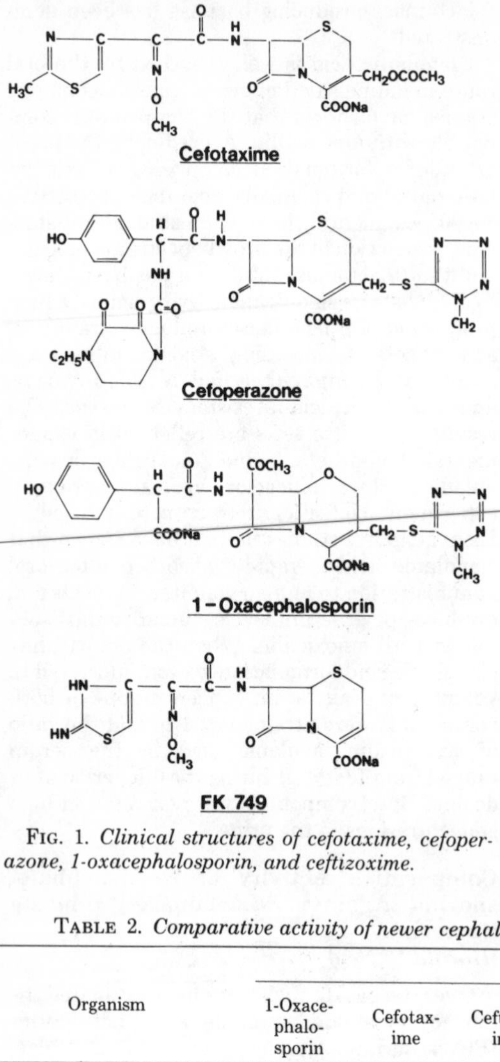

FIG. 1. *Clinical structures of cefotaxime, cefoperazone, 1-oxacephalosporin, and ceftizoxime.*

C. freundii, E. cloacae, P. morganii, P. rettgeri, etc., and *P. stuartii.* The activity of the compound against these species is only partly related to β-lactamase stability, but it is related also to its affinity for β-lactam receptor proteins involved in cell wall synthesis and to its ability to penetrate a complex gram-negative cell wall. Cefotaxime is a β-lactamase inhibitor of some of the Richmond type I β-lactamases and is a more effective inhibitor of these β-lactamases than is cefoxitin.

Cefoperazone has markedly increased activity against *P. aeruginosa* but is less β-lactamase stable than is carbenicillin. Cefoperazone has greater β-lactamase stability than the older compounds such as cephalothin and cefazolin and may be more β-lactamase stable than cefamandole, but it is less stable than cefoxitin or cefuroxime. Some *E. coli* spp. and many *B. fragilis* spp. can hydrolyze the compound.

Replacement of the sulfur at position 1 of the cephem nucleus with an oxygen, as well as the presence of the methoxy group at position 7, has provided a compound with both high intrinsic activity and β-lactamase stability, a 1-oxacephem. It is as resistant to hydrolysis by β-lactamases as is cefoxitin, but it inhibits microorganisms resistant to cefoxitin such as *E. cloacae,* *C. freundii,* and even some *B. fragilis* spp. This agent, similar to cefotaxime, combines a β-lactamase stability with a high degree of intrinsic activity against bacteria since it is as active against organisms which produce large amounts

TABLE 2. *Comparative activity of newer cephalosporins against β-lactamase-resistant bacteria*[a]

Organism	MIC (μg/ml) of drug						
	1-Oxace-phalosporin	Cefotaxime	Ceftizoxime	Cefoperazone	Cefoxitin	Cefuroxime	Cefamandole
E. coli	0.1	0.05	0.1	50	12.5	3.1	100
K. pneumoniae	0.8	0.05	0.05	50	25	25	50
E. cloacae	0.1	0.1	0.1	>100	>400	12.5	200
E. hafnia	0.8	0.8	0.4	0.4	200	50	25
S. marcescens	12.5	25	3.1	>100	>400	>400	>400
C. freundii	0.1	0.1	0.1	0.4	100	1.6	12.5
S. typhimurium	0.05	0.05	0.05	0.8	1.6	3.1	12.5
S. sonnei	0.2	1.6	0.2	100	100	12.5	50
P. mirabilis	0.1	0.1	0.05	>100	>100	>100	>100
P. morganii	6.3	3.1	6.3	12.5	12.5	100	25
P. rettgeri	0.1	0.05	0.005	12.5	1.6	1.6	0.8
P. vulgaris	0.05	0.01	0.005	1.6	1.6	200	200
P. stuartii	1.6	3.1	0.8	50	12.5	12.5	100
A. anitratus	50	50	25	>100	>400	>400	>400
P. aeruginosa	6.3	12.5	25	1.6	>400	>400	>400
B. fragilis	12.5	50	50	100	6.3	>100	>100

[a] Resistant to cephalothin and carbenicillin, MIC ≥ 200 μg/ml.

of β-lactamase as it is against bacteria in which a β-lactamase cannot be detected by routine means.

The most recent β-lactamase-resistant cephalosporin is ceftizoxime. This agent has structural features similar to cefotaxime. The in vitro activity of the agent is also similar to that of cefotaxime and the 1-oxacephalosporin. It is stable against β-lactamases of most of the *Enterobacteriaceae* as well as those found in a number of *Bacteroides* spp. and in *P. aeruginosa*. Like the aforementioned agents, this compound is as active in vitro against bacteria which possess β-lactamases as it is against those which do not have these enzymes, indicating that the other factors mentioned, receptor affinity and entry, are important in explaining its extremely broad activity.

It will be intriguing to see whether new β-lactamases or alteration in receptor sites will evolve as a mechanism of resistance to these powerful new drugs.

Animal Models as Predictors of Therapeutic Efficacy in Bacterial Infections in Man

H. H. GADEBUSCH
Chairman

Merck Institute for Therapeutic Research
Rahway, New Jersey 07065, U.S.A.

M. P. GLAUSER
Co-Chairman

Centre Hospitalier
Universitaire Vaudois
Lausanne, Switzerland

J. E. PENNINGTON

Peter Bent Brigham Hospital and Harvard University
Boston, Massachusetts 02115, U.S.A.

M. A. SANDE

University of Virginia
School of Medicine
Charlottesville, Virginia 22901, U.S.A.

J. G. BARTLETT

VA Hospital and Tufts University School of Medicine
Boston, Massachusetts 02130, U.S.A.

R. J. McRIPLEY

Squibb Institute for Medical Research
Princeton, New Jersey 08540, U.S.A.

The treatment of bacterial infections until the beginning of the 20th century was largely empirical, relying for the most part on successful past experience directly in the target species. Human and ethical considerations have gradually imposed greater restrictions on the evaluation of new therapeutic agents in man. It has thus become necessary to interpose testing in one or more subhuman animal species between discovery of a new drug in the laboratory and demonstration of its clinical utility.

The choice of an animal model that will provide information about the outcome of a human infection, when both are treated with the same chemotherapeutic agent, has been the subject of several symposia as well as numerous papers and informal discussions. Basically, the selection process is an exercise in both comparative pathogenesis and comparative pharmacology in which the experimenter plays the role of arbiter. It is he who must decide, based on a knowledge of the aforementioned, which test animal(s) and microorganism is most appropriate and the conditions under which he wishes to study the protective effects, if any, of the drug. Since bacteria invade, colonize, and may cause infection in various locations in the body, requiring different modalities of therapy, participants in this symposium have focused on the site-organism relationship in their discussion of drug-parasite interaction.

Bacteremia
(*H. H. Gadebusch*)

Even though experimentally induced bacteremia/septicemia in laboratory animals is quite different from the acquired disease in man, a great deal of useful information with qualitative relevance for man can be derived from such studies, including data in the following areas: acute and subacute toxicity, therapeutic efficacy, comparative efficacy among structurally related compounds, potential for oral absorption, pharmacological behavior, pharmacokinetic profile, effects of drug-inactivating enzymes generated by bacteria, changes in gastrointestinal flora, and multiple drug interactions.

It is unlikely that data derived from animal studies can be applied to humans in the following areas: drug idiosyncrasy, hypersensitivity reactions, and dosage regimen of drug.

No new anti-infective agent would be developed without a thorough study of its antimicrobial, pharmacokinetic, and potential toxicological properties in laboratory animals. Of these, the results of early chemotherapeutic studies, conducted against a background of comparative pathogenesis and pharmacology and which seek to define the attributes/liabilities of the new agent, often are the major determinant in the future course of drug development. Such confidence would be ill-placed if animal studies represented a poor parallel of human disease.

Urinary Tract Infections and Kidney Damage
(*M. P. Glauser*)

Uncomplicated urinary tract infections occur in the vast majority of patients by the ascending route, and only in exceptional cases do they cause permanent kidney damage, usually when obstruction or underlying renal disease is present.

In the presence of obstruction, reflux, or underlying renal disease, infection of the urinary tract may be devastating and may lead to acute obstructive pyelonephritis, and eventually to bacteremia, septic shock, and death. The kidney may be destroyed by the infectious process. Many different animal models have been proposed for studying the pathogenesis and the treatment of acute and chronic pyelonephritis. Some of these models use the hematogenous route of infection, with or without obstruction. In others, the bacteria are injected directly into the kidney parenchyma. But only a few of them mimic severe human kidney infection: bacteria arriving in the kidney by the ascending route in the presence of obstruction.

Chronic pyelonephritis is the end result of the infectious destruction of the kidney. Its pathogenesis has been the subject of considerable interest for many years, and the experimental studies of its treatment have aimed at establishing the best antibiotic regimen that would sterilize the kidney. When a combination of β-lactam and aminoglycoside antibiotics is synergistic in vitro against the infecting microorganism, sterility of the obstructed pyelonephritic kidney is achieved faster and more reliably with the synergistic combination than with either drug alone. It is necessary to sterilize the kidney in the presence of persisting obstruction, because severe infection and acute pyelonephritis may recur under these circumstances even if very few viable microorganisms remain in the kidney parenchyma (M. P. Glauser et al., J. Infect. Dis. **139**:133, 1979).

Most studies of the treatment of acute obstructive pyelonephritis were not designed with the purpose of establishing when and how the antibacterial treatment would be most effective in preventing kidney damage. Recent experimental evidence in the rat strongly suggests that the kidney damage of chronic *Escherichia coli* pyelonephritis results from scarring and shrinkage secondary to suppuration and necrosis that occurs early during the acute phase of infection. It has been shown that antibiotic treatment started early in the course of the inflammatory process due to infection completely prevented kidney destruction, e.g., chronic pyelonephritis. On the contrary, even the best available synergistic combination of antibiotics was not able to prevent kidney destruction (chronic pyelonephritis) if it was given after the full inflammatory process due to infection and obstruction had appeared. In these experiments, the scars of chronic pyelonephritis evolved from acute obstructive pyelonephritis even after sterilization of the tissue (M. P. Glauser et al., J. Clin. Invest. **61**:403, 1978). These observations, therefore, clearly show that, although it is important to administer the best antibiotic regimen in obstructive kidney infections, the prevention of renal damage depends on giving antibiotics early enough in the course of the disease so as to prevent inflammation and consequent scarring.

There is other experimental evidence which suggests that diminishing inflammation and suppuration is more important in preventing renal scarring in kidney infections than merely suppressing infection. For example, the evolution from acute obstructive pyelonephritis to chronic pyelonephritis did not develop in the rat even in the presence of persisting infection, provided inflammation was suppressed with a short course of antibiotic during the acute obstructive phase. Furthermore, aminoglycosides, antibiotics which accumulate and persist in the kidney parenchyma, not only diminish the frequency of acute obstructive pyelonephritis when given before infection (M. P. Glauser et al., J. Infect. Dis. **139**:172, 1979), but also protect against chronic pyelonephritis in those animals which do develop acute obstructive pyelonephritis. This protection is in direct proportion to the diminution of inflammation during the acute phase. It appears, therefore, that, even in the continued presence of infection, irreversible kidney damage can be prevented by the suppression of inflammation and that antibacterial agents prevent kidney damage by diminishing the bacterial load below a suppurative level.

Respiratory Infections
(J. E. Pennington)

The use of antimicrobial agents for treatment of lower respiratory tract bacterial infections is not uniformly successful. In fact, the mortality rate for gram-negative bacillary pneumonias is often high, particularly for infections with *Pseudomonas aeruginosa*. This lecture described how animal models might be used for evaluation of: (i) antibiotic delivery to the lung; (ii) antibiotic efficacy to increase survival from infection; and (iii) antibiotic effect on bacterial clearance from the lungs. Throughout these studies, continuity was provided by the underlying clinical question, "Why is mortality from *Pseudomonas* pneumonia so high and what might be the best method to treat this infection?"

Since the early studies by J. R. May (Br. J. Tuberc. **49**:166, 1955), the value of achieving concentrations of antibiotics in bronchial fluids which exceed the minimal inhibitory concentration (MIC) for an infecting bacterium has been well known. To evaluate both the delivery and the patterns of clearance of anti-*Pseudomonas* antibiotics in bronchial fluids, normal dogs were anesthetized and intubated, and concomitant serum and bronchial fluid specimens were obtained. Gentamicin and tobramycin levels in the bronchial fluids were about 40% of those in serum over most time intervals (up to 3 h). Others (Wieser et al., Dtsch. Med. Wochenschr. **96**:870, 1971) have shown that inflammation does not increase gentamicin penetration into bronchial fluids. For carbenicillin, the bronchial level was only 20% of that in serum. Thus, these concentrations in bronchial fluids were below the MIC of many clinical *Pseudomonas* isolates and may partially explain the difficulty in treating *Pseudomonas* bronchopneumonia when a component of bronchial mucosal infection exists.

To evaluate the various efficacies of anti-*Pseudomonas* antibiotics for the therapy of active parenchymal lung infection, a guinea pig model of acute hemorrhagic pneumonia was established. An intratracheal inoculum of 10^8 colony-forming units (CFU) of our challenge strain of *Pseudomonas* produced 100% mortality in normal guinea pigs. Infected animal groups were treated with either gentamicin, tobramycin, carbenicillin, ticarcillin, or gentamicin plus ticarcillin. A saline-treated control group was included. The MICs of gentamicin (0.75 μg/ml), tobramycin (1.50 μg/ml), carbenicillin (64 μg/ml), and ticarcillin (32 μg/ml) were routinely exceeded by peak serum levels in treated animals. The challenge strain of *Pseudomonas* did not exhibit in vitro synergy for any of the combination regimens in this study. Survival rates from infection were: controls, 0%; carbenicillin, 0%; ticarcillin, 0%; gentamicin, 39%; tobramycin, 67%; combination regimens, 60% (range 45–73%). Other groups were electively sacrificed 3 h after infection and lungs were cultured quantitatively. The clearance of viable *Pseudomonas* from lungs in each group correlated closely with the survival data.

Our conclusions from these studies were as follows. (i) The penetration of anti-*Pseudomonas* antibiotics in lung secretions often fails to achieve local levels above the MIC encountered in *Pseudomonas* isolates. (ii) Aminoglycosides (in particular, tobramycin) may be more effective than β-lactam agents in *Pseudomonas* pneumonia. (iii) Combination regimens of an aminoglycoside plus β-lactam agent may not be more effective than aminoglycosides alone, if the infecting pathogen lacks in vitro synergy for this combination.

Endocarditis and Meningitis
(*M. A. Sande*)

Animal models have been effectively utilized to predict factors that influence the treatment of endocarditis and meningitis. A rabbit model of endocarditis has been used to demonstrate that bactericidal antibiotics with a high initial peak and sustained activity were necessary to prevent endocarditis caused by strains of viridans streptococci and enterococci (*Streptococcus faecalis*). Utilizing the same model, it has been found that the rate at which antimicrobial agents kill viridans streptococci, enterococci, and *S. aureus* in broth is predictive of the relative rate the drugs alone or in combination eradicate the microorganisms from cardiac vegetations in vivo. Treatment with the synergistic combination of benzylpenicillin and streptomycin achieved sterility of vegetations in one-third the time required for penicillin alone in *S. sanguis*-induced endocarditis. A peak serum bactericidal titer of ≤1:8 was necessary for maximal effectiveness for viridans streptococcal endocarditis and activity of ≤1:2 for 50% of each treatment interval was necessary for successful treatment of experimental *S. aureus* endocarditis.

In experimental meningitis, similar studies have been reported. Drugs that are bactericidal in vitro produce a more rapid reduction in bacterial counts in cerebrospinal fluid (CSF) in vivo than bacteriostatic agents and are more effective in curing animals with *S. pneumoniae* meningitis. Synergistic combinations of ampicillin and gentamicin produced a more rapid bactericidal effect in vivo than ampicillin alone in *Listeria monocytogenes* meningitis. Chloramphenicol antagonized the bactericidal action of gentamicin in vitro and reduced the latter drug's effectiveness in experimental *Proteus mirabilis* meningitis. The reduction in CSF pH found in experimental meningitis may significantly reduce the activity of aminoglycosides in gram-negative bacillary meningitis.

Infections of the Peritoneum
(*J. G. Bartlett*)

Intraabdominal sepsis usually involves multiple bacterial species derived from the colonic flora. Bacteriological studies of 72 patients with generalized peritonitis or intraabdominal abscesses in our laboratory showed an average of five microbial species per specimen, with the dominant isolates belonging to the *B. fragilis* group (62 isolates) and *E. coli* (42 isolates). The polymicrobic flora at infected sites poses a therapeutic dilemma due to uncertainty regarding which organisms represent pathogens and thus require antimicrobial treatment.

An animal model was designed to simulate intraabdominal sepsis following colonic perforation. Wistar rats were challenged with an intraperitoneal implant of gelatin capsules containing an inoculum of pooled rat stool. Initial studies in untreated animals showed a biphasic disease. In the first stage, the animals had generalized peritonitis with *E. coli* bacteremia and a 43% mortality; all animals which survived the first 7 days had the second phase characterized by indolent intraabdominal abscesses in which *B. fragilis* was the numerically dominant isolate. Thirty-one antimicrobial regimens were tested in this model using doses based on preliminary pharmacokinetic studies in healthy Wistar rats. Groups of 30 to 60 animals were then challenged with the pooled stool inoculum, and the test agents were given at 8-h intervals for 10 days starting 4 h after implantation. Surviving animals were sacrificed at 12 days after challenge for necropsy. Results were evaluated by mortality rates and the incidence of intraabdominal abscesses at necropsy. Cure was defined as the absence of either mortality or abscess(es).

The results of these studies showed that all antimicrobials which demonstrated activity in vitro against *E. coli* reduced mortality rates in untreated controls from 35 to 45% to 0 to 18%. Drugs active against the *B. fragilis* strain in the inoculum reduced the incidence of abscesses in surviving animals from 100% to 5 to 15%. The highest cure rates were achieved with the following regimens: doxycycline + gentamicin (80% cured); metronidazole (82%); rosamicin + gentamicin (87%); clindamycin + gentamicin (87%); carbenicillin + gentamicin (90%); and cefoxitin (93%). Chi-square analysis showed no statistically significant differences for cure with these six regimens.

Wound Infections
(R. J. McRipley)

Animal models of bacterial wound infections and their ability to predict therapeutic efficacy in man, from the literature and our own experience, were reviewed. Preclinical efficacy testing of candidate antibacterial agents usually includes animal models based on the site-organism concept, but few models of wound infections have been extensively employed in recent years for chemotherapeutic efficacy studies. Those model infections used, mainly in rodents, have ranged from simple surgical incisions to massive traumatic wounds and have been utilized to evaluate the efficacy of topical and systemic antibacterial agents as well as antibiotic solutions for irrigation. Only a few candidate drugs have actually been tested in these models prior to clinical studies; the models have been utilized mainly for retrospective studies with clinically proven drugs. Analysis of data obtained from the evaluation of various chemotherapeutic

agents in models of bacterial wound infections has revealed that the pharmacokinetics of the drug, the mode of therapy (oral, parenteral, local), the type and severity of the wound, and the nature of the causative organism all have a profound effect upon the rate of resolution of the lesion. A true assessment of the predictive values of the models reviewed is not possible because of the paucity of comparative efficacy data from animal and clinical studies. There is, however, suggestive evidence that the models may provide some measure of confidence in the selection of candidate drugs for clinical studies where the final decision concerning therapeutic efficacy must be made.

Conclusions

Bacterial infections in animals as models of human disease have been shown to be useful both during the early evaluation of prospective new therapeutic agents and later in furnishing information about the potential clinical utility of the drug in various site/organism situations. Optimization of the results of experimental studies requires a thorough familiarity with the comparative pathogenesis of the disease condition, the nature of the inciting pathogen, and the pharmacology of the drug. In recent years, chemotherapists have been very successful in extrapolating data derived from animal studies to man and have identified those areas where this has not been possible.

Of prime importance to medicine is the prevention of infectious disease; short of that goal must be the limitation of tissue damage. This aspect has been convincingly demonstrated by Dr. Glauser who showed that prevention of renal damage (inflammation and scarring) in obstructive kidney disease depends upon early therapy with preferably bactericidal antibiotics. A similar theme was echoed by Dr. McRipley who advocated aggressive intervention with oral or parenteral agents (in preference to local therapy) to control superficial wound infections and thereby limit tissue damage. Bactericidal antibiotics are also preferred in serious and often life-threatening infections such as bacteremia (Dr. Gadebusch), meningitis, and endocarditis (Dr. Sande), because of their ability to rapidly reverse an otherwise lethal process. The adequate delivery of a microbiologically active agent to the site of infection in meaningful concentrations and the influence of inflammation upon therapy were studied by Dr. Pennington in respiratory infections due to *Pseudomonas aeruginosa*. He concluded that inability to penetrate to the site of infection and intrinsic activity of the antibiotic used were principal factors in failure to control infection of the lung. Mixed infections due to aerobic and anaerobic bacteria in the peritoneum apparently respond best to agents (Dr. Bartlett) that possess activity against both categories of microorganisms, e.g., cefoxitin, with activity against anaerobes seemingly more important. All investigators agreed that combinations of antibiotics are often more effective than the single agent alone, but only when synergy can be demonstrated in vitro.

Human Infection with *Chlamydia trachomatis*

JULIUS SCHACHTER
  Co-Chairman

Department of Epidemiology and
George Williams Hooper Foundation
University of California at San Francisco
San Francisco, California 94122, U.S.A.

J. DAVID ORIEL
  Co-Chairman

Department of Genitro-Urinary Medicine
University College Hospital
London, England

CHANDLER R. DAWSON

Department of Ophthalmology and
Francis I. Proctor Foundation
University of California at San Francisco
San Francisco, California 94143, U.S.A.

KING K. HOLMES

Department of Medicine
University of Washington
Division of Infectious Diseases
U.S. Public Health Service Hospital
Seattle, Washington 98114, U.S.A.

MARC O. BEEM

Department of Pediatrics
University of Chicago
Chicago, Illinois 60637, U.S.A.

This symposium was organized as a result of the recent exciting advances in our knowledge of human chlamydial infections. In the past few years these agents have been shown to cause a number of diseases of public health significance. Although the diseases produced and the epidemiological patterns may differ in developing countries as compared with industrial countries, it is abundantly clear that chlamydiae are among the most ubiquitous of human pathogens and major causes of morbidity, worldwide.

Chemotherapy of Endemic Trachoma
(Chandler R. Dawson)

Trachoma is still the leading cause of preventable blindness in the world, particularly in underdeveloped rural areas of developing countries. The chronic inflammation of the external eye in trachoma produces scarring with painful inturned eyelids and eventually blindness. It is produced by eye infection with *Chlamydia trachomatis* often associated with ocular bacterial pathogens (*Haemophilus* sp., pneumococcus, *Neisseria* sp.) that spread from eye to eye in young children by close personal contact and eye-seeking flies.

Public health programs to control active trachoma now consist of the application of antibiotic ointment (usually a tetracycline) to the eyes of all children in endemic communities. Controlled trials of such topical chemotherapy with tetracyclines, erythromycin, and rifampin have shown only a temporary effect, with a recurrence of disease in 12 to 20 weeks. The recrudescent disease is attributed to reinfection from untreated cases in the community.

C. trachomatis is also a common infection in industrialized countries, where the sexually transmitted agent is the main cause of nongonococcal urethritis in men and chronic cervicitis in women. About half of the infants born of infected mothers acquire chlamydial infection and develop some disease, such as inclusion conjunctivitis and pneumonia or intestinal infection.

Since infants in hyperendemic trachoma areas also develop chlamydial infection by eye-to-eye spread, it appeared likely to us that they might also have respiratory and intestinal infection. Indeed, we have recovered chlamydiae from the nasopharynx and rectum of children with severe endemic trachoma living in Egyptian and Tunisian villages. Thus the chlamydial infection at extraocular sites could be the endogenous source of ocular reinfection following topical antibiotic treatment. This generalized chlamydial infection might also lead to pneumonia and possibly diarrhea, important causes of morbidity and mortality among children of developing countries.

There is a clear rationale, then, for the use of systemic chemotherapy for endemic trachoma. The relative lack of side effects makes erythromycin (excluding the estolate) or other macrolides the apparent choice for community-wide (blanket) treatment of children in endemic trachoma areas. The major drawback is the frequent dosage (four times daily) needed to maintain therapeutic levels with the presently available preparations. Doxycycline might be a useful alternative because of the once-daily dose; moreover, tooth staining (a major contraindication) is minimal with this drug, even in neonates.

Nongonococcal Urethritis and Other Genital Infections
(King K. Holmes)

In adults the newly defined clinical spectrum of sexually transmitted *C. trachomatis* infections is easily memorized because it parallels exactly the spectrum of gonococcal infections (Table 1). Although the causal role of *C. trachomatis* is not firmly established, both agents have been associated with urethritis, epididymitis, mucopurulent cervicitis, acute salpingitis, Bartholinitis, the Fitz-Hugh and Curtis syndrome (perihepatitis), and both can be associated with systemic complications, particularly with arthritis. The etiological significance of *C. trachomatis* infection in certain of these syndromes, such as the Fitz-Hugh and Curtis syndrome and Reiter's syndrome, requires further study. The possibility that *C. trachomatis* is a cause of proctitis in women and in homosexual men remains to be defined.

Genital infections other than lymphogranuloma venereum (LGV) are caused by *C. trachomatis* immunotypes D through K. Although data are lacking, the incidence of genital *C. trachomatis* infection is undoubtedly increasing, since the incidence of nongonococcal urethritis (NGU) has risen dramatically over the last two decades, and *C. trachomatis* has consistently been isolated from 30 to 50% of men with NGU. The peak age incidence of genital *C. trachomatis* infections occurs in the late teens and early twenties, resembling other sexually transmitted infections. Sexual transmission is further evi-

denced by a rising prevalence of serum antibody to *C. trachomatis* in relation to the increased numbers of sex partners of infected individuals. The prevalence of *C. trachomatis* in the cervix of pregnant women is 5 to 10 times higher than that of *N. gonorrhoeae* in the United States. The prevalence of genital infection with either agent is highest in individuals who are indigent, nonwhite, unmarried, and between ages 18 and 24. The ratio of chlamydial to gonococcal urethritis is highest for heterosexual men and those with high socioeconomic status, and lowest for homosexual men and indigent populations. The ratio of symptomatic to asymptomatic infections appears to be lower for *C. trachomatis* than for *N. gonorrhoeae* infections, as does the clinical severity of symptomatic infections. However, because the total number of *C. trachomatis* infections exceeds that of *N. gonorrhoeae* infections in industrialized countries, the total morbidity caused by *C. trachomatis* genital infections is comparable to that caused by *N. gonorrhoeae*. The prevalence of *C. trachomatis* is higher than that of *N. gonorrhoeae* in industrialized countries, in part because measures such as treatment of sex partners and routine cultures for case detection in asymptomatic individuals are being applied much more effectively for gonorrhea control than for control of *C. trachomatis* infection.

NGU is a diagnosis of exclusion, given to men with symptoms or signs of urethritis who do not have gonorrhea. Postgonococcal urethritis (PGU) refers to NGU which commonly develops 2 to 3 weeks after treatment of gonococcal urethritis in men. *C. trachomatis* causes 30 to 50% of cases of NGU and PGU. The cause of the remainder is uncertain, although evidence suggests that *Ureaplasma urealyticum* causes an additional 30 to 40%.

The most suitable method for diagnosis of *C. trachomatis* urethritis is isolation of the agent in tissue cell culture. It is necessary to insert an endourethral swab 1 to 2 cm into the urethra to obtain an adequate specimen, since cultures of expressed exudate are insensitive. Unfortunately, direct Giemsa-stained or immunofluorescent (IF)-stained smears are insensitive. Serological techniques are as difficult to perform as culture, and serological diagnosis by micro-IF testing of serum requires demonstration of IgM antibody (lacking in the many patients who have previously experienced infection with the same immunotype) or a fourfold rise in antibody titer in paired sera. (Because *C. trachomatis* infections are often mild, many patients do not seek therapy until it is too late to demonstrate a rise in antibody titer.) Serological techniques, therefore, often cannot differentiate current from past

TABLE 1. *Similarity of clinical manifestations of sexually transmitted infections caused by Neisseria gonorrhoeae and Chlamydia trachomatis*

Site of infection	N. gonorrhoeae	C. trachomatis
Male		
Urethra	Urethritis	Urethritis
Epididymis	Epididymitis	Epididymitis
Systemic	Disseminated gonococcal infection	Reiter's syndrome
Female		
Cervix	Cervicitis	Cervicitis
Salpinx	Salpingitis	Salpingitis
Urethra	Urethritis	Urethral syndrome
Bartholin's gland	Bartholin's gland abscess	Bartholin's gland abscess

infection. Where culture is not available, it is current practice to diagnose NGU by documentation of a leukocytic urethral exudate and by exclusion of gonorrhea by Gram stain or culture, but not to pursue a specific etiological diagnosis of NGU. *C. trachomatis* urethritis is generally less severe than gonococcal urethritis. Symptoms include urethral discharge, dysuria, or urethral itching. Signs include meatal erythema and tenderness and a urethral exudate which is often demonstrable only by stripping the urethra in the morning before voiding. A substantial proportion of men with *C. trachomatis* urethral infection have no demonstrable signs or symptoms. An estimated 5 to 10% of male sexually transmitted diseases clinic patients have asymptomatic *C. trachomatis* urethral infection. Such patients frequently have first-glass pyuria (≥ 15 leukocytes per 400× microscopic field in the sediment of first-voided early morning urine) or an increased number of leukocytes on Gram-stained smear prepared from a urogenital swab inserted 1 to 2 cm into the anterior urethra. An average of ≥ 4 leukocytes in five 1,000× (oil immersion) fields is indicative of urethritis and is correlated with recovery of *C. trachomatis*.

C. trachomatis is also a cause of epididymitis in sexually active males. In a recent study, *C. trachomatis* infection was found by cultures of the urethra, urine, semen, or epididymal aspirate or by serology in 11 of 13 men under 35, but in none of 10 over 35 years of age who presented with epididymitis. (Coliform bacteria or *Pseudomonas aeruginosa* are the most common cause of epididymitis in men over 35.) In recent studies, *C. trachomatis* has been recovered from the urethra from up to 70% of men with untreated Reiter's syndrome who have associated urethritis. This is a striking association, which is as yet unexplained. As with gonococcal infection, *C. trachomatis* has been isolated from the cervix of 20 to 60% of women with gonorrhea, or contact with gonorrhea, from 10 to 20% of women attending sexually transmitted diseases clinics who do not have a history of contact with a partner with urethritis, and from about 5% of U.S. college students, or young women attending gynecology clinics or prenatal clinics in recent studies.

Although many women with *C. trachomatis* cervical infection have a normal cervix or only nonspecific changes, there is a significant correlation of this infection with endocervicitis, manifested by mucopurulent exudate in the cervical os. A distinctive pattern of hypertrophic (edematous and congested) cervical erythema and increased friability also may be seen. Herpes simplex virus causes inflammation and ulceration of the exocervix, rather than of the endocervix

alone, but can be confused with gonococcal or chlamydial cervicitis. The presence of mucopurulent endocervicitis suggests the presence of *C. trachomatis* or *N. gonorrhoeae* infection. If tests for gonorrhea are negative, nongonococcal endocervicitis should be treated with tetracycline, and male sex partners should be examined for NGU.

C. trachomatis has recently been implicated as a cause of acute salpingitis. In one study, it was isolated from the cervix of 19 of 53 women with laparoscopy-verified acute salpingitis; it was recovered from the fallopian tubes of 6 of 7 who had *C. trachomatis* in the cervix and displayed no other pathogens. A related development is the demonstration of IgM antibody to *C. trachomatis*, suggestive of recent infection, in 7 of 11 women with acute peritonitis and/or perihepatitis (Fitz-Hugh and Curtis syndrome) suggesting an association with recent *C. trachomatis* infection. *C. trachomatis* has also been isolated from the rectum of 10% of women with genital chlamydial infection and from pus expressed from Bartholin's gland in association with Bartholinitis. Our own unpublished data suggest *C. trachomatis* is a cause of some cases of the urethral syndrome in women.

Management of Chlamydial Infections of the Genital Tract
(J. David Oriel)

Chlamydial infections of the genital tract have a reputation for being difficult to treat. Should *C. trachomatis* infection of the genital tract be treated at all? The answer must be "yes" in order to protect infected patients and their consorts from complications and to reduce the level of infection in the community. Most clinical studies are derived from NGU and cervicitis, as these are the most common infections and specimen collection is relatively easy.

Several points arise from recent laboratory studies on the action of antimicrobial agents against *C. trachomatis*. (i) Some agents, e.g., tetracyclines and erythromycin, have a low MIC with sharp, reproducible endpoints, and passage shows little difference between MIC and minimal chlamydicidal concentration (MCC). (ii) Other agents, e.g., pentothenes and cephalosporins, induce abnormal inclusions, and the endpoints are erratic and hard to define. (iii) Others, e.g., chloramphenicol and thiamphenicol, show an apparently low MIC, but passage reveals a wide difference between MIC and MCC. (iv) Some agents, e.g., gentamicin, have virtually no antichlamydial activity. (v) By varying the experimental conditions, e.g., by adding antimicrobial agents to cells which are already infected, different results may be obtained; e.g., minocycline is far more effective than tetracyclines under these conditions, whereas, if cultures are infected simultaneously with the application of the agents, their MICs are very similar.

In vitro experiments provide general guidance for the clinician, but the results should not be extrapolated into clinical situations. By general agreement the tetracyclines and erythromycin preparations are the agents of choice for treating *C. trachomatis* infections.

Clinical studies have been mostly on NGU, which is not an ideal disease to study in this regard, because its multiple etiology lends to noncorrespondence of clinical and laboratory results, presumably because other factors are not affected by the drug being investigated.

Data are available on short-term follow-up of men with chlamydial NGU treated with tetracycline/oxytetracycline. *C. trachomatis* was reisolated in 1 week after completing therapy as follows: 250 mg q.i.d. for 14 days (2/35, Oriel et al., 1977); 500 mg q.i.d. for 7 days (0/10, Handsfield et al., 1977); 500 mg q.i.d. for 7 days (1/28, Oriel et al., unpublished data). Data for minocycline are: 100 mg b.i.d. for 21 days (0/33, Oriel et al., 1975); 200-mg start, then 100 mg b.i.d. for 6 days (1/12, Prentice et al., 1976); 50 mg b.i.d. for 7 days (0/16, Oriel et al., unpublished data). Erythromycin stearate, 500 mg b.i.d. for 14 days (1/30, Oriel et al., 1977), but erythromycin, 500 mg b.i.d. for 10 days (5/23, Johannisson, 1979). Similar data for women are as follows: oxytetracycline, 250 mg q.i.d. for 14 days gave reisolates in 2/70 (Oriel et al., 1977); oxytetracycline, 500 mg q.i.d. for 7 days gave reisolates in 1/45 (Oriel et al., unpublished data); minocycline, 100 mg b.i.d. for 21 days (0/24, Oriel et al., 1975); erythromycin stearate, 500 mg b.i.d. for 14 days (0/70, Oriel et al., 1979).

As the period of follow-up lengthens and pressure of reinfection increases, reisolation of *C. trachomatis* can often be demonstrated as to reinfection. Contact-tracing studies showed that this had occurred in 3 of 5 women who yielded *C. trachomatis* up to 3 months after treatment with a 2-week course of oxytetracycline, 250 mg q.i.d. Prolonged follow-up of a group of 68 women by Rees et al. for up to 18 months showed reisolation of *C. trachomatis* in only about 10%.

It is concluded that tetracycline preparations, and probably erythromycin as well, cure *C. trachomatis* of the genital tract, and that a course of treatment probably need not exceed 1 week. Shorter courses are often found to be followed by reisolation of *C. trachomatis*, but the prolonged courses of 2 to 3 weeks are probably unnecessarily long for the eradication of *C. trachomatis*, although they may be desirable for other reasons.

Treatment of sexual contacts is an essential part of management. Our unpublished data show that 30/36 (83%) of *source* contacts, and 33/69 (48%) of *secondary* contacts of men with *C. trachomatis*-positive NGU yield cervical isolates. Contact-tracing studies of a group of women with "unsuspected" *C. trachomatis* infection showed that 26/47 (55%) of their current male partners had urethral infection with *C. trachomatis*.

It is concluded that patients with *C. trachomatis* infection of the genital tract should be treated as follows: (i) tetracycline, 500 mg q.i.d. for 1 week, or equivalent dosage of other tetracycline preparations such as minocycline; (ii) abstinence from intercourse during therapy; (iii) at least two follow-up examinations during the 4 weeks after completing therapy; (iv) similar treatment for sexual contacts (treatment of both partners can be extended to 2 weeks if this provides better overlap); (v) women who are pregnant or lactating should be treated with erythromycin stearate, 500 mg b.i.d. for 2 weeks.

Some *C. trachomatis* infections of the genital tract are mixed with other infecting agents. Many cases of *C. trachomatis*-negative NGU are responsive to tetracyclines and erythromycin, but some of these infections (whose etiology is uncertain at present) are unresponsive; this is why some men treated for *C. trachomatis*-positive NGU still show evidence of urethritis after therapy despite the elimination of *C. trachomatis*.

Several studies have shown that 20 to 25% of men with gonorrhea are infected with *C. trachomatis*, and the proportion may be higher in women. Currently recommended treatment schedules for gonorrhea with penicillin, ampicillin, and spectinomycin do not eradicate *C. trachomatis*. There is no antimicrobial agent which will cure both infections in single dosage. Possibilities appear to be: (i) treating gonorrhea with tetracycline, 500 mg q.i.d. for 1 week, or (ii) treating gonorrhea with ampicillin-probenecid, thereby retaining the advantage of single-dose therapy, followed the next day by a 1-week course of tetracycline, 500 mg q.i.d. I have treated 150 men with gonorrhea in this way. PGU has been virtually eliminated, and *C. trachomatis* has been isolated from no patient so far during a follow-up period of 2 weeks.

It is concluded that effective therapy for *C. trachomatis* infections of the genital tract is available but that the problems of treating mixed infections are more complex.

Chlamydial Pneumonia of Early Infancy
(Marc O. Beem)

Respiratory tract involvement in natally acquired chlamydial infection occurs very commonly, perhaps it is "the rule." Although this infection may be clinically inapparent, a syndrome of afebrile pneumonia has been observed in infected infants. It seems likely that other respiratory syndromes may result from infection. The evidence linking *C. trachomatis* infection with pneumonia in infants includes: (i) cross-sectional studies comparing the incidence of chlamydial infection in infants with pneumonia with various control groups; (ii) identification of *C. trachomatis* in lung biopsies of several infants with pneumonia; (iii) apparent clinical improvement of infants with chlamydia-associated pneumonia when they are treated with antimicrobial agents that terminate the chlamydial infection. The clinical and laboratory profile of chlamydial pneumonia of early infancy is outlined in Table 2. The natural course of this illness tends to be protracted but relatively benign, although occasional infants experience episodes of sudden severe respiratory distress. We believe that infants benefit from treatment and that those with significant symptomatology should be hospitalized for supportive care (chest physical therapy, supplemental O_2) during the initiation of treatment. Specific systemic antichlamydial treatment with erythromycin or sulfisoxazole usually is followed by clinical improvement that begins within 3 to 5 days and progresses to complete return to normality.

TABLE 2. *Clinical and laboratory characteristics of chlamydial pneumonia of infants*

Profile	Indications
Age	2–12 weeks[a]
Onset	Gradual
Systemic	Absence of fever[a]
	Minimal malaise
	Poor weight gain
Eye	Inclusion conjunctivitis (chronic phase)
Ear	Secretory otitis media
Respiratory	Tachypnea
	Cough (sometimes in staccato paroxysms)
	Lung findings:[a]
	Auscultation:
	Good breath sounds
	Inspiratory crepitant rales
	Absent or minimal expiratory wheezing
	X-ray:
	Interstitial infiltrates
	Hyperexpansion
Laboratory	Blood eosinophils $\geq 300/mm^3$
	Blood gas values $\downarrow$ PaO_2, normal $PaCO_2$
	Serum immunoglobulins elevated:[a]
	IgA—sometimes
	IgG—usually
	IgM—always
	Chlamydia cultures:[a]
	Nasopharyngeal secretions positive
	Chlamydia serum antibody values:[a, b]
	Sustained high, or rising

[a] Characteristics that we believe are essentially invariable components of this illness.

[b] Measured by indirect microimmunofluorescence to lymphogranuloma venereum type 1.

Use of Antibiotics in Special Clinical Situations

HAROLD C. NEU
  Chairman

Columbia University
New York, New York 10032, U.S.A.

JOHN KOSMIDIS
  Co-Chairman

University of Athens
Athens, Greece

GEORGE H. McCRACKEN, JR.

University of Texas
Southwestern Medical School
Dallas, Texas 75235, U.S.A.

TOM BERGAN

University of Oslo
Oslo, Norway

JEAN KLASTERSKY

Institut Jules Bordet
Brussels, Belgium

RUEDI LÜTHY

University of Zurich
Zurich, Switzerland

MICHAEL BARZA

Tufts University
Boston, Massachusetts 02111, U.S.A.

There are a number of clinical situations in which the optimal method to use antimicrobial agents is undergoing reevaluation in light of information concerning the pharmacology of these drugs. This symposium is directed at reviewing what information is extant and at pointing out areas in which more information is needed.

Use of Antibiotics in Neonates
(George H. McCracken, Jr.)

For more than two decades the aminoglycosides have been used as first-line drugs for treatment of serious infections in five areas of pediatrics: the newborn nursery, cystic fibrosis, oncology, surgery, and burns. Of these, aminoglycoside therapy in newborn infants is most critical because of the frequently overwhelming nature of the bacterial disease and because dosage schedules must be tailored to the constantly changing physiological and metabolic processes that occur during the newborn period. As pediatric pharmacology has gained recognition as a specialized field, the pharmacokinetics of antibiotics have been defined in the neonate and related to gestational and chronological ages. Failure to adjust dosage schedules has resulted in the past in irreversible ototoxicity because of excessive dosages or to clinical and bacteriological failures because of subtherapeutic regimens.

The principles that apply to one aminoglyco-side drug in this age group apply to all the agents in this class. The first exposure to these drugs may occur during intrauterine life as a result of maternal therapy. Transplacental passage of aminoglycosides appears to be greater in the first and third trimesters than in the second trimester. The concentrations of aminoglycosides in cord serum have ranged from 15 to 70% of the peak maternal serum values. Relatively large concentrations of tobramycin and amikacin have been measured in fetal kidney and urine, suggesting selective binding of these agents to renal tissue during intrauterine development. The only documented instances of toxicity in infants and children resulting from antepartum administration of aminoglycosides has been ototoxicity after prolonged administration of streptomycin or dihydrostreptomycin for therapy of tuberculosis.

The glomerulus in a full-term infant is only one-third of its eventual adult diameter, and creatinine clearance values correlate directly with gestational age, increasing from 0.45 ml/min in infants less than 34 weeks to 2.2 ml/min in those greater than 38 weeks gestational age. Renal plasma flow and glomerular filtration rates are small at birth but increase substantially by 3 days of age.

The half-life of aminoglycosides has been inversely correlated to birth weight and gestational age. The volume of drug distribution was largest in low-birth-weight babies of younger gestational and chronological ages, a finding that reflects the increased extracellular fluid volume characteristic of these immature infants. Accordingly, peak concentrations of aminoglycosides in serum were smaller in these babies and increased with increasing maturity and chronological age as the volume of extracellular fluid decreased.

It is apparent that the pharmacokinetics of aminoglycosides are constantly changing during the newborn period and that there are large variations in serum values when small premature infants at birth are compared to older, term infants. If these factors are not taken into consideration when formulating dosages, the resulting serum concentrations may be either excessively large and potentially toxic or too small and subtherapeutic in some infants.

The observations that concentrations of aminoglycosides may exist for long periods in the urine may have important implications in neonates. The prolonged excretion of subinhibitory concentrations of an aminoglycoside in urine may exert selective pressure for development of resistant strains of *Enterobacteriaceae* that reside in the environment of intensive care units for high-risk, low-birth-weight infants. The potential nephrotoxicity in infants who require either prolonged or repeated antimicrobial therapy during their nursery stay also may be greater.

Ventriculitis is present in approximately 75% of neonates with coliform meningitis. However, we have been unable to show a beneficial effect of systemic plus lumbar intrathecal gentamicin therapy in these patients. In the second Cooperative Study initiated in 1976, we evaluated intraventricular gentamicin therapy in infants with meningitis and ventriculitis. Gentamicin administered intraventricularly produces cerebrospinal fluid (CSF) concentrations that greatly exceed the MIC values for most coliforms causing meningitis and the drug diffuses rapidly and completely throughout the CSF space. Despite these pharmacological results, the mortality rate in those treated with intraventricular therapy has been significantly greater than that after systemic therapy only.

Aminoglycosides are administered orally to some infants for therapy of diarrheal disease caused by enteropathogenic strains of *Escherichia coli* and for prophylaxis and therapy of necrotizing enterocolitis. Infants with necrotizing enterocolitis who received oral plus parenteral gentamicin therapy had significantly higher serum concentrations of gentamicin than did comparably ill, randomly selected infants with enterocolitis who received parenteral therapy only, and concentrations were in the potentially ototoxic range.

Kanamycin administered orally to newborn infants for prophylaxis of necrotizing enterocolitis produced emergence of resistant enteric bacilli. Thus, orally administered aminoglycosides cannot be recommended for prophylaxis because of the extreme selective pressure exerted by such management for development of resistant *Enterobacteriaceae*.

The two major potential toxic effects of aminoglycosides in newborns are nephrotoxicity and ototoxicity. In a 4-year follow-up study of neonates who were treated with kanamycin or gentamicin or who received no antimicrobial therapy during the first month of life, no substantial sensorineural hearing loss or vestibular dysfunction was identified in these patients that could be attributed to aminoglycoside therapy.

Pharmacokinetics of Antimicrobial Agents in Cystic Fibrosis
(Tom Bergan)

Patients with cystic fibrosis require frequent therapy with antibacterial agents because of the respiratory tract infections caused by *Staphylococcus aureus* and *Pseudomonas aeruginosa*.

Low serum levels have been found in cystic fibrosis even when antibiotics are injected directly intravenously.

In 1966, Huang, Sheng, and Basavanand studied doxycycline in cystic fibrosis patients. The peak levels were not significantly different from normals, but doxycycline disappeared with a serum half-life of 7 h in the cystic fibrosis patients compared to 16 to 18 h in normal adults. This may be due to altered hepatobiliary excretion.

The aminoglycosides examined in cystic fibrosis patients have been tobramycin and gentamicin. After intravenous doses, lower peak serum levels were obtained than in normal adults. A similar trend was seen after intramuscular doses.

Observations made with dicloxacillin in cystic fibrosis patients ranging from 9 to 22 years and matched with comparable healthy volunteers revealed that serum levels were considerably lower in the cystic fibrosis group. The mean peak was less than half and the overall serum concentrations more than 2.5 times smaller than in normal subjects. Since cystic fibrosis entails physiological changes of the gastrointestinal tract, it would not have been unexpected if reduced absorption could explain the lower cystic fibrosis levels. This does not appear to be the case, since urinary recoveries of dicloxacillin were equal or greater in cystic fibrosis patients and the times of peak levels were similar in the two subject groups. Renal elimination was faster in cystic fibrosis patients which may be related to lower protein binding of the highly bound penicillin.

Azlocillin produced serum levels considerably lower in cystic fibrosis patients than in normal subjects. The serum half-life was the same in cystic fibrosis as in healthy subjects, i.e., 0.9 to 1.0 h.

Endotracheal Therapy with Aminoglycosides for Gram-Negative Bacillary Bronchopneumonias in Tracheotomized Patients
(Jean Klastersky)

Patients with tracheostomies, especially when they are unconscious and cannot cooperate in obtaining adequate bronchial drainage, have a high incidence of bronchopulmonary infections caused by *P. aeruginosa* and other gram-negative enteric bacilli. Morbidity and mortality are high under these circumstances. Aminoglycosides have been used for therapy, but the clinical results are poor perhaps due to the inadequate penetration of aminoglycosides into the bronchial secretion and to partial inactivation of these antibiotics within the bronchial lumen.

Inactivation of aminoglycosides occurs in acidic pH, under anaerobic conditions, in the presence of some cations, and purulent material can bind aminoglycosides extensively.

Since systemic administration of aminoglycosides results in low levels of antibacterial activity in bronchial secretions, we have administered aminoglycosides directly into the bronchial tree. After both aerosol and endotracheal injection, very high levels within the sputum can be obtained; blood levels, on the other hand, remain quite low, indicating a relatively poor absorption from the bronchi into the blood. Usually 15 to 20% of the dose administered endotracheally can be recovered in the urine during the 24 h after tracheal injection.

In a controlled study, 43 tracheostomied neurosurgical patients received endotracheally gentamicin (3 times, 40 mg daily) and 42 patients were treated with placebo. Pulmonary infections were more frequent in patients receiving placebo, 17 versus 5. Among these 17 infections, 5 resulted in gram-negative septicemia. Among the patients who received endotracheal gentamicin, two deaths were related to bronchopulmonary infections and four such deaths were seen in the control group. Thus endotracheal gentamicin was effective in preventing gram-negative bronchopneumonia in tracheotomized

unconscious patients. However, the emergence of gentamicin-resistant strains caused us to use a rotating regimen with endotracheal antibiotics in order to minimize this selection of resistant microorganisms.

We also studied the clinical efficacy of endotracheal therapy with aminoglycosides in patients receiving optimal systemic therapy in whom the possible role of the endotracheal injection was adequately controlled. The study was limited to tracheotomized neurosurgical patients, all of whom received carbenicillin plus sisomicin systemically. One group received sisomicin endotracheally and the other group received endotracheal placebo. Only patients with clinical and radiological evidence of bronchopneumonia were analyzed. Infection was due to a sisomicin-susceptible microorganism, most often *P. aeruginosa*. Bronchopneumonia responded more often in patients who received the endotracheal sisomicin than in the controls. However, bacteriological results did not necessarily parallel the clinical results, but in no patient receiving endotracheal sisomicin did the number of pathogens within the bronchial secretions increase during therapy. Not only did the bronchopneumonia respond more often (75%) among the patients who were treated endotracheally, as compared to the controls (45%), but no infectious deaths were observed in those patients. Thus, the endotracheal injection of aminoglycosides might represent the ideal adjunct to systemic antimicrobial therapy for the management of gram-negative bronchopneumonias.

The emergence of aminoglycoside-resistant microorganisms might be feared as a serious complication of endotracheal administration of aminoglycosides. We suggest that endotracheal therapy should be reserved only for patients with documented gram-negative bronchopneumonias. Careful bacteriological monitoring of the patients receiving antibiotics endotracheally is indicated to quickly detect the possible emergence of resistant strains. Isolation of the patients who are receiving endotracheal therapy might also prevent the spread of emerging resistant microorganisms throughout the hospital. Use of endotracheal antibiotics to prevent infection by gram-negative rods should not be used routinely on a large-scale basis unless alternating drug regimens can be developed and be used without much selection of resistant strains.

Use of Antibiotics in Patients with Renal Failure
(John Kosmidis)

Patients in renal failure are particularly susceptible to infections. Defective chemotaxis and phagocytosis, altered cellular and humoral immunity, and frequent hospitalization involving repeated parenteral procedures are the main predisposing factors. Furthermore, the infecting organisms often include opportunistic pathogens which require prolonged antimicrobial therapy.

Clinicians must be able to select appropriate dosage of an antibiotic for a patient in renal failure. For dosage calculation they need simple, easy to remember methods. Instructions to nursing personnel must be easy to carry out. One cannot give 3/8 of a tablet or a 1.18 ml of an injectable solution. However, simplicity must not jeopardize effectiveness and safety.

In formulating recommendations for antibiotic dosage in renal failure, the most important parameters are the relative contribution of renal versus extrarenal elimination for a particular drug, the mechanism of renal excretion, and the therapeutic margin needed to achieve therapeutic success without toxicity. Protein binding and changes in renal failure, the mode of action of the antibiotic and the need of intact phagocytic mechanisms for a better effect, the formation of metabolites and their possible accumulation in renal failure, and alterations in distribution volume are other factors that may assume importance for some drugs in renal failure. Other factors, unrelated to renal failure, such as liver function, anemia, and age, are also important. Adequate concentration in urine in renal failure is mandatory for the treatment of urinary tract infection. Finally, nephrotoxicity itself may be a limiting factor.

On the basis of the above, the antibacterial agents can be divided into four groups: (i) drugs with mainly extrarenal elimination, for which no dosage alteration is necessary even in end-stage renal failure; (ii) drugs that are either partly removed by extrarenal mechanisms or are mainly excreted by the kidney, but have a very broad therapeutic margin (for these drugs, dosage reduction is not necessary unless renal failure is severe and even then simple rules are adequate); (iii) drugs that are best avoided in renal failure (these will produce damage to the kidney or other organs, and those that are mainly used for urinary tract infections but will not concentrate adequately in urine in the presence of renal failure); (iv) those agents that are excreted mainly by the kidney, mostly via glomerular filtration, have a narrow therapeutic margin and often are nephrotoxic.

Before calculating dosage, an accurate estimate of the degree of renal failure is necessary. Several dosage recommendations are based on the value of serum creatinine. However, the latter is dependent not only on renal function

but also on production rate, which is altered depending on age, sex, weight, and the presence of disease. The serum creatinine may not correspond to the existing degree of impairment at the time of measurement, especially in acute or rapidly changing renal failure, since a long time is needed before achieving a steady state. On the other hand, measurements of various clearances necessitate accurate collection of urine, which requires cooperation from the patient and the nursing staff.

Two approaches have been recommended for dosage reduction. The first is to administer the same dose at prolonged intervals and the second is to give diminished doses at the usual intervals. The former may result in very prolonged dosage intervals in patients with severe renal failure which may lead to inadequate serum levels so that at the latter part of the interval the patient is exposed to the risk of bacteremia. On the other hand, dosage reduction may result in impracticable results such as 3/8 of a tablet. Sometimes a mixture of the two approaches is necessary to satisfy all the requirements.

During hemodialysis and peritoneal dialysis dosage is either diminished according to instructions based on knowledge of the elimination rate of the drug during the procedure or, with peritoneal dialysis, antibiotic is added to the dialysis fluids, especially in the presence of peritonitis. The amount added is calculated so that it gives local levels similar to those desired in the serum. Systemic dosage is calculated according to the patient's degree of renal failure.

Use of Antimicrobial Agents in Patients with Severe Hepatic Insufficiency
(Ruedi Lüthy)

Hepatic drug elimination is controlled by hepatic blood flow, metabolic clearance, drug binding, and anatomical changes in hepatic circulation. Only severe hepatitis and advanced cirrhosis cause enough damage to the liver to interfere with oxidative metabolism or drug binding, or to produce changes in the vascular structures resulting in decreased hepatic blood flow, portosystemic shunting, or chronic biliary obstruction. The complexity of liver damage becomes even more evident when factors such as microsomal enzyme induction by lipophilic drugs or genetic differences are considered. No single laboratory value such as albumin or bilirubin concentration can quantitatively predict drug elimination in patients with liver disease, and none of the liver function tests can differentiate and quantitate the major determinants of hepatic drug clearance.

Despite the lack of predictability between laboratory evidence of hepatic disease and drug elimination, the use of half-life to characterize the behavior of a drug in a patient with hepatic insufficiency is the best method. The three variables determining half-life ($T_{1/2}$) are volume of distribution (V_D), renal clearance (Cl_R), and hepatic clearance (Cl_H) = $T_{1/2}$ = 0.693 $V_D/(Cl_R + Cl_H)$. Hepatic clearance is determined by blood flow (Q), protein binding (f), and instrinsic clearance (Cl_{int}) of that drug: $Cl_H = fCl_{int}/(Q + fCl_{int})$. Thus the half-life of a drug in liver disease is controlled by a number of independent parameters subject to considerable changes in various hepatic diseases.

Gross ascites leads to an increase of 10 liters or more of extracellular fluid. For example, the volume of distribution of ampicillin in cirrhotic patients with ascites is 300% higher than in normals, but there is a high interindividual variability not correlated with the volume of ascites.

Renal clearance is frequently decreased in patients with hepatic failure. Carbenicillin half-life in patients with combined hepatic and oliguric renal failure compared to oliguria alone is increased, suggesting a negative synergism of combined liver and kidney disease. A qualitative estimate of hepatic clearance must take into account blood flow, protein binding, and intrinsic clearance. Blood flow may decrease in severe cirrhosis and remain normal or even increase in acute hepatitis. Plasma protein concentrations only vaguely reflect the degree of protein binding. In addition to hypoalbuminemia and competitively bound ligands such as bilirubin and unknown factors determine the increased availability of the non-protein-bound antibiotic. A practical conclusion is that severe hypoalbuminemia and jaundice will increase the free drug. Due to an increase in the volume of distribution, total drug concentrations may be low, but the non-protein-bound concentration may well be within normal limits.

Qualitative assessment of intrinsic hepatic metabolic clearance is even more difficult. The enzyme system catalyzing the oxidation metabolism of lipid-soluble drugs such as erythromycin, rifampin, or fusidic acid is drastically reduced in a patient with fulminant hepatic failure. However, drug metabolism is inhibited only in severe hepatitis and advanced cirrhosis of the liver. But even in these patients, lipid-soluble drugs like barbiturates, meprobamate, phenytoin, and rifampin are capable of inducing the drug-hydroxylating enzyme system in the endoplasmic reticulum of the liver which may increase the clearance of these or other drugs primarily metabolized by the same enzyme system. These factors may be of little practical

value to the practicing physician; nevertheless, they illustrate that too many variables are involved in hepatic elimination of drugs to justify a formula relating albumin or bilirubin concentration or transaminase activity to intrinsic clearance, protein binding, hepatic flow, or volume of distribution.

Table 1 shows a classification of drugs according to half-lives and association with hepatotoxicity.

Intraocular Penetration of Antibiotics
(Michael Barza)

Many studies of this subject are carried out in rabbits' eyes. This species differs from humans

TABLE 1. *Classification of antibiotics for use in patients with severe hepatic insufficiency*

Category	Antibiotics
I. Antibiotics with little or no change in half-lives	Aminoglycosides Aminopenicillins Cephalosporins Isoxazolyl-penicillins Methicillin Ethambutol Nalidixic acid Nitrofurantoin Penicillin G Sulfonamides Tetracyclines Thiamphenicol Trimethoprim Vancomycin
II. Antibiotics with significantly prolonged half-lives	Carbenicillin Chloramphenicol Clindamycin Isoniazid Lincomycin Nafcillin Rifampin
III. Antibiotics predictably associated with hepatotoxicity	Erythromycin, estolate and propionyl esters Isoniazid (fast acetylators) Pyrazinamide Talampicillin Tetracycline hydrochloride (>2 g i.v./day) Rifampin
IV. Antibiotics rarely associated with hepatotoxicity	Aminopenicillins Amphotericin B Carbenicillin Cefazolin Cefuroxime Cephradine Chloramphenicol Clindamycin Fluorocytosine Fusidic acid Lincomycin Pyrimethamine Sulfonamides Trimethoprim

do not exist, e.g., that chloramphenicol should not be employed in pregant women because it causes "gray" syndrome in the newborn. To my knowledge, this has never been reported, and it represents misunderstanding of maternal fetal interaction during pregnancy.

During pregnancy, the placenta is an efficient organ of exchange between fetus and mother. This permits transfer of various fetal waste products to the mother to be handled by the maternal kidney or liver for clearance. A good example of the differences between intrauterine environment for the fetus and the nursery environment in the newborn is erythroblastosis fetalis. During pregnancy, the transfer of maternal antibody across the placenta results in destruction of fetal red cells. Elevated free bilirubin levels in the fetus is not a problem, for the free bilirubin is transferred across the placenta to the mother; it is then transported to the liver for conjugation and elimination. The major intrauterine fetal problem is anemia, and this is the reason for the use of intrauterine transfusion in seriously affected infants. After delivery of these affected babies, the situation dramatically changes. These infants may be anemic and have all of the clinical difficulties associated with that. More important, they are now dependent upon their own immature livers to conjugate and eliminate bilirubin. The major clinical concern is now directed towards reducing bilirubin levels so that kernicterus can be avoided. This is the justification for the exchange transfusion employed in these patients.

A similar situation exists when antibiotics such as chloramphenicol are employed during pregnancy. There is exchange of the free drug across the placenta and the drug is eliminated by the mother. The situation alters after birth when the liver of the newborn must conjugate and clear drugs like chloramphenicol. The inability of livers of newborns to handle these demands with repeated antibiotic dosing in the nursery results in excessively high serum levels and toxicity characterized by the "gray" syndrome. Similar difficulties can occur with sulfas which compete for the same conjugation system in the liver as does bilirubin. If long-acting sulfas have been employed in the mother, then residual levels in the newborn can cause a problem in clinical situations in which elevated bilirubin levels can be a problem. These observations do not support the indiscriminate use of these antibiotics in pregnant women, but they do suggest that some of the prohibitions have been too absolute. If a pregnant woman has a bacterial infection best treated by chloramphenicol or short-acting sulfas, I believe these drugs could and should be employed. Concerns about the safety for the newborn can be eased by discontinuing the drugs to the mother if labor ensues. This should permit sufficient elimination of the antibiotics so that toxic effects on the newborn will not be seen.

Global Deployment of Antibiotic Resistance Genes

THOMAS F. O'BRIEN
Chairman

Department of Medicine
Peter Bent Brigham Hospital
  and Harvard Medical School
Boston, Massachusetts 02115, U.S.A.

JACQUES F. ACAR
Co-Chairman

Département de Microbiologie
Hôpital Saint Joseph
Université Pierre et Marie Curie
Paris, France

STANLEY FALKOW

Microbiology Department
University of Washington
Seattle, Washington 98105, U.S.A.

E. JOHN THRELFALL

Division of Enteric Pathogens
Central Public Health Laboratory
London, N.W.9, 5HT, England

RICHARD W. LACEY

West Norfolk and King's Lynn
  General Hospital
King's Lynn, Norfolk, PE 30, 5QD, England

CLYDE THORNSBERRY

Bacteriology Division
Bureau of Laboratories
Center for Disease Control
Atlanta, Georgia 30333, U.S.A.

An antibiotic resistance gene could spread through the bacterial flora of the world in one strain of bacteria, or transfer on a plasmid and spread in multiple strains, or transpose from one plasmid to another and spread in multiple plasmids in multiple strains. In vitro studies over the past two decades have greatly increased our understanding of the mechanisms available for dissemination of resistance genes. We have also come to realize that the result of the spreading processes, that is, the eventual distribution of the various resistance genes in the world's bacterial flora, ultimately determines how effective each of the antibiotics will be.

Besides understanding the mechanisms in vitro, however, there are many observations we need to make before we can understand the workings of the global antibiotic resistance system. How many resistance genes are there? How many are widely distributed? Does the number of genes greatly exceed the number of known distinctive phenotypic mechanisms of resistance (e.g., two TEM genes code for products that are functionally nearly indistinguishable)? Has each resistance gene arisen singly at one time and place or has each (or some) had multiple origins? What mechanisms of spread are used by each and does this differ from one species of bacteria to another? How efficient is the spread of each

relative to the amount of selection pressure exerted by antibiotic usage? This symposium explores these issues by reviewing available data on the deployment of antibiotic resistance genes in several clinically important bacterial species and genera.

Salmonella, Plasmids Linked to Strains
(E. John Threlfall)

The worldwide deployment of plasmid-encoded antimicrobial drug resistance in the normal enterobacterial flora is a consequence of the injudicious use of antimicrobial drugs in human and veterinary medicine. The dissemination of these plasmids to pathogenic enterobacteria has resulted in the appearance of multiresistant strains of salmonellae and shigellae which have caused protracted outbreaks of enteric fever, salmonellosis, and shigellosis in many countries.

In Britain, *S. typhimurium* is the predominant serotype in human food poisoning, and cattle are the primary source of human infection with this serotype. Thus, the appearance of drug resistance in human *S. typhimurium* is frequently subsequent to resistance plasmid acquisition in cattle. The proportion of multiresistant *S. typhimurium* isolated from both cattle and humans in Britain has increased dramatically in the last 2 years. This increase has followed the acquisition of resistance plasmids, in the bovine host, by a strain of *S. typhimurium* phage type 204. The new multiresistant lines then spread epidemically in cattle in Britain and have also caused infections among calves on the continent of Europe. The widespread distribution of infected calves has been a major factor in the dissemination of these strains. Antimicrobial drugs have been used in attempts to control the spread of infection and to treat infected animals, and the use of these agents may have assisted the establishment of the multiresistant strains in calf herds. These strains have entered the food chain, and there have been many human isolations.

A situation similar to that in Britain exists in several countries in northern Europe, where food animals are the primary source of human *S. typhimurium*. For example, pigs were the animal host of a tetracycline-resistant strain of phage type 194, which has caused many infections in humans in Belgium, France, and Germany since 1968, and cattle have provided the reservoir of a strain of phage type 207, which carries a plasmid coding for resistance to six antimicrobial drugs. Antimicrobials have been used extensively in animal husbandry in the countries concerned.

Multiresistant strains of salmonellae have caused serious outbreaks of salmonellosis in many developing countries in recent years. These outbreaks are nosocomial and are generally confined to pediatric wards. Septicemia is a frequent complication. Several serotypes are implicated, although *S. typhimurium* is the most common. Outbreaks caused by the dissemination of a single clone of the pathogens have frequently occurred in widely separated geographical areas. Resistances in the strains are plasmid encoded, and the strains involved are unusual in that there is no obvious animal source. Examples of outbreaks include those caused by a multiresistant strain of *S. wien*, which has spread from North Africa to France and Italy, *S. typhimurium* type 208 in many Middle Eastern countries, *S. saint-paul* in Venezuela, and *S. typhimurium* in other South American countries.

The resistance plasmids in these strains have been characterized and classified, and there are distinct patterns of the predominance of plasmids on both a strain basis and a regional basis. For example, plasmids of the $F_I me$ group were distributed throughout the Middle East because of the dissemination of a clone of *S. typhimurium* phage type 208 that caused outbreaks of salmonellosis in pediatric wards in several countries. In addition, $F_I me$ plasmids were present in the strain of *S. wien* mentioned earlier and in strains of *S. typhi* and *S. isangi* isolated in North Africa.

One of the consequences of indiscriminate use of chloramphenicol is the appearance of plasmid-encoded chloramphenicol resistance in *S. typhi* and *Shigella dysenteriae* 1, and since 1968 there have been a number of large, protracted outbreaks of *Shigella* dysentery and typhoid fever, with a high rate of mortality. The most serious of these have been the pandemic of *S. dysenteriae* 1 in Central America in 1968–1970 and the prolonged outbreak of chloramphenicol-resistant *S. typhi* in Mexico in 1972–1973.

The plasmids carried by chloramphenicol-resistant *S. dysenteriae* 1 and *S. typhi*, which have been isolated in outbreaks in different parts of the world, frequently code for the same spectrum of resistance. However, *S. dysenteriae* 1 appears to have an affinity for plasmids of compatibility group B, whereas group H_I plasmids are most common in *S. typhi*.

Multiresistant salmonellae and shigellae are now a threat to the health of individuals in many countries, and the use of antimicrobial drugs has encouraged the proliferation and establishment of these drug-resistant pathogens. A critical assessment of the use of antimicrobials in both human and veterinary medicine is long overdue, and more prudent administration is essential if the incidence of drug-resistant enterobacterial pathogens is to be reduced.

Staphylococcus aureus, Mechanisms for Abrupt Widespread Shifts in Resistance
(Richard W. Lacey)

It has hitherto been thought that plasmids spread between strains of *S. aureus* by generalized transduction in which the plasmid in the donor cell is occasionally accidentally incorporated into a bacteriophage upon its assembly within the donor. The resultant defective bacteriophage can then insert the plasmid in question into a recipient cell. This form of transfer is inefficient, requiring the destruction of the donor cell and the protection of the recipient against lysis by the predominant intact phage population. Evidence is presented that prophages are involved in a further form of gene transfer, described as phage-mediated conjugation, which occurs at frequencies of greater than 10^{-1} and does not require death of the donor. In this transfer, bacteriophages in either the donor or the recipient can permit plasmid transfer, presumably by effecting cell-to-cell adhesion. Bacteriophages can also inhibit this process; some plasmid elements can promote their own transfer. Because of the ease of the dissemination of resistant staphylococci from the body surface, there is every expectancy that resistant cocci will continue to be disseminated globally. It is suggested that important antibiotics for treating serious systemic infections (particularly gentamicin) should not be used on the body surface.

Gentamicin Resistance in *Enterobacteriaceae*; Opportunity to Trace the Global Spread of Two Genes?
(Thomas F. O'Brien)

The common resistance genes have been widely disseminated for so long that it is extremely difficult to trace their further spread. The introduction of a new antibiotic for which there are initially few if any detectable resistance genes, such as gentamicin a decade ago, is thus an opportunity to observe spread of distinctive resistance genes when and if they appear.

Witchitz and Chabbert (14) observed in a hospital in Paris dissemination in many species of *Enterobacteriaceae* of plasmid-mediated resistance to gentamicin which appears in retrospect to have been due to the aminoglycoside-acetylating enzyme, AAC(3). In 1970 Martin and his colleagues (5) observed in Washington, D.C., a nosocomial outbreak of *Klebsiella* type 22 with plasmid-mediated resistance to gentamicin apparently due to the 2″ aminoglycoside nucleotidyltransferase AAD(2″). The same enzyme appeared to be involved in *Enterobacter* in an outbreak of gentamicin-resistant *Klebsiella* which began in 1973 in a New York hospital (9). At about the same time, the same enzyme appeared involved in an outbreak in a Nashville hospital (13). It was at first exclusively in *Serratia marcescens* but later in *Klebsiella*. The *Serratia* then appeared to spread to three other hospitals in Nashville (12). Similar outbreaks with multiple strains carrying one or the other of the enzymes were reported in Toronto (8), Los Angeles (6), London (2), Melbourne (3), and Johannesburg (1). Data from an international survey of antibiotic resistance (7) suggests that one or the other of these enzymes is now either prevalent or almost completely absent in species of *Enterobacteriaceae*, particularly *Klebsiella* and *Serratia*, in different hospitals in different parts of the world. Transposition of what appears to be the gene for AAC(3) has recently been reported (10).

Two outbreaks occurring within a few months of each other in hospitals in widely separated cities in the United States are notable for their similarity (4, 11). Each involved the AAD(2″) enzyme. Each began with an outbreak of a single serotype of *Klebsiella* (one 30 and one 2) that circulated widely for several months and then virtually disappeared. By that time, however, the plasmid that mediated gentamicin resistance had appeared in a number of other nosocomial strains and species of *Enterobacteriaceae* in which it tended to persist. The plasmids in each outbreak appeared to have carried the same resistance gene, were of nearly the same molecular weight, and yielded approximately the same number of fragments on *Eco*RI endonuclease digestion.

TEM β-Lactamase in *Haemophilus influenzae* and *Neisseria gonorrhoeae*: Global Consequences of Rare Historic Genetic Events
(Clyde Thornsberry)

Before 1974, *H. influenzae* and *N. gonorrhoeae* were considered to be universally susceptible to ampicillin and penicillin, respectively, the drugs of choice for treating patients infected with these organisms. In 1973, a strain of *H. influenzae* was isolated from the spinal fluid of a child in Germany who later died with meningitis. This organism was resistant to ampicillin and other penicillins because it produced β-lactamase. The β-lactamase was mediated by a plasmid. Within a short period of time, β-lactamase-producing strains were isolated in all parts of the world. The incidence of β-lactamase-producing *H. influenzae* within a community varies, but until recently it generally remained at less than 10%. In the latest survey by the Center for Disease Control, however, the incidence in the United States was 18%. It is possible that the latter figure was influenced by selective reporting of β-lactamase-positive strains.

During the period of 1950 to 1970, *N. gonorrhoeae* strains became progressively more resistant to penicillin. This relative resistance was chromosomally mediated. In 1976, however, β-lactamase-producing strains of *N. gonorrhoeae* were isolated in the Far East and England, and subsequently on all continents. Although the incidence of β-lactamase-positive gonococci in selected groups of patients to gonorrhea (e.g., prostitutes) may be as high as 40%, the overall incidence in general has remained quite low and in selected areas is usually 0 to 2%. In the United States the overall incidence is much less than 1% of the total number of gonorrhea cases. Two different types of β-lactamase-positive *N. gonorrhoeae* have been recognized. The Far East strains are generally auxotypically wild types and have a larger plasmid than the English-African strains, which generally require at least arginine.

The β-lactamase produced by both of these organisms is of the TEM type, which is the most common β-lactamase produced by enteric bacteria. The plasmids of β-lactamase-positive *H. influenzae* and *N. gonorrhoeae* share a common DNA segment with the plasmid of TEM and *Escherichia coli*. These common segments of DNA contain the genes for production of TEM β-lactamase. Although it is not certain, it is probable that β-lactamase production in *H. influenzae* and *N. gonorrhoeae* resulted from the insertion of transposable DNA segments from plasmids of enteric bacteria into indigenous plasmids of these two organisms.

1. **Block, C. S.** 1978. Gentamicin-resistant gram-negative bacilli in hospital patients. Part I. Preliminary epidemiological assessment. S. Afr. Med. J. **53**:391–394.
2. **Casewell, M. W., M. Webster, M. T. Dalton, and I. Phillips.** 1977. Gentamicin-resistant *Klebsiella aerogenes* in a urological ward. Lancet **i**:444–445.
3. **Davey, R. B., and J. Pittard.** 1977. Plasmids mediating resistance to gentamicin and other antibiotics in *Enterobacteriaceae* from four hospitals in Melbourne. Aust. J. Exp. Biol. Med. Sci. **55**:299–307.
4. **Gerding, D. N., A. E. Buxton, R. A. Hughes, P. P. Cleary, J. Arbaczawski, and W. E. Stamm.** 1979. Nosocomial multiply resistant *Klebsiella pneumoniae*: epidemiology of an outbreak of apparent index case origin. Antimicrob. Agents Chemother. **15**:608–615.
5. **Martin, C. M., N. S. Ikari, J. Zimmerman, and J. A. Waitz.** 1971. A virulent nosocomial Klebsiella with a transferable R factor for gentamicin: emergence and suppression. J. Infect. Dis. **124**:S24–S29.
6. **Meyer, R. D., J. Halter, R. P. Lewis, and M. White.** 1976. Gentamicin-resistant *Pseudomonas aeruginosa* and *Serratia marcescens* in a general hospital. Lancet **i**:580–583.
7. **O'Brien, T. F., R. A. Norton, R. L. Kent, and A. A. Medeiros.** 1977. International surveillance of prevalence of antibiotic resistance. J. Antimicrob. Chemother. **3**:59–66.
8. **Rennie, R. P., and I. B. R. Duncan.** 1977. Emergence of gentamicin-resistant *Klebsiella* in a general hospital. Antimicrob. Agents Chemother. **11**:178–184.
9. **Richmond, A. S., J. J. Rahal, M. S. Simberkoff, and S. Schaefler.** 1975. R factors in gentamicin-resistant organisms causing hospital infection. Lancet **ii**:1176–1178.
10. **Rubens, C. E., W. F. McNeill, and W. E. Farrar, Jr.** 1979. Transposable plasmid deoxyribonucleic acid sequence in *Pseudomonas aeruginosa* which mediates resistance to gentamicin and four other antimicrobial agents. J. Bacteriol. **139**:877–882.
11. **Sadowski, P. L., B. C. Peterson, D. N. Gerding, and P. P. Cleary.** 1979. Physical characterization of ten R plasmids obtained from an outbreak of nosocomial *Klebsiella pneumoniae* infections. Antimicrob. Agents Chemother. **15**:616–624.
12. **Schaberg, D. R., R. H. Alford, R. Anderson, J. J. Farmer III, M. A. Melly, and W. Schaffner.** 1976. An outbreak of nosocomial infection due to multiply resistant *Serratia marcescens*: evidence of interhospital spread. J. Infect. Dis. **134**:181–188.
13. **Thomas, F. E., R. T. Jackson, M. A. Melly, and R. H. Alford.** 1977. Sequential hospitalwide outbreaks of resistant *Serratia* and *Klebsiella* infections. Arch. Intern. Med. **137**:581–584.
14. **Witchitz, J. L., and Y. A. Chabbert.** 1972. Resistance transferable a la gentamicine. II. Transmission et liaisons due caractere de resistance. Ann. Inst. Pasteur Paris **122**:367–378.

Newer Instrumental Techniques of Structural Elucidation and Purification of Antibiotics

JOHN C. GREENFIELD
Moderator

Infectious Diseases Research
The Upjohn Company
Kalamazoo, Michigan 49001, U.S.A.

TOMOHISA TAKITA
Moderator

Department of Chemistry
Institute of Microbial Chemistry
Tokyo, Japan

KENNETH L. RINEHART, JR.

School of Chemical Sciences
Roger Adams Laboratory
University of Illinois
Urbana, Illinois 61801, U.S.A.

NORBERT NEUSS

Lilly Research Laboratories
Eli Lilly and Company
Indianapolis, Indiana 46206, U.S.A.

DAN W. URRY

Laboratory of Molecular Biophysics
University of Alabama Medical Center
Birmingham, Alabama 35294, U.S.A.

MORTON E. MUNK

Department of Chemistry
Arizona State University
Tempe, Arizona 85281, U.S.A.

Recent Developments in the Study of Antibiotics by Mass Spectrometry
(Kenneth L. Rinehart, Jr.)

Each of the components of a mass spectrometer—inlet system, ion source, analyzer, detector, and recorder—is important to its performance. The usual methods of sample introduction—a gas chromatograph for the most volatile compounds, a batch inlet (gas bulb) system for less volatile materials, and a direct probe for still less volatile materials—require that the sample first volatilize into the vapor state, where it can be ionized by electron impact (EI), chemical ionization, or field ionization.

Two techniques for ionizing compounds in the solid state have been developed recently and these have proved especially valuable in extending the range of applicability of mass spectrometry to polar compounds of low volatility, a description which applies to most antibiotics. Of these two techniques, californium-252 radiation (plasma desorption) mass spectrometry (PDMS) appears more successful with the most intractable molecules, providing molecular ions from even heptaene antibiotics and bleomycin. The technique involves applying the sample to a thin foil and irradiating the foil with high-energy particles from ^{252}Cf, which leads to very

high but very localized temperatures, ionization in the solid state, and rapid desorption of the ions. The procedure, studied mainly in the laboratory of R. F. Macfarlane at Texas A & M University, has been employed only with a time-of-flight mass spectrometer and the resolution obtainable is still relatively modest. Another hindrance to use of the technique is the potential danger of working with ^{252}Cf.

A more widely used technique is field desorption (FD) mass spectrometry (FDMS), which involves adding a solution of the sample under study to a specially prepared emitter wire and applying a high field (ca. 12,000 V) to ionize the compound in the solid state. FD also gives abundant molecular ions with nonvolatile compounds, is useful for qualitative and rough quantitative analysis of mixtures, can provide excellent high-resolution data, and requires samples as small as 10 ng. Fragmentation ions are normally weak but can be enhanced by running spectra at higher emitter wire currents. Recent attempts to enhance further the utility of the technique include use of lasers instead of emitter current as a source of heat for the samples and use of phosphazenes as mass markers to m/e 3,000.

The principal applications of mass spectrometry to the study of antibiotics can be categorized as structure determination, characterization, molecular weight determination, and isotope ratio studies, which will be discussed in reverse order. Stable isotope studies can be employed both for quantitating physiological levels of antibiotics and their metabolites and for establishing the degree of incorporation of precursors into antibiotics in fermentations.

Probably the most common and obvious use of mass spectrometry as a tool in antibiotics research is in the determination of molecular weights and molecular formulas. Our laboratory long ago established the value of FD relative to EI and chemical ionization in giving molecular ions for antibiotics, and we subsequently demonstrated high-precision mass measurements above m/e 1,800 to assign molecular formulas for some antibiotics. Although not a high-resolution technique, PDMS does give molecular ions for some compounds that do not give molecular ions by FDMS; e.g., the polyenes aureofungins A and B.

For purposes of characterization of known antibiotics, EIMS is optimal in providing the multitude of fragment ions which can serve to distinguish one compound from another, even when the molecular ion is absent, as illustrated by the EI spectrum of alamethicin. Alternatively, minimal chemical evidence coupled with FDMS can serve to characterize complex molecules, as illustrated by the hydrolysis of alamethicin to a mixture of amino acids identified by FDMS or the periodate oxidation of fungichromin to two fragments identified by FDMS.

In a different sense, we recently studied early characterization of antibiotics in fermentation broths by adding samples of the antibiotics streptolydigin and streptovaricin to their fermentation media at concentrations typical of those found in the broth (ca. 100 µg/ml) and then attempting to observe the molecular ions in FD mass spectra. Dipping the emitter wire in the medium itself was unsuccessful, but extracting with 1-butanol or methylene chloride, concentrating, and dipping the emitter wire in the concentrate gave recognizable molecular ions for the antibiotics without purification. For unknown antibiotics, the technique should be augmented with high-resolution measurements.

Applications of mass spectrometry to structural assignments of antibiotics are too numerous to review but have been summarized elsewhere. Two especially valuable uses of mass spectrometric techniques can be noted. One is the determination of the carbon skeletons of polyene antibiotics by conversion of the backbone to saturated hydrocarbons or saturated methyl esters, as illustrated for dermostatin. The other is establishing sequences of small units,

for example in oligosaccharides and polypeptides. The sequencing of known discrete small fragments in polypeptides is perhaps the most powerful application of mass spectrometry to structure assignment in that it allows the greatest use of mass spectrometry and requires the least use of other spectroscopic and chemical techniques. Use of an FD-intensive procedure in assigning structures to polypeptide antibiotics was recently summarized elsewhere, but the procedure can be summarized as follows: (1) Total hydrolysis of the antibiotic to amino acids, identified by (a) high-resolution FDMS (HRFDMS), (b) derivatization and HREIMS, and (c) derivatization and gas chromatography (GC) retention times on a chiral column; (2) quantitation of the amino acids by GC and amino acid analyzer; (3) assignment of a molecular formula to the antibiotic by molar ratios of amino acids and by HRFDMS on the molecular ion; (4) assignment of a partial sequence to the antibiotic from fragment peaks in its HREI mass spectrum; (5) partial hydrolysis of the antibiotic to oligopeptides, identified by (a) derivatization and GC/HREIMS and GC/field ionization mass spectrometry, and (b) HRFDMS; (6) overlapping of the oligopeptides, combined with HREIMS on the intact antibiotic, to assign the structure.

High-Performance Liquid Chromatography of β-Lactam Antibiotics
(Roger D. Miller and Norbert Neuss)

The technique of high-performance liquid chromatography has enjoyed an enormous popularity in the last decade. The dramatic increase in its use is due mainly to availability of excellent instrumentation and improvements in the efficiency of a variety of packing materials. The presence of many β-lactam-containing antibiotics, including partially synthetic and naturally occurring compounds, required a search for chromatographic systems with great selectivity as well as high column efficiency and preparative methods to obtain some of the observed metabolites produced by fungi and streptomycetes.

Many of these compounds are amphoteric substances. Therefore, we have selected microbonded propylamine columns based upon two considerations. First, the stationary phase is much more polar than the octadecyl function present in reversed-phase adsorbents such as C_{18}/Porasil II and C_{18}/Porasil 3 (Waters Associates), thus allowing for better retention of metabolites not extractable into organic solvents. Second, the amino function acts as a weak anion exchanger at low pH, affording an additional parameter of selectivity. A thorough study of different ratios of acetic acid-methanol in relation to acetonitrile-water led to a ratio with a remarkably efficient separation power as shown in Fig. 1 and 2.

The use of a larger column permitted a direct isolation of 8 mg of cephalosporin C from 1.3 ml of filtered broth. This procedure is illustrated in Fig. 3.

Finally, we were able to correlate peaks in the UV recording with inhibition zones (bioautography) by diverting a portion of the eluent from the column during chromatography of the fermentation broth and applying it to an absorbent paper at the same rate as the recording of the

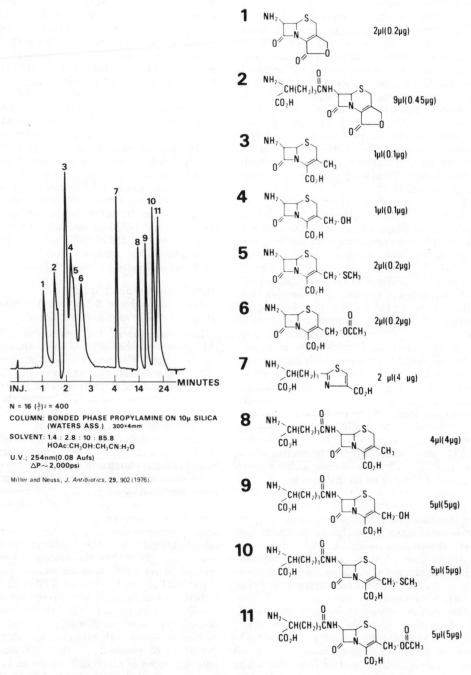

N = 16 $(\frac{5}{1})_2$ = 400

COLUMN: BONDED PHASE PROPYLAMINE ON 10µ SILICA (WATERS ASS.)   300×4mm

SOLVENT: 1.4 : 2.8 : 10 : 85.8
HOAc:CH₃OH:CH₃CN:H₂O

U.V.: 254nm(0.08 Aufs)
ΔP~2,000psi

Miller and Neuss, J. Antibiotics, 29, 902(1976).

FIG. 1. *Separation of different cephem derivatives. From Miller and Neuss, J. Antibiot.* **29**:*902, 1976.*

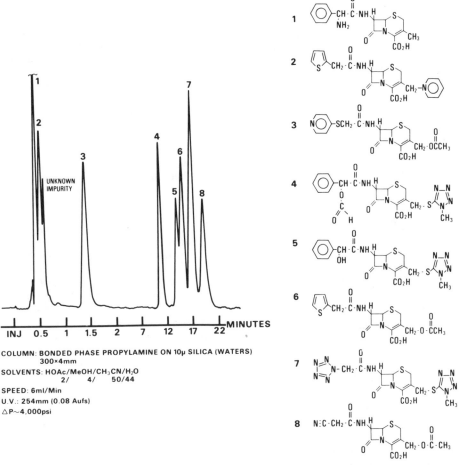

FIG. 2. *Structures: 1, cephalexin (0.5 μg); 2, cephaloridine (0.4 μg); 3, cephapirin (1.5 μg); 4, cefamandole nafate; 5, cefamandole (10.0 μg); 6, cephalothin (15 μg); 7, cefazolin (20 μg); 8, cephacetrile (30 μg). From Miller and Neuss, J. Antibiot. 29:902, 1976.*

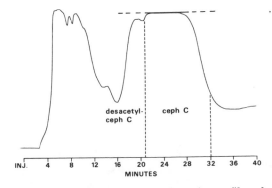

FIG. 3. *Cephalosporium acremonium filtered broth (1.3 ml). UV range, 254 nm; chart speed, 6.35 mm/min; flow rate, 4 ml/min; column size, 8 by 600 nm; packing, 10 μ NH_2 bonded phase propylamine on 10 μ silica (Waters); solvent, 2:4:7.5:86.5, HOAc-CH_3OH-CH_3CN-water; lb/in², 2,000. From Miller and Neuss, J. Antibiot. 29:902, 1976.*

· UV absorption. A typical separation of *Cephalosporium acremonium* fermentation broth is shown in Fig. 4.

High-performance liquid chromatographic bioautography has been further developed by the use of Systec microprocessor permitting unattended sample handling. Operations include gradient elution as well as column washing procedures with two solvents. The inclusion in the system of WISP (Waters) autoinjector provides programmable injections of 48 samples.

Sodium-23 and Nitrogen-15 Magnetic Resonance of Membrane-Active Peptide Antibiotics (Gramicidin A and Gramicidin S)

(Dan W. Urry, M. A. Khaled, A. Spisni, C. M. Venkatachalam, and R. D. Harris)

Sodium-23 magnetic resonance of the gramicidin A ion channel. While there is gen-

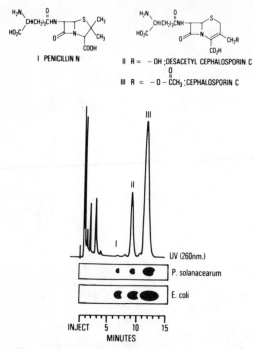

FIG. 4. *Typical separation of Cephalosporium acremonium fermentation broth. From Miller and Neuss, J. Antibiot.* **31:**1142, 1978.

eral agreement as to the nuclear magnetic resonance (NMR) results of ion interaction studies with cellular constituents, the interpretations of the results are lacking. Since ion movement through the gramicidin A channel, (HCO-L·Val$_1$-Gly$_2$-L·Ala$_3$-D·Leu$_4$-L·Ala$_5$-D·Val$_6$-L·Val$_7$-D·Val$_8$-L·Trp$_9$-D·Leu$_{10}$-L·Trp$_{11}$-D·Leu$_{12}$-L·Trp$_{13}$-D·Leu$_{14}$-L·Trp$_{15}$-NH CH$_2$CH$_2$OH)$_2$, has been thoroughly characterized as a function of [Na] and transmembrane potential by electrical studies which measure sodium ion current passing through gramicidin A doped planar bilayers, the question as to whether the NMR-characterized binding processes are compatible with that ionic current provides a critical test of ^{23}Na-NMR data interpretation.

The phenomena of temperature dependence of sodium-23 line width and T$_1$ (the longitudinal relaxation time), of Ag$^+$ and Tl$^+$ competitive blocking of ^{23}Na interaction, and of associated lipid core mobility decreases allow argument for the packaging of gramicidin channel structures in lysolecithin micelles. The NMR-characterized interaction of ^{23}Na with the channel distinguishes two binding processes. By means of sodium concentration dependence—of chemical shift, of T$_1$ and of T$_2$ (the transverse relaxation time)—a tighter site is observed with a forma-

tion constant, K_f^t, of about 100 M^{-1} and a weaker site with a K_f^w of about 5 M^{-1}. Off rate constants for the two binding processes were approximated from the fitting of the line width versus chemical shift data to obtain $k_{off}^t (\simeq 10^5$ s^{-1}) and directly from the inverse of the correlation time at high ion concentrations to obtain $k_{off}^w (\simeq 4 \times 10^8$ s^{-1}).

Utilizing X-ray diffraction data of the Stryer group as a guide for the positioning of tight and weak binding sites, deriving steady-state equations for two-, three-, and four-site models, and employing Eyring rate theory to add voltage dependence to the NMR-derived rate constants, it has been possible to calculate single-channel currents as a function of sodium ion concentration in the 10^{-3} M to 10 M range and for 50-, 100-, 150-, and 200-mV transmembrane potentials. A comparison of the experimental and calculated values for 100 mV is given in Fig. 5 for the two-site model. Recognizing the variability of the experimental single-channel currents with lipid, temperature, etc., this comparison provides a most stringent test of the validity and relevance of the NMR-derived constants.

Nitrogen-15 magnetic resonance and peptide structure. Gramicidin S, cyclo-(-L-Val-L-Orn-L-Leu-D-Phe-L-Pro)$_2$, has been used as a model in the development of methods for determining conformational detail. This model was used to show, with proton magnetic resonance, that temperature and solvent dependence

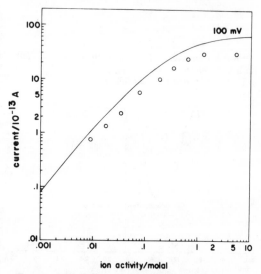

FIG. 5. *Calculated single-channel current for gramicidin A as a function of ion concentration for 100-mV transmembrane potential. Circles denote experimental data taken from S. B. Hladky, B. W. Urban, and D. A. Haydon, in Membrane Transport Processes, vol. 3, Raven Press, New York, 1979.*

of peptide N<u>H</u> chemical shift could be used to identify hydrogen-bonded NH moieties and, with carbon-13 magnetic resonance, that solvent dependence of peptide <u>C</u>=O chemical shift could be used to identify the carbonyl to which the NH is hydrogen bonded. It is now possible with nitrogen-15 magnetic resonance to determine those peptide moieties whose carbonyls are exposed by means of a dimethylsulfoxide-trifluoroethanol solvent titration as shown in Fig. 6A. Note the gramicidin S structure in Fig. 6B.

Additionally, it is possible to obtain information on distortions from planarity of the peptide moiety on the basis of the magnitude of the $^1J(^{15}N\text{-}^1H)$ coupling constant. In the *trans* state, $\omega = 180°$, the coupling constant is 95 Hz and only a few degrees distortion from *trans* causes a substantial drop in the magnitude of the coupling constant as shown in Fig. 6C. Thus, with nitrogen-15 magnetic resonance it is possible to further delineate polypeptide secondary struc-

ture and to assess distortions from planarity of the peptide moiety.

Computer-Assisted Structure Elucidation
(C. A. Shelley and Morton E. Munk)

The value of computers in chemical and spectral data acquisition, storage, and retrieval is well established, but it has only recently been shown that they also can assist in the process of structure elucidation based on the interpretation of such chemical and spectral data. This paper focuses on the CASE program.

In the early development of the CASE program, the "manual" process of structure elucidation was analyzed and dissected into its three major components: (i) the reduction of the chemical and spectral properties of the unknown to their structural implications and the expression of this information as a "partial structure" (interpretation); (ii) the expansion of the "partial structure" into some or all of the complete molecular structures compatible with the "partial

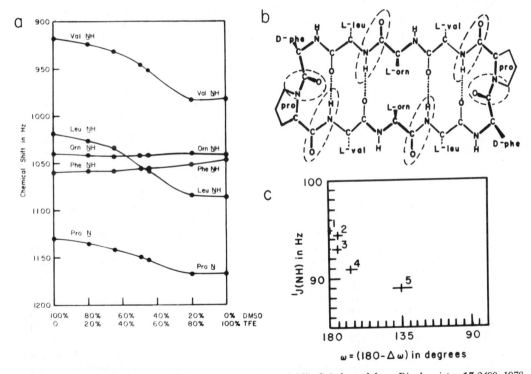

FIG. 6. *(A) Solvent titration of* ^{15}N *resonances of gramicidin S (adapted from Biochemistry **17**:2490, 1978 utilizing the assignments for Phe N, Orn N and Leu N resonances in DMSO as appeared in* ^{15}N*-NMR by Levy and Lichter, Wiley International, p. 199, 1979). (B) Gramicidin S structure with exposed C=O groups are encircled together with the H-bonded or solvent-shielded NH groups. (C) Plot of* $^1J(^{15}N\text{-}^1H)$ *versus the torsion angle* ω *(with permission from Int. J. Quantum Chem., QBS **4**:97, 1977). Numbers in the figure are: 1 for Pro-Gly trans peptide bond in Boc Pro-Gly-OMe, 2, 3, and 4 for peptide bonds in Ac-Gly$_1$-Val$_2$-Gly$_3$-OMe, and 5 for Val$_1$-Gly$_2$ peptide bond in Ac-Val$_1$-Gly$_2$-OMe.*

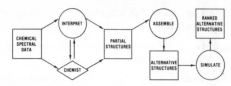

FIG. 7. *Graphic presentation of the CASE program.*

structure" (molecule assembly); and (iii) the prediction of the chemical and/or spectral properties of the compatible molecular structures followed by ranking or pruning on the basis of the fit between predicted and observed properties (simulation). Thus, the three major program modules of CASE are INTERPRET, ASSEMBLE, and SIMULATE. Figure 7 provides an overview of the system.

At the present stage of development, the reduction of the chemical and spectral properties of an unknown compound to their structural implications is shared by INTERPRET and the chemist. An infrared spectrum interpreter (INFRARED) is at an advanced but not final state of development. The artificial intelligence program was developed with two requirements in mind: the program must make decisions about a large number of functional groups, and it must be able to treat the complex spectra of multifunctional compounds. At the present time 53 major classes of functional groups are considered. The program reports subclass assignments for 22 of these classes. Several hundred spectra of varying complexity have been analyzed by INFRARED; however, additional testing and program refinement are planned. The interpretation of other types of spectral data must be chemist generated at this time.

The combined structural information is expressed as a "partial structure," which comprises the input to ASSEMBLE. As used here, the "partial structure" consists of: the molecular formula, nonoverlapping structural fragments known to be present, and constraints, that is, pieces of structural information that cannot be conveniently expressed as nonoverlapping structural fragments, e.g., the unknown possesses a total of three cyclopropyl hydrogens.

ASSEMBLE is unique in approach and designed to expand a "partial structure" into *all* structural isomers compatible with it. The interface to ASSEMBLE provides for the precise and convenient entry of the "partial structure." The molecular formula is entered in conventional format. Structural fragments are input by means of a generally applicable linear code that closely resembles conventional structural representation, e.g., CH_3CHOH, a 1-hydroxyethyl group with residual valence at the 1-position. Atom tags, which directly follow an atom of the structural fragment and are not counted as part of the structural fragment, may be used to provide the following additional information about the local environment of constituent atoms: the nature of neighboring atoms, the presence or absence of conjugation, the presence or absence of the tagged atom in a cycle or cycles of specified size, the presence or absence of vicinal hydrogens, and the atom composition of branches.

Structural information not specific to structural fragments (constraints) is entered by a series of routines that may be called by the user. Some routines treat information frequently obtained from spectral data, e.g., the number and kinds of different atoms, including their hybridization (coordination number) and hydrogen multiplicity; and the number and kinds of protons (cyclopropyl, vinyl/aromatic, etc.). The number (or a range) and kinds of multiple bonds and cycles may be input. The presence or absence of any specified substructure may be required. A strain detector in ASSEMBLE prospectively eliminates the construction of molecules with strained skeletons.

SIMULATE is at an early stage of development. One operational routine, SPRUNE, predicts the number of signals expected in the broad-band decoupled ^{13}C-NMR spectrum of a given molecular structure and compares the value to the observed number of signals.

CASE is interactive and is designed to complement, not replace, the talents of the chemist. At any stage in the structure determination, CASE can express the available evidence in terms of the molecular structures compatible with it. In contrast to the chemist, CASE possesses no preconceived ideas of structure type; therefore, the entire spectrum of plausible structures is constructed. Finally, at each stage of the structure elucidation, including that of final assignment, there is the assurance that no equally valid structure has been overlooked.

Sources of New Antibiotics

MARVIN J. WEINSTEIN
Chairman

Schering-Plough Corporation
Bloomfield, New Jersey 07003, U.S.A.

D. JOHN FAULKNER

Scripps Institution of Oceanography
University of California
San Diego, California 92105, U.S.A.

ASHIT K. GANGULY

Schering-Plough Corporation
Bloomfield, New Jersey 07003, U.S.A.

CLAUDE NASH

Smith Kline & French Laboratories
Philadelphia, Pennsylvania 19101, U.S.A.

HANS ZÄHNER

Universität Tübingen
Institut für Biologie II
Tubingen, Federal Republic of Germany

ARNOLD L. DEMAIN

Massachusetts Institute of Technology
Cambridge, Massachusetts 02139, U.S.A.

Chemical Ecology and Antibiotics from Marine Sponges
(D. John Faulkner)

During the past decade, many unusual chemicals have been isolated from marine organisms. The impetus for marine natural products research has been the expectation that new pharmaceuticals, particularly antimicrobial compounds, could be isolated from organisms living in the marine environment. It was argued that the secondary metabolites found in marine organisms have evolved as a response to their environment. Marine organisms, particularly the lower invertebrates, are likely to produce antibacterial compounds as a response to a constant contact with marine bacteria. The production of halogenated metabolites is likewise a response to the chemical composition of the marine environment.

Any successful program to find new pharmaceuticals from marine organisms is ultimately dependent on the choice of organisms to be studied. One cannot usually afford to collect large quantities of all the organisms at any particular collecting site. In order to obtain the greatest number of physiologically active compounds from marine organisms, we have adopted two collecting strategies, which we refer to as the screening approach and the ecological approach.

The screening approach requires a bioassay that can be performed in the field. The antimicrobial assay is ideally suited for this approach since it can be performed at most marine laboratories and on most research vessels. During a typical collection trip marine sponges are collected using SCUBA, and ethanolic extracts of a small sample of each organism are screened against test microorganisms. Those organisms that give positive assay results are then recollected in sufficient quantity for chemical studies. This approach has led to the discovery of many new antimicrobial compounds, including some classes of compounds that are uniquely marine in their source. The disadvantage of the screening approach is that the type of pharmaceutical agent found is predetermined by the assay used during the collection.

The ecological approach to the discovery of potential drugs from marine organisms is based on observations of the behavior and interactions of marine organisms in their natural environment. The literature abounds with reports of toxic and venomous marine organisms. Less frequently one encounters reports of organisms that use chemical deterrents to predation, but investigations of these reports are more likely to yield useful compounds that are physiologically active yet nontoxic. Field observations can also yield useful pointers to the presence of physiologically active compounds. For example, we have observed a negative correlation between fouling of sponges by epibionts and antimicrobial activity. The observation that one organism overgrows and kills another often indicates the presence of active compounds. Marine organisms that are soft-bodied, sessile or slow-moving, and which do not appear to have predators, may be suspected of using a chemical defense mechanism that involves physiologically active compounds.

Our collaboration with both ecologists and pharmacologists has led us to examine assays that might result in data of interest to both groups. The substitution of marine bacteria for pathogenic bacteria in the antimicrobial assay is a simple example. The ecologist is interested in antifouling or antilarval assays that indicate an organism's ability to withstand the pressures of overgrowth by epibionts and predation. The relevance of these assays to pharmacology is tenuous at best. However, the assay for compounds that inhibit cell division in fertilized sea urchin eggs has been shown to detect compounds that inhibit microtubule assembly and may provide a very sensitive assay for potential antineoplastic agents.

When we have isolated pure compounds, usually through a bioassay-directed isolation procedure, we identify the compounds and have the pure samples screened for pharmacological activity other than antimicrobial activity. The results are quite promising. We have identified more than 50 compounds with in vitro antimicrobial activity, and more than half the compounds submitted for pharmacological screening have shown activity in at least one assay. The active compounds that have been identified include terpenoid isonitriles and carbonimidic dichlorides; many halogenated terpenoids and particularly brominated phenols; several indole derivatives; some hydroquinones and quinones, including an isoquinoline-quinone; and some simple sulfur-containing heterocycles.

Everninomicins, a New Class of *Micromonospora*-Produced Antibiotics
(Ashit K. Ganguly)

Micromonospora spp. have been reported to produce many novel antibiotics, e.g., aminoglycosides (gentamicin, sisomicin, etc.), macrolides (rosaramicin, megalomicin), ansamycin (halomicin, rifamycin), peptides (68-1147), etc. Some of these compounds have proven to be extremely important in the clinic and others are at various stages of development. We discuss here the chemistry and microbiological activities of yet another novel class of antibiotics produced by micromonospora, i.e., oligosaccharides (everninomicins).

The oligosaccharide group of antibiotics represent complex structures and possess many centers of asymmetry. So far, only four members of this group of antibiotics have been isolated. These are everninomicin, curamycins, avilamycins, and flambamycins. Among these, everninomicins are produced by *Micromonospora* spp. and the other three by *Streptomyces*. Extensive chemical degradations and spectroscopic evidence have led to the structural elucidation of everninomicins B, C, D, and 2. Following the degradation methods established in the above structural studies, the structures of flambamycins, avilamycins, and curamycins have been established.

Everninomicins are highly active against a wide variety of gram-positive aerobes and anaerobes as well as *Neisseria* and *Mycobacterium*. They are active against a variety of strains of *Staphylococcus, Streptococcus, Bacillus,* and *Mycobacterium* (mean MIC ~ 0.05 to 0.5 μg/ml). The above strains include ones resistant to β-lactams, macrolides, tetracycline, lincomycin, and vancomycin. These antibiotics (i) are bactericidal for group A streptococci and bacteriostatic for other organisms and (ii) lack cross-resistance with other antimicrobials. Everninomicins show excellent in vivo activities in experimental animals, for example ED_{50}'s were less than 5 mg/kg for protection against infection caused by gram-positive organisms.

Everninomicins possess the following unique features in their structures: (i) evernitrose (the first example of a naturally occurring nitro sugar); (ii) a dichloroisoeverninic acid residue; (iii) two ortho ester carbons; (iv) one methylene dioxy group; (v) everninose, a disaccharide linked $1 \rightarrow 1$.

Elucidation of structures of everninomicins involved extensive chemical degradation and use of spectroscopy. A summary of the methodology developed in our laboratories to elucidate structures of everninomicins is presented.

We chemically modified everninomicins to obtain compounds with retention of the high activity of the parent antibiotic while improving their pharmacokinetics. Everninomicin D on electrochemical reduction yielded everninomicins 2, 3, and 7. All these compounds possess high antibacterial activity and everninomicin 7 shows good blood level when administered to rats.

On chemical reduction, everninomicin D is converted into aminoeverninomicin D and hydroxylaminoeverninomicin D. The latter compound possessed high antibacterial activity and yielded excellent blood level with the desired half-life (1.44 h). However, hydroxylaminoeverninomicin D was easily oxidized in alkaline solution to the corresponding nitroso compound which yielded poor blood level when administered to animals. The stability of the hydroxylaminoeverninomicin D was vastly improved by converting it to nitrones. Among a large number of nitrones prepared, acetaldehyde nitrone possessed the most desirable activity and pharmacokinetics. Hydroxylaminoeverninomicin D, like other everninomicins, has high LD_{50} values, e.g., >2,000 i.p., 1,600 s.c., >2,000 oral. Aminoeverninomicin D was alkylated and acylated. A variety of derivatives were prepared, among which N-acetyleverninomicin D possessed high antimicrobial activity, gave excellent blood level (80 μg/ml) when administered to rats (i.m.; 60 mg/kg), and showed a half-life of 1.4 h.

Flambamycin, curamycin, and avilamycin show many structural features similar to those of everninomicins. Everninomicins, unlike the other members of this group, possess a nitro sugar which is amenable to further modification to produce antibiotics with good spectrum of activity and improved pharmacokinetics.

Protoplast Fusion, Plasmids, and Recombinant DNA Applied to Antibiotic Discovery
(Claude Nash)

The search for new antibiotics has depended almost exclusively upon the isolation of genetically diverse microbes from soil. Conventional antibiotic screening programs have relied heavily on isolation of large numbers of microbes, ability to identify known groups of antibiotics, and manipulation of fermentation conditions. In recent years, emphasis has been placed on the application of automated systems, the development of sensitive and specific test systems, and the improvement of soil isolation procedures. With the advent of a series of "new genetic tools," a dramatic change in the drug discovery process is on the horizon. Rather than relying on evolutionary diversity, research scientists will utilize genetic techniques—such as protoplast fusion, in vitro and in vivo recombinant DNA, transposable elements and plasmids—to construct or discover novel antibiotics.

Interspecific recombination should become practical using protoplast fusion or in vitro recombinant techniques. The fusion of cells in the presence of polyethylene glycol appears to be generally applicable and permits exchange of the complete genome. This method may be limited by the need for considerable DNA homology between strains in order for recombination to occur. However, the high frequency of intraspecific recombination observed with various actinomycetes is extremely encouraging. Recombinant DNA technology takes advantage of autonomous replication of the hybrid DNA and therefore does not depend on DNA homology. Once suitable vector and host systems have been developed for antibiotic-producing microbes, this technology should be able to extend markedly the scope of achievable recombinations between diverse antibiotic-producing strains. Both protoplast fusion and recombinant DNA techniques should permit the construction of "hybrid" antibiotics and possibly new chemical classes. Although "hybrid" antibiotics have been formed by feeding chemically altered intermediates to blocked mutants, genetic methods circumvent the need to synthesize analogs and the potential problems associated with transport and activation. Because of the biochemical diversity, the likelihood of constructing new chemical classes of antibiotics would be enhanced by recombination between different genera.

The distribution of plasmids which code for either specific biosynthetic enzymes or elements which control antibiotic production probably contributes to the frequent occurrence of certain antibiotics. For example, curing experiments suggest the existence of a plasmid-borne structural gene for deoxystreptamine, which may account for its frequent occurrence as a constituent of aminoglycoside antibiotics produced by diverse actinomycetes. Plasmids which "control" the synthesis of antibiotics by some general mechanisms provide the opportunity to enhance the expression of genes found in natural isolates. For example, if a plasmid were found which nonspecifically enhances the excretion of antibiotics, it could provide a method of rapidly increasing the yield of a new antibiotic and, in turn, facilitate recovery of the active molecule.

Transposable elements may be responsible for the genetic variability commonly encountered with actinomycetes. If these elements exist in antibiotic-producing strains, they could be used to facilitate recombination between strains with only limited DNA homology and to construct tandem repeats.

In addition to the construction of new antibiotics, microbial genetics provides the tools for rapidly identifying groups of antibiotics, isolating diverse species, increasing genetic diversity, and developing unique testing procedures. The latter approach could be the most crucial to the discovery of new antibiotics.

New Ways to New Antibiotics
(Hans Zähner)

If the search for new antibiotics is not to be a work of Sisyphus we have to look for new ways. These can be found in four different methods: (i) by feeding in new groups of microorganisms not so far screened for antibiotic formation or by feeding in genetically modified microorganisms;

(ii) by modifying existing antibiotics by chemical, microbial, and genetic methods or a combination of them; (iii) by the use of other methods for the recognition of antibiotics; (iv) by possible alternatives of the antibiotic concept. The first two methods will be the subject of other lectures and are discussed here only briefly.

The new β-lactams are very good examples of the importance of the recognition methods. No new β-lactam was reported from 1956 to 1971, and it seemed that all β-lactams in existence had been found. The scene changed completely in 1972 after the introduction of β-lactam-supersensitive strains into the screening and the search for inhibitors of β-lactamases and for sulfur-containing compounds. A new series of β-lactams was discovered and the pool of β-lactams is by no means exhausted.

The classical screening uses for the primary test microorganisms that are as closely as possible correlated to the latter application, and modern developments using certain cell-free systems are based on the same principles. We should dispense with this direct correlation because it is not as accurate as expected, in many cases a correlation cannot be found, and without the restriction caused by the need of this correlation we would have a much larger choice of recognition methods. We could then choose tests that reduce the problems of identification of the activities discovered.

Some new compounds include the tetracenomycins, an example of what can be found using unusual microorganisms for screening. These antibiotics stand from the chemical point of view between the tetracyclines and the anthracyclinones. The nikkomycins Z and X were found in a test with *Mucor mihei*; they demonstrate greater activity in the formation of zygospores than in the growth of mycelium. These antibiotics inhibit the chitin synthase and are perhaps useful for plant protection against fungi, insects, or mites.

Some new compounds were also found in screening by thin-layer chromatography as a method. It should be possible to find 2 to 20 new compounds of 100 strains in screening with combined new methods for recognition and isolation, and probably all of the new compounds would show biological activity as well.

The study of antibiotic transport could lead to an alternative method of producing new antimicrobial agents. If we would know more about the way in which antibiotics enter the cells, we would be able to design new drugs. Some very interesting results were reported recently by the group at Roche in England (Ringrose et al.).

Based on knowledge of transport and splitting of small peptides by bacteria, they designed a group of new drugs with a peptide part as a vehicle and the aminoethylphosphonic acid as a warhead. Additional research will probably identify other vehicles, such as sideramines or polyamines, and also some other warheads. Perhaps the trend toward mass screening or with autoanalyzers should be changed to screening in a more academic and sophisticated way.

Role of the Microbiologist in Obtaining New Antibiotics
(Arnold L. Demain)

Screening of natural populations is not the only way to obtain new antibiotic compounds. The microbiologist can accomplish the same thing by either environmental or genetic modifications. The environmental manipulations include directed biosynthesis by addition of novel precursors or by the addition of precursors. New penicillins, bleomycins, polyoxins, tetracyclines, lincomycins, streptomycins, and others have been produced by these techniques.

Another environmental method is that of bioconversion of known antibiotics, which has yielded new macrolides, aminocyclitols, and lincomycins, among others. Genetic manipulations involve the use of certain types of mutants with or without special supplements. The most popular method, mutational biosynthesis, involves feeding idiotrophic mutants analogs of the antibiotic moiety which they cannot make. This method has led to the production of new aminocyclitols, macrolides, and novobiocins. Another procedure is to add to the media of auxotrophic mutants analogs of their requirement. Thus, feeding L-*S*-carboxymethylcysteine to a Lys⁻ *Cephalosporium acremonium* culture yielded a new penicillin, and feeding ethionine to a Met⁻ *Penicillium griseofulvum* gave a new griseofulvin. Auxotrophs have also been obtained which produce new antibiotics without special supplementation; these antibiotics include derivatives of tetracycline, rubradirin, penicillin N, and celesticetin.

Another mutant category is that of mutants blocked in production of the normal antibiotic which do not respond to feeding of the missing moiety, i.e., they are not idiotrophs. These sometimes produce a new antibiotic, often an antibiotically active intermediate or shunt metabolite. These have included cephalosporins, macrolides, tetracyclines, and rifamycins. There are unblocked mutants that produce a new antibiotic alongside the old one; these include a cephalosporin, an anthracycline, and aminocyclitols, among others. Mixtures of mutants or the addition of a mutant accumulation product to a producer of a different antibiotic have yielded new tetracyclines, a new anthracycline, and a new macrolide.

Genetic recombination of different species appears to be yielding new antibiotics, but no new product has yet been reported via the protoplast fusion technique.

A. New Agents

Synergy of LY127935 (Shionogi Compound 6059-S) with Aminoglycoside and β-Lactam Antibiotics Against Multiple-Antibiotic-Resistant Gram-Negative Isolates

GORDON L. BRIER,* HENRY R. BLACK, RICHARD S. GRIFFITH, AND JAMES D. WOLNY

Lilly Laboratory for Clinical Research, Wishard Memorial Hospital, Indianapolis, Indiana 46202, U.S.A.

Hospital-acquired infections due to gram-negative organisms are an increasing problem in hospitalized patients. Aminoglycoside antibiotics have been used to treat these infections successfully in the past. However, outbreaks of hospital-acquired infection due to multiple-antibiotic-resistant gram-negative organisms are becoming more frequent. Although the newer cephalosporin antibiotics—cefamandole, cefuroxime, and the cephamycin antibiotic cefoxitin—have a broader spectrum of activity than currently available cephalosporins, especially among the gram-negative organisms, they are not active against multiple-antibiotic-resistant gram-negative isolates or pseudomonads.

LY127935 is a new β-lactam antibiotic that has an extended gram-negative spectrum which includes both *Pseudomonas* species and multiple-antibiotic-resistant gram-negative isolates. It has been shown that LY127935 possesses a high degree of activity against most multiple-antibiotic-resistant isolates for which it has been tested. Whether LY127935 would be used as a single agent in treating the infections caused by these isolates is yet to be determined; however, at the present time, an aminoglycoside antibiotic is commonly used in combination with either a cephalosporin or a penicillin with the purpose being either to increase the spectrum of activity of the antibiotic or to take advantage of any synergistic effect the antibiotic combination might have.

An unwanted effect of antibiotic combinations can be antagonism of antibacterial activity of the antibiotic being used in some combinations. Combinations of LY127935 with the newer penicillins—piperacillin and ticarcillin—were tested for synergy, as was the combination of LY127935 with tobramycin and amikacin. Piperacillin and ticarcillin were chosen because of their broad spectrum of activity, which includes *Pseudomonas*. Amikacin was chosen because it possessed some activity against many of the multiple-antibiotic-resistant isolates tested, and tobramycin was chosen because it was active against many of the multiple-antibiotic-resistant *Pseudomonas* isolates.

The organisms tested included multiple-antibiotic-resistant isolates of *P. aeruginosa, Ser-*

TABLE 1. *Effect of tobramycin, amikacin, and piperacillin in combination with LY127935*

Combination and organism	No. of isolates	FIC <1	FIC 1	FIC >1
LY127935 with tobramycin				
P. aeruginosa	11	10	1	0
P. maltophilia	3	3	0	0
Acinetobacter	5	5	0	0
S. marcescens	9	9	0	0
E. cloacae	5	5	0	0
E. coli	4	2	0	0
K. pneumoniae	6	6	0	0
P. rettgeri	5	3	0	2
P. stuartii	5	2	0	3
P. mirabilis	2	2	0	0
LY127935 with amikacin				
P. aeruginosa	5	4	0	1
P. maltophilia	3	2	0	1
Acinetobacter	5	3	0	2
S. marcescens	5	5	0	0
E. cloacae	5	4	0	1
E. coli	4	2	2	0
K. pneumoniae	5	3	1	1
P. rettgeri	5	4	0	1
P. stuartii	5	2	0	3
P. mirabilis	3	0	0	3
LY127935 with piperacillin				
P. aeruginosa	11	11	0	0
P. maltophilia	3	1	0	2
Acinetobacter	5	4	0	1
S. marcescens	5	3	0	2
E. cloacae	6	2	0	4
E. coli	4	3	1	0
K. pneumoniae	5	2	0	3
P. rettgeri	5	0	0	5
P. stuartii	5	0	0	5
P. mirabilis	2	1	0	1

ratia marcescens, Enterobacter cloacae, Escherichia coli, Proteus mirabilis, P. rettgeri, Klebsiella pneumoniae, Providencia stuartii, and P. vulgaris. Other isolates tested were those clinical isolates that are not normally considered susceptible to β-lactam antibiotics. They included isolates of P. maltophilia and Acinetobacter sp.

The effect of the various antibiotic combinations was determined by use of a broth-microdilution checkerboard technique. Mueller-Hinton broth was used to make the antibiotic dilutions, and the diluted plates were inoculated with dropping pipettes (Cooke Engineering Co.) that were calibrated to deliver 50 µl per drop. The inoculum was prepared from an overnight broth culture that had been diluted to contain 10^5 colony-forming units. The plates used had eight rows of 10 wells and were obtained from MicroMedia, Inc. The antibiotic dilutions were made with an Autotiter IV.

The MIC for each isolate was determined for each of the antibiotics individually at the same time that the MICs for the antibiotics in combination were determined. A fourfold decrease in the MIC of each of the combined drugs from the MIC of the individual drug was considered synergy.

An alternate method for reporting synergism is the use of the fractional inhibitory concentration (FIC), which is determined by dividing the MIC of the antibiotic present in the combination by the MIC of the individual antibiotics. The sum of the FICs (FIC = FIC of antibiotic A + FIC of antibiotic B) can be used to determine whether or not a compound is synergistic. Sums of <1 indicate a synergy, 1 indicates additive, and >1 indicates antagonism. The effect of tobramycin, amikacin, and piperacillin in combination with LY127935 is shown in Table 1.

LY127935 with ticarcillin showed less synergism than any of the four combinations tested. Of the 47 isolates tested for synergism with this combination, only 21% showed any degree of synergism; the remaining 79% showed antagonism. Combinations of LY127935 with amikacin and piperacillin yielded synergistic response in 71% and 55%, respectively, of the isolates tested. The combination of tobramycin with LY127935 yielded a synergistic response with 90% of the isolates tested.

In Vitro Activity of 6059-S (LY 127935) Compared with Those of Cefotaxime and Other β-Lactam Antibiotics

PRAMOD M. SHAH,* SCHLOMO STANCHOWSKI, AND WOLFGANG STILLE

Zentrum der Inneren Medizin, J. W. Goethe-Universität, D 6 Frankfurt am Main 70, Federal Republic of Germany

6059-S (LY127935) is a new cephalosporin with a broad spectrum of activity against both gram-positive and gram-negative bacteria, including Pseudomonas aeruginosa. In this study we present the results of in vitro comparison of the activities 6059-S with those cefotaxime, cefazolin, cefuroxime, and cefoxitin against Staphylococcus aureus, Escherichia coli, Klebsiella pneumoniae, and Enterobacter and Proteus species. The activity of 6059-S against P. aeruginosa was compared with those of cefotaxime, cefsulodin, piperacillin, azlocillin, and carbenicillin.

MICs were determined by using the agar dilution technique (1). The inoculum was adjusted to 10^5 colony-forming units per ml. The effect of inoculum on the in vitro activity of 6059-S was studied, using 10^3, 10^5, and 10^7 colony-forming units per ml, against a selected number of strains. Cross-resistance with cefotaxime was evaluated with some Enterobacter strains.

Viable counts at 0, 0.5, 1, 2, and 4 h were performed to determine the bactericidal activity of 6059-S. The effect of concentration on the bactericidal activity of 6059-S was evaluated after exposing the test strain to serial twofold dilutions of the antibiotic for 2 and 4 h. The method has been described explicitly in previous papers (2, 3).

Table 1 gives the concentrations needed to inhibit 50 and 90% of the strains. Against E. coli and K. pneumoniae, 6049-S and cefotaxime were more active than the other cephalosporins. Against S. aureus, 6059-S was found to be the least active. Both 6059-S and cefotaxime were found to be more active than carbenicillin against P. aeruginosa, cefsulodin being the most active. Concentrations of ≦16 µg of 6059-S and

TABLE 1. *MICs needed to inhibit 50 and 90% of the strains of various species*

Species	Strains		MIC (µg/ml)								
	No.	% Inhibited	6059-S	Cefotaxime	Cefazolin	Cefuroxime	Cefoxitin	Cefsulodin	Piperacillin	Azlocillin	Carbenicillin
E. coli	49	50	0.12	0.03	0.2	4	4				
		90	0.5	0.5	64	16	16				
K. pneumoniae	37	50	0.12	0.03	8	4	2				
		90	0.5	0.5	128	32	64				
Proteus species	43	50	0.12	0.03	4	2	4				
		90	16	2	>128	16	128				
Enterobacter species	34	50	0.12	1	128	64	128				
		90	64	≧128	>128	≧128	>128				
S. aureus	41	50	4	1	<0.25	0.5	4				
		90	≧16	2	8	8	16				
P. aeruginosa	41	50	10	10				1.25	2.5	5	60
		90	20	20				2.5	5	5	60

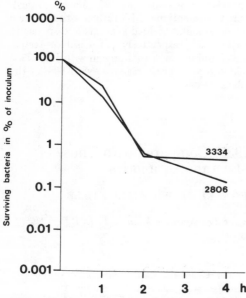

FIG. 1. *Kinetics of bactericidal activity of 40 µg of 6059-S against P. aeruginosa strains 3334 and 2806 (MIC for both strains, 20 µg/ml).*

cefotaxime per ml inhibited 41 and 34, respectively, of 51 cefoxitin-resistant strains. Both 6059-S and cefotaxime were found to be sensitive to rise in inoculum, especially against *P. aeruginosa*. Against selected strains of *Enterobacter* species, no cross-resistance was seen between

6059-S and cefotaxime. When the inocula were exposed to twice the MICs, the time needed to kill 99% ranged from 95 to 220 min. Figure 1 shows a typical curve of kinetics of bactericidal activity. Similar curves were derived for other tested strains. Increasing the concentration of 6059-S to more than twice the MIC did not show a proportional increase in bactericidal activity.

6059-S and cefotaxime were found to be highly active against gram-positive and gram-negative clinical isolates, especially against cefoxitin-resistant strains. Both compounds were more active than carbenicillin on a weight basis. This activity was, however, influenced negatively by inoculum size.

Using the membrane filtration technique, it could be clearly shown that 6059-S is a bactericidal drug. Whereas the "Eagle effect" of cefotaxime was observed when the concentration was raised, no such effect was seen for 6059-S (3).

The present study showed that 6059-S is active in vitro against clinical isolates, and controlled clinical trials are recommended to evaluate the efficacy of this compound.

1. **Reeves, D. S., I. Phillips, J. D. Williams, and R. Wise.** 1978. Laboratory methods in antimicrobial chemotherapy. Churchill Livingstone, London.
2. **Shah, P. M., and H. Bender.** 1978. Bactericidal activity of cefoxitin and cefuroxime. J. Antimicrob. Chemother. 4:163–168.
3. **Shah, P. M., G. Troche, and W. Stille.** 1979. Effect of concentration on bactericidal activity of cefotaxime. J. Antimicrob. Chemother. 5:419–422.

Antibacterial Activity of 6059-S, a New 1-Oxacephem, Against Clinical Isolates of *Enterobacteriaceae* and Nonfermenters

L. VERBIST

Diagnostic Microbiology Laboratory, St. Rafaël Hospital, University of Louvain, B-3000 Louvain, Belgium

In recent years a number of new cephalosporins have been developed which have remarkable stability against β-lactamases and enhanced activity against gram-negative microorganisms. One of the latest developments is a cephalosporin-like compound, 6059-S (LY127935), which was recently shown to have similar features (S. Matsuura, T. Yoshida, K. Sugeno, Y. Harada, M. Harada, and S. Kuwahara, Program Abstr. Intersci. Conf. Antimicrob. Agents Chemother. 18th, Atlanta, Ga., abstr. no. 152, 1978). This semisynthetic compound bears an α-methoxy group in C_7, as do the cephamy-

cins, but the sulfur in the 1 position has been replaced by an oxygen. Therefore, the compound may be designated a 1-oxacephem (1-OXA).

The purpose of this study was to compare the in vitro activity of 1-OXA with that of cefotaxime (CTX), cefuroxime, cephalothin (CLT), piperacillin (PIP), and tobramycin (TOB) against a wide variety of *Enterobacteriaceae*, and in addition with that of cefsulodin (CSL) against *Pseudomonas*. The MICs for 453 *Enterobacteriaceae* and of 107 *Pseudomonas* and *Acinetobacter* isolates were determined. All were clinical isolates cultured from pathological specimens in

TABLE 1. *Comparative activity of antibiotics against gram-negative organisms*

Species (no. of isolates)	Percent inhibited	MIC for 50% and 90% of the isolates (μg/ml)						
		1-OXA[a]	CTX	CFU	CLT	PIP	TOB	CSL
E. coli (60)	50	0.12	0.06	4	8	2	0.5	
	90	0.25	0.12	8	32	>128	1	
K. pneumoniae (60)	50	0.12	0.06	4	16	128	0.5	
	90	0.5	0.25	16	128	>128	2	
Enterobacter spp. (30)	50	0.12	0.25	8	>128	2	0.5	
	90	4	4	>128	>128	128	0.5	
S. marcescens (30)	50	0.25	0.5	>128	>128	8	2	
	90	0.5	1	>128	>128	>128	4	
Salmonella spp. (30)	50	0.06	0.06	4	2	2	0.5	
	90	0.06	0.12	8	8	4	1	
Shigella spp. (29)	50	0.06	0.03	0.5	4	0.5	1	
	90	0.12	0.03	2	8	2	1	
Y. enterocolitica (22)	50	0.12	0.12	2	128	2	0.5	
	90	0.25	0.25	4	>128	8	1	
C. freundii (15)	50	0.12	0.25	8	128	4	0.5	
	90	8	4	32	>128	>128	4	
P. mirabilis (59)	50	0.06	0.03	1	4	0.25	0.25	
	90	0.06	0.03	2	4	8	0.5	
P. vulgaris (33)	50	0.12	0.06	128	128	0.5	0.25	
	90	0.12	0.25	>128	>128	2	1	
P. morganii (35)	50	0.03	0.03	32	>128	0.5	1	
	90	0.03	0.03	32	>128	16	2	
P. rettgeri (19)	50	0.03	0.03	0.25	16	0.5	0.5	
	90	0.03	0.06	4	>128	64	2	
P. inconstans (31)	50	0.03	0.06	2	64	32	2	
	90	0.03	0.25	16	>128	64	8	
P. aeruginosa (60)	50	16	32	>128	>128	8	1	2
	90	32	64	>128	>128	16	64	4
Pseudomonas spp. (28)	50	4	8	>128	>128	16	64	64
	90	64	>128	>128	>128	>128	>128	128
Acinetobacter spp. (19)	50	32	16	32	>128	16	2	
	90	64	32	64	>128	32	32	

[a] 1-OXA, 1-oxacephem; CTX, cefotaxime; CFU, cefuroxime; CLT, cephalothin; PIP, piperacillin; TOB, tobramycin; CSL, cefsulodin.

TABLE 2. *Inhibitory and bactericidal effect of β-lactam antibiotics on microorganisms in Mueller-Hinton broth*

Species (no. of isolates)	Antibiotic[a]	Cumulative no. of isolates inhibited (MIC)/killed (MBC) at a concn (μg/ml) of:											
		0.015	0.03	0.06	0.12	0.25	0.5	1	2	4	8	16	32
E. coli (16)	1-OXA	0	3/3	12/11	14/13	15/15	16/16						
	CTX	0	13/13	15/15	15/15	16/16							
	PIP				0	2/2	7/6	15/13	16/16				
K. pneumoniae (16)	1-OXA			0	3/3	13/13	15/15	16/16					
	CTX	16/16											
	PIP						0	1/0	2/2	16/15	16/15	16/16	
P. mirabilis (16)	1-OXA			0	5/5	16/16							
	CTX	16/16											
	PIP			0	8/7	16/13	16/16						
S. marcescens (16)	1-OXA			0	1/0	10/7	14/14	14/14	15/15	16/16			
	CTX				0		1/0	2/0	8/0	10/3	16/15	16/16	
	PIP				0		2/0	9/9	11/11	15/15	15/15	15/15	16/16
P. aeruginosa (16)	1-OXA							0	2/0	6/4	7/5	15/12	16/16
	CTX							0	3/0	4/3	8/6	15/10	16/16
	PIP					0	2/0	4/2	5/5	11/7	16/16		

[a] 1-OXA, 1-oxacephem; CTX, cefotaxime; PIP, piperacillin.

my laboratory. MIC determinations by the agar dilution method were performed in Mueller-Hinton agar, with a multipoint inoculator and over a range of concentrations between 0.015 and 128 μg/ml.

The comparative MICs for 50 and 90% of the isolates in the different species are shown in Table 1. 1-OXA and CTX were equivalent in activity and by far the most active antibiotics against the *Enterobacteriaceae*. 1-OXA and CTX inhibited 90% of the *Escherichia coli*, *Klebsiella pneumoniae*, *Salmonella*, *Shigella*, *Yersinia enterocolitica*, and *Proteus* species at 0.5 μg or less/ml and at 0.25 μg or less/ml, respectively, and even 100% of the same species at 1 μg or less/ml and 2 μg or less/ml, respectively. Ninety percent of the *Serratia marcescens* and 75% of the *Enterobacter* and *Citrobacter freundii* isolates were inhibited by 0.5 μg of 1-OXA/ml and by 1 μg of CTX/ml. The next best antibiotic against the *Enterobacteriaceae* was TOB, with 90% inhibition between 0.5 and 8 μg/ml. Within the β-lactam antibiotics, CSL was the most active against *P. aeruginosa*, followed by PIP, 1-OXA, and CTX. But 1-OXA showed the highest activity against the other *Pseudomonas* species, especially as a result of its good performance against *P. maltophilia*, a species resistant to almost all antibiotics.

The MBCs for 16 selected isolates of *E. coli*, *K. pneumoniae*, *Proteus mirabilis*, *S. marcescens*, and *P. aeruginosa* were tested in Mueller-Hinton broth with the microtiter system and by subculturing 1 μl of the content of the inhibited wells on Mueller-Hinton agar (Table 2). The MBCs of 1-OXA were very similar to its MICs with the five species tested. The same applied to PIP and to CTX, except with *S. marcescens*, for which the MBCs of CTX were often four to eight times higher than the MICs. The activity of 1-OXA in broth was nearly the same as in agar with all five species. In contrast, the activity of CTX against the same isolates of *Klebsiella* and *P. mirabilis* was four times higher in broth than in agar, but against *S. marcescens* its activity was six times lower.

The inoculum effect on the MIC and MBC of 1-OXA for five isolates of the same species was studied. Between an inoculum of 10^3 colony-forming units (CFU)/ml and 10^5 CFU/ml, only a slight increase in MIC and MBC was observed (zero- to fourfold). With an inoculum of 10^7 CFU/ml, the increase in MIC and MBC of 1-OXA was slight for *Klebsiella* isolates (on average, 4 times), moderate for *E. coli* (average, 10 times) and *P. aeruginosa* (average, 12 times), high for *S. marcescens* (average, 25 times), and very high for *P. mirabilis* (average, 500 times). Surprisingly, all these *P. mirabilis* isolates were very susceptible to CLT. The addition of 10% and 50% serum to the Mueller-Hinton broth had a rather enhancing effect on the MIC and MBC of 1-OXA against *E. coli*, *Klebsiella*, *P. mirabilis*, and *S. marcescens*, and caused a slight decrease of the activity against *P. aeruginosa*.

It can be concluded that the activity of 1-OXA

is almost equivalent to that of CTX: the differences are generally limited to one dilution in favor of one compound or the other according to the different species, and at the very low concentrations needed to inhibit 90% or more of the isolates these differences seem to be irrelevant. Both new cephalosporins are markedly more active than cefuroxime and PIP, one of the most active broad-spectrum penicillins. They were also more active than TOB against all species of the *Enterobacteriaceae*. It will be difficult to give preference to either 1-OXA or CTX on the basis of their in vitro performance; probably the pharmacological properties will decide in favor of one or the other.

In Vitro Antibacterial Activity of Cefoperazone and LY127935 Against Aerobic Isolates

M. C. RUBIO-CALVO* AND R. GOMEZ-LUS

Department of Microbiology, School of Medicine, Zaragoza, Spain

Cefoperazone (T-1551) is a new semisynthetic injectable third-generation cephalosporin with a wide antibacterial spectrum, high resistance to β-lactamases, and favorable pharmacokinetic properties. LY127935 (Shionogi compound 6059-S) is a new β-lactam antibiotic with an expanded spectrum against gram-negative organisms, including those resistant to other antibiotics.

In this study, 1,336 strains of *Enterobacteriaceae*, *Pseudomonas aeruginosa*, *Acinetobacter calcoaceticus*, and *Staphylococccus* species were tested. All were isolated from patients hospitalized between March 1978 and March 1979 at the University Hopsital of Zaragoza, School of Medicine. The strains of *P. aeruginosa*, *Serratia marcescens*, and *Enterobacter* species had been bacteriocin typed. In vitro agar-dilution tests were performed in the conventional manner by using Mueller-Hinton agar. Plates were inoculated with a Steers-Foltz replicating device adjusted to deliver approximately 10^3 to 10^4 viable units of each organism to the agar surface.

Drugs were obtained from the manufacturers: cefoperazone from Pfizer International Inc. and LY127935 from Eli Lilly & Co.

The susceptibilities of gram-negative bacilli and staphylococci to cefoperazone are shown in Table 1. Cefoperazone was active against a wide range of gram-negative organisms. *Escherichia coli* showed a fairly uniform susceptibility, with 90.23% susceptible to 4 µg/ml and 95.41% susceptible to 15 µg/ml. Cefoperazone at a concentration of 4 µg/ml inhibited 81.76% of *Klebsiella pneumoniae* strains, and at a concentration of 16 µg/ml it inhibited 94.56%. A concentration of 16 µg/ml inhibited 86.63% of *Enterobacter aer-*

TABLE 1. *Susceptibility of 1,336 clinical isolates to cefoperazone*

Organism (no. of strains)	Cumulative % inhibited at a concn (µg/ml) of:										
	0.12	0.25	0.5	1	2	4	8	16	32	64	128
E. coli (482)	30.08	45.22	61.61	75.92	86.50	90.23	92.30	95.41	96.86	98.10	100
K. pneumoniae (203)	33.0	44.33	61.57	72.90	77.82	81.76	87.67	94.56	95.54	97.01	100
E. cloacae (52)	36.53	46.14	63.44	67.28	71.12	73.04	73.04	80.73	86.49	94.18	100
E. aerogenes (30)	26.66	46.66	59.99	66.65	69.98	73.31	79.97	86.63	89.96	96.62	100
C. freundii (11)	9.09	36.36	45.45	63.63	72.72	81.81	90.9	90.9	100		
H. alvei (2)		100									
S. marcescens (102)		1.96	5.88	7.84	9.80	15.68	35.28	41.16	70.76	74.68	100
P. mirabilis (21)	4.76	9.52	28.56	38.08	80.93	90.45	95.21	100			
P. vulgaris (18)		11.11	27.77	38.88	66.65	77.76	94.42	100			
P. morganii (17)		5.88	23.52	35.28	58.8	64.68	70.56	88.2	100		
P. rettgeri (20)		10.0	25.0	35.0	45.0	55.0	70.0	85.0	90.0	95.0	100
P. inconstans (2)						50.0	100				
A. calcoaceticus (17)					5.88	23.52	23.52	23.52	47.04	70.56	100
P. aeruginosa (246)			0.40	0.80	9.74	47.13	67.04	89.8	94.67	97.1	100
S. aureus (80)		1.25	3.75	36.25	65.0	73.75	78.75	78.75	78.75	78.75	100
S. epidermidis (33)		3.03	15.15	51.51	81.81	87.87	96.96	100			

TABLE 2. *Susceptibility of 1,013 clinical isolates to LY127935 (6059-S)*

Organism (no. of strains)	Cumulative % inhibited at a concn (µg/ml) of:										
	0.12	0.25	0.5	1	2	4	8	16	32	64	128
E. coli (440)	91.58	97.94	98.62	99.07	99.52	99.52	99.74	100			
K. pneumoniae (204) . . .	73.03	93.61	99	99	99	99	99	100			
E. cloacae (44)	84.08	88.62	93.16	95.43	95.43	95.43	95.43	97.70	100		
E. aerogenes (21)	95.23	95.23	95.23	100							
C. freundii (10)	100										
H. alvei (2)		100									
S. marcescens (63)	46.03	85.71	90.47	95.23	98.40	98.40	98.40	98.40	98.40	98.40	100
P. mirabilis (17)	88.23	94.11	100								
P. vulgaris (10)	80.0	90.0	100								
P. morganii (11)	90.90	90.90	100								
P. rettgeri (8)	100										
P. inconstans (2)	100										
A. calcoaceticus (21) . . .	4.76	9.52	9.52	9.52	9.52	14.28	19.04	28.56	52.36	61.88	100
P. aeruginosa (43)						20.93	51.16	72.09	88.36	93.01	100
S. aureus (15)		1.33	2.66	15.99	49.32	62.65	67.98	75.98	75.98	85.31	100
S. epidermidis (42)		2.38	4.76	21.42	52.37	59.51	71.41	85.69	88.07	92.83	100

ogenes and 80.73% of *E. cloacae.* Cefoperazone at a concentration of 16 µg/ml inhibited 90.9% of *C. freundii* isolates. Two strains of *Hafnia alvei* were inhibited by 0.25 µg/ml. *S. marcescens* isolates showed a variable resistance pattern: 41% of 102 strains were inhibited by 16 µg/ml, but 58.81% of the remaining isolates required concentrations equal to or higher than 32 µg/ml. All *Proteus mirabilis* and *P. vulgaris* strains were susceptible to 16 µg or less/ml. Cefoperazone at a concentration of 16 µg/ml inhibited 88.2% of *P. morganii* isolates and 85% of *P. rettgeri* strains. One strain of *P. inconstans* was inhibited by 4 µg/ml and the other isolate required 8 µg/ml. Only 23.52% of *A. calcoaceticus* strains were inhibited by 16 µg/ml, and against 76.45% of the isolates MICs of cefoperazone were equal to or higher than 32 µg/ml. Of the *S. aureus* strains tested, 73.75% were inhibited by 4 µg/ml and 78.75% by 16 µg/ml. In contrast, all *S. epidermidis* isolates were susceptible to 16 µg of cefoperazone per ml.

The percentage of strains susceptible to LY127935 is summarized in Table 2. LY127935 was highly effective against a wide variety of gram-negative bacilli. All *E. coli* and *K. pneumoniae* strains were susceptible to 16 µg or less/ml, and 97% of *E. cloacae* isolates were inhibited by 16 µg/ml. All *Citrobacter freundii* strains were susceptible to 0.12 µg/ml. LY127935 at a concentration of 1 µg/ml inhibited 100% of *E. aerogenes* isolates. Two isolates of *H. alvei* were susceptible to 0.25 µg/ml. A concentration of 2 µg/ml inhibited 95.23% of *S. marcescens* isolates, and only 11.60% of those remaining required concentrations equal to or higher than 32 µg/ml. All *P. mirabilis, P. vulgaris,* and *P. morganii*

strains were susceptible to 0.5 µg/ml. Eight isolates of *P. rettgeri* and two isolates of *P. inconstans* were inhibited by 0.12 µg/ml. Activity of LY127935 against *A. calcoaceticus* was variable. A concentration of 16 µg/ml inhibited only 28.56% of the isolates, and 71.44% of the remaining isolates required concentrations equal to or higher than 32 µg/ml. The MIC for 20.93% of *P. aeruginosa* strains was 4 µg/ml, and 72.09% were susceptible to 16 µg/ml. The MIC of LY127935 for *S. aureus* was 0.25 to 128 µg/ml, with 75.98% inhibited by 16 µg/ml. A concentration of 4 µg/ml inhibited 59.51% of *S. epidermidis* strains, and 85.69 were susceptible to 16 µg/ml.

The in vitro activity of cefoperazone and LY127935 was investigated. Cefoperazone was highly active against gram-negative bacilli, with geometric mean MIC values (gmmv) as follows: *E. coli,* 0.605; *K. pneumoniae,* 0.725; *E. aerogenes,* 1.023; *E. cloacae,* 1.055; *C. freundii,* 1.065; *P. mirabilis,* 1.438; *P. vulgaris,* 1.782; *P. morganii,* 2.887; *P. rettgeri,* 3.732; and *P. aeruginosa,* 7.626. The activity against *Enterobacter* species, indole-positive *Proteus* species, and *P. aeruginosa* was remarkable. Cefoperazone was less active against *S. marcescens* (gmmv, 23.730) and *A. calcoaceticus* (gmmv, 33.332). With respect to gram-positive cocci, cefoperazone showed more activity against *S. epidermidis* (gmmv, 1.554) than against *S. aureus* (gmmv, 4.141).

As can be seen from the gmmv, LY127935 was highly effective against the following organisms: *C. freundii,* 0.120; *P. rettgeri,* 0.120; *E. coli,* 0.131; *E. aerogenes,* 0.133; *P. mirabilis,* 0.136; *P. morganii,* 0.137; *P. vulgaris,* 0.149; *K. pneumoniae,* 0.158; *E. cloacae,* 0.169; *S. marcescens,*

0.215; and *H. alvei*, 0.250. The activity against indole-positive *Proteus* species, *Enterobacter* species, and *S. marcescens* was notable. LY127935 was less active against *P. aeruginosa* (gmmv, 13.400) and *A. calcoaceticus* (gmmv, 27.988). Regarding 112 strains of staphylococci, LY127935 showed more activity against *S. epidermidis* (gmmv, 4.641) than against *S. aureus* (gmmv, 6.176).

LY127935 (6059-S): a Novel β-Lactam Antibiotic

CHRISTINE C. SANDERS,* W. EUGENE SANDERS, JR., MARK A. DYKSTRA, AND LAUREL C. PREHEIM

Creighton University School of Medicine, Omaha, Nebraska 68178, U.S.A.

LY127935 is a new β-lactam antibiotic containing unusual substitutions both within and around its ring structure. In vitro studies were performed with LY127935, cefotaxime (HR-756), and a variety of other antibiotics to evaluate the following characteristics of the new drugs: (i) spectrum of antibacterial activity, (ii) in vitro potency, (iii) bactericidal activity, (iv) susceptibility to β-lactamases, (v) induction of β-lactamase, and (vi) selection of resistant mutants. The in vitro activity of each antibiotic was determined by serial twofold dilution in 3 ml of Mueller-Hinton broth (aerobic and facultative strains) or Wilkins-Chalgren agar (anaerobes). An inoculum of 10^5 colony-forming units (CFU)/ml (broth) or 10^5 CFU/cm^2 (agar) was used. The MIC was defined as the lowest concentration preventing macroscopic growth. Subcultures were made of each clear tube, and the minimal bactericidal concentration (MBC) was defined as the lowest concentration preventing growth on subculture. Data are presented as MIC$_{50}$ (MIC for 50% of strains tested) or MIC$_{90}$ (MIC for 90% of strains tested). The kinetics of bacterial killing were examined by inoculating isolates into Mueller-Hinton broth containing drug. At 0, 2, 4, 6, 8, and 24 h of incubation, samples were removed and the number of viable bacteria was determined by agar dilution plate counts. Residual drug in the broth was measured by bioassay with *Bacillus subtilis* ATCC 6633. β-Lactamase activity before and after induction was determined by a UV spectrophotometric method described previously (1).

In tests with 300 aerobic and facultative gram-negative isolates, the activity of LY127935 was generally equal to or greater than that of the other β-lactam antibiotics tested. It was active against many strains, including *Pseudomonas*, that were resistant to other cephalosporins, cephamycins, and penicillins (Table 1). Most *Haemophilus* and *Neisseria* strains, including those producing β-lactamases, were inhibited by 1 µg or less of LY127935 or cefotaxime per ml. Against 50 obligate anaerobes, LY127935 was the most active β-lactam antibiotic tested, but it was generally less active than clindamycin or chloramphenicol (Table 1). MBCs of LY127935 were usually similar to MICs, except in tests with nonfermentative gram-negative bacilli. The

TABLE 1. *In vitro activity of LY127935 (LY), cefotaxime (HR), and various commonly used antibiotics against 338 clinical isolates*

Organism (no. of isolates)	MIC$_{90}$ (µg/ml) of indicated drug		
	LY	HR	Other drugs[a]
Serratia/Enterobacter (65)	1.0	2.0	CM, >64; CX, >64; GM, 1.0
Indole-positive *Proteus/Providencia* (53)	1.0	1.0	CM, >64; CX, 16; GM, 2.0
Other *Enterobacteriaceae* (100)	0.25	0.25	CM, 8.0; CX, 16; CZ, 32
Bacteroides fragilis (29)	16	>32	CB, >32; CHL, 8.0; CLN, 2.0
Other gram-negative anaerobes (12)	32	>32	CB, >32; CHL, 8.0; CLN, 1.0
Gram-positive anaerobes (9)	1.0	2.0	PEN, ≤0.5; CHL, 4.0; CLN, ≤0.5
Pseudomonas aeruginosa (50)	64	64	PIP, 16; CB, 256; TM, 0.5; GM, 1.0
Other nonfermenters (20)	32	64	PIP, 128; CB, >256; TM, 64; GM, >64

[a] CM, Cefamandole; CX, cefoxitin; CZ, cefazolin; GM, gentamicin; TM, tobramycin; PEN, penicillin G; CB, carbenicillin; PIP, piperacillin; CHL, chloramphenicol; CLN, clindamycin.

TABLE 2. *β-Lactamase activity in gram-negative bacteria before and after induction by growth on drug-containing agar*

Strain	Cell prepn	Amt (nmol) of substrate[a] inactivated/ 10^9 cells			
		CM	CX	HR	LY
E. aerogenes	Uninduced	0	0	0	0
	Induced, CX	34	31	9	5
	Induced, HR	0	4	3	3
	Induced, LY	0	2	3	5
E. cloacae	Uninduced	0	0	0	0
	Induced, CX	81	51	8	16
	Induced, HR	19	2	0	0
	Induced, LY	0	2	0	0
P. morganii	Uninduced	78	11	10	0
	Induced, CX	76	33	10	4
	Induced, HR	82	24	12	0
	Induced, LY	81	31	10	0
E. coli	Uninduced	82	74	6	0
	Induced, CX	100	97	27	10
	Induced, HR	88	67	9	4
	Induced, LY	80	92	4	0
P. aeruginosa	Uninduced	0	0	0	0
	Induced, CX	29	7	6	3
	Induced, HR	0	0	2	0
	Induced, LY	0	0	0	0

[a] CM, Cefamandole; CX, cefoxitin; HR, cefotaxime, LY, LY127935.

ratio of the MBC$_{50}$ to the MIC$_{50}$ for LY127935 against these strains was greater than eight; however, the same ratio was obtained with cefotaxime against these strains. The inoculum size affected the in vitro activity of both drugs. Increasing the inoculum from 10^3 CFU/ml to 10^5 CFU/ml increased the MIC$_{50}$ for both drugs only twofold. However, increasing the inoculum to 10^7 CFU/ml increased the MIC$_{50}$ over 256-fold.

Quantitative studies revealed the initial rate of bacterial killing by LY127935 to be similar to that observed with other β-lactam antibiotics, with onset of killing coincident with entrance of the cells into logarithmic growth. However, kill-ing by LY127935 was usually complete within 24 h in contrast to other β-lactam antibiotics such as cefamandole, cefoxitin, or piperacillin, with which killing was either (i) slow and incomplete at 24 h or (ii) partial, followed by regrowth of the bacteria to drug-free control levels.

LY127935 was the most resistant to inactivation by a variety of β-lactamases when compared with cefotaxime, cefoxitin, cefamandole, and cephalothin (Table 2). Both LY127935 and cefotaxime induced β-lactamase production; however, these enzymes were generally only weakly active against the inducing drug. Neither was as effective an inducer as cefoxitin. Resistance to LY127935 or cefotaxime could be selected in several strains by overnight exposure of 10^5 CFU/ml to superinhibitory concentrations (30 μg/ml) of the drugs in broth. However, resistance was much more readily selected for by cefotaxime than by LY127935. Cells selected with cefotaxime showed parallel resistance to LY127935. Incubation of the resistant cells in broth containing 60 μg of LY127935 or cefotaxime per ml revealed that the cells either were capable of growth or had increased survival in each drug. Inactivation of LY127935 by these cells was not detected. Partial or complete inactivation of cefotaxime was observed with some strains, but this inactivation often occurred after growth of the cells. Thus, the resistance of the cells to LY127935 and cefotaxime did not appear to be mediated primarily by β-lactamases.

In summary, LY127935 compared very favorably with cefotaxime in vitro. Although both drugs have a similar broad spectrum, LY127935 was more potent than cefotaxime against various genera. Several strains were found that were resistant to cefotaxime but susceptible to LY127935. LY127935 was slightly more resistant to β-lactamase inactivation than was cefotaxime; it was also less likely than cefotaxime to select for resistance to itself. Further studies on this new β-lactam antibiotic are clearly indicated.

1. **Sanders, C. C., and W. E. Sanders, Jr.** 1979. Emergence of resistance to cefamandole: possible role of cefoxitin-inducible beta-lactamases. Antimicrob. Agents Chemother. **15:**792–797.

Characterization of *Proteus morganii* Cephalosporinases and Evaluation of Their Role in LY127935 (6059-S) and HR-756 (Cefotaxime) Antimicrobial Activities

ANTOINE KAZMIERCZAK,* MONIQUE BOLLE, ELIANE SIEBOR, PIERRE POTHIER, AND ROGER LABIA

Laboratoire de Bactériologie, Faculté de Médecine, 21033 Dijon, and *CNRS-CERCOA, 94320 Thiais, France*

In preliminary laboratory experiments with LY127935 (6059-S), a 1-oxacephalosporin, we found that this first representative of a new class of β-lactam antibiotics shows a very efficient antibacterial effect against all species of the *Enterobacteriaceae,* including those which are very resistant to the first generation of cephalosporins. It was thus of interest to determine whether or not the antibiotic activity of LY127935 is in particularly good correlation with its stability to β-lactamases. We also compared it with HR-756 (cefotaxime), a new cephalosporin which to date appears to be the best β-lactam antibiotic, being generally effective against all species of the *Enterobacteriaceae,* even those which are β-lactamase producers (2, 6).

As the resistance of the members of the *Enterobacteriaceae* to the first generation of cephalosporins is mainly related to cephalosporinase production, this study had to cover only the strains which produce this type of β-lactamase. Therefore, as an example, 50 *Proteus morganii* isolates from human infections were selected for study. All strains present a resistance to β-lactam antibiotics related only to cephalosporinase production, i.e., resistance to cephalothin and ampicillin and susceptibility to carbenicillin, which excludes any β-lactamase production (penicillinase) mediated by an R factor.

Evaluation of cephalosporinase production. Cephalosporinases are generally inducible enzymes, but constitutive cephalosporinases are not an exception (3); thus, β-lactamase extractions were performed on induced and uninduced bacterial cultures (5). Cephalosporinase production was evaluated by the specific β-lactamase activity (4), which is expressed as the number of β-lactamase units contained per milligram of total proteins in a crude bacterial extract.

The range of cephalosporinase production was 0.5 to 2 U for 44 strains (mean value, 0.8 U) and 6 to 8 U for the other 6 strains (mean value, 7.1 U). A constitutive cephalosporinase was only observed for two strains which belong to the group of six strains producing a high level of cephalosporinase. For the other 48 strains cephalosporinase production was undetectable with-out the addition of the inducer (penicillin G, 500 µg/ml).

Characterization of cephalosporinases by analytical isoelectric focusing. Isoelectric focusing (4) showed eight different cephalosporinases with isoelectric points (pI) of 8.98 (1 strain), 8.38 (27 strains), 7.96 (4 strains), 7.28 (9 strains), 7.12 (4 strains), 6.93 (1 strain), 6.46 (3 strains), and 5.90 (1 strain).

It must be pointed out that, for the strains producing a high level of cephalosporinase, the pI was 8.38 for two inducible and two constitutive cephalosporinases and 7.28 for two inducible cephalosporinases.

Susceptibility to LY127935 and HR-756. The MICs of the β-lactam antibiotics LY127935 and HR-756 were determined as described previously (1).

Figure 1 shows that the range of MICs was narrow for LY127935 (0.06 to 0.5 µg/ml; mean, 0.14 µg/ml) and wide for HR-756 (0.015 to 16 µg/ ml; mean, 0.18 µg/ml). Thus, it appears that the antibacterial activity of LY127935 was not affected by the cephalosporinases of *P. morganii,* whatever the mode and the level of enzyme production may have been. On the other hand, different results were observed with HR-756. For the 44 strains which produce an inducible cephalosporinase level within normal limits (0.5 to 2 U; mean, 0.8 U), there was no correlation between HR-756 activity and cephalosporinase production. The wide range of HR-756 MICs (0.015 to 1 µg/ml) might be interpreted as a characteristic related to a modification of the bacterial permeability barrier to the antibiotic (2). But, for the 6 strains which are very high cephalosporinase producers (2 constitutive and 4 inducible strains), the HR-756 activity became 40 to 160 times lower than the mean value of HR-756 activity (0.10 µg/ml) for the 44 strains producing a normal level of cephalosporinase. This decrease of HR-756 activity might be interpreted as also related to a modification of the bacterial permeability barrier to the antibiotic or as related to the high level of cephalosporinase production.

Stability of LY127935 and HR-756 to

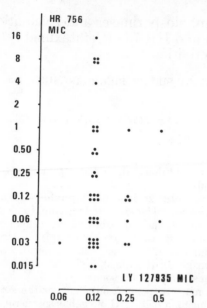

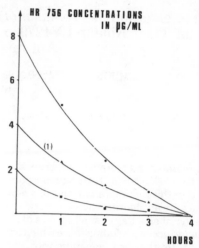

FIG. 2. *Hydrolysis kinetics of HR-756 in broth medium with strains producing a high level of cephalosporinase. Control shows no antibiotic inactivation. (1) Mean value for four strains.*

FIG. 1. *LY127935 MIC versus HR-756 MIC for 50 strains of Proteus morganii producing a cephalosporinase.*

cephalosporinase hydrolysis. The computerized microacidimetric method (4) shows that all *P. morganii* cephalosporinases hydrolyze LY127935 and HR-756. But hydrolytic activity is too low for quantitative analysis because one has to use crude bacterial extracts and not diluted ones, even those coming from strains which produce a high level of cephalosporinase. Nevertheless, it appears that HR-756 is more rapidly hydrolyzed than LY127935, and by a method described previously (5), the HR-756 hydrolysis can be observed in physiological conditions, but only for strains producing a high level of cephalosporinase.

After induction when an inducer was required, the strain to be studied was removed in antibiotic broth medium no. 3 (Difco) containing HR-756 to final concentration (in micrograms per milliliter) one-half the MIC. Every hour, the HR-756 concentration was determined in the supernatant by microbiological assay with *Escherichia coli* K-12 (HR-756 MIC, 0.015 µg/ml). Figure 2 shows that HR-756 hydrolysis occurred in physiological conditions for strains producing a high level of cephalosporinase.

In conclusion, LY127935 and HR-756 were rather resistant to hydrolysis by *P. morganii* cephalosporinases, but LY127935 was more resistant than HR-756. Frequently, cephalosporinases are inducible enzymes and their production

level in bacteria is not sufficient to affect the antibacterial activity of the two β-lactam antibiotics under study. Nevertheless, when *P. morganii* produces a high level of cephalosporinase (constitutive or, sometimes, inducible cephalosporinase), hydrolysis becomes efficient for HR-756 but not for LY127935. This points out that there is an important decrease in the antibacterial activity of HR-756.

1. **Barry, A. L., and L. D. Sabath.** 1974. Special tests: bacterial activity and activity of antimicrobics in combination, p. 431–435. *In* E. H. Lennette, E. H. Spaulding, and J. P. Truant (ed), Manual of clinical microbiology, 2nd ed. American Society for Microbiology, Washington, D.C.
2. **Chabbert, Y. A., and A. J. Lutz.** 1978. HR756, the *syn* isomer of a new methoxyimino cephalosporin with unusual antibacterial activity. Antimicrob. Agents Chemother. **14**:749–754.
3. **Fujii-Kuriyama, Y., M. Yamamoto, and Sugawara.** 1977. Purification and properties of beta-lactamase from *Proteus morganii.* J. Bacteriol. **131**:726–734.
4. **Labia, R., M. Guionie, J. M. Masson, A. Philippon, and M. Barthelemy.** 1977. Beta-lactamases produced by a *Pseudomonas aeruginosa* strain highly resistant to carbenicillin. Antimicrob. Agents Chemother. **11**:785–790.
5. **Labia, R., A. Kazmierczak, A. Philippon, F. Le Goffic, J. C. Faye, F. W. Goldstein, and J. F. Acar.** 1975. β-Lactamases de *Pseudomonas aeruginosa* et résistance à la carbénicilline. Ann. Microbiol. (Paris) **126A**:449–459.
6. **Neu, H. C., N. Aswapokee, P. Aswapokee, and K. P. Fu.** 1979. HR756, a new cephalosporin active against gram-positive and gram-negative aerobic and anaerobic bacteria. Antimicrob. Agents Chemother. **15**:273–281.

Comparative β-Lactamase Resistance and Inhibitory Activity of 1-Oxacephalosporin, Cefoxitin, and Cefotaxime

KWUNG P. FU AND HAROLD C. NEU*

Departments of Medicine and Pharmacology, College of Physicians and Surgeons, Columbia University, New York, New York 10032, U.S.A.

1-Oxacephalosporin, LY127935, is a new semisynthetic β-lactam antibiotic in which the sulfur at position one in the six-numbered ring of the cephem nucleus has been replaced with an oxygen. We have shown that it is highly active against a broad spectrum of microorganisms. It inhibited the majority of members of the *Enterobacteriaceae* at less than 0.8 μg/ml, and it was twice as active as cefotaxime against *Pseudomonas aeruginosa* and *Bacteroides fragilis* (1). Its β-lactamase stability and inhibitory activity were investigated and compared with that of cefoxitin and cefotaxime. Cephaloridine, cephalothin, and the 1-oxacephalosporin were obtained from Eli Lilly & Co. Cefotaxime was from Hoechst-Roussel Pharmaceuticals Inc., and cefoxitin was from Merck, Sharp & Dohme. Partially purified β-lactamases from *Escherichia coli, Citrobacter, Proteus, Providencia, Acinetobacter, Klebsiella, Pseudomonas, Shigella, Staphylococcus aureus,* and *Bacteroides* were obtained, representing β-lactamases of plasmid or chromosomal origin which were primarily cephalosporinases or enzymes which hydrolyzed both penicillins and cephalosporins. β-Lactamase stability was determined by a spectrophotometric method. Inhibition of hydrolysis of cephaloridine, determined spectrophotometrically, was used to determine β-lactamase inhibitory activity.

The MIC of 1-oxacephalosporin against the β-lactamase–producing bacteria was less than 1 μg/ml except for *P. aeruginosa, Acinetobacter, B. fragilis* subsp. *fragilis,* and *S. aureus* (Table 1). No significant hydrolysis of 1-oxacephalosporin could be detected by the spectrophotometric assay. The stability of the compound was the same as that of cefoxitin and cefotaxime for these different β-lactamases. The β-lactamase inhibitory activity of 1-oxacephalosporin was comparable to that of cefoxitin and cefotaxime. At equal molar concentrations of substrate and inhibitor, all compounds competitively inhibited the hydrolysis of cephaloridine. Cefoxitin and cefotaxime were more effective inhibitors than was the 1-oxacephalosporin against the *Providencia* enzyme, whereas cefotaxime and 1-oxacephalosporin were more effective inhibitors of a *Citrobacter* cephalosporinase (Fig. 1). The 1-oxacephalosporin had a K_i value of 7.5 μM against the *Providencia* enzyme and a K_i of 2.3 × 10^{-3} μM for the *Citrobacter* enzyme. The use of killing curves to determine whether there was synergy of 1-oxacephalosporin and cephaloridine against intact organisms showed that the extremely low inhibitory levels of the compound

TABLE 1. *Comparison of β-lactamase hydrolysis of 1-oxacephalosporin with that of cephaloridine, cephalothin, cefoxitin, and cefotaxime*

β-Lactamase types and sources	Relative hydrolysis rate[a]			MIC of 1-oxacephalosporin (μg/ml)
	Cephalothin	Cefoxitin, cefotaxime	1-Oxacephalosporin	
Escherichia coli[b]	82	5	10	0.05
Citrobacter freundii[c]	89	0	0	0.2
Proteus morganii[c]	160	0	0	0.1
Proteus stuartii[c]	30	0	0	0.05
Acinetobacter[d]	212	0	0	50
Providencia stuartii[d]	113	0	4	0.1
Klebsiella pneumoniae[b]	45	0	0	0.8
Pseudomonas aeruginosa[b]	30	0	0	12.5
Shigella sonnei[b]	45	0	0	0.2
Staphylococcus aureus[d]	0	0	0	3.1
Bacteroides fragilis subsp. *fragilis*[c]	85	8	12	>50

[a] The hydrolysis of cephaloridine is given a value of 100. The concentrations of all substrates are 0.1 mM.

[b] Cephalosporinase and penicillinase.

[c] Cephalosporinase.

[d] Penicillinase.

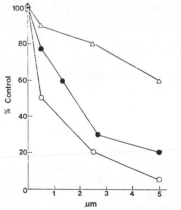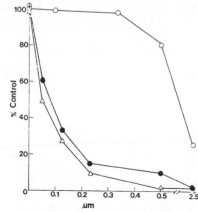

FIG. 1. *Comparative β-lactamase inhibitory activity of 1-oxacephalosporin (△), cefoxitin (○), and cefotaxime (●). The substrate was cephaloridine and the concentration was 0.01 mM. Left panel: Providencia β-lactamase. Right panel: Citrobacter enzyme.*

against most of the organisms made such synergy of no clinical significance when tested against *Pseudomonas, Acinetobacter*, and other bacteria. No antagonism of the activity of the 1-oxacephalosporin occurred in the presence of cephaloridine.

The competitive inhibition of hydrolysis of cephaloridine suggests that 1-oxacephalosporin competes with the substrate for the catalytic site in some β-lactamases. However, the fact that, like cefoxitin, this agent is neither a substrate

nor an inhibitor of some β-lactamases suggests that it may not enter the catalytic site. The activity of this agent against bacteria is related in part to its β-lactamase stability, but resistance may be related to other factors.

1. **Neu, H. C., N. Aswapokee, K. P. Fu, and P. Aswapokee.** 1979. Antibacterial activity of a new 1-oxacephalosporin compound with that of other β-lactam compounds. Antimicrob. Agents Chemother. **16:**141–149.

LY127935 and Cefoperazone Sodium (T-1551), Two β-Lactam Antibiotics with Anti-*Pseudomonas* Activity

MITCHELL V. BRODEY,* WILLIAM A. CRAIG, AND CALVIN M. KUNIN

Department of Medicine, William S. Middleton Memorial Veterans Hospital, Madison, Wisconsin 53705, U.S.A.

Cefoperazone (T-1551), a piperazine cephalosporin, and LY127935, a 1-oxacephalosporin, have been shown to have in vitro activity against *Pseudomonas aeruginosa* (1, 2). The in vitro activity of these two new compounds was compared with that of cefamandole, cefoxitin, carbenicillin, mezlocillin, and amikacin. The MIC for over 500 clinical isolates was determined by the agar dilution technique (3). Cefoperazone was fourfold more active than LY127935 against strains of *Staphylococcus aureus* and *Staphylococcus epidermidis*. However, both compounds were less active than cefamandole or amikacin against these organisms. Against strains of *Streptococcus pyogenes* and *S. pneu-*

moniae, cefoperazone was as active as cefamandole and more active than cefoxitin. Of the β-lactam antibiotics tested, mezlocillin had the lowest MICs, and LY127935 had the highest. Cefoperazone and carbenicillin inhibited 90% of strains of *S. faecalis* at concentrations of 16 µg/ml. LY127935 possessed no activity against enterococci at concentrations as high as 64 µg/ml, whereas mezlocillin inhibited all strains at concentrations of 2 µg/ml or lower.

LY127935, followed closely by cefoperazone, was the most active compound tested against the *Enterobacteriaceae*. Most strains of *Escherichia coli* were inhibited by both antibiotics at concentrations of 0.25 µg/ml. This same concentration of LY127935 inhibited 70% of the isolates of *Proteus mirabilis,* in contrast to 14% inhibited by cefoperazone. The majority of indole-producing strains of *Proteus* were inhibited by 0.25 μg of LY127935/ml. However, there were a substantial number of strains which required levels as high as 32 μg/ml. Cefoperazone, amikacin, and mezlocillin all possessed similar activity, but were less active than LY127935. Several indole-positive strains resistant to cefamandole and cefoxitin were inhibited by LY127935 and cefoperazone at concentrations of 8 μg/ml. Ninety percent of strains of *Klebsiella* were inhibited by LY127935 at concentrations of 0.25 μg/ml or lower. The same concentrations of cefoperazone inhibited only 50% of these organisms. Still, most strains of *Klebsiella* were susceptible to cefoperazone at concentrations severalfold lower than the inhibitory concentrations of cefamandole, cefoxitin, and amikacin. Carbenicillin and mezlocillin were the least active agents against *Klebsiella.* LY127935 was also the most effective antibiotic against *Enterobacter.* Cefoperazone was the next most active, followed by amikacin, cefamandole, and mezlocillin. Ninety percent of strains of *Serratia* were inhibited by LY127935 at 0.5 μg/ml. Cefoperazone, amikacin, and mezlocillin also possessed activity against a majority of these isolates, but at severalfold higher concentrations. Cefamandole, cefoxitin, and carbenicillin were the least active against *Serratia* isolates. LY127935 and cefoperazone were considerably more active against citrobacter than the other compounds tested. LY127935 appeared to be the most active compound tested against strains of *Providencia,* all isolates of which were inhibited by concentrations of 0.25 μg or less/ml. Cefoperazone and amikacin inhibited 90% of these strains at concentrations of 16 μg/ml and 249 μg/ml, respectively. *Acinetobacter* was relatively resistant to the action of LY127935 and cefoperazone, with only 10% and 30% of strains, respectively, being inhibited by concentrations of 16 μg/ml. Carbenicillin and mezlocillin possessed the lowest MIC against these strains of *Acinetobacter.* Amikacin, followed by cefoperazone and LY127935, was the most active drug tested against *Pseudomonas aeruginosa*; 80% of the strains were susceptible to concentrations of 4, 8, and 16 μg/ml, respectively. *Haemophilus influenzae* was highly susceptible to LY127935 and cefoperazone, with 80% of strains inhibited by 0.06 μg/ml. Cefamandole was the next most active compound against *Haemophilus,* inhibiting 80% of strains at 0.5 μg/ml; cefoxitin and amikacin were the least active, requiring concentrations of 4 μg/ml to inhibit the same percentage of isolates.

Representative isolates of *Klebsiella, Serratia, Proteus, Enterobacter,* and *Pseudomonas* were evaluated for the effect of growth conditions on the MIC and MBC. No consistent effects could be shown when susceptibility testing was done with Mueller-Hinton broth, Trypticase soy broth (BBL Microbiology Systems), nutrient broth, or a combination of Mueller-Hinton broth and heat-inactivated pooled human serum in equal proportions. There was no discernible effect over a pH range of 6 through 8. MICs determined by the agar dilution method were within one twofold dilution of those determined in broth for all 24 organisms tested. Against all five strains of *Pseudomonas aeruginosa,* the MBC of cefoperazone and LY127935 was within one twofold dilution of the MIC. Against two strains of *Pseudomonas,* the MBC of mezlocillin was fourfold higher than the MIC. However, when the inoculum was raised to 10^7 colony-forming units, an eightfold or greater increase in the MBC was noted for all three agents tested. This same inoculum effect was demonstrated for the seven strains of *Staphylococcus aureus* tested against cefoperazone, LY127935, and cefamandole.

On the basis of in vitro susceptibility testing, cefoperazone and LY127935 appear to be significant additions to the antibiotic armamentarium. Studies will be necessary to establish their clinical efficacy and safety.

1. **Neu, H. C., N. Aswapokee, K. P. Fu, and P. Aswapokee.** 1979. Antibacterial activity of a new 1-oxa cephalosporin compared with that of other beta-lactam compounds. Antimicrob. Agents Chemother. **16:**141–149.
2. **Neu, H. C., K. P. Fu, N. Aswapokee, P. Aswapokee, and K. Kung.** 1979. Comparative activity and β-lactamase stability of cefoperazone, a piperazine cephalosporin. Antimicrob. Agents Chemother. **16:**150–157.
3. **Washington, J. A., II, and A. L. Barry.** 1974. Dilution test procedures, p. 410–417. *In* E. H. Lennette, E. H. Spaulding, and J. P. Truant (ed.), Manual of clinical microbiology, 2nd ed. American Society for Microbiology, Washington, D.C.

In Vitro Evaluation of LY127935 (6059-S) in Comparison with 11 Related β-Lactam Compounds and Two Aminoglycosides

ARTHUR L. BARRY,* CYLDE THORNSBERRY, RONALD N. JONES, AND E. HUGH GERLACH

University of California (Davis) Medical Center, Sacramento, California 95817*; Center for Disease Control, Atlanta, Georgia 30333; Kaiser Foundation Hospitals (Oregon Region), Portland, Oregon 97217; and St. Francis Hospital, Wichita, Kansas 67214, U.S.A.

LY127935 (Eli Lilly & Co.; Shionogi 6059-S) is a new semisynthetic β-lactam antibacterial agent. Its in vitro activity was evaluated by testing 645 bacterial isolates by means of a microdilution procedure with cation-supplemented Mueller-Hinton broth. The antibacterial activity of LY127935 was compared to that of cefotaxime (HR-756), cefoxitin, cefamandole, cefazolin, cephalothin, azlocillin, mezlocillin, piperacillin, ticarcillin, carbenicillin, ampicillin, amikacin, and gentamicin. The results of tests with 14 antimicrobics are summarized in Tables 1 and 2 as the minimal concentration required to inhibit at least 50% of the strains within each subgroup of isolates.

Both LY127935 and cefotaxime demonstrated marked activity against the 289 Enterobacteriaceae isolates that were tested; i.e., modal MICs for both drugs were ≤0.5 µg/ml against all species. LY127935 and cefotaxime demonstrated nearly identical spectra of activity, except that LY127935 was somewhat less active against streptococci, Staphylococcus aureus, and Acinetobacter sp. Both were moderately active against Pseudomonas aeruginosa; i.e., activity was similar to that of ticarcillin. Streptococcus faecalis isolates were all resistant to LY127935 and cefotaxime.

Acinetobacter sp. and Pseudomonas spp. (other than P. stutzeri and P. aeruginosa) were relatively resistant to all of the β-lactam compounds, but the aminoglycosides were effective against most strains. The aminoglycosides were relatively inactive against Streptococcus pyogenes and S. pneumoniae; the penicillins were uniformly effective. Gentamicin-resistant gram-negative bacilli were often susceptible to the newer β-lactam compounds, especially LY127935 and cefotaxime. Most cephalothin-resistant strains were susceptible to the newer β-lactam compounds.

Tests with 105 Pseudomonas aeruginosa isolates included 37 gentamicin-resistant (MIC >8 µg/ml) strains. Amikacin was active against half of the gentamicin-resistant strains. The only cephalosporins with activity against P. aeruginosa were LY127935 and cefotaxime; both were similar to ticarcillin. Piperacillin was the most active β-lactam antibiotic tested; i.e., the modal MIC was 4 µg/ml, and 95% of the strains were

TABLE 1. Antimicrobial activity of 14 compounds against selected genera

Antimicrobial agent	Minimal concn (µg/ml) required to inhibit 50% of strains tested								
	Esche-richia (52)[a]	Salmo-nella (20)	Klebsiella (28)	Entero-bacter (54)	Serratia (31)	Provi-dencia (25)	Proteus spp.		Acineto-bacter (15)
							P. mi-rabilis (25)	Other spp. (35)	
LY127935	≤0.1	≤0.1	≤0.1	≤0.1	0.5	≤0.1	≤0.1	≤0.1	32
Cefotaxime	≤0.1	≤0.1	≤0.1	≤0.1	0.5	≤0.1	≤0.1	≤0.1	8
Cefamandole	0.5	0.5	1.0	2.0	>64	1.0	0.5	16	64
Cefoxitin	4.0	2.0	2.0	>64	16	2.0	2.0	4.0	64
Cefazolin	2.0	1.0	2.0	>64	>64	>64	4.0	>64	>64
Cephalothin	16	2.0	4.0	>64	>64	64	2.0	>64	>64
Azlocillin	16	32	64	32	64	16	2.0	32	32
Mezlocillin	4.0	8.0	16	4.0	8.0	4.0	≤0.5	4.0	32
Piperacillin	2.0	4.0	16	4.0	4.0	2.0	≤0.5	2.0	16
Ticarcillin	4.0	4.0	256	4.0	8.0	≤0.5	≤0.5	4.0	8
Carbenicillin	8.0	4.0	>256	4.0	16	1.0	≤0.5	2.0	8
Ampicillin	8.0	1.0	256	256	256	32	1.0	256	16
Amikacin	2.0	2.0	1.0	1.0	2.0	2.0	4.0	1.0	2.0
Gentamicin	0.5	0.5	0.2	0.2	0.5	4.0	1.0	0.5	0.5

[a] Number of isolates tested.

TABLE 2. *Antimicrobial activity of 14 compounds against selected species*[a]

Antimicrobial agent	Minimal concn required to inhibit 50% of strains tested									
	Streptococcus		S. aureus		H. influenzae		N. gonorrhoeae		Pseudomonas	
	S. faecalis (10)[b]	Other spp. (39)	Pen-S (29)	Pen-R (27)	Amp-S (20)	Amp-R (20)	Pen-S (25)	Pen-R (25)	P. aeruginosa (105)	Other spp. (32)
LY127935	>64	1	8	8	≤0.06	≤0.06	≤0.01	0.03	16	32
Cefotaxime	>64	≤0.06	1	2	≤0.06	≤0.06	≤0.01	≤0.01	16	32
Cefamandole	32	≤0.06	≤0.1	0.5	0.2	0.2	0.3	0.2	>64	>64
Cefoxitin	>64	0.5	2	4	2.0	1.0	0.1	0.5	>64	>64
Cefazolin	32	≤0.06	0.2	0.5	4.0	4.0	0.2	0.5	>64	>64
Cephalothin	>32	≤0.06	≤0.1	0.2	2.0	2.0	0.1	0.5	>64	>64
Azlocillin	1	≤0.2	≤0.1	4	≤0.2	16	<0.01	0.5	8.0	32
Mezlocillin	1	≤0.2	1	4	≤0.2	8.0	<0.01	0.06	32	64
Piperacillin	4	≤0.2	≤0.5	8	≤0.2	2.0	<0.01	0.06	4.0	16
Ticarcillin	32	≤0.2	≤0.5	4	≤0.2	2.0	0.02	4.0	16	256
Carbenicillin	32	≤0.2	≤0.5	4	≤0.2	2.0	0.02	4.0	64	>256
Ampicillin	1	≤0.2	≤0.5	2	≤0.2	64	<0.01	4.0	>256	>256
Amikacin	256	64	1.0	1	8.0	4.0	8.0	8.0	8.0	2.0
Gentamicin	16	8	≤0.1	0.2	1.0	1.0	2.0	2.0	8.0	2.0

[a] Pen-S and -R, penicillin-susceptible and -resistant; Amp-S and -R, ampicillin-susceptible and -resistant.
[b] Number of isolates tested.

inhibited by 64 μg/ml. In contrast, cefotaxime and LY127935 demonstrated modal MICs of 16 μg/ml, with about one-quarter of the isolates having MICs ≥64 μg/ml. Azlocillin was two to four times more active than mezlocillin, but both drugs inhibited most strains at achievable concentrations. Mezlocillin and carbenicillin had similar activity against *P. aeruginosa*; ticarcillin was twice as active. Whether these β-lactam antibiotics will be effective in treating *P. aeruginosa* infections will depend largely upon the pharmacology of each drug. With the newer drugs, further clinical experience will be needed to support evaluation of in vitro studies and to define "resistant" and "susceptible" populations.

Methicillin-resistant strains of *S. aureus* were relatively resistant to all β-lactam antibiotics, but most were susceptible to the aminoglycosides. Relative susceptibility to staphylococcal β-lactamase can be assessed by comparing modal MICs for penicillin-susceptible strains to those observed with β-lactamase–producing strains. The cephalosporins all appeared to be relatively resistant to the β-lactamases, since penicillin-resistant and penicillin-susceptible strains were equally susceptible to the cephalosporins. The penicillins, on the other hand, were less active against penicillin-resistant strains than against penicillin-susceptible strains. The most active cephalosporin against *S. aureus* was cephalothin; LY127935 was the least active cephalosporin.

Neisseria gonorrhoeae isolates were all susceptible to the β-lactam compounds, but β-lac-

tamase–producing strains were less susceptible than penicillin-susceptible strains. On the other hand, the penicillins appeared to be susceptible to the β-lactamase activity of ampicillin-resistant *Haemophilus influenzae*. The cephalosporins were equally effective against both types of *H. influenzae*.

In our experience (in press), LY127935 is at least as active as cefoxitin against anaerobic microorganisms, including many strains of *Bacteroides fragilis*. Neu et al. (1) recently reported similar results with LY127935. They also demonstrated minimal synergy when LY127935 was combined with aminoglycosides or carbenicillin. We have also observed a bactericidal activity of all the β-lactam compounds against most of the isolates that were tested.

In conclusion, LY127935 and cefotaxime appear to be promising antimicrobial agents with remarkable in vitro activity against most of the common bacterial pathogens; *S. faecalis* is the only species uniformly resistant to both drugs. Cefotaxime has somewhat greater activity against staphylococci and streptococci. Both drugs might be effective in treating infections due to many *P. aeruginosa* strains, if the pharmacology can be manipulated to achieve concentrations in excess of 32 μg/ml.

1. Neu, H. C., N. Aswapokee, K. P. Fu, and P. Aswapokee. 1979. Antibacterial activity of a new 1-oxa cephalosporin compared with that of other β-lactam compounds. Antimicrob. Agents Chemother. **16**:141–149.

In Vitro Activities of Cefotaxime (HR-756) and LY127935 Against *Pseudomonas aeruginosa* and Other Nonfermentative or Oxidase-Positive Gram-Negative Bacilli

J. H. JORGENSEN,* S. A. CRAWFORD, AND G. A. ALEXANDER

Department of Pathology, The University of Texas Health Science Center, San Antonio, Texas 78284, U.S.A.

Pseudomonas aeruginosa and other aerobic gram-negative nonfermentative or oxidase-positive bacilli are becoming increasingly important as causative agents of nosocomial infections. Treatment of patients infected with these organisms is often made difficult by intrinsic resistance to commonly used antibiotics, including aminoglycosides. At times, combination antibiotic therapy must be used to effectively treat infections due to these organisms.

Cefotaxime (HR-756) and LY127935 are two new β-lactam class antibiotics which demonstrate an extremely broad spectrum of antimicrobial activity, in large part due to their resistance to β-lactamase hydrolysis (1, 3). This study compares the in vitro activities of these two new compounds with those of cefoxitin, cefamandole, cefuroxime, cephalothin, and carbenicillin against 252 isolates of aerobic gram-negative nonfermentative or oxidase-positive fermentative bacilli. Susceptibility tests were performed by the WHO-ICS agar dilution technique with

TABLE 1. *MIC_{50}'s obtained for seven β-lactam antibiotics against commonly isolated nonfermentative or oxidase-positive fermentative gram-negative bacilli*

Organisms (no. of isolates)	MIC_{50} (μg/ml)						
	LY127935	Cefotaxime	Cefoxitin	Cefamandole	Cefuroxime	Cephalothin	Carbenicillin
Pseudomonas aeruginosa (53)	16	16	>128	>128	>128	>128	64
P. maltophilia (12)	>128	32	>128	>128	>128	>128	256
P. putida (10)	64	16	>128	>128	>128	>128	512
P. putrefaciens (4)	1	0.125	4	32	2	>128	128
Acinetobacter anitratus (22)	32	16	64	64	32	>128	16
A. lwoffi (15)	4	1	4	8	1	16	1
Comamonas terrigena (5)	0.5	2	1	32	32	>128	256
Achromobacter xylosoxidans (4)	4	64	128	>128	>128	>128	8
Moraxella spp. (4)	<0.06	<0.06	0.25	0.125	0.125	0.06	<0.06
Aeromonas hydrophila (8)	<0.06	<0.06	4	0.5	0.25	32	128
Pasteurella spp. (5)	<0.06	<0.06	0.25	<0.06	<0.06	<0.06	0.25
Vibrio spp. (4)	<0.06	<0.06	4	1	0.25	1	128

TABLE 2. *Comparative MIC ranges of seven β-lactam antibiotics against less frequently isolated aerobic gram-negative bacilli*

Organisms (no. of isolates)	MIC (μg/ml)						
	LY127935	Cefotaxime	Cefoxitin	Cefamandole	Cefuroxime	Cephalothin	Carbenicillin
Alcaligenes odorans (1)	<0.06	0.5	1	0.25	32	1	8
Bordetella bronchiseptica (2)	1	64	128->128	16	>128	8	16
CDC-EF-4 (3)	0.125–0.25	0.25	8	4–8	32	64	0.5–1
CDC-Ve-2 (1)	16	8	>128	>128	64	>128	64
CDC-III-F (4)	0.5–16	0.125–16	0.25–1	0.5–8	1–64	0.125–16	0.25–4
CDC-IVC-2 (1)	16	128	64	>128	64	>128	>512
CDC-IVe (3)	0.06	<0.06–0.5	0.5–1	0.25–0.5	1–2	0.25–0.5	<0.06–0.125
Flavobacterium sp. (1)	32	64	16	>128	>128	>128	>512
Pleisiomonas shigelloides (2)	<0.06	<0.06	1–2	<0.06	<0.06–0.06	0.5	16–32
Pseudomonas cepacia (1)	2	1	16	32	16	64	8
P. denitrificans (1)	0.5	0.5	4	8	16	32	2
P. diminuta (1)	64	4	32	64	32	32	64
P. fluorescens (3)	128->128	16–64	>128	>128	>128	>128	32->512
P. pseudoalcaligenes (2)	<0.06–0.06	0.125–0.25	0.5	0.25–0.5	2	1	1
P. stutzeri (1)	8	4	16	64	128	>128	16

Mueller-Hinton agar and an inoculum of 10^4 microorganisms (2).

Table 1 depicts the results obtained with *P. aeruginosa* and other commonly isolated nonfermentative or oxidase-positive fermentative organisms. Both cefotaxime and LY127935 demonstrated in vitro activity against *P. aeruginosa*, in contrast to the other cephalosporin or cephamycin class antibiotics which failed to show inhibition. Cefotaxime proved to be slightly superior to LY127935 against *Pseudomonas maltophilia*, *Pseudomonas putida*, *Pseudomonas putrefaciens*, and *Acinetobacter* species. Conversely, LY127935 demonstrated greater activity than cefotaxime against *Comamonas terrigena* and *Achromobacter xylosoxidans*. *Moraxella*, *Aeromonas*, *Pasteurella*, and *Vibrio* isolates were exquisitely susceptible to both of the new agents. Thus, both agents were equivalent to or markedly more active than the existing β-lactam compounds against these more commonly encountered isolates.

With the exception of *Pseudomonas fluorescens* and one isolate of *Flavobacterium meningosepticum*, cefotaxime and LY127935 proved highly active when tested against a variety of less commonly encountered species (Table 2). Cefotaxime showed greater inhibition of *Pseu-*

domonas diminuta, *Pseudomonas stutzeri*, *Pseudomonas cepacia*, and CDC-Ve-2, whereas LY127935 was more active against *Alcaligenes odorans*, *Bordetella bronchiseptica*, and CDC-IVC-2.

Both cefotaxime and LY127935 were very highly active against those isolates showing susceptibility to the other β-lactam compounds, as expected. The greatest potential usefulness of these new agents would be against those organisms which are not effectively inhibited by cephalosporins or carbenicillin. In this regard, both drugs seem promising for single-drug therapy of infectious processes which involve organisms such as *P. aeruginosa* and certain isolates of *P. maltophilia*, *P. putida*, *Achromobacter* spp., and *Acinetobacter* spp.

1. **Barza, M., F. P. Tally, N. V. Jacobus, and S. L. Gorbach.** 1979. In vitro activity of LY 127935. Antimicrob. Agents Chemother. **16:**287–292.
2. **Ericsson, H. M., and J. C. Sherris.** 1971. Antibiotic sensitivity testing. Report of an international collaborative study. Acta Pathol. Scand. Sect. B Suppl. **217:**1–90.
3. **Neu, H. C., N. Aswapokee, P. Aswapokee, and K. P. Fu.** 1979. HR-756, a new cephalosporin active against gram-positive and gram-negative aerobic and anaerobic bacteria. Antimicrob. Agents Chemother. **15:**273–281.

Comparison of LY127935 and Cefotaxime (HR-756) for In Vitro Activity Against Anaerobic Bacteria

J. H. JORGENSEN,* G. A. ALEXANDER, AND S. A. CRAWFORD

Department of Pathology, The University of Texas Health Science Center, San Antonio, Texas 78284, U.S.A.

An increased awareness of the importance of anaerobic bacteria in infectious processes has emphasized the need for new antimicrobial agents which are effective in their treatment. In recent years, considerable effort has gone into development of β-lactam antibiotics which show improved activity by virtue of resistance to β-lactamases produced by many species of aerobic and anaerobic bacteria. Two such compounds are LY127935 and cefotaxime (HR-756). Both of these antibiotics appear to possess extremely broad spectra (1, 2) which may prove useful in therapy of both aerobic and anaerobic bacterial infections.

The present study compares LY127935 and cefotaxime for in vitro activity with cefoxitin, cefamandole, cefuroxime, carbenicillin, and penicillin against 130 isolates of various species of anaerobic bacteria. The proposed National

Committee for Clinical Laboratory Standards agar dilution susceptibility method was employed, using Wilkins-Chalgren agar (3) with GasPak (BBL Microbiology Systems) incubation for 48 h.

LY127935 proved to be the most active agent tested against isolates of *Bacteroides fragilis* and *B. thetaiotaomicron*, as well as other members of the *B. fragilis* group (Table 1). Cefotaxime and cefoxitin showed similar inhibition of *B. fragilis*, which was two to four times greater than that of the remaining drugs. However, against other members of the *B. fragilis* group, cefotaxime was essentially similar in activity to the currently available antibiotics. LY127935 and cefotaxime were found to be similar in activity to the other drugs against the remaining species of *Bacteroides* and *Fusobacterium* tested (Table 1).

TABLE 1. *Comparative activities of seven β-lactam antibiotics against Bacteroides and Fusobacterium species*

Organism (no. of isolates)	Antibiotic	MIC$_{50}$ (μg/ml)	MIC$_{90}$ (μg/ml)	MIC range (μg/ml)
B. fragilis (28)	LY127935	0.5	1	0.25–4
	Cefotaxime	8	16	2–32
	Cefoxitin	8	8	4–16
	Cefamandole	32	32	16–64
	Cefuroxime	16	32	4–>128
	Penicillin	16	32	2–32
	Carbenicillin	16	32	0.25–64
B. thetaiotaomicron (13)	LY127935	8	8	4–16
	Cefotaxime	64	64	16–128
	Cefoxitin	32	32	8–64
	Cefamandole	64	64	64–128
	Cefuroxime	64	>128	32–>128
	Penicillin	32	32	16–64
	Carbenicillin	32	64	16–64
B. fragilis group, other (7)	LY127935	1	32	0.5–64
	Cefotaxime	8	16	0.5–16
	Cefoxitin	8	16	1–32
	Cefamandole	16	>128	16–>128
	Cefuroxime	16	16	4–32
	Penicillin	2	16	1–32
	Carbenicillin	2	16	0.5–32
Bacteroides spp., other (14)	LY127935	1	16	0.125–32
	Cefotaxime	0.25	32	<0.06–32
	Cefoxitin	1	8	0.06–16
	Cefamandole	0.5	32	0.125–64
	Cefuroxime	0.5	64	0.125–128
	Penicillin	0.125	32	<0.06–64
	Carbenicillin	2	32	0.25–64
Fusobacterium spp. (5)	LY127935	0.06	0.5	<0.06–8
	Cefotaxime	0.06	0.5	0.06–>128
	Cefoxitin	0.06	0.125	<0.06–8
	Cefamandole	0.06	0.06	<0.06–8
	Cefuroxime	0.06	0.5	<0.06–>128
	Penicillin	0.06	0.06	<0.03–1
	Carbenicillin	0.06	0.25	<0.06–2

TABLE 2. *Comparative activities of seven β-lactam antibiotics against Clostridium species and anaerobic gram-positive cocci*

Organism (no. of isolates)	Antibiotic	MIC$_{50}$ (μg/ml)	MIC$_{90}$ (μg/ml)	MIC range (μg/ml)
C. perfringens (19)	LY127935	0.125	0.5	<0.06–1
	Cefotaxime	0.5	2	<0.06–4
	Cefoxitin	0.5	1	0.125–1
	Cefamandole	0.5	2	<0.06–2
	Cefuroxime	1	4	<0.06–4
	Penicillin	0.06	0.125	0.03–0.25
	Carbenicillin	0.25	0.5	0.125–0.5
C. sordellii (5)	LY127935	2	2	1–2
	Cefotaxime	0.25	0.5	0.125–0.5
	Cefoxitin	0.5	0.5	0.25–0.5
	Cefamandole	0.5	1	0.5–1
	Cefuroxime	0.5	0.5	0.25–0.5
	Penicillin	0.06	0.06	0.03–0.06
	Carbenicillin	0.5	0.5	0.5–1
Clostridium spp., other (14)	LY127935	1	64	0.125–128
	Cefotaxime	4	8	0.125–128
	Cefoxitin	1	64	0.125–64
	Cefamandole	1	16	0.06–32
	Cefuroxime	4	16	0.25–>128
	Penicillin	0.125	8	0.06–16
	Carbenicillin	1	8	0.25–32
Anaerobic gram-positive cocci (11)	LY127935	0.25	0.5	0.06–8
	Cefotaxime	0.25	0.25	<0.06–2
	Cefoxitin	0.125	0.25	0.06–1
	Cefamandole	0.5	1	0.06–2
	Cefuroxime	0.125	0.5	0.06–1
	Penicillin	0.03	0.125	0.015–1
	Carbenicillin	0.25	0.5	0.06–2

Penicillin was the most effective drug tested against species of *Clostridium* and anaerobic gram-positive cocci (Table 2). LY127935 was slightly more active than the remaining drugs against *Clostridium perfringens*, but was equivalent to or slightly less active than the other antibiotics against the remaining clostridia and anaerobic gram-positive cocci (Table 2).

A concentration of 0.5 μg of cefotaxime or 2 μg of LY127935 per ml inhibited all isolates of *Actinomyces* sp., *Propionibacterium* spp., and *Veillonella* spp. tested. However, equivalent results were obtained with the remaining antibiotics against these three genera. Interestingly, from 1 to 8 μg of either LY127935 or cefotaxime per ml was required to inhibit *Eubacterium lentum* isolates which were susceptible to 1 μg or less of penicillin per ml. Cefoxitin, cefamandole, cefuroxime, and carbenicillin were similar in activity against *E. lentum*, but less active than penicillin.

We conclude from these data that both LY127935 and cefotaxime show promising activity against anaerobic bacteria. LY127935 was strikingly active against *B. fragilis* and showed good activity against other members of the *B. fragilis* group. Cefotaxime was at times more active than LY127935, although such isolates were frequently also susceptible to penicillin.

1. **Barza, M., F. P. Tally, N. V. Jacobus, and S. L. Gorbach.** 1979. In vitro activity of LY 127935. Antimicrob. Agents Chemother. **16:**287–292.
2. **Neu, H. C., N. Aswapokee, P. Aswapokee, and K. P. Fu.** 1979. HR-756, a new cephalosporin active against gram-positive and gram-negative aerobic and anaerobic bacteria. Antimicrob. Agents Chemother. **15:**273–281.
3. **Wilkins, T. D., and S. Chalgren.** 1976. Medium for use in antibiotic susceptibility testing of anaerobic bacteria. Antimicrob. Agents Chemother. **10:**926–928.

Comparative Inhibition of β-Lactamase–Producing *Haemophilus* Strains by Newer Cephalosporins

WAHEED N. KHAN,* BETHANN WILLERT, SHAMA AHMAD, WILLIAM J. RODRIGUEZ, AND SYDNEY ROSS

Microbiology Section, Research Foundation of Children's Hospital National Medical Center, and Department of Child Health and Development, The George Washington University School of Medicine, Washington, D.C. 20010, U.S.A.*

Haemophilus species are among the most frequent causes of bacterial infections in children. According to the most recent United States estimates, approximately 65% of all cases of bacterial meningitis and 25% of suppurative otitis media in children between the ages of 2 months and 5 years are caused by these pathogens. Bacterial infections secondary to *Haemophilus* species in older children are relatively uncommon, although we have seen otitis media and meningitis due to this organism in children 8 to 14 years of age.

In early 1974, ampicillin-resistant β-lactamase–producing strains of *H. influenzae* causing systemic infections in children were reported in the Washington, D.C., area (1). Since then, there have been numerous reports describing serious infections due to β-lactamase-producing *Haemophilus* strains from North America, Europe, and Australia. Furthermore, there is substantial evidence now that an increasing number of strains, both encapsulated and nonencapsulated, of *H. influenzae* and *H. parainfluenzae* have become β-lactamase positive. These strains can cause severe systemic diseases in children (5). Ampicillin has been the drug of choice for the treatment of infections due to *Haemophilus* during the past 12 years (2). Since ampicillin may lose its clout and effectiveness in the foreseeable future, the evaluation of new antibiotics with predictable effectiveness and potential value in the treatment of infections due to *Haemophilus* is of first importance. It was considered of interest to compare the MICs of the newer cephalosporins against these ampicillin-resistant and β-lactamase–positive *Haemophilus* species.

MICs of ampicillin, cefaclor, cefoxitin, cefamandole, cefuroxime, cefotaxime (HR-756, Hoechst-Roussel Pharmaceuticals Inc.), and LY127935 (Eli Lilly & Co.) were determined for 300 β-lactamase–producing ampicillin-resistant *Haemophilus* strains isolated from children whose meningitis, otitis media, pneumonitis, and septicemia were due to *Haemophilus* species. These disease-causing isolates occurred in widely separated areas of the United States, and a few strains were collected from Canada, Eng-

land, and New Zealand. Of the 300 strains, 30 (10%) were *H. parainfluenzae* and 270 (90%) were *H. influenzae*. Among the *H. influenzae* strains, 4 (1.5%) were type A, 103 (38%) were type B, 3 (1%) were type E, and 160 (59.5%) were nontypable. The source of these isolates was as follows: 42 (14%) from throat, 78 (26%) from nasopharynx, 6 (2%) from blood, 42 (14%) from middle ear, 45 (15%) from cerebrospinal fluid, and 87 (29%) from miscellaneous sources such as lungs and tonsils. The in vitro activity (MICs) of ampicillin and six new cephalosporins was established by the agar dilution method with the use of a Steers replicator. The medium used was brain heart infusion agar with 5% Fildes enrichment (Difco), with 10^5 colony-forming units as inoculum.

Susceptibility tests illustrating MICs for these seven antibiotics are summarized in Fig. 1. All the isolates were ampicillin resistant, with MICs ranging from 3.12 to 100 µg/ml. The six cephalosporins had similar antimicrobial effectiveness, although cefaclor and cefoxitin were somewhat less inhibitory; at 3.12 µg/ml, 93% and 90% of strains were inhibited by cefaclor and cefoxitin, respectively. By way of comparison, at 1.56 µg/ml, 96% of isolates were inhibited by cefamandole. Cefuroxime was uniformly effective, with MICs ranging from 0.19 to 3.12 µg/ml for all the strains tested. LY127935 was more inhibitory, with MICs ranging from 0.006 to 0.095 µg/ml for 95% of the isolates. HR-756 was the most effective of all the cephalosporins, inhibiting 100% of the strains at 0.095 µg/ml (Table 1).

Ideally, an antibiotic for use against ampicillin-resistant *Haemophilus* strains should be bactericidal, nontoxic, capable of crossing the blood-brain barrier, and freely excreted into the middle ear, tears, and saliva for optimal effect against serious diseases caused by *Haemophilus*. In addition, it should be uniformly effective against *Haemophilus*, β-hemolytic streptococci, and *Streptococcus pneumoniae*.

All six of the new generation of cephalosporins show great promise in being effective against *Haemophilus*. Although cefoxitin shows comparatively less in vitro effectiveness against *Hae-*

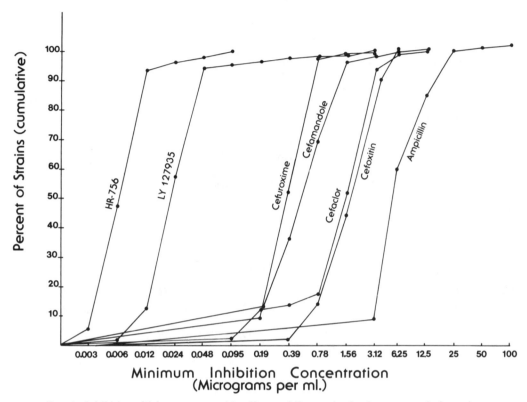

FIG. 1. *Inhibition of β-lactamase–positive Haemophilus strains by the newer cephalosporins.*

TABLE 1. *MICs of the newer cephalosporins for ampicillin-resistant Haemophilus isolates*

ANTIBIOTICS	# of Strains Tested	0.003	0.006	0.012	0.024	0.048	0.095	0.19	0.39	0.78	1.56	3.12	6.25	12.5	25	50	100 mcg/ml
Ampicillin %	289											34 11.8	138 47.8	73 25.3	39 13.5	4 1.4	1 0.35
Cefuroxime %	293						25 8.5	127 43.3	136 46.4	4 1.4	1 0.3						
Cefamandole %	260						30 11.5	64 24.6	84 32.3	72 27.6	4 1.5	3 1.2	3 1.2				
Cefoxitin %	308							4 2	36 12	92 30	146 46	30 10					
Cefaclor %	277						5 1.9	29 10.2	2 0.7	11 4	99 35.7	110 40	19 6.8	2 0.7			
LY 127935 %	287		4 1.4	30 10.4	131 45.6	104 36.2	5 1.7	4 1.4	2 0.7	2 0.7	0 0	5 1.7					
HR-756 %	283	14 4.9	117 41.2	134 47.1	13 4.6	4 1.4	1 0.4										

mophilus, it represents a big improvement when compared to the earlier cephalosporins. Cefaclor, an oral preparation which was approved recently by the Food and Drug Administration for use against respiratory pathogens such as *Haemophilus* and other susceptible organisms, has been declared the drug of choice by some investigators (3). Our data on cefaclor do not warrant this optimism. Cefamandole is quite effective in vitro, but does not traverse the blood-cerebrospinal fluid barrier in sufficient quantities to make it useful for serious systemic disease (4). Cefuroxime, a new drug under clinical investigation in this country, was uniformly effective against these ampicillin-resistant *Haemophilus* strains. LY127935, also under clinical investigation in this country, was more inhibitory in vitro than the other cephalosporins discussed so far. The most effective cephalosporin in these in vitro trials was HR-756, which inhibited 100% of strains tested at the extremely low concentration of 0.095 µg/ml. The members of this new generation of cephalosporins possess excellent in vitro activity which, if paralleled by in vivo performance, should make this family of antibiotics one of the most important in our armamentarium.

1. **Khan, W., S. Ross, W. Rodriguez, et al.** 1974. *Hemophilus influenzae* type B resistant to ampicillin. J. Am. Med. Assoc. **227**:298–301.
2. **Khan, W., S. Ross, and E. A. Zarcuba.** 1967. Comparative inhibition of *Haemophilus influenzae* by eight antibiotics, p. 393–396. Antimicrob. Agents Chemother. 1966.
3. **Nelson, J. D.** 1979. Pocketbook of pediatric antimicrobial therapy, 3rd ed., p. 7–14. Hill Printing & Stationery Co., Waco, Tex.
4. **Rodriguez, W., S. Ross, W. N. Khan, and R. Goldenberg.** 1978. Clinical and laboratory evaluation of cefamandole in infants and children. J. Infect. Dis. **137**: S150–S154.
5. **Schwartz, R., W. Rodriguez, W. Khan, and S. Ross.** 1978. The increasing incidence of ampicillin-resistant Haemophilus influenzae: a cause of otitis media. J. Am. Med. Assoc. **239**:320–323.

In Vitro Activity of β-Lactam Antibiotics Against *Bordetella pertussis*: Unusually High Anti-*B. pertussis* Activity of Piperazine β-Lactams

HARUMI SHISHIDO,* KEIZO MATSUMOTO, KIWAO WATANABE, AND YOSHIO UZUKA

Department of Internal Medicine, Institute for Tropical Medicine, Nagasaki University, Nagasaki 852, Japan

Bordetella pertussis causes whooping cough, or pertussis, which is a common acute infection of childhood; adults too are often susceptible. In Japan more patients with pertussis have been reported due to the lowered rate of pertussis vaccination in recent years. *B. pertussis*, like *Haemophilus influenzae*, is a small gram-negative nonmotile rod with rather fastidious growth requirements, which made it difficult to determine the in vitro activity of antimicrobial agents against various species. To overcome this problem, we have established a modified method for measuring MICs of antimicrobial agents against *B. pertussis* and *H. influenzae* by use of an agar dilution technique.

In the past, the only β-lactam antibiotics used against both *B. pertussis* and *H. influenzae* were ampicillin and its derivatives. Recently, certain newly developed β-lactams have been found to be more active than ampicillin against *H. influenzae*. Thus, assuming that β-lactams with high anti-*H. influenzae* activity may possess high activity against *B. pertussis*, a comparative study was made of the in vitro activity of various antimicrobial agents, particularly β-lactams, against *B. pertussis* and *H. influenzae*.

The MICs of 25 antimicrobial agents, including β-lactams, against 23 strains of *B. pertussis* isolated from patients with whooping cough were determined by the agar dilution method, using Bordet-Gengou broth (2.5 g of soluble starch, 10 g of peptone, 5 g of NaCl, and 10 ml of glycerol per liter supplemented with 15% defibrinated horse blood) for preparation of inocula and Bordet-Gengou agar, in which one of the 25 antimicrobial agents was incorporated. The Bordet-Gengou broth inoculated with a loopful of *B. pertussis* contained about 10^8 colony-forming units (CFU)/ml after 18 h of incubation at 37°C. The inoculum size had almost no effect on the MICs of antimicrobial agents against *B. pertussis* except for those of piperacillin.

To compare the in vitro activity against *B. pertussis* and *H. influenzae*, the MICs of corresponding antimicrobial agents against clinical isolates of *H. influenzae* regarded as causative pathogens of respiratory infections (1) were determined by the agar dilution method, using Fildes broth (brain heart infusion broth containing 5% Fildes extract) and Fildes agar. The MIC was defined as the lowest concentration of antimicrobial agent that completely inhibited visible growth after 18 (*H. influenzae*) or 72 (*B. pertussis*) h of incubation at 37°C.

The following comparisons were made of the in vitro activities of various antimicrobial agents against *B. pertussis* and *H. influenzae*, using the MICs with an inoculum consisting of a loopful

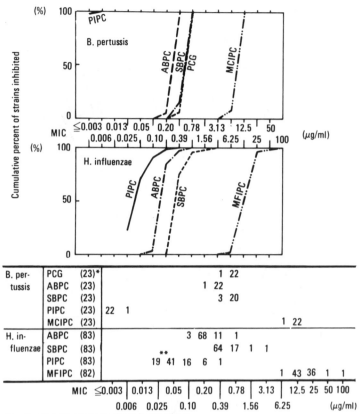

B. per-tussis	PCG	(23)*							1	22				
	ABPC	(23)							1	22				
	SBPC	(23)							3	20				
	PIPC	(23)	22	1										
	MCIPC	(23)										1	22	
H. in-fluenzae	ABPC	(83)					3	68	11	1				
	SBPC	(83)			**			64	17	1	1			
	PIPC	(83)			19	41	16	6	1					
	MFIPC	(82)										1	43 36	1 1
	MIC	≤0.003	0.013	0.05	0.20	0.78	3.13	12.5 25 50 100						
			0.006	0.025	0.10	0.39	1.56	6.25					(µg/ml)	

*: No. of strains tested are shown in parentheses.
**: ≤0.025
penicillin G (PCG), ampicillin (ABPC), sulbenicillin (SBPC), piperacillin (PIPC), cloxacillin (MCIPC), flucloxacillin (MFIPC)

FIG. 1. *MICs of penicillins against B. pertussis compared with those against H. influenzae. Inoculum size: one loopful of 10^6 CFU/ml.*

of 10^6 CFU/ml. The in vitro activities of penicillins against *B. pertussis* were compared with those against *H. influenzae* (Fig. 1). Piperacillin showed the highest activity against *B. pertussis* as well as *H. influenzae.* All of the 23 strains of *B. pertussis* were inhibited at concentrations as low as 0.006 µg/ml. Piperacillin was at least 64-fold more active than ampicillin against *B. pertussis,* and it was approximately fourfold more active than ampicillin against *H. influenzae.* Ampicillin was more active than sulbenicillin or isoxazolyl penicillins against *B. pertussis* and *H. influenzae.* Against both species, the mean MICs of sulbenicillin and isoxazolyl penicillins were 0.39 and 12.5 µg/ml, respectively. The geometric mean MIC of ampicillin was 0.38 µg/ml against *B. pertussis* and 0.22 µg/ml against *H. influenzae.*

Comparison of the MICs of cephalosporins, including an oxacephem, against *B. pertussis* and *H. influenzae* indicated that piperazine cephalosporin, (syn)methoxyimino cephalosporins, and the oxacephem were highly active against both *B. pertussis* and *H. influenzae* (Fig. 2). Whereas all of the older cephalosporins had low activities against *H. influenzae* and *B. pertussis,* cefoperazone (T-1551), SCE-1365, 6059-S, and cefotaxime (HR-756), which were recently developed, had higher activities against both species. Of these, T-1551 was the most active against *B. pertussis,* with an MIC of 0.006 to 0.013 µg/ml, and SCE-1365 was the most active against *H. influenzae,* with an MIC of ≤0.003 to 0.013 µg/ml. All of the four (syn)methoxyimino cephalosporins tested, i.e., cefuroxime, HR-756, FK-749, and SCE-1365, were more active against *H. influenzae* than the older cephalosorins, whereas only two of them, SCE-1365 and HR-756, had higher activities than ampicillin against *B. pertussis.* Anti-*B. per-*

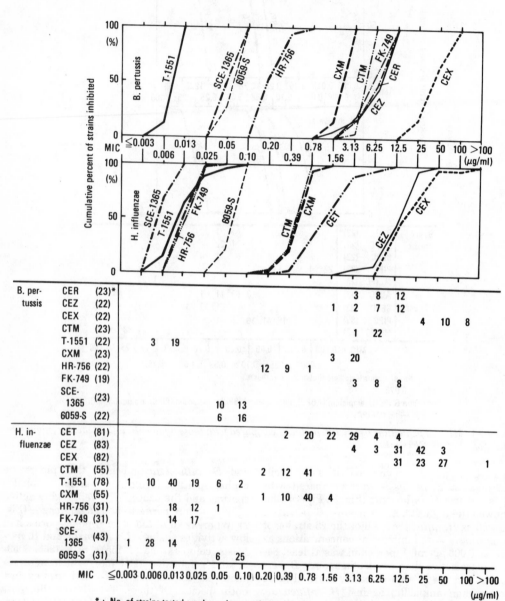

B. per- tussis			≤0.003	0.006	0.013	0.025	0.05	0.10	0.20	0.39	0.78	1.56	3.13	6.25	12.5	25	50	100	>100
B. per- tussis	CER	(23)*											3	8	12				
	CEZ	(22)									1	2	7	12					
	CEX	(22)													4	10	8		
	CTM	(23)											1	22					
	T-1551	(22)		3	19														
	CXM	(23)								3	20								
	HR-756	(22)					12	9	1										
	FK-749	(19)									3	8	8						
	SCE- 1365	(23)			10	13													
	6059-S	(22)			6	16													
H. in- fluenzae	CET	(81)								2	20	22	29	4	4				
	CEZ	(83)											4	3	31	42	3		
	CEX	(82)													31	23	27		1
	CTM	(55)						2	12	41									
	T-1551	(78)	1	10	40	19	6	2											
	CXM	(55)							1	10	40	4							
	HR-756	(31)			18	12	1												
	FK-749	(31)			14	17													
	SCE- 1365	(43)	1	28	14														
	6059-S	(31)				6	25												

MIC   ≤0.003 0.006 0.013 0.025 0.05 0.10 0.20 0.39 0.78 1.56 3.13 6.25 12.5   25   50   100 >100
(µg/ml)

* : No. of strains tested are shown in parentheses

cephaloridine (CER), cephalothin (CET), cefazolin (CEZ), cephalexin (CEX), cefotiam (CTM)

FIG. 2. *MICs of cephalosporins including an oxacephem against B. pertussis compared with those against H. influenzae. Inoculum size: one loopful of 10^6 CFU/ml.*

tussis activities of the remaining two were similar to those of the older cephalosporins. In addition, 6059-S, a newly synthesized β-lactam with a cephalosporin-like oxacephem ring, inhibited all the strains of both species at a concentration of 0.10 μg/ml.

Josamycin, with an MIC of 0.05 to 0.20 μg/ml, was approximately fourfold more active than erythromycin against *B. pertussis*. The in vitro anti-*B. pertussis* activities of two tetracyclines, minocycline and doxycycline, with geometric mean MICs of 0.18 and 0.41 μg/ml, respectively, were superior to those of chloramphenicol, gentamicin, dibekacin, sulfamethoxazole-trimethoprim (5:1), nalidixic acid, and miloxacin.

These data suggest that two piperazine β-lactams, piperacillin and T-1551, are more active than other antimicrobial agents tested against *B. pertussis* as well as *H. influenzae* and that further in vivo and clinical studies of *B. pertussis* infections are warranted.

1. **Matsumoto, K.** 1978. Importance of *Hemophilus influenzae* on chronic respiratory infectious diseases. Jpn. J. Med. 17:269–270.

Activity of Three Cephalosporins and an Oxa-β-Lactam Compound Against *Pseudomonas aeruginosa*

R. J. WILLIAMS* AND J. D. WILLIAMS

The London Hospital Medical College, London, England

The aim of this investigation was to compare the in vitro activity of three cephalosporins, cefotaxime, cefsulodin (CGP 7174/E), and cefoperazone (T-1551/CP52640), and a closely related oxa-β-lactam compound, LY127935 (6059-S). These compounds represent a development in the cephalosporin group of antibiotics since all four compounds have activity against *Pseudomonas aeruginosa* at concentrations likely to be achievable therapeutically in humans. At present, the aminoglycosides and carbenicillin are the antibiotics of choice for the treatment of *P. aeruginosa* infections, but the increasing incidence of strains resistant to these antibiotics makes the investigation of new agents even more important.

LY127935 (6059-S) differs structurally from the three cephalosporins in having an oxygen atom in place of the sulfur atom normally present in the cephem nucleus. All four compounds have large chemical groupings substituted at the 7 position of the cephalosporin nucleus, and this is usually associated with stability to β-lactamase attack. A comparison of the β-lactamase susceptibility of these four compounds forms part of this study.

Activity of cefotaxime, cefsulodin, cefoperazone, and LY127935 against *P. aeruginosa*. The agar dilution technique, using antibiotic solutions incorporated into DST agar (Oxoid CM 261), was used to determine the MICs of the four antibiotics for 100 clinical isolates of *P. aeruginosa*. Strains of *P. aeruginosa* resistant to gentamicin and/or carbenicillin were included in the collection because the activity of these cephalosporins against such strains is of particular interest. A multipoint inoculator was used to deliver a standardized inoculum of 10^3 organisms/ml (other inocula were also tested). The susceptibility of the *P. aeruginosa* strains to carbenicillin and gentamicin was also determined for comparison.

As can be seen in Table 1, cefsulodin and cefoperazone, with mode MICs of 2 μg/ml, were the most active of the four cephalosporin-type compounds tested. LY127935, with a mode MIC of 8 μg/ml, was slightly less active. When the strains of *P. aeruginosa* which were resistant to carbenicillin (46 strains; MIC, 64 μg/ml) were analyzed separately, the mode MICs of cefotaxime, cefsulodin, cefoperazone, and LY127935 were 16, 4, 16, and 32 μg/ml, respectively. Thus, the mode MIC of cefotaxime remained unchanged, and those of cefsulodin, cefoperazone,

TABLE 1. *MICs of cefotaxime, cefsulodin, cefoperazone, and LY127935 (6059-S) for Pseudomonas aeruginosa*

Antibiotic	No. of *P. aeruginosa* strains inhibited by a concn (μg/ml) of:								
	0.5	1	2	4	8	16	32	64	128	128
Cefotaxime	0	1	0	4	26	32	14	11	11	1
Cefsulodin	1	16	34	22	10	10	4	2	1	0
Cefoperazone	1	1	30	28	15	12	11	2	0	0
LY127935	0	1	0	13	27	22	22	9	4	2
Carbenicillin	1	0	0	0	0	2	22	29	24	22
Gentamicin	43	24	8	6	9	3	2	2	2	1

TABLE 2. *MICs of cefotaxime, cefsulodin, cefoperazone, and LY127935 (6059-S) compared with those of gentamicin and carbenicillin for a variety of gram-negative bacilli*

Bacterial sp.	Antibiotic	No. of strains inhibited by a concn (µg/ml) of:									
		0.5	1	2	4	8	16	32	64	128	>128
Providencia sp. (15)[a]	Cefotaxime	15									
	Cefsulodin		1					7	4		3
	Cefoperazone	1		9	5						
	LY127935	14	1								
Proteus vulgaris (5)	Cefotaxime	5									
	Cefsulodin								1	1	3
	Cefoperazone	1		2		2					
	LY127935	4		1							
P. mirabilis (4)	Cefotaxime	4									
	Cefsulodin						1		3		
	Cefoperazone		1	3							
	LY127935	4									
Serratia sp. (9)	Cefotaxime	8	1								
	Cefsulodin									4	5
	Cefoperazone			2	3	4					
	LY127935	2	3	4							
Citrobacter freundii (6)	Cefotaxime	1	5								
	Cefsulodin										6
	Cefoperazone				4	1		1			
	LY127935	1		3		2					
Escherichia coli (4)	Cefotaxime	4									
	Cefsulodin					1					3
	Cefoperazone	1				2	1				
	LY127935	4									
Enterobacter cloacae (14)	Cefotaxime	4	9		1						
	Cefsulodin										14
	Cefoperazone			1	3	6	1	2		1	
	LY127935	2	8	3			1				
Klebsiella aerogenes (8)	Cefotaxime	7	1								
	Cefsulodin								1		7
	Cefoperazone	1		2	2			1	1		1
	LY127935	5	3								
Acinetobacter sp. (11)	Cefotaxime		1	2	4	2		2			
	Cefsulodin		1	1	3	1	1	1		1	2
	Cefoperazone				4	5		1		1	
	LY127935					7	1		2	1	
Alcaligenes sp. (2)	Cefotaxime			1				1			
	Cefsulodin				1		1				
	Cefoperazone		2								
	LY127935	1	1								

[a] Number of strains tested.

and LY127935 were increased two- or fourfold. Using different inocula had little or no effect on the MICs.

Activity of cefotaxime, cefsulodin, cefoperazone, and LY127935 against resistant gram-negative bacilli. Using the technique described above, we determined the MICs of the four antibiotics for a variety of gram-negative bacilli other than *P. aeruginosa* (Table 2). The test organisms were selected because they were resistant to gentamicin, and many were also resistant to carbenicillin. Cefsulodin was outstanding in its complete lack of activity against the gram-negative bacilli tested, with the exception of a few strains of *Acinetobacter* sp. Cefotaxime and LY127935 were both very active against the majority of strains tested, although less so against *Acinetobacter* sp. Cefoperazone was slightly less active, with MICs falling between those of cefotaxime and cefsulodin, in the range from 2 to 32 μg/ml.

Stability of cefotaxime, cefsulodin, cefoperazone, and LY127935 to hydrolysis by β-lactamases. The stability of the four compounds to hydrolysis by various β-lactamases was compared with that of cephaloridine. The enzymes, designated R_{TEM}, RP1, K1, and P99, were prepared by a method based on that of O'Callaghan et al. (3). The absorption spectrum of a 0.1 mM solution of each antibiotic was determined by using a Unicam SP 1700 spectrophotometer and scanning over the range from 210 to 320 nm. A 20-μl volume of enzyme preparation was added to the antibiotic solution in the cuvette (1.5 ml) and mixed well. Hydrolysis was allowed to proceed at room temperature for 30 min. After this time the spectrum of the hydrolyzed compound was superimposed exactly over that of the unhydrolyzed antibiotic. The wavelength of maximum difference between the two spectra was determined. At this wavelength, the rate of hydrolysis was determined by measuring the decrease in optical density with time as hydrolysis proceeded.

For purposes of comparison, the rate of hydrolysis of cephaloridine was taken to be 100 and the rates of hydrolysis of the other compounds were compared with this. Cefoperazone was the only one of the four test compounds that was hydrolyzed by R_{TEM} and RP1, and the rate of hydrolysis by these enzymes was 73% and 58%, respectively, of the rate of hydrolysis of cephaloridine by the same enzymes. Cefotaxime, cefsulodin, and LY127935 were unaffected by R_{TEM} and RP1, and none of the compounds (except cephaloridine) was detectably hydrolyzed by K1 or P99 enzymes.

In conclusion, considering each antibiotic in turn, cefotaxime was the least active of the four antibiotics when tested against *P. aeruginosa*, but it showed marked activity against other gram-negative bacilli, and its resistance to hydrolysis by β-lactamases may in part be responsible for this. Cefsulodin was remarkable in its lack of activity against gram-negative bacilli (other than *P. aeruginosa*) despite complete resistance to hydrolysis by the β-lactamases tested. This is in keeping with the findings of other workers, e.g., Goto et al. (2). Cefsulodin's lack of activity may be due to its failure to permeate the cell walls of these gram-negative bacilli or to its low affinity for the target sites.

Cefoperazone was equal to cefsulodin in its activity against *P. aeruginosa*, but it was less stable to β-lactamase hydrolysis, and this was reflected in its lower activity against resistant gram-negative bacilli, many of which are β-lactamase producers. This supports the theory put forward by other workers, e.g., Garber and Friedman (1), that intrinsic resistance is probably a major factor in *P. aeruginosa*'s defense against β-lactam antibiotics, whereas β-lactamase production plays a minor role.

LY127935 was similar to cefotaxime in its β-lactamase stability and its activity against gram-negative bacilli. It was slightly more active than cefotaxime against *P. aeruginosa* but less active than cefoperazone and cefsulodin.

1. **Garber, N., and J. Friedman.** 1970. Beta-lactamase and the resistance of *Pseudomonas aeruginosa* to various penicillins and cephalosporins. J. Gen. Microbiol. **64:** 343–352.
2. **Goto, S., M. Ogawa, Y. Kaneko, S. Kuwahara, K. Tsuchiya, M. Kondo, T. Nishi, and H. Nagatomo.** 1978. SCE-129, a new antipseudomonal cephalosporin; in vitro and in vivo antibacterial activity, p. 835–838. *In* Current chemotherapy, Proceedings of the 10th International Congress of Chemotherapy. American Society for Microbiology, Washington, D.C.
3. **O'Callaghan, C. H., P. W. Muggleton, and G. W. Ross.** 1969. Effects of β-lactamase from gram-negative organisms on cephalosporins and penicillins, p. 57–63. Antimicrob. Agents Chemother. 1968.

Comparative Antibacterial Activity of the Cephalosporins LY127935 (a 1-Oxacephem), Cefotaxime (HR-756), and Cefoperazone (T-1551)

WENDELL H. HALL,* BONNIE OPFER, AND DALE N. GERDING

Veterans Administration Medical Center, Minneapolis, Minnesota 55417, U.S.A.

Since 1975 we have seen more than 200 patients in our hospital who were either infected with or colonized by multiply resistant, gram-negative enteric bacilli. As recently reported by Gerding et al. (1), the resistant species included at first only strains of *Klebsiella pneumoniae*, which seem to have been introduced into the hospital by a suspected index case. The multiply resistant *Klebsiella* strains were resistant to many aminoglycosides, including gentamicin and tobramycin (but not amikacin), as well as to ampicillin, chloramphenicol, and cephalothin. The resistance was shown to be mediated by a plasmid transferable in vitro to *Escherichia coli* K-12.

More recently, in our hospital multiply resistant strains of *Serratia marcescens* and *Pseudomonas aeruginosa* (with similar resistance patterns) have become more frequent, but multiply resistant *Klebsiella* have continued to be present.

Three new "third generation," broad-spectrum cephalosporins, including a 1-oxacephem (LY127935), cefotaxime (HR-756), and cefoperazone (T-1551), have been compared for their in vitro growth-inhibiting activities against these multiply resistant bacterial strains. We have also tested the three new cephalosporins against other less resistant 1979 isolates of gram-negative enteric bacilli from our hospital patients. Their antibacterial activity was compared with that of ticarcillin, a broad-spectrum carboxypenicillin, like carbenicillin, but more active than carbenicillin against most gram-negative enteric bacilli. The recently marketed broad-spectrum cephalosporin known as cefamandole was also included for comparison.

A review of the chemical structure of the three new cephalosporins shows some interesting relationships. They share with cephalothin, the first cephalosporin to be marketed, the common core 7-aminocephalosporanic acid. In cefotaxime (HR-756) the amide-linked side chain has been replaced by aminothiazolyl and methoxyimino groups. With cefoperazone (T-1551) the amide-

linked side chain contains dioxo-1-piperazine, and the acetate group has been replaced by thiomethyl- and methyl-tetrazole groups. In the 1-oxacephem (LY127935) we have a dicarboxy cephalosporin resembling the dicarboxy penicillin, ticarcillin. However, with LY127935 in the cephalosporanic acid nucleus a sulfur atom is replaced by oxygen. As in cefoperazone, the acetate is also replaced by thiomethyl- and methyl-tetrazole groups.

The method we used for determining the MICs of the antibiotics was the agar dilution method of Washington. Mueller-Hinton agar plates were poured with doubling antibiotic dilutions from 128 down to 0.03 µg/ml. Each of the antibiotic plates was spot inoculated with about 10,000 bacteria in broth with a Steers replicating device and incubated for 18 h at 35°C.

In Table 1 we show the geometric means of the MICs of the three new cephalosporins and also of ticarcillin for each of nine species of gram-negative aerobic enteric bacilli, including the three multiply resistant species (defined as gentamicin resistant, ≥8 µg/ml). *P. aeruginosa* was the least susceptible species tested, but here cefoperazone was by far the most active of the four antibiotics. Cefotaxime and the 1-oxacephem (LY127935) were definitely the most active antibiotics for both the *Serratia* and the *Klebsiella* groups, especially for the multiply resistant strains. The three new cephalosporins were all more active than ticarcillin for the common enteric bacilli *E. coli*, *Enterobacter*, *Proteus*, and *Citrobacter*. The less frequent *Providencia* spp. were most susceptible to the 1-oxacephem (LY127935) and cefotaxime.

In conclusion, all three new broad-spectrum

TABLE 1. *Geometric means of MICs of cephalosporins and ticarcillin*

Species	No. of strains	Geometric mean of MIC[a] (µg/ml) of:			
		LY[b]	T	HR	TIC
Pseudomonas aeruginosa	63	25.68	7.09	26.83	24.04
Gentamicin susceptible	47	23.48	6.23	24.54	21.49
Gentamicin resistant	16	33.42	10.37	34.90	39.74
Serratia marcescens	61	1.06	7.14	0.56	65.79
Gentamicin susceptible	18	0.76	2.62	0.42	10.48
Gentamicin resistant	43	1.21	10.87	0.63	>128
Klebsiella pneumoniae	61	0.31	3.58	0.07	121.15
Gentamicin susceptible	29	0.34	0.61	0.08	103.23
Gentamicin resistant	32	0.28	18.69	0.07	>128
Escherichia coli	114	1.18	1.29	1.13	4.44
Enterobacter sp.	49	0.34	0.48	0.22	5.92
Proteus mirabilis	30	0.09	0.17	<0.03	0.52
Proteus (non-*P. mirabilis*)	86	0.15	0.42	<0.03	1.29
Providencia stuartii	28	0.16	2.69	0.16	2.39
Citrobacter sp.	50	0.27	0.82	0.19	23.44

[a] Agar dilution susceptibility method.

[b] LY, LY127935 (a 1-oxacephem); T, T-1551 (cefoperazone); HR, HR-756 (cefotaxime); TIC, ticarcillin.

cephalosporins are at present more active than the established cephalosporins and the most active broad-spectrum penicillin, ticarcillin, against most species of aerobic gram-negative enteric bacilli. Against multiply resistant strains, cefoperazone was notably effective against *P. aeruginosa,* and cefotaxime and the 1-oxacephem (LY127935) were effective against *Serratia* and *Klebsiella.* All three new cephalosporins were active against *E. coli, Enterobacter, Proteus,* and *Citrobacter* species. Their usefulness in serious infections caused by these troublesome organisms remains to be established. They may be especially useful in people who are allergic to the penicillins.

1. Gerding, D. N., A. E. Buxton, R. A. Hughes, P. P. Cleary, J. Arbaczawski, and W. E. Stamm. 1979. Nosocomial multiply resistant *Klebsiella pneumoniae*: epidemiology of an outbreak of apparent index case origin. Antimicrob. Agents Chemother. **15**:608–615.

In Vitro Activity of the New Cephalosporins HR-756, LY127935, and T-1551

JESUS MARTINEZ-BELTRAN,* MARIA A. LEDESMA, ELENA LOZA, EMILIO BOUZA, AND FERNANDO BAQUERO

Microbiology Service and Infectious Disease Unit, Centro Especial "Ramon y Cajal," Madrid, Spain

Aminoglycosides are still essential in the treatment of severe gram-negative infections. The toxicity of these drugs justifies the active search for new β-lactam drugs with a high degree of resistance to enzymatic inactivation.

The activity of the new cephalosporins HR-756 (HR), LY127935 (LY), and T-1551 (T) was tested against 360 recent clinical isolates and compared with that of the better-known cefazolin (Cfz), cefamandole (Cfm), and cefoxitin (Cfx). The synergistic effect of clavulanic acid (CA) with the three new cephalosporins was tested against 47 selected microorganisms, 36 of which were β-lactamase producers.

Recent clinical isolates were identified according to standard criteria (3); they included *Enterobacteriaceae* (230), *Pseudomonas aeruginosa* (50), *P. cepacia* (10), *Staphylococcus aureus* (50), and *Streptococcus faecalis* (20). The standard reference strains *Escherichia coli* ATCC 25922, *P. aeruginosa* ATCC 27853, and *S. aureus* ATCC 25923 were always used as internal controls. Standard reference powders of the different antibiotics were obtained from the manufacturers [HR (Roussel), LY (Eli Lilly, Indiana), and T (Pfizer)]. MICs and MBCs were determined in Mueller-Hinton agar and broth according to the procedure reported by Ericsson and Sherris (2). For all antibiotics tested, the concentration ranged from 128 to 0.06 µg/ml in a twofold dilution. Checkerboard agar dilution was used for synergy studies. The β-lactamase activity was tested by the chromogenic cephalosporin method (5).

Comparative activities of the new and of the better-known cephalosporins against 360 recent clinical isolates are shown in Table 1. Reference strains had the following susceptibilities (expressed in µg/ml) to the newer cephalosporins: *E. coli* ATCC 25922 (HR, 0.06; LY, 0.125; T, 0.125), *P. aeruginosa* ATCC 27853 (HR, 16; LY, 16; T, 4), and *S. aureus* ATCC 25923 (HR, 1; LY, 4; T, 1).

HR and LY were the most active against *E. coli,* inhibiting all the strains with 1 µg/ml or less. T was more active than Cfz, Cfm, and Cfx, but one isolate had an MIC of 128 µg/ml. The activity of HR against *Klebsiella* was similar to that of LY. All isolates were inhibited by 2 µg/ml or less. It is noteworthy that 31 of the 40 *Klebsiella* isolates were resistant to 32 µg of gentamicin per ml. All 40 *Enterobacter* isolates had MICs lower than 8 to 16 µg/ml for LY and HR. Six of them, with an MIC of 2 µg/ml for both drugs, showed MICs higher than 128 µg/ml for Cfz, Cfm, and Cfx. T showed greater activity than Cfm, the most active drug among the already well-known cephalosporins. Against *Serratia,* HR and LY had the same high activity, although it was slightly lower against other members of *Enterobacteriaceae.* T is less active than HR and LY but more effective than Cfx. All 20 isolates of *Salmonella typhi* were uniformly susceptible to 0.06 µg of HR and LY per ml. All isolates had an MIC of 0.25 µg/ml against ampicillin. Fifteen isolates of *Yersinia enterocolitica* (resistant to ampicillin, carbenicillin, and Cfz) showed uniformly descending levels of susceptibility to HR, LY, T, Cfx, and Cfm, in that order. The three newer cephalosporins were also very active against all indole-positive *Proteus* strains.

T was the most active cephalosporin in the 50 strains of *P. aeruginosa* tested. With 4 µg/ml, 50% were inhibited. An unexpected result was found in 10 isolates of gentamicin-resistant *P. cepacia,* which showed a uniform susceptibility pattern to 8 µg of HR, 16 µg of T, and 32 µg of LY per ml. The in vitro activity of the experimental cephalosporins against *S. aureus* isolates was inferior to those already on the market. Regarding *S. faecalis,* the same undesirable results were found.

MBC/MIC ratios of HR, LY, and T against 70 strains of *Enterobacteriaceae* and *P. aerugi-*

nosa selected on the basis of their different patterns of susceptibility are presented in Table 2. LY and HR exerted powerful bactericidal activity, slightly superior in LY, against all the tested *Enterobacteriaceae.* In *P. aeruginosa,* this bactericidal effect was significantly reduced. Five strains tested against HR and 4 strains against LY, showed an MBC/MIC ratio of 8. The bactericidal activity of T was comparatively greater.

Different concentrations (0.1, 1, 10, 20 µg/ml) of the β-lactamase inhibitor drug CA were assayed in combination with HR, LY, and T against strains of the following microorganisms: *E. coli* (5), *Klebsiella* (4), *Enterobacter* (10),

TABLE 1. *HR-756, LY127935, and T-1551 versus other cephalosporins against clinical isolates*

Organism	Strains inhibited (%)	Concn (µg/ml) required to inhibit given % of strains					
		CFZ[a]	CFM	CFX	HR-756	LY127935	T-1551
E. coli (45)[b]	50	2	2	2	≤0.06	≤0.06	1
	90	32	128	8	0.125	0.25	16
Klebsiella sp. (40)	50	32	64	4	≤0.06	0.125	16
	90	128	128	8	0.125	0.25	64
Enterobacter sp. (40)	50	>128	4	128	0.125	≤0.06	1
	90	>128	64	>128	4	2	32
S. marcescens (40)	50	>128	128	32	0.5	0.5	8
	90	>128	>128	64	2	1	32
Citrobacter sp. (10)	50	64	1	64	≤0.06	≤0.06	0.25
	90	128	4	128	0.125	≤0.06	0.5
S. typhi (20)	50	1	0.125	0.25	≤0.06	≤0.06	0.25
	90	1	0.25	0.5	≤0.06	≤0.06	0.5
Y. enterocolitica (15)	50	128	4	4	≤0.06	0.25	2
	90	>128	8	4	≤0.06	0.25	2
Indole-positive *Proteus* (20)	50	>128	2	8	≤0.06	≤0.06	1
	90	>128	32	16	0.25	0.125	4
P. aeruginosa (50)	50				16	32	4
	90				64	64	16
P. cepacia (10)	50				8	32	16
	90				8	32	16
S. aureus (20)	50	0.5	0.5	2	2	8	4
	90	1	1	2	2	8	4
S. faecalis (20)	50	16	16	>128	32	>128	16
	90	32	32	>128	128	>128	32

[a] Abbreviations: CFZ, cefazolin; CFM, cefamandole; CFX, cefoxitin.
[b] Total number tested.

TABLE 2. *Comparison of MBC to MIC*

Organism	No. tested	No. of isolates for each MBC/MIC ratio											
		HR-756				LY127935				T-1551			
		1	2	4	8	1	2	4	8	1	2	4	8
Escherichia coli	10	6	4			6	4						
Klebsiella sp.	10	2	8			8	2						
Enterobacter sp.	10	5	4	1		4	5	1					
S. marcescens	10	8	1	1		6	4						
S. typhi	10	4	6			8	2						
Indole-positive *Proteus*	10	4	4	2		6	4						
P. aeruginosa	10	2	2	1	5	1	2	3	4	3	3	2	2

Serratia (10), *Proteus morganii* (1), *P. vulgaris* (1), *S. aureus* (5), and *P. aeruginosa* (11). All microorganisms, except one strain of *S. aureus* and 10 strains of *P. aeruginosa,* showed β-lactamase production and were selected on the basis of the different susceptibility patterns to the new cephalosporins. The MIC of CA against all strains referred to was higher than 20 μg/ml. The combination of HR plus CA uniformly reduced one-half the MIC values in five *E. coli* strains, one *Klebsiella,* and one *P. morganii.* All of them were susceptible to less than 0.5 μg of HR per ml. No enhancing effect was observed on those *Enterobacter, Serratia,* and *Pseudomonas* strains showing different levels of susceptibility. The MIC for HR was reduced in all strains of *S. aureus* (mean 5.2 times) in the presence of 20 μg of CA per ml. Almost identical results were obtained with the LY plus CA combination, but the mean was decreased (mean 3 times) in four *Enterobacter* and two *Serratia* strains. In *S. aureus,* this combination caused a drop of MIC in the tested strains to 1/35th of the original level. Association of T with 20 μg of CA per ml led to an important decrease in the MIC values of T for all the *Enterobacteriaceae* strains except in one *P. morganii* strain (RYC 7159/79) and one *Serratia* strain (RYC 45502/78). The mean value of decrease in MIC in *E. coli* strains was 1/282, 1/220 in *Klebsiella,* 1/55 in *Enterobacter,* and 1/38 in *Serratia* strains. No effect was observed in *P. aeruginosa* strains

and only a slight drop in MIC values in *S. aureus* (1/32) was detected.

Our tests with the in vitro activity of HR and LY revealed that a significant step in the development of new cephalosporins has been taken. Against *Enterobacteriaceae,* HR and LY are very active and superior to T, Cfz, Cfm, and Cfx (1, 4, 6). T-1551 is the most active agent tested against *P. aeruginosa.* The poor results with the combination of CA with HR-756 and LY127935 on the relatively resistant strains suggest that the mechanisms of inactivation for those drugs could also be mediated by a type I β-lactamase.

1. **Chabbert, Y. A., and A. J. Lutz.** 1978. HR-756, the syn isomer of a new methoxyimino cephalosporin with unusual antibacterial activity. Antimicrob. Agents Chemother. **14:**749–754.
2. **Ericsson, H. M., and J. C. Sherris.** 1971. Antibiotic sensitivity testing. Report of an international collaborative study. Acta Pathol. Microbiol. Scand. Sect. B Suppl. **217:**1–90.
3. **Lennette, E. H., E. H. Spaulding, and J. P. Truant** (ed.). 1974. Manual of clinical microbiology, 2nd ed. American Society for Microbiology, Washington, D.C.
4. **Neu, H. C., N. Aswapokee, P. Aswapokee, and K. Fu.** 1979. HR-756, a new cephalosporin active against gram-positive and gram-negative aerobic and anaerobic bacteria. Antimicrob. Agents Chemother. **15:**273–281.
5. **O'Callaghan, C. H., A. Morris, S. M. Kirby, and A. M. Shingler.** 1972. Novel method for the detection of β-lactamase by using a chromogenic cephalosporin substrate. Antimicrob. Agents Chemother. **1:**283–288.
6. **Wise, R., T. Rollason, M. Logan, J. M. Andrews, and K. A. Bedford.** 1978. HR-756, a highly active cephalosporin: comparison with cefazolin and carbenicillin. Antimicrob. Agents Chemother. **14:**807–811.

Comparative In Vitro Activity of LY127935 and Cefoperazone with Other Beta-Lactam Antibiotics Against Anaerobic Bacteria

JAVIER AZNAR, RUFINO JIMÉNEZ, FERNANDO GARCÍA, MARIA V. BOROBIO, AND EVELIO J. PEREA*

Department of Microbiology, University of Sevilla, Medical School, Seville, Spain

The in vitro activity of two new antibiotics, LY127935 {(6R,7R)-7-[(carboxy(4-hidroxyphenyl)acetyl] amino)-7-methoxy-3-[[(1-methyl-1H-tetrazole-5-yl)thio] methyl]-8-oxo-5-oxa-1-azabicyclo [4.2.0] oct-2-ene-2 carboxylic acid, disodium salt} and cefoperazone {sodium 7-[D-(−)-α-(4-ethyl-2,3-dioxo-1-piperazine-carboxamido)-α-(4-hidroxyphenyl acetamido]-3-[1-methyl-1H-tetrazol-5-yl)-thiomethyl]-3-cephem-4-carboxylate} (T-1551), is compared with that of cefoxitin (CX), cefuroxime (CFI), cefsulodin (CFS), cefotaxime (CTX), and cefaclor (CFC) against 85 anaerobic bacteria: 30 *Bacteroides* (fragilis group), 30 *Clostridium* spp., and 25 *Pep-*

tococcaceae spp. using the agar dilution method. Additionally, two different culture media were used: brucella agar (BA) and Wilkins-Chalgren (WC). β-Lactamase production was determined in all *Bacteroides* strains by the plate method (3).

The median MIC values and cumulative percentages of MICs of three different groups of anaerobic bacteria against seven antibiotics in BA and WC are summarized in Tables 1–3.

It is well known that, of anaerobic bacteria, the *Bacteroides* group is most resistant to antibiotics. Of the two new β-lactams, LY127935 showed excellent activity, inhibiting at 1 μg/ml

TABLE 1. *Bacteroides fragilis group (30 strains)*

Antibiotic	Media[a]	Median values of MIC (µg/ml)	Cumulative % of isolates inhibited at MIC (µg/ml) of:													
			0.06	0.12	0.25	0.5	1	2	4	8	16	32	64	128	256	512
LY127935	BA	0.8			3.3	80	90			93	97	100				
	WC	0.7	3.3	13.3	37	90	93			97		100				
Cefoperazone	BA	96								10	27	43	57	97	100	
	WC	73.1								10	27	43	90	97	100	
Cefoxitin	BA	6.5						10	73	97		100				
	WC	3.8					17	53	73	100						
Cefuroxime	BA	3.5					40	53	60	77	87	100				
	WC	7.7						3.3	53	90	93	97	100			
Cefsulodin	BA	6.7					3.3	13.3	67	77	83	93	97	100		
	WC	8				3.3	27	30	50	73	83	97	100			
Cefotaxime	BA	13.1						13.3	27	63	70	93		97	100	
	WC	14.5						10	20	57	73	93		97	100	
Cefaclor	BA	108.4							3.3		10	20	63	70	87	100
	WC	91.4									7	37	60	87	100	

[a] BA, Brucella agar; WC, Wilkins-Chalgren.

TABLE 2. *Clostridium (30 strains)*

Antibiotic	Media[a]	Median values of MIC (µg/ml)	Cumulative % of isolates inhibited at MIC (µg/ml) of:								
			0.06	0.12	0.25	0.5	1	2	4	8	16
LY127935	BA	2		7		13	50	80	100		
	WC	1.6		3.3	7		30	63	90	100	
Cefoperazone	BA	3				3.3	10	30	70	100	
	WC	1.2	17	23		30	43	77	100		
Cefoxitin	BA	0.09	97	100							
	WC	0.09	100								
Cefuroxime	BA	0.16	27	100							
	WC	0.10	80	100							
Cefsulodin	BA	0.47	10	13	53	87	100				
	WC	0.10	83	93		100					
Cefotaxime	BA	3.17				3.3	10	27	67	90	97	100
	WC	2.50					7	40	80	93	100
Cefaclor	BA	1.4			10	23	90	100			
	WC	0.7	3.3	7	23	90	100				

[a] BA, Brucella agar; WC, Wilkins-Chalgren.

the majority of strains of this group, but T-1551 was less active, with MIC values ranging from 8 to 128 µg/ml.

Of the other cephalosporins, CX was the most active, inhibiting 100% of strains at 8 µg/ml, as previously reported (4). CFI has not been extensively studied against anaerobic bacteria. Our results showed good activity in both culture media on *Bacteroides,* inhibiting all strains at 32 µg/ml. CFS has not previously been tested

TABLE 3. *Peptococcaceae (25 strains)*

Antibiotic	Media[a]	Median values of MIC (μg/ml)	Cumulative % of isolates inhibited at MIC (μg/ml) of:									
			0.06	0.12	0.25	0.5	1	2	4	8	16	>16
LY127935	BA	27.6								20	64	100
	WC	30.2								20	56	100
Cefoperazone	BA	0.83	4	24	44	56	72	88	92	100		
	WC	0.46		16	60	68	80	92	100			
Cefoxitin	BA	0.175	28	80	88	96	100					
	WC	0.225	24	56	84	92	96	100				
Cefuroxime	BA	0.11	8	44	64	88	92	100				
	WC	0.11	8	28	64	88	92	96	100			
Cefsulodin	BA	2.25	16		20	28	48	80	96		100	
	WC	0.8	80	84	96		100					
Cefotaxime	BA	0.35	8	44	64	88	92	100				
	WC	0.42	8	28	64	88	92	96	100			
Cefaclor	BA	1.75	4	16	28	40	56	72	80	92	96	100
	WC	0.93		12	28	56	76	80	92	96		100

[a] BA, Brucella agar; WC, Wilkins-Chalgren.

against anaerobes, and on *Bacteroides* it showed the same activity as CFI in our tests. Our results with CTX were similar to those of CFS and CFI, with MICs higher than those obtained by Hamilton-Miller et al. (1) and lower than those obtained by Neu et al. (2).

Among the 30 *Bacteroides* strains, only 4 of them failed to produce β-lactamase. There were no significant differences between the median values of MIC of the producers and those of the nonproducers with most of the antibiotics tested. The antibiotic that appeared to be affected by *B. fragilis* β-lactamase was T-1551, with MIC values of 64 μg/ml in the producer group and 8 μg/ml in the nonproducers. No conclusion can be obtained from this because of the small number of nonproducers.

All antibiotics showed excellent activity against clostridia, and 0.12 μg of CX or CFI per ml inhibited all strains. CFS and CFC required concentrations of 1 μg/ml whereas T-1551 and LY127935 required concentrations of 4 μg/ml to inhibit 100%. The least active was CTX. In the case of CX, the results were similar to those previously reported by us (4).

Against *Peptococcaceae*, good activity was found with all antibiotics tested except for LY127935 and CFC, which required more than 16 μg/ml to inhibit all the strains. All other cephalosporins at 2 to 4 μg/ml inhibited all strains and their median values were below 1. Differences in species susceptibility were not found among the *Bacteroides fragilis* group, nor among the *Clostridium* species or *Peptococcaceae*.

There were no significant differences between MIC values obtained in BA or WC; however, in WC these values were in general slightly lower than in BA with most of the antibiotics. An exception was CFI against *Bacteroides,* which showed higher median values in WC (7.7) than in BA (3.5). In general, the slight differences found in MIC values in the two different media are not significant because they generally fell within the range of the experimental error of procedure.

Considering the achievable serum levels after i.m. administration of 1 g of each antibiotic, we can conclude theoretically that LY127935 would inhibit all *Bacteroides* and *Clostridium* strains tested and possibly half of the *Peptococcaceae*. T-1551 would inhibit almost half of *Bacteroides* and all strains of *Clostridium* and *Peptococcaceae*. CX would inhibit all three groups tested. Two thirds of *Bacteroides* and all clostridia and *Peptococcaceae* would be inhibited by CFI, CFS, or CTX. Finally, CFC would not be useful in treatment of *Bacteroides* infections, but would appear to be useful in infections produced by *Peptococcaceae* and clostridia.

1. **Hamilton-Miller, J. M. T., W. Brumfitt, and A. V. Reynolds.** 1978. Cefotaxime (HR-756) a new cephalo-

sporin with exceptional broad-spectrum activity in vitro. J. Antimicrob. Chemother. 4:437–444.
2. **Neu, H. C., N. Aswapokee, P. Aswapokee, and K. P. Fu.** 1979. HR 756, a new cephalosporin active against gram-positive and gram-negative aerobic and anaerobic bacteria. Antimicrob. Agents Chemother. 15:273–281.
3. **O'Callaghan, C. H., A. Morris, S. M. Kirby, and A. H. Shingler.** 1972. Novel methods for detection of β-lac-

tamases by using a chromogenic cephalosporin substrate. Antimicrob. Agents Chemother. 1:283–288.
4. **Perea, E. J., J. Aznar, M. C. Garcia-Iglesias, and M. V. Borobio.** 1978. Cefoxitin sodium activity against anaerobes: effect of the inoculum size, pH variation and different culture media. J. Antimicrob. Chemother. 4(Suppl. B):55–60.

In Vitro Comparison of Three New Cephalosporins: LY127935, Cefotaxime, and Cefoperazone

GARY M. TRAGER,* G. WESLEY WHITE, VICTORIA M. ZIMELIS, DEBORAH A. BRYK, AND ANAND P. PANWALKER

University of Illinois Hospital,* Abraham Lincoln School of Medicine, and University of Illinois College of Medicine, Chicago, Illinois 60612, U.S.A.

Alterations of the basic cephalosporin nucleus and its substituents have resulted in the development of several new antibiotics which have an expanded spectrum of activity and a remarkable stability against hydrolysis by β-lactamases when compared to older agents. Various in vitro properties of three new cephalosporins, LY127935 (LY), cefotaxime (CTX), and cefoperazone (CFP), are compared in this report.

Two hundred and eighty-nine clinical aerobic isolates were tested for antimicrobial susceptibility using the microdilution technique with Mueller-Hinton broth. The inoculum size was 10^5 to 10^6 organisms/ml and the MIC and MBC values were measured as described in an earlier report (4). Thirteen strains of *Bacteroides fragilis* were tested using the agar dilution method of Sutter et al. (3). A chromogenic cephalosporin substrate, nitrocefin, was used to qualitatively determine β-lactamase production on all study isolates (2). Combinations of the three cephalosporins with gentamicin (GM) were studied against selected strains of *Pseudomonas aeruginosa* to assess synergy. The MIC of each agent was assigned a value of one. When two drugs were tested in combination, synergy was defined as existing when the sum of the fractional MICs was less than one (1).

The results of the susceptibility tests are shown in Table 1. The three cephalosporins had similar activity against *Staphylococcus aureus,* with the MIC90 being 6.2 µg or less of drug per ml. Against *Escherichia coli* and *Proteus mirabilis,* CTX had an MIC90 of 0.1 µg/ml while the other compounds were two- to fourfold less inhibitory. This pattern was also observed for *Klebsiella* spp. and indole-positive *Proteus* spp. For these organisms, however, CFP was clearly less active than either LY or CTX.

LY and CTX were highly active against GM-susceptible *Enterobacter* spp., and all isolates were resistant to CFP. For GM-resistant *Enterobacter* strains, LY was 16-fold more inhibitory than CTX, whereas CFP was ineffective. CFP had moderate activity against GM-susceptible *Serratia* spp. (MIC90 = 32 µg/ml) but was inactive against GM-resistant isolates. LY and CTX inhibited 90% of GM-susceptible *Serratia* at 2.0 and 4.0 µg/ml, respectively, and 90% of GM-resistant *Serratia* at 16.0 µg of drug per ml. CFP had fourfold more activity against GM-susceptible *P. aeruginosa* when compared to LY and CTX. However, it was ineffective against GM-resistant *P. aeruginosa*. All 13 strains of *B. fragilis* were inhibited by the three cephalosporins, although LY was fourfold more active than CTX and CFP. The presence of β-lactamase had no effect on the susceptibilities to any cephalosporin for any organism. The MBCs were two- to fourfold greater than the MICs in every instance.

Increasing the size of the inoculum from 10^1 to 10^5 organisms/ml had no effect on the MICs. However, at higher inocula, the MICs to these three agents against *E. coli, P. mirabilis, Enterobacter* spp., *Serratia* spp., and *P. aeruginosa* began to increase. The susceptibilities of the *Klebsiella* strains were unaffected by the inoculum size. The inhibitory activity of the three compounds increased two- to fourfold with a change in the pH of the medium from 7.3 to 5.0. In Mueller-Hinton broth with an NaCl content of 4%, the MICs of *E. coli, Enterobacter* spp. and *Serratia* spp. were reduced severalfold, while there were only minor changes for the other organisms.

Combination studies with a strain of *P. aeruginosa* resistant to GM, LY, CTX, and CFP

TABLE 1. *Comparative in vitro activity of LY127935 (LY), cefotaxime (CTX), cefoperazone (CFP), and gentamicin (GM)*

Organism (no. of isolates)	Antibiotic	MIC (μg/ml)			
		Range	50%	75%	90%
S. aureus (24)	LY	6.2–25.0	6.2	6.2	6.2
	CTX	1.5–3.2	1.5	3.2	3.1
	CFP	1.5–6.2	3.1	3.2	6.2
E. coli (20)	GM	1.0–4.0	2.0	2.0	2.0
	LY	0.1–0.4	0.1	0.2	0.2
	CTX	0.05–0.2	0.05	0.1	0.1
	CFP	0.1–>50.0	0.2	0.2	0.4
Klebsiella spp. (21)	GM	1.0–2.0	1.0	1.0	2.0
	LY	0.1–0.4	0.2	0.2	0.4
	CTX	>0.02–0.1	0.05	0.05	0.1
	CFP	0.4–50.0	0.4	3.1	6.2
P. mirabilis (20)	GM	<0.25–16.0	4.0	4.0	8.0
	LY	<0.025–0.8	0.2	0.2	0.2
	CTX	<0.025–1.5	<0.025	<0.025	0.1
	CFP	<0.025–0.8	0.4	0.4	0.4
Indole-positive *Proteus* (30)	GM	1.0–32.0	2.0	4.0	4.0
	LY	<0.25–1.0	<0.25	0.25	0.5
	CTX	<0.25–32.0	<0.25	<0.25	0.25
	CFP	<0.25–>500	1.0	1.0	16.0
Enterobacter spp. (25) Gentamicin susceptible	GM	1.0–4.0	1.0	2.0	2.0
	LY	<0.25–64	<0.25	0.5	1.0
	CTX	<0.25–125	0.5	1.0	2.0
	CFP	<0.25–>500	2.0	500	>500
Enterobacter spp. (7) Gentamicin resistant	GM	8.0–64	16.0	32.0	64
	LY	<0.25–4.0	0.5	2.0	2.0
	CTX	0.5–125	2.0	2.0	32.0
	CFP	500–>500	>500	>500	>500
Serratia spp. (17) Gentamicin susceptible	GM	1.0–4.0	2.0	2.0	4.0
	LY	0.5–4.0	0.5	1.0	2.0
	CTX	<0.25–32	0.25	1.0	4.0
	CFP	1.0–250	2.0	4.0	32
Serratia spp. (26) Gentamicin resistant	GM	8.0–500	32	125	250
	LY	<0.25–125	1.0	4.0	16
	CTX	<0.25–125	1.0	4.0	16
	CFP	4.0–>500	>50	>500	>500
P. aeruginosa (68) Gentamicin susceptible	GM	0.5–4.0	1.0	2.0	2.0
	LY	8.0–250	16	32	64
	CTX	2.0–250	32	32	64
	CFP	2.0–125	8.0	8.0	16
P. aeruginosa (31) Gentamicin resistant	GM	16–>500	500	>500	>500
	LY	2.0–>500	16	16	32
	CTX	8.0–250	32	32	64
	CFP	2.0–500	32	64	125
B. fragilis (13)	LY	0.5–8.0	1.0	1.0	4.0
	CTX	2.0–>16	4.0	4.0	16.0
	CFP	4.0–>16	8.0	16.0	>16.0

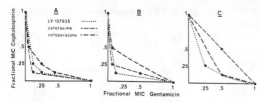

FIG. 1. *Isobolograms derived from checkerboard studies of Pseudomonas aeruginosa with either LY127935, cefotaxime, or cefoperazone combined with gentamicin (GM) for a cephalosporin and GM-resistant isolate (A), a cephalosporin-susceptible and GM-resistant isolate (B), and a cephalosporin- and GM-susceptible isolate (C).*

showed synergy (Fig. 1A). This was also true for a GM-resistant and cephalosporin-susceptible isolate (Fig. 1B). When a strain of *P. aeruginosa* susceptible to all four agents was examined, synergy was demonstrated for the combination of

GM and LY or CFP (Fig. 1C), while an additive effect was noted with GM and CTX.

As demonstrated by these studies, these three new cephalosporins have a remarkably wide spectrum of activity against most *Enterobacteriaceae* when compared to older agents. More interesting is their activity against GM-resistant *Enterobacteriaceae*, *P. aeruginosa*, and *B. fragilis*. This enhanced activity could herald an important advance in antimicrobial chemotherapy.

1. **Berenbaum, M. C.** 1978. A method of testing for synergy with any number of agents. J. Infect. Dis. **137**:122–130.
2. **O'Callaghan, C. H., A. Morris, S. M. Kirby, and A. H. Shingler.** 1972. Novel method for detection of beta-lactamases by using a chromogenic cephalosporin substrate. Antimicrob. Agents Chemother. **1**:283–288.
3. **Sutter, V. L., V. L. Vargo, and S. M. Finegold.** 1975. Wadsworth anaerobic bacteriology manual, 2nd ed. Extension Division, University of California, Los Angeles.
4. **Trager, G. M., G. W. White, V. M. Zimelis, and A. P. Panwalker.** 1979. LY-127935: a novel beta-lactam antibiotic with unusual antibacterial activity. Antimicrob. Agents Chemother. **16**:297–300.

Comparison of Four Anti-*Pseudomonas* Cephalosporin-Like Antibiotics with Cephalothin

MARCIA R. MOODY,* MAUREEN J. MORRIS, VIOLA YOUNG, AND STEPHEN C. SCHIMPFF

Baltimore Cancer Research Program, National Cancer Institute, University of Maryland Hospital, Baltimore, Maryland 21201, U.S.A.

A number of new cephalosporin-like antibiotics with reported activity against *Pseudomonas aeruginosa* as well as stability to a wide range of β-lactamases have been introduced for clinical use. As there is a need for agents with such enlarged spectra of activity, we became interested in evaluating the in vitro antibacterial spectra of four such agents and comparing them with the spectrum of a standard cephalosporin. Four agents that were chosen were LY127935 (Eli Lilly), LY; HR-756 (Hoechst-Roussel), HR; T-1551 (Pfizer), T; and C7174/E (Ciba-Geigy), C; the standard agent was cephalothin.

Five hundred and fifteen bacterial strains that were isolated from clinical specimens from cancer patients were used as test organisms. They were collected consecutively from February 1979 through April 1979, but no more than one of a bacterial species from an individual patient was included in the test strains. MICs were determined by a microtechnique (MIC 2000, Dynatech Laboratories, Alexandria, Va.). The MBCs were determined. All tests were performed in

duplicate and at two different concentrations, 10^3 colony-forming units (CFU) and 10^6 CFU per well.

One hundred and thirty-three strains of *P. aeruginosa* were tested. C had the highest degree of activity, and T was only slightly less active. HR and LY had similar activity but were about fourfold less active than C or T. Cephalothin had no activity. Eighteen strains had MICs of 128 μg/ml or greater for LY, 16 for HR, and 3 for C. An MIC inoculum effect on a single agent occurred most often with HR, but strain responses to two or more agents were most frequently associated with HR and LY (Table 1). The MBC inoculum effect was again most frequently observed with HR and LY.

HR and LY were equally effective against the 53 test strains of *Serratia*, all of which were resistant to cephalothin. T was slightly less active than HR and LY, and C had little activity. No MIC inoculum effect was observed for any strain. Increased MBCs were seen in 27 strains for T alone as compared to none for the other

TABLE 1. *Effect of inoculum concentration on the MIC and MBC of P. aeruginosa*

Agent	Inoculum effect[a]		Increased MBC[b]	
	>1[c]	1[c]	>1	1
C7174	0	1	2	0
T-1551	1	2	2	4
HR-756	8	6	23	3
LY127935	7	2	24	3

[a] Higher MIC at 10^6.
[b] Higher MBC at 10^6.
[c] >1 = more than 1 agent; 1 = single agent.

agents, and increased MBCs were seen in 9 strains to T as well as to one or more of the other agents.

Thirty-one *Enterobacter cloacae* strains and 19 *E. aerogenes* strains were tested. Both species were quite susceptible to LY, HR, and T. C was more effective against *E. cloacae* than cephalothin, whereas the reverse was true for *E. aerogenes*. An MBC inoculum effect to HR was seen in 13% of *E. cloacae* strains.

Fifty-seven strains of *Proteus mirabilis* and 21 strains of indole-positive *Proteus* spp. were tested. HR was most active against *P. mirabilis* whereas LY was most active against the indole-positive group. For both groups, T was approximately eightfold less active than LY or HR. All strains of *P. mirabilis* were susceptible to cephalothin whereas the indole-positive group was resistant. C was also more effective against the former than against the latter.

Fifty-one strains of *Klebsiella pneumoniae* and 13 strains of *K. oxytoca* were tested. All were inhibited by very low concentrations of HR, LY, and T. Cephalothin was also active whereas C was the least active. The MBC inoculum effect was seen in two strains of *K. pneumoniae*.

Fifty-seven strains of *Escherichia coli* were tested. HR and LY were equally effective against this organism and T was only slightly less so.

Cephalothin was more effective than C. Three strains had an MBC inoculum effect to T.

Forty-seven strains of *Staphylococcus aureus* were tested. Of the five agents, cephalothin was the most effective. HR and T were less active than cephalothin but were fourfold more active than LY and C. Against the 33 strains of enterococci tested, cephalothin was also most active, with T only slightly less so. HR and LY had little or no activity and C had none.

Of 515 bacterial strains tested in this study, 52% had MICs of 64 μg or greater to C (some strains from all test species except *S. aureus*). Thirty-four percent, including strains from all test species except *S. aureus* and *P. mirabilis*, had MICs in this range to cephalothin. While the percentages for LY, HR, and T were 9, 8, and 8%, respectively, the exclusion of enterococci reduced these to 3, 2, and 2%, respectively. The majority of these strains were *P. aeruginosa*. T was affected most often when the inoculum concentration was increased, and the organism most often affected was *Serratia* (80% of 47 strains).

In conclusion, C was most effective against *P. aeruginosa* but relatively inactive against the other test species except *S. aureus* and *P. mirabilis*. HR and LY had similar inhibitory concentration ranges and were most effective against enterobacteria, especially cephalothin-resistant strains; they also were active against *P. aeruginosa* and *S. aureus*. They had dual responses to changes in inoculum concentrations of certain strains, especially *P. aeruginosa*. T had antipseudomonas activity that was similar to C, and of the test agents had the most activity against ticarcillin-resistant pseudomonas strains; it was also active against enterobacteria, *S. aureus*, and enterococci. Cephalothin was the most effective against *S. aureus* and enterococci. These results indicate that HR, LY, and T have broad in vitro spectra against both gram-negative and gram-positive bacteria, but that C is mainly an antipseudomonas agent.

Susceptibility Testing with LY127935 (Shionogi 6059-S): Proposals for Disk Content and Interpretive Criteria

D. A. PRESTON,* M. A. SURPRENANT, AND L. C. HAWLEY

Lilly Research Laboratories, Indianapolis, Indiana 46206, U.S.A.

LY127935 (6059-S) is a member of a new class of β-lactam antibiotics that have a unique spectrum of antibacterial activity, including most strains of *Haemophilus influenzae*, *Neisseria* meningitidis, *N. gonorrhoeae*, *Pseudomonas aeruginosa*, *Staphylococcus aureus*, *S. epidermidis*, *Streptococcus pyogenes*, *Streptococcus pneumoniae*, most species within the family *En-*

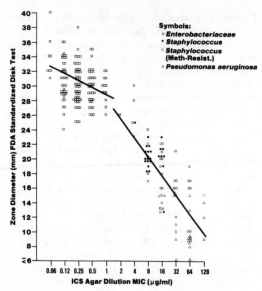

FIG. 1. *Relationship between MIC and zone diameter for 248 bacterial isolates. LY 127935 (6059-S), 30-μg disks.*

terobacteriaceae, and most anaerobic pathogens, particularly *Bacteroides fragilis.*

Determination of bacterial susceptibility by the FDA standardized disk test is usually limited to nonfastidious, rapidly growing, aerobic bacterial pathogens, such as *Enterobacteriaceae*, staphylococci, and *Pseudomonas*. Two hundred forty-eight (248) isolates of this group were used to evaluate the performance of test disks containing LY127935 and to correlate the zone responses with MICs for the same antibiotic. The bacteria were tested in batches of strains simultaneously by the ICS agar dilution method (1) and by the FDA standardized disk method (2) using disks containing 30, 10, 5, and 1 μg of LY127935.

The disk mass most appropriate for routine testing is that which produces moderate inhibition zones (15 to 17 mm) on organisms considered to be of intermediate susceptibility to the agent. On the basis of early human pharmacology studies with LY127935, an MIC of 32 μg/ml has been proposed as indicative of intermediate susceptibility. Within the group of 248 isolates tested for MIC, there were 17 strains that had MICs of 32 μg/ml. None of these had inhibition zones around the 1-μg disks; only two had zones around the 5-μg disks; and 16 had zones less than 12 mm around the 10-μg disks. The 30-μg disks produced zones of 14 to 17 mm on 11 of 17 strains; of the zones with the remaining 6 strains, one was larger than 18 and 5 were smaller than 13 mm. These results suggested that the 30-μg

disk contained sufficient activity to allow discrimination between bacterial isolates having an MIC of <32 μg/ml and those having an MIC of >32 μg/ml.

A scatter plot of zone diameters against $\log_2$ MIC revealed a biphasic correlation characterized by a steep slope for *P. aeruginosa* and staphylococci and a shallow slope for *Enterobacteriaceae* (Fig. 1).

Utilizing a standard curve technique as suggested by Ericsson and Sherris (1), slopes of standard curves of representative organisms from the two areas of the original plot, the highly susceptible organisms exhibited a shallow slope and the less susceptible organisms exhibited a steep slope. The former organisms (mostly *Enterobacteriaceae*) grow rapidly under the conditions of the disk test, usually becoming visible macroscopically within 3 to 5 h. The latter (mostly staphylococci and *Pseudomonas*) usually appear as visible growth within 7 to 9 h. This difference in growth rate is most likely the reason for the differences in slope between the plots of the two groups of organisms. Experiments were designed to simulate acceleration or retardation of growth of several of the cultures. This was accomplished by preincubating the plates prior to placing the disks, or by prediffusing the antibiotic in the plates in the refrigerator prior to incubating the plates. The absolute values of the slopes of the resulting standard curves

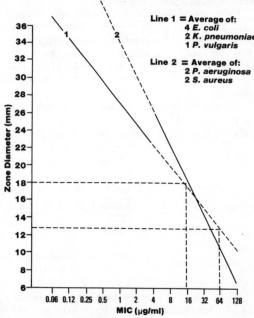

FIG. 2. *Selection of susceptibility criteria for LY127935 (6059-S), 30-μg disks.*

shifted toward smaller values (shallower) when plates were preincubated and toward larger values (steeper) when the antibiotics were prediffused. These results gave strength to the argument that it was the relatively slower rate of growth of the less susceptible organisms that caused the steeper slope in that area of the scatter plot.

For the purpose of selecting zone diameter criteria for use with the 30-μg disks of LY127935, two regression lines were plotted on the same axes: one characteristic of the very susceptible, rapidly growing organisms, and the other characteristic of the less susceptible, relatively slower growing organisms (Fig. 2). MIC criteria chosen to represent susceptible and resistant organisms ($\geq$16 and $\leq$64 μg/ml) were applied to the lines. Choosing the larger zone diameter indicated by one of the lines at each limit of susceptibility, the following interpretive criteria for disk testing were selected: resistant, $\leq$14 mm; susceptible, $\geq$18 mm. Rates of error, i.e., false susceptible or

false resistant interpretations, were calculated by the method of Metzler and DeHaan (3) for this population of organisms. False susceptible (zone, $\geq$18 mm; MIC, >32 μg/ml) occurred with a frequency of 0.4%; false resistant (zone, $\leq$14 mm; MIC, <32 μg/ml) occurred with a frequency of 2%. The suggested criteria should be considered tentative standards for susceptibility testing with 30-μg disks of this new antibiotic. If new data should indicate that MIC breakpoints other than those suggested here are more appropriate, then the zone diameter criteria would have to be modified accordingly.

1. **Ericcson, H. M., and J. C. Sherris.** 1971. Antibiotic sensitivity testing, Report of International Collaborative Study. Acta Pathol. Microbiol. Scand. Sect. B, Suppl. no. 217.
2. **Food and Drug Administration.** 1972. Rules and regulations. Fed. Regist. **37**:20525–20529.
3. **Metzler, C. M., and R. M. DeHaan.** 1974. Susceptibility tests of anerobic bacteria: statistical and clinical considerations. J. Infect. Dis. **130**:588–594.

Effect of LY127935 (6059-S) on Human Fecal Flora

STEPHEN D. ALLEN,* JEAN A. SIDERS, MORRIS D. CROMER, JOHN A. FISCHER, JAMES W. SMITH, AND KAREN S. ISRAEL

Department of Clinical Pathology, Indiana University Medical Center, Indianapolis, Indiana 46223, and Lilly Laboratory for Clinical Research, Wishard Memorial Hospital, Indianapolis, Indiana 46202, U.S.A.*

LY127935 (LY), or compound 6059-S (Shionogi Research Laboratories, Osaka, Japan), is a new beta-lactam antibiotic with a broad spectrum of in vitro activity against many *Enterobacteriaceae*, *Pseudomonas aeruginosa*, and obligate anaerobes, including *Bacteroides fragilis* (Lilly Research Laboratories and Shionogi Research Laboratories, unpublished data). The microbiologically active drug, as parent compound, appears in feces after intravenous administration (G. L. Brier, personal communication). The object of this study was to determine the effect of LY on the fecal flora of healthy volunteers.

LY was given intravenously to 10 male volunteers, 25 to 48 years of age. Each had received no antimicrobial agent for 3 months and underwent history, physical, and laboratory studies to exclude abnormalities. Statements of consent were signed. A dietary protocol was followed. There were two treatment groups given either 0.5 or 2 g of LY intravenously every 8 h for 10 days. Fecal specimens from both groups were collected on days 0 (pretreatment), 3, and 9; for

the 2-g group, specimens were collected 4 days after the last dose had been administered.

Specimens were placed in an anaerobic chamber within 5 min of collection and then homogenized with a Stomacher. Serial 10-fold dilutions in buffered gelatin were done in a glove box. Various selective and nonselective plating media were surface inoculated for quantitative enumeration of aerobes, facultative anaerobes, and obligate anaerobes, using techniques described elsewhere (1). Isolates were identified by standard procedures (2, 3).

LY was tolerated relatively well except that four volunteers on the 6-g-daily dose and one of five receiving 1.5 g per day experienced brief periods of diarrhea characterized by one to three loose to watery stools per day for 1 to 5 days, but the diarrhea resolved spontaneously before treatment was stopped (K. S. Israel, H. R. Black, R. S. Griffith, G. L. Brier, and J. D. Wolny, this volume).

The stool culture changes observed during administration of LY are given in Table 1. The total number of anaerobic bacteria per gram (dry weight) of feces was approximately 10^{11} (median) for the 10 pretreatment stools. Striking decreases in the counts for the five former subspecies of *B. fragilis*, for the other species of *Bacteroides*, and for *Fusobacterium* sp. were seen. *B. fragilis* concentrations were $>10^{10}$ colony-forming units (CFU) per g (dry weight) in the pretreatment stools. *B. fragilis* disappeared from the stools of one subject on the lower-dose regimen and from those of four subjects receiving the higher dose. Other *Bacteroides* and *Fusobacterium* disappeared from one subject on

the low dose and from all five subjects receiving the higher dose. These were not detected in the 4-day posttreatment stools. Anaerobic cocci, lactobacilli, *Bifidobacterium*, and *Eubacterium* were eliminated from some stools. The anaerobic bacteria which most commonly remained after LY treatment were species of *Clostridium*. The concentration of *Clostridium* was relatively unchanged in eight volunteers, but did show a >4-log decrease in two volunteers on the high-dose regimen. Clostridia detected in highest number during and after administration were C.

TABLE 1. *Changes in the concentrations of microorganisms in the stools of 10 volunteers treated with LY127935*

Organism	5 Volunteers, 1.5 g daily				5 Volunteers, 6.0 g daily				Return, 4 days post-treatment[e]
	Pre-treat-ment[a]	$\geq$4-log de-crease[b]	4-log in-crease[c]	No sig-nificant change[d]	Pre-treat-ment	$\geq$4-log de-crease	4-log in-crease	No sig-nificant change	
Total anaerobes	5	0	0	5	5	2	0	3	1
B. fragilis group	5	2	0	3	5	4	0	1	0
Bacteroides and Fuso-bacterium	5	2	0	3	4	4	0	1	0
Anaerobic cocci	4	4	1	0	3	3	2	0	2
Lactobacillus	3	2	0	1	5	3	1	1	1
Clostridium	5	0	0	5	5	2	0	3	1
Total aerobes	5	0	1	4	5	0	1	4	0
E. coli	5	4	0	1	5	5	0	0	1
Other Enterobacteria-ceae	0	0	0	0	1	0	3	1	1
Pseudomonas	0	0	2	3	0	0	0	5	0
Enterococci	2	0	5	0	4	0	5	0	0
Candida	3	1	0	4	3	0	2	3	1

[a] Number of pretreatment stools containing organisms.
[b] Number of stools collected during or after treatment with $\geq$4-log decrease or disappearance of organism.
[c] Number of stools collected during or after treatment with 4-log increase or gain of organism.
[d] Number of stools with no significant change compared with pretreatment samples.
[e] Number of stools in which organism returned to pretreatment concentration 4 days after last dose.

TABLE 2. *Susceptibility of fecal flora isolates to LY127935*

Organisms	Low dose, 1.5 g daily				High dose, 6.0 g daily				4 Days posttreat-ment	
	Pretreat-ment		9 Days		Pretreatment		9 Days			
	No.	MIC[a] (μg/ml)	No.	MIC (μg/ml)	No.	MIC (μg/ml)	No.	MIC (μg/ml)	No.	MIC (μg/ml)
B. fragilis group	15	4	6	>64	17	8	2	>64	1	>64
Bacteroides and Fusobacterium sp.	5	1	6	8	4	0.25	0		0	
Lactobacillus	1	8	1	>64	3	>64	1	>64	3	>64
C. perfringens	3	4	0		6	$\leq$0.125	0		4	16
C. innocuum	4	>64	4	>64	1	>64	2	>64	3	>64
Clostridium sp.	5	1	1	0.5	10	2	0		8	>64
E. coli	5	$\leq$0.5	2	4	4	1	0		0	
Other Enterobacteriaceae	0		0		0		0		4	16
P. aeruginosa	0		2	32	0		0		0	
Enterococci	2	>64	6	>64	4	>64	8	>64	6	>64

[a] Expressed as 50% or median MIC.

innocuum and *C. ramosum.* Their concentrations reached 10^{11} CFU/g in a few stools. *C. difficile* was detected in one stool at a concentration of $10^{3.6}$ CFU/g (dry weight) on day 9 in a volunteer receiving 1.5 g of LY daily. Although the isolate was toxic for WI-38 cells, toxin was not detected in a cell-free filtrate of that individual's stool diluted 1:2. This subject briefly had diarrhea which subsided spontaneously after 2 days. *C. difficile* was not detected in his stool 4 months later.

Escherichia coli was eliminated in seven and returned to base-line levels in only one individual's stool 4 days after the drug was stopped. Other *Enterobacteriaceae* were acquired in three of five volunteers receiving the higher-dose regimen. *P. aeruginosa* was acquired in three stools ($<10^7$ CFU/g [dry weight]) and lost in one of them. There was a 4- to 5-log increase in the enterococci of all subjects (median count, $\sim10^{10}$/g [dry weight]) at day 9. *Candida* sp. was gained by three subjects and lost by two.

The in vitro activity of LY against certain bacteria isolated from the stools was determined by a microtiter broth dilution technique. The antibiotic was diluted in Mueller-Hinton broth for facultative anaerobes. Wilkins-Chalgren broth was used for anaerobes. The in vitro susceptibility results are summarized in Table 2. The 50% MIC for the *B. fragilis* strains isolated from pretreatment stools was 8 µg/ml. However, >64 µg/ml was required to inhibit >80% of the strains isolated from posttreatment stools and stools collected during administration of the drug. Eight relatively resistant *B. fragilis* strains (25% of 32 tested) were present in the pretreatment stools. In general, LY was not particularly active against *C. innocuum, C. ramosum,* and certain other *Clostridium* species found in the pretreatment and posttreatment stools or in stools cultured during treatment. Activity against *C. perfringens* varied. The single *C. difficile* isolate was inhibited by 16 µg/ml. LY was highly active against *E. coli.* The other *Enterobacteriaceae* which replaced *E. coli,* two strains of *Klebsiella pneumoniae,* one of *Enterobacter cloacae,* and one of *Citrobacter freundii,* were moderately resistant.

The results indicate that LY127935 caused major changes in the stool concentration of certain bacteria, especially in volunteers receiving the higher-dose regimen.

1. **Allen, S. D., G. D. Dunn, D. L. Page, and F. A. Wilson.** 1977. Bacteriological studies in a patient with antibiotic-associated pseudomembranous colitis. Gastroenterology **73:**158–163.
2. **Dowell, V. R., Jr., and T. M. Hawkins.** 1974. Laboratory methods in anaerobic bacteriology, CDC manual. Department of Health, Education, and Welfare publication no. (CDC) 74-8272. Center for Disease Control, Atlanta.
3. **Koneman, E. W., S. D. Allen, V. R. Dowell, Jr., and H. M. Sommers.** 1979. Color atlas and textbook of diagnostic microbiology. J. B. Lippincott Co., Philadelphia.

Treatment of Experimental *Haemophilus influenzae* Meningitis with LY127935 (Shionogi 6059-S)

CYNTHIA S. CORDERA* AND ROBERT S. PEKAREK

The Lilly Research Laboratories, Indianapolis, Indiana 46206, U.S.A.

The isolation of increasing numbers of ampicillin-resistant (AR) *Haemophilus influenzae* has been observed in patients with bacterial meningitis (2, 3). This trend suggests that ampicillin may no longer be appropriate as the drug of choice for this infection. Although chloramphenicol is often used for treatment of AR *H. influenzae* meningitis, its potential toxicity presents a major drawback. Currently, there is no single antibiotic or combination of antibiotics available to treat AR *H. influenzae* meningitis which offers the combined characteristics of uncomplicated administration and ability to enter the cerebrospinal fluid (CSF) in therapeutic concentrations and which has minimal toxicity. The present communication describes a new type of β-lactam broad-spectrum antibiotic, LY127935 (Shionogi 6059-S), which meets the above criteria in an animal model and treats experimental AR *H. influenzae* meningitis.

This compound is extremely active against AR strains of *H. influenzae,* exhibiting MICs as low as 0.06 µg/ml (Lilly Research Laboratories, unpublished data). LY127935 also has the ability to cross the blood-brain barrier and to achieve therapeutic levels in the CSF. LY127935 was administered subcutaneously to normal rats and rats with meningitis (Table 1). Antibiotic levels in blood and CSF were determined by a seeded agar microwell technique at 15, 30, and 60 min after administration of the drug. LY127935 penetrated into the CSF of both normal animals and animals with inflamed meninges to approximately 10% of the corresponding blood levels. Ampicillin given at the same dose achieved higher concentrations in the CSF of animals with meningitis than in normal animals. However, the peak concentration of LY127935 in the CSF was at least 100 times the MIC for the AR *H. influenzae* strain, whereas even the peak ampicillin concentration was 3-fold below the MIC (>64 μg/ml) for the AR strain.

From these results, it appeared that LY127935 might show therapeutic efficacy in treating bacterial meningitis even when administered at a lower dose. To determine this, an experimental AR *H. influenzae* meningitis was produced in infant rats, using a previously established model (4, 5). Briefly, 4-day-old Sprague-Dawley rats were inoculated intranasally with 10^8 AR *H. influenzae* organisms. One day later, blood cultures were taken and rats which demonstrated bacteremia were retained for treatment studies. A positive blood culture for *H. influenzae* always resulted in a concomitant meningitis. The infected rats were initially treated subcutaneously with 50 mg/kg three times a day (t.i.d.) for 2 days, as shown in Table 2. Blood and CSF samples were taken 1 and 5 days after the termination of therapy and tested for the presence of *H.*

TABLE 1. *Antibiotic concentration in blood and CSF from normal and infected infant rats*

Antibiotic tested[a]	Animal	Sample	Concn (μg/ml)[b]		
			15 min[c]	30 min	60 min
LY127935	Normal	Blood	57.0 ± 3.0	67.0 ± 3.0	43.0 ± 3.0
		CSF	4.4 ± 2.0	3.8 ± 0.7	3.9 ± 0.6
LY127935	Infected	Blood	80.0 ± 6.0	103.0 ± 16.0	95.0 ± 18.0
		CSF	5.6 ± 2.0	9.0 ± 3.0	3.3 ± 0.7
Ampicillin	Normal	Blood	71.0 ± 6.0	58.0 ± 8.0	48.0 ± 3.0
		CSF	1.0 ± 0.4	2.2 ± 0.2	1.7 ± 0.2
Ampicillin	Infected	Blood	130.0 ± 21.0	109.0 ± 11.0	100.0 ± 14.0
		CSF	22.0 ± 6.0	18.0 ± 3.2	15.0 ± 7.0

[a] Antibiotic administered subcutaneously at 100 mg/kg.
[b] Mean ± SE of 5 to 10 animals per time period.
[c] Time post-administration of antibiotic.

TABLE 2. *Treatment of ampicillin-resistant H. influenzae meningitis in infant rats*

Antibiotic	Treatment[a]	Days post-treatment	Cured animals/total animals	Avg CFU/ml[b]
LY127935	50 mg/kg t.i.d. (2 days)	1	Blood 7/7	0
			CSF 7/7	0
		5	Blood 10/10	0
			CSF 10/10	0
LY127935	10 mg/kg t.i.d. (2 days)	1	Blood 9/9	0
			CSF 9/9	0
		5	Blood 9/9	0
			CSF 9/9	0
Ampicillin	10 mg/kg t.i.d. (2 days)	1	Blood 1/5	2.0×10^4
			CSF 1/5	1.0×10^6
		5	Blood 0/3	4.8×10^5
			CSF 0/3	1.1×10^6
Untreated		1	Blood 0/10	2.0×10^7
			CSF 0/10	1.0×10^8
		5	Blood 0/10	2.0×10^4
			CSF 0/10	2.0×10^5

[a] Administered subcutaneously. t.i.d., Three times a day.
[b] CFU, Colony-forming units.

influenzae. Samples from all of the animals tested were free of *H. influenzae* organisms. The control group of untreated infected animals showed positive blood and CSF *H. influenzae* cultures when assayed on corresponding days, with titers of up to 10^8 colony-forming units/ml.

Since the cure rate was 100% at this dose level, the amount of LY127935 was decreased to 10 mg/kg t.i.d. for 2 days. Again, *H. influenzae* organisms were not detected in blood or CSF samples of any animal at 1 or 5 days posttreatment. In contrast, only a single animal treated with ampicillin at 10 mg/kg t.i.d. for 2 days had negative blood and CSF cultures 1 day posttreatment. Furthermore, at 5 days posttherapy, blood and CSF samples from three additional rats showed numbers of *H. influenzae* organisms equal to or greater than the numbers of organisms in the untreated infected controls.

These studies illustrate that LY127935 is effective in treating experimental AR *H. influenzae* meningitis. This success is due in part to the ability of LY127935 to penetrate into the CSF at therapeutic levels. Results here indicate that this compound can cross the blood-brain barrier and achieve concentrations in the CSF many times the MIC (0.06 μg/ml) of a variety of strains of *H. influenzae* even when the meninges are intact and no inflammation is present. In contrast, ampicillin given at an equivalent dose was unable to effectively treat this infection.

In addition to the low MIC for *H. influenzae,* LY127935 has excellent in vitro activity against *Neisseria meningitidis* (MIC, <0.01 μg/ml) and *Streptococcus pneumoniae* (MIC, 1 μg/ml) (Lilly Research Laboratories, unpublished data). These organisms are also significant pathogens in bacterial meningitis (1). The combination of potent activity against these bacteria and the ability to enter the CSF as shown in an animal model makes LY127935 a candidate for potential use in the treatment of bacterial meningitis in clinical situations.

1. **Carpenter, R. R., and R. G. Petersdorf.** 1962. The clinical spectrum of bacterial meningitis. Am. J. Med. **33:**262–275.
2. **Clymo, A. B., and I. A. Harper.** 1974. Ampicillin resistant *H. influenzae* meningitis. Lancet i:143.
3. **Khan, W., S. Ross, W. Rodriguez, et al.** 1974. *H. influenzae* Type B resistant to ampicillin: a report of two cases. J. Am. Med. Assoc. **229:**288–301.
4. **Moxon, E. R., and P. T. Ostrow.** 1977. *H. influenzae* meningitis in infant rats: role of bacteremia in pathogenesis of age-dependent inflammatory responses in cerebrospinal fluid. J. Infect. Dis. **135:**303–307.
5. **Moxon, E. R., A. L. Smith, D. R. Averill, and D. H. Smith.** 1974. *H. influenzae* meningitis in infant rats after intranasal inoculation. J. Infect. Dis. **129:**154–162.

Pharmacokinetics and Bacteriological Efficacy of LY127935, Netilmicin, and Ampicillin in Experimental Gram-Negative Enteric Bacterial Meningitis

URS B. SCHAAD, GEORGE H. McCRACKEN, JR., CHRISTINE A. LOOCK, AND MARION L. THOMAS

Department of Pediatrics, The University of Texas Health Science Center at Dallas, Southwestern Medical School, Dallas, Texas 75235, U.S.A.

The mortality rate of gram-negative bacillary meningitis in newborn infants is from 15 to 30%, and sequelae are found in approximately one-third of survivors. Results from the two Neonatal Meningitis Cooperative Studies indicate that neither lumbar intrathecal nor intraventricular gentamicin administration combined with systemic therapy has a beneficial effect on outcome from coliform meningitis when compared to results with systemic antimicrobial therapy alone (2, 3). Moreover, an increasing percentage of *Escherichia coli* strains isolated from the cerebrospinal fluid (CSF) of newborns are resistant to ampicillin, which together with gentamicin represents the currently recommended initial therapeutic regimen for neonatal bacterial meningitis.

LY127935, a new semisynthetic oxacephalosporin, was found to be active in vitro against greater than 95% of 128 gram-negative enteric strains isolated from the CSF of newborn infants. The concentration of LY127935 required to inhibit 50% of the strains was 0.06 μg/ml, whereas that for 90% was 0.5 μg/ml. By contrast, the MIC_{90} values for gentamicin and ampicillin were 2.5 and >20 μg/ml, respectively.

The purpose of the present study was to evaluate the pharmacokinetics and bacteriological efficacy of this new cephalosporin in the lapine meningitis model, using five strains of gram-negative bacteria (two different *E. coli* K1 strains, *Citrobacter diversus, Klebsiella pneumoniae, Salmonella saint-louis*) isolated from the CSF of neonates with purulent meningitis.

CSF penetration and bacteriological efficacy of LY127935, netilmicin (an investigational aminoglycoside), and ampicillin were studied in 2- to 3-kg New Zealand white rabbits which were prepared according to the method described by Dacey and Sande (1).

Mean values ± SD for serum concentration, CSF concentration, and percent penetration into CSF, observed in the different animal categories according to pathogen and drug regimen, are listed in Table 1. The antibiotic levels were determined by microbioassay technique. The percent penetration into CSF is defined as the CSF concentration expressed as a percentage of the concurrent serum concentration. Antibiotic regimens were given by constant intravenous infusion over 9 h, starting 15 to 18 h after production of meningitis. Dosages were chosen to attain serum levels comparable to those observed in humans. Serial blood and CSF samples were collected at 0, 3, 6, and 9 h of therapy.

Drug concentrations in CSF. CSF penetration in normal rabbits ranged from 0.9 to 2.3%

(mean, 1.4%) for LY127935 and from 1.7 to 11.8% (mean, 6.1%) for netilmicin. The mean CSF penetration through inflamed meninges was 23% (range, 8 to 44%) for LY127935, 25% (10 to 45%) for netilmicin, and 11% (5 to 20%) for ampicillin. The concentrations of LY127935 in CSF ranged from 6.6 to 68.5 µg/ml, with a mean of 22.1 µg/ml.

Bacteriostatic and bactericidal titers in CSF against the individual pathogens were determined by microtiter technique in Mueller-Hinton broth, using an inoculum of 5×10^5 organisms. The median titers measured in the different animal groups are shown in Table 1. With LY127935 the average CSF bactericidal titer was 1:64, and the range was from 1:16 to 1:256. By contrast, the range of bactericidal titers for netilmicin and ampicillin was from <1:2 to 1:16 and from <1:2 to 1:8, respectively, with a median titer of 1:4 for both.

Bacteriological efficacy. The mean changes in CSF bacterial counts (Δ $\log_{10}$ bacteria per milliliter) ± SD after the 9-h period of therapy, compared to the initial titer before therapy, are shown in Table 1. All 27 untreated, infected rabbits showed stable or increasing CSF colony counts, with a range from 0.0 to +2.4 logs. In-

TABLE 1. *Pharmacological and bacteriological data in rabbits with experimental gram-negative enteric bacterial meningitis*

Pathogen	Antibiotic	No. of animals	Mean ± SD			Median CSF titer		Mean Δ $\log_{10}$ bacteria/ml in CSF ± SD over 9 h
			Serum concn (µg/ml)	CSF concn (µg/ml)	CSF/serum penetration (%)	Bacteriostatic	Bactericidal	
None	LY127935	5	74.3 ± 18.3	1.0 ± 0.4	1.4 ± 0.4			
	Netilmicin	4	13.9 ± 4.4	0.8 ± 0.3	6.1 ± 2.6			
E. coli K1 (AR)[a]	None (controls)	9						+1.48 ± 0.63
	LY127935	5	102.6 ± 22.3	20.4 ± 6.1	20.5 ± 6.5	1:128	1:64	−4.47 ± 0.46
	Netilmicin	5	10.4 ± 1.7	2.7 ± 1.0	26.1 ± 9.1	1:4	1:2	−2.73 ± 0.90
	LY plus netilmicin	5	92.5 ± 17.7	19.7 ± 4.1	21.6 ± 3.5	1:128	1:64	−4.84 ± 1.14
			10.6 ± 1.8	2.6 ± 0.6	24.8 ± 5.0			
E. coli K1 (AS)[b]	None (controls)	4						+0.31 ± 0.17
	LY127935	6	82.6 ± 26.4	21.6 ± 8.1	26.7 ± 8.5	1:64	1:64	−3.95 ± 0.84
	Ampicillin	6	84.2 ± 23.3	11.1 ± 4.4	12.4 ± 3.1	1:4	1:2	−1.95 ± 1.08
	LY plus ampicillin	5	113.5 ± 29.0	32.1 ± 15.4	27.3 ± 8.0	1:128	1:128	−4.36 ± 2.09
			125.1 ± 32.9	12.9 ± 4.5	10.4 ± 2.2			
C. diversus (AR)	None (controls)	4						+1.37 ± 0.61
	LY127935	4	96.6 ± 24.0	19.5 ± 8.2	20.2 ± 6.1	1:64	1:64	−3.73 ± 1.04
	Netilmicin	4	10.3 ± 1.8	2.6 ± 0.4	26.3 ± 6.3	1:4	1:4	−2.14 ± 0.84
K. pneumoniae (AR)	None (controls)	6						+0.53 ± 0.70
	LY127935	5	88.5 ± 22.0	16.3 ± 5.7	18.5 ± 4.7	1:128	1:128	−4.78 ± 0.87
	Netilmicin	4	12.0 ± 2.8	2.5 ± 0.7	21.4 ± 5.5	1:16	1:8	−2.93 ± 0.83
S. saint-paul (AS), group B	None (controls)	4						+0.74 ± 0.67
	LY127935	4	110.5 ± 19.0	24.3 ± 11.3	21.6 ± 8.4	1:128	1:64	−5.34 ± 0.54
	Netilmicin	4	9.9 ± 1.8	2.3 ± 1.0	22.9 ± 5.8	1:8	1:8	−3.50 ± 0.76
	Ampicillin	4	118.4 ± 36.0	10.3 ± 3.4	8.9 ± 1.5	1:8	1:4	−2.70 ± 0.47

[a] AR, Ampicillin resistant.
[b] AS, Ampicillin susceptible.

fected animals treated with LY127935 demonstrated a significantly greater reduction in CSF bacterial titers (mean, −4.5 logs) over the 9-h therapy period than observed with netilmicin (mean, −2.8 logs) or ampicillin (mean, −2.3 logs) ($P < 0.05$). No definite in vivo additive or synergistic effect of LY127935 plus netilmicin against *E. coli* K1 (ampicillin resistant) and LY127935 plus ampicillin against *E. coli* K1 (ampicillin susceptible) was seen in these experiments.

LY127935 shows excellent in vitro activity against gram-negative enteric bacteria that cause meningitis in neonates. The penetration of this investigational cephalosporin into CSF of infected rabbits exceeds that for any cephalosporins and for the penicillins. The CSF concentrations achieved with serum levels that appear safe for humans result in a median bactericidal titer of 1:64 against the five coliform organisms

used in these experiments. LY127935 was consistently more effective than netilmicin or ampicillin in reducing the bacterial colony counts and in sterilizing the CSF of experimentally infected rabbits. These results suggest that LY127935 has theoretical advantages over netilmicin and ampicillin for therapy of gram-negative bacillary meningitis in newborn infants.

1. **Dacey, R. G., and M. A. Sande.** 1974. Effect of probenecid on cerebrospinal fluid concentration of penicillin and cephalosporin derivates. Antimicrob. Agents Chemother. **6**:437–441.
2. **McCracken, G. H., Jr., and S. G. Mize.** 1976. A controlled study of intrathecal antibiotic therapy in gram-negative enteric meningitis of infancy. Report of the Neonatal Meningitis Cooperative Study Group. J. Pediatr. **89**:66–72.
3. **McCracken, G. H., Jr., et al.** 1979. Intraventricular therapy of neonatal meningitis caused by gram negative enteric bacilli. Report of the Second Neonatal Meningitis Cooperative Study Group, in press.

Pharmacology of LY127935 (Shionogi Compound 6059-S) in Humans

KAREN S. ISRAEL,* HENRY R. BLACK, RICHARD S. GRIFFITH, GORDON L. BRIER, AND JAMES D. WOLNY

Lilly Laboratory for Clinical Research, Wishard Memorial Hospital, Indianapolis, Indiana 46202, U.S.A.

LY127935 (Shionogi compound 6059-S) is a member of a new class of β-lactam antibiotics which has an expanded spectrum of antibacterial activity against cephalosporin-susceptible and multiple-antibiotic-resistant gram-negative microorganisms. We wish to report the pharmacology of this drug when administered intramuscularly (i.m.) and intravenously (i.v.).

Seventy-three adult healthy male volunteer subjects, between 23 and 60 years of age, were admitted to the Lilly research ward and underwent histories, physical examinations, and clinical laboratory examinations to exclude abnormalities. Signed statements of consent were obtained. Five subjects were administered single doses of 0.25, 0.5, 1, and 2 g i.v. over 20 min in 125 ml of 5% dextrose and water. Thirty-nine subjects (five per dose) received multiple doses of 0.25, 0.5, 1, and 2 g i.v. over 20 min in 100 ml of 5% dextrose and water every 8 or 12 h for 10 days. Fecal samples from five subjects who received 2 g i.v. every 8 h for 10 days were collected, diluted with gelatin, homogenized with a Stomacher, and centrifuged at 2,500 rpm for 20 min. Five microliters of supernatant and 1 μl (1 μg) of standard were spotted on a thin-layer chromatography plate. The plate was developed

using solvent system no. 20 (methanol, 6 parts; *n*-propanol, 2 parts; and water, 1 part). The plate was air dried, placed face down on an agar plate seeded with *Escherichia coli* ATCC 4157. After 20 min, the plate was removed, the seeded plate was incubated at 35°C for 18 h, and the chromatogram was read. In addition, the fecal flora of the samples was examined before, during, and after drug, and results have been reported in a previous paper (S. D. Allen, J. A. Siders, M. D. Cromer, J. A. Fischer, J. W. Smith, and K. S. Israel, this volume). Five subjects were given single doses of 0.25, 0.5, and 1 g i.m., and 25 subjects (four to five per dose) received 0.25 g i.m. every 8 h and 0.5 and 1 g i.m. every 8 or 12 h for 10 days. On study days, the subjects were kept fasting until 1.5 h after termination of the infusion or injection.

Serum or plasma concentrations of drug, obtained at appropriate times, were determined microbiologically, using a standard agar well diffusion assay, and urines, which were obtained at 2-h intervals and then at 12 to 24 h, were assayed using a turbidimetric assay (Autoturb). *E. coli* ATCC 4157 was the indicator organism.

The serum half-life and mean serum concentrations after single 20-min i.v. infusions of 0.25,

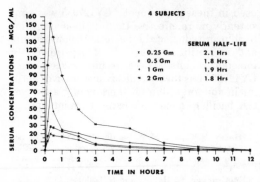

FIG. 1. *Mean serum concentrations after single 20-min i.v. infusions of 0.25, 0.5, 1, and 2 g of LY127935 (6059-S).*

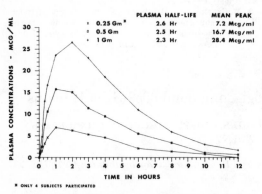

* ONLY 4 SUBJECTS PARTICIPATED

FIG. 2. *Mean plasma concentrations after single i.m. doses of 0.25, 0.5, and 1 g of LY127935 (6059-S) given to five subjects.*

0.5, 1, and 2 g are shown in Fig. 1. Urinary excretion of drug was highest in the first 2 h after administration of these doses: 55 mg (170 μg/ml) after 0.25 g; 174 mg (446 μg/ml) after 0.5 g; 402 mg (1,820 μg/ml) after 1 g; and 716 mg (4,220 μg/ml) after 2 g. At 10 to 12 h, there were urinary concentrations of 2 mg (14 μg/ml) after a 0.25-g dose and 30 mg (156 μg/ml) after a 2-g dose. The overall mean 24-h urine recoveries ranged from 50 to 92% for these doses.

The plasma half-life and mean plasma concen-

trations after i.m. administration of 0.25, 0.5, and 1 g are shown in Fig. 2. Urinary excretion of drug was highest in the 2- to 4-h collection period: 55 mg (347 μg/ml) after 0.25 g; 129 mg (469 μg/ml) after 0.5 g; and 199 mg (586 μg/ml) after 1 g. At 10 to 12 h, urinary concentrations of 3 mg (18 μg/ml) after 0.25 g and 21 mg (89 μg/ ml) after 1 g were observed. The overall mean 24-h urine recoveries ranged from 55 to 65%. Peak mean plasma concentrations ranged from 20 to 25, 35 to 58, 94 to 150, and 201 to 246 μg/ ml after multiple i.v. doses of 0.25, 0.5, 1, and 2 g for 10 days. LY127935 was excreted into the feces as a microbiologically active compound, as parent drug, in subjects who received 2 g i.v. every 8 h for 10 days. Peak plasma concentrations were 6 to 11, 13 to 18, and 22 to 35 μg/ml at 1 to 2 h after multiple i.m. doses of 0.25, 0.5, and 1 g for 10 days. No plasma accumulation was observed after the i.v. or i.m. multiple doses.

The kidney appears to be the primary route of excretion of drug, with some excretion into the feces, presumably via the biliary pathway. Single and multiple i.v. doses up to 6 g daily and single and multiple i.m. doses up to 3 g daily were tolerated well for 10 days. No phlebitis was observed. No significant adverse reactions were observed, except a few subjects who received multiple i.v. doses experienced brief periods of diarrhea characterized by an average of one to three very loose to watery stools per day for 1 to 5 days, but the diarrhea resolved during drug administration. In one subject, the course of diarrhea was more protracted, lasting 8 days; therefore, a sigmoidoscopy was performed and revealed no evidence of colitis or pathological abnormalities except for a sessile polyp. The diarrhea did not appear to be dose related and was infrequent with the multiple i.m. doses. Three subjects had some elevation in serum glutamic oxalic transaminase (SGOT) and serum glutamic pyruvic transaminase (SGPT) poststudy. After multiple i.m. doses, two subjects had slight elevations in SGOT only. A direct relationship between these elevations and drug could not be established.

Renal Excretion of 6059-S, a New Semisynthetic Beta-Lactam Antibiotic

J. SHIMADA,* Y. UEDA, T. YAMAJI, Y. ABE, AND M. NAKAMURA

Jikei University School of Medicine, Tokyo*; Osaka City University Medical School, Osaka; and Shionogi Research Laboratory, Shionogi & Company, Ltd., Osaka, Japan

The mechanism of renal excretion of 6059-S, a new semisynthetic β-lactam antibiotic, was investigated in beagle dogs, using the stop-flow and renal clearance methods.

In addition, serum levels, serum half-life, and renal excretion of 6059-S were examined both in healthy human volunteers and in volunteers with various degrees of reduced renal function. The effects of hemodialysis, peritoneal dialysis, and probenecid were also examined.

Healthy beagle dogs, 12 months of age, with body weights of 9 to 10 kg, were anesthetized with pentobarbital sodium and prepared for the stop-flow and renal clearance studies as described previously (1).

In the studies in human subjects, 1 g of 6059-S dissolved in 20 ml of 20% glucose was injected intravenously over a 5-min period. Concentrations of 6059-S were determined by bioassay, using *Escherichia coli* 7437 as the test organism.

In the stop-flow studies, no specific peak or trough was observed for 6059-S (Fig. 1). With the administration of probenecid, the peak of *p*-aminohippuric acid disappeared, whereas there

was no significant change in the pattern of 6059-S levels.

Glomerular filtration of 6059-S was calculated by multiplying the plasma concentration of free 6059-S (which was obtained by assuming that the protein-binding ratio of 6059-S in beagle plasma was 40%) by the inulin clearance. The glomerular filtration of 6059-S thus calculated was nearly equal to the urinary excretion of 6059-S actually determined at various plasma concentrations (Fig. 2).

When 6059-S was infused at the rate of 8.0 mg/kg of body weight per h, the ratio of free 6059-S clearance to inulin clearance was 0.98 ± 0.09. This ratio was 1.14 ± 0.10 when probenecid was used, which was not significantly different from the value without probenecid. In the crossover study in four healthy human volunteers, there was no significant difference between serum levels, serum half-life, and urinary recovery with or without probenecid. These findings suggested that the renal excretion of 6059-S took place mainly through glomerular filtration, and there was little tubular excretion.

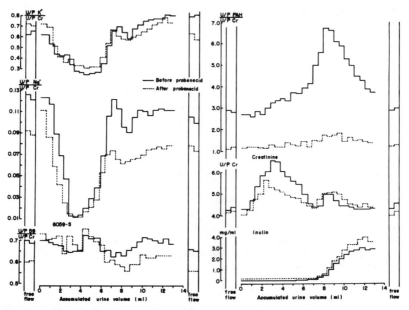

FIG. 1. *Stop-flow pattern in dogs. 6059-S was given at a priming dose of 10 mg/kg of body weight followed by a sustaining dose of 5.0 mg/kg of body weight per h.*

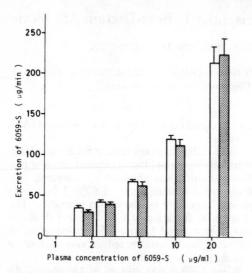

FIG. 2. *Urinary excretion of 6059-S in beagle dogs (n = 4). Average of four experiments (dog 1-dog 4). Symbols:* □, *urinary excretion;* ▧, *glomerular filtration.*

When 6059-S was administered intravenously by slow bolus injection, the peak serum level was 201 ± 39.6 µg/ml, the half-life was 6.3 ± 1.8 min (alpha phase) and 96.0 ± 18.1 min (beta phase), and cumulative urinary excretion up to 8 h was 86.7 ± 7.1%.

The values for cefazolin in a crossover study in the same volunteers were 147.6 ± 25.4 µg/ml, 9.2 ± 0.9 min, 102.9 ± 14.1 min, and 83.0 ± 7.2%,

respectively, and were very similar to those for 6059-S.

When 500 mg of probenecid was administered orally 30 min before the intravenous administration of 1 g of 6059-S, the peak serum level was 154.2 ± 48.1 µg/ml, the half-life was 6.5 ± 2.9 min (alpha phase) and 107.8 ± 25.5 min (beta phase), and urinary recovery up to 8 h was 74.3 ± 13.6%. These values were not significantly different from those without probenecid.

In cases with compromised renal function, serum levels were not different from those in healthy volunteers until 15 min after intravenous administration. However, serum levels 30 min after administration were higher in patients with markedly reduced renal function than in healthy subjects. Serum levels 6 h after intravenous administration were 8.1, 16.0, 17.3, 22.0, 30.8, and 46.0 µg/ml for creatinine clearance values of 82.6, 59.4, 40.8, 29.0, 8.2, and 4.0 ml/min, respectively. The serum half-life (beta phase) in subjects with a creatinine clearance value of 10 ml/min or less was 295 min and markedly prolonged. With hemodialysis, the half-life (beta phase) was shortened to 214.3 min. In patients undergoing peritoneal dialysis, the recovery of 6059-S in dialysate was 17.8%, and cumulative urinary recovery was 2.8%, both up to 12 h. Since 6059-S may accumulate in the plasma of patients with impaired renal function, investigations are continuing.

1. Higashio, T., et al. 1978. J. Pharmacol. Exp. Ther. 207: 212.

Human Pharmacokinetics of 6059-S

JIRO KURIHARA, KEIZO MATSUMOTO, YOSHIO UZUKA, HARUMI SHISHIDO, TAKESHI NAGATAKE, HIDEO YAMADA,* TADASHI YOSHIDA, TAKAYOSHI OGUMA, YASUO KIMURA, AND YOSHIHIRO TOCHINO

Kitano Hospital, Osaka; School of Medicine, Nagasaki University, Nagasaki; and Shionogi Research Laboratory, Shionogi & Company, Ltd., Osaka, Japan*

Compound 6059-S, discovered by Shionogi Research Laboratory, Osaka, Japan, is a new semisynthetic β-lactam antibiotic having a unique chemical structure in which sulfur is replaced with oxygen at position 1 of the six-membered ring of the conventional cephem nucleus (1). This novel 1-oxacephem derivative was reported to be highly active against a variety of pathogenic microorganisms, including genera resistant to other β-lactam antibiotics (T. Yoshida, M. Narisada, S. Matsuura, W. Nagata, and S.

Kuwahara, Program Abstr. Intersci. Conf. Antimicrob. Agents Chemother. 18th, Atlanta, Ga., abstr. no. 151, 1978).

This paper deals with the pharmacokinetic properties of 6059-S in normal adult male volunteers.

The first group, consisting of four volunteers, was administered single doses of 0.5 and 1 g dissolved in 20 ml of 5% dextrose by intravenous injection over 2 min. The second group, consisting of four volunteers, was administered single doses of 0.5, 1, and 2 g in 500 ml of 5% dextrose by intravenous slow infusion over 2 h and 1 g in 250 ml of 5% dextrose by intravenous slow infusion over 1 h. The third group, consisting of four volunteers, was given single doses of 0.25 and 0.5 g in 2 ml of 0.5% lidocaine by intramuscular injection. Each single dose was separated by an interval of 1 week.

The fourth group, consisting of five volunteers, was given multiple doses of 1 g in 20 ml of 5% dextrose by intravenous injection over 2 min at 12-h intervals for 5 days.

Plasma samples were obtained at 0, 15, and 30 min and 1, 2, 4, and 8 h after dosing. Urine specimens were collected every 1 or 2 h for 12 h and then during a 12- to 24-h interval. The plasma and urine samples were assayed by the agar diffusion method, using *Escherichia coli* 7437, and analyzed pharmacokinetically.

The plasma concentration obtained after single administration was approximately proportional to the dose. Figure 1 shows the plasma concentrations after intravenous slow infusion of 6059-S. Almost all of the dose, about 90% or more, was recovered in the 24-h urine.

Results obtained from examination by thin-layer chromatographic bioautography indicate that there was no active metabolite in the plasma and urine after administration of 6059-S.

The individual and mean plasma concentration data obtained after single intravenous injections were well fitted to a two-compartment open model. The mean elimination half-life was 5 to 8 min in the α-phase and 79 to 98 min in the β-phase.

A two-compartment open model with a constant infusion process fitted well to the individual and mean plasma concentrations obtained after intravenous slow infusion. The mean elimination half-life was 17 to 38 min in the α-phase and 100 to 154 min in the β-phase.

After intramuscular injection of 0.25 and 0.5 g, peak mean plasma levels of 13.3 and 21.0 μg/ml, respectively, were observed at 1 h after administration. The plasma concentration data on each dose by intramuscular injection were fitted to a one-compartment model with a first-order absorption process and a first-order elimination process. The half-life of the mean elimination curve was 147 to 167 min. The α-phase cannot be observed in the case of intramuscular injection, because it overlaps the absorption phase.

In the multiple dosing of 1 g by intravenous injection, the plasma concentrations after the first dose were fitted to a two-compartment model, and the pharmacokinetic parameters were obtained; then the sequential plasma levels were calculated using these parameters. This simulation curve indicates no accumulation, as

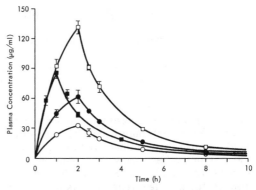

FIG. 1. *Plasma concentration of 6059-S during and after intravenous slow infusion in healthy volunteers (n = 4, cross-over). Symbols:* ○, *0.5 g/2 h;* ●, *1 g/2 h;* □, *2 g/2 h;* ■, *1 g/1 h.*

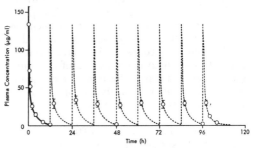

FIG. 2. *Plasma concentration of 6059-S after multiple intravenous injection in healthy volunteers (1 g every 12 h; n = 5). Symbols:* ——, *fitted curve;* ...., *simulation curve;* ○, *observed value.*

shown in Fig. 2, and it is in good agreement with the observed plasma concentration. From these results, no change and no accumulation were observed in plasma concentration after intravenous multiple injections of 1 g at every 12 h for the 5-day period.

Equations for prediction of plasma level of 6059-S in adults with normal renal function were derived by using the pharmacokinetic parameters obtained from the studies mentioned above. The predicted plasma levels using the equations were in agreement with actual plasma concentrations of 6059-S observed in other volunteer studies. This agreement supports use of these simple models for analyzing the plasma concentration of 6059-S.

1. **Narisada, M., T. Yoshida, H. Onoue, M. Ohtani, T. Okada, T. Tsuji, I. Kikkawa, N. Haga, H. Satoh, H. Itani, and W. Nagata.** 1979. Synthetic studies on β-lactam antibiotics. 10. Synthesis of 7β-[2-carboxy-2-(4-hydroxyphenyl)-acetamido]-7α-methoxy-3-[[(1-methyl-1H-tetrazol-5-yl)-thio]-methyl]-1-oxa-1-dethia-3-cephem-4-carboxylic acid disodium salt (6059-S) and its related 1-oxacephem. J. Med. Chem. **22:**757–759.

Clinical Evaluation of 6059-S, a New Active Oxacephem

KEIZO MATSUMOTO,* YOSHIO UZUKA, TSUYOSHI NAGATAKE, AND HARUMI SHISHIDO

Department of Internal Medicine, Institute for Tropical Medicine, Nagasaki University, Nagasaki 852, Japan

Since it is well recognized that the side-chain modification of naturally occurring antibiotics could improve their antibacterial and pharmacological properties, many new semisynthetic penicillins and cephalosporins have been developed. In the past few years, efforts have been made to modify the penicillin and cephalosporin "nuclei" themselves. 6059-S, an oxacephem newly synthesized by Shionogi & Co., Osaka, Japan, is the first compound that has a new cephalosporin-like nucleus; it has broad antibacterial activity and high stability against β-lactamase. This compound has several side chains, such as 7-methoxy-, 4-hydroxyphenyl-, and D-α-carboxyphenyl groups, which have been recently developed through studies of structure-activity relationships. These new side chains seem to give superior antibacterial and pharmacological properties to the compound. Therefore, we performed the following studies to evaluate the clinical applications of 6059-S.

In vitro susceptibility tests. The in vitro antibacterial activity against 159 respiratory pathogenic organisms was measured by the agar dilution method and compared with activities of the older cephalosporins and penicillins. All isolates were causative organisms of lower respiratory tract infections as determined by our quantitative sputum culture method. 6059-S was less active than the other cephalosporins and penicillins against *Streptococcus pneumoniae*, but inhibited most isolates of *S. pneumoniae* at concentrations of less than 3.13 μg/ml. Only one of 50 isolates was resistant to 6059-S and was inhibited at a concentration of 50 μg/ml.

Against the other respiratory pathogens tested in this study, 6059-S was more active than the other cephalosporins and penicillins. Thirty-one isolates of *Haemophilus influenzae*, 27 isolates of *Klebsiella pneumoniae*, and 10 isolates of *Escherichia coli* were inhibited at concentrations 0.20 μg/ml or less. Therefore, against these species, 6059-S was 8- to 256-fold more active than cefazolin, cephaloridine, and other compounds tested. The MICs of 6059-S against 33 isolates of *Pseudomonas aeruginosa* ranged from 1.56 to 50 μg/ml; against 8 isolates of *Enterobacter* species, MICs ranged from 6.25 to 50 μg/ml. From these results, it was concluded that 6059-S was less active against isolates of gram-positive bacteria than were the older cephalosporins, but much more active against isolates of gram-negative bacteria. 6059-S inhibited almost all isolates of respiratory pathogenic bacteria at clinically available concentrations.

Clinical studies. 6059-S was given to 54 patients. Four had acute bronchitis, 15 had pneumonia, 17 had chronic bronchitis, 4 had chronic bronchiolitis, 4 had bronchiectasis, 2 had meningitis, 1 had sepsis, 5 had acute cholecystitis, and 2 had urinary tract infections. The dosage level was 0.25 to 3 g administered intravenously two or three times a day, and most of the patients were administered less than 2 g daily, which was two- to threefold less than the ordinary dose of cefazolin.

Pharmacokinetic study. The concentrations of 6059-S in serum, urine, sputum, and cerebrospinal fluid were measured in nine patients by a cup-plate assay procedure, using *E. coli* 7437. A dose of 1 g administered intravenously in 5 min resulted in serum peak concentrations of 92 to 103 μg/ml; 2 g infused in 60 min resulted in serum peak concentrations of 141 to 176 μg/ml. The serum half-lives of 6059-S ranged from 100 to 145 min; this value is one of the longest of all cephalosporins and penicillins. Total urinary recovery of administered doses ranged from 68 to 93% (0 to 8 h and 0 to 12 h). The sputum peak levels reached 1.8 to 2.1 μg/ml, and the ratio of sputum peak levels to serum peak levels ranged from 1.4 to 2.3% in four patients (1). A dose of 3 g infused intravenously in 60 min resulted in a cerebrospinal fluid concentration of 4.1 μg/ml at 30 min after administration in a patient with meningitis due to *H. influenzae*.

From theses results, it was concluded that the pharmacokinetic properties of 6059-S were similar to those of cefazolin, and correlation with the results of in vitro studies suggested that 6059-S would inhibit most gram-positive and gram-negative bacteria at these doses.

Clinical results. Clinical cures were obtained in 40 (93%) of 43 patients with respiratory tract infections and in all 10 patients with meningitis, sepsis, cholecystitis, or urinary tract infections (Table 1). In one patient with bronchiectasis, clinical efficacy was not determined because the treatment was stopped after only 1 day due to

TABLE 1. *Clinical response to 6059-S treatment*

Diagnosis	No. of cases	No. with response of:					% of satisfactory clinical response
		Excellent	Good	Fair	Poor	Undetermined	
Respiratory tract infections	44	8	32	1	2	1	93
Acute bronchitis	4	1	3				100
Acute pneumonia	15	4	10		1		93
Chronic bronchitis	17	1	15	1			94
Chronic bronchiolitis	4	2	2				100
Bronchiectasis	4		2		1	1	67
Meningitis	2	1	1				100
Sepsis	1		1				100
Acute cholecystitis	5		5				100
Urinary tract infection	2	1	1				100
Total	54	10	40	1	2	1	94

TABLE 2. *Bacteriological response to 6059-S treatment*

Species	No. of strains	No. of strains:				% of bacteriological cure
		Eradicated	Decreased	Persisting	Superinfecting	
Staphylococcus aureus	2	2				100
Streptococcus pneumoniae	7	7				100
Streptococcus haemolyticus	1	1				100
Streptococcus faecalis	1				1	0
Haemophilus influenzae	27	27				100
Haemophilus parahaemolyticus	1	1				100
Escherichia coli	4	4				100
Klebsiella pneumoniae	5	4	1			100
Enterobacter cloacae	1	1				100
Serratia marcescens	2	2				100
Pseudomonas aeruginosa	3			2	1	0
Total	54	44	1	2	2	93

skin rash, but his pathogenic bacteria, *H. influenzae* and *Serratia marcescens*, were eradicated. Three patients who showed fair or poor clinical response were associated with bacteriological failures; i.e., the organisms were resistant before the therapy, or superinfections of resistant organisms developed. One tracheostomized patient with pneumonia and cerebral bleeding responded poorly to 6059-S treatment because of persisting *P. aeruginosa* infection (MIC, 12.5 µg/ml) and superinfection with *S. faecalis*. Another patient with chronic bronchitis was partially respondent because the superinfection with *P. aeruginosa* (MIC, 50 µg/ml) occurred after eradication of the initial pathogen, *H. influenzae*. The other patient with bronchiectasis responded poorly because of persisting *P. aeruginosa* infection (MIC, 25 µg/ml). All causative bacteria isolated from 44 patients with clinical cure were eradicated. Forty-nine (96%) of 51 initial infecting bacteria were eradicated,

but superinfection occurred in two patients (Table 2).

Clinical effects were excellent in 10 patients, good in 40, fair in 1, poor in 2, and undetermined in 1.

Skin rash and mild eosinophilia were observed in one patient, and mild elevation of serum transaminases was observed in two. Adverse reactions were less frequent than with other cephalosporins such as cefazolin and cephaloridine.

From this study, it is concluded that 6059-S is one of the most effective and useful antibiotics for the treatment of both gram-positive and gram-negative bacterial infections.

1. **Matsumoto, K., and Y. Uzuka.** 1976. Concentrations of antibiotics in bronchiolar secretions of the patients with chronic respiratory infections, p. 73–76. *In* J. D. Williams and A. M. Geddes (ed.), Chemotherapy, vol. 4. Plenum Publishing Co., New York.

Pharmacokinetic Studies and Results of a Clinical Trial with Cefotaxime (HR-756)

DIETMAR H. WITTMANN,* HANS H. SCHASSAN, AND VOLKER FREITAG

I. Department of Surgery and Department of Bacteriology, Hamburg Altona General Hospital, and Institute of Immunology and Medical Bacteriology, University of Hamburg, Hamburg, Federal Republic of Germany

The aim of the present pharmacokinetic study as well as the clinical trial with 121 patients was to assess the concentrations of cefotaxime (HR-756) in the serum and various peripheral compartments and to correlate these data with the inhibitory concentrations for the less susceptible pathogens and the clinical results. Cefotaxime was chosen because of its marked stability to most β-lactamases and its good antimicrobial spectrum against almost all pathogenic bacteria, including a certain activity against *Pseudomonas aeruginosa* and *Streptococcus faecalis*.

All pharmacokinetic studies were conducted on hospitalized patients, under therapeutic conditions.

Serum. The antimicrobial concentration in the serum after intravenous bolus injection of 2 g of cefotaxime was determined in 43 patients with a mean age of 61 years (Fig. 1). The average level after 30 min was 81 mg/liter and after 60 min was 41 mg/liter. After 8 h a concentration of 1.7 mg/liter was observed, and after 12 h the concentration was 0.3 mg/liter.

Bone. Bone samples were obtained from 19 patients undergoing hip joint replacement surgery. Special care was taken not to contaminate the bone sample with blood, and samples with measurable hemoglobin content were excluded from the calculations. At 30 to 60 min after administration of 2 g of cefotaxime, the bone level was 5.4 mg/kg for cortical and spongious bone. By 2 h after the injection the concentration decreased to 4.4 mg/kg in spongiosa and to 2.1 mg/kg in corticalis.

At this concentration achieved in bone, 100% of our *Klebsiella* sp., *Proteus mirabilis*, and penicillin-susceptible *Staphylococcus aureus* and 89 to 100% of the penicillin-resistant *S. aureus* strains were inhibited. The mean values for *Escherichia coli*, indole-positive *Proteus*, and *Enterobacter* sp. were 68 to 87%. Only 14% of *P. aeruginosa* and *S. faecalis* were inhibited at the highest concentration achieved in bone.

Altogether, the concentration achieved in bone was sufficient to inhibit the typical bacteria causing bone infections. The results of our clinical trial correspond well with these data. Nine patients were treated with satisfactory results.

All bacteria, including one strain of *P. aeruginosa* and one of *S. faecalis*, were eliminated by therapy with cefotaxime.

Tissue fluid. Tissue fluid is defined as the secretion in postsurgical wounds after hip joint replacement arthroplasty. The fluid was collected by suction from the chamber around the polyethylene cup from the first postoperation day onwards when further hematoma formation was unlikely. We have evidence that this fluid is similar to that obtained from subcutaneously implanted tissue cages. A total of 117 samples from 17 patients were collected at 2-h intervals. Samples with a hematocrit of more than 5% were rejected. The peak concentration of 20.8 mg/liter was achieved after 2.3 h. One-fourth of this concentration was maintained for 7.6 h in this fluid. All of the isolates of most pathogens were inhibited at this concentration. From 71 to 90% of the isolates of indole-positive *Proteus*, *E. coli*, and *Enterobacter* sp. were inhibited. The rate of inhibition for *S. faecalis* was 12 to 54%, and for *P. aeruginosa* it was 12 to 32%.

These findings correspond well with the results of our clinical trial. Of 30 patients with soft tissue infection, 29 were cured. In two cases *S. faecalis* was isolated after therapy without any sign of infection. Three cases of infection due to *P. aeruginosa* were successfully treated. The other organisms most commonly isolated before

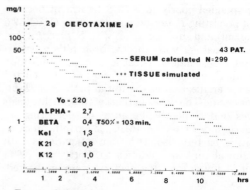

FIG. 1. *Calculated serum concentration after intravenous bolus injection of 2 g of cefotaxime (open two-compartment model).*

therapy were *S. aureus* (16 times), *Streptococcus* sp. (9 times), *Proteus* sp. (4 times), *Klebsiella* sp. (2 times), and anaerobes (3 cases).

Peritoneal fluid. In this study peritoneal fluid is defined as the fluid secreted through the transcutaneous drainage tubes from the peritoneal cavity after abdominal surgery. Most of the samples were obtained from patients with chemical peritonitis after ulcer perforation. Sampling was carried out in eight patients at 1-h intervals.

For the 2-g dosage the concentration as a function of time is shown in Fig. 2. After the mean calculated time of 2.4 h, the peak concentration reached 28.6 mg/liter. During 6.5 h 25% of the maximal concentration was maintained in this fluid.

With this concentration, 100% of *Klebsiella* sp., *P. mirabilis*, and penicillin-susceptible and -resistant *S. aureus* were inhibited. The percentages were 71 to 89% for *E. coli* and indole-positive *Proteus* as well as for *Enterobacter* sp., 12 to 54% for *S. faecalis*, and 12 to 31% for *P. aeruginosa*.

These pharmacokinetic data correlate with the results of the clinical trial. Seventeen patients were treated for severe diffuse secondary peritonitis. After therapy three strains of *Enterobacter* sp. and *E. coli* were isolated in the patients who were not cured. *S. faecalis* infection was treated successfully once. In one patient *Pseudomonas aeruginosa* was the cause of the therapeutic failure.

T-drain bile. Hourly samples were taken in 18 patients 176 times and were frozen with phosphate buffer immediately after sampling before being assayed. The half-life in bile was 118 min,

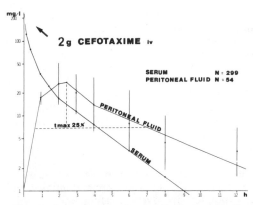

FIG. 2. *Serum and peritoneal fluid concentration after intravenous bolus injection of 2 g of cefotaxime. One-fourth of the peak concentration achieved is indicated by t max 25%. The serum samples were from 43 patients, and the peritoneal fluid samples were from 8 patients.*

the concentrations being 15.4 mg/liter after 2 h, 4.7 mg/liter after 4 h, and 1.2 mg/liter after 10 h. One-fourth of the peak concentration was maintained for 3.4 h. This time was shorter than that observed with tissue fluid and peritoneal fluid. The explanation for this is that no rediffusion into the serum took place; the bile was excreted directly.

At the concentrations found between the peak and 25% of the peak, most pathogens were inhibited. The inhibition of *E. coli* ranged from 86 to 89%; 79 to 92% of indole-positive *Proteus*, 75 to 82% of *Enterobacter* sp., and of 18 to 68% of *S. faecalis* strains were inhibited. In *P. aeruginosa* infection (18 to 35% of the strains were inhibited in bile with 2 g intravenously), a higher dosage was necessary. In our clinical trial with cefotaxime all 17 patients with severe biliary infections were treated successfully.

Clinical trial. A group of 121 patients were treated with 2 g of cefotaxime every 12 h. The mean age was 55 years, and the average duration of therapy was 10 days. One patient received cefotaxime for 67 days without any side effect. The indications for antibiotic treatment were (i) severe pneumonia with positive X-ray findings in 25 patients, (ii) severe soft tissue infections in 10 patients and ENT infections in 20 patients, (iii) urinary tract infections (UTI) in 20 patients (pyelonephritis in 7, acute UTI in 8, and UTI after prostatectomy in 5), (iv) secondary osteomyelitis in 8 patients and empyema of the shoulder joint in 1, (v) severe secondary peritonitis after perforation of the alimentary tract in 17 patients, and (vi) biliary tract infections with septicemia in 17 patients. Allergic skin reactions developed in four patients between the 6th and 10th days of therapy. In one patient colitis proven by fiberscope colonoscopy developed after therapy. *Clostridium novii* was isolated from the stools, but we failed to find an antitoxin. The patient recovered. Other side effects such as thrombocytosis (six times), elevation of liver enzymes (six times), and alkaline phosphatase (four times) could not be clearly related to cefotaxime therapy.

E. coli was the most commonly isolated organism, being found 13 times in peritonitis, 10 times in UTI, 8 times in biliary infections, and once in pneumonia, soft tissue infection (STI) and bone and joint infections. After therapy, this organism was isolated from 7 patients. In 4 of these it was responsible for therapeutic failures. *S. aureus* was isolated from 19 patients before therapy, mostly in STI and bone and joint infections. All of these patients were treated successfully. *S. faecalis* was isolated from 17 patients before therapy and was responsible for 3 therapeutic failures. *P. aeruginosa,* isolated from 10 patients before therapy, was treated successfully in 5. It had been a problem in our UTI since 4 failures were due to this organism. However, all 4 patients had severe coincidental diseases such as leukemia and paraplegia and 1 had a vesical stone. *Enterobacter* sp. was isolated 5 times (4 in peritonitis and 1 in UTI) and was responsible for therapeutic failures in 3 cases of peritonitis, once together with *Bacteroides fragilis.* All other infections due to anaerobes, *Proteus* sp., *Klebsiella* sp., *Streptococcus* sp., *Diplococcus pneumoniae, Neisseria* sp., and other organisms were treated successfully. Satisfactory results were obtained in 100% of biliary, ENT, and bone and joint infections. Results were satisfactory in 90% of the soft tissue infections, 88% of the pneumonias, 76% of the peritonitises, and 70% of the UTI. The quick disappearance of the inflammatory symptoms was remarkable.

In summary cefotaxime fulfilled most of the promises of earlier bacteriological investigations as the most active cephalosporin tested to date. Low toxicity, good pharmacokinetic behavior, and high cure rates are characteristics of this antibiotic. In the case of infections due to *P. aeruginosa* and *S. faecalis,* a higher dosage of 4 to 6 g every 12 h is advised.

Pharmacokinetic Parameters of Cefotaxime After Intravenous and Intramuscular Administration of Single and Multiple Doses

IRWIN HO,* PRASIT ASWAPOKEE, KWUNG P. FU, CHARLES MATTHIJSSEN, AND HAROLD C. NEU

Department of Medical Research, Hoechst-Roussel Pharmaceuticals, Inc., Somerville, New Jersey 08876, and Division of Infectious Diseases, Department of Medicine and Pharmacology, College of Physicians and Surgeons, Columbia University, New York, New York 10032, U.S.A.

Cefotaxime (HR-756) is a new cephalosporin antibiotic with an unusually broad spectrum of antibacterial activity that includes both gram-positive and -negative aerobic and anaerobic bacteria (1). The pharmacokinetic properties of cefotaxime were studied in normal subjects after intravenous and intramuscular administration of the drug. Serum and urine samples were assayed by the agar dilution technique, with a susceptible strain of *Escherichia coli* (≥0.16 µg/ml) as assay organism.

Intravenous injection—single dose. Fifteen normal males were given 500, 1,000, and 2,000 mg of cefotaxime intravenously by random allocation according to a Latin-square design with a 1-week period between study days. All doses were injected over a period of 5 min. Blood samples were collected at 0 min (just prior to injection) and at 5, 15, 30, 45, 60, 90, 120, 180, and 240 min after the start of the injection. Total urine specimens were collected before the drug was injected and at intervals ending at 2, 4, 6, 12, and 24 h after the start of the injection.

The serum levels were evaluated kinetically by use of a first-order, two-compartment, open model. To account for the brief injection time, the coefficients of the model were adjusted for calculating the kinetic parameters. For urinary concentrations of cefotaxime, the cumulative amounts of unchanged drug, the percentage of the administered dose recovered, and the renal clearance were calculated. Nonlinear weighted regression analysis was used to fit the serum levels. The weight was the inverse of the squared serum level. The univariate analysis of variance for a Latin-square design was employed to compare the mean differences among the dose groups.

The estimates for the pharmacokinetic parameters are given in Table 1. Of the 15 normal males who participated in this study, 4 were excluded from the analysis as a result of failure to complete various aspects of the study. After adjusting the exact dose given to each subject, the mean serum peaks were 38.9 ± 2.2 µg/ml for 500 mg, 101.7 ± 7.4 µg/ml for 1,000 mg, and 214.4 ± 17.3 µg/ml for 2,000 mg. The alpha-phase half-lives for the three dose groups ranged from 3.9 to 26.1 min. The mean alpha-phase half-life was 1 h for all three doses. Total serum clearances for all doses were similar and did not change with dose. The peak serum levels, the area under the curve (AUC) between zero and infinity, and the total urinary levels of cefotaxime showed a linear relationship for the three dose groups, indicating that the kinetics of cefotaxime were independent of dose. The average overall urinary recovery of unchanged drug was 50 to 60%. Differences among the mean values generally occurred only between the 500-mg group and

TABLE 1. *Pharmacokinetic parameters of cefotaxime administered by rapid (5-min) infusion (mean ± SE)*

Parameter	Dose (mg)		
	500	1,000	2,000
Peak level, μg/ml	37.9 ± 2.1	102.4 ± 9.9	214.1 ± 18.7
Level at 4 h, μg/ml	1.0 ± 0.1	1.9 ± 0.1	3.3 ± 0.4
Area under curve, μg/ml per h	30.6 ± 2.2	70.4 ± 3.9	134.1 ± 8.4
		$(35.6)^a$	$(34.4)^a$
Elimination rate constant, h^{-1}	0.69 ± 0.04	0.68 ± 0.03	0.84 ± 0.05
K_{12}, h^{-1}	1.71 ± 0.44	0.79 ± 0.15	1.56 ± 0.28
K_{21}, h^{-1}	2.41 ± 0.45	1.22 ± 0.09	2.18 ± 0.32
K_{10}, h^{-1}	1.46 ± 0.08	1.66 ± 0.13	1.87 ± 0.17
Alpha-phase half-life, h	0.19 ± 0.03	0.26 ± 0.03	0.18 ± 0.03
Beta-phase half-life, h	1.04 ± 0.07	1.04 ± 0.06	0.86 ± 0.05
V_c, liters/1.73 m^2	11.8 ± 0.8	9.1 ± 0.7	8.5 ± 0.8
V_t, liters/1.73 m^2	7.3 ± 0.7	5.2 ± 0.8	5.5 ± 0.6
$V_{d,\,ss}$, liters/1.73 m^2	19.1 ± 1.2	14.3 ± 0.9	14.0 ± 1.0
V_d, area, liters/1.73 m^2	25.6 ± 3.0	21.8 ± 1.8	18.1 ± 0.9
Serum clearance, ml/min per 1.73 m^2	245.3 ± 19.5	206.8 ± 13.1	215.1 ± 14.1
Renal clearance, ml/min per 1.73 m^2	146.8 ± 18.6	104.0 ± 9.7	110.4 ± 10.7
Total urinary levels (24 h), mg	293.8 ± 24.8	502.9 ± 42.1	991.8 ± 71.4

^{a} Value after dose normalization.

the two higher dose groups. No significant differences were found between the 1,000- and 2,000-mg groups.

Intravenous infusion—multiple doses. Sixteen normal males were infused with 1,000 mg of cefotaxime at a constant rate over 30 min through small-bore needles. Three subjects did not complete the study and were, therefore, excluded from the analysis. Cefotaxime was administered every 6 h for 14 days, with the final dose administered on day 15. Blood samples were drawn prior to the infusion and at 25, 45, 60, 75, 90, 120, 180, and 240 min after the start of the infusion on days 1 and 15. On days 2, 3, 4, 6, and 10, blood samples were drawn 5 min before the infusion and 25 min after the start of the infusion. Urine samples were collected before the infusion, at the end of 2, 4, and 6 h on day 1, and at the same intervals as well as at the end of 12 and 24 h after the infusion on the final day. The elimination rate constant, β, was calculated by the least-squares method for the terminal points. The AUC was calculated by the trapezoidal rule. The one-factor analysis of variance with repeated measures was used to compare the mean differences between the first day and the last day. Regression analysis was used to fit the serum concentrations of each subject at 5 min prior to the start of the infusion on the days between the first and last day. A significant positive slope would indicate drug accumulation.

Significant mean differences for serum concentrations were found during the distribution phase but not the elimination phase. The mean difference between the first and last days for AUCs was 20% (57.4 μg/ml per h and 68.9 μg/ml per h, respectively). The elimination rate constants and biological half-lives did not differ significantly on days 1 and 15. The mean half-lives were 1.16 and 1.03 h, respectively. Serum clearance, renal clearance, and percentage of drug excreted in the urine were similar on days 1 and 15, i.e., 259 and 219 ml/min per 1.73 m^2, 154 and 133 ml/min per 1.73 m^2, and 59 and 61%. No trend for drug accumulation was observed during the study period. However, minimal amounts of cefotaxime (1.33 to 2.12 μg/ml) were present in the sera of all subjects on each day before the start of the first infusion.

Intramuscular injections—multiple doses. Fifteen normal males were injected intramuscularly with 500 mg of cefotaxime every 8 h for 10 days. The final dose was injected on day 11. Blood samples were drawn on day 1 and day 11 at 5 min prior to injection and 30, 60, 90, 120, 180, 240, and 360 min thereafter. On days 2, 3, 4, and 6, samples were obtained 5 min prior to, and 30 min and 60 min after, the first dose. Urine specimens were collected immediately before the injection of the drug, at the end of 2, 4, and 6 h on day 1, and at the end of 2, 4, 6, 12, and 24 h on day 11. The pharmacokinetic and statistical methods were the same as those applied to the multiple-dose infusion study.

The elimination rate constants and half-lives on day 1 and day 11 showed no significant mean differences (0.93 and 0.92 h, respectively). Differences were noted for the AUC between 0 and 8 h, the fractional serum clearance, and the renal clearance, i.e., 24 and 20 μg/ml per h, 305 and

377 ml/min per 1.73 m^2, and 194 and 147 ml/min per 1.73 m^2 on day 1 and day 11, respectively. However, these differences were within the expected range of experimental error. No trend for drug accumulation was noted. The mean serum levels at 8 h on day 2 through day 8 ranged from 0.08 to 0.55 µg/ml.

These studies demonstrate that cefotaxime given by intravenous infusion every 6 h or by intramuscular injection provided serum and urine levels well in excess of the concentrations needed to inhibit the majority of clinically important bacteria for which this agent would be appropriate therapy (1).

1. Neu, H. C., N. Aswapokee, P. Aswapokee, and K. P. Fu. 1979. HR 756, a new cephalosporin active against gram-positive and gram-negative aerobic and anaerobic bacteria. Antimicrob. Agents Chemother. **15**:273–381.

Comparison of the Activity of the Desacetyl Metabolite of Cefotaxime (HR-756) with That of Cefotaxime and Other Cephalosporins

RICHARD WISE,* JENNIFER M. ANDREWS, DOROTHY HAMMOND, PETER J. WILLS, ALISDAIR M. GEDDES, AND MICHAEL W. McKENDRICK

Department of Medical Microbiology, Dudley Road Hospital, and Department of Communicable and Tropical Diseases, East Birmingham Hospital, Birmingham, England*

The novel cephalosporin cefotaxime (HR-756, CEF) has been shown by in vitro studies to be a potent antimicrobial (1) and is at present under clinical evaluation. It is known that CEF, like cephalothin, undergoes desacetylation in vivo, but unlike cephalothin, the desacetyl cefotaxime (DES) is said to have antibacterial activity. From our clinical and pharmacological studies it appears that the serum levels of DES 15 min after an intravenous injection are 10 to 20% of the concomitant levels of CEF (Fig. 1). As the apparent serum half-life of DES is longer than that of CEF, about 4 h postadministration the levels of DES are greater than those of CEF. Approximately 30 to 40% of the administered dose is excreted as DES. It is therefore important to understand the antimicrobial activity of both compounds, as the DES metabolite will contribute a significant proportion of the activity of an administered dose of CEF.

In this study the activities of CEF and DES were compared with those of three other cephem compounds, cefazolin, cefuroxime, and cefoxitin.

The 60 strains tested were all recent clinical isolates identified by the API (API Laboratory Products Ltd., Farnborough, United Kingdom) method.

Susceptibility testing was performed by an agar dilution procedure using Isosensitest agar, pH 7.2 (Oxoid, Basingstoke, United Kingdom) as previously described (1) and with two inocula, 10^3 and 10^6 colony-forming units (CFU) per µl of inoculum.

Table 1 summarizes the results obtained with the five antimicrobials when they were tested at an inoculum of 10^3 CFU.

It is interesting to note that DES was consistently more active than cefoxitin, cefuroxime, or cefazolin against these strains but about one-tenth as active as the parent compound. In particular, DES was 10- to 20-fold more active than cefazolin, cefoxitin, and cefuroxime against *Proteus mirabilis*. The susceptibility of the indole-positive *Proteus* spp. to DES was more variable: the MIC for one strain of *Proteus morganii* was 128 µg/ml but for another it was 0.5 µg/ml. Two strains of *Enterobacter* spp. (MIC of DES, 0.5 and 1 µg/ml), three strains of *Providencia stuartii* (MIC of DES, 2, 0.06, and 0.06 µg/ml) and two strains of *Serratia marcescens* (MIC of DES, 0.5 and 1 µg/ml) were more susceptible to DES than to cefoxitin, cefuroxime, and cefazolin. The 10 strains of *P. aeruginosa* were uniformly resistant to DES, yet they were moderately susceptible to CEF.

Although the activity of CEF against *Staphylococcus aureus* was comparable to that of cefoxitin and cefuroxime, DES was considerably less active. One strain of *Streptococcus pneumoniae* was susceptible to 0.06 µg of DES/ml, one strain of *S. pyogenes* (Lancefield group A) was susceptible to 0.03 µg/ml, and one strain of Lancefield group D streptococcus was inhibited by >128 µg/ml.

The 10 strains of *Bacteroides fragilis* showed a wide variability of susceptibility to DES and CEF, more consistent activity being noted with cefoxitin.

TABLE 1. *MICs of five antimicrobials tested against 60 clinical isolates at an inoculum of 10^3 CFU*

Organism (no. of strains tested)	Geometric mean MIC (μg/ml)[a]				
	Cefotaxime	Desacetyl cefotaxime	Cefoxitin	Cefuroxime	Cefazolin
E. coli (10)	0.056 (0.03–0.12)	0.5 (0.25–1)	1.46 (1–2)	1.6 (1–4)	1.0
Klebsiella spp. (10)	0.053 (0.015–0.25)	0.15	1 (0.5–2)	1.74 (0.25–16)	2.8 (1–128)
Proteus mirabilis (5)	0.019 (0.015–0.03)	0.09 (0.06–0.12)	2.0	1.0	1.8 (1–2)
Indole-positive *Proteus* spp. (5)	0.04 (0.015–0.5)	1.5 (0.12–128)	2.8 (1–4)	16 (4–64)	90 (64–256)
P. aeruginosa (10)	8.6 (4–32)	>128	>128	>128	>128
S. aureus (10)	1.6 (1–4)	24.3 (8–64)	2.3 (2–4)	1.1 (0.25–2)	0.3 (0.12–1)
B. fragilis (10)	4 (1–64)	12.9 (2–256)	5.6 (4–16)	8 (4–128)	26 (4–256)

[a] The range is given in parentheses.

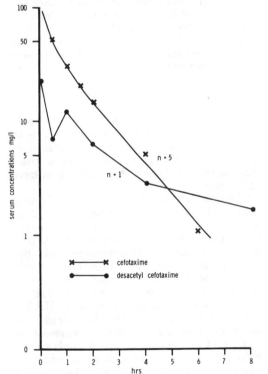

FIG. 1. *Serum levels of cefotaxime and desacetyl cefotaxime.*

An increase in inoculum to 10^6 CFU was accompanied generally by a zero- to twofold decrease in susceptibility to DES among the *Esch-*

erichia coli, Klebsiella, and *Proteus mirabilis* strains tested, although approximately 50% of such strains were known β-lactamase producers, as ascertained by the nitrocefin test. This indicated that DES possesses stability to the β-lactamase of these organisms. The two strains of *Proteus morganii* susceptible to DES at the inoculum of 10^3 CFU were resistant (MIC, >128 μg/ml) at the higher inoculum.

It therefore appears that, although CEF is biologically less stable than many other compounds of this class, the desacetyl metabolite itself exhibits an in vitro antimicrobial activity against the clinically important gram-negative pathogens comparable to that of the recently introduced compounds cefoxitin and cefuroxime. It is interesting to note that in those pathogens which are relatively less susceptible to CEF (*S. aureus, B. fragilis,* and *P. aeruginosa*) the desacetyl metabolite shows little clinically useful activity.

It is possible that in certain diseases, for example, renal failure, or in certain organs where the desacetyl metabolite is concentrated, such as the biliary tree (M. W. McKendrick, A. M. Geddes, and R. Wise, Antimicrob. Agents Chemother., in press), the activity of this metabolite may assume considerable clinical importance.

1. **Wise, R., T. Rollason, M. N. Logan, J. M. Andrews, and K. A. Bedford.** 1978. HR756, a highly active cephalosporin: comparison with cefazolin and carbenicillin. Antimicrob. Agents Chemother. **14:**807–811.

Penetration of HR-756 (Cefotaxime) in Lung Tissu e and Bronchial Secretions

G. GIALDRONI GRASSI,* R. DIONIGI, A. FERRARA, AND E. POZZI

University of Pavia, Pavia, Italy

The presence of adequate concentrations of antibiotic at the site of infection is considered necessary to achieve a therapeutic result. Hence, there is a growing interest in the pharmacokinetics of antibacterial drugs. A number of studies have been devoted to the determination of the antibiotic concentrations that can be achieved in bronchial secretions, on the assumption that efficient penetration in this area is important to obtaining therapeutic results in bronchial infections. Therefore, in pharmacokinetic studies of any new antibiotic the determination of penetration in bronchial secretions is considered useful in gaining a more complete profile of the antibiotic's behavior (3, 4).

HR-756 (cefotaxime) is a new semisynthetic derivative of cephalosporin endowed with a very high intrinsic antibacterial activity against gram-positive and gram-negative bacteria and a remarkable resistance to β-lactamases. It is the most active compound against *Enterobacteriaceae* and β-lactamase–producing *Neisseria gonorrhoeae* and *Haemophilus influenzae* (2). In the present study we determined the concentrations that HR-756 can reach in bronchial secretions, sputum, and pulmonary and bronchial tissues after administration by intravenous and intramuscular routes.

The study was performed in 30 patients (22 males, 8 females) with bronchopulmonary infections admitted to the Intensive Care Unit or to the Clinic of Respiratory Diseases. Antibiotic assays were carried out contemporaneously in serum and in bronchial secretion obtained through an inserted tracheal cannula or by fiberoptic bronchoscopy. In 12 patients the antibiotic content was measured in sputum. Patients were treated either with 2 g intravenously (as a bolus injection) or with 1 g intramuscularly every 8 h. Samples of serum and bronchial secretions were taken at 15 and 30 min and at 1, 2, 4, 6, and 8 h after one single intravenous or intramuscular injection or at the same time intervals after administration of 1 g intramuscularly every 8 h. Sputum specimens were collected at 2-h intervals and more frequently in the case of intravenous injections. All of them were frankly mucopurulent. They were homogenized mechanically by means of a Stomacher apparatus and kept at −22°C until assayed. Antibiotic assay was performed by the cup plate method of Grove and Randall (1), with *Escherichia coli* ISM as test microorganism. The sensitivity of the method was 0.12 µg/ml.

In six patients who underwent pulmonary surgery for lung cancer, a single dose of 2 g of HR-756 was injected before operation to make it possible to obtain specimens of bronchial and pulmonary tissue 1 h after administration. The tissues were ground, diluted in buffered saline (pH 6.8), and then assayed for content of antibiotic.

The results are shown in Table 1. After administration of 2 g intravenously, very high serum levels were achieved, the peak being at 15 min with mean values of 266.6 µg/ml. After intramuscular injection of 1 g, the peak was reached after 30 min to 1 h. Peaks in bronchial secretions and sputum were usually obtained 2 h after intravenous injection, whereas after intramuscular administration they were usually reached after 2 to 4 h. Antibiotic assay performed after four doses of 1 g intramuscularly at 8-h intervals did not reveal any substantial modifications in serum concentrations, but in bronchial secretions there was a tendency to have higher peaks.

The bronchial secretion/tissue ratio shows a clear tendency to increase with time, that is, when serum concentrations were at the lowest levels (from 0.01 to 0.02 at 30 min to 0.25 to 0.53 at 8 h). In bronchial and pulmonary tissues the contents of antibiotic were high, being a little more elevated in bronchial than in pulmonary tissue (a mean value of 7.5 µg/g versus 5.3 µg/g).

Conclusions. The concentrations of HR-756 found in bronchial secretions after intramuscular or intravenous administration represent, as do those of all other cephalosporins, only a small percentage of the concentrations in serum. In any case, however, they are in the range of concentrations active on the common respiratory pathogens as well as on many *Enterobacteriaceae, Providencia, Serratia*, and, to a certain extent, on *Pseudomonas aeruginosa* organisms. If we consider the high intrinsic antibacterial activity of HR-756, peak concentrations achieved in bronchial secretions were manyfold higher than the MIC (approximately 5- to 20-fold higher) for the susceptible strains, and even the trough levels were superior to the MIC.

Even if at lower levels the curve of drug con-

TABLE 1. *Mean concentrations of HR-756 in serum, bronchial secretions, and sputum after administration by the intravenous or intramuscular route*

Time (h)	Mean concn (μg/ml) after indicated treatment[a]									Ratios[b]					
	Serum			Bronchial secretions			Sputum			B/S			Sp/S		
	A	B	C	A	B	C	A	B	C	A	B	C	A	B	C
0.25	266 ±82.6			0.24 ±0.33						0.0009					
0.5	137 ±61.3	33.9 ±11.3	31.8 ±8.7	1.52 ±1.4	0.28 ±0.26	0.58 ±0.41	0.17 ±0.20			0.01	0.008	0.02	0.001		
1	105 ±50.5	26.9 ±8.3	27.6 ±6.5	2.96 ±1.65	0.74 ±0.38	0.96 ±0.38	1.19 ±1.01			0.03	0.03	0.03	0.01		
2	48 ±26.8	17.5 ±3.9	17.2 ±4.2	1.60 ±0.7	1.58 ±1.37	2.46 ±0.94	2.91 ±2.08	0.25[c] ±0.30	0.46[c] ±0.23	0.03	0.09	0.14	0.06	0.01	0.02
4	22.5 ±9	8.2 ±3.1	7.6 ±2.2	0.94 ±0.40	1.52 ±0.97	2.30 ±0.99	1.34 ±1.31	1.33[c] ±0.43	2.80[c] ±0.89	0.04	0.18	0.30	0.05	0.16	0.34
6	3.19 ±2.1	3.3 ±8.6	3.2 ±1	0.48 ±0.34	0.80 ±0.44	0.86 ±0.48	0.29 ±0.10	1.30[c] ±0.88	1.46[c] ±0.55	0.15	0.24	0.26	0.09	0.39	0.45
8	0.68 ±0.4	1.2 ±0.4	0.79 ±0.4	0.17 ±0.28	0.37 ±0.23	0.42 ±0.28	0.12 ±0.11	0.30[c] ±0.26	0.84[c] ±0.44	0.25	0.31	0.53	0.17	0.25	1.06

[a] Treatment groups were as follows: (A) 2 g intravenously; (B) 1 g intramuscularly; (C) 1 g intramuscularly every 8 h (assay performed after the fourth administration). Concentrations in serum are for 10 patients in each treatment group; those in bronchial secretions are for 7 patients in treatment group A, 6 patients in group B, and 5 patients in group C; and those in sputum are for 3 patients in group A, 4 in group B, and 5 in group C.

[b] Ratios: B/S, bronchial secretion/serum ratio; Sp/S, sputum/serum ratio.

[c] Sputum samples collected at 2-h intervals.

centrations in bronchial secretions and sputum roughly has the same trend as serum levels, nevertheless, the peak is reached with some delay and shows a certain delay in elimination, as the higher bronchial secretion/serum ratio in the last hours of observation indicate.

In the present experience the concentrations of antibiotic in bronchial secretions and sputum correlate quite well. The difference between them consists mainly in a delay in reaching the highest concentrations in sputum. It seems that, at least in this case, the determination of antibiotic concentrations in sputum, which is usually regarded as misleading, can give some reliable information. It can be observed that the increase in dosage and correspondingly in serum concentrations was followed by an increase in bronchial secretions that was not proportional to the variations observed in serum levels. It could be probably inferred from this observation that, according to the present concepts on the passage of antibiotics through the "blood-bronchus barrier," HR-756 may pass into bronchial secretions by a mechanism of active transport, which prob-

ably has a maximum capacity that cannot be surpassed. In bronchial and pulmonary tissue, however, the concentrations of HR-756 are high, demonstrating that the drug easily diffuses in bronchial and pulmonary parenchyma. It can be concluded that HR-756 promptly reaches active concentrations in secretions and parenchyma of the respiratory tract, and it can reasonably be expected that it exerts an efficacious therapeutic effect.

1. Grove, D. C., and W. A. Randall. 1955. Assay methods of antibiotics. Medical Encyclopedia, New York
2. Neu, H. C., N. Aswapokee, P. Aswapokee, and K. P. Fu. 1979. HR 756, a new cephalosporin active against gram-positive and gram-negative aerobic and anaerobic bacteria. Antimicrob. Agents Chemother. 15:273–281.
3. Pennington, J. E. 1970. Kinetics of penetration and clearance of antibiotics in respiratory secretion, p. 355–374. In C. H. Kirkpatrick and H. Y. Reynolds (ed.), Immunologic and infectious reactions in the lungs. M. Dekker Inc., New York.
4. Puchelle, E., and Q. T. Pham. 1976. La concentration en antibiotiques de la secretion bronchique au cours des traitment de l'infection respiratoire, p. 59–66. In Voisin (ed.), Sécrétions and excretions bronchiques. Expansion Scientifique Francaise, Paris.

Therapeutic Effectiveness and Pharmacokinetic Results of Cefotaxime (HR-756) in Human Infections Due to Multiresistant Bacteria

N. CLUMECK,* R. VANHOOF, Y. VANLAETHEM, AND J. P. BUTZLER

Departments of Internal Medicine and Microbiology, St. Pierre Hospital, 1000 Brussels, Belgium

The occurrence of antibiotic resistance among gram-negative bacilli is alarming. This high prevalence of isolates with grouped resistance to a large number of antibiotics has serious clinical implications, and in some patients sepsis caused by these organisms becomes nearly untreatable. The discovery of a new class of cephalosporins resistant to the β-lactamases represents, therefore, great progress. Among the new cephalo-

in a dose varying from 500 to 1,500 mg/24 h. Serum concentrations of cefotaxime were determined after administration of 1,000 or 500 mg intravenously or 500 mg intramuscularly (Table 1). For patients with normal renal function, the half-life was 1.14 h, determined after administration of 1 g intravenously. In patients with a creatinine clearance lower than 30 ml/min, the half-life was 2.64 h, determined after administra-

TABLE 1. *Serum concentrations of cefotaxime in patients with normal renal function or renal failure*

Dose (mg)	Route[a]	Creatinine clearance (ml/min)	Cefotaxime concn in serum (µg/ml)					Half-life (h)
			0.5 h	1 h	2 h	4 h	8 h	
1,000 ($n = 6$)	i.v.	Normal (>80)	46 (36–52)[b]	29 (8–34)	3 (5–23)	6 (3.6–9.4)	0.66 (0–2.1)	1.14
500 ($n = 7$)	i.m.	Normal	8.8 (3.8–13)	8.8 (4.9–15)	5.7 (2.9–9.6)	2.8 (0–6.2)	0.5 (0–2.5)	1.80
500 ($n = 5$)	i.m.	30–60	12.3 (0–24)	21.3 (15.5–31)	17.1 (13–24.5)	NT[c]	3.7 (1.5–6.7)	2.84
500 ($n = 4$)	i.v.	<30 >10	40.3 (20–87)	27.3 (21–38)	22.6 (13.5–31)	NT	5.6 (2–8.6)	2.64

[a] i.v., Intravenous; i.m., intramuscular.
[b] Mean (and range).
[c] NT, Not tested.

sporins, cefotaxime (HR-756) is probably the most potent. Indeed, in vitro studies have shown cefotaxime to be 100 to 1,000 times more active than cefuroxime and cefoxitin against cephalosporin-resistant species (1). This clinical study was undertaken to evaluate the effectiveness of this highly potent drug.

Eighteen adult patients of whom 6 had a bacteremia and 12 had a urinary tract infection (UTI) were treated with cefotaxime. The causative agents were all members of the *Enterobacteriaceae* and all were resistant to ampicillin and cephalotin. In addition, 11 strains were resistant to gentamicin and 5 were also resistant to tobramycin. One strain was resistant to all antibiotics except colistin. All isolates were susceptible to cefotaxime. Patients with UTI received 500 mg intramuscularly three times a day, and bacteremic patients received 2 to 4 g per day intravenously. Nine patients with renal failure (serum creatinine > 1.2 mg/100 ml) received cefotaxime

tion of 500 mg intravenously. In 16 patients the infection was cured, and 2 patients improved. In one case a colonization with *Pseudomonas aeruginosa* occurred. No cefotaxime resistance developed during treatment. In all nine patients with renal failure, renal function remained stable during treatment. In one patient without renal failure, renal function was impaired transiently. In conclusion, cefotaxime is a very potent antibiotic which has been life saving in hospitalized patients infected with multiresistant *Enterobacteriaceae*. Since an extended and uncontrolled use of antibiotics leads to the emergence of resistant strains, it is advisable to reserve the use of cefotaxime for life-threatening infections due to multiresistant *Enterobacteriaceae*.

1. **Hamilton-Miller, J. M. T., W. Brumfit, and A. V. Reynolds.** 1978. Cefotaxime, a new cephalosporin with exceptional broad-spectrum activity in vitro. J. Antimicrob. Chemother. 4:437–444.

Clinical Experience with Cefotaxime (HR-756)

MICHAEL W. McKENDRICK,* ALISDAIR M. GEDDES, AND RICHARD WISE

East Birmingham and Dudley Road Hospitals, Birmingham, England

Cefotaxime is a new semisynthetic cephalosporin antibiotic for parenteral use. It is resistant to hydrolysis by many β-lactamases and has a broad spectrum, with a particularly high degree of activity against gram-negative organisms. Its spectrum is remarkable in including many problem organisms such as *Pseudomonas aeruginosa* and *Serratia marcesens* (2).

We have studied 61 patients treated with cefotaxime of whom 58 had acute bacterial sepsis. The patients were aged between 16 and 88 years and all were treated in hospital. Fifty-four had a positive bacterial isolate, and seven patients with clinical and radiological evidence of bacterial pneumonia were also included. Twenty-five patients had septicemia, 18 had renal tract infection, 13 had respiratory tract infection, 2 had intra-abdominal sepsis, 1 had skin sepsis, 1 had tonsillitis, and 1 had osteomyelitis. The dosage used ranged from 0.375 to 8 g daily, the usual dose being 1 g every 8 h. *Pseudomonas* infection at sites other than the urinary tract was treated with 2 g every 6 h. The total dose for a course of treatment was between 1.87 and 56 g. All patients had routine hematological and biochemical monitoring before, during, and after treatment. Samples of serum and other body fluids were taken from selected patients to study the distribution and excretion of cefotaxime. Cefotaxime was measured by a microbiological method, using a *Proteus morganii* strain resistant to the desacetyl metabolite (see below). The metabolite was measured using high-pressure liquid chromatography. Desacetyl cefotaxime has considerable microbiological activity and is particularly active against gram-negative organisms, notable exceptions being *P. morganii* and *P. aeruginosa*. Clean venesection and rapid separation and freezing of serum samples were performed to prevent further desacetylation occurring after blood withdrawal.

Forty-two patients (71%) were clinically cured. A further eight (14%) improved clinically but remained culture positive during therapy or relapsed subsequently, and nine (15%) failed to respond to therapy. Two patients who died within 2 h of admission were unassessable.

Rapid recovery was seen in most patients on cefotaxime, particularly with infections related to the respiratory, renal, and biliary tracts. Four patients with infective endocarditis were treated, of whom one was cured (β-hemolytic streptococcus), one improved but was changed to conventional therapy at 48 h (*Staphylococcus aureus*), and two failed to respond and both required urgent cardiac surgery (*Escherichia coli* and β-hemolytic streptococcus). Seven patients were treated for *P. aeruginosa* infections. Three had asymptomatic urinary tract infections (two cured, one relapsed after treatment), two patients on ventilators had pneumonia (one improved, one died), one patient had sternal osteomyelitis after cardiac surgery (cured with surgery), and one had bronchiectasis (improved). Two patients with typhoid fever failed to respond clinically to cefotaxime by 5 and 12 days despite becoming culture negative. One failure occurred in a patient with an *E. coli* urinary tract infection, and the three others were in association with severe intra-abdominal sepsis.

All primary bacterial isolates were susceptible to cefotaxime. Forty-one of 54 strains tested were inhibited by less than 0.1 mg of cefotaxime per liter. The mean MIC for 25 strains of *E. coli* was 0.04 mg/liter, and of these, 11 were resistant or only moderately susceptible to ampicillin and 4 were resistant to co-trimoxazole. The mean MIC of eight strains of *Klebsiella aerogenes* was 0.024 mg/liter, with three strains resistant to ampicillin and one resistant to co-trimoxazole. The mean MIC of seven strains of *P. aeruginosa* was 11 mg/liter. Only one strain, a nonhemolytic streptococcus isolated from the blood of a man with cholangitis, was resistant to gentamicin (MIC of cefotaxime, 0.004 mg/liter).

Complications with cefotaxime were rarely encountered. Two patients developed a penicillin-type rash, and transient pain on intramuscular injection of 500 mg (2 ml) occurred in three. Bacterial superinfection occurred in six patients by the end of treatment (*Proteus, Pseudomonas* [two], *Enterobacter* spp., and *Streptococcus faecalis* [two]), and four of these strains were resistant to cefotaxime. Resistant strains of the infecting organism were isolated from two patients during treatment (*Pseudomonas, Acinetobacter*). Seven patients developed candidiasis, of whom four required treatment.

No serious toxicity was observed. Transient elevation of transaminases occurred in seven patients (maximum, 53 IU/liter) and of alkaline phosphatase in four (maximum, 317 IU/liter).

TABLE 1. *Levels of cefotaxime and metabolite in body fluids*

Fluid	Dose (g)	Time post-dose (h)	Cefotaxime (mg/liter)	Desacetyl cefotaxime (mg/liter)	Serum cefotaxime (mg/liter)
Common duct					
Bile	1.0	1.3	36	243	19.2
Gall bladder					
Bile	1.0	1.3	16	193	19.2
Cerebrospinal fluid	1.0	2	0	NT[a]	20
Pus	0.5	2	7.4	NT	15.5
Sputum	1.0	6	0.6–23.4	NT	<1

[a] NT, Not tested.

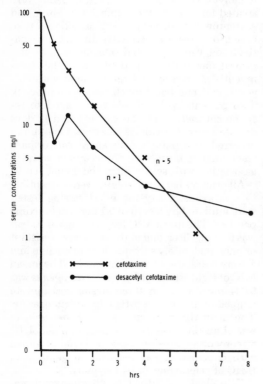

FIG. 1. *Serum levels of cefotaxime and desacetyl cefotaxime after a dose of 1 g intravenously.*

None developed a positive Coombs test, but two had mild eosinophilia (maximum, 550×10^9/liter). No deterioration in renal function occurred in any patient, including two treated concurrently with furosemide. Transient granular casts were noted in one patient and transient proteinuria was noted in another.

The serum half-life of cofotaxime in five patients with normal renal function after a dose of 1 g intravenously was 63 min, and serum levels of up to 78 mg/liter were recorded at 15 min. Serum levels >1 mg/liter were found up to 6 h, and the serum level of the desacetyl metabolite exceeded that of the parent compound by about

5 h (Fig. 1). The mean urinary recovery of cefotaxime over 6 h was 56% with levels in excess of 1,000 mg/liter at 0 to 2 h and in excess of 500 mg/liter at 2 to 4 h. Table 1 shows the level of cefotaxime and desacetyl metabolite in different body fluids. The antibacterial activity of the desacetyl metabolite is important in biliary infection as considerable concentration occurs at this site. No level of cefotaxime or metabolite was detectable in the cerebrospinal fluid of two patients with uninflamed meninges at 2 or 4 h after 1 g intravenously, although levels of 0.3 to 15 mg/liter have been reported in three patients with bacterial meningitis by Shah et al. (1). The serum half-life of cefotaxime in four volunteers after 1 g intravenously was 45 min, which compares with cefamandole, 43 min, and cefuroxime, 90 min, in the same subjects.

Cefotaxime is a safe, nontoxic antibiotic which is well tolerated intravenously. Its broad spectrum is illustrated by the fact that all primary bacterial isolates were susceptible, and it is evident from this series that it is effective in the treatment of patients with serious infection. It does have a particular weakness in lacking activity against *S. faecalis*, and though it is active in vitro against *P. aeruginosa* strains, its value in serious *Pseudomonas* infection, particularly in the immune compromised host, requires further study. Activity against *B. fragilis* is also variable, and assessment from this study is not possible. The MIC of cefotaxime against *S. aureus* is 1 to 2 mg/liter, and more active antibiotics should be used for the treatment of serious staphylococcal infection. The failure of cefotaxime in enteric fever probably reflects the intracellular nature of this infection and the lack of penetration by cefotaxime. Poor penetration of uninflamed meninges was noted, and lack of penetration may be a factor in the limited success in the treatment of endocarditis.

The place of cefotaxime in clinical practice is determined by its broad spectrum of activity. It is particularly useful for the initial treatment of serious bacterial sepsis. Therapy may then be altered, depending on clinical response, after the identification of the infecting agent (change in therapy was required in three patients in this study). The efficacy of cefotaxime in the treatment of sepsis in immune compromised hosts, where its broad spectrum would be particularly valuable, awaits further study.

1. **Shah, P. M., E. B. Helm, and W. Stille.** 1979. Clinical experience with cefotaxime, a new cephalosporin derivative. Med. Welt **30:**298–301.
2. **Wise, R., T. Rollason, J. M. Andrews, and K. A. Bedford.** 1978. HR 756, a highly active cephalosporin: comparison with cefazolin and carbenicillin. Antimicrob. Agents Chemother. **14:**807–811.

Clinical Studies with Cefotaxime

S. W. B. NEWSOM,* JULIE MATTHEWS, S. J. CONNELLAN, AND V. R. PEARCE

Addenbrooke's Hospital, Cambridge CB2 2QQ, United Kingdom

Cefotaxime (HR-756) is a parenteral cephalosporin with a broad spectrum and remarkable antibacterial activity, especially against gram-negative bacteria including β-lactamase producers. This paper reports clinical and laboratory studies with cefotaxime in 36 patients, aimed at testing the relevance of laboratory findings to clinical results, especially in chest and urinary tract infection (i) by using a range of doses and relating urine antibiotic levels to the MICs of cefotaxime for the infecting microbes and (ii) by treating chest infections with ampicillin-resistant *Haemophilus*, enterobacteria, and *Pseudomonas*.

Thirty-five patients had proven microbial infection before therapy. One patient was treated blindly for rigors, which proved to be due to raised intracranial pressure, not infection. All were given cefotaxime alone. Ages ranged from 3 to 96, and renal function ranged from normal to nil. Two were allergic to penicillin. Assays of blood, urine, sputum, cerebrospinal fluid, or pleural fluid cefotaxime levels were done as appropriate, using *Escherichia coli* as an indicator. Bacteria in sputum or urine were counted daily, the urine being taken directly into sample bottles containing β-lactamase to neutralize the cefotaxime. Fecal and throat flora were examined for cefotaxime-resistant microbes. Renal and liver function was monitored, and patients asked about the acceptability of injections.

Results. (i) Urinary tract infection. Seven patients were given two 500-mg doses intramuscularly (i.m.) each day for 5 days. *E. coli* caused five infections (four ampicillin resistant), *Klebsiella* caused one, and a Providence-enterococcal mixture caused one. All but the mixed infection cleared with rapid disappearance of bacteria and pus cells from the urine, which contained up to 9 mg of cefotaxime per ml (compared with MICs of <0.06 to 1.25 μg/ml for the infecting microbes).

Because of these high levels, 11 patients were given two 50-mg i.m. doses per day for 5 days. *E. coli* caused 10 infections (four ampicillin resistant); the 11th was due to a mixture of *Enterobacter aerogenes* and staphylococci. All but the mixed infection cleared as before, and the urine contained up to 250 μg of cefotaxime per ml (compared with MICs of <0.04 to 2.5 mg/ml for the infecting microbes). However, one patient relapsed a week later. The two immediate failures were both in mixed infections related to in-dwelling urinary catheters; the failure underlines the inadequacy of systemic antibiotics for such cases.

(ii) Chest infections. Thirteen patients received 1 g of cefotaxime three times daily by intravenous bolus doses. Six had bronchitis associated with *Haemophilus influenzae* strains, five of which were ampicillin resistant, but all were inhibited by 0.05 to 0.1 μg of cefotaxime per ml. In all six the sputum cleared rapidly, although one patient relapsed 6 weeks later. Four patients had postoperative chest infections (pneumonia-2, bronchopleural fistula, and empyema). These patients also had inhalations of cefotaxime (1 g). Two were caused by *Klebsiella*, and two were caused by *Proteus mirabilis* (MICs of 0.04 to 0.1 μg/ml). One had an associated bacteremia. All responded well. Two patients had cystic fibrosis with *Pseudomonas* chest infection. Although one improved clinically on an increased dose of 200 mg/kg (9 g per day), the improvement was not maintained, and in neither case was the infecting *Pseudomonas* in the sputum reduced in count. Treatment was changed in both cases.

(iii) Miscellaneous infections. Four miscellaneous infections included: subphrenic abscess and septicemia in a liver transplant (due to multiply antibiotic-resistant *E. coli*); perirenal abscess around a failed kidney transplant (given 500 mg daily), also caused by *E. coli*; infected heart pacemaker wires discharging *Proteus mirabilis*-laden pus in a submammary sinus (of 9 years' duration); and vulvovaginitis in a 3-year-old girl due to non-β-lactamase-producing gonococci which were resistant to penicillin (2 μg/ml) but susceptible to cefotaxime (0.1 μg/ml). Six weeks of prior therapy with cotrimoxazole and then erythromycin failed, but 3 days of cefotaxime at 50 mg/kg per day eradicated the organism.

Pharmacokinetics. Blood levels showed that the older patients had a delayed excretion; the 500-mg dose in the anephric patient produced a level of 18 μg/ml after 12 h and therefore seemed about the correct daily dose for the anuric patient. Sputum levels reached up to 3.7 μg/ml except in the two cystic fibrosis patients, in whom no cefotaxime was found. Inhalation produced levels up to 150 μg/ml in sputum.

Acceptability. Intramuscular doses above 500 mg were too painful, and on occasion patients complained of the 500-mg dose. Larger doses were those always given intravenously and were well tolerated, as were i.m. doses of 50 mg.

One patient developed transient decrease of an already poor renal function on doses of 200 mg/kg; otherwise no change in renal or liver function or in hematological parameters occurred.

Cefotaxime-resistant bacteria only rarely appeared in the throat and feces, but candida organisms were found; two patients required later therapy for oral candidiasis.

In summary, cefotaxime proved highly active against gram-negative infections (*Pseudomonas* excepted) and should be useful for therapy of β-lactamase-producing strains (especially *Haemophilus* and *Neisseria* spp.) and for infections in sites that antibiotics cannot readily penetrate, such as the bronchi, urethra, and possibly the meninges.

In Vitro, Pharmacokinetic, and Clinical Evaluation of Cefotaxime

CLAUDE REGAMEY* AND ANNE LAVANCHY

Hôpital de Zone, Aigle, and Division of Infectious Diseases, University of Geneva, Geneva, Switzerland

We compared the antibacterial activity of cefotaxime (HR-756) with that of cephalothin and cefamandole against clinically relevant gram-negative rods, studied the stability of cefotaxime against *Staphylococcus aureus* in comparison with cephalothin, and studied the activity of cefotaxime against *Pseudomonas aeruginosa*. In the clinical evaluation of cefotaxime, we looked at the Coombs effect and the human pharmacokinetics of this cephalosporin. Two clinical failures in treating *P. aeruginosa* infections motivated some complementary studies.

As expected, recently collected strains of gram-negative bacilli from clinically isolated infectious material showed cefotaxime MICs and MBCs of ≤0.5 μg/ml for *Escherichia coli, Proteus vulgaris, P. mirabilis,* and *Citrobacter* and ≤1.0 μg/ml for *Klebsiella pneumoniae* and *Enterobacter cloacae* when tested in Mueller-Hinton (M-H) broth with an inoculum of 10^6 colony-forming units (CFU)/ml. All zone sizes around a 30-μg disk were ≥29 mm when tested by the Kirby-Bauer method. The superiority of cefotaxime in comparison with cephalothin and cefamandole was evident; of a small series of clinically relevant gram-negative rods (excluding *P. aeruginosa*) prospectively collected, 55% were susceptible to cefamandole and 100% were susceptible to cefotaxime.

Cefotaxime was active, but less potent against *S. aureus* than against gram-negative bacilli. With inocula of 10^4 and 10^5 CFU/ml incubated in M-H broth at 30 and 37°C, MICs were ≤2 μg/ml and MBCs were ≤4 μg/ml, with zone sizes ≥23 mm around the cefotaxime disk.

Cefazolin, cephalothin, and sometimes cefamandole seemed more active than cefotaxime against *S. aureus*. Inocula of 10^4 to 10^7 CFU/ml were destroyed at similar rates in the presence of 64 μg of cephalothin or cefotaxime per ml; 10.2 and 11.7%, respectively, of the inoculum survived after 4 h, and 1.2 and 1.75%, respectively, survived after 8 h. After 24 h the bactericidal action of cephalothin was almost complete (>99.9%); it was incomplete with cefotaxime (99.7%). In no case was there any regrowth. No destruction of cefotaxime by *S. aureus* β-lactamases could be detected. The spontaneous loss of cefotaxime activity was 39.4% after 24 h; it was the same in the presence of a large inoculum of penicillinase-producing *S. aureus*.

Whereas all of our *P. aeruginosa* strains were completely resistant to cephalothin and cefamandole, cefotaxime had antibacterial activity against these strains; MICs varied between 0.5 and 16 μg/ml, and MBCs varied between 1 and 32 μg/ml. But an inoculum effect was found: with one strain from a clinical failure, the MICs

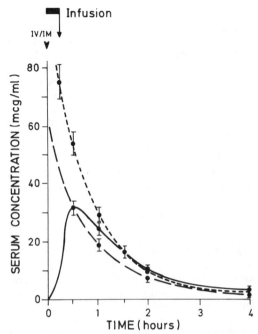

FIG. 1. *Serum concentrations (± SEM) of cefotaxime after administration of a single dose of 15 mg/kg (approximately 1 g) as a 15-min infusion, an i.v. bolus, and an i.m. injection.*

and MBCs were 4 and 8 μg/ml with inocula of 10^2 and 10^4 CFU/ml, and they increased abruptly to 64 and 128 μg/ml with an inoculum of 10^6 CFU/ml and over 512 μg/ml with 10^8 CFU/ml. This sudden increase between 10^4 and 10^6 CFU/ml could be shown for all of our strains and did not depend on pH or the calcium or magnesium content of the M-H broth.

A positive direct Coombs reaction has been observed in patients receiving cephalosporins, especially cephalothin. Rare cases of hemolytic anemias are known. This phenomenon is explained by two mechanisms. One is immunological. Antibodies against the cephalosporin are fixed by the erythrocyte membrane; the repeatedly administered cephalosporin, acting as an antigen, will react with the anti-cephalosporin antibodies fixed on the erythrocytes. The second, more important mechanism is not immunological. By this mechanism, nonspecific plasma proteins are absorbed by the erythrocyte membrane, which has been sensitized by the cephalosporin, giving a positive direct Coombs reaction. We studied this last mechanism for cefotaxime in comparison with cephalothin in vitro by determining the minimal concentration of cephalosporin necessary to obtain a positive direct Coombs test. With nonspecific antisera against human plasma proteins (from rabbits),

6.25 or 25 mg of cephalothin per ml elicited a positive test, whereas 80 or 150 mg of cefotaxime per ml was necessary for the same effect. With a specific anti-human albumin, three times more cefotaxime (80 mg/ml) than cephalothin was necessary to obtain a positive reaction. The minimal concentrations of the two cephalosporins giving hemolysis were 25 mg of cephalothin and 80 mg of cefotaxime per ml. These high concentrations of cefotaxime necessary for a positive Coombs reaction and hemolysis make it unlikely that they will occur in clinical situations.

To study the pharmacokinetics of cefotaxime, a single dose of 15 mg/kg (approximately 1 g) was administered to the same four healthy volunteers as a 15-min infusion, an intravenous (i.v.) bolus, and an intramuscular (i.m.) injection (Fig. 1). The serum concentrations were 75 μg/ml 5 min after the end of the infusion, 54 μg/ml at 30 min, 8 μg/ml at 2 h, and 1.7 μg/ml at 4 h. We measured 32 μg/ml 30 min after the i.v. bolus injection, 7 μg/ml at 2 h, and 1.7 μg/ml at 4 h. The i.m. injection gave the same serum level at 30 min as after the i.v. bolus injection of 32 μg/ml. The serum concentrations were slightly more sustained with 2.1 μg/ml at 4 h. The $t_{1/2}$ calculated during the elimination phase was 75 min. Comparison with cephalothin and cefaman-

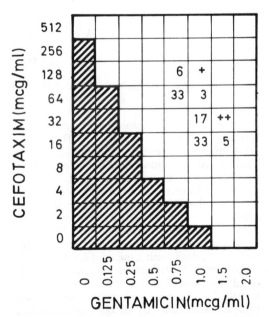

FIG. 2. *Checkerboard for the study of inhibitory and bactericidal activity of the combination cefotaxime/gentamicin against a strain of P. aeruginosa. Inoculum was 5×10^6 CFU/ml. Checkerboard shows unpredictable killing with evidence of some antagonism. Symbols: (+) >100 CFU/ml; (++) >200 CFU/ml.*

dole administered at the same dosage as a short infusion showed: cephalothin had a lower peak and more rapid disappearance from the serum; cefamandole and cefotaxime had an identical first phase of distribution; but cefotaxime was present in slightly higher and more prolonged blood concentrations due to its longer $t_{1/2}$ (75 min versus 40 min for cefamandole).

These studies indicate that this new cephalosporin can be prescribed for patients admitted with severe infections, including sepsis. For infections due to susceptible organisms, the clinical response to monotherapy with cefotaxime prescribed at 6-h intervals was favorable. Possible side effects included allergic skin reactions, phlebitis, modification of hepatic enzymatic tests, and transient leucopenia. Two cases of *P. aeruginosa* infections did not respond: one with an acute exacerbation of a chronic pyelonephritis and a girl with an osteomyelitis.

We studied the synergism of cefotaxime and gentamicin for the *P. aeruginosa* strain isolated from the osteomyelitis. With a large inoculum of 5×10^6 CFU/ml, the MICs were 512 μg of cefotaxime and 1.5 μg of gentamicin per ml (Fig. 2); with a smaller inoculum of 5×10^4 CFU/ml, the MICs were 64 and 1.0 μg/ml, respectively.

After combining the two antibiotics and determining the MICs for both inocula, we found obvious synergism: inhibition was achieved with 8 μg of cefotaxime and 0.5 μg of gentamicin per ml or 4 and 0.75 μg/ml, respectively. But studying the bactericidal activity in a checkerboard (Fig. 2) showed some surprises. In subculturing the clear tubes, we noticed that killing did not occur in a predictable way. When we recovered 3 to 33 CFU/loop, there had been a 99.9% killing; but in some tubes there were more than 100 or 200 CFU/loop, e.g., $>4 \times 10^3$ CFU/ml. There was even some evidence of antagonism. With 1.5 μg of gentamicin alone per ml, there was bactericidal action; after adding 32 μg of cefotaxime per ml, we recovered $>4 \times 10^3$ CFU/ml.

In conclusion, cefotaxime is certainly a promising cephalosporin antibiotic of a new generation: it has a broad spectrum and does not easily produce a Coombs effect, and its pharmacokinetics in humans are similar to those of cefamandole. We would be very careful in using it for *P. aeruginosa* infections because of its inoculum effect in vitro and some unpredictable antagonism with gentamicin in checkerboard studies.

Cefotaxime in Pediatrics

HELMUT F. HELWIG

St. Hedwig Children's Hospital, D-7800 Freiburg i.Br., Federal Republic of Germany

Because of its extraordinary antibacterial spectrum and activity, cefotaxime (HR-756) is of great interest for pediatric patients (2, 3, 5, 6). The effectiveness and tolerance of cefotaxime were evaluated in a prospective study of 49 patients in different age groups (26 infants, 11 of them less than 1 week old). The antibiotic was administered to all patients by slow intravenous injection in a dose of 50 mg/kg every 12 h, resp. 24 h in neonates. The maximum treatment period was 25 days, with a mean of 6.9 days.

Indications for treatment were different bacterial infections (Table 1). Twenty-five bacterial isolates from the sites of infection were susceptible to cefotaxime. In all but one controlled case, these bacteria could be eliminated. Only in one patient with purulent chronic otitis media was the causative organism (*Pseudomonas aeruginosa*) not eradicated; however, later treatment with azlocillin did eliminate the bacteria. Another patient with *Pseudomonas* uri-

nary tract infection showed recurrence of infection 1 week after cefotaxime treatment was stopped.

Kinetic studies were performed in eight patients, seven of them infants and three of them neonates. Determinations of plasma concentrations were performed by K. Seeger of Hoechst Laboratories, Frankfurt, Federal Republic of Germany, in capillary whole-blood samples on Mueller-Hinton broth, using *Escherichia coli* V 6311/65. These studies (Table 2) demonstrated great variation in values among patients. For all patients, the elimination curve came close to ideal values for a two-phase elimination as shown by r^2 of 1.0. Except for the neonates, the plasma half-life of the β-phase (0.96 h) was in the same range as for adults (1, 4). In two full-term babies, $t_{1/2}$ was prolonged to about 3 h; in one premature baby, in 1st day of life the $t_{1/2}$ was prolonged to more than 8 h. These newborn babies also had effective plasma concentrations

TABLE 1. *Diagnoses and results*

Patients	Infection[a]						
	ORL	RTI	GTI	UTI	STI	S	O
Total	5	19	3	9	6	6	2
No. of cures	4	16	2	8	6	1	1
No. of failures	1	1	1	1		1	
No. not evaluated		2				4	1

[a] Abbreviations: ORL, otorhinolaryngeal infection; RTI, respiratory tract infection; GTI, gastrointestinal tract infection; UTI, urinary tract infection; STI, soft-tissue infection; S, septicemia; O, osteomyelitis.

TABLE 2. *Plasma concentrations of cefotaxime after one intravenous injection of 50 mg/kg*

Patient no.	Age	Concn (mg/liter)				
		0.5[a]	1	2	4	6
36	1 day	26		30	26	
39	3 days	79	64	52	35	
48	5 days	55	40	23	23	
46	14 wk	90	60	34	14	4.4
7	5 mo	95	59	30	9	2.3
8	6 mo[b]	21	15	7.8	2.1	1.3
10	8 mo	184	84	44	2.2	0.9
13	4 yr	39	19	7.1	0.9	0.5
Mean						
All patients		73.6	48.7	28.5	14	1.88
No. 36, 39, 48		53	52	35	28	

[a] Hours after administration.
[b] Dose was only 32 mg/kg.

12 to 24 h after a single injection. Studies of urine elimination provided too few reliable data. Area under the curve varied with individual plasma concentrations (range, 86 to 585 μg × h/ml).

Clinical results of therapeutic studies, even in cases of severe bacterial infections, need very rigid criteria. Therefore, it seems more justifiable to analyze cases where the initiated therapy failed. Favorable results in otorhinolaryngeal, respiratory tract, gastrointestinal tract, and soft-tissue infections may have been produced with less potent drugs and therefore do not prove the superiority of the antibiotic used. Failure of treatment in these groups is far more interesting.

Pseudomonas infection of the middle ear, as mentioned before, did not respond to cefotaxime administered for 8 days. One very small premature baby treated for pneumonia died on the 2nd day of life in spite of therapy. This failure could not be attributed to inadequate treatment alone.

Salmonella enteritis in a 4-year-old girl was eradicated after cefotaxime treatment, but *Salmonella* excretion in the feces continued, as would be expected. Therapy initially was begun because of the septic condition of the patient.

Urinary tract infections are much better suited for therapeutic studies than other infections, since the causative microorganisms can easily be checked at any time during and after treatment. There was only one failure in this group, caused by recurrence of *Pseudomonas* infection in a case of bladder exstrophy shortly after cefotaxime treatment was stopped.

Cefotaxime was used in six neonates, most of them premature, for certain or suspected septicemia. One very small baby died in spite of therapy after only 1 day of life. Four cases could not be evaluated since septicemia could not be confirmed by identification of causative organisms. One child with suspected osteomyelitis manifested as gross lesions could not be evaluated, whereas the child with confirmed osteomyelitis showed good response.

Favorable results in 38 out of 49 treated cases are not overwhelming; most successes were achieved by treatment before the susceptible causative organisms were identified.

Tolerance was controlled by routine blood and urine tests performed before, during, and after treatment, including corpuscular elements, liver enzymes, blood urea nitrogen, and urinalysis. There were no obvious adverse reactions in these tests. Six patients complained of repeated pain during injection by the skin vein infusion method. However, there was no case of thrombophlebitis.

More studies are necessary to prove the superiority and tolerance of cefotaxime in children of all ages. There are as yet no data showing that this antibiotic presents a higher risk for children than for adults.

1. Lüthy, R., H. J. Bheno, R. Munch, and W. Siegenthaler. 1978. Clinical pharmacology of HR 756, a new cephalosporin. Program Abstr. Intersci. Conf. Antimicrob. Agents Chemoth. 18th, Atlanta, Ga., abstr. no. 83.
2. Naumann, P., and H. Rosin. 1978. Fortschritte in der antibakteriellen Chemotherapie. Internist 19:664–671.
3. Neu, H. C., N. Aswapokee, P. Aswapokee, and K. P. Fu. 1979. HR 756, a new cephalosporin active against gram-positive and gram-negative aerobic and anaerobic bacteria. Antimicrob. Agents Chemother. 15:273–281.
4. Shah, P. M., E. B. Helm, and W. Stille. 1979. Klinische Erfahrungen mit Cefotaxim, einem neuen Cephalosporin-Derivat. Med. Welt 30:298–301.
5. Shah, P. M., G. Troche, and W. Stille. 1978. In vitro activity of HR 756, a new cephalosporin compound. J. Antibiot. 31:1170–1174.
6. Sosna, J. P., P. M. Murray, and G. Medoff. 1978. Comparison of the in vitro activities of HR 756 with cephalothin, cefoxitin, and cefamandole. Antimicrob. Agents Chemother. 14:876–879.

Clinical Pharmacology of Cefotaxime in Bronchopulmonary Infections

B. KEMMERICH,* H. LODE, G. GRUHLKE, G. DZWILLO, P. KOEPPE, AND I. WAGNER

Klinikum Steglitz, Freie Universität Berlin, West Berlin, Federal Republic of Germany

Twelve patients with chronic mucopurulent bronchitis or chronic infected bronchiectasis participated in a comparative study evaluating sputum and serum levels of cefazolin and cefotaxime (HR-756). They were between 32 and 72 years old (average, 52 years); body weight ranged from 52 to 91 kg (average, 70.6 kg). Cefazolin (1.0 g) and cefotaxime (1.0 and 2.0 g) were administered intravenously (i.v.) over 30 min. Serum levels were measured over a period of 8 h after infusion. Sputum samples were collected in four 2-h periods over the first 8 h, followed by one 16-h period up to 24 h after infusion. The daily sputum amounted to a mean volume of 45 ml. The sputum, preponderantly purulent, was homogenized in an ultrasonic apparatus. The agar diffusion cup-plate method was used for bioassay, with *Bacillus subtilis* (ATCC 6633) and *Sarcina lutea* (ATCC 9341) as test strains. The antibiotic content was determined by using homologous activity-free media as standards.

The serum concentration curves of the two cephalosporins showed the typical high concentrations of cefazolin over a long period (average, 7.6 ± 4.2 mg/liter even after 8 h) and a more rapid decrease of cefotaxime in serum (with 1.0 g i.v., 0.25 ± 0.16 mg/liter; with 2.0 g i.v., 0.78 ± 0.22 mg/liter after 8 h).

The corresponding sputum concentrations are shown in Fig. 1. Cefazolin concentrations increased from 2.4 mg/liter after 2 h to 3.0 mg/liter in the 8- to 24-h interval. Cefotaxime concentrations after 1.0 g i.v. were in a very low range (between 0.18 and 0.7 mg/liter) during the entire period. After 2.0 g i.v., the maximal average concentration was 5.4 mg/liter in the first 2-h period and decreased continuously to 3.0 mg/liter in the 4- to 6-h period and to 1.2 mg/liter in the 8- to 24-h period.

In agreement with Lambert (3), the antibiotic sputum concentrations showed considerable individual fluctuations. No close correlation between the percentage of penetration into the bronchial mucus and protein binding could be seen. In contrast, cefazolin, which has a high protein-binding value of 86%, had a considerably higher sputum concentration after an i.v. dose of 1.0 g than cefotaxime, an agent with a much lower protein-binding value (33%). There was no close relationship between serum and bronchial concentrations of cefotaxime given in doses of

1.0 and 2.0 g with quite different serum/sputum ratios. The relatively high sputum concentrations after a 2.0-g dose are surprising considering the low levels achieved after a 1.0-g dose. Possibly these observations can be explained by bronchial clearance mechanisms with a limited capacity, intrabonchial metabolism, or degradation. In summary, there are numerous factors influencing antibiotic transport from blood to bronchus. In many cases, the penetration is unpredictable.

Pleural fluid concentrations. In six patients with exudative pleurisy, serum and concomitant pleural fluid concentrations of cefazolin and cefotaxime were studied. The patients, seven females and five males, 37 to 82 years old (average, 61 years) and weighing 41 to 78 kg, suffered from histologically or cytologically proven malignant pleural effusion. All but one had an exudate with a pleural fluid-to-serum protein ratio greater than 0.5. Renal function was normal in all patients. Cefazolin and cefotaxime were administered as i.v. bolus injections in a dose of 1.0 g. Serum and pleural fluid samples were collected simultaneously 1, 3, 6, and 9 h after application. The concentrations were determined by the agar diffusion procedure with homologous standards.

Pleural fluid concentrations of cefazolin (Fig. 2) increased rather slowly compared with high serum levels and reached an average peak of 8.1 ± 2.4 mg/liter after 3 h. The pleural

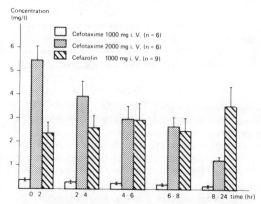

FIG. 1. *Mean sputum concentrations ± SD of cefazolin and cefotaxime in patients with chronic bronchitis.*

concentration (mg/l)

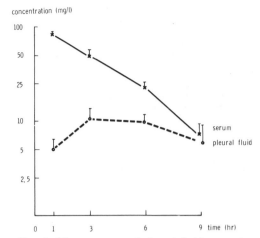

FIG. 2. *Mean serum and pleural fluid concentrations ± SD after cefazolin (1.0 g i.v. over 9 h).*

concentration (mg/l)

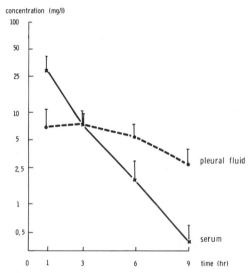

FIG. 3. *Mean serum and pleural fluid concentrations ± SD after cefotaxime (1.0 g i.v. over 9 h).*

concentration curve also declined slowly and reached the serum level after 9 h.

Cefotaxime serum levels declined more rapidly (Fig. 3) due to the shorter half-life (75 min compared with 120 min for cefazolin). At the end of the 9-h period, only 0.7 ± 0.8 mg/liter was detectable. Pleural peak levels, measured after 3 h, averaged 7.2 ± 3.1 mg/liter and decreased more slowly than serum concentrations, which averaged 2.7 ± 1.2 mg/liter even after 9 h. The intersection of pleural and serum concentration curves lay between 1 and 3 h after application.

Our results show good passage of the two cephalosporins into pleural fluid, with little de-

pendence on protein binding. Gerding et al. (2) did not find an inverse correlation between the percentage of binding to serum and the degree of penetration of various cephalosporins into peritoneal and interstitial capsular fluid. According to Meinardi et al. (4), the extravascular penetration of cephalosporins depends mainly on the rate of elimination of an agent and its area under the curve; dependency on protein binding is negligible. Other factors influencing the extravascular antibiotic concentration are concentration gradient from serum to extravascular fluid, lipid solubility, and ionization state. There is a general pattern of slow accumulation and elimination of the drug from extravascular fluid. Cole and Pung (1) found higher pleural fluid concentrations of cefazolin than we did. Their results had a wide range, and determinations of antibiotic concentration were not performed with a homologous standard. Data on body weight and kidney function were missing.

Pleural fluid is an extravascular space comparable to other experimental models. It probably gives better information on antibiotic concentrations at the inflamed tissue than do sputum concentrations.

Clinical studies. Cefotaxime was used in 19 patients (13 males and 6 females) with serious bronchopulmonary and pleural infections. The patients were 36 to 82 years old, with a mean body weight of 67 kg. Cefotaxime was administered i.v. over 30 min in a dose of 2.0 g every 8 h for 7 to 32 days (average, 12 days). The diagnoses were pneumonia in eight cases, lung abscess in one, exacerbation of chronic bronchitis in six, bronchiectasis in one, and pleural empyema in three. The clinical outcome was favorable in 14 patients; 4 patients did not respond to antibiotic treatment. Two suffered from a far-advanced stage of chronic bronchitis and died. In one patient, severe bronchopneumonia with fatal outcome occurred after neurosurgical treatment. An alcoholic with an extensive lung abscess probably due to aspiration became more ill while under cefotaxime treatment. Local and systemic tolerance were good in the majority of patients. Mild diarrhea occurred in two cases; in one case of allergic exanthem, treatment had to be discontinued. Laboratory tests of blood, kidney, and liver functions were not altered by therapy.

From these studies, we conclude that cefotaxime is an effective and well-tolerated cephalosporin for treatment of serious bronchopulmonary infections. Because it has greater antibacterial activity than known cephalosporins, including potentially useful activity against *Pseudomonas aeruginosa*, cefotaxime may become a valuable agent for treatment of serious hospital infections caused by multiresistant pathogens.

1. Cole, D. R., and J. Pung. 1977. Penetration of cefazolin into pleural fluid. Antimicrob. Agents Chemother. **11:** 1033–1035.
2. Gerding, D. N., W. N. Hall, E. A. Schierl, and R. E. Manion. 1976. Cephalosporin and aminoglycoside concentrations in peritoneal capsular fluid in rabbits. An-

timicrob. Agents Chemother. **10:**902–911.
3. **Lambert, H. P.** 1978. Clinical significance of tissue penetration of antibiotic in the respiratory tract. Scand. J. Infect Dis. **14** (Suppl.):262–266.
4. **Meinardi, G., G. Monti, S. Grasso, V. Tamassia, and I. de Carneri.** 1978. Penetration of cephalosporins into extravascular fluids: role of protein binding and elimination rate, p. 379–381. *In* Current chemotherapy, Proceedings of the 10th International Congress of Chemotherapy. American Society for Microbiology, Washington, D.C.

Cefotaxime in the Treatment of Septicemia

DIANA M. D. RIMMER

Hillingdon Hospital, Uxbridge, Middlesex UB8 3NN, England

The blind therapy for patients with serious infection is commonly a combination of an aminoglycoside and a penicillin. Such patients frequently have disturbances of renal function, so that difficulties are experienced with the dosage of the aminoglycoside. The newer cephalosporins have a broad spectrum comparable to that of the aminoglycoside-penicillin combination. In this study cefotaxime was used instead of the combination in the treatment of serious undiagnosed infections.

Cefotaxime is a semisynthetic cephalosporin with the structure 3-acetoxymethyl-7 (2-(2-amino-4-thiazolyl)-2-methoxyimino-acetyl)-amino)-ceph-3-em-4-carboxyl, sodium salt. The compound is more active than cefuroxime and cefoxitin against a wide range of pathogens and more active than carbenicillin against strains of *Pseudomonas aeruginosa.*

Thirty-six patients admitted to Hillingdon Hospital with serious infections were treated with cefotaxime. Dosage and duration of treatment depended on the severity of infection. Twenty-eight patients received 3 g/day, five patients had doses varying between 4.5 and 6.0 g/day, and three patients initially received only 2 g/day. Of these last three patients, poor response to treatment resulted in increasing the dose to the standard 3 g/day with ultimate success.

Hematological parameters, liver function tests, and renal function tests were performed before, during, and after treatment with cefotaxime. None of the patients received an additional antibiotic.

Ten of the patients had bacteriologically proven septicemia. The organisms isolated were as follows: *Escherichia coli*, 3; *Klebsiella pneumoniae*, 5; *Enterobacter cloacae*, 2. The MICs for these organisms ranged from 0.01 to 10 mg/liter. At the end of the course of treatment all 10

patients were clinically free from symptoms, and posttreatment blood cultures were sterile.

Two patients with enteric fever (both *Salmonella paratyphi* A) were treated for 14 days with cefotaxime. Although they responded clinically to the antibiotic initially, the response was slow. One of the patients subsequently became stool positive, and the other patient relapsed 1 week after completion of the course, with positive blood cultures. The MIC of cefotaxime for both *Salmonella* isolates was 0.06 mg/liter.

Eight patients with severe urinary tract infection were included in the series. Of these there was only one failure, a paraplegic with an indwelling catheter and an infection with *P. aeruginosa*. The cefotaxime MIC for the *Pseudomonas* isolate was 10.0 mg/liter. Three patients with severe wound infections due to *Staphylococcus aureus*, *E. coli*, and *Proteus mirabilis* were all successfully treated.

Only two proven chest infections were included. One patient with severe corpulmonale had an infection with an unidentifiable gram-negative rod. Although her sputum became clear of the organism after a course of cefotaxime, her clinical improvement was minimal. The second patient had a pneumonia caused by *K. pneumoniae*. This patient responded extremely well to the minimal dose of 2 g of cefotaxime per day.

Three "miscellaneous" cases deserve special note. One patient with acute lymphatic leukemia presented with an enormous peritonsillar swelling and a history of allergy to penicillins. Within 24 h of initiation of treatment with cefotaxime, the swelling subsided, thus obviating the necessity for tracheostomy. A patient aged 85 years with purulent peritonitis following ruptured diverticular abscess was cured. The peritoneal pus grew *E. coli* and a *Klebsiella* sp. One partial failure is also worthy of note. A patient on peritoneal dialysis developed peritonitis with micrococci and *Streptococcus faecalis*, to the extent of the dialysis tubes becoming completely blocked with pus. The patient was given cefotaxime, 50 mg/liter of dialysate, together with intermittent parenteral doses. Clinically the condition improved, but we continuously isolated the *S. faecalis* (MIC > 10.0 mg/liter) from the dialysate.

Serum levels were measured in all patients immediately before a dose and 0.5 to 1 h postdose. The range of trough levels was 0.5 to 2.2 mg/liter. The range of peak serum levels was 16.0 to 42.0 mg/liter.

Adverse reactions were infrequent. Two patients developed a rash during treatment. Many patients, however, complained of pain at the site of intramuscular injection. No reactions were seen associated with intravenous therapy.

Overall, 31 of 34 (91%) patients with serious infection were clinically and bacteriologically cured of their surgical infection. This compares favorably with the attenuative combination therapy with an aminoglycoside and a penicillin. The two patients with enteric fever were both classified as failures. Further work must be done with this disease to determine the true picture.

Cefotaxime Elimination in Patients with Renal and Liver Dysfunction

NOEL WRIGHT* AND RICHARD WISE

Departments of Medicine and Medical Microbiology, Dudley Road Hospital, Birmingham, England

Cefotaxime is a semisynthetic cephalosporin. It has a broad spectrum of activity and considerably greater activity against gram-negative organisms than previously marketed preparations. It is administered parenterally, so the most obvious clinical application is in serious gram-negative infection. With this in mind, the pharmacokinetic properties of the preparation in patients relatively acutely ill with diminished renal and hepatic function were investigated.

Patients with a variety of illnesses causing renal dysfunction were, after consent had been obtained, included in the study. All had recently suffered acute illness, including urinary tract infection, malaria, and hypertensive renal disease. Only patients who had taken paracetamol in overdosage were included in the study of kinetics in acute hepatic damage.

Blood and urine samples were obtained at intervals after administration of 1 g of cefotaxime intravenously over a 5-min period. The study was continued for 8 h in patients with moderate renal impairment and for 24 h in those with severe injury.

The drug was assayed by two methods. *Proteus morganii* was used as the test organism on Isosensitest agar (Oxoid, Basingstoke, United Kingdom) at pH 7.2 in a microbiological assay of unchanged cefotaxime. *Bacillus subtilis* ATCC 6633 was used as the indicator organism for assay of cefotaxime and the deacetylated derivative.

The drug levels and metabolites were also assayed by a high-pressure liquid chromatographic method. The sample was extracted into acetonitrile, using a 2:1 ratio. The resultant extract was centrifuged; the supernatant was added to a solution consisting of 20% methanol and 1% acetic acid in water. Internal standard was next added, and an aliquot was chromatographed on a 25 Partisil 10 ODS column, using the Applied Chromatography system consisting

TABLE 1. *Cefotaxime elimination in varying degrees of renal failure*

Subjects	Half-life (h)	Vol distribution (liters)	Drug clearance (ml/min)	Urine excretion (mg)
Normal volunteers ($n = 5$)	0.82	27.25	383	680
Creatinine clearance				
<30 > 5 ml/min	1.87	19.94	123	210
($n = 5$)				
<5 > 0 ml/min ($n = 4$)	4.2	19.2	53	147
0 ml/min ($n = 3$)	6.2	16.2	30	0
Acute hepatic necrosis				
Mean creatinine clearance = 42 ml/min				
($n = 4$)	1.31	22	193	

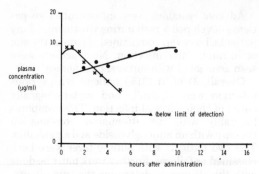

FIG. 1. *Comparison of serial plasma concentrations of desacetyl cefotaxime taken from one normal subject (×), one patient with severe renal failure (●), and one patient with severe liver damage (▲).*

of a 750/03 pump and a 750/ii UV detector with a 254-nm filter.

No patients experienced any adverse effects from the drug either at the time of administration or at any time later. There was good agreement between the different methods of drug assay.

Cefotaxime elimination fell progressively as the creatinine clearance became smaller. When glomerular filtration was effectively zero, the drug half-life was 6.2 h (Table 1). At these very low glomerular filtration rates the desacetyl metabolite accumulated (Fig. 1). Cefotaxime elimination was not increased by peritoneal dialysis in four subjects but was increased by a mean of 43%, reducing the drug half-life to 2.2 h in a further three subjects undergoing hemodialysis.

Desacetyl cefotaxime formation was markedly reduced by the presence of hepatic necrosis (Fig. 1). The extent of damage appeared to correlate with the severity of reduction of hepatic metabolism as measured by the plasma paracetamol half-life and peak serum enzyme activities.

Cefotaxime is a useful new cephalosporin antibiotic. However, the dose regime will need to be modified in the presence of renal failure. The parent drug will not accumulate to a great extent if the dosing interval is extended to 8 h when the glomerular filtration rate (GFR) is between 20 and 50 ml/min, 12 h when the GFR is between 10 and 20 ml/min, and 24 h when the GFR is between 5 and 10 ml/min.

Further work needs to be done on the toxicity and accumulation of desacetyl cefotaxime before this dose regime can be safely accepted.

Clinical and Pharmacokinetic Study of Cefotaxime (HR-756) in Infants and Children

DIMITRIS A. KAFETZIS,* JOHN KANARIOS, CONSTANTINOS A. SINANIOTIS, AND CONSTANTINOS J. PAPADATOS

Second Department of Pediatrics, Athens University School of Medicine, Athens, Greece

Cefotaxime is a new semisynthetic cephalosporin which has been shown by in vitro studies to be several times more active against most gram-negative bacteria than "first- and second-generation" cephalosporins (3). Moreover, it has an extended antibacterial spectrum covering many strains of *Enterobacteriaceae*, which are resistant to the older cephalosporins, some *Pseudomonas* strains, and most *Haemophilus influenzae* strains (1, 2). Its spectrum renders the compound very suitable for "high-risk" pediatric patients. This report summarizes our experience with the use of cefotaxime in pediatric bacterial infections.

After informed consent was obtained from the parents, cefotaxime was administered to 41 patients of the "Aglaia Kyriakou" Children's Hospital in Athens. Twelve of these patients were infants (6 males and 6 females) and 29 were children (13 males and 16 females) aged 1 to 12 years. All patients were hospitalized for serious infections, and 39 of the 41 patients included had been under unsuccessful antimicrobial therapy. Patient diagnoses are shown in Table 1. Appropriate cultures were obtained from all patients before, during, and after therapy. All pathogens isolated from our patients were tested for susceptibility to antibiotics by use of the Bauer-Kirby disk-agar diffusion technique, and the drug was administered when pathogen was susceptible to cefotaxime. Fifty-four pathogens were isolated from 39 patients. In one patient with liver abscess, who was under unsuccessful treatment with gentamicin plus ampicillin, no pathogen was isolated. Pathogens isolated are shown in Table 1. In all cases treatment with cefotaxime was started with a dosage of 100 mg/kg per day divided into four doses every 6 h. In

TABLE 1. *Analysis of cases treated with cefotaxime*

Diagnosis	No. of patients	Bacteria isolated	No. of cases	MIC (mg/liter)	Cured	Improved	Failed
Peritonitis	14	E. coli	5	<0.06, <0.06, <0.06, 0.06, 0.12	5		
		E. coli plus S. faecalis	2	<0.06, <0.06 NT[a]	1	1	
		E. coli plus B. fragilis	4	<0.06, <0.06, <0.06, 0.06 NT	4		
		Klebsiella spp.	2	0.06, 0.06	2		
		Klebsiella spp. plus P. mirabilis	1	<0.06 <0.06	1		
Pneumonia	5	H. influenzae	2	NT	2		
		H. influenzae plus S. pneumoniae	2	NT NT	2		
		Klebsiella spp.	1	<0.06	1		
Urinary tract infection	5	E. coli	2	<0.06, <0.06	2		
		P. mirabilis	1	<0.06	1		
		Proteus, indole positive	1	<0.06	1		
		P. aeruginosa	1	0.5	1		
Septicemia	2	Enterobacter spp.	1	0.06	1		
		S. marcescens	1	0.06		1	
Infected burns	3	P. aeruginosa	1	1.0	1		
		P. aeruginosa plus Klebsiella spp.	1	8.0 0.06		1	
		Enterobacter spp.	1	0.06	1		
Osteomyelitis	2	P. aeruginosa	1	4.0	1		
		Salmonella spp.	1	0.06	1		
Liver abscess	2	Enterobacter spp.	1	0.12			1
		None	1		1		
Infected hydatid cyst (liver)	1	P. aeruginosa plus P. mirabilis	1	2.0 <0.06		1	
Infected hydatid cyst (lung)	2	S. marcescens	1	0.06	1		
		P. aeruginosa	1	2.0	1		
Pleural effusion	1	S. marcescens	1	0.06	1		
Omphalitis	2	E. coli plus S. aureus	2	<0.06, <0.06 NT	2		
Infected Leiner's disease	1	P. aeruginosa plus Proteus, indole positive	1	8.0 0.06		1	
Otitis media	1	H. influenzae	1	NT	1		

[a] NT, Not tested.

TABLE 2. Mean serum concentrations of cefotaxime in infants and children after intramuscular (i.m.) or intravenous (i.v.) injection of 25 mg/kg

Route of administration	No. of patients	Serum concn[a] (mg/liter) at indicated times after dose:							Mean serum half-life (h)
		5 min	30 min	1 h	2 h	3 h	4 h	6 h	
i.m.	7		25.6 ± 4.6[a] (18.9–30.0)	21.9 ± 5.6 (14.2–31.0)	12.1 ± 3.1 (8.6–17.5)	5.0 ± 1.1 (3.3–6.3)	2.16 ± 0.5 (1.6–2.9)	0.61 ± 0.28 (<0.4–1.1)	0.98 ± 0.15 (0.85–1.26)
i.v.	26	51.3 ± 10.3 (38.4–72.0)	23.8 ± 5.5 (16.8–37.5)	13.4 ± 5.5 (6.6–27.5)	6.1 ± 3.1 (2.8–13.5)	3.2 ± 2.3 (1.1–9.1)	1.71 ± 1.1 (0.7–4.5)	0.51 ± 0.4 (<0.4–1.6)	1.0 ± 0.16 (0.77–1.32)

[a] ± standard deviation; numbers in parentheses are ranges.

the case of a 4-year-old boy with osteomyelitis due to *Pseudomonas aeruginosa*, the dosage was increased to 200 mg/kg per day on day 3 of treatment. The duration of therapy ranged from 7 to 28 days. The route of administration of the drug was intramuscular in 7 patients and as an intravenous bolus injection in 34. Surgical procedures were performed when indicated. All patients were carefully observed for side effects, and suitable laboratory tests were performed before and after therapy to detect hemopoietic, hepatic, and renal toxicity. The kinetics of cefotaxime were studied in 33 infants and children, 26 receiving the drug intravenously and 7 intramuscularly. Blood was drawn by heel prick before and at 5 min and 0.5, 1, 2, 3, 4, and 6 h after one dose during the first 24 h of treatment. Urine was collected before and at 0 to 2, 2 to 4, and 4 to 6 h postdose. Concentrations of cefotaxime were measured by an agar well-plate technique, with a strain of *Escherichia coli* as the indicator organism.

All 54 pathogens isolated from our patients were found to be susceptible to cefotaxime. All *Enterobacteriaceae*, *P. aeruginosa*, and *Staphylococcus aureus* strains were also found to be susceptible to amikacin, but 9 strains of the above organisms were found to be resistant to gentamicin, 15 strains to carbenicillin, 18 strains to cephalothin, and 25 strains to ampicillin. One of the five isolated strains of *H. influenzae* was ampicillin resistant. Susceptibility tests to *Streptococcus faecalis*, *S. pneumoniae*, and *Bacteroides fragilis* were not performed. Of the 41 patients, 35 were cured and 5 improved; treatment failed only in one patient. This was a 9-year-old girl with liver abscess and bacteremia. *Enterobacter cloacae* isolated from blood was found to be resistant to all antibiotics tested, except cefotaxime and amikacin. Treatment with cefotaxime resulted in a fast regression of temperature and eradication of the pathogen from the blood. On day 5 of treatment, fever appeared again, whereas blood cultures remained sterile. Treatment was changed and cefotaxime was replaced by amikacin. In 36 of the 40 patients, pathogens were eradicated. In four patients, two with indwelling catheters and two with skin infections, bacteria from those sites persisted or changed. Cefotaxime was very well tolerated. No toxic effects were noticed, and the abnormal finding observed in five patients was a mild, transient eosinophilia.

Serum concentrations of cefotaxime in infants and children after intramuscular or intravenous injections are shown in Table 2. Peak blood levels were obtained 0.5 h after intramuscular and 5 min after intravenous injection and averaged 25.3 ± 4.7 and 53.3 ± 10.3 mg/liter, respectively. Bactericidal serum levels were present for at least 4 h after injection with both routes of administration but were more sustained for up to 6 h after intramuscular injections. The serum half-life averaged 0.98 ± 0.15 h after intramuscular and 1.0 ± 0.16 h after intravenous administration. Urinary excretion of cefotaxime averaged 44.9 ± 10.7% of the intramuscularly and 56.6 ± 10.0% of the intravenously injected amount in 6 h. Most drug was excreted in the first 2 h after administration, with a mean percentage of 29.7 ± 10.0 after intramuscular and 49.3 ± 9.2 after intravenous injection. Urine concentrations were bactericidal for the whole 6-h period. This study has shown that cefotaxime, with its high antimicrobial activity against bacteria commonly affecting pediatric patients, its clinical effectiveness, its very low incidence

of side effects, and its pharmacokinetic properties suitable for treatment in pediatrics, is a very promising new antimicrobial agent. It may be used successfully for the treatment of infections of infants and children. However, more experience is needed to fully evaluate this compound in the pediatric field.

1. **Chabbert, Y. A., and A. J. Lutz.** 1978. HR-756, the syn isomer of a new methoxyimino cephalosporin with unusual antibacterial activity. Antimicrob. Agents Chemother. **14**:749–754.
2. **Drasar, F. A., W. Farrell, A. J. Howard, C. Hince, and J. D. Williams.** 1978. Activity of HR-756 against Haemophilus influenzae, Bacteroides fragilis and gram-negative rods. J. Antimicrob. Chemother. **4**:445–450.
3. **Shah, P. M., G. Troche, and W. Stille.** 1978. In vitro activity of HR-756, a new cephalosporin compound. J. Antibiot. **31**:1170–1174.

Serum and Urine Levels of Cefotaxime (HR-756) and Desacetylcefotaxime in Patients with Various Degrees of Renal Function

YOSHIMARU USUDA,* OSAMU SEKINE, NOBUKI AOKI, TAKEAKI SHIMIZU, YOSHIHEI HIRASAWA, TADAO AOKI, MIKIO OMOSU, AND KAZUHIRO KASAI

Shinrakuen Hospital, Niigata City, 950-21, and Development Laboratories, Hoechst Japan Ltd., Kawagoe City, Japan*

Cefotaxime is a new semisynthetic cephalosporin antibiotic which shows a high degree of β-lactamase stability and possesses broad-spectrum antibacterial activity (1, 2). We have studied the administration method of cefotaxime for patients with renal dysfunction by examining the changes in blood and urine concentrations of both the drug itself and its main metabolite, desacetylcefotaxime.

The in vivo dynamics of cefotaxime were investigated by giving single i.v. injections of 1,000 mg of the drug into each of 10 patients with various types of renal dysfunction [creatinine clearance (Ccr) of 0 to 77 ml per min/1.48 m²]. The mean body weight of 10 patients was 48.9 kg, and their ages were between 34 and 80 years. In 2 of 10 patients, hemodialysis was performed during the study. Blood and urine samples were taken at various intervals ranging from 0 to 24 h after injection, and drug concentrations were measured by both bioassay and high-pressure liquid chromatography (HPLC). Bioassay was carried out by the thin-layer cup method using *Micrococcus luteus* ATCC 9341 as the test organism. HPLC was performed using a JASCO Trirotar chromatograph, a stainless steel column

of 4.6 mm by 12.5 cm, SC-02 as a filler, a determining wavelength of UV 254 nm, and solvent containing a 5:1 ratio of 0.2% ammonium acetate and methanol for the serum or solvent containing a 78:22 ratio of 1.0% acetic acid and methanol for the urine. A flow rate of 1.0 ml/min was adopted.

As shown in Tables 1 and 2, in the patient whose Ccr was 77, the greater part of the injected 1,000 mg of cefotaxime was rapidly excreted into the urine without undergoing any metabolism, whereas a part of the drug was metabolized into desacetylcefotaxime and also rapidly excreted into the urine. Since high blood concentrations of cefotaxime persisted with intensification of renal dysfunction, the half-life of cefotaxime was prolonged and high blood concentrations of desacetylcefotaxime persisted for an extended period of time. Due to the prolonged urinary excretion of cefotaxime with intensification of renal dysfunction, the amount excreted into the urine decreased. On the other hand, the urinary excretion of desacetylcefotaxime increased, although its urinary excretion was prolonged with intensification of renal dysfunction. In patients with more severe renal dysfunction (Ccr: below

TABLE 1. *Serum levels of cefotaxime and its metabolite after single i.v. injection of 1,000 mg in patients with various degrees of renal function*

Patient (kidney function)[a]	Assay method for CTX and dCTX[b]	Serum level (μg/ml) at time after dosing (h):					
		1	2	4	6	8	24
1. (Ccr 77)	CTX (Bioassay)	14.0	8.1	1.8	0.3		ND[c]
	CTX (HPLC)	16.8	6.1	1.3	ND		ND
	dCTX (HPLC)	4.4	3.4	1.3	ND		ND
2. (Ccr 44)	CTX (Bioassay)	27.0	16.2	6.6	4.4		ND
	CTX (HPLC)	26.8	13.9	5.5	1.9		ND
	dCTX (HPLC)	3.4	3.8	2.2	1.3		ND
3. (Ccr 40)	CTX (Bioassay)	40.0	24.0	12.0	3.3		ND
	CTX (HPLC)	44.7	25.1	5.4	1.6		ND
	dCTX (HPLC)	9.6	8.7	4.6	2.1		ND
4. (Ccr 24)	CTX (Bioassay)	40.0	24.0	17.5	10.8		ND
	CTX (HPLC)	53.4	30.9	13.3	6.3		ND
	dCTX (HPLC)	6.6	11.4	9.9	9.3		ND
5. (Ccr 25)	CTX (Bioassay)	33.0	19.8	12.0	6.6		ND
	CTX (HPLC)	39.1	18.4	7.0	2.8		ND
	dCTX (HPLC)	9.1	9.2	12.4	9.7		ND
6. (Ccr 9)	CTX (Bioassay)	50.0	36.0	26.0	26.0		2.5
	CTX (HPLC)	44.2	34.1	20.7	11.1		ND
	dCTX (HPLC)	3.9	9.8	18.9	21.6		10.3
7. (Ccr 4)	CTX (Bioassay)	40.0	36.0	26.0	17.5		1.7
	CTX (HPLC)	51.9	37.0	20.7	11.5		ND
	dCTX (HPLC)	4.9	12.0	19.9	21.1		7.6
8. (Ccr 5)	CTX (Bioassay)	60.0	43.5	31.5	31.5		2.7
	CTX (HPLC)	64.7	45.5	28.0	14.8		ND
	dCTX (HPLC)	5.8	11.0	19.3	19.9		11.8
9. (Ccr 0.7 + HD)	CTX (Bioassay)		30.0	19.8	10.0	6.6	0.63
	CTX (HPLC)		36.0	13.5	3.8	1.4	ND
	dCTX (HPLC)		28.0	31.4	24.5	17.4	3.7
10. (Ccr 0 + HD)	CTX (Bioassay)		44.0	24.0	17.5	10.0	3.7
	CTX (HPLC)		23.2	10.9	6.3	2.6	ND
	dCTX (HPLC)		6.9	6.9	10.3	6.4	3.9

[a] Ccr, Creatinine clearance, ml/min per 1.48 m^2; HD, patients 9 and 10 received 5-h hemodialysis from 3 to 8 h after administration.

[b] CTX, cefotaxime; dCTX, desacetylcefotaxime; HPLC, high-pressure liquid chromatography.

[c] ND, Not detected.

20), cefotaxime could not be detected either in the blood or in the urine 15 to 20 h after its i.v. injection, while desacetylcefotaxime was continuously excreted into the urine in only small increments. Accordingly, desacetylcefotaxime was not completely excreted into the urine 24 h after the injection of cefotaxime. Hemodialysis reduced blood concentrations of both cefotaxime and desacetylcefotaxime.

Cefotaxime and desacetylcefotaxime were mainly excreted into the urine. Urinary excretion of these substances decreased with intensification of renal dysfunction and, as a result,

reduction in their blood concentration was delayed.

The half-lives of cefotaxime measured by the bioassay were 0.9 h for Ccr 77, 1.9 h for Ccr 44, 2.26 h for Ccr 25, and 4.3 h for Ccr 4. Its half-life during hemodialysis was about 3 h. As compared with cephalosporin antibiotics that are excreted mainly into the urine without having undergone in vivo metabolism, the prolongation of the half-life of cefotaxime was relatively small even when renal function was greatly reduced, because cefotaxime in the blood was successively metabolized into desacetylcefotaxime, which possesses

TABLE 2. *Urine levels and recovery of cefotaxime and its metabolite after single i.v. injection of 1,000 mg in patients with various degrees of renal function*

Patient (kidney function)[a]	Time of collection (h)	Urine vol (ml)	Bioassay[b]: cefotaxime		High-pressure liquid chromatography[b]			
					Cefotaxime		Desacetylcefotaxime	
			Level (µg/ml)	Recovery (mg)	Level (µg/ml)	Recovery (mg)	Level (µg/ml)	Recovery (mg)
1. (Ccr 77)	0–2.5	200	2,739.6	547.9	3,079.8	616.0	815.5	163.0
	2.5–4.5	240	236.3	56.7	184.6	44.3	97.4	23.4
	4.5–6.2	200	45.2	9.0	44.6	8.9	ND	0
	6.2–8.8	220	11.9	2.6	14.8	3.3	ND	0
	8.8–10.8	270	2.0	0.6	ND	0	ND	0
	10.8–20.8	770	ND	0	ND	0	ND	0
2. (Ccr 44)	0–4.2	180	1,728.8	311.2	2,208.2	397.5	824.8	148.5
	4.2–8.5	240	1,049.7	251.9	890.1	213.6	510.6	122.5
	8.5–20.5	200	70.4	14.1	278.2	55.6	108.0	21.6
3. (Ccr 40)	0–1	110	824.1	90.7	793.5	87.3	154.7	17.0
	1–4	130	3,347.8	435.2	3,134.2	407.4	1,021.1	132.7
	4–6.3	120	530.0	63.6	681.7	81.8	463.3	55.6
	6.3–9.5	100	76.8	7.7	59.5	6.0	95.6	9.6
	9.5–11.3	300	24.0	7.2	ND	0	51.3	15.4
	11.3–24.0	140	3.6	0.5	ND	0	19.3	2.7
4. (Ccr 24)	0–1	50	3,332.5	166.6	3,764.6	188.2	1,256.5	62.8
	1–4	50	2,080.9	104.0	4,220.9	211.0	1,997.5	99.9
	4–6	60	1,928.9	115.7	1,863.3	111.8	1,594.8	95.7
	6–10	133	404.5	53.8	418.8	55.7	794.7	105.7
	10–16.5	290	25.9	7.5	23.8	6.9	131.7	38.2
	16.5–20.5	280	11.8	3.3	6.4	1.8	75.7	21.2
	20.5–24.0	153	7.8	1.2	ND	0	56.2	8.6
5. (Ccr 25)	0–1	125	1,160.7	145.1	1,181.1	147.6	284.8	35.6
	1–2	180	327.7	58.9	590.6	106.3	255.3	46.0
	2–4	540	225.4	121.7	164.8	89.0	150.6	81.3
	4–6	380	86.7	32.9	68.5	26.0	240.6	91.4
	6–24	1,100	3.4	3.7	10.7	11.7	147.3	162.0
6. (Ccr 9)	0–1	180	361.9	65.1	365.4	65.8	88.9	16.0
	1–2	190	252.2	47.9	250.5	47.6	110.7	21.0
	2–4	220	161.9	35.2	186.8	41.1	177.8	39.1
	4–6	155	168.7	26.1	158.1	23.7	268.4	41.6
	6–10	450	49.6	22.3	42.0	18.9	165.8	74.6
	10–14.5	285	40.7	11.6	21.4	6.1	184.9	52.7
	14.5–20.5	305	24.9	7.6	6.9	2.1	179.7	54.8
	20.5–24.0	110	10.8	1.2	ND	0	107.1	11.8
7. (Ccr 4)	0–1	90	120.0	10.8	102.7	9.2	ND	0
	1–2	50	159.9	8.0	142.7	7.1	33.1	1.7
	2–3.8	60	161.9	9.7	160.1	9.6	90.5	5.4
	3.8–8.8	140	86.3	12.1	81.5	11.4	113.5	15.9
	8.8–12.2	300	22.3	6.7	27.3	8.2	71.3	21.4
	12.2–15.7	320	5.9	1.9	11.9	3.8	55.0	17.6
	15.7–24.0	520	3.3	1.7	ND	0	33.8	17.6

[a] Ccr, Creatinine clearance, ml/min per 1.48 m^2.
[b] ND, Not detected.

only a weak antibacterial action against *M. luteus* ATCC 9341. Therefore, the prolongation of the half-life of cefotaxime became smaller according to HPLC rather than bioassay. The half-lives of cefotaxime determined by HPLC were 0.8 h for Ccr 77, 1.34 h for Ccr 44, 1.43 h for Ccr 25, 2.4 h for Ccr 4, and about 1.5 h for Ccr less than 1 during hemodialysis.

For the reason mentioned above, it is possible to reduce the dose of cefotaxime for patients with renal dysfunction, and there may be cases that require such reduction. The dose reduction of cefotaxime could be smaller than that of non-metabolized cephalosporin agents, but, from the viewpoint of safety, the similar reduction is preferable until the effect of desacetylcefotaxime on the human body is clarified. We consider that, in hemodialysis patients with little renal function, daily administration of 1,000 mg of cefotaxime supplemented with an additional 250 to 500 mg of the drug during hemodialysis would be effective for controlling even severe infections.

1. **Hamilton-Miller, J. M. T., W. Brumfitt, and A. V. Reynold.** 1978. Cefotaxime (HR 756) a new cephalosporin with exceptional broad-spectrum activity *in vivo.* J. Antimicrob. Chemother. **4:**437–444.
2. **Heymes, R., A. Lutz, and E. Schrinner.** 1978. Experimental evaluation of HR 756, a new cephalosporin derivative, p. 823–824. *In* Current chemotherapy, Proceedings of the 10th International Congress of Chemotherapy, American Society for Microbiology, Washington, D.C.

Bactericidal Activity of Serum in Volunteers Receiving Cefotaxime (HR-756) with or Without Amikacin

C. BERNARD,* L. COPPENS, G. MOMBELLI, AND J. KLASTERSKY

Department of Medicine, Institut Jules Bordet, Brussels, Belgium

Overwhelming bacterial infections commonly occur in granulocytopenic patients. The microorganisms most frequently involved under these conditions are gram-negative bacilli (*Escherichia coli, Klebsiella* species, *Pseudomonas aeruginosa*) and *Staphylococcus aureus* (2). Early empiric antimicrobial therapy for febrile granulocytopenic patients is widely accepted: a β-lactam antibiotic and an aminoglycoside are most often combined. The emergence of strains resistant to commonly used antibiotics makes it necessary to study new drugs and new combinations. The present study deals with a new semisynthetic cephalosporin, cefotaxime (HR-756) (CEF), in combination with amikacin (A).

Six volunteers free of any hepatic or renal impairment received on 3 consecutive days: CEF (15 mg/kg), A (7.5 mg/kg), and CEF plus A. Antibiotics were infused over 15 min in 50 ml of 5% glucose. Serum samples were obtained 1 h and 6 h after infusion.

Ten strains of *E. coli* (MIC of CEF, 0.007 to 0.03 μg/ml; MIC of A, 0.7 to 3 μg/ml), 10 of *Klebsiella* (Cef, 0.007 to 0.07; A, 0.7 to 3), 10 of *P. aeruginosa* (Cef, 6 to 25; A, 0.3 to 3), and 10 of *S. aureus* (Cef, 0.15 to 25; A, 0.7 to 6) were obtained from a variety of clinical isolates at the clinical microbiology laboratory at the Institut Jules Bordet; MIC values were measured by a broth dilution technique with tryptic soy broth (TSB).

Concentrations of antibiotics were measured

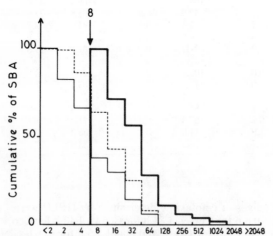
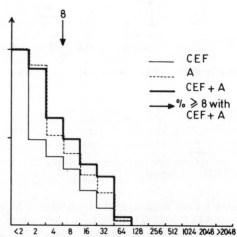

FIG. 1. *Cumulative percentage of serum bactericidal activity (reciprocal) against P. aeruginosa 1 h (left) and 6 h (right) after antibiotic injection.*

TABLE 1. *Serum bactericidal activity 1 and 6 h after injection of cefotaxime or amikacin or both antibiotics*

| Organism | Time (h) | Antibiotic (SBA[a]) | | | | | |
| | | Cefotaxime | | Amikacin | | CEF + A | |
		Median	% ⩾ 1/8	Median	% ⩾ 1/8	Median	% ⩾ 1/8
E. coli	1	512	100	16	93	512	**100**
	6	32	88	2	0	32	98
Klebsiella	1	1024	100	16	98	1024	**100**
	6	32	77	4	18	32	97
P. aeruginosa	1	4	38	8	63	32	**100**
	6	<2	32	2	41	4	47
S. aureus	1	4	37	16	86	16	**86**
	6	<2	0	<2	18	<2	24

[a] SBA = serum bactericidal activity (reciprocal).

in serum samples obtained after administration of each antibiotic alone, using the agar diffusion technique of Bennett (1). For CEF, peak concentration was 14.5 ± 4 μg/ml and trough concentration was 0.8 ± 0.5 μg/ml; for A, peak and trough concentrations were 21 ± 4 μg/ml and 4 ± 2 μg/ml.

Serum bactericidal activity (SBA) of the 36 serum samples was determined against the 40 selected strains by titration with TSB; the strains were grown in TSB with a final concentration of 10^4 gram-negative bacilli per ml or 10^6 staphylococci per ml. Reciprocal of median SBA and percentage of specimens with SBA ⩾1:8 are presented in Table 1. In Fig. 1, the same data are presented for *P. aeruginosa* as cumulative percentages of SBA.

It is well accepted that SBA has an important role in the management of patients with bacterial sepsis, and it has been demonstrated that peak SBA ⩾1:8 correlates with a good cure rate in patients with bacterial infections (3). Thus, for *E. coli* and *Klebsiella*, SBA with CEF was quite high and CEF plus A provided no increase

in SBA. For *P. aeruginosa*, CEF alone did not result in adequate SBA, but CEF plus A was significantly more active than CEF or A alone ($\chi^2 = 24.5$, $P < 0.001$ for percentage of peak SBA ⩾1:8 with CEF for A compared with A). Satisfactory rates of bacterial killing were achieved with this combination. Against *S. aureus*, peak SBA with A was adequate and the addition of CEF did not increase SBA.

The results of this study suggest that the combination of cefotaxime and amikacin might be valuable empiric treatment for febrile neutropenic patients.

1. Bennett, J. V., J. L. Brodie, E. J. Benner, and W. M. M. Kirby. 1966. Simplified, accurate method for antibiotic assay of clinical specimens. Appl. Microbiol. **14:** 170–177.
2. E.O.R.T.C. International Antimicrobial Therapy Project Group. 1978. Three antibiotic regimens in the treatment of infection in febrile granulocytopenic patients with cancer. J. Infect. Dis. **137:**14–29.
3. Klastersky, J. A., D. Daneau, G. Swings, and D. Weerts. 1974. Antibacterial activity in serum and urine as a therapeutic guide in bacterial infections. J. Infect. Dis. **129:**187–193.

Laboratory Investigations of the Susceptibility of Hospital Microorganisms to Cefotaxime (HR-756) and Seven Other Cephalosporins, and Three Anti-*Pseudomonas* Drugs

BRYAN C. STRATFORD* AND SHIRLEY DIXSON

St. George's Hospital, Medical School at St. James' Hospital, Balham, London SW12 8HW, U.K., and St. Vincent's Hospital, Fitzroy, Victoria 3065, Australia*

A glance at the contents of this book shows the enormous interest worldwide in the latest generation of cephalosporins. Some variation in

the results of our antipodean work reflects particular problems with multiply antibiotic-resistant organisms, some of which, e.g., *Serratia marcescens*, have caused substantial outbreaks of hospital sepsis (3). At present, the major problem at St. Vincent's Hospital, Melbourne, is epidemic sepsis due to *Staphylococcus aureus* resistant to all conventional antibiotics except rifampin, vancomycin, and fusidic acid. Therefore, the fact that most are susceptible to cefotaxime is one of immediate relevance.

Disk susceptibility testing was performed by the ICS method (1), and MICs were determined in duplicate using both the broth and agar dilution techniques (2), which we found to be in substantial agreement. Table 1 shows the results of disk testing of 630 isolates against cefotaxime and 7 other cephalosporins (cefoxitin being here loosely described as a cephalosporin) and also the results against gentamicin, amikacin, and carbenicillin. Results against tobramycin are not included, as in our hands, where an organism appeared susceptible by disk, it often showed an MIC >20 µg/ml. With carbenicillin against *S. marcescens*, most of our isolates proved resistant, possessing a group L plasmid (3). The results of cefotaxime against gram-negative rods were excellent, and those against *S. aureus* were more than acceptable. No other cephalosporin tested gave comparable results, and no other was active against *Pseudomonas aeruginosa*. Cefuroxime gave good overall results but was totally inactive against *S. marcescens*; cefoxitin was better, except against *S. aureus*. Amikacin seems the best aminocyclitol aminoglycoside, but it has toxicity problems. Nonetheless, clinicians are (despite contrary advice) using fusidic acid alone, not in combination, so that the problem of early resistance to the latter drug is a very real one. Until now, in Australia, vancomycin and fusidic acid have been used rarely against the time when a resistance problem might arise.

The MICs against different organisms are shown in Table 2. We took 3.1 µg/ml as a base line because we had little of the drug available even for laboratory use. It is easily seen that (excluding *P. aeruginosa*), with the exception of two isolates of *Klebsiella aerogenes* and a small number of *S. aureus*, all organisms tested were susceptible to cefotaxime at <3.1 µg/ml. No other cephalosporin gave comparable results, although amikacin was at least as active as cefotaxime.

Table 2 also details the results with 80 isolates of *P. aeruginosa*. Here, as in Table 1, cefotaxime had a definite range, but the median was either 6.25 or 12.5 µg/ml, concentrations easily attainable in the serum with conventional dosage. It is interesting (although the numbers are small) that 1967 isolates and those which are either

TABLE 1. *Numbers and percentages (in parentheses) of organisms susceptible by disk method*

Organism	No.	Cefotaxime	Cefazolin	Cephalothin	Cefamandole	Cefuroxime	Cephaloridine	Cefalexin	Cefoxitin	Gentamicin	Amikacin	Carbenicillin
S. aureus	238	222 (93)	230 (97)	236 (99)	232 (97)	222 (93)	238 (100)	182 (76)	194 (82)	156 (66)	234 (98)	NT[a]
E. coli	150	150 (100)	144 (96)	138 (92)	150 (100)	148 (99)	140 (93)	138 (92)	144 (96)	150 (100)	150 (100)	NT
K. aerogenes	44	44 (100)	40 (91)	38 (86)	38 (86)	40 (91)	34 (77)	42 (95)	42 (95)	40 (91)	42 (95)	NT
S. marcescens	20	18 (90)	0	0	8 (40)	0	0	0	14 (70)	6 (30)	20 (100)	NT
P. mirabilis	98	98 (100)	96 (98)	92 (94)	86 (88)	94 (96)	78 (80)	82 (84)	98 (100)	98 (100)	98 (100)	NT
P. aeruginosa	80	60 (75)	NT	NT	NT	NT	NT	NT	NT	72 (90)	40 (100)	70 (88)

[a] NT = not tested.

TABLE 2. *MICs against different organisms tested by dilution and tube methods*

Organism (no. tested)	Antibiotic	MICs	
		Range	Median
S. aureus (40)	Cefotaxime	<3.1–12.5	<3.1
	Cefuroxime	<3.1–25	<3.1
	Cephalothin	<3.1	<3.1
	Amikacin	<3.1–12.5	<3.1
	Gentamicin	<1.5–25	<1.5
E. coli (20)	Cefotaxime	<3.1	<3.1
	Cefuroxime	<3.1	<3.1
	Cephalothin	<3.1	<3.1
	Amikacin	<3.1	<3.1
	Gentamicin	<1.5–25	<1.5
K. aerogenes (31)	Cefotaxime	<3.1–64[a]	<3.1
	Cefuroxime	<3.1–8[b]	<3.1
	Cephalothin	<3.1–64	<3.1
	Amikacin	<3.1	<3.1
	Gentamicin	<1.5–50	50
S. marcescens (20)	Cefotaxime	<3.1	<3.1
	Cefuroxime	12.5–>100	12.5
	Cephalothin	>100	>100
	Amikacin	3.1–6.25	6.25
	Gentamicin	50–>100	50
P. aeruginosa (80)	Cefotaxime	6.25–100	6.25
13 strains isolated in 1967	Amikacin	<3.1–3.1	<3.1
	Gentamicin	<1.5	<1.5
	Carbenicillin	31–500	62
7 gentamicin-resistant strains (1976–77)	Cefotaxime	6.25–12.5	6.25
	Amikacin	<3.1	<3.1
	Carbenicillin	31	31
10 carbenicillin-resistant strains (1976–77)	Cefotaxime	6.25–50	6.25
	Amikacin	<3.1	<3.1
	Gentamicin	<1.5	<1.5
50 routine isolates (1976–77)	Cefotaxime	6.25–>50	12.5
	Amikacin	<3.1–12.5	<3.1
	Gentamicin	<1.5–3.1	<1.5
	Carbenicillin	31–250	31

[a] 0.025 to 0.25, except two isolates.
[b] Two isolates >64.

carbenicillin or gentamicin resistant from 1976 to 1977 show the lower median.

The MICs of cefotaxime, cefuroxime, and cefoxitin against 20 isolates each of almost totally antibiotic-resistant *S. aureus* and *K. aerogenes* were compared, but the results are not shown here. Cefotaxime was shown to be unquestionably the best of the three drugs; but to achieve a serum level in excess of 32 μg/ml reliably requires bolus i.v. injection of the drug (1 g i.m. gives a serum peak of about 24 μg/ml, whereas i.v. bolus peaks at about 110 μg/ml). In contrast,

all strains of *K. aerogenes* were exquisitely susceptible and should be well covered by a 250-mg i.m. injection which gives a serum peak of about 5 μg/ml. As others have noted, this drug is exceedingly active against gram-negative bacteria (2), but it is a perplexing yet happy situation that seemingly the more resistant an organism is to other antibiotics, the more susceptible it is to cefotaxime.

The question will inevitably arise in the clinical situation as to whether combined therapy should be used, either for the patient's benefit (sic) or to protect cefotaxime against the emergence of resistance. There is a definite case for using the drug on its own in high i.v. dosage, but if it is to be combined, then our results suggest unequivocally that amikacin should be the second drug. This presupposes that such a combination be not nephrotoxic. One may speculate that, once clavulanic acid or a similar derivative proves itself clinically, it will become the obvious drug of second choice.

In summary, our in vitro work shows cefotaxime to be the most active cephalosporin or cephamycin presently available, with the important additional property of being a new, presumably nontoxic antipseudomonas drug.

1. **Ericsson, H. M., and J. C. Sherris.** 1971. Acta Pathol. Microbiol. Scand. Suppl. 217.
2. **Hamilton-Miller, J. M. T., W. Brumfitt, and A. V. Reynolds.** 1978. Cefotaxime (HR 756) a new cephalosporin with exceptional broad-spectrum activity in vitro. J. Antimicrob. Chemother. 4:437–444.
3. **Stratford, B. C., S. Dixson, B. G. Clarke, and B. F. Stratford.** 1978. Epidemic of hospital-acquired infection due to Serratia marcescens: report of 104 cases, p. 442–445. In Current chemotherapy, Proceedings of the 10th International Congress of Chemotherapy. American Society for Microbiology, Washington, D.C.

Activity and Beta-Lactamase Susceptibility of Cefotaxime: Comparison with Six Other Cephalosporins

R. PETER MOUTON,* GER P. A. BONGAERTS, AND MARIETTE VAN GESTEL

Department of Medical Microbiology, University Hospital, Leiden, The Netherlands

Cefotaxime (HR-756) is a new cephalosporin with high activity against *Enterobacteriaceae* (2, 3). The activity of this new antibiotic against randomly selected strains of *Enterobacteriaceae, Staphylococcus aureus, Haemophilus influenzae, Pseudomonas aeruginosa*, and enterococci was compared with six other cephalosporins (cefuroxime, cefamandole, cefoxitin, cefazolin, cephradin, and cephalothin). Comparison was performed by means of agar dilution tests on Isosensitest agar (Oxoid) and an inoculum of 10^3 CFU per spot.

Cefotaxime showed the lowest MIC values for *Enterobacteriaceae*, 90% of the strains being inhibited by concentrations ranging from 0.06 µg/ml (*Proteus* spp.) to 0.5 µg/ml (*Enterobacter* spp.). Fifty percent of *P. aeruginosa* strains were inhibited by 16 µg/ml, of enterococcus by 8 µg/ml, and of *H. influenzae* by 0.004 µg/ml; all other cephalosporins were less active against these species. *S. aureus* was most susceptible to cephalothin; cefamandole and cefazolin were the next most active against this species.

For five enterobacterial species, a comparison was made between MIC values of cefotaxime and three other new cephalosporins (cefamandole, cefuroxime, and cefoxitin) with two groups of strains, e.g., randomly selected and cephalothin-resistant strains, respectively (Table 1). The effect of cephalothin resistance on median MIC values was small. MIC_{50} and MIC_{90} values showed some increase for all antibiotics tested, but all MIC_{90} values of cefotaxime for cephalothin-resistant (and presumably β-lactamase positive) strains were well within the therapeutic range. This did not hold for the other three cephalosporins, of which MIC_{90} values frequently were higher than the borderline concentration of susceptibility (16 µg/ml). Second to cefotaxime was cefamandole for *Enterobacter, E. coli*, and indole-negative *Proteus*, cefuroxime for *Klebsiella*, and cefoxitin for indole-positive *Proteus*.

The effect of the inoculum size on the MIC values of a β-lactam antibiotic often is a good parameter for β-lactamase susceptibility. This inoculum effect on cephalosporin activity was determined by calculating the ratio of the MIC obtained with an inoculum of 10^6 CFU/ml and of the MIC obtained with an inoculum of 10^3 CFU/ml. This ratio was calculated for two strains each of the same five enterobacterial species. The geometric means of the ratios for 10 strains were 3.48, 2.93, and 2.83 for cefotaxime, cefuroxime, and cefoxitin, respectively. For cefamandole it was 5.28, pointing to higher β-lactamase susceptibility than of the other three cephalosporins tested. However, the difference was just short of statistical significance.

The in vitro β-lactamase susceptibility of the same four cephalosporins and of cephalothin was assayed according to the UV spectrophotometric method of O'Callaghan et al. (4). For this test, cell-free extracts of cephalothin-resistant strains were prepared by overnight shake culture in brain heart infusion (BHI) and subsequently 1 ml was used for inoculation of 300 ml of BHI. After 2 h of incubation, 25 µg of cephalothin/ml was added to induce β-lactamase production. After another 3 h of incubation, cells were harvested, washed, and subsequently treated by sonic disruption. The supernatants of the centrifuged sonic extracts (which were stored at $-20°C$) were used for assay. Optimal wave-lengths for the cephalosporin antibiotics were determined before assay of β-lactamase susceptibility. These were 262 nm for cephalothin, cefuroxime, and cefotaxime, and 272 nm for cefamandole. For cefoxitin, which was not hydrolyzed, a wavelength of 262 nm was chosen. Sep-

TABLE 1. *MIC values of cefotaxime (CTX), cefuroxime (CXM), cefoxitin (CXT), and cefamandole (CMD) which inhibit 50% and 90%, respectively, of five organisms*

Organism (no. of strains)		Group[a]	Antibiotic							
			CTX		CXM		CXT		CMD	
			MIC_{50}	MIC_{90}	MIC_{50}	MIC_{90}	MIC_{50}	MIC_{90}	MIC_{50}	MIC_{90}
E. coli	(30)	RA	0.06	0.12	4	16	4	16	2	16
	(22)	CR	0.12	2	16	32	16	64	16	32
Enterobacter	(20)	RA	0.12	0.5	8	16	128	>128	2	16
	(22)	CR	0.12	0.5	8	32	>128	>128	2	32
Klebsiella	(30)	RA	0.03	0.12	4	16	4	16	8	32
	(17)	CR	0.12	0.5	16	32	32	128	16	64
Indole[+] *Proteus*	(18)	RA	0.03	0.06	64	128	4	16	4	32
	(20)	CR	0.03	0.06	64	128	4	16	8	32
Indole[−] *Proteus*	(20)	RA	0.015	0.06	2	16	4	16	2	8
	(13)	CR	0.03	0.03	16	128	4	16	4	16

[a] RA, randomized strains; CR, cephalothin-resistant strains (MIC $\geq$ 16 μg/ml).

TABLE 2. *Beta-lactamase activity of cell-free extracts of cephalothin-resistant strains against cephalothin, cefotaxime, cefuroxime, cefamandole, and cefoxitin*

Strain	Antibiotic				
	Cephalothin activity[a]	Cefotaxime activity[b] (MIC)	Cefuroxime activity[b] (MIC)	Cefamandole activity[b] (MIC)	Cefoxitin activity[b] (MIC)
Klebsiella					
D2982	0.120	0.25 (0.5)	6.7 (32)	200 (32)	tr[c] (32)
E6148	0.060	11.6 (0.06)	8.3 (4)	133 (64)	0 (32)
8105	0.019	0 (0.12)	0 (16)	58 (32)	0 (>128)
Enterobacter					
101164	0.060	0 (1)	0 (32)	183 (32)	0 (>128)
AZL1	0.037	0 (1)	0 (8)	0 (4)	0 (128)
E. coli					
L123	0.580	0.1 (1)	0.5 (64)	64 (16)	tr[c] (64)
104050	0.390	0 (2)	0 (32)	0.5 (16)	0 (32)
E3320	0.110	0.9 (0.06)	2.7 (64)	336 (16)	0 (8)
D8808	0.060	0 (4)	1.7 (64)	167 (>128)	0 (>128)
Proteus vulgaris					
2566	0.970	0.4 (12)	0.6 (8)	23 (8)	0 (2)
B1392	0.200	10 (0.06)	10 (64)	195 (32)	tr[c] (64)
P. mirabilis M7	0.0820	0 (0.03)	0 (32)	2.4 (4)	0 (16)
Whatman beta-lactamase	2.4	58	62	187	0

[a] Calculated as micromoles per minute per milligram of protein.
[b] Calculated as micromoles per minute per milligram of protein, but given as a percentage of activity against cephalothin (100%).
[c] Trace.

arate sonicates of 12 strains of 5 genera were prepared. The results are given in Table 2, in which the specific enzyme activities are given as a percentage of activity against cephalothin, after calculation as micromoles per minute per milligram of protein. Comparison of these data with the MIC values of the same strains shows that a correlation between MIC values and β-lactamase susceptibility is lacking for cefotaxime, cefoxitin, and cefuroxime. This is in agreement with earlier reports concerning this phenomenon (1, 5). However, for cefamandole there seems to be some indication for a relationship between the two values for each strain, higher MIC values usually being found for strains with high β-lactamase activity and low MIC values for those in which β-lactamase activity is negligible. This observation correlates with the finding of the relatively large inoculum effect of cefamandole as compared with the three other new cephalosporins.

In conclusion, cefotaxime is the most active of the cephalosporins tested, except against S. au-

reus. Inactivation of this antibiotic by β-lactamase of *Enterobacteriaceae* is rare and when present is minimal.

1. **Fu, K. P., and H. C. Neu.** 1978. A comparative study of the activity of cefamandole and other cephalosporins and analysis of the β-lactamase stability and synergy of cefamandole with aminoglycosides. J. Infect. Dis. **137** (Suppl.): S38–S48.
2. **Hamilton-Miller, J. M. T., W. Brumfitt, and A. V. Reynolds.** 1978. Cefotaxime (HR 756) a new cephalosporin with exceptional broad-spectrum activity *in vitro*. J. Antimicrob. Chemother. **4**:437–444.
3. **Neu, H. C., N. Aswapokee, P. Aswapokee, and K. P. Fu.** 1979. HR 756, a new cephalosporin active against gram-positive and gram-negative aerobic and anaerobic bacteria. Antimicrob. Agents Chemother. **15**:273–281.
4. **O'Callaghan, C. H., P. W. Muggleton, and G. W. Ross.** 1968. Effects on β-lactamase from gram-negative organisms on cephalosporins and penicillins, p. 57–63. Antimicrob. Agents Chemother. 1967.
5. **Ott, J. L., J. R. Turner, and D. F. Mahoney.** 1979. Lack of correlation between β-lactamase production and susceptibility to cefamandole or cefoxitin among spontaneous mutants of *Enterobacteriaceae*. Antimicrob. Agents Chemother. **15**:14–19.

Activity of Cefotaxime Against Pathogens from Hospitals and the General Community

J. C. GOULD,* B. WATT, AND O. YOUNG

Central Microbiological Laboratories, Western General Hospital, Edinburgh, Scotland

The results quoted in this presentation refer to those obtained at the Central Microbiological Laboratories, Edinburgh, Scotland, and therefore represent that geographical locality. The figures may not be strictly comparable with those obtained in other parts of the world and other clinical situations. They do, however, cover the complete range of clinical sources within the given locality.

Ninety percent of the significant isolates in this general clinical laboratory are found to belong to a limited range of bacterial species within the groups *Staphylococcus, Streptococcus, Haemophilus,* and the gram-negative coliform bacilli. Many antibacterial agents effective against these organisms are available, but the cephalosporins are of interest in being active against a high proportion of isolates.

With earlier available cephalosporins, however, a significant proportion of isolates has been found to be relatively resistant in vitro, e.g., penicillinase-producing staphylococcus, *Streptococcus faecalis,* some strains of *Haemophilus* spp., and increasingly among some strains of

Escherichia. Pseudomonas, Serratia, Enterobacter, Providencia, and some *Proteus* spp. are also usually resistant, although it must be stated that these in vitro findings do not always correspond with the clinical response using cephalosporins in treatment.

A higher proportion of these cephalosporin-resistant strains has been isolated in hospital practice, which has discouraged the more widespread use of cephalosporins in the treatment of patients with severe clinical infection. Also, other organisms involved in serious infections in hospital patients, such as the anaerobic bacteria, are less susceptible to the cephalosporins, e.g., *Bacteroides* spp. Accordingly, it was with great interest that a detailed study of the in vitro susceptibility of a large and unselected sample of isolates in our laboratory was examined to assist in determining the usefulness of this new cephalosporin, cefotaxime.

This presentation shows the experimental results with several thousand consecutive fresh isolates. These results are intended to be essentially comparative with what are accepted as standard susceptible strains simultaneously tested. We feel that this is of first importance in the clinical application of susceptibility results and recommend that the term "coefficient of resistance" (CR) be returned to general use in preference to absolute figures denoting susceptibility which depends very much upon the technique used and uncontrollable variables in the test system. Thus, an organism may be of similar susceptibility to a known susceptible control organism and have a CR equal to 1: if it is more susceptible, the CR will be less than 1, and if less sensitive, the CR will be greater than 1.

Clinical experience will determine the significance to be attached to the coefficient of resistance, e.g., experience with susceptibility testing of *Mycobacterium tuberculosis* has attached great significance to a CR greater than 4 in relation to most antituberculous drugs. We consider that any organism 10 times more resistant than the susceptible control should not be regarded as amenable to treatment, but this ratio may vary from species to species, and probably also with the nature of the lesion. This may be related to a wider range of antibiotic concentration available at the site of infection, e.g., in the urinary tract where there are high concentrations of the antibacterial agent in the urine.

The diffusion test, when carried out with suitable control of variables such as thickness of the medium, water content of agar, size of inoculum, etc., can be made quantitative (1–3).

Alternatively, serial dilution methods in fluid or solid media may be used to determine the MIC. These may be more accurate and reproducible in the experimental sense, but whether or not such results are more relevant to the clinical situation remains controversial. Whichever method is used, cefotaxime performs well in vitro and inhibited the great majority of the common pathogens tested. The results are summarized in Table 1.

Activity against anaerobes. Organisms of the *Bacteroides fragilis* group such as *B. fragilis* and *B. thetaiotaomicron* were resistant to cefotaxime with MICs greater than 5 μg/ml. On the other hand, *Bacteroides* spp. such as *B. melaninogenicus* were susceptible, with MICs in the range 0.15 to 0.3 μg/ml. These values were obtained using an agar dilution technique with DST agar to which 10% horse blood was added at a pH of 7.2 and using an inoculum of approximately 10^5 CFU.

Clostridia in general were found to be relatively susceptible. Strains of *C. welchii* (*perfringens*) had MICs of 0.15 to 0.5 μg/ml. Other clostridia such as *C. tetani* and *C. septicum* were somewhat less susceptible, with MICs within the range 1.25 to 2.5 μg/ml.

Anaerobic cocci have a wide distribution of susceptibilities. A few strains were more resistant, with MICs greater than 5 μg/ml, but the majority had MICs within the range 0.3 to 0.6 μg/ml.

Preliminary experiments with the disk diffusion test have given an indication of increased activity between cefotaxime and cefoxitin against anaerobic bacteria, particularly those of the *B. fragilis* group. This phenomenon was not found with all organisms but occurred most regularly with β-lactamase-producing strains of *Bacteroides* spp. Further experiments with checkerboard titration using agar dilutions confirmed that, for such strains, synergy occurred

TABLE 1. *Sensitivity to cefotaxime of 3,000 strains tested*

Organism	No. of strains	% of strains with MIC (μg/ml):					
		<0.05	<0.1	<1.0	<2	<5	<25
Escherichia coli	850	2.8	55	95	97	100	
Proteus mirabilis	120	0	29	91	98	100	
P. vulgaris	30	0	0				
Klebsiella	23	0	47	100			
Providencia	7	0	14	94	100		
Citrobacter	11	0	80	100			
Other coliform bacilli	41	7	36	97	100		
Serratia	12	0	0	74	100		
Pseudomonas	150	0	0	2	27	45	96
Salmonella typhi	10		50	100			
Shigella sonnei	45		30	100			
Staphylococcus aureus	400	0	0	2	44	72	94
α and β streptococci	100	25	59	85	94	100	
Pneumococcus	60	67	100				
Streptococcus faecalis	105	0	0	0	23		100
Other streptococci	115	30	47		77		100
Haemopilus influenzae	220	73	88	100			

between the two antibiotics with an FIC index less than 0.3. So far, there is no evidence of synergy occurring with the anaerobic cocci nor with clostridia, but the phenomenon has been noted with β-lactamase-negative strains of *Bacteroides* spp.

Synergism can be frequently demonstrated in vitro, but there is difficulty in reconciling the results with clinical experience. The interpretation of any such in vitro results must therefore be made with caution and circumspection. During the tests described above, activity greater than might be expected from the sum of the arithmetic content of concentrations of the two antibiotics was observed using cefotaxime and a number of other cephalosporins.

On this evidence, cefotaxime is likely to be a useful antibiotic in the treatment of many infections, particularly serious gram-negative infections where the organism is resistant to other antibiotics, and severe respiratory infections involving *Haemophilus influenzae* and pneumococci. In patients in whom both aerobic and anaerobic bacteria are present, cefotaxime may become a useful alternative to the amino-sugars

or amoxicillin when combined with a second antibacterial agent such as metronidazole effective against anaerobic bacteria. A further use could be in compromised patients infected with opportunistic organisms such as *Serratia*; however, our results with *Pseudomonas* are not very encouraging in this respect.

As cefotaxime is available only for parenteral administration, its clinical use will be restricted; this may reduce its misuse and the antibiotic could be useful in helping to limit the spread of bacteria resistant to multiple antibiotics within the hospital community.

1. Bauer, A. W., W. M. M. Kirby, J. C. Sherris, and M. Turck. 1966. Antibiotic susceptibility testing by a standardized single disc method. Am. J. Clin. Pathol. 45:493–496.
2. Ericsson, H. M., and J. C. Sherris. 1971. Antibiotic sensitivity testing. Report of an international collaborative study. Acta Pathol. Microbiol. Scand. Sect. B Suppl. 217.
3. Gould, J. C., and J. H. Bowie. 1952. The determination of bacterial sensitivity to antibiotics. Edin. Med. J. 59:178–179.

Evaluation of So-Called Bone Levels for Instance for Cefotaxime (HR-756) Concentrations in Bone Under Critical Conditions

HARRY ROSIN* AND WOLFGANG UPHAUS

Institute for Medical Microbiology and Virology, University of Düsseldorf, D-4000 Düsseldorf, Federal Republic of Germany

To prove the suitability of an antibiotic in the treatment of osteomyelitis, it is common to provide analysis of "antibiotic levels in bone." Reports of investigations on osteomyelitic bone specimens are rare. However, many brochures announcing new antibiotics quote drug concentrations obtained on healthy bone specimens. As our investigation shows, the concentration of cefotaxime (HR-756) in healthy bone, which served as our model, cannot provide guidance in the therapy of osteomyelitis. It is therefore necessary to examine chronically infected bone specimens. When noninflamed bone is examined, only experimental data taken on compact bone specimens yield relevant information about the permeation of the antibiotic into the bone. This conclusion is based on an analysis of the most important components of bone specimens and their relative volumina for distribution of the antibiotics.

Compact bone. Compact bone contains primarily solid tissue, some blood, few cells (osteoblasts, osteoclasts), and interstitial fluid (ISF). The solid tissue is heavy and not diffusible by antibiotics. Measuring the hemoglobin concentration in the eluate and in the blood of the patient permits measurement of the blood content in the supernatant fluid after homogenization. The volume of intracellular liquid is very small. For this reason, the volume of the ISF can be determined with adequate precision by heating the homogenized bone sediment and total vaporization of the water. After considering the relation between the total volume of the eluate, the blood content, and the volume of ISF, concentration of the antibiotic in the ISF can be determined. This value represents the actual permeation of antibiotic into the extravascular liquid space of bone.

Yellow spongy bone. Yellow spongy bone

consists of solid tissue, some blood, much fat, a minor amount of watery intracellular liquid, and ISF. Here again, the portion of the blood can be determined by means of the hemoglobin concentration. The fatty portion does not evaporate below 120° C. By vaporizing the water, the total volume of the intracellular liquid and the ISF can be determined. Concentration of the antibiotic in the eluate and the resulting volume permit reasonably accurate measurement of permeation of the antibiotic into the bone.

Red spongy bone. When red spongy bone is homogenized, the eluate obtained is quantitatively not definable. It contains buffer solution, plasma, intracellular liquid of the blood and marrow cells, and ISF. The portion of the blood in the red spongy bone can be determined neither by measuring the hemoglobin nor by measuring the IgM. Red spongy bone is rich in extravascular preerythrocytic cells which contain hemoglobin like the intravascular erythrocytes and is also rich in extravascular plasma cells, which contain IgM as do the intravascular plasma cells and the serum.

Figures 1 and 2 illustrate these principles with

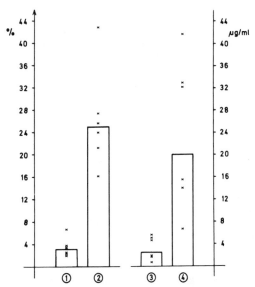

FIG. 2. *Cefotaxime (HR-756) concentrations in human compact bone. Columns 1 and 3 show each data point and the mean cefotaxime concentrations in percentages of the serum levels (1) and as absolute values (3) contained in the eluate of compact bone specimens after subtraction of the amount of retained blood. Columns 2 and 4 show the respective values after additional consideration of the weight of the solid tissue.*

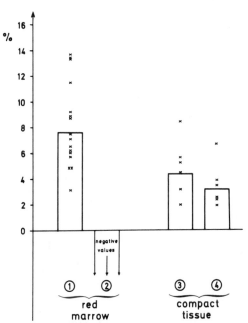

FIG. 1. *Cefotaxime (HR-756) concentrations in human bone specimens in percentages of simultaneously taken serum levels. Columns 1 and 3 show each data point and the mean cefotaxime concentrations in percentages of the serum levels contained in the eluate of red spongy bone (1) and compact bone (3). Columns 2 and 4 show respective values after subtraction of the retained blood by measuring the hemoglobin concentration.*

cefotaxime data in bone tissue. We used bone specimens from 10 patients operated on for osteotomy or arthroplasty of the hip. During the operation one or several bone specimens were removed, and simultaneously two blood samples were taken. One was used to obtain serum, and the other was placed in an EDTA-coated tube for determination of the hemoglobin. Immediately after surgery the bone samples were separated, as well as possible, into compact, yellow spongy and red spongy bone and then homogenized in phosphate-buffer solution (pH 6.5). After centrifugation on the following day, the cefotaxime activity of the extraction fluids and the serum samples was estimated by the agar diffusion test using a very susceptible (MIC = 0.078 μg/ml) *E. coli* strain; the minimal detectable quantity was <0.1 μg of cefotaxime per ml.

Column 1 in Fig. 1 shows the geometric mean and each data point of the cefotaxime concentrations expressed in percentages of the respective serum levels in the eluate of the red spongy bone specimens, as is common in the literature about "antibiotic levels in bone." After allowing for the hemoglobin concentration in the eluate, negative values were obtained as shown in column 2 because there is extravascular hemoglobin in the preerythrocytic cells of the red marrow which, together with the intravascular hemoglobin of the erythrocytes, yields to computation of a falsely high portion of blood in the bone specimens. Columns 3 and 4 show the geometric means and each data point of the cefotaxime concentration in the eluate of compact bone specimens before (column 3) and after (column 4) subtracting the blood portion.

Column 1 in Fig. 2 is consistent with column 4 of Fig. 1. Cefotaxime concentrations in the compact bone specimens were in the order of 3% of the respective serum concentrations after allowing for the blood portion. Due to the method employed, the values were low, since the weight of the solid substance brought about an attenuation effect. When the measured concentrations were related to the original volume of the ISF, the values increased on the average to 25% (column 2). Analogous to the percentages in columns 1 and 2, columns 3 and 4 show the absolute concentrations (in micrograms per milliliter). Considering the mean value of 20 µg/ml,

the cefotaxime concentrations in the ISF of the compact bone were relatively high. They are indicative of a good and easy mass transfer between the blood and the perivascular space in the bone. The marrow sinuses, e.g., belong to capillary type III according to the classification by G. Majno (Am. Physiol. Soc. 1965:2253–2375). They have endothelial gaps and their subepithelial membrane is discontinuous or even absent. Also indicative of normally good penetration of antibiotics into the ISF of the bone are the good chemotherapeutic results in cases of acute osteomyelitis. The inadequate permeability of antibiotics into bone in case of chronic osteomyelitis is not a consequence of their physical-chemical properties but rather a result of disturbances of the microcirculation caused by the inflammation and a result of the peculiarities of vessel structure in bone. Thus, for relevant evidence about the therapy of osteomyelitis, investigations on chronically infected bone specimens are indispensable.

Azlocillin and Ticarcillin in Combination with Cefoxitin and Cefotaxime (HR-756): an In Vitro Study

JENNIFER M. ANDREWS, KEITH A. BEDFORD, RICHARD WISE,* AND ADRIAN P. GILLETT

Department of Medical Microbiology, Dudley Road Hospital, Birmingham B18 7QH, U.K.

Azlocillin (AZ) and ticarcillin (TIC) have similar antibacterial properties, being broad-spectrum penicillins with marked antipseudomonal activity. As both these agents are hydrolyzed by many of the prevalent β-lactamases, including Tem, it is probable that these agents will be used in combination with another agent in the treatment of severe sepsis.

Synergy between β-lactams and aminoglycosides is well documented (1). As potent and β-lactamase-stable cephems (which should be less toxic than aminoglycosides) are becoming available, it is possible that AZ or TIC could be used clinically with a cephalosporin.

In this study we investigated the in vitro effect of combining both penicillins with each of cefoxitin (CEF) and cefotaxime (HR-756 [HR]). Both bacteriostatic, checkerboard procedures and a viable count method were used.

The agar plate dilution checkerboard was designed so that the following combinations were studied: AZ + CEF, AZ + HR, TIC + CEF and TIC + HR.

The strains tested are shown in Table 1. The medium used was Isosensitest (Oxoid), pH 7.2,

supplemented with 10% lysed horse blood for *Bacteroides fragilis.*

In the viable count investigation, the strains given in Table 2 were studied.

The organisms were inoculated into Isosensitest broth, pH 7.2, at an initial viable count of 10^3 to 10^4 colony-forming units/ml. The broth contained the above combinations of antibiotic and each alone, each agent being at a concentration of 0.5 MIC. An antibiotic-free control was used.

Subcultures and dilutional procedures to determine the viable count were performed at time 0, 0.5, 1, 2, 4, 6, and 24 h.

The checkerboard results were analyzed by determining the fractional inhibitory concentration (FIC) of each agent at the point of maximal interaction and then noting the ΣFIC. Synergy was defined as ΣFIC of ≤0.6 µg/ml, with the MIC of each agent at the point of interaction being ≤32 µg/ml; this was arbitrarily defined as outside the clinical range. Indifference was considered to be present if the FIC was >0.6 and <2 µg/ml.

The viable counts were plotted semilogarith-

Organism and strain	ΣFIC at high (H) and low (L) inoculum								No. of strains showing synergy/total (ΣFIC < 0.6)							
	AZ + CEF		AZ + HR		TIC + CEF		TIC + HR		AZ + CEF		AZ + HR		TIC + CEF		TIC + HR	
	L	H	L	H	L	H	L	H	L	H	L	H	L	H	L	H
P. aeruginosa																
1	ID[a]	OC[b]	ID	ID	ID	OC	ID	ID								
2	ID	ID	ID	0.56	ID	OC	ID	ID								
3	ID	ID	ID	0.5	ID	OC	ID	0.25	0/4	0/4	1/4	3/4	0/4	0/4	0/4	0/4
4 (Tem⁺)	OC	ID	0.51	0.53	OC	OC	OC	OC								
E. coli																
1	ID	0.5	0.56	0.5	ID	ID	ID	ID								
2	0.5	0.4	ID	0.4	ID	0.5	ID	ID								
3	0.5	0.5	0.5	0.25	ID	0.25	ID	0.25	1/5	3/5	3/5	4/5	2/5	3/5	1/5	2/5
4	ID	ID	0.07	0.03	0.56	OC	0.15	OC								
5	ID	ID	ID	ID	0.5	0.56	ID	ID								
K. pneumoniae																
1	0.5	ID	0.56	ID	0.56	OC	0.6	OC								
2	OC	0.5	OC	OC	OC	OC	OC	OC	3/4	2/3	1/4	1/3	1/4	0/3	0/4	0/3
3	0.5	NT	ID	NT	ID	NT	OC	NT								
4	0.5	0.51	ID	0.56	ID	OC	OC	OC								
S. aureus																
1	0.56	0.28	ID	ID	ID	0.38	0.3	0.25								
2	0.38	0.25	ID	0.5	0.38	0.5	0.56	OC	4/4	4/4	0/4	2/4	3/4	4/4	3/4	2/4
3	0.38	0.25	ID	0.51	0.38	0.5	0.5	0.56								
4	0.38	0.38	ID	ID	0.38	0.25	ID	ID								
P. mirabilis																
1	0.31	0.5	0.56	ID	ID	ID	ID	ID								
2	0.25	0.38	0.5	0.5	ID	ID	ID	ID	3/3	3/3	2/3	2/3	3/3	0/3	0/3	0/3
3	ID	0.5	ID	0.5	ID	ID	ID	ID								
Proteus, indole positive																
1	ID	0.3	0.5	ID	ID	ID	ID	0.5								
2	OC	OC	0.15	0.25	ID	ID	ID	ID	0/4	1/4	2/4	2/4	0/4	1/4	0/4	2/4
3	ID	OC	ID	ID	ID	ID	ID	0.56								
4	ID	ID	ID	0.56	ID	0.38	OC	ID								
Total excluding B. fragilis									10/24	13/23	9/24	14/23	9/24	8/23	4/24	6/23
Mean % showing synergy									50	52.4	45	42	37	38	22	20
B. fragilis																
1	ID	ID	ID	ID	ID	ID	ID	ID								
2	0.31	0.31	OC	OC	0.5	0.5	0.5	OC	3/4	3/4	0/4	0/4	2/4	2/4	1/4	0/4
3	0.37	0.31	ID	ID	ID	ID	ID	ID								
4	0.25	0.13	ID	ID	OC	0.38	OC	OC								
Grand total mean % showing synergy									52.4		42		38		20	

[a] ID, Indifference.
[b] OC, Outside clinical range.

TABLE 2. *Summary of viable count study*

Organism and strain	AZ + CEF	AZ + HR	TIC + CEF	TIC + HR
P. aeruginosa				
Tem$^+$ (2 strains)	2-log reduction at 6 h	2-log reduction at 4 h		
Tem$^-$	Delay in regrowth	No regrowth		
E. coli				
β^-	1-log reduction at 3 h	1-log reduction at 6 h		1-log reduction at 6 h
β^+	Slight delay in regrowth	Slight delay in regrowth	1-log reduction at 3 h	Slight delay in regrowth
K. pneumoniae				
1	2-log reduction at 3 h	1-log reduction at 4 h	2-log reduction at 4 h	Slight delay in regrowth
2	2-log reduction at 3 h	2-log reduction at 4 h	1-log reduction at 4 h	Slight delay in regrowth

mically against time and analyzed by noting the following: (i) failure to yield a 1-log reduction in initial inoculum; (ii) time for growth or regrowth to at least 1 log greater than initial inoculum.

Checkerboard study. The results of the checkerboard study are shown in Table 1. In the case of *Pseudomonas aeruginosa* no synergy was noted with AZ + CEF and TIC + HR and only minimal synergy was noted with AZ + HR. Against *Escherichia coli* the most synergistic combination was AZ + HR, TIC + HR being the least. AZ + CEF was the only combination showing significant synergy against *Klebsiella* spp., and the most consistent results against *Staphylococcus aureus* were seen with AZ + CEF. Against *Proteus mirabilis* AZ + CEF was again the most successful combination, but no combination was consistently synergistic against the indole-positive *Proteus* spp. AZ + CEF was again the most successful combination against *B. fragilis*, where the most marked synergy of all the bacterial strains tested was seen, and AZ + HR was the least. Analyzing the overall results, 52% of the strains tested at the two inocula showed synergy with AZ + CEF, 42% with AZ + HR, 38% with TIC + CEF, and 20% with TIC + HR.

Viable count study. The results of the viable count study are summarized in Table 2. The Tem$^+$ strain of *P. aeruginosa* showed some effect of AZ + CEF and AZ + HR interaction, where there was a marked fall in the viable count and delay (as in the case of AZ + HR, no regrowth) in regrowth. TIC + CEF and TIC +

HR showed no interaction, but no synergy was seen against the Tem$^-$ strain. The β-lactamase-negative strain of *E. coli* showed an interaction (an increase in killing) in all but the TIC + CEF. The usual effect in the β^+ strain was a slight delay in regrowth of the combination compared with each agent alone. The most synergistic combination against the two strains of *Klebsiella* was AZ + CEF, with a 2-log reduction at 3 h. The least synergistic was TIC + HR, when only a slight delay in growth to 1 log greater than the initial count was observed.

The overall results of the viable count study showed that of the six strains tested, there was a 99% reduction in viable count (i.e., a 2-log kill) in 50% of the strains tested to the AZ + CEF combination, 33% to the AZ + HR, 17% to TIC + CEF, and 0% to TIC + HR combinations.

It would appear from these two studies that if AZ and TIC are to be combined with one of the broad-spectrum cephalosporins such as CEF or cefotaxime, a combination of AZ and CEF might be superior.

In both the checkerboard and viable count studies about one-half of the strains tested showed a significant interaction with AZ + CEF. The other combinations showed a discrepancy between the viable counts and agar dilution study, but TIC + HR was the least effective combination.

1. **Smith, C. B., P. E. Dans, J. N. Wilfert, and M. Finland.** 1969. Use of gentamicin in combination with other antibiotics. J. Infect. Dis. **119:**370–377.

Separation and Assay of Cefotaxime (HR-756) and Its Metabolites in Serum, Urine, and Bile

L. O. WHITE,* H. A. HOLT, D. S. REEVES, M. J. BYWATER, AND R. P. BAX

Department of Microbiology, Southmead Hospital, Bristol, and Roussel Laboratories Limited, Wembley Park, Middlesex, England*

Cefotaxime (HR-756), a new semisynthetic cephalosporin with a broad spectrum including antipseudomonal activity, is partially metabolized in vivo. The desacetyl metabolite (DACM) is less microbiologically active than cefotaxime and has a different spectrum (R. Wise, J. M. Andrews, D. Hammond, P. J. Wills, A. M. Geddes, and M. McKendrick, this volume). The lactone form of DACM is also microbiologically active.

Cefotaxime and DACM have different pharmacokinetics; therefore, pharmacokinetic data for cefotaxime obtained from the results of microbiological assays with DACM-susceptible indicator organisms will be incorrect, especially in uremic patients where cephalosporin metabolites accumulate (2).

This paper describes specific assays for cefotaxime and DACM and reports the results of some investigations using them.

Specific microbiological assay of cefotaxime. A DACM-resistant strain of *Proteus morganii*, selected from a number of clinical isolates, was inoculated onto Penassay agar (Difco). Standard solutions of cefotaxime (2.5 to 40 mg/liter, in pooled human serum [phosphate buffer, pH 6.6] for the assay of plasma [urine] samples) and samples were applied to the agar on paper disks (6-mm diameter). Incubation was for 18 h at 37°C. Zone sizes were measured with a zone reader (Leebrook Co. Ltd.), and the results were computed by Bennett's method (1).

High-performance liquid chromatographic (HPLC) assays. A Waters Associates liquid chromatograph with two pumps (model 6000A, controlled by a model 660 flow programmer), a U6K injector, and a model 440 UV detector (254 nm) set at 0.005 AUFS was used. The analytical column (Microbondapak C_{18}) was protected by a guard column (C_{18} Corasil). For urine assays the mobile phase was water-methanol (93:7), containing paired-ion reagent B7 (Waters Associates). For plasma and bile assays the mobile phase was acetic acid (1% in water)-methanolic acetic acid (1%), 70:30. The solvent flow rate was 2 ml/min. Bile and urine samples were diluted before injection, plasma proteins were precipitated with acetonitrile (50%), and

the supernatant was injected. Injection volumes were 5 to 20 µl.

High-voltage electrophoresis (HVE)/bioautography. Samples of body fluids or standard solutions, or both, were applied to wells in an agarose slab gel (40 by 32 by 0.2 cm in Tris-malic acid buffer, pH 5.6) and electrophoresed at 1,000 to 1,200 V/200 mA for 3 h. Subsequently the agarose was overlaid with DST agar (Oxoid), seeded with *Bacillus subtilis*, and incubated at 37°C overnight. The developed plates were photographed, and the migration of the zones of inhibition was measured. Alternatively, a single sample was applied to every well in the agarose and, after electrophoresis, the bioautograph using *B. subtilis* was confined to the two strips (4 cm wide) along the edges of the plate between the electrodes. The central area of agarose was cut into strips orientated perpendicular to the current flow which were removed and frozen. Gel-free fluid from the thawed strips was analyzed by HPLC.

Results and discussion. In the HPLC plasma assay the retention times were 3.0 (DACM) and 6.5 (cefotaxime) min. No interfering peaks were seen in blank plasma or bile samples, but they were present in urine samples and prevented accurate assay of DACM. The inclusion of heptane sulfonic acid (paired-ion reagent) in the mobile phase resulted in the separation of DACM from interfering urine peaks. In this system retention times were 8.5 (DACM) and 30 (cefotaxime) min.

Results of the HPLC assay correlated well with the results of the microbiological assay using *P. morganii* (correlation coefficient, 0.99; regression equation, $Y = 0.9916X - 0.65$).

The concentrations of cefotaxime in the blood of an anuric volunteer at intervals after receiving 1 g intravenously were measured by HPLC and microbiological assays using various indicator organisms. The results are shown in Fig. 1. HPLC and *P. morganii* assays generated similar results. The other microbiological assays gave falsely elevated cefotaxime concentrations in samples taken 4 h or more after the dose due to the metabolite levels being relatively high compared with those of cefotaxime.

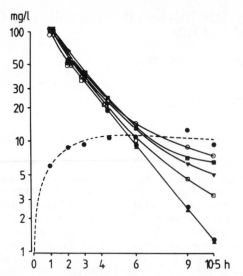

FIG. 1. *Comparison of observed blood concentrations of cefotaxime in an anuric volunteer obtained by assays using HPLC (●) or microbiological methods with various indicator organisms: ▲, P. morganii, ■, B. subtilis; ▼, E. coli (UC 1020); □, E. coli (local strain); ○, Klebsiella sp. (NCTC 10896). ●– – –●, DACM (HPLC).*

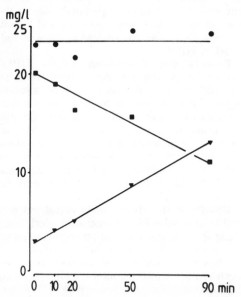

FIG. 2. *Conversion of cefotaxime (■) to DACM (▼) in plasma containing lysed blood; experiment conducted at 22°C. ●, Both cefotaxime and DACM.*

Stability of cefotaxime in water and plasma was studied by HPLC assay. In plasma and water in vitro cefotaxime was significantly de-

graded in 24 h at 37°C. Thus, in water 20 mg of cefotaxime per liter fell to 11.7 mg/liter; the DACM level rose from 0 to 4.1 mg/liter. In serum the corresponding figures were 20 to 3.1 (cefotaxime) and 0 to 2.7 (DACM) mg/liter. Cefotaxime was not significantly degraded in 24 h at 4°C. In contrast, in plasma tinged with lysed blood cefotaxime was rapidly and quantitatively deacetylated (Fig. 2). This finding indicates that hemolysis must be avoided in samples from clinical trials or volunteer studies.

HVE/bioautography of both cefotaxime and DACM supplied as reference samples produced two zones of antibiotic antivity (one anodal, one cathodal). HPLC analysis of the cathodal zones revealed an unidentified substance (named "component X") with an HPLC retention time of 3.5 min (plasma assay). The anodal zones comprised cefotaxime or DACM, both of which had similar electrophoretic mobilities. A sample of pure DACM-lactone (supplied by Roussel Laboratories Limited) behaved identically to component X in HPLC and had the same mobility in HVE. HPLC analysis of reference samples of cefotaxime and DACM confirmed that they contained traces of lactone.

HVE/HPLC of body fluids showed the presence of lactone in bile and some urines, although the major component of bile was DACM. Thus, in one patient concentrations were: cefotaxime, 39.7 mg/liter, and DACM, 101.2 mg/liter; in another patient concentrations were: cefotaxime, 77.4 mg/liter, and DACM, 78.6 mg/liter. In addition, these biles showed other zones of antimicrobial activity in HVE and other peaks in HPLC. This may indicate the presence, in bile, of further degradation products of cefotaxime.

HPLC and HVE/bioautography have proved very powerful tools for the study of cefotaxime and its metabolites and should find similar application in the study of other cephalosporins. Our results demonstrate the importance of using specific assays in pharmacokinetic studies and of taking particular care to avoid lysis in blood samples for cefotaxime assay.

1. **Bennett, J. V., J. L. Brodie, E. J. Benner, and W. M. M. Kirby.** 1966. Simplified, accurate method for antibiotic assay of clinical specimens. Appl. Microbiol. **14:** 170–177.
2. **Nilsson-Ehle, I., and P. Nilsson-Ehle.** 1979. Pharmacokinetics of cephalothin: accumulation of its deacetylated metabolite in uremic patients. J. Infect. Dis. **139:** 712–716.
3. **Reeves, D. S., and H. A. Holt.** 1975. Resolution of antibiotic mixtures in serum samples by high-voltage electrophoresis. J. Clin. Pathol. **28:**435–442.

Pharmacokinetics of Cefotaxime and Its Desacetyl Metabolite

R. BAX,* L. WHITE, D. REEVES, R. INGS, M. BYWATER, AND H. HOLT

Southmead Hospital, Bristol; Roussel Laboratories, Wembly Park,* and Hoechst Pharmaceutical Research Laboratories, Milton Keynes, England

Cefotaxime (HR-756) is a novel and highly effective broad-spectrum antibiotic with considerable advantages over other cephalosporins. A pharmacokinetic study was initiated with three main objectives: (i) to determine the dose dependency of the kinetics of cefotaxime; (ii) to determine the interaction of probenecid on the kinetics of intravenously administered cefotaxime; and (iii) to determine the interaction of lidocaine on the kinetics of intramuscularly administered cefotaxime.

For the dose range study, three volunteers each received three incremental intravenous doses of cefotaxime of 0.5, 1, and 2 g. When

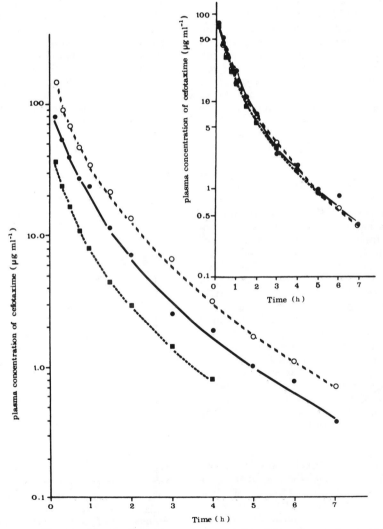

FIG. 1. *Plasma profiles of cefotaxime in subjects given incremental intravenous doses of 0.5 (■), 1.0 (●), and 2.0 (○) g of the compound. The inset shows the same plasma profiles normalized to a 1.0-g dose.*

studying the interaction of cefotaxime with probenecid, six volunteers received cefotaxime (1 g)
intravenously with and without concomitant
doses of probenecid. Finally, for the lidocaine
interaction study, three volunteers received cefotaxime (1 g) intramuscularly administered
with and without lidocaine.

Plasma and urine were collected at predetermined times and assayed for parent cefotaxime,
using both a microbiological (*Proteus morganii*)
and a high-pressure liquid chromatographic
analysis. The methods were in excellent agreement with each other, although the high-pressure liquid chromatographic method had the
advantage of also measuring the desacetyl metabolite of cefotaxime (DACM).

Each of the plasma profiles of cefotaxime and,
where possible, DACM were curve fitted, using
an iterative least-squares curve-fitting program.
Pharmacokinetic parameters of half-life, clearance, renal clearance, volume of distribution calculated from area, and initial distribution volume were also calculated (1). The statistical
tests of split-plot analysis, two-way analysis of
variance, paired *t* test, and 95% confidence limits
were applied as appropriate.

In all cases where cefotaxime was administered intravenously, the plasma concentrations
of the drug declined in two phases, with approximate half-lives of 0.2 to 0.4 h for the initial
phase and 0.9 to 1.7 h for the terminal phase.
When cefotaxime was given intramuscularly,
only one phase could be identified for the decline, with a half-life very similar to that observed for intravenous cefotaxime. The proportion of an intravenous dose excreted as unchanged cefotaxime was 61 ± 14%, although an
additional 24 ± 10% of the dose was also found
in urine as DACM. Plasma profiles of DACM
were generally more difficult to curve fit, although the half-life of this metabolite was found
to be longer (approximately 2 to 3 h) than that
of parent cefotaxime (0.9 to 1.7 h) and was,
therefore, elimination rate limited.

Before it is possible to make any meaningful
pharmacokinetic predictions, especially relating
to the design of a dosage regimen and how it
may be adjusted during disease states or drug
interactions, it is necessary to establish the linearity of kinetics. The dose range study demonstrated conclusively that the plasma levels of
cefotaxime increased in direct proportion to dose
and were superimposable when normalized for
dose (Fig. 1). A direct proportionality with dose
was also observed for area under the curve and
for the urinary excretion of unchanged cefotaxime. Furthermore, the pharmacokinetic parameters of plasma clearance (273 ± 52 ml min⁻¹),

renal clearance (164 ± 37 ml min⁻¹), initial distribution volume (10.7 ± 2.7 liters), and initial
(0.29 ± 0.10 h) and terminal (1.14 ± 0.22 h) half-
lives all remained constant with dose. The kinetics of cefotaxime were, therefore, considered
to be dose independent and linear.

Coadministration of probenecid increased and
sustained the levels of cefotaxime, as well as
DACM, in subjects given the compound intravenously when determined by split-plot analysis.
In addition, the area under the plasma level of
cefotaxime versus time curve was significantly
increased (79.7 ± 21.5 to 101.1 ± 24.6 μg ml⁻¹
h⁻¹), whereas clearance was significantly decreased (223 ± 60 to 174 ± 47 ml min⁻¹). Moreover, even though there was no significant
change in half-life and renal clearance when
measured by analysis of variance, the confidence
interval approach did indicate a definite trend
of increasing half-life (1.65 ± 0.87 to 2.40 ± 1.35
h) and decreasing renal clearance (153 ± 43 to
111 ± 45 ml min⁻¹) of cefotaxime with probenecid. It was perhaps striking that none of the
statistical tests detected any change in volume
of distribution. This is important when considering the mechanism of action of probenecid, for
Gibaldi and Schwartz (2) have proposed that
probenecid acts primarily by altering the distribution of the antibiotic, which in turn reduces
its apparent volume of distribution. No evidence
could be found to substantiate this for cefotax-

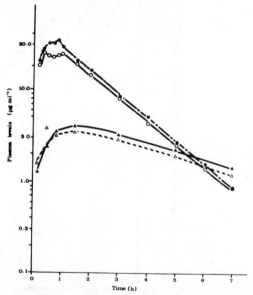

FIG. 2. *Mean plasma levels of parent cefotaxime
(○, ●) and DACM (△, ▲) in subjects given the drug
intramuscularly with and without lidocaine, respectively.*

ime, and it was concluded that for this drug, probenecid acts by inhibiting renal tubular secretion, resulting in a reduction of renal and total clearance.

To minimize any pain on intramuscular injection of cefotaxime, it has been proposed that the cephalosporin be formulated with a local anesthetic, lidocaine. Although no statistically significant difference in the plasma kinetics of intramuscular cefotaxime could be found with and without 1% lidocaine, the mean maximum plasma levels of the drug were reduced slightly with lidocaine (22.6 ± 4.6 µg ml^{-1} with lidocaine and 35.9 ± 6.2 µg ml^{-1} without lidocaine). Overall, the plasma levels of unchanged cefotaxime and DACM, with and without lidocaine, appeared to be very similar (Fig. 2). A slight but

significant increase in the renal clearance was observed when lidocaine was coadministered.

Thus it has been shown that (i) the kinetics of cefotaxime are linear and independent of dose, (ii) concomitant probenecid increases and sustains plasma levels of cefotaxime, primarily by inhibiting tubular secretion and decreasing the clearance of the drug, and (iii) lidocaine has a marginal, if any, effect on the absorption and elimination kinetics of cefotaxime.

1. **Gibaldi, M., and D. Perrier.** 1975. *In* J. Swarbrick (ed.), Pharmacokinetics. Marcel Dekker Inc., New York.
2. **Gibaldi, M. and M. A. Schwartz.** 1968. Apparent effect of probenecid on the distribution of penicillins in man. Clin. Pharmacol. Ther. **9:**345–349.

Synergy Between Cefotaxime, Cefsulodin, Azlocillin, Mezlocillin, and Aminoglycosides Against Carbenicillin-Resistant or -Susceptible *Pseudomonas aeruginosa*

EVELIO J. PEREA,* MARÍA C. NOGALES, JAVIER AZNAR, ESTRELLA MARTÍN, AND MERCEDES C. GARCÍA-IGLESIAS

Department of Microbiology, University of Seville Medical School, Seville, Spain

The present report presents an in vitro evaluation of four new β-lactam antibiotics with antipseudomonal activity. Two new cephalo- sporins, cefsulodin (SCE 129 or CGP 7174 [CGP]) (5) and cefotaxime (HR-756 [HR]) (1), and the ureido penicillin derivates azlocillin (AZ)

TABLE 1. *Antimicrobial activity (MIC) of cefotaxime (HR), cefsulodin (CGP), azlocillin (AZ), mezlocillin (MZ), gentamicin (GM), tobramycin (TM), sisomicin (SSM), amikacin (AMK), and dibekacin (DKB) against 50 P. aeruginosa (25 CAR^r and 25 CAR^s) strains*

Test agent	Strain group[a]	Median MIC (µg/ml)	% of inhibited test strain at MIC (µg/ml) of:													
			<0.25	0.25	0.5	1	2	4	8	16	32	64	128	256	512	>512
HR	CAR^r	40							12	44	76	92			100	
	CAR^s	23.6							12	92	100					
CGP	CAR^r	6.7				8	36	60	80		88		100			
	CAR^s	4.6				16	48	76	84	88	100					
AZ	CAR^r	8						20	52	64	84	96	100			
	CAR^s	17.8					4	12	24	60	84	88	96	100		
MZ	CAR^r	80					8			12	40	88	96	100		
	CAR^s	61.3								8	56	100				
GM	CAR^r	3.5		12	16		64	88	92							100
	CAR^s	5				24	48	64	68	84	88	96	100			
TM	CAR^r	0.92		12	60	88		92					100			
	CAR^s	0.92		8	60	64	76		80		96	100				
SSM	CAR^r	2.9		4	12	24	60	92								100
	CAR^s	6			4	24	44	60	72		80	84	96	100		
AMK	CAR^r	6.9		8				20	64	84	88	100				
	CAR^s	5.8					4	36	72	84	92	96		100		
DKB	CAR^r	2.9		8	12	32	76	92						100		
	CAR^s	2			8	44	52	56	68		72	76	80	96	100	

^{a} See text.

and mezlocillin (MZ) were evaluated alone and in combination with five aminoglycosides, gentamicin (GM), tobramycin (TM), dibekacin (DKB), sisomicin (SSM), and amikacin (AMK), against 50 *Pseudomonas aeruginosa* (25 carbenicillin resistant, MIC ≥ 128 µg/ml [CAR^r], and 25 carbenicillin susceptible, MIC < 128 µg/ml [CAR^s]) strains, 11 of which were resistant to aminoglycosides.

MICs were determined by the agar dilution method. So-called checkerboard MIC studies with two drug combinations were performed simultaneously on Mueller-Hinton agar with CGP, HR, AZ, MZ, and GM, TM, SSM, DKB, and AMK by the agar plate dilution method, using a Steers replicator (2). Results of the interaction are expressed by the fractional inhibitory concentration index (2).

The activities of these antibiotics against the 50 *P. aeruginosa* strains and the median MICs are shown in Table 1. At low concentrations, CGP was the most active β-lactam antibiotic. At 32 µg/ml, CGP, HR, and AZ showed similar activities. MZ was the least active. No significant differences were encountered in the MICs obtained with the groups of CAR^s and CAR^r strains. Only at low concentrations did HR and AZ show more activity in the CAR^s than in the CAR^r group. Schassan et al. (3) found MZ to be less active against GM-resistant than against GM-susceptible strains. We obtained similar MICs with aminoglycoside-resistant and -susceptible *P. aeruginosa*.

Among the aminoglycoside antibiotics, TM was the most active. All the aminoglycosides showed more activity on the CAR^r strains than on the CAR^s strains. The only exception was AMK, which showed the same MICs in both groups.

Resistance to both aminoglycosides and carbenicillin was not frequently encountered.

The results of the interactions of CGP, HR, AZ, and MZ with the five aminoglycosides against the 50 *P. aeruginosa* strains are shown in Table 2. The most favorable interactions (synergy and addition) of CGP were with SSM and GM. There were no significant differences between the CAR^r and CAR^s strains except for combinations containing TM and GM, which showed more synergism in the CAR^s group.

With HR, combinations containing DKB and GM showed more favorable interactions and were significantly more synergistic on the CAR^s than on the CAR^r strain group. Combinations of HR showed the least antagonism of all.

The interactions of the aminoglycosides with AZ and MZ on CAR^r and CAR^s strain groups

TABLE 2. *Interactions of cefsulodin (CGP), cefotaxime (HR), azlocillin (AZ), mezlocillin (MZ), and five aminoglycosides against 50 P. aeruginosa strains*

Test agent combination	No. of strains exhibiting:			
	Synergy (≤0.75)^a	Addition (0.75–1.0)	Indifference (>1.0)	Antagonism (>2.0)
CGP + GM	31	4	11	4
TM	20	7	19	4
SSM	34	3	12	1
AMK	28	7	14	1
DKB	24	9	13	4
HR + GM	34	5	10	1
TM	23	5	20	2
SSM	30	0	18	2
AMK	32	4	13	1
DKB	35	6	9	0
AZ + GM	26	4	11	9
TM	16	3	24	7
SSM	34	2	11	3
AMK	21	1	25	3
DKB	24	4	18	4
MZ + GM	39	5	3	3
TM	24	9	16	1
SSM	45	3	1	1
AMK	32	0	15	3
DKB	33	2	13	2

^{a} Number in parentheses is fractional inhibitory concentration index.

behaved similarly, with no significant differences between them.

The combinations of AZ + TM and AZ + GM showed the highest antagonism with seven and nine strains, respectively.

MZ showed more favorable interaction than AZ with the five aminoglycosides, especially with SSM (96% favorable interactions).

The 11 aminoglycoside-resistant strains showed results similar to those of the aminoglycoside-susceptible strains with all of the various combinations. The most synergistic combinations were those containing SSM. Combinations with AZ showed more antagonism than any other combination.

The MZ + SSM combination showed the highest number of favorable interactions of all the combinations tested. Similar results were obtained in the aminoglycoside-resistant group.

These results are in disagreement with those of Schassan et al. (3), who found better activity of MZ + TM and MZ + AMK against *P. aeruginosa*, but these authors used only subinhibitory concentrations of the aminoglycosides in their tests for interactions and did not use all the combinations we used.

If we examine the results of all the possible combinations of these β-lactam antibiotics with the aminoglycosides, we find that the favorable interactions (synergy and addition) were those of MZ (76.8%), HR (69.6%), CGP (66.8%), and AZ (54%). Even though MZ was the β-lactam which showed the least activity on its own, in combination with aminoglycosides MZ showed the most synergy and addition.

With the exceptions of CGP + TM and HR + DKB, which showed more synergism with the CAR[s] group, the behavior of the combinations was independent of the carbenicillin MIC for the strains.

In the aminoglycoside-resistant group, combinations containing SSM, DKB, and GM showed more synergy. The results with this group are similar to those obtained with the aminoglycoside-susceptible *P. aeruginosa*. There appears to be no correlation between degree of susceptibility to aminoglycoside and ability to predict synergy.

1. **Neu, H. C., N. Aswapokee, P. Aswapokee, and K. P. Fu.** 1979. HR 756, a new cephalosporin active against gram-positive and gram-negative aerobic and anaerobic bacteria. Antimicrob. Agents Chemother. **15:**273–281.
2. **Perea, E. J., M. A. Torres, and M. V. Borobio.** 1978. Synergism of fosfomycin-ampicillin and fosfomycin-chloramphenicol against *Salmonella* and *Shigella*. Antimicrob. Agents Chemother. **13:**705–709.
3. **Schassan, M. H., K. Kopersky, and H. Sheerf.** 1978. Mezlocillin: a new acyl ureido-penicillin. Antimicrobial activity and combination effects with four aminoglycoside antibiotics. Chemotherapy **24:**134–142.
4. **Stewart, D., and C. P. Bodey.** 1977. Azlocillin: in vitro studies of a new semisynthetic penicillin. Antimicrob. Agents Chemother. **11:**865–870.
5. **Tosch, W., F. Kradolfer, E. A. Konopka, J. Regös, W. Zimmermann, and O. Zak.** 1978. In vitro characterization of CGP 7174/E, a cephalosporin active against *Pseudomonas*, p. 843–844. *In* Current chemotherapy, Proceedings of the 10th International Congress of Chemotherapy. American Society for Microbiology, Washington, D.C.

Serum, Urine, and Bile Levels of Cefoperazone (T-1551)

NOBUKI AOKI,* OSAMU SEKINE, YOSHIMARU USUDA, TAKEAKI SHIMIZU, YOSHIHEI HIRASAWA, AND TADAO AOKI

Shinrakuen Hospital, Niigata City, 950-21, Japan

Cefoperazone (T-1551) is a new cephalosporin antibiotic for parenteral use that has been developed in the Toyama Research Laboratory. Since T-1551 has high resistance to β-lactamase, the antibacterial spectrum of this antibiotic is considerably broader in vitro and in vivo than that of the parent cephalosporin. In vitro and in vivo studies have indicated that T-1551 is active against indole-positive *Proteus, Enterobacter, Pseudomonas aeruginosa*, and *Serratia marcescens*, as well as against all the bacterial pathogens usually susceptible to the cephalosporins. In addition, T-1551 is active against many strains of gram-negative bacteria that have become resistant to the other β-lactam antibiotics (3, 6).

Two studies of T-1551 were carried out. First, its concentrations in blood and urine were determined in patients with various degrees of renal dysfunction. Second, its concentration in the bile juice and the influence of bile acid metabolism on antibiotic excretion were investigated.

In the first study, antibiotic concentrations were measured after intravenous (i.v.) injection (for 5 min) of 1,000 mg of T-1551 into each of five patients with various degrees of renal dysfunction (creatinine clearances between 0 and 74.5 ml/min per 1.48 m^2). In the uremic cases, hemodialysis was not performed during the study. Blood samples were taken 0.5, 1, 2, 4, 6, and 24 h after administration. Urine samples were collected at various time periods after the injection: 0 to 1, 1 to 2, 2 to 4, and 4 to 6 h. Drug concentrations were determined by bioassay performed by the thin-layer cup method, using *Bacillus subtilis* PCI 219 as the test strain.

In the second study, T-tube drainage was performed for three patients with pancreas cancer, biliary tract cancer, or choledocholithiasis. The T-tube was left open for 7 days after the operation, making the bile flow out freely. The tube was clamped on the 10th postoperative day, in order to establish the complete enterohepatic circulation, and was removed on the 22nd postoperative day. Antibiotic excretion into the bile juice was determined on the day of operation and on the 7th and 21st postoperative days. A 500-ml amount of 5% glucose solution mixed with 2,000 mg of T-1551 was administered to the patients by constant i.v. drip infusion for 2 h. Bile and serum specimens were collected at various intervals, ranging from 0 to 10 h, and the concentrations were determined by the method used in the first study. In addition, the concentrations of cefazolin, cefamandole, and cefuroxime in the bile juice were similarly determined by bioassay. Simultaneously, the concentrations of bile acids were measured by gas chromatography.

The blood concentration and urinary excretion of T-1551 are shown in Fig. 1. The T-1551 blood concentration was 90 μg/ml 1 h postinjection in two uremic cases and about 50 μg/ml in three cases with creatinine clearance above 32.9 ml/min. Regardless of the degree of renal dysfunction, however, there was little difference in the blood concentrations of T-1551 among all cases from 2 to 6 h postinjection. The serum concentrations of T-1551 declined to an undetectable level 24 h postinjection. Thus, in the cases with the more severely impaired renal functions, the serum half-lives of T-1551 were prolonged but not markedly. Urinary excretion decreased in parallel with the degree of renal dysfunction: the urinary excretions were 2.0 and 0.39%, respectively, in two uremic cases and were below 30% in the other cases by the 6th hour. These results show that the urine excretion of T-1551 is considerably less than that of other cephalosporins which are mainly excreted into the urine (1, 2).

The peak concentration of T-1551 in the bile juice on the day of operation and the 21st postoperative day was observed 5 h after the i.v. drip infusion, and the decrease in concentration was

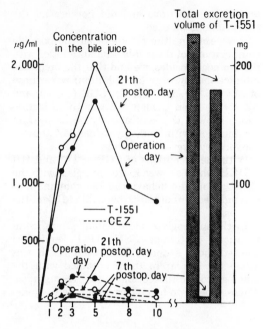

FIG. 2. *Concentrations of T-1551 and cefazolin in the bile juice after a 2,000-mg i.v. drip infusion for 2 h*

relatively slow (Fig. 2). The concentration of this antibiotic was more than 10-fold greater than that of the other cephalosporins (4, 5). However, the concentration on the 7th postoperative day was significantly lower than on the day of operation or on the 21st postoperative day. The concentration of bile acids in the bile juice, especially chenodeoxycholic acid, deoxycholic acid, ursodeoxycholic acid, and lithocholic acid, decreased significantly ($P < 0.001$) on the 7th postoperative day and recovered to the initial level on the 21st postoperative day. Biliary excretion of the antibiotics showed the same tendency. Levels of the bile juice components, such as lecithin, cholesterol, bilirubin, potassium, sodium, and chloride, were changed very slightly. The peak level of the antibiotics in the bile juice on the 7th postoperative day decreased about 97% for T-1551, 80% for cefamandole, 84% for cefazolin, and 56% for cefuroxime, compared with the levels on the day of operation. The total amount of biliary excretion of these antibiotics during 8 h also decreased significantly. The peak antibiotic levels in the bile juice again recovered nearly to the initial level on the 21st postoperative day.

In conclusion, elevation of serum levels and prolongation of serum half-lives of T-1551 cor-

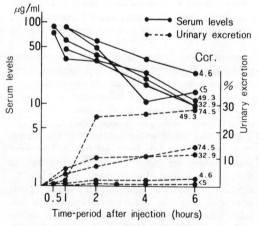

FIG. 1. *Serum levels and cumulative urinary excretion after a 1,000-mg i.v. injection in patients with various renal functions.*

related more with the degree of liver dysfunction than with the degree of renal failure. Antibiotic excretion into the bile juice depended upon bile acid metabolism. When the enterohepatic circulation of bile acid was disturbed, it was difficult to obtain the effective level of antibiotics in the bile juice.

1. **Gimbrére, J. S. F., J. C. M. Hafkensheid, R. van Dalen, and T. B. Vree.** 1979. Determination of plasma and renal clearance of cefuroxime and its pharmacokinetics in renal insufficiency. J. Antimicrob. Chemother. **5:**281–292.
2. **Fillastre, J. P., M. Godin, G. Humbert, A. Leroy, and**

C. **Van Winzum.** 1979. Pharmacokinetics of cefoxitin in normal subjects and in patients with renal insufficiency. Rev. Infect. Dis. **1:**118–125.
3. **Mitsuhashi, S., N. Matsubara, S. Minami, T. Muraoka, T. Yasuda, and T. Saikawa.** 1978. Program Abstr. Intersci. Conf. Antimicrob. Agents Chemother. 18th, Atlanta, Ga., abstr. no. 158.
4. **Ratzan, K. R., C. Ruiz, and T. L. Irvin III.** 1974. Biliary tract excretion of cefazolin, cephalothin, and cephaloridine in the presence of biliary tract disease. Antimicrob. Agents Chemother. **6:**426–431.
5. **Powis, S. J. A., and M. Severn.** 1979. Biliary excretion and tissue levels of cefuroxime. J. Antimicrob. Chemother. **5:**183–188.
6. **Ueda, Y., A. Saito, M. Ohmori, K. Shiba, T. Yamasu, and H. Ihara.** 1978. Program Abstr. Intersci. Conf. Antimicrob. Agents Chemother. 18th, Atlanta, Ga., abstr. no. 153.

Protein Binding of T-1551

Y. WATANABE,* H. TAKASHITA, E. TAKADA, T. HAYASHI, T. YASUDA, I. SAIKAWA,
AND K. SHIMIZU

Research Laboratory of Toyama Chemical Company, Ltd., Toyama, and Department of Internal Medicine,
Tokyo Women's Medical College, Tokyo, Japan

T-1551, a new semisynthetic cephalosporin with a broad antibacterial spectrum, has a high serum level, a long biological half-life, and high protein-binding rates, much like cefazolin (CEZ).

Approximately 15 to 30% of the administered dose of T-1551 is recovered in the urine in humans; however, urinary excretion of CEZ is more than 90%. It is of pharmacological interest to clarify the difference in the excretion of these two drugs. Therefore, we investigated the protein binding of T-1551, which seems to influence its pharmacokinetics.

At first, high-pressure liquid chromatography (HPLC) was undertaken to determine the concentrations of T-1551 and CEZ, since it is difficult to determine simultaneously by bioassay more than two kinds of antibiotics having a broad antibacterial spectrum.

The extent of protein binding, number of binding sites, and association constant to human serum albumin determined by the centrifugal ultrafiltration technique and the formulation of Klotz et al. (1) were 90.4%, 0.87, and 2.16×10^4 (M^{-1}) for T-1551 and 89.2%, 0.78, and 2.46×10^4

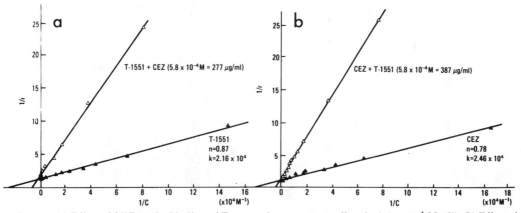

FIG. 1. *(a) Effect of CEZ on the binding of T-1551 to human serum albumin (5.8×10^{-4} M, 4%). (b) Effect of T-1551 on the binding of CEZ to human serum albumin (5.8×10^{-4} M, 4%). C = free drug concentration; γ = moles of drug bound per mol of albumin; n = number of binding sites; k = association constant. A molecular weight of 69,000 for albumin was assumed in the calculations.*

(M^{-1}) for CEZ, respectively. The mode of the binding of T-1551 to serum protein was similar to that of CEZ. It also seemed that T-1551 and CEZ competed for the same binding site on albumin, since in the presence of CEZ, less T-1551 was bound to albumin; similarly, in the presence of T-1551, the binding of CEZ to albumin was decreased (Fig. 1a and b).

The T-1551 or CEZ serum curve during the entire course in simultaneous administration to rabbits (i.e., 20 mg of each drug per kg was coadministered intravenously) was below that of each drug in a single administration. The serum levels of T-1551 at 15 and 30 min were statistically different ($P < 0.05$). Urinary and biliary excretions in the simultaneous administration were 59.2 and 12.8% within 4 h for T-1551 and 86.7 and 0.80% for CEZ, respectively, whereas in a single administration they were 44.4 and 19.7% within 4 h for T-1551 and 81.3 and 0.33% for CEZ, respectively. Urinary excretion of T-1551 in the first 15 min with the simultaneous administration was significantly higher than that with a single administration ($P < 0.05$). When 1 g of

T-1551 and 1 g of CEZ were coadministered intravenously to humans, the serum level of T-1551 was lower than that with the single administration. Although the serum level of CEZ before 30 min with the simultaneous administration was below that with the single administration, the CEZ serum curve after 60 min was similar to that with the single administration (Fig. 2).

Urinary excretions of T-1551 and CEZ for the simultaneous administration were 30.3 and 91.0% within 4 h and those for a single administration were 22.0 and 80.4%, respectively. Especially, the urinary excretion rate of T-1551 for the simultaneous administration in the first 1 h was 20.4%, which was significantly different from 11.5% with the single administration ($P < 0.01$). The serum level data obtained in rabbits and humans were analyzed by using the open two-compartment pharmacokinetic model. α, K_{12}, K_{13}, and V_d of T-1551 with the simultaneous administration showed higher values in comparison with those for a single administration. Similar results were obtained with CEZ.

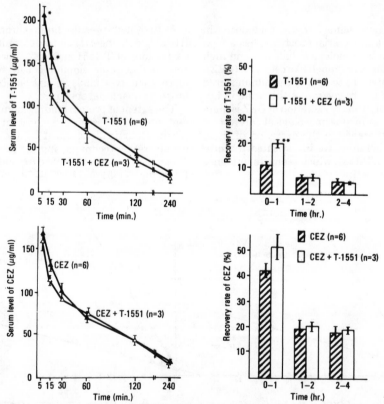

FIG. 2. *Effect of simultaneous administration of T-1551 and CEZ on serum level and urinary excretion in humans. Dose: 1 g of each drug per person intravenously. * Significant difference at $P < 0.1$. ** Significant difference at $P < 0.01$.*

These results suggest that concomitantly administered drugs influenced one another's binding to serum protein in vivo and an increase in the concentration of unbound drug in the serum made the drug available for glomerular filtration. It seemed that the high protein binding of

T-1551 to serum protein was an important factor affecting its pharmacokinetics.

1. **Klotz, I. M., H. Triwush, and F. M. Walker.** 1948. The binding of organic ions by proteins. Competition phenomena and denaturation effects. J. Am. Chem. Soc. **70:**2935–2941.

Antibacterial Activity of Cefoperazone (T-1551) and Resistance to β-Lactamases from Gram-Negative Bacteria

S. MINAMI, N. MATSUBARA, T. MURAOKA, A. YOTSUJI, T. YASUDA, I. SAIKAWA,
AND S. MITSUHASHI*

Department of Microbiology, School of Medicine, Gunma University, Maebashi, and *Research Laboratory of Toyama Chemical Co., Ltd., Toyama, Japan*

The new semisynthetic cephalosporin cefoperazone (T-1551), sodium 7-[D(−)-α-(4-ethyl-2,3-dioxo-1-piperazinecarboxamido)-α-(4-hydroxyphenyl)acetamido]-3-[(1-methyl-1H-tetrazol-5-yl)thiomethyl]-3-cephem-4-carboxylate, has been shown to have a broad antibacterial spectrum and potent activity against *Pseudomonas aeruginosa* and *Serratia marcescens* (1). The spectrum of antibacterial activity of T-1551 against standard strains of gram-positive and gram-negative bacteria was compared with that of cefazolin (CEZ) and cefamandole (CMD). T-1551 was active against gram-positive bacteria, and its MICs against most of the gram-positive bacteria were on a level with those of CEZ and CMD, inhibiting the growth at concentrations ranging from 0.2 to 25 μg/ml when an inoculum of one loopful of 10^6 colony-forming units (CFU) per ml was used. T-1551 also showed potent antibacterial activity against gram-negative bacteria, inhibiting the growth of the strains tested at concentrations lower than those of CEZ and CMD. A remarkable characteristic of T-1551 was its high antibacterial activity against *P. aeruginosa, S. marcescens*, indole-positive *Proteus* species, and *Enterobacter cloacae*, which were resistant to CEZ and CMD.

The distribution of the MICs of T-1551 against about 1,300 clinical isolates of gram-positive and gram-negative bacteria was examined at an inoculum size of 10^6 CFU/ml (Table 1). T-1551 was less active against *Staphylococcus aureus* than CEZ and CMD, but it was more active against *Escherichia coli, Klebsiella pneumoniae*, and *Proteus mirabilis* strains, most of which were susceptible to CEZ and CMD. The MICs of T-1551 against 75% of the indole-positive *Proteus* and *Citrobacter freundii* strains were 3.52 and 4.00 μg/ml, respectively, whereas

those of CEZ were more than 100 μg/ml. T-1551 was also highly active against *P. aeruginosa, S. marcescens*, and *E. cloacae*, which were resistant to various cephalosporins including CEZ and CMD, and the peaks of the MIC value distributions of T-1551 against these species of bacteria were located at 3.1 to 6.25, 3.1, and 0.2, respectively. It is notable that T-1551 has a particularly potent activity against *P. aeruginosa*, which is little affected by the cephalosporins now used for chemotherapy.

The excellent antibacterial activity of T-1551 described above may be based on its high resistance to β-lactamases, high affinity to a target site(s), and good penetrability into bacterial cells. To clarify the mode of action of T-1551, we investigated the enzymological properties of T-1551 on β-lactamases from gram-negative bacteria.

We purified cephalosporinases produced by gram-negative bacteria including *Enterobacteriaceae, P. aeruginosa, S. marcescens*, etc., by means of column chromatography using carboxymethyl-Sephadex and gel filtration. All purified enzymes gave a single protein band upon polyacrylamide gel electrophoresis. β-Lactamase activity was determined spectrophotometrically (2). The Michaelis constant (K_m), maximum rate of hydrolysis (V_{max}), and the dissociation constant of the enzyme-inhibitor complex (K_i) were determined (Table 2). T-1551 was more stable to typical cephalosporinases from *E. cloacae, E. coli, S. marcescens, P. morganii, P. rettgeri*, and *P. aeruginosa* than were cephaloridine, CEZ, cephalothin, cephalexin, and cefotiam, and the V_{max} values of T-1551 by these typical cephalosporinases were smaller than 5.0, taking the V_{max} of cephaloridine as 100. Among the cephalosporins, except for cefoxitin, T-1551

TABLE 1. *Antibacterial activity of T-1551 against clinical isolates of bacteria*

Organism (no. of strains)	$MIC_{50}{}^a$ (µg/ml)			$MIC_{75}{}^a$ (µg/ml)		
	T-1551	CMD[b]	CEZ[b]	T-1551	CMD	CEZ
E. coli (200)	0.19	1.10	1.46	0.77	2.09	2.68
K. pneumoniae (100)	0.21	1.56	1.81	1.05	7.34	3.00
P. aeruginosa (200)	3.60	>100	>100	5.46	>100	>100
S. marcescens (200)	5.40	50.0	>100	45.8	>100	>100
Indole-positive *Proteus* (200) ..	1.80	18.4	>100	3.52	100	>100
Indole-negative *Proteus* (100) .	0.76	1.54	4.90	1.09	3.05	6.80
C. freundii (52)	0.47	1.31	18.0	4.00	6.29	>100
E. cloacae (200)	0.16	3.60	>100	0.62	50.0	>100
S. aureus (100)	1.20	0.33	0.21	1.75	0.51	0.32

[a] MIC_{50} and MIC_{75} indicate the concentrations required to inhibit the growth of 50 and 75%, respectively, of the total number of strains used.

[b] CMD, Cefamandole; CEZ, cefazolin.

TABLE 2. *Substrate profiles of β-lactamases from gram-negative bacteria[a]*

Cephalosporinase producer	Relative rate of hydrolysis[b]									
	T-1551	CER	CEZ	CET	CEX	CTM	CMD	CXM	CFX	PCG
E. coli GN5482	4 (51)[c]	100	311	269	29	88	5	<1	<1	63
E. cloacae GN7471	1 (202)	100	100	189	14	29	<1	<1	<1	12
S. marcescens GN10857	2 (7.2)	100	198	88	6	16	<1	<1	<1	3
P. morganii GN5407	1 (167)	100	20	46	4	8	<1	<1	<1	16
P. rettgeri GN4430	<1 (3.5)	100	99	85	8	4	<1	<1	<1	3
P. aeruginosa GN10362	5 (23)	100	222	139	64	12	<1	<1	<1	29
P. vulgaris GN7919	15 (—)	100	387	173	274	351	381	1,140	<1	20
P. cepacia GN11164	10 (5.0)	100	156	323	58	161	452	239	<1	161

[a] CER, Cephaloridine; CEZ, cefazolin; CET, cephalothin; CEX, cephalexin; CTM, cefotiam; CMD, cefamandole; CXM, cefuroxime; CFX, cefoxitin; PCG, penicillin G.

[b] Relative rate of hydrolysis is expressed by taking the V_{max} of cephaloridine as 100.

[c] Numbers in parentheses indicate the K_i values (micromolar) of T-1551.

was the most stable to β-lactamases produced by *Proteus vulgaris* and *Pseudomonas cepacia*, which could easily hydrolyze cefuroxime and CMD, although cefuroxime and CMD were highly resistant to typical cephalosporinases. The K_m and K_i of T-1551 were smaller than those of cephaloridine, CEZ, etc., and larger than those of cefoxitin and cefuroxime. From the above observations, we conclude that T-1551 is very stable to β-lactamases and its affinity to β-lactamases is rather low.

We also studied the affinity of T-1551 to penicillin-binding proteins (PBPs). Using the method described by Spratt (3), we prepared inner membrane protein fractions from *E. coli* JE1011 and *P. aeruginosa* NCTC10490. The affinity of T-1551 to PBPs was estimated by measuring the competition of unlabeled T-1551 with ^{14}C-penicillin G for binding to PBPs. Among the PBPs, T-1551 had higher affinities to PBP-3, a protein supposed to be concerned in septum formation, and also a high affinity to PBP-1Bs (*E. coli*) and PBP-1A (*P. aeruginosa*). PBP-1Bs of *E. coli*, which are thought to cor-

respond to PBP-1A of *P. aeruginosa*, are supposed to be related to cross-linking in peptidoglycan synthesis. The results of these competition experiments on the binding of T-1551 to PBPs are in good agreement with the observations that, over a wide range of concentrations, T-1551 can induce the formation of filamentous cells of *E. coli* and *P. aeruginosa*.

The excellent antibacterial activity of T-1551 can be partly explained by both its high resistance to β-lactamase and its high affinity to PBPs, which are essential for cell growth and cell division.

1. **Matsubara, N., S. Minami, T. Muraoka, I. Saikawa, and S. Mitsuhashi.** 1979. In vitro antibacterial activity of cefoperazone (T-1551), a new semisynthetic cephalosporin. Antimicrob. Agents Chemother. **16:**731–735.
2. **Samni, A.** 1975. A direct spectrophotometric assay and determination of Michaelis constants for β-lactamase reaction. Anal. Biochem. **63:**17–26.
3. **Spratt, A.** 1977. Properties of the penicillin binding proteins of *Escherichia coli* K 12. Eur. J. Biochem. **72:** 341–352.

Clinical Studies on Cefoperazone (T-1551) in the Field of Internal Medicine

Y. UEDA, A. SAITO,* M. OHMORI, AND K. SIBA

Department of Internal Medicine, The Jikei University School of Medicine, Tokyo, Japan

Cefoperazone (T-1551), a new cephalosporin derivative developed in Japan, has a broad antibacterial spectrum against gram-positive and gram-negative bacteria and shows excellent antibacterial activity, especially against indole-positive *Proteus* spp., *Enterobacter cloacae, Pseudomonas aeruginosa, Haemophilus influenzae*, and anaerobic bacteria. Serum levels of cefoperazone were found to be almost the same as those of cefazolin, and the transfer of cefoperazone into bile was excellent, which seems to be one of the specific characteristics of cefoperazone (New Drug Symposium, 27th Congress of the Japan Society of Chemotherapy, Fukuoka, 1979).

A total of 1,277 patients treated with cefoperazone were reported in Japan by June 1979. In the field of internal medicine, 521 cases have been reported. Since other antibiotics were used concurrently in 55 patients, the clinical results for 466 of the 521 patients were summarized.

Among these 466 patients, the most frequent daily dose was 4 g, which was administered in 53% of the total; 2 g was administered in 35%. The number of administrations was two times in 92% of the patients and was more than three times in only 4%. The most frequent route of administration was intravenous drip infusion, used in 74%; intravenous injection was used in 14%, and intramuscular injection was used in 7%.

The clinical efficacy of cefoperazone is shown in Table 1. In respiratory tract infections, excellent or good efficacy was observed in 253 of 316 cases, and the effective rate was 80.1%. Effective rates were 77.1% in hepatobiliary tract infections, 83.1% in urinary tract infections, 62.5% in

septicemia, and 77.8% in other infections. The high effective rate of 79.6% was observed for all patients.

Among the respiratory tract infections, cefoperazone showed an effective rate of 84.9% in 152 cases of pneumonia, 73.9% in 19 cases of pulmonary abscess, and 100% in 11 cases of pyothorax. Cefoperazone also showed high clinical efficacy in chronic respiratory tract infections.

Bacteriological efficacy of cefoperazone is shown in Table 2. The rates of eradication of the isolated organisms were 80.0% for 60 strains of *Klebsiella* spp., the most frequently isolated organism, 51.0% for 49 strains of *P. aeruginosa*, 97.9% for 48 strains of *Escherichia coli*, 92.9% for 42 strains of *H. influenzae*, 100% for 15 strains of *Proteus* spp., and 72.7% for 11 strains of *Enterobacter*. Among gram-positive bacteria, 94.7% of 19 strains of *Streptococcus pneumoniae*, 100% of 11 strains of *S. faecalis*, and 70% of 10 strains of *Staphylococcus aureus* were eradicated; 83.3% of 6 anaerobic bacteria were eradicated. The total rate of eradication was 78.9% (254 of 322), and this rate was almost the same as the clinical effective rate.

It is noteworthy that more than 90% of *E. coli* and *H. influenzae* strains were eradicated and that more than 50% of *P. aeruginosa* strains were eradicated in spite of the fact that cefoperazone is a cephalosporin derivative.

Since the transfer of cefoperazone into bile is favorable, good clinical efficacy was expected in hepatobiliary tract infections, and its clinical effective rate in these infections was 77.1%. The 27 strains isolated from bile included 1 strain of *S. faecalis*, 6 strains of *E. coli*, 2 strains of *P. aeruginosa*, 12 strains of *Klebsiella* spp., 2

TABLE 1. *Clinical efficacy of cefoperazone in various infections*

Infection	No. of patients	No. with indicated result				Total excellent or good	Effective rate (%)
		Excellent	Good	Fair	Poor		
Respiratory tract infections	316	50	203	33	30	253	80.1
Hepatobiliary tract infections	48	7	30	5	6	37	77.1
Urinary tract infections	77	23	41	4	9	64	83.1
Septicemia	16	5	5	3	3	10	62.5
Other infections	9	2	5	1	1	7	77.8
Total no.	466	87	284	46	49	371	79.6
Percent		18.7	60.9	9.9	10.5		

TABLE 2. *Bacteriological efficacy of cefoperazone*

Organism isolated	No. of patients	Eradicated	Decreased	No change	Rate of eradication (%)
Staphylococcus aureus	10	7	2	1	70.0
S. epidermidis	4	3	1		75.0
Alpha-hemolytic streptococcus	2	1	1		50.0
Beta-hemolytic streptococcus	1	1			100.0
Streptococcus pneumoniae	19	18	1		94.7
S. faecalis	11	11			100.0
Micrococcus	1	1			100.0
Other gram-positive cocci	5	3		2	60.0
Subtotal	53	45	5	3	84.9
Haemophilus influenzae	42	39	3		92.9
Haemophilus sp.	2	2			100.0
Escherichia coli	48	47		1	97.9
Klebsiella	60	48	5	7	80.0
Enterobacter	11	8	3		72.7
Serratia	10	3	3	4	30.0
Citrobacter	4	4			100.0
Proteus mirabilis	6	6			100.0
P. morganii	3	3			100.0
P. vulgaris	4	4			100.0
P. rettgeri	2	2			100.0
Alcaligenes	1	1			100.0
Salmonella	1	1			100.0
Pseudomonas aeruginosa	49	25	7	17	51.0
P. cepacia	2	1		1	50.0
Pseudomonas	12	6	2	4	50.0
Acinetobacter	2	2			100.0
Other gram-negative bacilli	3	1		2	33.3
Neisseria	1	1			100.0
Subtotal	263	204	23	36	77.6
Bacteroides	1	1			100.0
Peptococcus	2	2			100.0
Peptostreptococcus	2	1	1		50.0
Propionibacterium	1	1			100.0
Subtotal	6	5	1		83.3
Total	322	254	29	39	78.9

strains of *Serratia*, 1 strain of *Enterobacter*, 2 strains of *Citrobacter*, and 1 strain of *Bacteroides*. Among these organisms, only 2 strains of *Klebsiella* spp. and 1 strain of *Serratia* were unaffected; all other organisms were eradicated. The rate of eradication was 89%, and this result supported the concept that good transfer into bile is a specific characteristic of cefoperazone.

In 205 patients who showed poor results after other antibiotic therapy, the effective rates for cefoperazone were 77.8% (70 of 90) after other cephalosporins, 63.2% (36 of 57) after penicillins, and 56.9% (33 of 58) after other antibiotics.

Among 1,277 patients treated with cefoperazone, eruption in 2.2%, fever in 1.0%, diarrhea in 0.4%, and other side effects in 0.4% were observed. No serious side effect has been observed to date. Transient elevation of serum transaminase in 3.1% and eosinophilia in 1.4% of the patients were observed, but these values returned to normal immediately after the cessation of cefoperazone therapy.

As mentioned above, cefoperazone showed high clinical efficacy and no serious side effect in the field of internal medicine. It might be a useful cephalosporin derivative for serious infections caused by gram-negative bacilli such as *Klebsiella* spp., *Enterobacter* spp., *Proteus* spp., *P. aeruginosa*, and *H. influenzae*. Since the excretion of cefoperazone into bile is favorable, it might also be used clinically against hepatobiliary tract infections.

Placental Transfer of Cefoperazone (T-1551) and a Clinical Study of Its Use in Obstetrics and Gynecological Infections

S. MATSUDA,* M. TANNO, T. KASHIWAGURA, AND H. FURUYA

Juntendo University, Tokyo, Japan

Cefoperazone (T-1551), a parenteral cephalosporin developed by Toyama Chemical Co., Ltd., has a broad spectrum of antibacterial activity against gram-positive bacteria and gram-negative bacilli. T-1551 is more active than other cephalosporins, especially against *Pseudomonas aeruginosa, Enterobacter*, indole-positive *Proteus*, and *Serratia*.

Furuya and Matsuda (1) compared the placental transfer and clinical efficacy of several cephalosporins. We have studied maternofetal transfer and clinical applications of T-1551 in the field of obstetrics and gynecology (New Drug Symposium, 27th Congress of the Japan Society of Chemotherapy, Fukuoka, 1979).

Experimental method. For studies on placental transfer, 1.0 g of T-1551 was given intravenously or intramuscularly. The serum levels and the transfers into umbilical cord blood and amniotic fluid were measured by means of a thin-layer cup method with *Micrococcus luteus* ATCC 9341 as the test strain.

In the clinical application, the effect by administration route (intravenous injection, intravenous drip infusion, and intramuscular injection) and the bacteriological effect were investigated against 20 cases of various infections (pelvic infection, sepsis, urinary tract infections, and puerperal mastitis) in the field of obstetrics and gynecology.

Placental transfer. As for the maternofetal transfer of T-1551, the transfer to umbilical cord blood was 34.4% of the mother's serum level at an intravenous dose of 1 g and was 33.2% at an intramuscular dose of 1 g. The transfer into amniotic fluid within 6 h after administration was about 3 to 4 µg/ml. In the group (five cases) that was given 1 g of T-1551 intravenously two to four times every 12 h and from whom samples were collected at 1 to 5 h after the last administration, the transfer rate into umbilical cord blood via the placenta increased, the value being 40 to 48%. The transfer to amniotic fluid was 3.8 to 8.8 µg/ml, which also showed a significant increasing tendency (Table 1).

Little difference was observed in the transfer

TABLE 1. *Placental transfer of T-1551*

Treatment[a]	Patient no.	Sampling time after the last dosing	T-1551 concn (µg/ml) in:			U/M[b] (%)
			Mother's blood	Umbilical cord blood	Amniotic fluid	
Single administration of 1.0 g, i.m.	1	50 min	64.4	16.0	2.2	24.9
	2	1 h 10 min	68.3	20.2	2.0	29.6
	3	1 h 30 min	52.8	17.4		33.3
	4	2 h 45 min	44.5	19.1	2.2	45.1
	5	3 h 30 min	31.6	10.5	1.8	33.2
	6	4 h 50 min	11.2	3.8	2.6	33.9
Single administration of 1.0 g, i.v.	1	40 min	82.2	26.3		31.9
	2	55 min	74.0	26.5	2.0	35.8
	3	1 h 20 min	65.7	24.8	2.6	37.7
	4	2 h 20 min	40.5	13.0	1.8	32.1
	5	3 h 30 min	19.5	8.2		42.1
	6	4 h 20 min	9.3	3.6	4.8	38.7
	7	6 h 40 min	5.7	2.6	3.0	45.6
Continuous administration						
1.0 g × 3, i.v.	1	1 h 15 min	64.2	31.0	6.3	48.3
1.0 g × 3, i.v.	2	1 h 45 min	56.4	21.5	6.0	38.1
1.0 g × 4, i.v.	3	2 h 30 min	48.0	20.3	8.8	42.3
1.0 g × 2, i.v.	4	3 h 40 min	26.7	12.4	4.8	46.4
1.0 g × 3, i.v.	5	5 h 20 min	8.1	3.3	3.8	40.7

[a] Six patients received a single dose of 1.0 g intramuscularly (i.m.), and seven patients received a single dose of 1.0 g intravenously (i.v.). The five patients in the continuous administration group received 1.0 g intravenously two, three, or four times during a 12-h period.

[b] Concentration in umbilical cord blood/concentration in mother's blood.

TABLE 2. *Clinical effect of T-1551 classified by diagnosis*

Diagnosis	No. of cases	Clinical effect			Effective rate (%)
		Excellent	Good	Poor	
Pelvic infection					
Puerperal fever	2		1	1	1/2 ⎫
Puerperal sepsis	1			1	0/1 ⎪
Septic abortion	1		1		1/1 ⎬ (72.7)
Endometritis	2	1	1		2/2 ⎪
Adnexitis	4	1	2	1	3/4 ⎪
Pelveoperitonitis	1		1		1/1 ⎭
Urinary tract infection					
Pyelonephritis	4	2	2		4/4 ⎫ (85.7)
Cystitis	3	1	1	1	2/3 ⎬
Other infections					
Bartholinitis	1		1		1/1 ⎫ (50.0)
Puerperal mastitis	1			1	0/1 ⎬
Total	20	5	10	5	15/20 (75.0)

rate of several cephalosporins into umbilical cord blood; however, generally one-half to one-fourth of the mother's serum level was detected in the fetus. The rates of transfer to the umbilical cord blood were analyzed after division into two groups: the rates measured up to 3 h and those measured at 3 to 8 h after administration of the drugs. In the latter group, there was a tendency toward elevation of the rates with a decrease in the mother's serum level.

Transfer of T-1551 to amniotic fluid had no definite pattern when compared with the transfer of other cephalosporins. When T-1551 was given to mothers in the early stage of pregnancy (within 12 weeks of pregnancy), about one-sixth to one-tenth of the mother's serum level was detected in the villus tissue.

Clinical result. T-1551 was administered in a daily dose of 2 g to a total of 20 patients: 10 with pelvic infection (puerperal fever, endometritis, adnexitis, and pelveoperitonitis), 1 with puerperal sepsis, 1 each with Bartholinitis and puerperal mastitis, and 7 with urinary tract in-

fection (pyelonephritis and cystitis). The effective rate was 75% (15 cases). Among these 20 patients, T-1551 was effective against 8 of 11 cases of pelvic infection and against 6 of 7 cases of urinary tract infection (Table 2). In this study intravenous injection (intravenous drip infusion and intravenous injection) was first choice. The clinically effective rates based on the isolated organisms were 72.2% in the single infections and 80.0% in the mixed infections.

No noteworthy side effect was observed except for one case of diarrhea.

Conclusion. T-1551 showed rather good maternofetal transfer, and the transfer of T-1551 into amniotic fluid seemed to increase with the passage of time. Clinically, T-1551 is primarily indicated for pelvic infection and urinary tract infection which is characterized by the presence of a specific pattern of causative organisms in the field of obstetrics and gynecology.

1. **Furuya, H., and S. Matsuda.** 1974. Placental transfer of antibiotics. World Obstet. Gynecol. **26:**1307–1314.

Clinical and Laboratory Evaluation of Cefoperazone (T-1551) in Respiratory Infections

KEIZO MATSUMOTO, YOSHIO UZUKA,* HARUMI SHISHIDO, TSUYOSHI NAGATAKE, AND
HIROSHI SUZUKI

*Department of Internal Medicine, Institute for Tropical Medicine, Nagasaki University,
Nagasaki 852, Japan*

With the advance of antibiotic therapy, the causative bacteria of infectious diseases have changed, and severe infections caused by gram-negative bacteria resistant to older antibiotics have come to the fore. Against this movement, thousands of naturally occurring and semisynthetic antibiotics have beeen examined in an effort to find compounds with superior antibacterial and pharmacological properties. Especially in this decade with the advance of the studies on structure-activity relationships, new semisynthetic penicillins and cephalosporins superior to natural substances have been developed by the side-chain modification. T-1551 (cefoperazone) is one such cephalosporin antibiotic newly synthesized by Toyama Chemical Co. in Japan, and it has the same side chain, a piperazine group, as that of piperacillin (T-1220), which has antibacterial activity superior to that of the older penicillins. T-1551 is the first cephalosporin that has strong and broad antibacterial activity against both gram-positive and gram-negative bacteria, even against *Haemophilus influenzae* and *Pseudomonas aeruginosa*. Since the major pathogens of lower respiratory tract infections determined by our quantitative sputum culture study from 1971 to 1978 were, in order of frequency, *H. influenzae*, *Streptococcus pneumoniae*, *P. aeruginosa*, and *Klebsiella pneumoniae*, and since T-1551 is active against all of these bacteria, it may be an all-around antibiotic for the treatment of respiratory infections. Therefore, we performed the following clinical and laboratory evaluation of T-1551 in respiratory infections.

In vitro susceptibility tests. The in vitro antibacterial activity of T-1551 was tested against 218 isolates of respiratory pathogenic bacteria by the agar dilution method, and the results were compared with those for older cephalosporins. All of these bacteria were isolated as more than 10^7 colony-forming units/ml by our quantitative sputum culture method and were determined to be the causative organisms of lower respiratory tract infections. The MICs of T-1551 ranged from 0.025 to 1.56 μg/ml against 54 isolates of *S. pneumoniae*, from 0.003 to 0.10 μg/ml against 78 isolates of *H. influenzae*, from

0.20 or less to 6.25 μg/ml against 27 isolates of *K. pneumoniae*, from 0.20 or less to 50 μg/ml against 11 isolates of *Escherichia coli*, and from 1.56 to 12.5 μg/ml against 11 isolates of *Enterobacter* species; 176 (97.2%) of these 181 isolates were inhibited at concentrations of ≤ 3.13 μg/ml. The MIC against 35 of 37 isolates of *P. aeruginosa* ranged from 0.78 to 50 μg/ml, and 2 isolates were resistant to T-1551 (MIC more than 100 μg/ml). T-1551 was more active than the older cephalosporins, i.e., cefazolin, cephalothin, cefoxitin, cefuroxime, and so on, against almost all isolates tested in this study, and especially against *H. influenzae* and *P. aeruginosa*. T-1551 was 128- to 1,024-fold more active than the others, and most isolates of respiratory pathogens were inhibited at clinically achievable concentrations.

Clinical studies. T-1551 was given to 33 patients with lower respiratory tract infections: acute bronchitis in 1, pneumonia in 15, lung abscess in 3, chronic bronchitis in 7, chronic bronchiolitis in 3, and bronchiectasis in 4. The dosage level was 0.5 to 3 g administered intravenously one to three times a day, and daily doses ranged from 1 to 6 g. Ordinary doses were 0.5 to 1 g twice a day against *S. pneumoniae* and *H. influenzae*, 1 to 2 g twice a day against *Staphylococcus aureus*, *E. coli*, and *K. pneumoniae*, and 2 to 3 g twice a day against *P. aeruginosa*.

Pharmacokinetic studies. The concentrations of T-1551 in serum and sputum were measured in six patients by a cup-plate assay procedure with the use of *Proteus mirabilis* ATCC 21100. Doses of 0.5 g infused intravenously in 60 min resulted in peak serum concentrations of 31 to 53 μg/ml, a 2-g dose infused in 60 min resulted in a peak serum concentration of 145 μg/ml, and a 3-g dose infused in 30 min resulted in a peak serum concentration of 317 μg/ml. The serum half-lives were about 120 min. Peak levels in sputum ranged from 0.08 to 0.41 μg/ml after the administration of 0.5 g of T-1551 and from 1.1 to 2.0 μg/ml after a 2-g dose; a peak concentration of 6.1 μg/ml was reached after a 3-g dose. The ratios of sputum peak levels to serum peak levels ranged from 0.2 to 1.4%, a value almost the same

TABLE 1. *Clinical response to T-1551 treatment*

Infection	No. of patients	Excellent	Good	Fair	Poor	Percent with clinical response
Acute bronchitis	1	1				100
Acute pneumonia	15		13	2		87
Lung abscess	3	1	1	1		67
Chronic bronchitis	7	1	5	1		86
Chronic bronchiolitis	3		2	1		67
Bronchiectasis	4		3	1		75
Total	33	3	24	6	0	82

TABLE 2. *Bacteriological response to T-1551 treatment*

Organism	No. of strains	Eradicated	Decreased	Persisting	Superinfecting	Percent bacteriological cure
Staphylococcus aureus	1	1				100
Streptococcus pneumoniae	4	4				100
Haemophilus influenzae	10	10				100
Klebsiella pneumoniae	4	2	1		1	75
Escherichia coli	1	1				100
Pseudomonas aeruginosa	8	4	2	2		75
Total	28	22	3	2	1	89

as those of cefazolin and cephaloridine (1). In one patient with chronic bronchiolitis, the concentrations of T-1551 in four specimens of intrabronchial secretions about 1 h after a 3-g dose infused in 30 min were measured and found to be 1.3, 3.1, 10, and 39 μg/ml (1).

From these results, T-1551 appears to be able to inhibit most gram-positive and gram-negative bacteria in these doses.

Clinical results. Clinical cures were obtained in 27 (82%) of 33 patients with lower respiratory tract infections, and the other 6 patients were partially improved by T-1551 treatment (Table 1). Three of the six patients who partially responded were associated with bacteriological failures, that is, persisting infections due to *P. aeruginosa*. In two of the six patients, their initial pathogens (*H. influenzae* and *E. coli*) were eradicated, but clinical improvement seemed to be disturbed by their underlying diseases, i.e., silicotuberculosis, cor pulmonale, and chronic pulmonary emphysema, and the causa-

tive agents in the remaining patient could not be determined. Of 27 initial infecting bacteria, 25 (93%) were eradicated or suppressed; in 2 patients *P. aeruginosa* persisted (Table 2). In one patient with bronchiectasis, superinfection with *K. pneumoniae* occurred because the sputum levels of T-1551 were reduced to less than the MIC against the organisms (0.78 to 1.56 μg/ml) after 20 days of treatment.

All patients tolerated T-1551 therapy well, and only transient and mild elevations of serum transaminases were observed in two patients.

In conclusion, T-1551 appears to be an effective and useful antibiotic for the treatment of respiratory infections.

1. **Matsumoto, K., and Y. Uzuka.** 1976. Concentrations of antibiotics in bronchiolar secretions of the patients with chronic respiratory infections, p. 73–76. *In* J. D. Williams and A. M. Geddes (ed.), Chemotherapy, vol. 4. Plenum Publishing Co., New York.

Pharmacokinetics of the Cephalosporin T-1551 (Cefoperazone) in Normal Men and in Men with Renal Failure, and Behavior in Tissues of Rats

J. FABRE,* A. F. ALLAZ, M. RUDHARDT, P. DAYER, AND L. BALANT

Policlinique Universitaire de Médecine, Geneva, Switzerland

Cefoperazone (T-1551) is a cephalosporin with an antibacterial spectrum that extends to *Pseudomonas aeruginosa*, *Enterobacter*, and *Serratia*. Before the present study, its pharmacokinetics had been documented only in Japanese volunteers (Y. Ueda, A. Saito, M. Ohmori, K. Shiba, T. Yamaji, and H. Ihara, Program Abstr. Intersci. Conf. Antimicrob. Agents Chemother. 18th, Atlanta, Ga., abstr. no. 158, 1978), and as a consequence it seemed important to characterize the kinetics of this drug in Caucasian subjects before its administration to a wider patient population could be envisioned. In addition, the fact that cefoperazone seemed to be relatively little excreted in the urine prompted us to study its behavior in patients with kidney diseases.

Eight adult male volunteers (mean weight, 71.8 kg) with no known disease were selected. At time t_0 they received a 2-h intravenous infusion of 2 g of sodium cefoperazone diluted into 500 mg of 5% dextrose (Infusomat pump). Ten hours after the end of the first infusion (t_{12}), they received a second 2-g infusion of cefoperazone. The volunteers remained hospitalized during the whole experiment. Blood samples were obtained at the times indicated in Fig. 1. The serum was separated after coagulation and kept at −18°C until assayed. Fractionated urine collections were obtained, and portions were frozen until assayed.

The results obtained in three patients with renal insufficiency and one patient with obstruction of the bile ducts are included in this report. These results are part of a larger study. The patients received only one infusion of 2 g of cefoperazone.

Male Wistar rats weighing around 300 g received a single intraperitoneal injection of 100 mg of cefoperazone/kg. They were sacrificed and the organs were dissected. Serum and urine samples were also obtained.

Cefoperazone concentrations were measured by a bioassay (1). The test organism was *Sarcina lutea*. The values are the mean of six measurements of the same sample, each at two dilutions. The results presented in this report are based on standards made from one injection vial.

Cefoperazone serum concentrations after intravenous infusion to eight healthy volunteers are shown in Fig. 1. At the end of the two infusion periods, mean serum levels of 134 ± 17 µg/ml for the first infusion and of 143 ± 17 µg/ml for the second were measured. The decrease of the serum concentration-time curves was biexponential (Fig. 1), with a mean apparent half-life of elimination ($t_{1/2}$) for the terminal phase of 1.66 ± 0.25 h and 1.72 ± 0.36 h, respectively. At the end of each 12-h period, mean serum concentrations of 1.4 and 2.1 µg/ml were found. The area under the serum concentration-time curves calculated for the first infusion from time zero to infinity was 434 ± 88 µg/ml per h. The total clearance of cefoperazone, based on serum concentrations, measured 78 ± 15 ml/min. A volume of distribution of 11.4 ± 0.7 liters was calculated.

In the three patients with renal insufficiency maximal serum levels at 2 h measured 260 µg/ml (patient 1, 47 kg), 268 µg/ml (patient 2, 34 kg), and 167 µg/ml (patient 3, 47.5 kg). The half-lives of elimination were 2.9 h (patient 1; glomerular filtration rate [GFR], 17 ml/min), 2.8 h (patient 2; GFR, 14 ml/min), and 1.3 (patient 3; GFR, 9 ml/min). The practical consequence of this finding is that there should be no need, from a pharmacokinetic point of view, to modify the dosage regimen of cefoperazone, even in patients with a severe reduction of the renal functions.

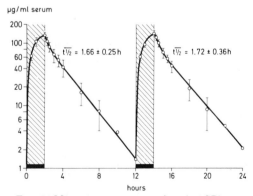

FIG. 1. *Mean serum concentrations (± 1 SD) measured in eight normal volunteers after the infusion of 2 g of cefoperazone for 2 h on two different occasions.*

For the patient with obstruction of the bile ducts, the maximal serum concentration was 146 μg/ml, the half-life was prolonged to 14 h, and 24 h after the beginning of the single 2-g infusion serum concentrations of 31 μg/ml were still measured. Clearly, no conclusions can be drawn from our single patient with biliary obstruction.

In the healthy volunteers the total amount of biologically active cefoperazone eliminated in the urine for the two infusion periods did not differ since 23.6 ± 3.7% of the dose and 23.3 ± 2.6%, respectively, were excreted after 12 h. The mean urinary concentrations of cefoperazone in the collection periods of 10 to 12 h after the beginning of the infusion were 44 and 52 μg/ml. The half-lives of elimination of cefoperazone estimated from the urinary excretion rates ($\Delta U / \Delta t$) versus time curves were 1.72 ± 0.23 and 1.93 ± 0.29 h for the two infusions. The renal clearance of cefoperazone calculated on the basis of total serum concentrations measured 18.3 ± 1.5 ml/min and 17.8 ± 2.4 ml/min, respectively.

In the three renal patients urinary excretion of cefoperazone was reduced to 8.4% of the dose (patient 1), 6.9% (patient 2), and 1.5% (patient 3) during the 12 h following the start of the infusion. In the last collection periods urinary cefoperazone concentrations were of the same order of magnitude as in the normal volunteers.

In the patient with a biliary obstruction, already more than 30% of the dose was excreted 20 h after the end of the infusion. At this time urinary concentrations were still higher than 400 μg/ml. Although the cumulative urinary recovery of cefoperazone was increased as compared to normal volunteers, the renal clearance was diminished to less than 10 ml/min.

The concentrations of cefoperazone in various tissues of rats 1 h after its intraperitoneal injection are given in Fig. 2. It is difficult to discuss,

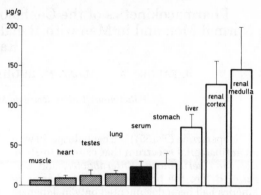

FIG. 2. *Mean tissue concentrations of cefoperazone (± SD) after its intraperitoneal administration to groups of six rats at a dose of 100 mg/kg.*

on the sole basis of serum concentrations, protein binding, or apparent volumes of distribution measured in humans, the potential advantages or disadvantages of closely related antibiotics. Clearly, more information is needed concerning the tissue-specific penetration of the drugs. In the case of cefoperazone it seems, at least in the animal model used in this study, that the apparent half-life of elimination measured in serum is a good indicator of the behavior of the drug in other tissue compartments and that cefoperazone penetrates well in most tissues (Fig. 2).

In conclusion, it appears that cefoperazone has interesting pharmacokinetic properties which might make it most useful as an antibiotic agent.

1. Fabre, J., P. Blanchard, and M. Rudhardt. 1977. Pharmacokinetics of ampicillin, cephalothin and doxycycline in various tissues of the rat. Chemotherapy (Basel) 23:129–141.

Fundamental and Clinical Studies of Cefoperazone (T-1551) in Otorhinolaryngological Infections

B. SAMBE,* K. JO, AND S. INAFUKU

Clinic of Otorhinolaryngology and Microbiological Laboratory, Kanto Teishin Hospital, Tokyo, Japan

The new semisynthetic cephalosporin cefoperazone (T-1551), sodium 7-[D(−)-α-(4-ethyl-2,3-dioxo-1-piperazine-carboxamido)-α-(4-hydroxyphenyl)acetamido]-3-[(1-methyl-1H-tetrazol-5-yl)thiomethyl]-3-cephem-4-carboxylate, has a broad antibacterial spectrum which appears to be wider than that of cefazolin. Of interest is its excellent activity against *Pseudomonas aeruginosa*, *Enterobacter* spp., and indole-positive *Proteus* spp., which are resistant to cephalosporins such as cefazolin and cephalothin (2, 4–6).

The MICs of T-1551 against 60 isolates of coagulase-positive staphylococci and 45 isolates of *P. aeruginosa* ranged from 0.78 to 6.26 µg/ml (peak MIC, 1.56 µg/ml) and 0.78 to 6.26 µg/ml (peak MIC, 1.56 µg/ml), respectively (3).

The bactericidal activities of T-1551 in serum were determined by inoculating 10^5 cells of *Staphylococcus aureus, Escherichia coli,* and *P. aeruginosa* in 10-fold diluted serum which was taken at 0.5, 1, 2, 4, and 6 h from patients who had received a single intramuscular injection of 500 mg. Results obtained by use of a biophotometer showed that T-1551 had a potent bactericidal effect against *S. aureus, E. coli,* and *P. aeruginosa*; however, T-1551 was shown to be inactive against *P. aeruginosa* in the serum at 6 h after injection (1).

The peak serum levels after a single intramuscular administration of 500 or 1,000 mg were obtained at 30 min and were 28.7 and 55.0 µg/ml, respectively, as determined by the thin-layer method with *Micrococcus luteus* ATCC 9341 as the test organism. The serum concentrations persisted through 8 h and were 3.7 and 6.5 µg/ml, respectively, at that time.

The concentrations of T-1551 in the serum and palatina tonsilla at 1 h after a 500-mg intramuscular injection were 31.5 and 3.4 µg/ml, respectively.

The concentrations of T-1551 in the serum, palatina tonsilla, mucous membrane of concha inferior, and mucous membrane of maxillar sinusitis at 1 h after the 1.0-g doses were 56.7 to 65 µg/ml, 6.0 µg/ml, 6.0 µg/ml, and 4.9 µg/ml, respectively.

The serum concentrations of T-1551 at 1, 2, and 3 h after a 2.0-g drip infusion injection were 185.0, 201.5, and 112.0 µg/ml, and the aural discharge concentrations were 3.2, 2.9, and 2.2 µg/ml, respectively. The concentration of T-1551 in the aural discharge was higher than the MIC for *P. aeruginosa* (peak, 1.56 µg/ml).

T-1551 was administered by means of drip infusion or intramuscular injection to 32 patients with various infections in the otorhinolaryngological area at the dosage of 1 to 6 g per day for 4 to 12 days. These patients included six with acute suppurative otitis media accompanying mastoiditis in two cases, eight with chronic suppurative otitis media accompanying mastoiditis in two cases, seven with acute tonsillitis, six with peritonsillitis and peritonsillar abscess, three with acute paranasal sinusitis, and one with phlegmon of the external ear and mouth floor. The effectiveness of T-1551 was excellent in 21 infections due to gram-positive bacilli, good in 8 infections due to gram-negative bacilli (*P. aeruginosa, Proteus mirabilis*), and poor in 2 patients. Administration was discontinued in one patient because of an unpleasant feeling. As

a whole, the efficacy rate of T-1551 was 93.5%.

Judged by causative organisms, T-1551 was effective in all of 11 infections caused by *S. aureus,* in the 1 infection caused by *S. epidermidis,* in 8 of 10 infections caused by *P. aeruginosa,* and in the 1 infection caused by *P. mirabilis.* The good antibacterial activities of T-1551 against these bacteria observed in vitro were confirmed by the clinical studies. It was especially worthy of note that the causative organism and the symptoms completely disappeared in four cases of incurable suppurative otitis media that accompanied mastoiditis due to *P. aeruginosa.*

The only side effect observed was an unpleasant feeling in one patient, and that returned to normal when drug administration was discontinued.

The following are three typical cases.

Case 1 was a 13-year-old male with acute suppurative otitis media (left) and acute mastoiditis. The disease began with the symptoms of headache, hardness of hearing, aural discharge, and febrile condition. Administration of cephalexin was ineffective. *S. aureus* and *P. aeruginosa* were detected in the aural discharge, and these isolates were susceptible to T-1551 concentrations of 3.13 and 1.56 µg/ml, respectively. A daily dose of 2 g was administered in two divided doses every 12 h by means of intravenous drip infusion. Pyretolysis took place on the third day at 37°C, and the aural discharge disappeared. The remarkable efficacy of T-1551 was shown by administering a total of 8 g during 4 days.

Case 2 was a 30-year-old male with acute exacerbation of chronic suppurative otitis media (right) and acute mastoiditis. There was profuse aural discharge, severe headache, and high fever after swimming in the sea. Administration of cephalexin did not show good efficacy. *S. aureus* and *P. aeruginosa* were detected in the aural discharge and were susceptible to T-1551 at 1.56 and 0.78 µg/ml, respectively. Although 4 g of T-1551 was administered daily by drip infusion in two divided doses, no effects were achieved. Pyretolysis, however, took place after daily doses of 6 g in three divided doses. A total of 50 g was administered during 9 days. Aural discharge stopped on the fifth day. Thus, satisfactory effects were obtained against a mixed infection due to *S. aureus* and *P. aeruginosa.*

Case 3 was a 26-year-old male with acute exacerbation of chronic suppurative otitis media (left) and acute mastoiditis. Profuse aural discharge began 1 month before presentation. He presented with severe headache on the left side and a febrile condition registering 38°C. A large volume of aural discharge occurred pulsatingly. *P. aeruginosa* was detected in the aural discharge, and it was susceptible to T-1551 at 1.56 µg/ml. The aural discharge was stopped by administering 4 g of T-1551 daily for a period of 7 days.

These cases show the efficacy of T-1551 in the treatment of acute mastoiditis due to *P. aeruginosa*.

1. **Jo, K., and B. Sambe.** 1970. Studies on the antibacterial, especially bacteriolytic action of cefazolin. Chemotherapy (Japan) 18:501-504.
2. **Kariyone, K., H. Harada, M. Kurita, and T. Takano.** 1970. Cefazolin, a new semisynthetic cephalosporin antibiotic. J. Antibiot. **23**:131-136.
3. **Mitsuhashi, S., N. Matsubara, S. Minami, T. Muraoka, T. Yasuda, and I. Saikawa.** 1978. Antibacterial activities of a new semisynthetic cephalosporin, T-1551. Program Abstr. Intersci. Conf. Antimicrob. Agents Chemother. 18th, Atlanta, Ga., abstr. no. 153.
4. **Murdoch, J. M., C. F. Speirs, A. M. Geddes, and E. M. Wallace.** 1964. Clinical trial of cephaloridine (Ceporin) a new broad-spectrum antibiotic derived from cephalosporin C. Br. Med. J. **2**:1238-1240.
5. **Sambe, B., H. Haruko, K. Nishizaki, and K. Jo.** 1970. Results of cefazolin treatment of various infection in otorhinolaryngological field. Chemotherapy (Japan) **18**: 831-835.
6. **Sambe, B., H. Murakami, K. Kobayashi, K. Jo, and S. Inafuku.** 1977. Fundamental and clinical study of T-1220 (piperacillin) in otorhinolaryngological field. Chemotherapy (Japan) **25**:1509-1518.

Pharmacokinetics of Cefoperazone (T-1551)

J. SASAKI,* J. GOTO, T. KONNAI, S. MIYACHI, Y. YAMADA, T. IMOTO, H. KOBUNE, AND K. TAKEYASU

Tokai University School of Medicine, Kanagawa, and Ashikaga Red Cross Hospital, Tochigi, Japan*

Cefoperazone (T-1551), a new semisynthetic cephalosporin derivative, has a broad antibacterial spectrum against gram-positive cocci and gram-negative bacilli, especially against *Klebsiella pneumoniae*, *Serratia marcescens*, *Enterobacter cloacae*, and *Pseudomonas aeruginosa*.

We have studied the absorption, excretion, and metabolism of T-1551 in comparison with cephaloridine (CER).

T-1551 was intravenously administered to healthy volunteers weighing between 65 and 83 kg (mean, 73 kg), and the blood levels and urinary excretion rates were measured. A crossover test was performed in which 2 g of T-1551 administered by drip infusion for 1 h was compared with dose administered for 2 h. The same experiment was done with the well-known cephalosporin antibiotic CER in the same volunteers.

Prior to the investigation, a physical examination including a medical history with attention to drug allergy, especially penicillin and cephalosporin allergy, was performed in each volunteer. The intravenous study was conducted in two different subjects on each of four experimental days. On each day, the subjects were admitted to the hospital at 7:00 a.m. after fasting from midnight until the finish of intravenous administration.

T-1551, 2 g in 500 ml of 5% glucose solution, and CER were infused for 1 and 2 h through a superficial forearm vein. Venous blood samples were obtained during the infusion at 0.25, 0.5,

and 1 h for 1-h infusion and at 0.25, 0.5, 1, and 2 h for 2-h infusion. The same samples were obtained after the infusion in bilateral groups at 0.5, 1, 2, 4, and 6 h. Urine samples were collected four times. The first samples were collected until the end of the intravenous infusion; the second, third, and fourth samples were collected through 2, 4, and 6 h after the infusion was completed.

The blood samples on each day were centrifuged. Serum specimens were collected and were stored at −80°C in a freezer until the experiment was performed. T-1551 and CER in serum were bioassayed, with *Micrococcus luteus* ATCC 9341 as the test organism. Standard curves for assaying blood samples were prepared in Monitrol 1, and urine samples were prepared in phosphate buffer solution at pH 7.0. The samples were dissolved at room temperature 1 h before the bioassay and were assayed by the cylinder method on Penassay seed agar for 18 h. As the major component of T-1551 in human serum was found to consist of a single constituent part, the antibacterial activity measured by this method was assumed to be related to unchanged T-1551.

The average blood level and urinary excretion are summarized in Fig. 1 and 2.

The disposition of T-1551 and CER infused intravenously for each subject was estimated by applying one- and two-compartment kinetic models. Two-compartment kinetic models were derived by use of an interactive least-square

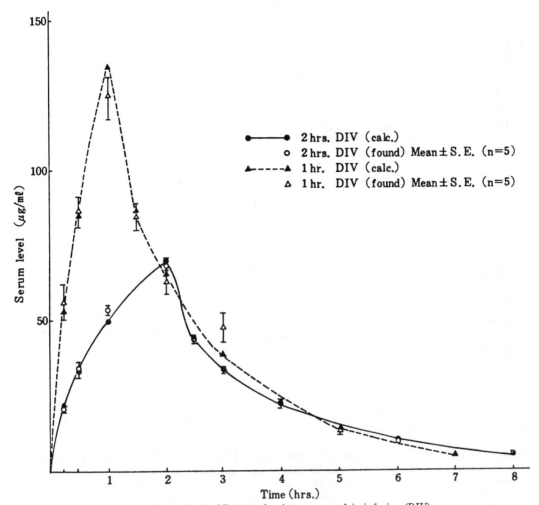

FIG. 1. *Serum level of T-1551 after intravenous drip infusion (DIV).*

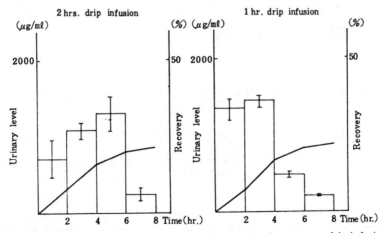

FIG. 2. *Urinary level and excretion rate of T-1551 after intravenous drip infusion.*

TABLE 1. *Pharmacokinetic parameters by one-compartment model*[a]

Treatment	V_d (liters)	K_{el} (h^{-1})	$t_{\frac{1}{2}}$ (h)	C_0 (μg/ml)	K_s (%/h)	C_s (ml/min)
T-1551, 2 g						
2-h DIV	36.05	0.4143	1.673	55.48	41.43	2,489
1-h DIV	22.24	0.5059	1.370	89.93	50.59	1,875
Cephaloridine, 2 g						
2-h DIV	54.55	0.5271	1.315	36.66	52.71	4,792
1-h DIV	26.62	0.5598	1.238	75.14	55.98	2,484

[a] DIV, intravenous drip infusion; V_d, apparent volume of distribution; K_{el}, first-order elimination rate constant; $t_{\frac{1}{2}}$, half-life; C_0, initial amount of drug in the body at endpoint of administration; K_s, percentage of first-order elimination rate constant; C_s, serum clearance.

TABLE 2. *Pharmacokinetics of T-1551 and cephaloridine by two-compartment models*[a]

$$A \rightarrow \boxed{\text{Compartment I}} \underset{k_{21}}{\overset{k_{12}}{\rightleftarrows}} \boxed{\text{Compartment II}}$$
$$\downarrow k_{13}$$
$$\alpha + \beta = k_{12} + k_{13} + k_{21}$$
$$\alpha \cdot \beta = k_{13} \cdot k_{21}$$

Treatment	V_d (liters)	k_{12} (h^{-1})	k_{21} (h^{-1})	k_{13} (h^{-1})	$t_{\frac{1}{2}}$ (h)	α (h^{-1})	β (h^{-1})
T-1551, 2 g							
2-h DIV	20.22	3.42	1.81	1.24	1.928	6.10	0.370
	±1.59	±1.36	±0.39	±0.22	±0.172	±1.86	±0.032
1-h DIV	13.08	4.31	4.57	1.19	1.343	9.53	0.527
	±2.02	±1.21	±0.65	±0.22	±0.096	±1.07	±0.042
Cephaloridine, 2 g							
2-h DIV	29.13	4.34	2.05	1.66	1.487	7.59	0.469
	±2.46	±1.48	±0.43	±0.22	±0.052	±2.07	±0.017
1-h DIV	15.96	3.84	1.74	2.07	1.402	7.15	0.504
	±1.22	±1.00	±0.34	±0.28	±0.102	±1.26	±0.034

[a] Calculation: computer Facom 230, Monte Carlo method + Simplex method. DIV, intravenous drip infusion; V_d, apparent volume of distribution; k_{12}, k_{21}, and k_{13}, transfer rate constants; $t_{\frac{1}{2}}$, half-life.

digital program on a Facom 230 computer. The rate constants for disposition and elimination and the volume of the central compartment were estimated directly from the one-compartment kinetic model. Results obtained with the one- and two-compartment kinetic models are summarized in Tables 1 and 2.

With T-1551, a twofold variation in the elimination half-lives was noted at approximately 1.3 to 1.7 h, with a mean log time for absorption of approximately 0.41 to 0.51 h. A computer-predicted plot of serum concentration over time after intravenous infusion using the mean derived kinetic parameters demonstrates an approximation to the observed serum concentration. Time and dose responses were also noted in this study.

In Vitro Activity and Laboratory Testing Considerations of Cefoperazone (T-1551)

DAVID F. WELCH,[1]* BARBARA J. SAXON, DONALD N. WRIGHT, AND JOHN M. MATSEN

Departments of Pathology and Pediatrics, University of Utah College of Medicine, Salt Lake City, Utah 84132, U.S.A.

The antibacterial spectrum of some recently developed β-lactam antimicrobials has been re-

[1] Present address: Division of Pediatric Infectious Diseases, University of Oklahoma Health Sciences Center, Oklahoma City, OK 73190.

markably extended to include most members of the *Enterobacteriaceae* and *Pseudomonas*, in addition to the aerobic gram-positive cocci. Because of the lower potential for toxicity when compared to the aminoglycosides, the availability of broader-spectrum β-lactam compounds for treatment of serious infections represents new therapeutic alternatives in the management of infectious diseases. Cefoperazone (T-1551) appears to be a potentially useful agent with activity against a wide range of gram-negative and gram-positive organisms (1). We have studied its spectrum of activity against commonly isolated bacteria of clinical origin and have further investigated this compound with respect to other in vitro characteristics.

Dilution and disk diffusion susceptibility testing methods were employed as described by the National Committee for Clinical Laboratory Standards.

Comparative agar dilution MICs for 237 *Enterobacteriaceae* isolates representing *Klebsiella, Escherichia coli, Salmonella, Shigella, Proteus, Providencia, Citrobacter, Enterobacter,* and *Serratia* demonstrated cefoperazone to be generally more active than other cepha compounds tested (Fig. 1A). Cefoperazone was the

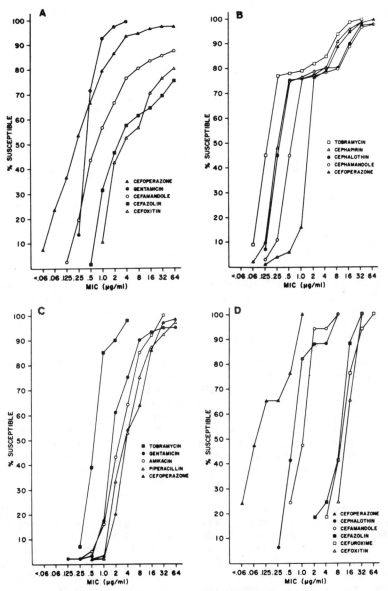

FIG. 1. *Cumulative percentage of (A) 237 strains of Enterobacteriaceae, (B) 96 strains of gram-positive cocci, (C) 59 strains of nonfermentative gram-negative organisms, and (D) 17 strains of Haemophilus influenzae inhibited.*

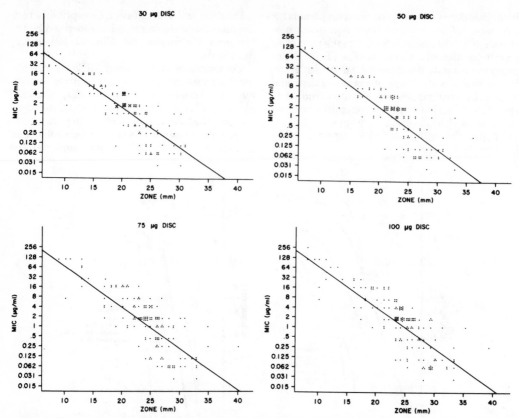

FIG. 2. *Regression analysis of MICs of cefoperazone and zones of inhibition produced by disk diffusion.*

only cepha compound tested which approached the activity of gentamicin and other aminoglycosides. Members of the *Enterobacteriaceae* having the highest cefoperazone MICs were encountered primarily within the *Klebsiella* group.

Ninety-six strains of gram-positive cocci representing enterococci, *Staphylococcus aureus*, and *S. epidermidis* were susceptible to cefoperazone at a concentration of 64 µg/ml (Fig. 1B). Although cefoperazone was less active than other agents, the highest MICs observed may be within therapeutically achievable serum concentrations. The highest concentrations required were almost exclusively those for enterococci.

The nonfermentative gram-negative organisms *Pseudomonas aeruginosa* and *Acinetobacter* (59 strains) were inhibited by cefoperazone at concentrations of 0.5 to 128 µg/ml (Fig. 1C). Cefoperazone was similar in activity to piperacillin, but markedly less active than the aminoglycosides, particularly tobramycin. The majority of organisms resistant to greater than 32 µg/ml were *Acinetobacter* strains.

Cefoperazone was the most active cepha compound tested against 17 strains of *Haemophilus*

influenzae, including three β-lactamase–producing strains (Fig. 1D). The MICs of five other cepha compounds for 50% of the isolates were approximately 8- to 150-fold greater than those of cefoperazone.

Comparisons of zones of inhibition produced by disk diffusion with MIC results were initially performed with 10, 20, 30, and 50 µg of cefoperazone per disk. However, more recent pharmacological information has suggested that the therapeutic serum levels may approximate 64 µg/ml. Additional testing was done with 30-, 50-, 75-, and 100-µg cefoperazone-containing disks. The results shown in Fig. 2 suggest that a disk containing 50 or 75 µg of cefoperazone may be appropriate.

Cefoperazone was bactericidal at concentrations equal to, or greater than, the MIC, but allowed regrowth of organisms after 4 to 6 h when tested in concentrations one-fourth or one-half the MIC. Gentamicin was generally more rapidly bactericidal than cefoperazone and the other β-lactam compounds against *E. coli*, *P. aeruginosa*, and *S. aureus*.

Minor inoculum effects on the MIC and MBC

were observed when 10^3 or 10^5 organisms were used. Increasing the inoculum size to 10^7 caused a marked effect on the MIC: a 10- to 100-fold increase in MICs for the gram-negative rods was observed, but less than 10-fold differences were observed with some staphylococci. The MBC was equal to, or within one twofold dilution of, the MIC for the majority of organisms tested.

Similar MIC ranges were observed for three groups of organisms when variation of the medium type was considered. Testing on nutrient agar resulted in a lower range and average MIC for *Enterobacteriaceae* but resulted in a higher range and average MIC for enterococcus and *Acinetobacter* in comparison to Mueller-Hinton agar. Slightly higher MICs were also obtained when enterococci were tested on heart infusion agar in contrast to results with Mueller-Hinton agar.

Cefoperazone in combination with various aminoglycosides resulted in the synergistic inhibition of 7 of 11 *Pseudomonas* strains and of one-fourth of the enterococci and *Enterobacter* strains tested.

1. **Neu, H. C., K. P. Fu, N. Aswapokee, P. Aswapokee, and K. Kung.** 1979. Comparative activity of cefoperazone, a piperazine cephalosporin. Antimicrob. Agents Chemother. **16:**150–157.

In Vitro Evaluation of Cefoperazone (T-1551), a New Semisynthetic Cephalosporin: Six-Center Collaborative Study

R. N. JONES,* P. C. FUCHS, A. L. BARRY, T. L. GAVAN, H. M. SOMMERS, AND E. H. GERLACH

Department of Pathology, Kaiser Foundation Hospitals, Portland, Oregon 97015; Department of Pathology, St. Vincent Hospital, Portland, Oregon 97225; Microbiology Laboratory, Sacramento Medical Center, Sacramento, California 95817; Department of Microbiology, The Cleveland Clinic Foundation, Cleveland, Ohio 44106; Department of Pathology, Northwestern Memorial Hospital, Chicago, Illinois 60611; and Department of Pathology, St. Francis Hospital, Wichita, Kansas 67214, U.S.A.*

Cefoperazone (CP; T-1551) is a new semisynthetic cephalosporin structurally similar to cefamandole and piperacillin. It has a broad spectrum of antimicrobial activity against *Pseudomonas aeruginosa*, *Enterobacter* species, *Klebsiella* species, and indole-positive *Proteus* species, as well as the usual organisms inhibited by this family of antimicrobials (S. Mitsuhashi, N. Matsubara, S. Minami, T. Muraoka, T. Yasuda, and T. Saikawa, Program Abstr. Intersci. Conf. Antimicrob. Agents Chemother., 18th, Atlanta, Ga., abstr. no. 153, 1978). In this six-laboratory collaborative study the in vitro antimicrobial activity of CP was compared with those of cephalothin (CF) and gentamicin (GM).

Experimental methods. CP-sodium was supplied by Pfizer Pharmaceuticals; cephalothin, by Eli Lilly Research Laboratories; and gentamicin, by Schering Corp. All three compounds were diluted in Mueller-Hinton broth supplemented with calcium (50 mg/liter) and magnesium (25 mg/liter) or included in Mueller-Hinton agar plates. A seven-dilution protocol was used for each antibiotic, ranging from 0.25 to 64 µg/ml.

The organisms used were consecutive clinical strains isolated during a 30- to 45-day period. Nearly 9,000 aerobic and facultative anaerobic organisms were tested and identified by previously described procedures (1). In addition, 248 anaerobic bacteria were tested by the National Committee for Clinical Laboratory Standards Wilkins-Chalgren reference procedure (Northwestern Memorial Hospital) or broth modification method (2) (Kaiser Foundation Hospitals).

The plastic microdilution broth susceptibility trays were prepared in three laboratories (Cleveland Clinic Foundation, Kaiser Foundation Hospitals, and Sacramento Medical Center) by use of a Dynatech MIC-2000 and Mueller-Hinton broth (Difco) as previously described (1). The MIC endpoint was defined as the lowest antimicrobial concentration totally inhibiting visible growth after 15 to 18 h of incubation at 35°C. Final inoculum size was adjusted to 10^5 colony-forming units/ml.

The agar dilution method was used in the other three centers, with media, inoculating methods, incubation, and interpretation closely controlled by use of standard performance characteristics, e.g., expected MIC modes on quality-control organisms, thus bringing agar and broth methods to parity (1).

Four or more quality-control organisms with known reproducible MICs were run daily in parallel with the unknown clinical isolates. Ac-

TABLE 1. *Comparative in vitro antimicrobial activity of cefoperazone (CP), gentamicin (GM), and cephalothin (CF) against 5,422 recent clinical isolates of Enterobacteriaceae*

Organism (no. of isolates)	Antibiotic	Cumulative % inhibited at a concn (μg/ml) of:						
		≤0.25	1	2	4	8	16	64
Citrobacter diversus (65)	CP	86	89	92	98		100	
	GM	52	92	94		95	98	100
	CF	2	24	76	85	97		98
C. freundii (98)	CP	65	85	86	87	88	89	97
	GM	12	94		95		96	98
	CF	5	6	8	10	17	33	69
Enterobacter aerogenes (234)	CP	71	85	90	92	94	98	100
	GM	11	89	95	97		98	99
	CF	4	5	7	11	12	15	44
E. cloacae (300)	CP	70	85	88	88	93	93	97
	GM	18	95	98	99			99
	CF		2		3	4	6	19
Escherichia coli (2,775)	CP	79	92	95	97	98	98	99
	GM	7	89	96	98	98	99	99
	CF	3	5	14	51	79	92	97
Klebsiella oxytoca (170)	CP	34	69	92	97	98		
	GM	11	99				99	100
	CF		15	45	71	86	92	94
K. pneumoniae (786)	CP	69	88	94	97	98	99	99
	GM	11	96	98	99	99	99	99
	CF	3	11	43	75	88	91	97
Morganella morganii (116)	CP	25	81	86	92	94	95	99
	GM	20	96					97
	CF	4	5	10			11	12
Proteus mirabilis (571)	CP	36	95	98	99	99	99	99
	GM	10	87	97	99	99		100
	CF	2	7	33	83	94	97	98
P. vulgaris (46)	CP	41	87	91		96	100	
	GM	37	91	93	98			
	CF			4			11	20
Providencia rettgeri (47)	CP	26	47	62	74	85		100
	GM	21	55	74	83	89	91	
	CF			2	6	11	13	30
P. stuartii (30)	CP	3	40	57	87		93	97
	GM	3	27	40	57	63	70	77
	CF			17		21	28	55
Serratia marcescens (184)	CP	16	64	80	86	88	93	97
	GM	8	79	88	90	93		95
	CF	3				5	6	14

ceptable and comparable results were obtained between laboratories and methods, with only 1% of endpoints beyond the ±1 dilution limits.

The statistical analysis of the differences in antimicrobial activity comparing the three anti-biotics or six institutions was done by means of Kalmozorov-Smironov two-sample (points on cumulative percentage curve) test.

Results and discussion. CP demonstrated significantly greater antimicrobial activity against the 5,422 strains of *Enterobacteriaceae* tested than did CF and GM (Table 1). The modal and median MICs were ≤0.25, 4, and 1 µg/ml for CP, CF, and GM, respectively. *Citrobacter freundii, Enterobacter aerogenes, E. cloacae, Morganella morganii, Proteus vulgaris, Providencia* species, and *Serratia* species were inhibited by CP but not by CF at ≤8 µg/ml. The in vitro efficacy of GM against these organisms ranged from 57 to 100% (≤4 µg/ml), with the lowest activity against the *Providencia* species. CP inhibited 85 to 100% of the species groups (≤16 µg/ml) and was also least active against *Providencia*.

Table 2 shows the comparative susceptibility to CP, CF, and GM of commonly isolated non-*Enterobacteriaceae* gram-negative bacilli and gram-positive bacteria. CP was comparable to GM in activity (by weight) against *Pseudomonas*, superior against *Pasteurella multocida*, and relatively inactive versus the *Acinetobacter* isolates.

Only 80% of current *P. aeruginosa* strains were inhibited by GM at ≤4 µg/ml. However, CP inhibited 93% of these isolates at ≤16 µg/ml (mode, 4 µg/ml), a clinically achievable concentration.

CF was more active than CP or GM against staphylococcal isolates, though all three drugs were highly effective at clinically obtainable concentrations. None of the compounds was active on the serogroup D streptococci. CP and CF were highly inhibitory against all other *Streptococcus* species, but the MICs of GM for 90% of these organisms were consistently within the resistant range.

CP inhibited 75% of *Bacteroides fragilis* isolates at ≤32 µg/ml (not shown). Comparable figures for other antimicrobials include: clindamycin, 96% at ≤2 µg/ml; chloramphenicol, 97% at ≤8 µg/ml; and cefoxitin, 100% at ≤16 µg/ml.

CP was very active against 100 CF-resistant and 50 aminoglycoside-resistant recent clinical isolates (not shown). The rank order of activity against CF-resistant isolates was as follows: amikacin, 92% at ≤16 µg/ml; CP, 87% at ≤32 µg/ml; piperacillin, 85% at ≤32 µg/ml; GM, 77% at ≤4 µg/ml; and cefoxitin, 42% at ≤16 µg/ml. Similarly, CP was very active against aminoglycoside-resistant organisms and superior to currently available cephalosporins and semisynthetic penicillins. CP inhibited 58 and 88% of this latter resistant population at 16 and 64 µg/ml, respectively.

In conclusion, the CP modal MIC for all strains of *Enterobacteriaceae* was ≤0.25 µg/ml.

TABLE 2. *Modal MIC and concentration inhibiting 90% (MIC₉₀) of 2,311 gram-positive cocci and 868 non-Enterobacteriaceae gram-negative bacilli*

Organism (no. of isolates)	Cefoperazone		Cephalothin		Gentamicin	
	Mode[a]	MIC$_{90}$[a]	Mode	MIC$_{90}$	Mode	MIC$_{90}$
Staphylococcus aureus (924)	2	4	≤0.25	1	≤0.25	1
S. epidermidis (586)	1	4	≤0.25	1	≤0.25	8
Micrococci (18)	≤0.25	16	≤0.25	2	≤0.25	8
Streptococcus faecalis (588)	64	64	64	64	16	64
Group D streptococci, not S. faecalis (26)	>64	>64	≤0.25	>64	8, 16	16
S. agalactiae (39)	≤0.25	1	≤0.25	≤0.25	8	16
S. pyogenes (18)	≤0.25	1	≤0.25	≤0.25	8	16
Beta-hemolytic streptococci not in groups A, B, and D (27)	≤0.25	1	≤0.25	≤0.25	≤0.25	8
S. pneumoniae (17)	≤0.25	1	≤0.25	2	≤0.25	8
Viridans group streptococci (37) . .	≤0.25	2	≤0.25	2	≤0.25	16
Other streptococci[b] (31)	≤0.25	4	≤0.25	8	≤0.25	8
Acinetobacter calcoaceticus var. anitratus (69)	64	64	>64	>64	1	8
A. calcoaceticus var. *lwoffi* (23) . .	64	>64	64	>64	1	8
Pseudomonas aeruginosa (718) . .	4	16	>64	>64	4	8
P. maltophilia (19)	4	>64	>64	>64	16	>64
Pseudomonas spp.[c] (16)	2	64	>64	>64	≤0.25	16
Other nonenteric bacilli[d] (33)	≤0.25	64	16, 64	>64	≤0.25	8

[a] Expressed in micrograms per milliliter.

[b] Includes various nonhemolytic ungroupable streptococci.

[c] Includes *P. cepacia* (2), *P. putida* (1), *P. putrefaciens* (1), and *Pseudomonas* sp. NOS (12).

[d] Includes *Aeromonas hydrophila* (4), *Achromobacter* sp. (2), *Alcaligenes denitrifaciens* (2), *Moraxella* species (3), group IV-2 (1), and *Pasteurella multocida* (11).

CP suppressed over 98% of these enteric gram-negative bacilli at ≤16 µg/ml and thus was significantly ($P < 0.001$) more active than either GM (≤4 µg/ml) or CF (≤8 µg/ml). Among the non-*Enterobacteriaceae* and gram-positive organisms, CP inhibited 86.0 and 84.6%, respectively. The overall (nearly 9,000 isolates) cumulative percentages were 93.3% inhibition at ≤16 µg/ml and 98.5% inhibition at ≤64 µg/ml. CP appears to be a very effective new cephalosporin with wide potential applications to infections caused by members of the *Enterobacteriaceae*, *Pseudomonas*, staphylococci, anaerobes, and certain *Streptococcus* species. These data support the performance of further in vitro and in vivo evaluations.

1. **Jones, R. N., A. L. Barry, P. C. Fuchs, T. L. Gavan, E. H. Gerlach, and H. Sommers.** 1978. 1-N-(S-3-amino-2-hydroxypropionyl) gentamicin B (SCH 21420): a collaborative in vitro susceptibility comparison with amikacin and gentamicin against 12,984 clinical bacterial isolates. Curr. Microbiol. 1:359–364.
2. **Jones, R. N., P. C. Fuchs, C. Thornsberry, and N. Rhodes.** 1978. Antimicrobial susceptibility tests for anaerobic bacteria. Comparison of Wilkins-Chalgren agar reference method and microdilution method, and determinations of stability of antimicrobics frozen in broth. Curr. Microbiol. 1:81–83.

Cefoperazone (T-1551), a New Semisynthetic Cephalosporin: Comparative In Vitro Study Against 630 Clinical Isolates

C. MOREL* AND N. MONROCQ

Centre Hospitalier Universitaire, Caen, 14040 Caen, France

T-1551 (cefoperazone) is a new semisynthetic cephalosporin that is freely soluble in water. The advent of a new antibacterial drug provides us with an opportunity to determine its activity against fresh clinical isolates and to compare it with other drugs of the same family. For this purpose, we have carried out an in vitro comparative study with T-1551 versus cephalothin, cefamandole, and cefotaxime (HR-756 or RU 24,756).

The organisms used were fresh clinical strains that had been isolated in the hospital's laboratory. Among the gram-negative bacteria were 428 isolates of *Enterobacteriaceae*, 100 of *Pseudomonas*, 15 of *Acinetobacter*, and 28 of *Haemophilus*. The gram-positive bacteria included 26 isolates of staphylococci, 22 of *Streptococcus faecalis*, and 11 of *Listeria* (Table 1). We also determined the MIC of the four drugs for 43 *Escherichia coli* K-12 strains carrying R factors which were mated with cephalothin-resistant enterobacteria at different levels (wild strains: *E. coli*, 9; *Klebsiella*, 16; *Enterobacter*, 11; *Serratia*, 4; and *Providencia*, 3). We did not study any anaerobic bacteria.

With concentrations of ≤0.12 and ≥64 µg/ml used as cut-off points, MICs were determined in Mueller-Hinton medium by the twofold agar dilution method. The inoculum used was about 10^4 colony-forming units/ml. The MBC is the concentration which killed 99.9% or more of the cells by 12 h after inoculation. The bactericidal activity of T-1551 versus seven isolates was determined by the broth dilution technique.

For ease, the results in Table 1 show the cumulative percentage of strains inhibited in relation to the MIC, in spite of the fact that there were few strains in some bacterial groups.

Gram-positive bacteria. Cephalothin remained the most active product against staphylococci; in our study there were no resistant strains. The least effective drug was cefotaxime; T-1551 took third place in the range of activity after cephalothin and cefamandole. Nevertheless, the highest MIC of T-1551 for cephalothin-susceptible staphylococcal strains was 16 µg/ml.

The activities of the four compounds against *Streptococcus faecalis* were similar, and cephalosporins did not appear to be the best treatment in such cases. *Listeria monocytogenes* was susceptible, and it appeared that T-1551 was the most active of the four drugs. However, we cannot say that the advent of T-1551 is a breakthrough in the fight against aerobic gram-positive bacteria.

Gram-negative bacteria. At the other extreme is T-1551's activity against gram-negative bacteria. Previous data had shown that cephalothin and cefamandole were effective, although a number of strains were still resistant; the latter, which is more active, should be considered a second-generation cephalosporin. A couple of years ago, cefotaxime appeared to be more active than the others, and only a few aerobic gram-

TABLE 1. *Susceptibility of gram-positive and gram-negative clinical isolates to cephalothin (A), cefamandole (B), cefotaxime (C), and T-1551 (D)*

Organism (no. of isolates)	Drug	Cumulative % inhibited by a concn (µg/ml) of:										
		≤0.12	0.25	0.5	1	2	4	8	16	32	64	>64
Gram-positive bacteria												
Staphylococcus (26)	A	0	8	69	80	100						
	B	4	8	35	58	73	96	100				
	C				0	15	42	77	92	100		
	D			0	4	24	70	74	100			
Streptococcus faecalis (22)	A	0	4	4	13	18	18	18	23	32	100	
	B			0	14	18	18	18	23	50	95	100
	C		0	9	18	18	22	31	45	50	55	100
	D	0	5	14	18	18	18	23	32	41	82	100
Listeria (11)	A					0	73	100				
	B				0	9	82	82	100			
	C					0	100					
	D		0	18	18	45	100					
Gram-negative bacteria												
Escherichia coli (100)	A				0	7	14	38	57	63	66	100
	B		0	8	42	56	85	100				
	C	48	58	89	97	98	99	99	100			
	D	7	59	90	98	99	100					
Klebsiella (80)	A				0	3	19	50	74	80	86	100
	B		0	1	16	42	52	91	97	100		
	C	77	93	99	100							
	D	8	13	46	85	95	99	100				
Enterobacter cloacae (50)	A					0	3	11	13	16	34	100
	B		0	15	41	61	74	89	92	92	97	100
	C	23	51	87	95	95	97	100				
	D	8	62	80	80	91	98	100				
Serratia (50)	A										0	100
	B			0	4	8	36	62	76	88	100	
	C	96	100									
	D	14	32	50	80	98	100					
Proteus, indole-negative (30)	A				0	3	27	27	94	94	97	100
	B	0	6	30	67	85	97	100				
	C	94	94	100								
	D	13	37	70	99	100						
Preoteus, indole-positive (57)	A		0	5	12	14	28	30	30	37	40	100
	B	0	9	16	60	83	95	100				
	C	58	77	94	100							
	D	21	58	72	74	92	100					
Providencia (50)	A						0	2	18	50	86	100
	B	0	6	38	64	80	92	98	98	98	100	
	C	2	68	94	94	98	100					
	D	0	12	38	50	76	90	100				
Pseudomonas (100)	A										0	100
	B										0	100
	C					0	31	73	87	94	100	
	D				0	6	39	88	95	95	96	100

TABLE 1—*Continued*

Organism (no. of isolates)	Drug	Cumulative % inhibited by a concn (μg/ml) of:										
		≤0.12	0.25	0.5	1	2	4	8	16	32	64	>64
Acinetobacter (15)	A				0	13	20	20	20	33	40	100
	B	0	6	12	18	18	24	30	42	48	60	100
	C	20	26	39	39	39	39	52	65	100		
	D	13	35	35	42	42	42	55	63	76	100	
Haemophilus (28)	A			0	25	92	100					
	B	0	7	25	57	100						
	C	0	43	82	93	100						
	D	0	57	93	100							
Salmonella (11)	A				18	36	73	100				
	B		63	91	100							
	C	100										
	D	73	91	100								

TABLE 2. *Bactericidal activity of T-1551*[a]

Organism	MIC	MBC
Escherichia coli	0.5	0.5
Klebsiella	16	16
Enterobacter cloacae	0.5	0.5
Serratia	0.5	1
Proteus morganii	16	32
Pseudomonas	1	2
Staphylococcus	0.5	2

[a] The MIC was determined by the broth dilution method. The MBC was the concentration that killed 99.9% or more of the cells by 12 h after inoculation. Initial cell concentration, about 1×10^4 to 3×10^4/ml.

negative strains were resistant, e.g., some *Pseudomonas* and *Acinetobacter* strains. In relation to its activity, cefotaxime was classed as a third-generation cephalosporin.

The T-1551 results achieved during our study may be compared with the previously obtained cefotaxime results. Cefotaxime appeared to be somewhat more active than T-1551 against *Serratia*, *Proteus*, and a few strains of *Klebsiella*; results against *E. coli*, *Enterobacter*, *Providencia*, and *Acinetobacter* were similar for the two drugs; and T-1551 was more effective against *Haemophilus*. The most important point was T-1551's activity against *Pseudomonas*: 73% of the strains were inhibited by cefotaxime, whereas 95% were susceptible to T-1551, at a concentration of 16 μg/ml (lowest concentration for resistant strains).

Bactericidal activity. As shown in Table 2,

concentrations of one to two times the MIC were bactericidal for gram-negative bacteria, but the MBC against staphylococci was four times the MIC.

Effect of inoculum size. We studied the effect of inoculum size on the MICs for four isolates (*E. coli*, *Proteus morganii*, *Pseudomonas*, and staphylococci), increasing the cell concentration from 10^2 to 10^5 or 10^6. There were no important effects: the MIC increased in a ratio of one dilution.

The NCCLS (National Committee for Clinical Laboratory Standards) and the Expert Committee on Biological Standards of the WHO (World Health Organization) recommend the following classification when using the agar diffusion method for cephalothin and other present-day cephalosporins (1977): MIC of ≥32 μg/ml as a "cut-off" for resistant strains and MIC of ≤10 μg/ml for susceptible strains. Those strains which have an intermediate susceptibility are between the two points. According to these reference criteria of the NCCLS and WHO, there were only a few clinical isolates which were resistant to cefotaxime or T-1551; this means that both of these can be considered third-generation cephalosporins. However, special mention should be made of the T-1551 activity against *Pseudomonas*, at "cut-off" point of resistance.

T-1551 needs further investigation. Pharmacokinetic aspects will be an important point for clinical use in humans.

Efficacy of Cefsulodin in Experimental *Pseudomonas* Pyelonephritis in Rats

ANNA BALACESCU* AND WOLFGANG RITZERFELD

Ciba-Geigy Ltd., Frankfurt am Main, and University of Münster, Münster, Federal Republic of Germany

CGP 7.174/E (proposed international nonproprietary name, cefsulodin) is the monosodium salt of 3-(4-carbamoyl-1-pyridiniomethyl)-7β-(D-α-sulphophenacetylamido)-ceph-3-em-4 carboxylate. It is the first cephalosporin antibiotic that is highly effective against *Pseudomonas aeruginosa*; its development is the result of collaborative research between Ciba-Geigy Ltd. and Takeda Chemical Industries Ltd.

The in vitro antibacterial activity of CGP 7.174/E, a narrow-spectrum antibiotic, includes, in addition to *Pseudomonas*, strains of staphylococci, β-hemolytic streptococci, *Streptococcus pneumoniae*, *Neisseriae*, and some obligate anaerobes. The drug has little or no effect on *Enterobacteriaceae*. The MICs of CGP 7.174/E were determined by the agar dilution method on DST agar or Mueller-Hinton agar. Of 161 clinical isolates of *P. aeruginosa*, 80% were inhibited by CGP 7.174/E at concentrations of 8 μg/ml or less, as compared with 7 and 17% inhibited by carbenicillin and ticarcillin, respectively, at the same concentration. The mean MIC value of CGP 7.174/E was found to be 4 μg/ml (4).

The compound binds to human serum protein to an extent equal to or less than 30%. In healthy, fasting subjects, intramuscular injections of 500 mg of CGP 7.174/E produced peak serum levels of 21 μg/ml within 30 min. After injection of 500 mg, the average peak value in urine was 2.420 μg/ml. After intravenous injection of 500 mg, the plasma half-life was found to be 1.5 h (1).

CGP 7.174/E proved to be highly active in a number of experimental animal infections, including some caused by organisms other than *P. aeruginosa*. In infections caused by *P. aeruginosa*, CGP 7.174/E was almost always superior to carbenicillin, ticarcillin, and azlocillin (2, 3).

The therapeutic indications for CGP 7.174/E comprise all types of infections with *P. aeruginosa* in patients of all ages, including newborn infants and the elderly. The bacteriological and clinical results obtained with CGP 7.174/E in a great variety of diseases, including life-threatening conditions caused by infection with *P. aeruginosa*, allow a very favorable evaluation of the compound, which proved to be well tolerated (1).

Materials and methods. CGP 7.174/E was tested for its activity in experimental acute occlusive pyelonephritis caused by *P. aeruginosa* A9532 in rats. By applying a ligature to the ureter of the left kidney for 4 h, retention of urine was produced which led to a lesion of the renal tissue. One hour after removal of the ligature, 1 ml of a suspension of 1.5×10^9 active *P. aeruginosa* per ml, isolated from fresh material obtained from a patient suffering from pyelonephritis, was given by intraurethral injection. The MIC of CGP 7.174/E against this strain was 1 μg/ml. Treatment with CGP 7.174/E was started 6 h after infection and continued for 3 days. The antibiotic, dissolved in sterile distilled water, was administered intramuscularly in doses of 10, 30, 50, 100, and 150 mg/kg three times daily, each dose being given to a group of 20 rats. The control group received 0.5 ml of physiological saline intramuscularly. After 2 days without treatment the rats were killed, and samples of tissue of the left (predamaged) and right (undamaged) kidneys and of the urine, partially obtained by puncture of the bladder, were transferred to the culture medium for bacterial counts.

The test regimen was as follows. On day 1, 6 h after the infection, therapy was started with 1 × 10 mg of CGP 7.174/E per kg intramuscularly. On day 2, treatment was continued with a dose of antibiotic or physiological saline every 8 h. On days 3 and 4, medication was as on day 2. On days 5 and 6, no medication was given. On day 7, the animals were killed and dissected, and specimens for cultivation of the microorganism were prepared. On day 8, *P. aeruginosa* colonies were counted and serological identity was checked; the bacterial counts were examined for statistical significance (Wilcoxon test).

Results. A significant difference in bacterial counts was found between control animals and animals treated with CGP 7.174/E (Fig. 1). At the lowest dose (10 mg/kg three times daily), the number of bacteria was already clearly reduced. With increasing doses of CGP 7.174/E, there was a continuous decrease in the number of bacteria. At the highest doses (100 and 150 mg/kg three times daily), only occasional bacterial growth was observed. The following daily doses were required to produce a comparable

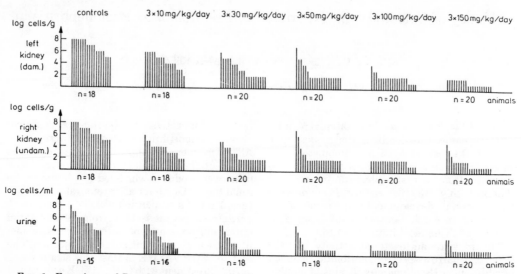

FIG. 1. *Experimental Pseudomonas pyelonephritis in rats. Results (bacterial cells counts) with cefsulodin after P. aeruginosa A9532 infection.*

effect with other *Pseudomonas*-active antibiotics under similar experimental conditions: gentamicin, 3 mg/kg; carbenicillin, 300 mg/kg; ticarcillin, 300 mg/kg; and azlocillin, 450 mg/kg (2, 3).

Conclusion. The results of our animal experiments indicate that the bacterial counts of the causative pathogen can be markedly reduced by using relatively low doses of cefsulodin (CGP 7.174/E). Even with the most critical evaluation of the experiment, we believe that cefsulodin can effectively be used in human *Pseudomonas* infections as well.

1. **Ahrens, T., W. Vischer, P. Imhof, J. Füllhaas, O. Zak, and F. Kradolfer.** 1979. Human pharmacology of CGP 7.174/E (SCE-129) and initial results of clinical trials in Europe. Drugs Exp. Clin. Res. **5:**61–70.
2. **Prat, V., M. Hatala, and W. Ritzerfeld.** 1974. Experimentelle Chemotherapie bei Harnwegsinfektionen. Zentralbl. Bakteriol. Parasitenkd. Infektionskr. Hyg. Abt. 1 Ref. **240:**326–330.
3. **Ritzerfeld, W.** 1975. Animal experiments on current antibiotics, p. 281–287. *In* Proceedings of the 9th International Congress of Chemotherapy, London.
4. **Zak, O., E. A. Konopka, W. Tosch, W. Zimmermann, T. Ahrens, and F. Kradolfer.** 1979. Experimental evaluation of CGP 7.174/E (SCE 129), a new injectable cephalosporin antibiotic active against *Pseudomonas aeruginosa.* Drugs Exp. Clin. Res. **5:**45–59.

Activity of Cefsulodin (CGP7174/E, SCE129) Against Anaerobic Bacteria: Synergy with Cefoxitin

BRIAN WATT* AND FIONA V. BROWN

Central Microbiological Laboratories, Western General Hospital, Edinburgh, Scotland

Most cephalosporins have a wide spectrum of antibacterial activity but are not active against strains of *Pseudomonas aeruginosa*. A new cephalosporin derivative, cefsulodin (CGP7174/E, SCE129) has recently been described as showing good in vitro activity against strains of *Pseudomonas* spp. We decided to investigate the in vitro activity of this compound against other organisms, both alone and in comparative studies with other cephalosporin derivatives. The present study reports on the in vitro activity of

cefsulodin against anaerobic bacteria of clinical interest.

A total of 212 clinical isolates and reference strains of anaerobic bacteria were tested (29 gram-positive bacilli, 58 anaerobic cocci, and 125 gram-negative bacilli). Disk sensitivity tests and MIC determinations were performed using DST agar (Oxoid) with 10% horse blood and two inoculum sizes (10^4 and 10^5 colony-forming units [CFU]). For MIC determinations, an agar dilution technique was used in conjunction with a

Denley multiple inoculator. Cultures were incubated using a standard anaerobic procedure (1) for 48 h at 37°C. The MIC was taken as the lowest concentration of the test compound that completely inhibited bacterial growth. In later studies, three antibiotics (cefsulodin, cephradine, and cefoxitin) were tested in parallel.

In preliminary studies, we found that cefsulodin was not significantly affected by alterations in medium pH: we standardized the surface pH of all of our media at 7.2. The compound was, however, significantly affected by change in inoculum size; for example, for *Bacteroides fragilis* NCTC 9343 the MIC to cefsulodin was 8 μg/ml with an inoculum size of 10^3 CFU but 128 μg/ml with an inoculum of 10^7 CFU. We decided to use two inoculum sizes (10^4 and 10^5 CFU) in our further studies.

We found cefsulodin to be stable at 4°C but to show a progressive loss of activity when incorporated into agar plates that were then incubated at 37°C. We used fresh dilutions for each experiment.

On the basis of disk sensitivity tests, it became clear that while many strains of clostridia and anaerobic cocci were susceptible to cefsulodin (zone diameter, >20 mm), most *Bacteroides* spp., especially those of the *B. fragilis* group (*B.*

TABLE 1. *Susceptibility of 124 strains of anaerobic bacteria to cefsulodin at two inoculum sizes*

Bacteria	No. of strains tested	Inoculum size (CFU)	Cumulative % susceptible to indicated concn (μg/ml):							
			2	4	8	16	32	64	128	>128
B. fragilis group[a]	60	10^4	2		5	28	40	50	55	100
		10^5		2		3	18	33	43	100
B. melaninogenicus	4	10^4				25	50		75	100
		10^5				25			75	100
Other *Bacteroides* spp.	11	10^4		21		53	58		68	100
		10^5		5		16	42	47	58	100
Fusobacterium spp.	3	10^4			33	67				100
		10^5						67		100
Anaerobic cocci	19	10^4	5			26	32	58	95	100
		10^5	5			21	26	58	95	100
C. perfringens	27	10^4		7	52	89	92	96	100	
		10^5			30	78	93	96	100	

[a] *B. fragilis*, *B. vulgatus*, *B. distasonis*, and *B. thetaiotaomicron*.

TABLE 2. *Comparative activity of cefsulodin, cephradine, and cefoxitin against organisms of the B. fragilis group*

Bacteria	No. of strains tested	Antibiotic[a]	Cumulative % susceptible to indicated concn[b] (μg/ml):							
			2	4	8	16	32	64	128	>128
B. fragilis	27	CFS		4		7	33	52	59	100
		CPR		4	11		44	56	67	100
		CFX		4	70	100				
B. distasonis	15	CFS					20	27	40	100
		CPR				7	27	67	73	100
		CFX			47	73	93	100		
B. thetaiotaomicron	1	CFS								100
		CPR								100
		CFX				100				
B. vulgatus	9	CFS						11		100
		CPR					11	33	67	100
		CFX		22	33	78			89	100

[a] CFS, Cefsulodin; CPR, cephradine; CFX, cefoxitin.
[b] Inoculum of 10^5 CFU.

fragilis, B. vulgatus, B. thetaiotaomicron, and *B. distasonis*) were resistant (zone diameter, <10 mm). These results were confirmed by the MIC determinations on 124 strains of anaerobic bacteria (Table 1). It is clear that although most strains of clostridia are inhibited by 16 µg of cefsulodin per ml, very few *Bacteroides* spp. are susceptible at this concentration; indeed, only about 50% of strains of the *B. fragilis* "group" are inhibited by levels as high as 128 µg/ml. The influence of inoculum size is especially noticeable in the case of these latter organisms.

We then tested a range of organisms in parallel against cefsulodin, cefoxitin, and cephradine. The results (Table 2) showed that, in general, cefsulodin was slightly less active than cephradine and markedly less active than cefoxitin for organisms of the *B. fragilis* group; although all strains of *B. fragilis* tested were susceptible to 16 µg of cefoxitin per ml, only 7% of strains were susceptible to this concentration of cefsulodin. Similar results were seen for the anaerobic cocci, where, for example, 100% of strains were inhibited by 8 µg of cefoxitin per ml, but only 71% of strains were inhibited by 8 µg of cephradine per ml and less than 14% by 8 µg of cefoxitin per ml. In the case of the clostridia, there was little difference in comparative activity among the three agents. However, from our results, it is clear that if we take 20 µg of cefsulodin per ml as the maximum achievable in vivo level after a 500-mg intramuscular dose, the majority of strains of anaerobic cocci and *Bacteroides* spp. would be resistant.

Studies with antibiotic disks had shown that, for some of our test strains, there appeared to be synergy between cefoxitin and cefsulodin. We did not observe synergy between cefsulodin and cefuroxime or cephradine. These findings were further investigated in a series of checkerboard titrations with doubling dilutions of cefoxitin and cefsulodin, singly and in combination. From these results it was possible to calculate the fractional inhibitory concentration index for each strain. An index of <0.3 was taken to indicate synergy. We found that synergy occurred in many of our strains of the *B. fragilis* group, 2 out of 20 test strains of anaerobic cocci, and one strain of *Eubacterium* spp. No synergy was demonstrated with any of the test clostridia. The synergy was very marked in several strains; even in relatively resistant strains, the MICs of the separate components were often reduced by 16-fold when in combination. The synergistic effect was not found in all strains of the *B. fragilis* group, nor was it associated with β-lactamase production, as determined by the chromogenic cephalosporin test (3).

We are hoping to study this synergy further and to determine the mechanism of the synergistic effect. However, our studies to date have shown that cefoxitin, added to cefsulodin, can result in a combination that not only covers a very wide antibacterial spectrum but also is highly active against many anaerobes, even those resistant in vitro to one antibiotic alone. Clinical studies are now necessary to evaluate the therapeutic potential of combinations of the two agents in the treatment of serious infections.

1. Collee, J. G., B. Watt, E. B. Fowler, and R. Brown. 1972. An evaluation of the Gaspak system in the culture of anaerobic bacteria. J. Appl. Bacteriol. 35:71–82.
2. Nomura, H., T. Fugono, T. Hitake, I. Minami, T. Axuma, S. H. Morimoto, and T. Masuda. 1974. Semisynthetic β-lactam antibiotics. 6. Sulfocephalosporins and their antipseudomonal activities. J. Med. Chem. 17:1312–1315.
3. O'Callaghan, C. H., A. Morris, S. Kirby, and A. H. Shingler. 1972. Novel method for detection of β-lactamases by using a chromogenic cephalosporin substrate. Antimicrob. Agents Chemother. 1:283–288.

In Vitro Antibacterial Activity of Cefsulodin, an Antipseudomonal Cephalosporin

KEVIN SHANNON,* ANNA KING, AND IAN PHILLIPS

St. Thomas's Hospital Medical School, London, SE1 7EH, England

MICs of cefsulodin (SCE-129, CGP 7174/E) and carbenicillin were determined for recent clinical isolates of *Pseudomonas aeruginosa* and other gram-negative bacteria by agar dilution (1). The medium used was Oxoid Diagnostic Sensitivity Test Agar (CM 261). Oxoid Iso-Sensitest Broth (CM 473) was used for the determination of MICs in liquid medium and of MBCs. The inoculum consisted of 10^4 colony-forming units (CFU) unless otherwise stated.

Cefsulodin, with MICs of 1 to 4 µg/ml for most isolates, was 16- to 32-fold more active than carbenicillin against *P. aeruginosa* (Table 1), but higher concentrations (8 to 64 µg/ml) were needed to inhibit the highly carbenicillin-resistant isolates. Increasing the inoculum from 10^4 to 10^6 CFU had little effect on MICs of cefsulodin and carbenicillin for *P. aeruginosa*. Rather more effect was seen with an increase in inoculum to 10^8 CFU, but mostly there was not more than a fourfold increase in the MIC of either antibiotic. However, larger increases occurred with some of the highly carbenicillin-resistant isolates. MICs determined in the liquid medium were not much different from those determined on the solid medium. MBCs were mostly the same as or twice the MICs for both cefsulodin and carbenicillin when the inoculum was 10^4 CFU, but MBCs increased more than MICs when larger inocula were tested.

The activities of cefsulodin and carbenicillin on species of *Pseudomonas* other than *P. aeruginosa* are also shown in Table 1. The two compounds were more or less equally active against *P. acidovorans* and *P. maltophilia*, but cefsulodin was more active against *P. fluorescens* and *P. putida*, whereas carbenicillin was more active against *P. cepacia*, *P. diminuta*, *P.*

TABLE 1. *Activity of cefsulodin and carbenicillin on gram-negative bacteria*

Organism	Antibiotic	No. of isolates	Cumulative % of isolates inhibited by (µg/ml):											
			0.5	1	2	4	8	16	32	64	128	256	512	>512
P. aeruginosa	Cefsulodin	131	2	22	55	77	92	98		100				
	Carbenicillin							9	34	60	75	84	86	100
P. acidovorans	Cefsulodin	12						8	17	25	50	83	100	
	Carbenicillin									25	42	58	100	
P. cepacia	Cefsulodin	12						17	83	92	100			
	Carbenicillin						17	50	83	92	100			
P. fluorescens	Cefsulodin	13								15	46	54	69	100
	Carbenicillin										8		15	100
P. maltophilia	Cefsulodin	10			20	40	60	80	100					
	Carbenicillin				30	50	70	90	100					
P. putida	Cefsulodin	27								7	19	67	100	
	Carbenicillin											11	48	100
Other species of *Pseudomonas*[a]	Cefsulodin	7		14				86			100			
	Carbenicillin				57	71	86			100				
Acinetobacter spp.[b]	Cefsulodin	11		9		55	64	73		100				
	Carbenicillin			18	64	73				91		100		
Enterobacteriaceae[c]	Cefsulodin	168						1	13	64	85	92	95	100
	Carbenicillin		5	17	24	44	53	55	57	59	64	74	79	100

[a] *P. paucimobilis* (3 isolates), *P. diminuta* (1), *P. pseudoalcaligenes* (1), *P. putrefaciens* (1), and *P. stutzeri* (1).

[b] *A. anitratus* (10 isolates), and *A. lwoffi* (1).

[c] *Citrobacter freundii* (5 isolates), *C. koserii* (7), *Enterobacter aerogenes* (6), *E. cloacae* (18), *Escherichia coli* (35), *Klebsiella aerogenes* (34), *K. ozaenae* (5), *Proteus mirabilis* (20), *P. morganii* (11), *P. rettgeri* (2), *P. vulgaris* (4), *Providencia stuartii* (11), and *Serratia marcescens* (10).

TABLE 2. *Substrate profiles of β-lactamases*

Enzyme type	Isolate	β-Lactamase activity[a]	Relative hydrolysis rate[b]					
			Cephaloridine	Cefuroxime	Cefsulodin	Benzylpenicillin	Ampicillin	Carbenicillin
TEM-1	*E. coli* TEM	9.1	100	<2	3.5	635	790	97
TEM-1	*P. aeruginosa* 69/1822	7.8	100	<2	2.6	564	696	88
TEM-2	*E. coli* 1725E	43.1	100	<2	4.3	682	907	95
Dalgleish-like	*P. aeruginosa* 625	1.0	100	<2	13	1,733	1,824	1,670
Cephalosporinase	*P. aeruginosa* NCTC 10662	2.5	100	<2	<2	152	12	<5
Cephalosporinase	*E. cloacae* 4.14.76	1.2	100	<2	<2	NT[c]	NT	NT
Cephalosporinase	*E. cloacae* 6.8.76	32.7	100	<0.2	1.2	NT	NT	NT
Cephalosporinase	*P. morganii* A131525	16.2	100	<0.3	11	NT	NT	NT
Cephalosporinase	*P. morganii* A181523	2.7	100	4	<2	NT	NT	NT

[a] nkat per mg of protein with cephaloridine as substrate.

[b] Relative to the rate of hydrolysis of cephaloridine.

[c] Not tested.

pseudoalcaligenes, P. paucimobilis, P. putre-faciens, and *P. stutzeri.* Cefsulodin was also less active than carbenicillin against *Acinetobacter* spp.

The *Enterobacteriaceae* showed a wide range of MICs of carbenicillin, but with cefsulodin the range was narrower, with most MICs falling in the range 64 to 512 µg/ml. Thus, although cefsulodin was less active than carbenicillin against the carbenicillin-susceptible isolates, it was more effective than carbenicillin against the carbenicillin-resistant organisms. These included most isolates of *Citrobacter koserii* and *Klebsiella aerogenes* as well as a proportion of the isolates from several other species.

The UV spectrophotometric method (2) was used to study the stability of cefsulodin and other β-lactam antibiotics to various β-lactamases (Table 2). Ten isolates of *P. aeruginosa* with carbenicillin MICs of ⩾2,048 µg/ml all produced a β-lactamase that resembled the enzyme produced by the Dalgleish strain of *P. aeruginosa* (4) and that focused at pH 5.2 in an Ampholine pH gradient (3); nine of these isolates were of the same pyocin type, which indicated probable though unsuspected cross-infection. Cefsulodin was a substrate of the Dalgleish-like enzyme and also of TEM-type enzymes, but it was hydrolyzed much more slowly than carbenicillin. Cefsulodin was also a substrate, but again a poor one, of the cephalosporinases from *Enterobacter cloacae* and *Proteus morganii.* However, neither it nor carbenicillin was hydrolyzed by the Sabath and Abrahams-type enzyme (4) induced in *P. aeruginosa* NCTC 10662 by growth in the presence of penicillin.

No detectable β-lactamase activity against carbenicillin, cefsulodin, or cephaloridine was found in cultures of five isolates of *P. aeruginosa* that were susceptible (three isolates; MIC 16 to 64 µg/ml) or moderately resistant (two isolates; MIC 128 to 256 µg/ml) to carbenicillin and that had been incubated for 5 h in the presence of one-quarter of their MIC of cefsulodin. An isolate for which the MIC of carbenicillin was 2,048 µg/ml and the MIC of cefsulodin was 64 µg/ml also failed to produce β-lactamase.

Although, as found earlier (5, 6), its useful activity was restricted to *P. aeruginosa* and a few other pseudomonads, we believe that cefsulodin would be a useful antibiotic for the treatment of infections with these organisms. Its slight susceptibility to TEM-type and Dalgleish-type β-lactamases probably accounts for the slightly reduced susceptibility of isolates of *P. aeruginosa* that produce one of these enzymes to cefsulodin.

We are grateful to Ciba Laboratories for providing cefsulodin and for financial support. We also thank Beecham Research Laboratories for ampicillin, benzylpenicillin, and carbenicillin; Glaxo Laboratories for cefuroxime, cephaloridine, and nitrocefin; E. J. Lowbury for TEM-1-producing isolates of *P. aeruginosa;* and R. B. Sykes for TEM-1- and TEM-2-producing strains of *E. coli.*

1. **Eykyn, S., C. Jenkins, A. King, and I. Phillips.** 1976. Antibacterial activity of cefuroxime, a new cephalosporin antibiotic, compared with that of cephaloridine, cephalothin, and cefamandole. Antimicrob. Agents Chemother. **9:**690–695.
2. **O'Callaghan, C. H., P. W. Muggleton, and G. W. Ross.** 1969. Effects of β-lactamase from gram-negative organisms on cephalosporins and penicillins, p. 57–63. Antimicrob. Agents Chemother. 1968.
3. **Phillips, I., and K. Shannon.** 1978. The activity of cephalosporins on β-lactamase-producing *Neisseria gonorrhoeae.* Scand. J. Infect. Dis. Suppl. **13:**23–26.
4. **Sykes, R. B., and M. Matthew.** 1976. The β-lactamases of gram-negative bacteria and their role in resistance to β-lactam antibiotics. J. Antimicrob. Chemother. **2:**115–157.
5. **Tsuchiya, K., and M. Kondo.** 1978. Comparative in vitro activities of SCE-129, sulbenicillin, gentamicin, and dibekacin against *Pseudomonas.* Antimicrob. Agents Chemother. **13:**536–539.
6. **Tsuchiya, K., M. Kondo, and H. Nagatomo.** 1978. SCE-129, antipseudomonal cephalosporin: in vitro and in vivo antibacterial activities. Antimicrob. Agents Chemother. **13:**137–145.

In Vitro Activity of Cefsulodin (CGP 7174/E) Compared with That of Five Antipseudomonal Beta-Lactams and Five Aminoglycosides Against *Pseudomonas aeruginosa*

PETER HOHL* AND VICTOR E. DEL BENE

Medical University of South Carolina, Charleston, South Carolina 29403, U.S.A.

The persistently unsatisfactory results in managing severe *Pseudomonas aeruginosa* infections and the more recent problem of increasing resistance of this organism to gentamicin and carbenicillin in our hospital prompted us to study the susceptibility of *P. aeruginosa* strains to cefsulodin, [3-(4-carbamoyl-1-pyridiniomethyl)-7β-(D-α-sulfophenylacetamido)-ceph-

TABLE 1. *Antimicrobial susceptibility of three groups of P. aeruginosa isolates*

Antibiotics	Antimicrobial susceptibility (µg/ml)											
	Consecutive clinical isolates (n = 68)				Gentamicin-resistant isolates (n = 23)				Carbenicillin-resistant isolates (n = 15)			
	Range	MIC$_{50}$	MIC$_{90}$	Geometric mean	Range	MIC$_{50}$	MIC$_{90}$	Geometric mean	Range	MIC$_{50}$	MIC$_{90}$	Geometric mean
β-Lactams												
Cefsulodin	1–128	4	8	4.5	4–16	8	16	6.7	4–256	8	32	11
Piperacillin	1–64	8	8	5.9	8–32	8	32	13.0	8–32	16	32	14
Azlocillin	1–64	16	32	12.0	8–64	16	32	18.1	8–256	16	128	29
Ticarcillin	2–>128	32	64	27	16–128	32	128	36	16–>256	64	256	81
Mezlocillin	4–>128	32	64	38	32–>128	64	128	57	32–>256	64	256	81
Carbenicillin ...	1–>128	64	128	48	32–>128	64	>128	95	64–>256	128	>256	154
Aminoglycosides												
Tobramycin	<1–128	2	4	2.6	1–32	4	16	4.8	<1–>128	2	>128	3.2
Sisomicin	<1–>128	4	8	3.5	2–128	16	32	12.6	1–>128	2	>128	3.7
Gentamicin	1–>128	8	32	9.5	4–>128	32	128	40.7	4–>128	8	64	11.5
Amikacin	1–128	16	32	9.6	4–64	32	64	24.4	2–>128	4	128	11.1
Netilmicin	1–>128	16	32	16.3	16–>128	64	>128	56.7	4–>128	8	>128	16.8

3-em-4-carboxylate monosodium salt], a new semisynthetic sulfacephalosporin with potent in vitro activity against *P. aeruginosa* (3).

The compound was compared to the five β-lactams piperacillin, azlocillin, ticarcillin, mezlocillin, and carbenicillin as well as to the five aminoglycosides gentamicin, tobramycin, sisomicin, netilmicin, and amikacin. Sixty-eight strains of *P. aeruginosa*, which had been consecutively isolated and identified at the Medical University Microbiology Laboratory, were tested. An additional 23 selected gentamicin-resistant and 15 selected carbenicillin-resistant clinical strains were also examined. Mueller-Hinton agar (Difco) with a magnesium content of 24 mg/liter and a calcium content of 72 mg/liter was used as medium. MICs were obtained in triplicate by agar dilution technique (WHO-ICS [1]) using a Steers replicating device. An inoculum of 10^5 CFU was employed. Plates were incubated at 37°C for 18 h. The MIC recorded was the minimal amount of drug that allowed for fewer than three colonies of growth.

The results of the susceptibility tests are summarized in Table 1. Among the β-lactam drugs, cefsulodin and piperacillin were the most effective. They both inhibited over 90% of consecutive clinical isolates at a concentration of 8 µg/ml. On average, azlocillin was 1 to 2, ticarcillin 3, mezlocillin 3, and carbenicillin 4 dilutions less active in all three groups of organisms. We did not find a correlation between the MICs of cefsulodin and carbenicillin. The presence of β-lactamase activity did not correlate with increased MICs of cefsulodin. Among the aminoglycosides, tobramycin and sisomicin were the most active and, on a weight basis, the two were

TABLE 2. *Effect of two inoculum sizes on MICs of antipseudomonal antibiotics and bactericidal activity against selected P. aeruginosa strains*

Antibiotic	MIC, (µg/ml)[a]		Bactericidal activity: difference between MBCs and MICs (µg/ml)[b]	
	Low inoculum (10^{2-3} CFU)	High inoculum (10^{6-7} CFU)	Low inoculum (10^{3-4} CFU)	High inoculum (10^{6-7} CFU)
Cefsulodin	7	81	128[d]	274[d]
Piperacillin	9	92	18[d]	73[d]
Azlocillin	39	144[c]	12[d]	49[d]
Ticarcillin	34	272[c]	8[d]	26[d]
Mezlocillin	36	316[c]	8[d]	17[d]
Carbenicillin	132	468[c]		
Tobramycin	4	12	1.7	1.9
Sisomicin	14	38	1.5	1.9
Amikacin	13	34		
Gentamicin	26	80	1.6	2.0
Netilmicin	50	168		

[a] Geometric means of 23 strains.
[b] Geometric means of 31 strains.
[c] Highest drug concentration tested, 1,024 µg/ml; these numbers underestimate the true rise.
[d] Highest drug concentration tested, 1,024 µg/ml. As most strains, particularly with the high inoculum showed growth at this concentration when bactericidal activity was assessed, these numbers underestimate the true rise. Therefore, they do *not* allow a relative rating among the β-lactam drugs.

the most active of all the compounds studied. Tobramycin inhibited 90% of the consecutive clinical isolates at 4 µg/ml or less and was two dilutions more active than gentamicin and amikacin (Table 1). Netilmicin was one dilution less active than the former and showed the highest degree of cross-resistance with gentamicin of all the aminoglycoside compounds evaluated.

All β-lactam antibiotics were subject to an inoculum effect (Table 2). An increase in inoculum size by 10^4 CFU raised the MICs approximately 10-fold.

At the higher inoculum of 10^6 to 10^7 CFU, cefsulodin remained the most active β-lactam, whereas both piperacillin and azlocillin were slightly less active but still comparable to cefsulodin, while the activities of ticarcillin, mezlocillin, and carbenicillin were distinctly weaker. Even though we used for these experiments a concentration of 1,024 μg of drug per ml, a large number of strains were not inhibited at this concentration with the latter three compounds mentioned.

In contrast, the aminoglycosides showed not nearly the large rises in MIC with an inoculum increase of 10^4 CFU. On average their MICs rose two- to fourfold and the relative increase was similar for each of the compounds tested. With the high inoculum, tobramycin again displayed the highest activity, followed in decreasing order by sisomicin, amikacin, gentamicin, and netilmicin.

The bactericidal activity of the β-lactams (Table 2) was inferior to that of the aminoglycosides. With the filter membrane technique (4), more than two-thirds of the strains were not killed ($\geq$99.9% reduction of an inoculum of 10^3 to 10^4 CFU) with the β-lactams at a concentration of 1,024 μg/ml. In those strains killed at lower

concentrations of the β-lactams, cefsulodin, piperacillin, and azlocillin appeared more active than the other drugs. At the high inoculum of 10^6 to 10^7 CFU, there were no differences between drugs with only few strains being killed at 1,024 μg/ml.

Although all (31/31) of our very resistant strains were β-lactamase producers (nitrocefin method), cefsulodin and the other β-lactams appeared remarkably stable to hydrolysis by the pseudomonal β-lactamases of these strains (alkalimetric titration method in a limited experience of five strains). This finding would confirm the hypothesis of others that the superior activity of cefsulodin against *P. aeruginosa* is not due solely to increased stability against pseudomonal β-lactamases but is also due to its superior intrinsic activity (2).

1. Ericsson, H. M., and J. C. Sherris. 1971. Antibiotic sensitivity testing. Report of an international collaborative study. Acta Pathol. Microbiol. Scand. Suppl. 217:1–90.
2. Okonogi, K., M. Kida, M. Yoneda, J. Itoh, and S. Mitsuhashi. 1978. SCE-129, a new antipseudomonal cephalosporin and its biochemical properties, p. 838–841. *In* Current chemotherapy, Proceedings of the 10th International Congress of Chemotherapy. American Society for Microbiology, Washington, D.C.
3. Tsuchiya, K., M. Kondo, and H. Nagatomo. 1978. SCE-129, antipseudomonal cephalosporin: in vitro and in vivo antibacterial activities. Antimicrob. Agents Chemother. 13:137–145.
4. Wick, W. E., and D. A. Preston. 1972. Biological properties of three 3-heterocyclic-thiomethyl cephalosporin antibiotics. Antimicrob. Agents Chemother. 1:221–234.

Activity of Cefsulodin, Cefotaxime, Azlocillin, Mezlocillin, Ticarcillin, Carbenicillin, and Cefoperazone Against *Pseudomonas aeruginosa*

D. DÁMASO,* B. ORDEN, G. ROYO, R. M. DAZA, AND M. MORENO-LÓPEZ

Service of Microbiology, Clínica Puerta de Hierro, Madrid, Spain

The "in vitro" antimicrobial activities of four penicillins and three cephalosporins against 50 strains of *Pseudomonas aeruginosa* were determined. Among the penicillins were included carbenicillin, ticarcillin, and the acyl-ureidopenicillins, azlocillin and mezlocillin. The cephalosporins tested were cefsulodin (CGP-7174/E = Takeda SCE 129), cefotaxime (HR 756), and cefoperazone (T-1551).

The bacteria tested for susceptibility had been the 13 indicator strains (1 to 8 and A to E) used for the pyocin typing technique as described by Gillies and Govan (1), 36 strains isolated from clinical material and typed in our laboratory

according to pyocin production, and, finally, NCTC strain 10662. The MICs were determined by using agar dilution tests, and the seven antibiotics were added aseptically to Mueller-Hinton medium (Oxoid) at final concentrations of 0.25 to 512 μg/ml. The agar plates were inoculated with the replicating device of Steers et al. (2) so that the number of organisms deposited on the plate surface was approximately 3×10^4 colony-forming units. The MIC was defined as the lowest concentration of antibiotic which prevented visible growth after incubation at 37°C for 18 h, when the readings were taken.

The results are shown in Table 1 and in Fig.

TABLE 1. *Susceptibilities of 50 strains of P. aeruginosa to newer cephalosporins and penicillins*

Antimicrobial agent	Cumulative percentage of strains susceptible to MIC (µg/ml) of:										
	1	2	4	8	16	32	64	128	256	512	>512
Cefsulodin	4	50	88	96	96	100					
Cefoperazone			6	82	96	96	100				
Azlocillin			16	66	76	96	96				
Cefotaxime			2	12	66	90	100				
Ticarcillin					34	88	92	96	96	96	100
Mezlocillin					12	38	82	96	96	96	100
Carbenicillin						14	82	90	94	94	100

1. Among all antibiotics tested, cefsulodin was the most active, inhibiting 50% of the strains at a concentration of 2 µg/ml. Forty-eight out of the 50 strains were inhibited by concentrations of 16 µg/ml or less, and the remaining 2 required 32 µg/ml; the MICs ranged between 1 and 32 µg/ml, and the mean MIC was 4.4 µg/ml. Second in activity came cefoperazone: 16 µg/ml inhibited the same percentage of strains (96%) as did 16 µg of cefsulodin per ml. However, at lower concentrations cefoperazone was less active; the MICs ranged from 4 to 64 µg/ml, and the mean MIC was 11.1 µg/ml, 2.5 times higher than that of cefsulodin. Azlocillin ranked third in activity: 76% of the strains were inhibited by 16 µg/ml; the MICs ranged from 4 to 256 µg/ml, and the mean MIC was 22.9 µg/ml, 5.2 times higher than that of cefsulodin. With cefotaxime, 66% of the strains were inhibited by 16 µg/ml; the MICs ranged between 4 and 64 µg/ml, and the mean MIC was 23.5 µg/ml, 5.3 times higher than that of cefsulodin. Therefore, azlocillin and cefotaxime appeared to be practically of equal activity.

The four antibiotics mentioned above inhibited our 50 strains (100%) with concentrations of 256 µg/ml or less; however, 3 strains were able to grow in the presence of 512 µg of carbenicillin per ml, and 2 of them were able to grow in the presence of the same concentration of ticarcillin or mezlocillin.

Moderate activity was shown by ticarcillin, which inhibited 34% of *Pseudomonas* strains at a concentration of 16 µg/ml; the MICs ranged from 16 to 128 µg/ml (two strains with MICs higher than 512 µg/ml), and the mean MIC was 31.7 µg/ml, 7.2 times higher than that of cefsulodin. Next in order of activity appeared mezlocillin, with 12% of the strains inhibited by 16 µg/ml; the MICs ranged from 16 to 128 µg/ml (two strains with MICs higher than 512 µg/ml), and the mean MIC was 58.7 µg/ml, 13.3 times higher than that of cefsulodin. Finally, the least activity was shown by carbenicillin, with no susceptibility demonstrated at a concentration of 16 µg/ml; MICs ranged from 32 to 256 µg/ml (three strains

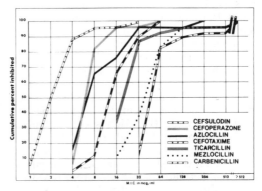

FIG. 1. *Susceptibilities of P. aeruginosa (50 strains) to cefsulodin, cefoperazone, azlocillin, cefotaxime, ticarcillin, mezlocillin, and carbenicillin.*

with MICs higher than 512 µg/ml), and the mean MIC was 72.8 µg/ml, 16.5 times higher than that of cefsulodin.

Two of the three strains susceptible to carbenicillin at very high concentrations (MIC > 512 µg/ml) showed evidence of cross-resistance to azlocillin, ticarcillin, and mezlocillin, decreased activities of cefsulodin and cefoperazone (MICs of 32 and 64 µg/ml, respectively), and indifference to cefotaxime (MICs of 8 and 16 µg/ml); the third carbenicillin-resistant strain did not show cross-resistance to the other six antibiotics.

Based on these MIC in vitro data, it can be concluded that, against *P. aeruginosa*, cefsulodin, cefoperazone, cefotaxime, and azlocillin—three new semisynthetic cephalosporins and an acyl-ureidopenicillin, respectively—show good antibacterial activities, particularly the strikingly superior results of cefsulodin.

1. **Gillies, R. R., and J. R. W. Govan.** 1966. Typing of *Pseudomonas pyocyanea* by pyocine production. J. Pathol. Bacteriol. **91**:339–345.
2. **Steers, E., E. L. Foltz, and B. S. Graves.** 1959. An inocula replicating apparatus for routine testing of bacterial susceptibility to antibiotics. Antibiot. Chemother. (Basel) **9**:307–311.

Cefsulodin, a New Cephalosporin with Marked Antipseudomonal Activity: In Vitro Studies

MARY P. E. SLACK,* D. B. WHELDON, JULIA D. BILLINGHAM, AND D. S. TOMPKINS

John Radcliffe Hospital, Oxford, England

Cefsulodin, a new semisynthetic cephalosporin (CGP 7174/E, Takeda SCE 129) is reported to have high intrinsic activity against *Pseudomonas* spp. We have examined the in vitro activity of this drug alone and in combination with gentamicin. The development of resistance to cefsulodin in vitro was also studied.

Susceptibility tests were carried out on (i) 253 *Pseudomonas* spp. and (ii) 100 strains of enterobacteria. The pseudomonads were identified by the method of King and Phillips (5), and the enterobacteria were identified by criteria derived from Cowan (1). MICs were determined by the International Collaborative Study agar incorporation technique (3) with Isosensitest agar (Oxoid). The strains were plated for purity and then inoculated into Eugonbroth (low-thymidine Eugonic broth, Pfizer). After 18 h of incubation at 37°C, the broth cultures were diluted to give standardized inocula of approximately 10^4 colony-forming units when delivered by an automatic multipoint inoculator (Dynatech). The plates were read after overnight incubation at 37°C. The in vitro activity of cefsulodin against these organisms is illustrated in Fig. 1. The mode MIC for the *Pseudomonas* strains was 1 mg/liter. Cefsulodin showed little activity against coliforms, the mode MIC being 64 mg/liter.

Studies on combinations of cefsulodin with gentamicin were performed with a chessboard arrangement on solid media. The fractional inhibitory concentrations (FIC) of each drug were determined, and the results were plotted graphically in the form of isobolograms. Significant synergy was defined as occurring when there was a concave isobol with a combined FIC (ΣFIC) at the point of maximum synergy < 0.6. This is equivalent to a 40% reduction in the concentration of each drug, a factor that exceeds the inherent error of doubling dilution methods. Antagonism was recorded if ΣFIC > 1.3; addition was noted if the FIC did not vary by more than ±0.3 around the central line; indifference was defined as a constant MIC of one drug in the presence of various amounts of the other drug.

Synergy was observed in 36% of 100 strains of *Pseudomonas aeruginosa* and addition was seen in a further 54%. Five percent of the strains were indifferent to the combination. A minimal degree of antagonism was noted in 5% of strains.

Qualitative studies of the interaction of cefsulodin and gentamicin in 12 strains of *P. aeruginosa* were carried out by a modification of the cellophane transfer method (4). As with other β-lactam antibiotics, a small proportion of inoculated organisms (<0.01%) persisted around the cefsulodin strip and grew after transfer to antibiotic-free media. In every case these persisting organisms were abolished by the combination of subinhibitory concentrations of gentamicin with cefsulodin.

Tests for acquired resistance to cefsulodin were carried out with 50 strains of *P. aerugi-*

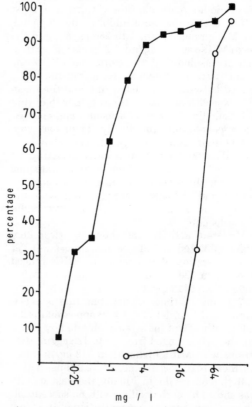

FIG. 1. *Cumulative MICs of cefsulodin. Symbols:* ■, *Pseudomonas;* ○, *enterobacteria.*

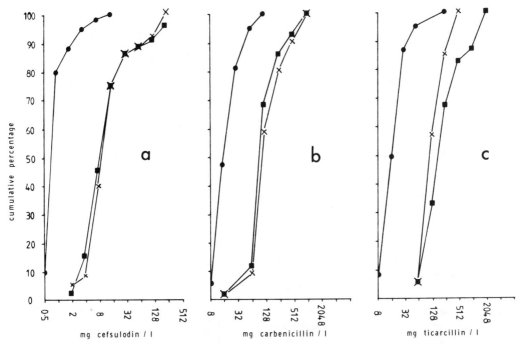

FIG. 2. *Effect of serial passage of 50 strains of P. aeruginosa on cefsulodin-containing media. Cumulative MICs of (a) cefsulodin, (b) carbenicillin, and (c) ticarcillin. Symbols:* ●, *Prepassage;* ■, *after eight passages;* ×, *after six further passages on antibiotic-free media.*

nosa. Each strain was serially passaged both on Columbia agar plates incorporating doubling dilutions of cefsulodin and on plates containing carbenicillin. After eight serial passages, all but two of the strains showed increased resistance (Fig. 2). Cross-resistance between cefsulodin and carbenicillin or ticarcillin was observed after passage. However no change in aminoglycoside susceptibility was detected. The resistance persisted during six serial passages on antibiotic-free media. It did not appear to be mediated by β-lactamase as detected by the chromogenic cephalosporin (6). However, pseudomonads are notoriously difficult organisms in tests for β-lactamase production.

A previous study (2) has shown that the cultural appearance, phage susceptibility and biochemical reactions of *P. aeruginosa* may alter after habituation experiments. Therefore, each strain was identified by biotyping, serotyping, and phage typing before and after serial passage. Twelve percent of the strains became nontypable (serotype and phage type) after passage, although their biochemical reactions remained unchanged. Furthermore, although no strain had been shown to produce pyorubrin on initial isolation, several strains produced this pigment after serial passage. Pyorubrin production has been associated with nontypability. Further studies to elucidate the mechanism of cefsulodin resistance in these strains are in progress.

Our results confirm that cefsulodin has marked in vitro activity against *P. aeruginosa.* It is 8 to 16 times more active than ticarcillin or carbenicillin. Ninety-three percent of strains were susceptible to a level of 16 mg of cefsulodin per liter, which is therapeutically achievable by intramuscular or intravenous injection. Cefsulodin appears to offer specific therapy for proven *Pseudomonas* infections. Resistant variants may be fairly readily selected out in vitro. Twenty-five percent of the strains had MICs > 16 mg/liter after the passage experiments. The combined use of an aminoglycoside may protect against this in vivo. However, if these resistant variants emerged in vivo during the course of therapy, the epidemiological markers of the organisms might be lost.

1. **Cowan, S. T.** 1974. Cowan and Steel's manual for the identification of medical bacteria, 2nd ed. Cambridge University Press, Cambridge.

2. **Dimitracopoulos, G., C. Intzes, and J. Paparassilou.**

1979. Characteristics of Pseudomonas aeruginosa in relation to laboratory induced resistance to gentamicin. J. Clin. Pathol. **32**:723-727.

3. **Ericsson, H. M., and J. C. Sherris.** 1971. Antibiotic sensitivity testing: report of an international collaborative study. Acta Pathol. Microbiol. Scand. Sect. B Suppl. no. 217, p. 11.

4. **Garrod, L. P., and P. M. Waterworth.** 1962. Methods of testing combined antibiotic bactericidal action and

the significance of the results. J. Clin. Pathol. **15**:328-338.

5. **King, A., and I. Phillips.** 1978. The identification of pseudomonads and related bacteria in a clinical laboratory. J. Med. Microbiol. **11**:165-176.

6. **O'Callaghan, C. H., A. Morris, S. M. Kirby, and A. H. Shingler.** 1972. Novel method for the detection of β-lactamases by using a chromogenic cephalosporin substrate. Antimicrob. Agents Chemother. **1**:283-288.

In Vitro Synergy of Cefsulodin (CGP 7174/E) and Mezlocillin, Ticarcillin, or Aminoglycosides Against *Pseudomonas aeruginosa*

JEAN-CHARLES RYFF,* LOTUS MOON-McDERMOTT, AND STEPHEN H. ZINNER

Roger Williams General Hospital, Brown University, Providence, Rhode Island 02908, U.S.A.

Cefsulodin (CS) is a recently developed cephalosporin active against *Pseudomonas aeruginosa* in vitro and in vivo. The present experiments were designed to test in vitro the synergistic effect of CS and either amikacin (AK), gentamicin (GM), tobramycin (TB), mezlocillin (MZ), or ticarcillin (TC) against *Pseudomonas aeruginosa*.

Fifteen strains of *P. aeruginosa* resistant by disk to one or more aminoglycosides (AGR) and 15 aminoglycoside-susceptible (AGS) strains were obtained from clinical specimens.

MICs of the antimicrobial agents alone or in combinations were determined by adding bacteria to serial dilutions of each antibiotic pair to a final concentration of 5×10^4 colony-forming units per ml. A microtiter checkerboard system was used. To insure thorough mixing, a 3-mm stirring bar was placed in each well. For MBCs, a replicator-type inoculator, adapted to the mi-

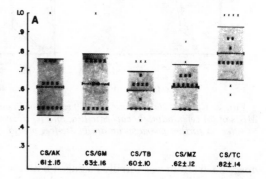

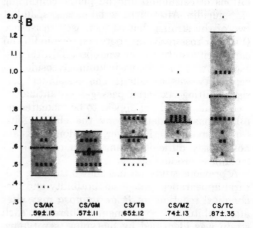

FIG. 1. *Distribution, mean, and standard deviation of FIC indexes for AGS (A) and AGR (B) strains.*

crotiter plate, was used to inoculate approximately 2 µl from each well onto antibiotic-free agar plates. These plates were incubated at 37°C for 18 h (1).

At the concentration of 0.375 µg of CS per ml, there was a fourfold mean decrease in MIC of

TABLE 1. *Geometric mean MIC (in micrograms per milliliter) against tested strains with and without 0.375 µg of CS per ml for AGS or 0.75 µg/ml for AGR strains*

	AGS [N=15]	AGR [N=15]
*AK	0.62 [0.36-1.06]	4.55 [1.42-14.59]
AK+CS	0.17 [0.09-0.31]	1.50 [0.36-6.30]
*GM	0.28 [0.17-0.46]	*3.46 [0.53-22.50]
GM+CS	0.07 [0.04-0.14]	0.86 [0.17-4.44]
*TB	0.19 [0.15-0.26]	1.09 [0.24-4.87]
TB+CS	0.06 [0.04-0.09]	0.39 [0.08-1.83]
*MZ	21 [12-36]	41 [22-75]
MZ+CS	6 [2-17]	20 [7-52]
*TC	14 [9-20]	32 [16-60]
TC+CS	7 [4-12]	16 [7-46]

95% CONFIDENCE LEVELS ARE GIVEN IN PARENTHESES
*P<0.001 FOR ALL PAIRS
*1 STRAIN HIGHLY RESISTANT TO GM [MIC 768µg/ml] BUT SENSITIVE TO CS [MIC 1.5µg/ml]

the aminoglycosides and approximately a two-fold decrease for the penicillins (Table 1). Similar data were found for MBCs.

Of 15 AGR strains, 14 (93%), including one that was highly GM resistant (MIC, 768 µg/ml), had an MIC < 15 µl of CS per ml. The geometric mean (with 95% confidence limits) of the MICs of CS against AGS strains was 1.18 (0.79 to 1.75) µg/ml, and that for AGR strains was 1.43 (0.95 to 2.16) µg/ml.

Fractional inhibitory concentration (FIC) indexes, when calculated for each drug pair against all strains tested, show synergistic or additive effects in all but one case: The CS-TC combination is indifferent (FIC index of 2) against one AGR strain (Fig. 1). If more stringent criteria (FIC index $\leq$ 0.5) are used, synergy is found against 45, 45, 40, 25, and 0% of the tested strains with CS and AK, GM, TB, MZ, or TC, respectively. There is no significant difference in mean FIC index for AGS or AGR strains. We conclude that CS has a good synergistic effect when combined in vitro with aminoglycosides.

When tested with either MZ or TC, this effect is less marked. CS alone is very active in vitro against AGS as well as against AGR *P. aeruginosa*. AGR strains have relatively higher MICs of this new cephalosporin.

1. **Parsley, T. L., R. B. Provonchee, C. Glicksman, and S. H. Zinner.** 1977. Synergistic activity of trimethoprim and amikacin against gram-negative bacilli. Antimicrob. Agents Chemother. **12:**349–352.

Diffusion of Cefsulodin (CGP 7174/E) into Human Tissues

ROLF R. WITTKE* AND D. ADAM

District Hospital, Achern, and Childrens Hospital of the University of Munich, Munich, Federal Republic of Germany*

The treatment of serious *Pseudomonas aeruginosa* infections is, because of the resistance of these organisms to most broad-spectrum antibiotics, one of the major problems in antibacterial chemotherapy, particularly in the treatment of nosocomial infections.

Of great interest was the development of CGP 7174/E (cefsulodin) which was the first a semi-synthetic cefalosporin with high efficacy against *P. aeruginosa*. Cefsulodin has excellent tolerance and low toxicity, like most cefalosporins. The antibacterial spectrum shows selectively high effects against *P. aeruginosa* (85% to 8 µg/ml about 97% to 32 µg/ml). In addition, its high bactericidal activity, one dilution above the MIC, is worth mentioning.

In our trial we had to examine how far the necessary serum levels and the corresponding tissue levels are therapeutically relevant. To 32 patients, 1 and 2 g of cefsulodin were administered preoperatively by the intravenous route. Serum was taken between 0.5 and 6 h. Samples of muscles, fascia, fat, and skin were taken between 0.5 and 2 h after injection, and exudate of wounds and peritoneal secretions were sampled on an antibiotic speculum postoperatively between 3 and 6 h after injection. Serum and tissue samples were deep-frozen immediately (−20°C) and examined by means of a biological dilution technique (1).

At a 1-g dosage, serum and tissue levels were insufficient for the treatment of *P. aeruginosa* infection. After injecting 2 g intravenously, serum levels of 50 to 90 µg/ml could be attained after 1 h. At 3 h, serum levels of 10 to 30 µg/ml were attained, and after 4 and 6 h serum levels of 10 and 5 µg/ml, respectively, were demonstrable. At a 2-g dosage, tissue levels more than 4 µg/ml were usually attained, whereas in skin, muscle, and fascia 8 µg/ml was mostly exceeded. Speculum examinations of fat were relatively inhomogeneous for reasons of variable blood circulation in fat and variable compression during the operation (see Table 1).

In peritoneal secretion and exudation of wounds, a concentration above 10 µg/ml was attained in all the cases, with a median of 20 µg/ml up to 6 h. Bile concentrations showed effective concentrations comparable to exudation of wound specula (see Table 1).

If the specula in serum and tissue as well as exudation of wounds are correlated with the regression line, organisms with a susceptibility of 8 µg/ml (85%) can be treated as fully susceptible, whereas organisms with susceptibility up to 32 µg/ml are of moderate susceptibility and require increased individual doses. As normal dosage regimen for the treatment of infections with *P. aeruginosa* 3 × 2 g are recommended. In the case of urinary tract infections, lower

TABLE 1. *Cefsulodin concentration after a 2-g bolus intravenous injection*

Material	Concn (µg/ml) after:							
	0.5	1	1½	2	3	4	5	6 h
Serum	88	64	34	27	20	12		4
	53	51	20	14	13	8		9
	34	60	42	16	13	12		3
	84	48	45	34	11	26		2
	88	30	19	34	29	10		6
	139	64	30	15	27			
	61	66	21	34				
		35		41				
		78						
Mean	78.2	55.1	30.2	26.9	18.9	13.6		4.8
Skin	5.8	4.9	21	16				
	14	4.4		17				
		13		5.2				
		12.6						
Mean	9.9	8.7	(21)	12.7				
Fat	24	18.3	5.3	4				
	15	3.6		2				
	5.4	8		5.6				
	14	10						
Mean	14.6	10.0	(5.3)	3.9				
Fascia	31	11	5.7	31				
		8	7	7				
		17		18				
		8.4		10				
		24						
	(31)	13.7	6.4	16.5				
Muscle	4.6	8.7	8.7	5.6				
	32	12	8.6	11				
		9	5	5				
		11		11				
Mean	18.3	10.2	7.2	8.1				
Peritoneal secretion					16	13	21	20
					20	21	9	20
					27			
					15			
Mean					19.5	17.0	15.0	20.0
Wound secretion					22	12	23	18
					22	12	9	
					26	21		
					17			
					21.8	15.0	16.0	18.0

dosage is possible because of increased levels in the urine.

Because of its high efficacy against *P. aeruginosa*, cefsulodin is an essential adjunct in the treatment of nosocomial infections. Normal dosage should be 3 × 2 g daily. With this dosage adequate antibacterial concentration can be attained in muscle, fascia, fat, and skin for the treatment of *Pseudomonas* infection. In the case

of moderately susceptible bacteria, the dosage has to be increased.

1. Bennett, J. V., J. L. Brodie, E. J. Benner, and W. M. M. Kirby. 1966. Simplified, accurate method for antibiotic assay for clinical specimens. Appl. Microbiol. 14: 170–177.
2. Füllhaas, J., P. R. Imhof, and W. A. Vischer. 1978. Clinical pharmacology of CGP 7174/E as compared to

carbenicillin, p. 848–849. *In* Current chemotherapy, Proceedings of the 10th International Congress of Chemotherapy. American Society for Microbiology, Washington, D.C.

3. **Konopka, E. A., H. C. Zoganas, E. R. Lasinski, E. F. Kimble, and H. Heymann.** 1978. CGP 7174/E, a novel cephalosporin derivative: activity in experimental *Pseudomonas* keratitis and burn-wound infections, p. 844–846. *In* Current chemotherapy, Proceedings of the 10th International Congress of Chemotherapy. American Society for Microbiology, Washington, D.C.

4. **Tosch, W., F. Kradolfer, E. A. Konopka, J. Regös, W.**

Zimmerman, and O. Zak. 1978. In vitro characterization of CGP 7174/E, a cephalosporin active against *Pseudomonas*, p. 843–844. *In* Current chemotherapy, Proceedings of the 10th International Congress of Chemotherapy. American Society for Microbiology, Washington, D.C.

5. **Zak, O., F. Kradolfer, E. A. Konopka, and E. Batt.** 1978. CGP 7.174/E (Takeda SCE 129): activity against systemic and urinary tract infections in mice and rats, p. 846–848. *In* Current chemotherapy, Proceedings of the 10th International Congress of Chemotherapy. American Society for Microbiology, Washington, D.C.

Clinical Evaluation of Cefsulodin (CGP 7174/E) in Urinary Tract Infections Caused by *Pseudomonas aeruginosa*

J. GUIBERT, M. D. KITZIS, AND J. F. ACAR

Service de Microbiologie Médicale, Hôpital Saint Joseph, Paris, France

Cefsulodin (CGP 7174/E) is a new semisynthetic cephalosporin with pronounced activity against *Pseudomonas aeruginosa* (1). This bacterium, resistant to most antibiotics, presents a difficult therapeutic problem: carbenicillin and aminoglycosides, widely used for the treatment of *Pseudomonas* infections, have become less effective because of increased resistance. An antibiotic active against strains of *P. aeruginosa* resistant to carbenicillin and gentamicin, less toxic than the aminoglycosides, and applicable in patients allergic to penicillin would be of great therapeutic value. Cefsulodin seems to provide the answer to these different problems (2).

The present study was designed to define the clinical activity of cefsulodin in *Pseudomonas* urinary tract infections.

Thirty-two patients were taken into the study, 20 males and 12 females. Their ages ranged from 2 to 80 years (mean age, 52 years). Twenty-nine patients had normal renal function, and three had chronic renal impairment.

The urinary tract infections in these patients were as follows: 20 chronic pyelonephritis (8 with renal lithiasis, 5 with hydronephrosis, 2 with nephrocalcinosis, 2 with cutaneous ureterostomy, 1 with hydronephrosis and nephrocalcinosis, 1 with lithiasis and cutaneous ureterostomy, and 1 with urological abnormality), 6 cystitis (3 after urethral catheterization and 3 with urethral or bladder abnormalities), and 7 prostatitis (4 after urethral catheterization and 3 after surgery).

Thus, all these infections were subsequent to urological catheterization or surgery. They were severe and lasted for many years, with an average of 5 years.

Cefsulodin was administered by the intramuscular route in two daily injections. The daily dosage was 2.0 g in 24 cases and 4.0 g in 8 cases, for 10 to 43 days (mean, 22 days). In a young child with renal impairment, 250 mg was administered in a single daily injection. Thirty treatments were administered in ambulatory patients, and three were administered in hospitalized patients.

Urinary cultures were obtained before therapy, on day 2 or 3 and then every 7 days during therapy, 2 to 3 days after therapy, and every month for 1 year. Results were evaluated as follows: cure was identified by negative urine culture during therapy and at least 4 weeks posttherapy; relapse was identified by reappearance of *Pseudomonas* in the posttherapy urine culture after apparent elimination during the treatment; in the other cases, there was no evidence of bacteriological activity.

Routine tests of renal, hepatic, and hematopoietic functions were carried out before, during, and after therapy.

Fifty-four strains of *P. aeruginosa* were isolated from the urine before treatment. Bacteriuria was $\geq 2 \times 10^4$ per ml of urine. Four types of colonies were identified and differentiated: smooth (*Escherichia coli*-like), rough, and mucoid and microcolonies. The MICs of cefsulodin were between 0.5 and 32 μg/ml (mean MIC, 4 μg/ml).

The clinical results of cefsulodin therapy are shown in Table 1. *P. aeruginosa* was eliminated in 12 cases, including 6 cases of chronic pyelonephritis. This was a very good therapeutic result, considering the chronic nature and the severity of these infections.

TABLE 1. *Results of cefsulodin therapy of urinary tract infections caused by P. aeruginosa*[a]

Indications	No. of treatments	Cures	Failures	
			No eradication	Relapse
Chronic pyelonephritis	20	6	4	10
Cystitis	6	5	1	
Prostatitis	7	1	1	5
Total	33	12	6	15

[a] Duration of follow-up: 4 weeks to 1 year.

Adverse reactions were minimal. Local tolerance was good in 24 treatments. Nine patients complained of pain at the site of injection, but in six of these cases the cefsulodin was dissolved in saline solution. Three allergic reactions were observed: two generalized rashes and one case of lipothymia. In these three cases cefsulodin was withdrawn. Hypereosinophilia was present in

four patients and raised transaminases in one. In all cases these transient abnormalities returned to normal.

To summarize, the antipseudomonal efficacy of cefsulodin seems equal to that of carbenicillin and the aminoglycosides. Like most of the other currently available cephalosporins, cefsulodin seems devoid of serious side effects.

1. Tosch, W., F. Kradolfer, E. A. Konopka, J. Regös, W. Zimmermann, and O. Zak. 1978. In vitro characterization of CGP 7174/E, a cephalosporin active against *Pseudomonas*, p. 843–844. *In* Current chemotherapy, Proceedings of the 10th International Congress of Chemotherapy. American Society for Microbiology, Washington, D.C.

2. Zak, O., F. Kradolfer, E. A. Konopka, S. Kunz, and E. Batt. 1978. CGP 7174/E (Takeda SCE 129): activity against systemic and urinary tract infections in mice and rats, p. 846–848. *In* Current chemotherapy, Proceedings of the 10th International Congress of Chemotherapy. American Society for Microbiology, Washington, D.C.

Cefsulodin (CGP 7174/E) in the Treatment of *Pseudomonas* Infections in Intensive-Care Patients

W. GRANINGER,* K. H. SPITZY, H. PICHLER, E. DIEM, J. SLANY, W. SCHERZER, A. GASSNER, AND S. BREYER

School of Medicine, University of Vienna, Vienna, Austria

Cefsulodin is a new parenteral semisynthetic cephalosporin derivative with a pronounced in vitro activity against *Pseudomonas aeruginosa*, about 10-fold greater than that of carbenicillin (2). It is also active against *Staphylococcus aureus* but has poor activity against *Enterobacteriaceae* compared with other cephalosporins (1).

The present study was conducted to assess the in vitro activity of cefsulodin against carbenicillin-resistant strains of *P. aeruginosa* and to evaluate the use of cefsulodin in the treatment of patients with serious infections.

Bacteriology. Seventy-two *P. aeruginosa* strains which were resistant to carbenicillin were isolated from 67 patients. Susceptibility testing was carried out by the impregnated-disk technique with disks containing 30 μg of cefsulodin, 100 μg of carbenicillin, 75 μg of ticarcillin, 30 μg of azlocillin, 30 μg of cefotaxime, 10 μg of gentamicin, and 10 μg of amikacin. Organisms with an inhibition zone of 18 mm or more in diameter with β-lactams and 16 mm or more in diameter with aminoglycosides were considered susceptible.

Of the 72 strains, 29 were susceptible (41%) to

ticarcillin, 46 were susceptible (64%) to azlocillin, 56 were susceptible (78%) to cefsulodin, 26 were susceptible (37%) to cefotaxime, 46 were susceptible (64%) to gentamicin, and 69 were susceptible (97%) to amikacin. Three strains of *Pseudomonas fluorescens* proved to be susceptible, and one strain of *Pseudomonas cepacia* was resistant to cefsulodin.

Clinical study. Nineteen patients with severe infections were studied from June 1977 to September 1979. They were selected on the basis of infections with carbenicillin-resistant pseudomonas strains (six), penicillin allergy (six), or ineffective treatment with carbenicillin-ticarcillin or gentamicin-tobramycin, or both (6). In two patients only intramuscular application was possible.

Cefsulodin was administered in doses of 15 to 60 mg/kg per day in urinary tract infections and of 40 to 200 mg/kg per day in septicemia or soft tissue infections. Application intervals were 12 and 8 h, respectively. The duration of therapy was from 4 up to 21 days (median, 13 days). In 12 patients cefsulodin was the sole antibiotic, in 4 cases it was combined with gentamicin or tobramycin, and in 4 cases with mixed infection, it was combined with cefotaxime. Frequent clinical assessment, multiple cultures, and determination of renal, hepatic, and hematological functions were performed.

Bacteriological success was assumed if follow-up cultures failed to demonstrate the infecting organism. Clinical success occurred if the patients became afebrile, the leukocyte count normalized, and signs at the infection sites resolved.

Nine female and ten male patients aged from 18 to 61 years were studied. Fifteen patients were admitted at intensive-care units because of wound infections after surgery (seven), burns (two), intoxications (one), pneumonia (two), agranulocytosis (one), and endometritis with septicemia (one). The remaining four patients suffered from obstructive urinary tract infections. Seventeen patients had infections with *P. aeruginosa*, one had an infection with *P. fluorescens*, and one was infected with *P. cepacia*. The results are shown in Table 1.

Patient 1 with agranulocytosis because of leukemia improved with a dose of 40 mg/kg per day, but septicemia due to *K. pneumoniae* occurred, and the patient died.

Patient 2 with extensive burns developed pneumonia and septicemia. The drug could be applied only intramuscularly because of infected subclavian catheters; furthermore, he was allergic to penicillin. Rapid recovery was seen with 50 µg/kg per day.

Patient 3 had received a prosthetic aortic valve, but developed a retrosternal abscess and septicemia. The organism was *P. cepacia*. The patient improved, but the drug was discontinued after the bacteria were found to be resistant to cefsulodin in vitro.

Patient 4 showed an initial response to the combination of cefsulodin and tobramycin, but superinfection with *K. pneumoniae* occurred. The patient was cured by combination of cefsulodin at 75 mg/kg per day and cefotaxime at 75 mg/kg per day.

Patient 5 died of congestive heart failure.

Patient 6, a juvenile diabetic, had been hospitalized for 6 months because of endometritis. *P. fluorescens* septicemia was treated effectively

TABLE 1. *Clinical and bacteriological results of cefsulodin therapy*

Infection	Patient No.	Sex	Age	Clinical diagnosis	Causative pathogens	Dose (mg/kg/day)	Duration (days)	Bacteriological results	Clinical response	Concomitant antibiotics
Septicemia	1	F	30	Leukemia agranulocytosis	*P. aeruginosa*	40	4	Superinfection	Died	Tobramycin
	2	M	39	Burn, pneumonia	*P. aeruginosa*	50	14	Elimination	Cured	Tobramycin
	3	F	39	Prosthetic heart valve	*P. cepacia*	75	7	Failure		
	4	M	53	Cancer of choledochus	*P. aeruginosa, K. pneumoniae*	50 75	16 16	Elimination, superinfection	Cured	Tobramycin Cefotaxime
	5	F	61	Burn	*P. aeruginosa*	120	9	Elimination	Died, CHF[a]	
	6	F	28	Endometritis, diabetes mell.	*P. fluorescens*	150	21	Elimination	Cured	
	7	F	49	Prosthetic atrial patch	*P. aeruginosa, Enterobacter cloacae*	150	7		Failure	Cefotaxime
Pneumonia	8	F	18	Pneumonia, intoxication	*P. aeruginosa*	150	7	Elimination	Cured	
	9	F	55	Pneumonia, bronchitis	*P. aeruginosa*	150	14	Failure, superinfection	Failure	Gentamicin
	10	M	50	Pneumonia	*P. aeruginosa*	100	7	Superinfection	Failure	
Postoperative wound infection	11	M	59	Hemihepatectomy	*P. aeruginosa, Enterobacter cloacae*	75	6	Elimination	Died	Cefotaxime
	12	M	18	Perforated appendix	*P. aeruginosa, E. coli*	75	14	Elimination	Cured	Cefotaxime
	13	F	50	Kidney transplant	*P. aeruginosa*	100	13	Elimination	Cured	
	14	M	32	Paraproct. abscess, paraplegia	*P. aeruginosa, E. coli*	100	7	Failure	Failure	

[a] CHF, Congestive heart failure.

with 150 mg/kg per day. The patient became afebrile within 2 days.

Patient 7 had an infected prosthetic atrial patch; the patient died in spite of a high-dose combination of cefsulodin and cefotaxime. A bacterial assessment could not be done because of missing follow-up cultures.

Patient 8 with aspiration pneumonia had been treated with high-dose cefotaxime for mixed *Klebsiella-Pseudomonas* infection without effect regarding *Pseudomonas*. The patient was cured rapidly by 150 mg/kg per day.

Patient 9 suffered from pneumonia. The organism showed a remarkable filamentous degeneration in vivo as shown by sputum smear, but could not be eradicated. Treatment had to be stopped when a new *Pseudomonas* strain resistant to cefsulodin emerged.

In patient 10, a cachectic diabetic, superinfection with a resistant *Proteus morganii* occurred.

Patient 11, hemihepatectomized because of hepatoma, died of surgical reasons.

Patient 12 with peritonitis after perforated appendicitis, as well as patient 13, with wound infection after kidney transplantation, both of whom had received azlocillin in combination with aminoglycosides without success despite in vitro susceptibility, responded well.

Patient 14 showed no response at all. One patient suffering from mucoviscidosis (not listed in Table 1) received 200 mg/kg per day; however, the organism could not be eliminated, but showed the same degeneration as in case 9.

Three of the patients with urinary tract infec-

tions were treated with 15 mg/kg per day but showed reappearance of *P. aeruginosa* after treatment. In one case with a bladder stone, the bacteria persisted in spite of 60 mg/kg per day.

Side effects consisted of eosinophilia in one patient. Urinalysis of the patient who received 200 mg/kg per day showed slight proteinuria and hyalin casts, which disappeared after discontinuation of the drug. Intravenous and intramuscular injections were tolerated well.

Conclusion. The intensive-care patients included in this study were hospitalized for at least 2 weeks and had received multiple antibiotic treatment which contributed with poor host resistance to the infection with highly resistant pseudomonas strains. In all these patients, carbenicillin treatment was not possible, due to resistance of bacteria, ineffective treatment with that compound, or allergy to penicillin. Cefsulodin was shown to be an effective alternative antibiotic. In intensive-care patients the combination of cefsulodin with an aminoglycoside or a broad-spectrum β-lactam antibiotic seems to be advisable because of mixed infections and the high risk of superinfection.

1. **Neu, H., and K. P. Fu.** 1979. In vitro antibacterial activity and β-lactamase stability of SCE-129, a new cephalosporin. Antimicrob. Agents Chemother. **15**:646–650.
2. **Tsuchiya, K., K. Kondo, and H. Nagatomo.** 1978. SCE-129, antipseudomonal cephalosporin: in vitro and in vivo antibacterial activities. Antimicrob. Agents Chemother. **13**:137–145.

Clinical, Bacteriological, and Pharmacokinetic Study of Cefsulodin in Serious *Pseudomonas aeruginosa* Infections

G. K. DAIKOS,* H. GIAMARELLOU, K. DISPIRAKI, K. HADJIPOLYDOROU, AND A. KOUMADITIS

First Department of Propedeutic Medicine, University of Athens Medical School, King Paul's Hospital, Athens 609, Greece

Cefsulodin is a new semisynthetic cephalosporin with marked antibacterial activity against clinical isolates of *Pseudomonas aeruginosa*, including carbenicillin- and gentamicin-resistant strains, whereas against other gram-negative bacteria it shows lower activity (2). Cefsulodin activity against carbenicillin-resistant strains has been attributed to its stability against hydrolysis by β-lactamase from carbenicillin-resistant *P. aeruginosa*. In experimental peritonitis in mice, cefsulodin was also found to be more active than carbenicillin (3). This report presents

an evaluation of cefsulodin in vitro against 150 *P. aeruginosa* strains in comparison with carbenicillin, azlocillin, and gentamicin and an in vivo evaluation of the effectiveness of cefsulodin against 40 serious infections due to *P. aeruginosa*.

In vitro study. Susceptibility tests were conducted on a total of 150 recent clinical isolates of *Pseudomonas* by the Bauer-Kirby method with the use of 30-μg disks of cefsulodin, as well as by applying a serial twofold dilution technique with a microtiter system in tryptose phosphate broth (Difco). The inoculum was adjusted to 10^5 bacteria/ml by a 10^{-3} dilution of an overnight growth. Comparative studies were performed simultaneously in quadruple. Strains exhibiting a zone size of 18 mm or more and an inhibitory concentration of 16 $\mu g/ml$ or lower were considered susceptible to cefsulodin. MICs are shown in Fig. 1. At a concentration of 64 $\mu g/ml$ or lower, azlocillin and carbenicillin inhibited 70% and 20% of the strains, respectively. Gentamicin, at a concentration of 8 $\mu g/ml$ or lower, inhibited 50% of the strains, whereas cefsulodin inhibited 92% of the strains tested. A good correlation was found between the two methods applied. MBCs of cefsulodin were rarely greater than a twofold dilution compared to MICs. The susceptibility patterns for all four antibiotics tested showed the following: (i) 40% of the strains were susceptible to cefsulodin but resistant to gentamicin, but only 6% were susceptible to gentamicin and resistant to cefsulodin; (ii) 65% were susceptible to cefsulodin but resistant to carbenicillin, while the reverse sensitivity pattern has not been observed; (iii) 28% were susceptible to cefsulodin but resistant to azlocillin without a reverse susceptibility pattern.

In vivo study. Since October 1978, 40 adult patients entered the study. Their ages ranged from 7 to 80 years, with an average of 50.3, and there were 35 males and 5 females. Bacterial cultures were obtained prior to the beginning of therapy and every 2 to 3 days thereafter, with a follow-up period of at least 1 month. Cefsulodin was administered as a 30-min intravenous (i.v.) infusion at a dose of 2 g every 8 h in systemic infections and 1 g intramuscularly (i.m.) every 8 h in urinary tract infections. Duration of treatment ranged from 10 to 30 days depending on the severity of the case. Pharmacokinetics in blood and urine as well as toxicity studies were performed as previously described by Daikos et al. (1). Measurements of cefsulodin levels were made by using an agar well diffusion technique with *P. aeruginosa* 10701 NCTC in brain heart infusion agar. Clinical and bacteriological results are shown in Table 1. In four patients, isolated *Pseudomonas* strains were resistant to amikacin, in 16 patients to gentamicin, in 26 to carbenicillin, and in 11 to azlocillin; cefsulodin was the only available antibiotic for treating 2 patients.

Results were best in urinary tract infections (93.7%), including several problem cases with multiresistant organisms and aggravating factors. Among them, a 72-year-old male patient developed septicemia after prostatectomy because of urinary tract infection. Isolated *Pseudomonas* strains from both blood and urine were susceptible only to amikacin and cefsulodin.

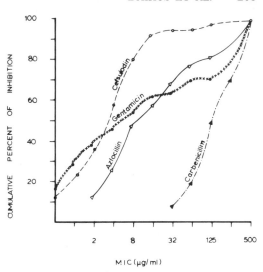

FIG. 1. *Cumulative percentage of 150 Pseudomonas aeruginosa strains inhibited by gentamicin, carbenicillin, azlocillin, and cefsulodin.*

However, while on amikacin he remained febrile and septic with positive cultures. His recovery after cefsulodin administration was prompt and remarkable. Another case of chronic symptomatic prostatitis due to a multiresistant *Pseudomonas*, in which all previous therapeutic schedules had failed, is also of great interest. The patient responded promptly to cefsulodin and was finally cured without relapse during a 9-month follow-up.

Respiratory infections either as bronchopneumonia or exacerbation of chronic bronchitis were serious. Five of the patients required intubation and mechanical ventilation. Two of them with multiresistant *Pseudomonas* were critically ill and would have died if cefsulodin had not been available. Another young patient with multiresistant *P. meningitis*, complicating a permanent shunt because of hydrocephalus, responded very promptly, thus showing strong evidence of an adequate cefsulodin concentration in the inflamed meninges. In patients with chronic osteomyelitis and malignant external otitis, a prolonged treatment course was considered necessary.

Bacteriological results were also very promising. In 29 of 40 patients (72.5%) *Pseudomonas* strains were eradicated, in 7 (17.5%) they persisted, and in 8 (20%) bacteria reappeared during the follow-up period, but no strain developed resistance to cefsulodin.

The following adverse reactions were observed during treatment: pain at the site of i.m. injection in seven patients, drug fever in two, sweat odor in one, and eyelid edema plus hoarse-

TABLE 1. *Clinical and bacteriological results of treatment with cefsulodin*

Diagnosis	No. of patients	Clinical		Bacteriological[a]		
		Excellent	Improvement	Eradication	Failure	Recurrence
Urinary tract infections						
Acute	3	3		3		
Chronic	12	11	1	11		5(5 S)
Chronic prostatitis	1	1		1		
Respiratory infections			6		5(4 R-1 S)	
Chronic bronchitis exacerbation	11	6	5	7	4(3 R-1 S)	
Bronchopneumonia	4	3	1	3	1(1 R)	
Osteomyelitis	4	1	3	2		2(2 S)
Meningitis	1	1		1		
Burn/septicemia	1		1		1(1 S)	
Malignant external otitis	2	1	1		1(1 R)	1(1 S)
Soft tissue phlegmon	1	1		1		

[a] R, Resistant; S, susceptible.

ness of voice in one. Abnormal but slight rise of blood urea and creatinine was observed in two patients, while in another seven patients mild serum glutamic pyruvic transaminase (SGPT) and serum glutamic oxalacetic transaminase (SGOT) elevations were observed during i.m. administration, attributed to local muscular irritation.

Peak serum concentrations of cefsulodin were 102 μg/ml (SD, ± 23.5) after 2-g 0.5-h infusion and sustained at bactericidal levels for 6 h or more but without danger of accumulation. Mean serum terminal half-life was 1.32 h. Urinary recovery averaged 60% of dose after i.v. infusion, with the main portion eliminated within 2 h after administration.

The data presented suggest that cefsulodin is a safe new cephalosporin with desirable pharmacokinetic properties and excellent clinical efficacy. It can be recommended for the treatment of *P. aeruginosa* infections particularly when confronted with multiresistant strains.

1. Daikos, G. K., H. Giamarellou, K. Hadjipolydorou, and K. Kanellakopoulou. 1977. In vitro and in vivo activity of azlocillin against *Pseudomonas aeruginosa*, p. 626–629. *In* Current chemotherapy, Proceedings of the 10th International Congress of Chemotherapy. American Society for Microbiology, Washington, D.C.
2. Kondo, M., and K. Tsushiya. 1978. Comparative in vitro activities of cefsulodin sulbenicillin and gentamicin against *Pseudomonas aeruginosa*. Antimicrob. Agents Chemother. 14:151–153.
3. Tsuchiya, K., M. Kondo, and H. Nagatomo. 1978. SCE-129, antipseudomonas cephalosporin: in vitro and in vivo antibacterial activities. Antimicrob. Agents Chemother. 13:137–145.

Cefsulodin in Treatment of Chronic Bronchitis Due to *Pseudomonas aeruginosa*

MASAO NAKATOMI,* MASARU NASU, TATSURO NAGASAWA, YOSHITERU SHIGENO, ATSUSHI SAITO, AND KOHEI HARA

The Second Department of Internal Medicine, Nagasaki University School of Medicine, Nagasaki City, Japan

Pseudomonas aeruginosa is well known as one of the opportunistic pathogens and has an important role in terminal infections which develop in patients with so-called immunosuppressive conditions such as malignant tumors, steroid therapy, and aging. It is quite difficult to handle pseudomonal infections because of the high MIC of current antimicrobial agents in addition to the retarded host factor.

Cefsulodin (CFS) is a newly developed cephalosporin antibiotic which has a narrow spectrum, being active only against *P. aeruginosa* with the peak MIC value of 1.56 μg/ml.

In this paper, serum and sputum levels of CFS

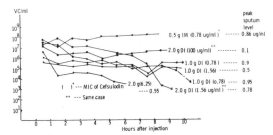

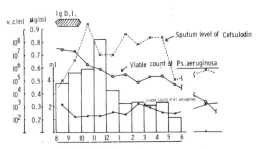

FIG. 1. *Viable count (VC) of P. aeruginosa in sputum of patients with chronic respiratory tract infection after cefsulodin injection.*

FIG. 2. *Viable count of P. aeruginosa in sputum after intravenous drip infusion of cefsulodin in a 68-year-old male.*

and trends of viable counts of *P. aeruginosa* in sputum after injection of CFS into patients with chronic bronchitis infected with *P. aeruginosa* are reported. Whole expectorated sputa were collected hourly from the patients with chronic bronchitis immediately after the start of CFS injection at about 10 h. Each sputum sample was liquefied by homogenization after adding less than 1% *N*-acetyl 1-cysteine. A serial 10-fold dilution was made from the treated sputum and a viable count of *P. aeruginosa* in sputum was done on BTB agar plates after overnight incubation. Serum and sputum levels of CFS were bioassayed by the thin-layer cup method. The test organism was *P. aeruginosa* NCTC 10490. MICs of CFS against *P. aeruginosa* isolated from the patients studied were examined by the agar plate method.

Serum levels of CFS. Peak serum levels of CFS after intravenous drip infusion for 1 to 2 h were 16 to 50 μg/ml at a dose of 1 g and 50 to 70 μg/ml at a dose of 2 g at termination of infusion. CFS of 2 to 3 μg/ml was still measurable 6 h after the termination of infusion.

Sputum levels of CFS. The peak sputum level was 0.78 μg/ml after intramuscular injection of 0.5 g. Peak sputum levels were 0.5 to 1.0 μg/ml after intravenous drip infusion at a dose of 1 g and 0.1 to 0.78 μg/ml at a dose of 2 g.

Trends of *P. aeruginosa* in sputum. Viable *P. aeruginosa* in sputum of four cases began to decrease in number around 4 to 5 h after injection (Fig. 1). MICs of CFS against *P. aeruginosa* isolated from these patients were 0.78, 0.78, 1.56, and 6.25 μg/ml, respectively. Peak sputum levels in these cases were 0.55, 0.78, 0.90, and 0.95 μg/ml and two of them exceeded the values of MICs

against *P. aeruginosa* isolated. Viable counts of *P. aeruginosa* in sputum of three cases were not changed after CFS treatment even though the sputum level in one case exceeded the MIC value for *P. aeruginosa*.

A female patient with chronic bronchitis was treated with CFS at a dose of 4 g per day in 1977 and again in 1979. In 1977, the MIC against *P. aeruginosa* was 1.56 μg/ml and the peak sputum level was around 0.78 μg/ml. *P. aeruginosa* was eliminated from the sputum. But in 1979, the MIC was 100 μg/ml and the peak sputum level was less than 0.1 μg/ml. Treatment was not successful the second time.

Figure 2 shows the results of successful treatment with CFS in a 68-year-old patient with chronic bronchitis. The viable count of *P. aeruginosa* cells in sputum began to decrease at 3 h after intravenous drip infusion at a dose of 1 g, after a peak sputum level of 0.95 μg/ml had been obtained. The number of *P. aeruginosa* cells decreased up to 10^4/ml from an initial 10^7 to 10^8/ml. This organism was eliminated from the sputum on the 5th day of therapy. The MIC of CFS against *P. aeruginosa* was 0.78 μg/ml, which was lower than the peak sputum concentration.

So far as success in treatment of chronic bronchitis is concerned, there are several factors to consider, such as MICs of drugs used against the causative organism, sputum penetration of drugs, stages of inflammation, and so on. These factors are important in judging the efficacy of the drugs. Sputum penetration and MIC seem to be the most important.

Clinical Experience with CGP 9000 in Japan

K. MASHIMO, O. KUNII,* J. ISHIGAMI, AND K. MATSUMOTO

Tokyo Kosei Nenkin Hospital, University of Tokyo, Tokyo*; University of Kobe, Kobe; and University of Nagasaki, Nagasaki, Japan

CGP 9000 (Fig. 1) is a new oral cephalosporin similar to cephalexin developed by Ciba-Geigy in 1972 (1). It possesses a stronger bactericidal action than cephalexin (2), and absorption into the intestine is not affected by eating. Clinical trials in various infections, mainly in outpatients, were carried out in internal medicine, surgery, urology, obstetrics and gynecology, otorhinolaryngology, and dermatology at 53 universities and public health hospitals from May 1978 to February 1979.

Phase II-III open clinical studies: patients and dosage. Of 1,459 cases studied, 1,430 were evaluated for efficacy of CGP 9000. The patients exempted were those whose indications were not included in the protocol, such as PAP, mycoplasma pneumonia, pulmonary fibrosis,

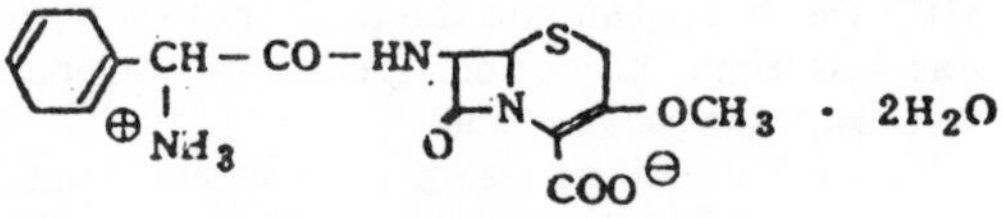

FIG. 1. *Structure of CGP 9000.*

etc., those who did not return for follow-up, and patients with uncertain symptoms of infection.

Data from all treated patients were included in the safety analysis. Among 1,430 patients, 691 had urinary tract infections and 398 had respiratory tract infections. There were 157 cases of surgical and dermatological infections, and 133 cases of otorhinolaryngological infections.

The ages of patients in each group ranged from 2 to 86 years. The dosage was 750 mg/day divided into three doses per os, with a maximum total dose of 42.0 g in one patient. The maximum duration of administration was 31 days.

Efficacy. Evaluation was made as to clinical symptoms and bacterial eradication (Table 1). Improvement of clinical symptoms was 88.9% (354/398) in respiratory tract infections, and 83.2% (575/691) in urinary tract infections. It was 82.0% (109/133) in otorhinolaryngological infections, 84.4% (151/179) in dermatological and ophthalmological infections, and 80.0% (12/15) in obstetrical and gynecological infections.

TABLE 1. *Clinical effect of CGP 9000 on several diseases*

	Disease	Cases for study	Clinical effect				Effective rate (excellent + good) (%)
			Excellent	Good	Fair	Poor	
Respiratory tract infection	Pharyngolaryngitis	74	9	58	1	6	67/74 (90.5)
	Tonsillitis	110	65	40	2	3	105/110(95.5)
	Acute bronchitis	71	17	51		3	68/71 (95.8)
	Chronic bronchitis	34	5	21		8	26/34 (76.5)
	Bronchiectasis	29	3	15	3	8	18/29 (62.1)
	Pneumonia	71	12	52	1	6	64/71 (90.1)
	Others	9		6	1	2	6/9 (66.7)
	Sub-total	398	111	243	8	36	354/398(88.9)
Urinary tract infection	Acute cystitis	446	313	107	9	17	420/446(94.2)
	Chronic cystitis	134	36	40	10	48	76/134(56.7)
	Acute pyelonephritis	35	14	18		3	32/35 (91.4)
	Chronic "	62	12	24	9	17	36/62 (58.1)
	Others	14	6	5		3	11/14 (78.6)
	Sub-total	691	381	194	28	88	575/691(83.2)
Otorhinolaryngo	Acute otitis media	51	27	17	1	6	44/51 (86.3)
	Chronic " "	27	11	7	1	8	18/27 (66.7)
	Furuncle of the ear	18	10	5	2	1	15/18 (83.3)
	Paranasal sinusitis	29	8	17	2	2	25/29 (86.2)
	Others	8	2	5	1		7/8 (87.5)
	Sub-total	133	58	51	7	17	109/133 (82.0)
Surgery, Dermatology, Ophthalmology	Biliary tract infection	5		4		1	4/5 (80.0)
	Wound infection	8	1	5		2	6/8 (75.0)
	Furunculosis. Carbuncle. Folliculitis	35	16	17		2	33/35 (94.3)
	Abscess	29	6	19	1	3	25/29 (86.2)
	Impetigo	16	12	4			16/16 (100)
	Conjunctivitis Hordeolum	14	3	9	1	1	12/14 (85.7)
	Keratitis, Corneal ulcer, Dacryocystis	8		4	3	1	4/8 (50.0)
	Others	64	22	29	2	11	51/64 (79.7)
	Sub-total	179	60	91	7	21	151/179 (84.4)
Obstetrics & Gynecology	Endometritis	2		2			2/2 (100)
	Adnexitis	5		3		2	3/5 (60.0)
	Others	8		7		1	7/8 (87.5)
	Sub-total	15		12		3	12/15 (80.0)
	Others	14	3	9	1	1	12/14 (85.7)
	Total	1,430	613	600	51	166	1,213/1,430(84.8)

TABLE 2. *Bacteriological effect of CGP 9000 on causative bacteria*

Name of bacteria	No. of cases	Cases of study	Bacteriological effect				Efficacy rate of elimination of bacteria (eliminated + Replaced) (%)
			Eliminated	Diminished	Replaced	No change	
S. aureus	152	107	91	8	4	4	95/107(88.8)
S. epidermidis	54	47	43		1	3	44/47 (93.6)
S. pneumoniae	19	16	16				16/16 (100)
S. pyogenes	32	21	18	2	1		19/21 (90.5)
S. haemolyticus	4	3	3				3/3 (100)
S. faecalis	4	3	3				3/3 (100)
Streptococcus	24	5	5				5/5 (100)
Other G.P.B.	13	7	4		1	2	5/7 (71.4)
E. coli	449	444	376	13	25	30	401/444(90.3)
K. pneumoniae	51	48	30	6	5	7	35/48 (72.9)
Klebsiella	18	17	10	1	2	4	12/17 (70.6)
H. influenzae	36	34	21	5		8	21/34 (61.8)
Haemophilus	5	5	4			1	4/5 (80.0)
P. mirabilis	26	25	20	2		3	20/25 (80.0)
P. morganii	1	1			1		1/1 (100)
P. vulgaris	1	1				1	0/1 (0)
Proteus	10	10	5		3	2	8/10 (80.0)
Enterobacter	13	12	2		1	9	3/12 (25.0)
Citrobacter	11	11	4		2	5	6/11 (54.5)
Acinetobacter	2	2	1		1		2/2 (100)
P. aeruginosa	14	12	1			10	1/12 (8.3)
Pseudomonas	9	7	2		2	3	4/7 (57.1)
Serratia	7	7			1	6	1/7 (14.3)
Neisseria	6	3	2	1			3/3 (100)
Other G.N.B.	11	8	5	2		1	6/8 (75.0)
Anaerobes	1	1				1	0/1 (0)
Mycoplasma	2	0					—
Fungi	2	1				1	0/1 (0)
Single infection Total	977	858	666	41	51	100	717/858 (83.6)
Mixed infection	126	99	53	12	12	22	65/99 (65.7)
Unknown	327	66	47	18		1	47/66 (71.2)
Total	1,430	1,023	766	71	63	123	829/1,023(81.0)

Appearance of other strains after complete elimination of the initial causative bacteria.

The total efficacy rate for each infection was 84.8% (1,213/1,430) in 1,430 cases.

Bacteriological examination revealed elimination of bacteria in 829 cases (81.0%) out of 1,023 in which causal bacteria could be identified. It was 88.8% (95/107) in *Staphylococcus aureus*, 90.3% (401/444) in *Escherichia coli*, 72.95% (35/48) in *Klebsiella pneumoniae*, and 80.0% (20/25) in *Proteus mirabilis* (Table 2).

Adverse reactions were found in only 28 (1.9%) of the 1,459 patients who were available for evaluation of adverse reactions after administration of CGP 9000. Their symptoms consisted mainly of exanthema and gastrointestinal disorders. Laboratory findings after administration of CGP 9000 showed elevation of SGOT, SGPT, and alkaline phosphatase, and each of these occurred in less than 1% of the cases.

Four double-blind trials are in progress at this time. These are in the urological field, with acute, uncomplicated cystitis as an indication for comparative study. CGP 9000 was given at 750 mg/day in three doses, and cephalexin was given at 1,000 mg/day in four doses for 3 days. The result was excellent in 85% (104/120) with CGP 9000 in contrast to 78% (93/118) with cephalexin. When excellent and effective cases are included, rate of efficacy is 98% (117/120) with CGP 9000 and 99% (117/118) with cephalexin.

Conclusion. Our results show that CGP 9000 is an effective, safe, and useful cephalosporin antibiotic for use against moderate cases of several infections in treatment on an outpatient basis.

1. **Castañer, J., and A. C. Playle.** 1977. CGP-9000, p. 574–578. Drugs of the future, vol. 2.
2. **Zak, O., W. A. Vischer, C. Schenk, W. Tosch, W. Zimmermann, J. Regös, E. R. Suter, F. Kradolfer, and J. Gelzer.** 1976. CGP-9000: a new orally active, broad-spectrum cephalosporin. J. Antibiot. **21**:653–655.

CGP 9000, a New Oral Cephalosporin: In Vitro and In Vivo Antibacterial Activities

RINTARO NAKAYA,* NOBUICHI GOTO, SANKICHI HORIUCHI, NOBORU OKAMURA, TOSHIO CHIDA, HARUMI SHIBAOKA, SADAYOSHI UEDA, IWAO ISHIZUKA, YOSHIKO SASAKI, AND MASANARI IKEDO

Department of Microbiology, Tokyo Medical and Dental University School of Medicine, and Institute of Environmental Science, Eiken Chemical, Ltd., Tokyo, Japan*

CGP 9000, 7β-[D-2-amino-2-(1,4-cyclohexadienyl)-acetamido]-3-methoxy-ceph-3-em-4-carboxylic acid, is a new orally absorbed semisynthetic cephalosporin. This study was undertaken to confirm results of previous studies of its chemical, antibacterial, and pharmacological properties, and to add data which compare the in vitro and in vivo antibacterial activities of CGP 9000 with those of similar oral cephalosporins, cephalexin (CEX) and cefatrizine (CFT).

In vitro tests consisted of determinations of the MICs against laboratory strains and a total of 465 clinical isolates of gram-positive and gram-negative bacteria, the effects of pH, type of media, and the addition of horse serum on the MICs, and its bactericidal and bacteriolytic effects. In vivo activity was evaluated by testing oral chemotherapeutic effects in mice challenged intraperitoneally with four drug-susceptible strains of gram-negative and gram-positive bacteria.

The in vitro antibacterial spectrum of CGP 9000 was similar to that of CEX and CFT. Clinical isolates of *Escherichia coli, Salmonella* spp., *Salmonella typhi, Shigella* spp., *Klebsiella pneumoniae, Proteus mirabilis,* and *Staphylococcus aureus* were found to be susceptible to CGP 9000 (Fig. 1). CGP 9000 was slightly more active than CEX against *E. coli, Shigella* spp., *K. pneumoniae,* and *P. mirabilis,* and the MICs of CFT were consistently lower than those of the other two drugs. *Enterobacter aerogenes* (1 strain), *Serratia marcescens* (32 strains), and *Pseudomonas aeruginosa* (40 strains) were resistant; *Enterobacter cloacae* (10 strains), *Proteus morganii* (16 strains), and *P. inconstans* A (4 strains) were of intermediate susceptibility; and *P. vulgaris* (26 strains), *P. rettgeri* (15 strains), and *P. inconstans* B (9 strains) were of intermediate resistance. Most of the CEX-resistant strains of *E. coli, Salmonella* spp., *S. marcescens, P. vulgaris,* and *P. mirabilis* showed cross-resistance to CGP 9000. The MICs of CGP 9000 and other reference drugs were only slightly, if at all, influenced by variations in the types of test media (eight types) or in the pH of the medium (heart infusion broth) between 6.0 and 8.5 or by the addition of 5 to 20% horse

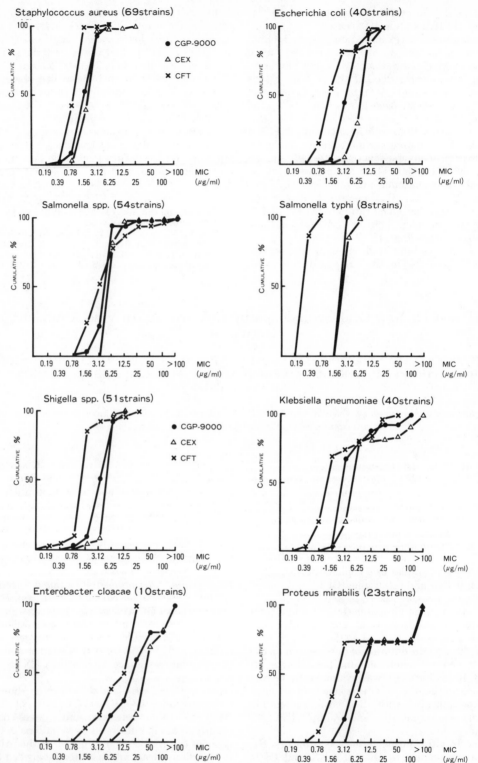

Fig. 1. *Comparative activity of CGP 9000, cefatrizine, and cephalexin against clinical isolates of various gram-positive and gram-negative bacteria.*

TABLE 1. *Chemotherapeutic activity of CGP 9000, cefatrizine, and cephalexin against infections due to gram-negative and gram-positive bacteria in mice[a]*

Infecting organism	Challenge dose (cells/ mouse)	CGP 9000		Cefatrizine		Cephalexin	
		MIC[b] (μg/ ml)	ED$_{50}$ (mg/kg)	MIC (μg/ ml)	ED$_{50}$ (mg/ kg)	MIC (μg/ ml)	ED$_{50}$ (mg/ kg)
Proteus mirabilis 32	1.0×10^7	6.25	8.8 (4.9–16)	1.56	0.69 (0.51–0.96)	6.25	62 (34–110)
Klebsiella pneumoniae 28	4.7×10^7	3.12	510 (83–3,100)	1.56	38 (16–91)	6.25	230 (110–470)
Escherichia coli 32	7.0×10^7	6.25	91 (34–180)	3.12	130 (63–250)	12.5	400 (190–870)
Staphylococcus aureus 76	3.3×10^7	1.56	1.2 (0.72–2.1)	0.78	0.70 (0.39–1.3)	3.12	4.1 (2.6–6.4)

[a] Mice (female, ICR) were infected by intraperitoneal inoculation of bacterial cultures suspended in 5% hog gastric mucin. The antibiotics were given orally to the mice 1 h after infection. The ED$_{50}$ was calculated by probit analysis and is indicated with 95% confidence limits.

[b] Inoculum size, 10^6/ml.

serum to the medium. CGP 9000 exhibited a bactericidal effect on *E. coli* at one MIC (6.25 μg/ml); a similar degree of effect was obtained with one MIC of CEX (12.5 μg/ml). Bacteriolytic activities of CGP 9000 (50 and 100 μg/ml) against *E. coli* and *K. pneumoniae* were most remarkable when added to an early exponential growth phase and were still noticed in the middle and late exponential growth phases. Retardation of initiation of bacterial growth was caused by addition of 2.5 and 5.0 μg of CGP 9000 per ml. The lag periods of these cultures were 2 to 6 h longer than those of control and CEX-containing cultures. No significant level of resistance to CGP

9000 was attained by successive cultivation of *E. coli* and *S. aureus* in drug-containing broth.

The oral protective effects of CGP 9000 in mice infected with *S. aureus, P. mirabilis,* and *E. coli* were very potent, with median effective doses of 1.2, 8.8, and 91 mg/kg, respectively; protection against infection due to *K. pneumoniae* was less potent (Table 1).

These experimental results indicated that CGP 9000 is consistently more active than CEX, particularly in vivo, though less active than CFT, and is a promising oral cephalosporin for clinical use.

Comparative Study on Different Assays of CGP 9000 and CGP 3940

I. NAKAYAMA,* H. KAWAGUCHI, AND S. ISHIYAMA

Nihon University School of Medicine, 1-8-13, Surugadai Kanda, Chiyoda-ku, Tokyo, Japan

CGP 9000, 7β-[D-2-amino-2(1,4-cyclohexadienyl)-acetamido]-3-methoxy-ceph-3-em-4-carboxylic acid, is a new semisynthetic broad-spectrum antibiotic which is derivative of cephalexin. CGP 9000 contains approximately 5% CGP 3940 as an admixture into the capsule of CGP 9000 in the production process. The chemical name of CGP 3940 is 7β(D-2-amino-2-phenylacetamide)-3-methyl-ceph-3-em-carboxylic acid.

The serum levels of CGP 9000 in three healthy adult volunteers after a single oral dose of 500 mg were determined by use of both the cylinder plate method with *Micrococcus luteus* ATCC 9341 as the test organism and high-pressure liquid chromatography (HPLC). Mean peak se-

rum levels of 10.55 μg/ml biologically and 11.52 μg/ml chromatographically were attained 1 h after a dose of 500 mg to fasting subjects. In the bioassay, measurable concentrations persisted and showed averages of 0.26 μg/ml 6 h after administration but no drug was detectable by HPLC after 6 h (Table 1).

The urinary concentration reached its peak 2 h after administration, averaging 5,083.3 μg/ml for bioassay and 3,577 μg/ml for HPLC. Then it gradually decreased to show average concentrations of 197.3 μg/ml for bioassay and 266 μg/ml for HPLC after at least 6 h. Of the dose given, 91.9% for the bioassay and 84.2% for HPLC were recovered from the urine samples taken over 6 h (Table 2).

TABLE 1. *Concentrations of CGP 9000 in serum determined by bioassay and by high-pressure liquid chromatography (HPLC)*

Volunteer no.	Time (h)	CGP 9000 concn (µg/ml)	
		Bioassay	HPLC
1 (6.94 mg/kg)[a]	0.25	Trace	ND[b]
	0.5	6.52	7.89
	1	11.55	13.68
	2	7.25	4.74
	4	1.38	ND
	6	0.24	ND
2 (8.20 mg/kg)	0.25	ND	ND
	0.5	1.04	ND
	1	5.60	5.77
	2	5.75	3.85
	4	1.81	1.92
	6	0.31	ND
3 (7.61 mg/kg)	0.25	3.69	5.04
	0.5	7.95	10.5
	1	14.50	15.12
	2	10.35	10.1
	4	1.34	ND
	6	0.23	ND
Average	0.25	1.23	1.68
	0.5	5.17	6.13
	1	10.55	11.52
	2	7.77	6.23
	4	1.51	0.64
	6	0.26	ND

[a] Dose per kilogram of body weight when a 500-mg oral dose was administered to patients in the fasting state.

[b] ND, Not detectable.

We also determined the CGP 3940 concentration by use of HPLC in both the serum and urine samples mentioned above. Mean peak serum levels of 1.16 µg/ml were obtained 1 h after a 500-mg oral dose of CGP 9000 to fasting subjects, and measurable concentrations that averaged 0.1 µg/ml were still present 6 h after administration.

The urinary concentration of CGP 3940 reached its peak 2 h after administration, averaging 121.7 µg/ml for HPLC. The urinary recovery of 14.84 mg of CGP 3940 within 6 h after administration was 59.4% of the total amount.

Pharmacokinetic parameters for the HPLC data were calculated by use of a computer and a one-compartment open-model method, with the following results: K_a, 1.12 h^{-1}; K_{el} (first-order elimination rate constant), 1.03 h^{-1}; $t_{1/2}$ (half-life), 2.11 h; V_d (apparent volume of distribution), 18.95 liters; t_{max} (time of the maximum drug concentration), 1.15 h; C_{max} (maximum amount of drug in the body), 10.09 µg/ml; and AUC (area under the curve), 25.5 µg/ml per h.

We also examined a bioautogram of the 0- to 6-h human urine for the purpose of studying the metabolites of CGP 9000 and CGP 3940. The examination was made by thin-layer chromatography and bioautography. The adsorbent used was Eastman Chromagram 6061 (silica gel), and the solvent system was composed of n-butanol-acetic acid–water (4:2:5). The test organism was *Micrococcus luteus* ATCC 9341.

In this study, one inhibition zone was obtained on the bioautogram. The position of the inhibition zone was identical to that obtained with the

TABLE 2. *Urinary excretion of CGP 9000 determined by bioassay and high-pressure liquid chromatography (HPLC) after administration of 500 mg orally to fasting volunteers*

Volunteer no.	Time (h)	Amt of urine (ml)	Drug concn in urine (µg/ml)		Amt of drug recovered (mg)	
			Bioassay	HPLC	Bioassay	HPLC
1	0.5	32	400	588	12.8	18.8
	1	26	2,270	4,353	59.0	113.2
	2	52	4,700	5,546	244.4	288.4
	4	94	1,380	546	129.7	51.3
	6	130	165	0	21.5	0
	Total				467.4 (93.5%)	471.7 (94.3%)
2	0.5	26	55	0	1.4	0
	1	22	1,100	504	24.4	11.1
	2	43	6,250	3,109	268.8	133.7
	4	62	2,800	3,193	173.6	197.9
	6	117	248	168	29.0	19.6
	Total				497.2 (99.4%)	362.3 (72.5%)
3	0.5	32	156	1,923	5.0	61.5
	1	21	1,980	4,154	41.6	87.2
	2	59	4,300	2,077	253.7	122.5
	4	45	2,120	2,100	95.4	94.5
	6	100	179	630	17.9	63
	Total				413.6 (82.7%)	428.7 (85.7%)

TABLE 2—*Continued*

Volunteer no.	Time (h)	Amt of urine (ml)	Drug concn in urine (μg/ml)		Amt of drug recovered (mg)	
			Bioassay	HPLC	Bioassay	HPLC
Average	0.5		203.7	837	6.4	26.8
	1		1,783.3	3,003.7	41.7	70.5
	2		5,083.3	3,577	255.6	181.5
	4		2,100.0	1,946	132.9	114.6
	6		197.3	266	22.8	27.5
	Total				459.4 (91.9%)	420.9 (84.2%)

standard CGP 9000 and CGP 3940. These results indicated that the active substance in the urine was unchanged CGP 9000 and CGP 3940 and suggested that there were no metabolites of CGP 9000 and CGP 3940 in collected human urine.

1. **Vischer, W. A., O. Zak, E. A. Konopka, H. Fehlmann, J. Regös, and W. Tosch.** 1978. Experimental evaluation of CGP 9000, a new orally active cephalosporin, p. 825–827. *In* Current chemotherapy, Proceedings of the 10th International Congress of Chemotherapy. American Society for Microbiology, Washington, D.C.

2. **Wirz, H., W. A. Vischer, J. Füllhaas, and P. R. Imhof.** 1978. Pharmacokinetics of CGP 9000, a new orally active cephalosporin, in healthy volunteers, p. 827–829. *In* Current chemotherapy, Proceedings of the 10th International Congress of Chemotherapy. American Society for Microbiology, Washington, D.C.

3. **Zak, O., W. A. Vischer, C. Schenk, W. Tosch, W. Zimmerman, J. Regos, E. R. Suter, F. Kradolfer, and J. Gelzer.** 1976. CGP-9000: a new orally active broad-spectrum cephalosporin. J. Antibiot. **21:**653–655.

Pharmacokinetics of a New Cephalosporin, CGP 9000, in Humans

J. HIRTZ,* J.-B. LECAILLON, A. GERARDIN, J.-P. SCHOELLER, G. HUMBERT, AND J. GUIBERT

Ciba-Geigy SA, Rueil-Malmaison; Hôpital Charles Nicolle, Rouen; and Hôpital Saint-Joseph, Paris, France*

CGP 9000, 7β-[D-2-amino-2-(1,4-cyclohexadienyl)acetamido-3-methoxy-3-cephem-4-carboxylic acid, is a new oral cephalosporin. Its pharmacokinetics were studied in humans by use of a new high-pressure liquid chromatography (HPLC) method which, in comparison with the microbiological technique, makes it possible to assay this antibiotic with greater sensitivity and accuracy. Deproteinized plasma or diluted urine are chromatographed on a 10-cm Lichrosorb RP 8 5-μm column, with orthophosphoric acid-methanol as the mobile phase. This column is preceded by a Permaphase ODS 10-cm precolumn. The UV detector is operated at 254 nm.

Intravenous (i.v.) administration. The pharmacokinetic study after i.v. administration was limited to a low dose because of the solubility of CGP 9000. Doses of 50 mg dissolved in 13 ml were administered to four healthy volunteers in 75 s. In two subjects the distribution of CGP 9000 in the total plasma volume was not completed in 2 min, and the plasma concentrations measured at times zero and 2 min after the end of the injection could not be used for calculations.

The plasma concentration-time curves showed three phases that are clearly apparent on a log-linear graph. The experimental data were fitted by nonlinear regression analysis using multi-exponential equations. Three-exponential equations could be used for only two subjects, the first phase being too fast and characterized by only one data point for the two others. Further calculations for the first two subjects were performed by assuming a three-compartment model with elimination from the central compartment. The apparent rate constants of the first two phases are high, so that they could be mixed into one single rate constant without significantly disturbing the other processes. This enables the plasma concentration-time profiles of all four subjects to be described in terms of a two-compartment model. The pharmacokinetic parameters derived from this model (k_e, V_c, and V_d) do not significantly differ from those obtained with a three-compartment model (Table 1).

Single-dose oral administration. Numerous plasma concentration data were available from pharmacokinetic studies in volunteers. The

TABLE 1. *Pharmacokinetic parameters of CGP 9000 after intravenous injection (50 mg in 75 s)*[a]

Subject	No. of compartments	k_e (h⁻¹)	k_{12} (h⁻¹)	k_{21} (h⁻¹)	k_{13} (h⁻¹)	k_{31} (h⁻¹)	Volumes (liters/kg)				Cl_T (ml/min)	Cl_r (ml/min)	$t_{\frac{1}{2}}$ (min)
							V_c (V_1)	V_2	V_3	V_d			
1	2	2.58	0.94	1.43	—	—	0.132	0.087	—	0.219	414	407	46
2	3	2.38	2.90	2.84	0.44	7.08	0.134	0.137	0.008	0.279	372	311	45
	2	2.32	3.04	2.92	—	—	0.137	0.143	—	0.280	372		45
3	3	2.92	0.92	1.60	2.00	5.65	0.085	0.049	0.030	0.164	285	267	42
	2	2.55	1.49	2.18	—	—	0.099	0.067	—	0.166	289		39
4	2	2.36	1.90	2.11	—	—	0.112	0.100	—	0.212	303	219	46

[a] Parameters: k_e, elimination rate constant; k_{12}, k_{21}, etc., transfer rate constants; V_c (V_1), volume of central compartment; V_2, V_3, volumes of distribution compartments; V_d, total volume of distribution; Cl_T, total body clearance; Cl_r, renal clearance; $t_{\frac{1}{2}}$, apparent elimination half-life.

areas under the plasma concentration-time curve (AUC) were measured for 118 subjects given various single doses of CGP 9000 and were corrected for body weight. The relationship between these corrected AUC values and the dose was found to be linear up to 1 g, with a correlation coefficient of $r = 0.913$. The regression line intercepts the dose axis almost at zero. This demonstrated that the pharmacokinetics of CGP 9000 are not dose dependent up to 1 g, and that results obtained with various doses may be pooled.

The plasma concentration data of six subjects, all given a single 1-g dose of CGP 9000 as an aqueous solution, were averaged and plotted as a log-linear graph. After the initial absorption phase, the plasma concentration decay exhibited two phases, with apparent half-lives of 53 and 82 min. The former was close to that found for the last disposition phase after i.v. administration (Table 1); the latter was significantly longer and corresponded to a process that appeared only around 4 to 5 h after oral administration and was not visible after a 50-mg i.v. dose. A three-compartment model is thus necessary to describe the pharmacokinetics of CGP 9000. On the other hand, the first disposition phase recorded shortly after i.v. administration is not visible after oral dosing.

The absorption rate constant was not calculated, but the absorption process was fast: the median values of the time corresponding to the maximum plasma concentration (T_{max}) ranged from 0.5 to 1.0 h after administration. Absorption appeared to be complete, since the AUC value calculated from the linear relationship between AUC and oral doses was in agreement with the experimental value following the administration of 50 mg i.v. Moreover, the fraction of the dose excreted unchanged in urine was, as

TABLE 2. *Mean pharmacokinetic parameters after intravenous administration*[a]

Drug	k_{12} (h⁻¹)	k_{21} (h⁻¹)	k_e (h⁻¹)	V_c (liters)	V_d[b] (liters)	$t_{\frac{1}{2}}$[c] (min)	Cl_T (ml/min)
CGP 9000	1.84	2.16	2.45	8.44	15.43	44	345
Cephalexin	1.27	2.68	1.62	10.90	16.40	45	294
Cephradine	2.39	1.73	2.12	10.20	19.02	49	364

[a] Data for CGP 9000 are mean values from the intravenous experiment; those for cephalexin and cephradine are taken from reference 1. Parameters: k_{12} and k_{21}, transfer rate constants; k_e, elimination rate constant; V_c, volume of central compartment; V_d, total volume of distribution; $t_{\frac{1}{2}}$, apparent elimination half-life; Cl_T, total body clearance.
[b] This was Vd_{ss} in reference 1.
[c] This was $t_{\frac{1}{2}\beta}$ in reference 1.

a mean ($\pm$ SD), 89.8% ($\pm$ 12.7) for 118 subjects given various doses. This fraction was independent of the dose administered. The urinary excretion was fast and was completed in around 10 h.

Repeated-dose oral administration. Healthy volunteers were given 250 mg of CGP 9000 four times a day for 6 days. A plasma concentration-time profile was obtained after the first and the last dose, and minimal concentrations were also measured on the intervening days just before administration. The AUC calculated over 6 h after the last dose was not found to be significantly different from the total AUC following the first dose. Also, the minimal plasma concentrations did not indicate any increase during the treatment.

Discussion. These various studies reveal that the pharmacokinetics of CGP 9000 are complicated. They may be described in terms of a three-compartment model in which the different transfers proceed at similar rates, so that it is difficult to differentiate them. Nevertheless, it is clear that CGP 9000 is rapidly distributed to extravascular compartments, from which it rapidly returns to the plasma.

The pharmacokinetic parameters of CGP 9000 may be compared to those of two structurally related cephalosporins, cephalexin and cephradine (Table 2). All three antibiotics appeared to behave in a similar fashion: the total body clearance of CGP 9000 was intermediary between that of cephalexin and that of cephradine, and

its apparent elimination half-life seemed to be slightly inferior to that of cephalexin, the value of which might have been slightly underevaluated in reference 1.

1. **Green, D. S., R. Quintiliani, and C. H. Nightingale.** 1978. Physiological perfusion model for cephalosporin antibiotics. I. Model selection based on blood drug concentrations. J. Pharm. Sci. **67**:191–196.

Antibacterial Effects of CGP 9000 in Human Urine In Vitro

W. TOSCH,* H. FEHLMANN, AND O. ZAK

Research Department, Pharmaceuticals Division, Ciba-Geigy Ltd., Basel, Switzerland

CGP 9000 is an orally active broad-spectrum cephalosporin derivative (3). Its antibacterial efficacy in human urine has been compared with that of cephalexin, cefadroxil, and cephradine in vitro.

The urine was collected from two volunteers in periods so chosen as to provide four pools of different osmolarities and pH values. MICs and MBCs were determined by the agar dilution technique, in medium containing 90% test urine and 10% agar (no. 11851, BBL Microbiology Systems). Otherwise, the agar dilution tests were performed under the conditions recommended by Ericson et al. (1) and by Steers et al. (2). The MBCs were determined by a membrane-transfer method (W. Tosch et al., Experientia, in press). The test organisms used comprised two laboratory strains each of *Escherichia coli, Klebsiella pneumoniae,* and *Proteus mirabilis* and 35 clinical isolates each of *E. coli, K. pneumoniae, P. mirabilis,* and *Salmonella* spp. The clinical isolates were obtained from two hospitals in Germany, one in Bangkok, and three in Switzerland.

Further investigations were made with an MS2 Research Device (Abbott Diagnostics Division), in which the turbidity of a large number of cultures in urine was measured and evaluated mathematically. In these experiments, the MIC was defined as the concentration at which the extinction coefficient does not exceed 0.2, which corresponds to the absence of turbidity upon visual inspection of the cuvettes. The rate of bacterial cell division was calculated with the help of a regression line indicating a bacterial count for each extinction value and by comparing the logarithms to the base 2 of the bacterial counts determined at various times. The calculated bacterial counts were checked in a Coulter

counter and by streak culture of dilutions on solid media.

The antibacterial action of all four substances against the laboratory strains was shown to be dependent on the pH of the urine. The MIC and MBC values were four to eight times higher in urine of pH 5.6 than in urine of pH 7.2. The same dependency was also evident when neutral urine was adjusted to pH 5.6 with HCl or acid urine to pH 7.2 with NaOH. Osmolarity in a range of 320 to 720 mosmol/liter seemed to have no effect on the activity of the substances, but the influence of acid pH was more pronounced at a high osmolarity of 720 mosmol/liter (increase in MICs by a factor of 3.3 to 8.7) than at a low osmolarity of 320 mosmol/liter (factor of 2.5 to 6.2).

The tests with the 140 clinical strains also showed the same dependency of the activity of the substances on the pH of the urine (Table 1). On the average, the substances were about five times less active in acid urine; the loss of activity was least pronounced in the case of *E. coli* (factor of 2.6 to 4.8) and most pronounced (factor of 6.6 to 8.4) with *K. pneumoniae.* Of the four cephalosporins tested, the most active was CGP 9000, the MICs of which for all four species in both acid and neutral urine were invariably lower than those of the other substances.

The results of the turbidimetric determinations made with the laboratory strain *E. coli* ATCC 25922 provided a possible explanation for the diminished activity of the four cephalosporins against *Enterobacteriaceae* in acid urine. As shown in Fig. 1, up to the 2nd h of incubation the bacteria multiplied more rapidly at pH 7.2 than at pH 5.6, which produced a higher bacterial count in neutral urine. After the

TABLE 1. *MICs of CGP 9000 and reference compounds for clinical isolates*

Organism[a]	pH of urine in agar	CGP 9000		Cephalexin		Cefadroxil		Cephradine	
		MIC[b]	f[c]	MIC	f	MIC	f	MIC	f
Escherichia coli	5.6	21.9	3.1	30.1	2.6	46.6	4.8	43.5	4.2
	7.2	7.1		11.6		9.7		12.8	
Klebsiella pneumoniae	5.6	28.5	8.4	30.8	7.9	47.9	6.6	59.2	8.2
	7.2	3.4		3.9		7.2		7.2	
Proteus mirabilis	5.6	61.6	4.8	76.1	4.1	87.1	4.4	• 109.7	3.4
	7.2	12.7		18.6		19.7		32	
Salmonella spp.	5.6	23.1	4.8	28.3	4.1	62.7	8.1	122.7	8.9
	7.2	4.8		6.9		7.7		13.8	

[a] The number of isolates tested for each organism was 35.
[b] $\bar{x}$ of $n = 35$ (micrograms per milliliter).
[c] Incremental factor: MIC ($\bar{x}$) at pH 5.6/MIC ($\bar{x}$) at pH 7.2.

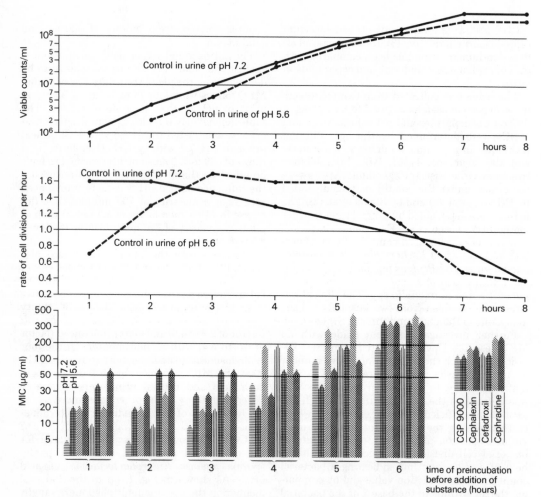

FIG. 1. *Viable counts, rate of cell division of E. coli ATCC 25922, and MICs of CGP 9000, cephalexin, cefadroxil, and cephradine, the drugs being added at various time intervals after the start of incubation.*

3rd h of incubation, however, the cell division rate decreased more rapidly at pH 7.2, so that proliferation was then greater at pH 5.6. When the antibiotics were added after different times of incubation, the MIC values showed a correlation with the corresponding growth rates of the control. After preincubation for up to 2 h, the MICs at pH 5.6 were higher and the bacterial growth rate was slower than at pH 7.2. After 3 h of preincubation, all MIC values were higher than when the bacteria were exposed immediately to the antibiotics, without preincubation, but they were then lower at pH 5.6 than at pH 7.2, corresponding to the growth rates.

On the basis of these results, the correlation between the MICs of the cephalosporins tested for *E. coli* ATCC 25922 and the pH of the urine can be attributed to differences in bacterial growth rate at varying pH values. Further data are needed, however, to support the theory that the activity of cephalosporins increases in parallel with the rate of bacterial proliferation.

Should it prove true that all slowly growing bacteria can only be inhibited by antibiotic concentrations significantly higher than those active against rapidly proliferating bacteria, new aspects would emerge that could call for modification of the therapeutic approach to chronic infections with slowly growing organisms.

Regardless of the underlying mode of action, these experimental results demonstrate that higher concentrations of the four cephalosporins are needed to inhibit bacterial growth in acid than in neutral urine. Although the antibiotic concentrations in the urine during treatment of urinary tract infections are very high, the loss of activity could be significant, inasmuch as the time elapsing until the concentrations decline to subinhibitory levels is presumably shorter in acid than in neutral urine.

1. **Ericson, H. M., and J. C. Sherris.** 1971. Antibiotic sensitivity testing. Acta Pathol. Microbiol. Scand. Sect. B, Suppl. 217 **76B:**1–90.
2. **Steers, E., E. L. Foltz, and B. S. Graves.** 1959. An inocula replicating apparatus for routine testing of bacterial susceptibility to antibiotics. Antibiot. Chemother. **9:**307–311.
3. **Zak, O., W. A. Vischer, C. Schenk, W. Tosch, W. Zimmermann, J. Regös, E. R. Suter, F. Kradolfer, and J. Gelzer.** 1976. CGP 9000: a new orally active, broad-spectrum cephalosporin. J. Antibiot. **29:**653–655.

Comparative Kinetics of CGP 9000 and Cephalexin After Simultaneous Administration in Humans

J. HIRTZ,* J. B. LECAILLON, W. THEOBALD, AND W. A. VISCHER

Ciba-Geigy SA, Rueil-Malmaison, France, and Research Department, Pharmaceuticals Division, Ciba-Geigy Ltd., Basel, Switzerland*

CGP 9000, 7β-[D-2-amino-2-(1,4-cyclohexadienyl)acetamido]-3-methoxy-3-cephem-4-carboxylic acid, is a new cephalosporin similar in structure to cephalexin. It was accordingly likely that the pharmacokinetics of the two antibiotics would not be very different. Making a statistically valid comparison of these pharmacokinetics by the usual crossover procedure, i.e., in a group of subjects given the two drugs successively, would have required a large number of volunteers. For this reason, we elaborated a new and discriminative analytical technique that makes it possible to assay each antibiotic in the presence of the other. We were thus able to compare their pharmacokinetic properties very precisely after their simultaneous administration to volunteers.

Two experiments were conducted. In the first, six subjects received 1,000 mg of both CGP 9000 and cephalexin orally as a solution (100 ml). In the second, six other subjects received 250 mg of each drug orally as a solution (100 ml), either with or without a copious breakfast, according to a crossover design. All amounts and concentrations are expressed as pure anhydrous compound (CGP 9000 and cephalexin).

The subjects were all males, aged between 22 and 49 years and weighing between 56 and 80 kg. They took the antibiotic solution at about 8 a.m. after an overnight fast. In the first experiment and in one of the two parts of the second, they were given 100 ml of water immediately after the administration of the substances and a light breakfast 2 h later. In the other part of the second experiment, they took the antibiotic solution 10 min after a copious breakfast. In all cases they had a light lunch 4 h after administration.

Blood samples were withdrawn at specific times into heparinized Vacutainers and centrifuged. Plasma was stored at −20°C, as was also the urine collected in portions over a period of 24 h.

CGP 9000 and cephalexin were simultaneously determined in plasma and urine by high-pressure liquid chromatography on a column of Lichrosorb RP 8 5-μm, with a mixture of ortho-phosphoric acid and methanol as the mobile phase. When low concentrations were to be determined, the deproteinized plasma was first purified on a column of Lichrosorb RP 8 10-μm (method to be published). It is possible to assay 100 ng per ml of plasma and urine with a coefficient of variation less than 16%.

Results and discussion. The results of the first experiment (1,000 mg) are depicted in Fig. 1. The plasma concentration curves of CGP 9000 and cephalexin are very much alike. The two antibiotics were absorbed at the same rate and produced similar peak concentrations (C_{max})

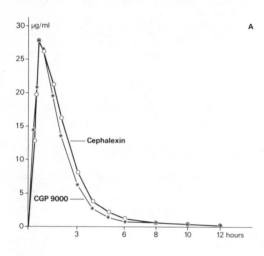

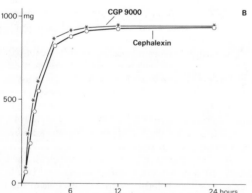

FIG. 1. *Plasma concentrations (A) and urinary excretion (B) of CGP 9000 and cephalexin after administration of 1 g of each simultaneously to six subjects (mean values).*

around the same time (T_{max}) after administration. CGP 9000 was eliminated from the plasma slightly faster than cephalexin, with the result that the area under the curve (AUC) was slightly smaller. Both drugs were eliminated almost exclusively by the kidneys, and similar percentages of the dose (UE %) were recovered unchanged in the urine. The renal clearance (Cl_r) of cephalexin was 85 to 88% of that of CGP 9000.

When in the second experiment (250 mg) the two drugs were given with food, there was a similar, slight reduction in their rates of absorption (Table 1). The two compounds were very similarly affected.

The absence of interaction between CGP 9000 and cephalexin when they are given simultaneously has not been checked directly. Nevertheless, this appears likely on the basis of the following observations.

When the plasma concentrations of CGP 9000 after administration alone and with cephalexin (corrected for the body weight of subjects) were compared, no statistically significant difference could be found.

The mean urinary excretion of CGP 9000, calculated from data on 110 subjects, was 89.80% (± 12.75%) of the dose. The value compares well with those recorded in the present experiment.

The results obtained after administration of 250 and 1,000 mg of each antibiotic were very similar. The pharmacokinetic data on cephalexin reported in the literature are also consistent with the findings presented here (1, 2).

TABLE 1. *Influence of food on absorption of CGP 9000 and cephalexin*[a]

Drug	Percentage of values in fasting subjects			
	C_{max}	T_{max}	AUC	UE
CGP 9000	−39	+75	−5	−11
Cephalexin	−42	+69	−10	−10

[a] C_{max}, Peak concentration; T_{max}, time after administration for maximum concentration; AUC, area under the curve; UE, urinary excretion.

TABLE 2. *Mean ratios of pharmacokinetic parameters of CGP 9000/cephalexin*[a]

Dose of each compound (mg)	C_{max}	T_{max}	AUC	UE	Cl_r
1,000	1.015	1.000	0.890	1.011	1.137
250	1.030	0.832	0.870	1.023	1.176
250 + food	1.041	0.861	0.915	1.003	1.096

[a] C_{max}, Peak concentration; T_{max}, time after administration for maximum concentration; AUC, area under the curve; UE, urinary excretion; Cl_r, renal clearance.

In a more recent experiment, in which 1,000 mg of two different cephalosporin formulations (CGP 9000 film-coated tablets of 500 mg and cephalexin capsules of 500 mg) were administered simultaneously to each test subject, it was shown that under these conditions as well CGP 9000 and cephalexin display very similar pharmacokinetic patterns.

Conclusion. Table 2 summarizes the results of the present experiments in the form of the mean ratios of CGP 9000/cephalexin. They clearly show that the two antibiotics are simi-

larly absorbed after oral administration and that CGP 9000 is eliminated at a slightly higher rate by renal excretion. CGP 9000 and cephalexin may thus be considered very closely similar from the pharmacokinetic point of view.

1. **Griffith, R. S., and H. R. Black.** 1971. Blood, urine and tissue concentrations of the cephalosporin antibiotics in normal subjects. Postgrad. Med. J. **47**(February Suppl.):32–40.
2. **Speight, T. M., R. N. Brogden, and G. S. Avery.** 1972. Cephalexin: a review of its antibacterial, pharmacological and therapeutic properties. Drugs **3**:9–78.

Concentrations of CGP 9000 in Plasma and Wound Secretions

C. ARMBRUSTER,* J. FUELLHAAS, AND M. GROETZINGER

*Florisdorf Hospital, Vienna, Austria, and CIBA-GEIGY Ltd., Basel, Switzerland**

CGP 9000, a new oral broad-spectrum cephalosporin, is an *N*-acyl derivative of 3 alkoxy-7-amino-3-cephem-4-carboxylic acid. CGP 9000 merits special attention, since in various experiments in vitro and in vivo it has displayed greater bactericidal activity than either cephalexin or cephradine (3, 4). The superior activity of CGP 9000 was clearly evident when the bactericidal effects of moderate concentrations of antibiotics on high bacterial counts were compared (2). In healthy volunteers given a single

dose of 500 mg of CGP 9000, the mean peak serum concentration was 14.1 µg/ml and the serum half-life was 0.95 h.

The objectives of this pharmacokinetic study were to determine the concentrations of CGP 9000 in plasma and wound secretions in patients with secreting surgical wounds. Patients were given either 500 mg (seven patients) or 1,000 mg (eight patients) in a single oral dose. In the group receiving 500 mg three patients were male and four were female, and the mean age was 53.6

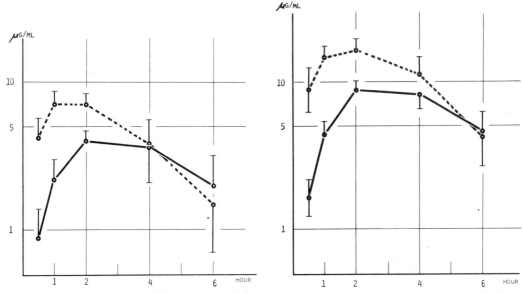

FIG. 1. *Concentrations of CGP 9000 ($\bar{x} \pm SEM_x$) in plasma (dashed line) and wound secretions (solid line). Mean values after a single oral dose of 500 mg (left panel) or 1,000 mg (right panel).*

years (range, 14 to 76 years). In the 1,000-mg group four patients were male and four were female, and the mean age was 59.5 years, ranging from 31 to 77 years. All patients were being treated in a surgical department for secreting surgical wounds, healing by second intention. This pharmacokinetic single-dose study was carried out between 4 and 21 days postsurgery.

The blood and wound secretion samples were taken 30 min and 1, 2, 4, and 6 h after administration of CGP 9000. A 5-ml amount of venous blood was withdrawn and centrifuged, and the heparinized plasma was immediately deep frozen. At the same time, five or six disks were placed on the wound until saturated with wound secretion, weighed, and deep frozen. The assay of the plasma was done by means of an agar-well diffusion test in Antibiotic Medium No. 1 (Oxoid) with *Bacillus subtilis* ATCC 6633. For the wound secretions the assay was made by means of a diffusion test (disks) on a nutrient agar with *Sarcina lutea* ATCC 9341.

After administration of 500 mg of CGP 9000 in a single oral dose, the maximum plasma concentration found was $7.10 \pm 1.5 \mu g/ml$, and after 1,000 mg in a single oral dose it was $16.6 \pm 3.0 \mu g/ml$. The maximum concentrations of CGP 9000 in wound secretion were $4.0 \pm 0.7 \mu g/ml$ after 500 mg and $8.8 \pm 1.4 kg/ml$ after 1,000 mg of CGP 9000. From 4 to 6 h after administration

the concentration of the drug in wound secretions was higher than that in plasma. Details are presented in Fig. 1.

With the MICs of CGP 9000 reached in wound secretions, the growth of 88.5% of the *Staphylococcus aureus* strains, 93.9% of the *S. epidermidis* strains, and 100% of the *Streptococcus pyogenes* strains can be inhibited. *S. aureus* and *S. pyogenes* are the most virulent and the most common microorganisms in hospital-acquired infections, both in compromised patients and in patients with an intact host defense mechanism (1).

CGP 9000 has proved to be of therapeutic value in the treatment of wound infections when an oral antibiotic is indicated.

1. **Keighley, B.** 1979. Antimicrobial prophylaxis in surgery, p. 9–11.
2. **Vischer, W. A., O. Zak, E. A. Konopka, H. Fehlmann, J. Regos, and W. Tosch.** 1978. Experimental evaluation of CGP-9000, a new orally active cephalosporin, p. 825–827. *In* Current chemotherapy, Proceedings of the 10th International Congress of Chemotherapy. American Society for Microbiology, Washington, D.C.
3. **Zak, O., W. Tosch, W. A. Vischer, and F. Kradolfer.** 1977. Comparative experimental studies on 3-methoxy and 3-methylcephems. Drugs Exp. Clin. Res. **3**:11–20.
4. **Zak, O., W. A. Vischer, C. Schenck, W. Tosch, W. Zimmerman, J. Regos, E. R. Suter, F. Kradolfer, and J. Gelzer.** 1976. CGP 9000: a new orally active broad-spectrum cephalosporin J. Antibiot. **29**:653–655.

Clinical Evaluation of Cefotiam in Complicated Urinary Tract Infections: a Comparative Study with Cefazolin by a Randomized Double-Blind Method

J. ISHIGAMI,* T. MITA, S. MOMOSE, AND J. KUMAZAWA

Kobe University, Kobe, and Kyushu University, Fukuoka, Japan*

Cefotiam, a new injectable cephalosporin synthesized at the Central Research Division of Takeda Chemical Industries Ltd., Japan, has been described as being several times more active against gram-negative rods than the previously introduced injectable cephalosporins and, moreover, to possess a broader antibacterial spectrum, including *Enterobacter*, *Citrobacter*, and indole-positive *Proteus*.

A double-blind controlled clinical trial of cefotiam was conducted to evaluate its efficacy and safety in the treatment of chronic, complicated urinary tract infections by intergroup comparison with cefazolin.

Treatment was carried out on a total of 191 patients, 95 on cefotiam and 96 on cefazolin. All

subjects were over 15 years of age and suffering from underlying urinary tract disease, with pyuria of 10 or more white cells per high-power field and bacteriuria of 1×10^4 or more viable organisms per ml. The daily dosages of cefotiam and cefazolin were 2 g and 4 g, respectively. Each dose in a vial was diluted with 300 ml of 5% xylitol solution and administered by drip infusion over approximately 1 h, twice daily (morning and evening), for 5 consecutive days.

Appraisal of the clinical response of each patient was made regarding (i) overall clinical efficacy, (ii) effect on pyuria, (iii) effect on bacteriuria, (iv) bacteriological effect, and (v) effect on pyrexia. Criteria for the judgment of (i), (ii), and (iii) were those of the Committee of Urinary

Tract Infections Study, Japan Society of Chemotherapy. In addition, data concerning body temperature were recorded, and the clinical response was rated on a three-point scale, i.e., normalized, improved, and unchanged.

Of the 191 patients admitted to the trial, 166 (86 on cefotiam and 80 on cefazolin) were eligible for efficacy evaluation and the remainder were excluded from the evaluation because conditions did not satisfy the criteria of the Committee aforementioned or, in some cases, patients were dropped due to discontinuation of the treatment. In the safety evaluation, however, the data from all, i.e., 191 patients, were included.

Background characteristics and patient factors in both treatment groups were found to be fairly equivalent.

(i) The overall clinical efficacy was excellent in 10 patients, good in 30, and poor in 46 on cefotiam, giving an efficacy rate of 46.5%. In the cefazolin group, there were 12 patients with excellent results, 15 with good, and 53 with poor, with an efficacy rate of 33.8%.

(ii) Pyuria was cleared in 17, decreased in 19, and unchanged in 50 cases in the cefotiam group. In the cefazolin group, pyuria was cleared in 14, decreased in 7, and unchanged in 59 cases. The cefotiam group showed a higher improvement (cleared plus decreased) rate (41.9%) than the cefazolin group (26.3%), $P < 0.1$.

(iii) Bacteriuria was eliminated in 26 patients, suppressed in 3, replaced with other organisms in 21, and unchanged in 36 in the cefotiam group, showing an improvement rate (eliminated plus suppressed) of 33.7%. The corresponding numbers were 21, 3, 14, and 42 in the cefazolin group, an improvement rate of 30.0%. The microbial replacement rate was 24.4% in the cefotiam group and 17.5% in the cefazolin group.

(iv) Bacteriological evaluation showed that the eradication of *Enterobacter*, *Citrobacter*, and *Serratia* occurred more frequently with cefotiam.

(v) Effect on pyrexia was assessed in 32 patients (18 on cefotiam and 14 on cefazolin) with pyelonephritis. The cefotiam group showed a higher improvement rate (cleared plus decreased) of 83.3% than the cefazolin group (71.4%).

The two treatment groups were compared as to overall clinical efficacy and effects on pyuria and bacteriuria in the patients classified according to group of diseases, indwelling catheter, type of infection, diagnosis, pyuria, urinary total bacterial count, and kinds of organisms (Fig. 1). Classified analyses favored cefotiam over cefazolin in most groups. Cefotiam especially was significantly superior to cefazolin in the improve-

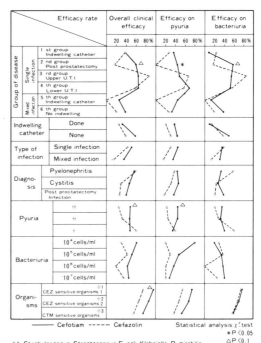

FIG. 1. *Comparison of the efficacy rates of cefotiam and cefazolin.*

ment rate of pyuria in patients with postoperative prostate infections ($P < 0.05$).

Two patients receiving cefotiam developed side effects, i.e., moderate eruption in one and moderate nausea and vomiting in the other, and administration of the drug was discontinued in both cases. In the cefazolin group, two patients recorded side effects: mild nausea in one and moderate chills and other sensations leading to the discontinuation of treatment.

All of these findings are, however, commonly observed in the course of cephalosporin treatment. Abnormal laboratory findings were noted in four patients on cefotiam and six patients on cefazolin, though all were found to have returned to normal after completion of treatment. In the cefotiam group, slight elevation of serum GPT or BUN, erythropenia, decreased hemoglobin content, and thrombocytopenia were noted, and the patients with lowered RBC and Hb showed this trend even before treatment, a factor which should be taken into consideration. In the cefazolin group, elevation of serum GOT, GPT, and Al-P were the main abnormal laboratory findings. The safety of cefotiam and cefazolin appeared to be essentially comparable.

The present study showed that cefotiam is a

more valuable chemotherapeutic agent than cefazolin for treatment of chronic, complicated urinary tract infections. Even with one-half the dose of cefazolin, cefotiam appears to have a higher efficacy rate, and safety evaluation showed no difference between the two drugs.

Double-Blind Comparison of Cefotiam (SCE-963) and Cefazolin in Postoperative Infections

YAEMON SHIRAHA,* NORIYUKI KAWABATA, AND JIRO YURA

Ashihara Hospital, Osaka, and Nagoya City University Medical School, Nagoya, Japan*

Cefotiam (CTM) is a new semisynthetic parenteral cephalosporin antibiotic (Fig. 1) developed by Takeda Chemical Industries, Ltd., Japan. The antimicrobial activities of cefotiam are about 10-fold more potent than the activities of cefazolin (CEZ) against gram-negative organisms. Furthermore, cefotiam is also active against indole-positive *Proteus*, *Citrobacter*, and *Enterobacter*, which are presumed to be resistant to those marketed cephalosporins in Japan (2).

We conducted a multicenter, double-blind comparison of cefotiam and cefazolin in the treatment of postoperative superficial purulent wound infections (trial A) and the treatment of postoperative localized peritonitis or dead-space infections (trial B). Patients received either 2 g of cefotiam or 4 g of cefazolin per day in two divided doses by intravenous drip infusion for 7 days in trial A and for 14 days in trial B.

Assessment of clinical response in trial A showed that cefotiam was effective in 89.1% (41/46) of the patients treated, and cefazolin was effective in 67.4% (29/43) of the patients treated. In trial B, cefotiam and cefazolin were effective, respectively, in 81.6% (31/38) and 70.7% (29/41) of the patients treated. These results significantly favored cefotiam over cefazolin.

Overall assessments of clinical results were made by each surgeon in charge on the 7th day of therapy in trial A and on the 14th day of therapy in trial B. In trial A, 87.2% (41/47) of the cefotiam-treated patients and 62.2% (28/45) of the cefazolin-treated patients showed moderate to significant improvement. In trial B, 69.8% (30/43) and 69.0% (29/42) of the patients treated with cefotiam and cefazolin, respectively, showed moderate to significant improvement. These results of overall assessment were significantly in favor of cefotiam in trial A. However, there was no difference between cefotiam-treated and cefazolin-treated patients in trial B.

Usefulness of the drugs in therapy was also evaluated by each investigator. The results showed that 62.2% (28/45) of cefotiam-treated patients and 45.2% (19/42) of cefazolin-treated patients were appraised as satisfactory with the therapy in trial A. These results from trial A were significantly in favor of cefotiam. In trial B, there was no difference between the two groups in the evaluation of usefulness of the drugs in the therapy. Both cefotiam (19/38) and cefazolin (22/44) achieved satisfactory therapy in 50% of the patients treated.

The progress of symptoms was analyzed according to the life table method and logrank test of Peto et al. (1). In trial A, cefotiam-treated patients showed a more rapid disappearance of suppurative discharge and faster improvement of local signs such as redness, swelling, induration, pain, and local heat (Fig. 2).

Among all patients treated in both trial A and trial B, cefotiam achieved 82.6% (76/92) eradication of organisms, while cefazolin achieved 65.1% (56/86). The difference between the two

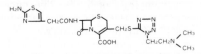

FIG. 1. *Chemical structure of cefotiam.*

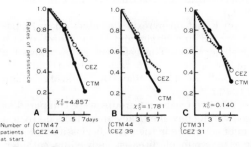

FIG. 2. *Comparison of the "rates of persistence" with respect to target symptoms and findings. Analyses were carried out by the life table method and logrank test of Peto et al. (1). A, Discharge; B, local signs (redness, swelling, induration, pain, local heat); C, fever. *P < 0.05.*

groups in eradication of organisms was statistically significant in favor of cefotiam.

Undesirable side effects were observed in 7 patients out of 92 treated with cefotiam in trials A and B. Of the 86 patients treated with cefazolin in trials A and B, 8 patients developed undesirable side effects. There was no significant difference between the two groups in the incidence of side effects, and no severe adverse reactions were observed.

The present investigation showed that cefotiam, with one-half of the daily dosage of cefazolin, achieved a better and/or equal clinical efficacy than cefazolin in the treatment of postoperative infections.

We are grateful to A. Sakuma, M. Akagi, K. Inokuchi, K. Orita, K. Sakai, K. Shibata, H. Shimura, T. Ishii, T. Taguchi, S. Tanaka, and Y. Tsuji for participating in this study.

1. **Peto, R., M. C. Pike, P. Armitage, and N. E. Breslow.** 1976. Design and analysis of randomized clinical trials requiring prolonged observation of each patient. I. Introduction and design. Br. J. Cancer **34**:585–612; 1977. II. Analysis and examples. **35**:1–39.
2. **Symposium on New Drugs.** 1978. SCE-963, the 26th Congress of the Japan Society for Chemotherapy.

Pharmacokinetics of Cefotiam (CGP 14 221/E) in Infected Animals

W. TOSCH,* O. ZAK, P. SCHNEIDER, AND E. BATT

Research Department, Pharmaceuticals Division, Ciba-Geigy Limited, Basel, Switzerland

Cefotiam is an injectable cephalosporin, highly active against a broad spectrum of gram-positive and gram-negative bacteria (1). In the present study an attempt has been made to assess the significance of the inactivation of cefotiam by TEM-β-lactamase in vivo on the basis of pharmacokinetic investigations in the infected mouse.

The antibiotic is hydrolyzed by the TEM enzyme in vitro at a rate of 75 nmol per unit of enzyme. The degree of inactivation is thus about 13 times less than that of penicillin G or cephaloridine, but greater than that of cefoxitin. To shed more light on the significance of this rate of hydrolysis, preliminary experiments were carried out in vitro and supplemented by pharmacokinetic studies in vivo in mice infected with the laboratory strain *Escherichia coli* 16, which synthesizes about three times as many units of enzyme per bacterial cell as the most productive TEM-β-lactamase synthesizing clinical isolates so far known to us.

In the in vitro experiments, the loss of microbiological activity of cefotiam in the presence of *E. coli* 16 was determined in ISO-Sensitest broth, in relation to the size of the inoculum and the time of exposure. We found that an inoculum of 10^7/ml was needed to cause a 50% loss of activity within 1 h. Inocula of less than 10^7/ml induced little loss of activity. Fifty percent inactivation took place in about 30 min, when the inoculum was increased to 10^8/ml, and within a few minutes at an inoculum of 10^9/ml. *E. coli* 16 cells destroyed by ultrasonication gave results similar to those obtained with intact cells, and

the residual of both the destroyed and intact cells showed only a fraction of the inactivation potency of whole suspensions. These results indicate that the greater part of the *E. coli* 16 enzyme is spontaneously discharged into the medium, so that, in animals infected with *E. coli* 16, the pharmacokinetics of the tested substance could presumably be altered.

In MIC determinations in vitro, in which cefotiam present in the solid nutrient medium is exposed for 18 to 24 h to TEM-β-lactamase from *E. coli* 16, small changes in the MIC values were demonstrated when the inoculum was $>10^3$/ml (Table 1).

The pharmacokinetic studies were performed in groups of female Tif: MF 2f, SPF mice infected intraperitoneally with *E. coli* 16 or, for comparison, the β-lactamase-negative strain *E. coli* 205, and in uninfected controls. The infective dose used in each case was a multiple of the LD_{100} (10^8 CFU per mouse). Cefotiam (30 mg/kg) was injected subcutaneously 30 min after infection. Blood samples were taken from the axillary veins under light anesthesia, and the organs were homogenized with water in a tissue grinder. Counts of viable bacteria were made by plating out dilutions of samples, and the concentrations of cefotiam were determined microbiologically by the agar diffusion method with *E. coli* 205 as test organism and Antibiotic Medium No. 2 as culture medium.

In the first experiments only the plasma of mice was examined. The concentrations found indicated that no inactivation of cefotiam had taken place: no difference was detectable between the infected animals and the controls, either in the peak plasma concentrations or in the apparent half-lives of the substance. The bacterial counts of *E. coli* 16 in the plasma were around 10^6/ml.

In the subsequent experiments, the liver and the kidneys were also examined and the infective dose was increased as much as possible. The maximum bacterial counts reached in the liver and kidneys were approximately 10^7 per g of

TABLE 1. *Rate of hydrolysis of cefotiam and reference compounds by TEM-β-lactamase, and MICs for the TEM-enzyme-producing laboratory strain E. coli 16*

Antibiotic	Rate of hydrolysis in nmoles per enzyme unit*	MIC (µg/ml) at inoculum indicated					
		10^7	10^6	10^5	10^4	10^3	10^2
Cefotiam	70	>128	64	8	4	1	1
Penicillin G	1000	>256	>256	>256	>256	>256	>256
Cephaloridine	770	>256	>256	256	128	128	128
Cefoxitin	<0.01	4	4	4	4	4	4

* 1 unit hydrolysis 10^3 nmoles Penicillin G per minute

tissue. As is evident from the results shown in Fig. 1, the concentrations of cefotiam in the plasma and kidneys of animals infected with *E. coli* 16 were not lower than in the controls, and the areas under the curve (AUCs) were in fact larger. The only difference observed was in the concentrations in the livers 15 min after infection, at which time those of the infected animals were about 30% lower than the control values; after 60 min, however, the concentrations in the infected and uninfected mice were in the same range. The AUCs of the liver concentrations were consequently smaller, but this was also found in the mice infected with *E. coli* 205. Elevated concentrations of cefotiam in the kidneys were also observed in mice infected with *E. coli* 205.

The alterations in the tissue contents of cefotiam are not attributable to the action of the TEM enzyme, but rather to the infectious disease, since the same changes occurred in mice infected with *E. coli* 16 as in those infected with

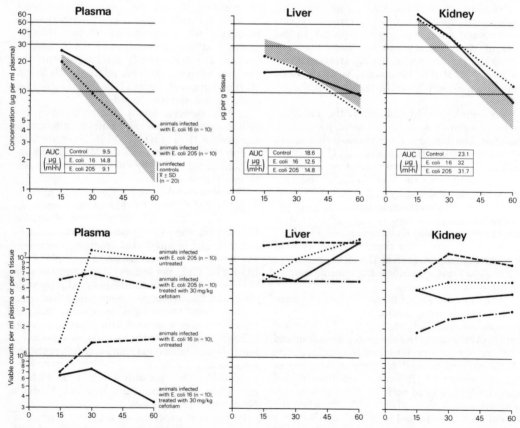

FIG. 1. *Concentrations of cefotiam in the plasma and tissues and corresponding viable counts after a single dose of 30 mg/kg s.c. in infected mice (n = 10, infection 30 min before treatment) and in uninfected mice (n = 20) as control.*

E. coli 205. At all events, the consistently elevated concentrations of cefotiam in the plasma of mice infected with *E. coli* 16 exclude any manifest inactivation of the substance. The assumptions made on the basis of the results obtained in vitro are thus confirmed, inasmuch as the pharmacokinetically relevant period of time is too short for any perceptible inactivation of cefotiam to occur at bacterial counts of 10^7/ml. On the other hand, bacterial counts significantly higher than 10^7/ml in the plasma or tissues could not be reached under our experimental conditions, so that it is hard to conceive of any inactivation sufficient to influence the pharmacokinetics of cefotiam occurring in the mouse.

In conclusion, whatever the significance of the hydrolysis of cefotiam by TEM-β-lactamase in vitro, at large inocula and long exposure times in vivo in infected mice, we were unable to establish any conditions under which significant inactivation of cefotiam could be shown to occur.

1. **Zak, O., W. Tosch, E. A. Konopka, and F. Kradolfer.** 1978. *In Vitro* characteristics of CGP 14 221/E (SCE 963), a new injectable cephalosporin. Abstr. Annu. Meet. Am. Soc. Microbiol. 1978, no. A21.

Experimental Studies of Cefotiam (CGP 14221/E)

O. ZAK,* E. A. KONOPKA, W. TOSCH, W. ZIMMERMAN, S. KUNZ, H. FEHLMANN, AND F. KRADOLFER

Research Department, Pharmaceuticals Division, Ciba-Geigy Limited, Basel, Switzerland, and Ciba-Geigy Corp., Summit, New Jersey 07901, U.S.A.

Cefotiam (CGP 14221/E, SCE-963) is a new injectable broad-spectrum cephalosporin now being jointly developed by Ciba-Geigy and Takeda. It is superior in its antibacterial activity to cephalothin, cephaloridine, and cefazolin (4). The present paper describes experimental comparisons of cefotiam with cefuroxime (CF), cefamandole (CM), cefoxitin (CX), and cefazolin (CZ).

MICs and MBCs. MICs were determined against 821 clinical isolates by the agar dilution method on Oxoid DST agar (with 1% Difco Supplement C for fastidious organisms) with an inoculum of 10^4 organisms. MBCs were measured by a modified membrane transfer technique (3). Cefotiam proved highly effective against all isolates of *Staphylococcus aureus* (*n* = 110), *Staphylococcus epidermidis* (36), *Streptococcus pyogenes* (48), *Streptococcus pneumoniae* (23), *Neisseria gonorrhoeae* (41), *Neisseria meningitidis* (18), and *Haemophilus influenzae* (37); the geometrical means of the MICs were 0.62, 0.5, 0.06, 0.12, 0.06, 0.08, and 0.71 µg/ml, respectively. In general, it was as active as CF and superior to CX. Against *Neisseria* spp., it was also superior to CM and CZ. Like the reference drugs, cefotiam displayed poor activity against enterococci and was inactive against *Pseudomonas aeruginosa*. Cefotiam was, in general, the most active drug tested against 508 isolates of *Enterobacteriaceae*, of which 50% were β-lactamase producers (111 *Escherichia coli*, 109 *Klebsiella pneumoniae*, 63 indole-positive *Proteus* spp., 106 *Proteus mirabilis*, 33 *Enterobacter* spp., 36 *Serratia* spp., 32 total *Salmonella* spp. and *Shigella* spp., and 18 additional *Enterobacteriaceae*): 80% of the isolates were inhibited by cefotiam at 1 µg/ml and by CF, CX, CM, and CZ at 8, 8, 16, and 128 µg/ml, respectively. Cefotiam inhibited 70 to 90% of the isolates of *P. mirabilis*, *E. coli*, *Klebsiella*, *Salmonella*, *Shigella*, and *Enterobacter* spp. at concentrations from 4 to >100 times lower than the reference drugs. Cefotiam is bactericidal; in 80% of the 120 different strains tested, the MBCs were equal or close to the corresponding MICs.

Penetration of the outer cell membrane. An indirect method (2) based on comparisons of the MICs for *E. coli* UB 1005, possessing normal cell-surface layers, and its mutant DC2 with a reduced permeation barrier was used. Cefotiam inhibited both strains at a concentration of 0.06 µg/ml; it therefore penetrates readily through the permeation barrier and is highly active at the target site. None of the other drugs tested combined both activities to such a degree. CF inhibited strain UB 1005 at 4 and strain DC2 at 0.125 µg/ml; CX, CM, and CZ inhibited UB 1005 and DC2 at 2 and 1, 0.5 and 0.06, and 2 and 2 µg/ml, respectively.

Experimental systemic infections. The chemotherapeutic efficacy of cefotiam was compared with that of CF, CM, and CZ in MF2 mice infected with 27 different bacterial strains, including 21 β-lactamase producers. The mice were infected intraperitoneally with 3 to 25 times the LD_{100} of the following organisms: *S. aureus* ($n = 3$), pyogenic streptococci (2), *E. coli* (7), *Serratia* (2), *Enterobacter cloacae* (1), *K. pneumoniae* (3), *Salmonella* (1), indole-positive *Proteus* spp. (7), and *P. mirabilis* (1). Antibiotics were given subcutaneously once (staphylococcal infections) or twice, immediately and 3 h after

TABLE 1. *Therapy of K. pneumoniae keratitis in guinea pigs[a]*

Antio-biotic	Dose (mg/kg)	No. of animals with keratitis (avg severity of ocular involvement[b]) on postinfection day:			Bacteriology, day 6 (no. positive/no. cultured)
		1	3	6	
Cefotiam	50	3 (5.0)	3 (3.0)	2 (0)	0/3
	10	3 (5.4)	3 (6.0)	3 (4)	2/3
CM	50	3 (7.0)	3 (8.0)	2 (7.5 1[c]	2/2
CF	50	3 (5.2)	3 (8.0)	3[c]	
Control	0	3 (7.7)	3 (8.7)	3 (10)	3/3

[a] Treatment was given intramuscularly 5 h after infection and then twice daily for 3 days.

[b] Parentheses indicate average severity of gross involvement in animals with keratitis only; the average severity (0 to maximum of 12) represents the sum of gradings of the percentage of corneal surface showing infiltration (0 = 0%; ++++ = 75 to 100%), density of infiltrate (0 to ++++), and vascularization, hemorrhaging, or both of the sclera/conjunctiva (0 to ++++).

[c] Number of animals dead on days 4 to 6 from penicillin-like toxicity.

infection. The ED_{50} values were calculated by probit analysis on day 5 after infection. Cefotiam was effective against all test infections. Against the gram-positive infections, it was as effective as CF, CM, and CZ. It was, however, superior to CF in 60% and to CM and CZ in 75% of the gram-negative infections; the geometrical mean of its ED_{50}'s was 5.6 mg/kg, and those of CF, CM, and CZ were 22.4, 29.2, and >40 mg/kg, respectively.

Experimental keratitis. The therapeutic potential of cefotiam was further investigated in guinea pigs with corneal infection due to *K. pneumoniae* by a modification of the method of Davis and Chandler (1). A volume of 20 μl of a washed suspension of *K. pneumoniae* (10^5 colony-forming units) was injected into the cornea. Antibiotics were administered subcutaneously at 0.5 or 5 h after infection and then twice daily for 3 days. The severity of infection was recorded daily for 6 days. Bacterial counts were made from homogenates of the entire excised cornea on day 6 of the infection. In all animals treated with 10 or 50 mg of cefotiam per kg, starting 0.5 h after infection, no keratitis developed. Cefotiam also proved highly effective when treatment was delayed 5 h after infection (Table 1). At a dose of 50 mg/kg, it produced a complete cure, and at 10 mg/kg, the severity of keratitis was significantly decreased; CM, at a dose of 50 mg/kg, was virtually ineffective.

Experimental pyelonephritis. Efficacy and renal concentrations of cefotiam were determined in a rat pyelonephritis model in which each of the kidneys was infected with a different *E. coli* strain. A suspension of 10^7 colony-forming

TABLE 2. *Renal concentrations of antibiotics and chemotherapeutic effect in experimental pyelonephritis in rats[a]*

Antiobiotic	Kidney	Avg drug concn (μg/ml) ± SD at posttreatment min[b]:					Avg log CFU ± SD after treatment[c]
		20	30	40	60	120	
Cefotiam	Left	60 ± 12	NE[d]	28 ± 11	19 ± 6	3.9 ± 3	2.87 ± 1.90
	Right	51 ± 11		27 ± 11	19 ± 4	3.6 ± 2	2.89 ± 2.02
CF	Left	NE[d]	38 ± 13	NE	29 ± 6	19 ± 7	2.80 ± 1.65
	Right		45 ± 13		31 ± 7	21 ± 15	3.04 ± 2.40
AM	Left	NE	14 ± 8	NE	11 ± 5	1.0	5.40 ± 0.45
	Right		51 ± 17		30 ± 10	5 ± 1	3.87 ± 0.48
Control	Left						5.32 ± 0.56
	Right						5.45 ± 0.54

[a] Pyelonephritis was due to β-lactamase-positive *E. coli* 2018 R^+_{TEM} in left kidney and β-lactamase-negative *E. coli* 2018 in right kidney

[b] Single dose of 30 mg/kg was administered intramuscularly on day 5 after infection.

[c] Treatment: once on day 1, 6 h after infection, twice daily on days 2 to 5, and once on day 6. Bacteriological examination was done on day 8. CFU, Colony-forming units.

[d] NE, Not examined.

units of *E. coli* 2018 producing no β-lactamase was injected into the parenchyma of the right kidneys; the left kidneys were infected with the corresponding β-lactamase-producing mutant (strain 2018 R^+_{TEM}). In the experiment in which the renal antibiotic concentrations were measured, the animals were given 30 mg of cefotiam, CF, or ampicillin (AM) per kg intramuscularly 5 days after infection and sacrificed thereafter at specified intervals. The kidney homogenates were centrifuged, and the drug concentrations were determined in the supernatants; assays were performed in antibiotic medium no. 1 (Oxoid) with *E. coli* 205 for cefotiam, *B. subtilis* ATCC 6633 for AM, and *Sarcina lutea* ATCC 9341 for CF. Cefotiam and CF produced identical concentrations in both kidneys. Cefotiam, however, was eliminated at a distinctly shorter half-life (30 min) than CF (≥70 min). On the other hand, the renal concentrations of AM in the left kidneys (β-lactamase-positive infection) were significantly lower (factor ≥ 3) than in the right kidneys. In therapeutic experiments, the animals were given intramuscular doses of 20 mg of cefotiam or CF per kg or 200 mg of AM per kg 5 h after infection, and then the same doses were given twice daily on days 2 to 5 and once on day

6. Thirty-six hours after the last treatment, bacterial recoveries were made separately on the homogenates of the left and right kidneys. Cefotiam and CF proved equally effective in both kidneys, reducing the bacterial populations by >2 log units as compared to those in untreated controls. AM, however, was only effective in the kidneys infected with the β-lactamase-negative strain (Table 2).

Cefotiam thus compares favorably with CF, CX, CM, and CZ in its antibacterial activity in vitro and in vivo.

1. **Davis, S. D., and J. W. Chandler.** 1975. Experimental keratitis due to *Pseudomonas aeruginosa*: model for evaluation of antimicrobial drugs. Antimicrob. Agents Chemother. **8:**350–355.
2. **Richmond, M. H., D. C. Clark, and S. Wotton.** 1976. Indirect method for assessing the penetration of β-lactamase nonsusceptible penicillins and cephalosporins in *Escherichia coli* strains. Antimicrob. Agents Chemother. **9:**307–311.
3. **Tosch, W., H. Fehlmann, R. Gisler, and O. Zak.** 1980. Studies of the bactericidal activity of antibiotics. Experientia **36:**153–154.
4. **Tsuchiya, K., M. Kida, M. Kondo, H. Ono, M. Takeuchi, and T. Nishi.** 1978. SCE-963, a new broad-spectrum cephalosporin: in vitro and in vivo antibacterial activities. Antimicrob. Agents Chemother. **14:**557–568.

Activity of Cefotiam (CGP 14 221/E) Against *Haemophilus influenzae*, *Neisseria gonorrhoeae*, and *Neisseria meningitidis*, Including β-Lactamase-Producing Isolates, In Vitro

I. BRAVENY* AND K. MACHKA

Institute of Medical Microbiology, Technical University Munich, D-8000 Munich 80, Federal Republic of Germany

Haemophilus influenzae and *Neisseria gonorrhoeae* are among the most common pathogens. In contrast to other gram-negative bacteria, they are extensively susceptible to antibiotics. Therefore, and also because of methodological problems with these fastidious organisms, it is not common practice to use susceptibility tests in routine laboratory procedures. However, the appearance of penicillin-resistant and ampicillin-resistant strains has led to therapeutic uncertainty. The β-lactamase of type III, which is mediated by plasmids, can hydrolyze these valued compounds. Furthermore, chloramphenicol-resistant and tetracycline-resistant strains of *H. influenzae* have appeared. These facts greatly emphasize the importance of the search for alternative therapy. Chief among the alternatives are the cephalosporins, because they generally

have greater β-lactamase stability but at the same time are as low in toxicity as penicillin. There are only a few reports on the antibacterial activity of the new injectable broad-spectrum cephalosporin cefotiam (2–4). We therefore determined the activity of cefotiam against *H. influenzae*, *N. gonorrhoeae*, and *Neisseria meningitidis* in vitro and compared this activity with that of cephalothin, cefazolin, cefamandole, cefuroxime, and cefoxitin.

Most of the organisms used in this study were recently isolated in Munich: 118 strains of *H. influenzae* (including 18 β-lactamase positive), 107 strains of *N. gonorrhoeae* (including 7 β-lactamase positive), and 39 *N. meningitidis* strains. Among the β-lactamase-positive strains, one *H. influenzae* and three *N. gonorrhoeae* strains were obtained from the Center for Disease Control, Atlanta, Ga. The MICs of the six antibiotics were determined by the microdilution method (1). The medium used for *H. influenzae* and *N. meningitidis* was Iso-Sensitest broth (Oxoid) with 0.1% nicotinamine adenine dinucleotide, 0.002% phenol red, and 5% horse blood. The medium used for *N. gonorrhoeae* was Mueller-Hinton broth with 0.4% glucose, 0.01% glutamine, 0.002% cocarboxylase (Merck), and 0.02% phenol red. The inocula, which were different for the three species, were photometrically adjusted to the following concentrations (colony-forming units [CFU] per ml): *H. influenzae*, 5×10^4; *N. meningitidis*, 5×10^5; *N. gonorrhoeae*, 10^7. The plates were incubated at 37°C for 24 h in 5% CO_2. This broth dilution

method permitted rapid determination of MICs; the endpoints, based on a change in color of the pH indicator, are clear without trailing growth.

Results of the susceptibility tests are summarized in Tables 1 and 2. Cefotiam was effective for both β-lactamase-positive and -negative strains of *H. influenzae*: all isolates were inhibited by a concentration of 2 mg/liter. At the same concentration, cefuroxime inhibited 88%, cephalothin inhibited 44%, cefoxitin inhibited 17%, and cefazolin inhibited 5% of the β-lactamase-negative isolates. Against β-lactamase-positive strains of *H. influenzae*, cefotiam was also substantially more active than cephalothin, cefazolin, and cefoxitin, comparable to cefamandole, and less active than cefuroxime.

TABLE 1. *Susceptibility of non-β-lactamase-producing H. influenzae, N. gonorrhoeae, and N. meningitidis*

Organism	Drug	Cumulative % inhibition at MICs (mg/liter) of:													
		0.007	0.015	0.03	0.06	0.12	0.25	0.5	1	2	4	8	16	32	64
H. influenzae (n = 100)	Cefotiam				3		7	21	84	100					
	Cephalothin					2	6	8	17	44	70	85	99	100	
	Cefazolin								1	5	9	27	67	87	100
	Cefamandole			1	5	8	14	60	98	100					
	Cefuroxime					2	6	14	43	88	97	100			
	Cefoxitin						1	2	8	17	68	96	100		
N. gonorrhoeae (n = 100)	Cefotiam	39	76	93	97	98		100							
	Cephalothin			7	17	31	50	66	90	98	100				
	Cefazolin			6	17	29	60	87	94	100					
	Cefamandole	33	73	75	82	95	97	100							
	Cefuroxime	77	91	94	97		99	100							
	Cefoxitin			1	4	31	88	96	98	100					
N. meningitidis (n = 39)	Cefotiam				92	100									
	Cephalothin						13	33	100						
	Cefazolin							15	100						
	Cefamandole					67	100								
	Cefuroxime				39	98	100								
	Cefoxitin						3	95	98	100					

TABLE 2. *Susceptibility of β-lactamase-producing H. influenzae and N. gonorrhoeae*

Organism	Drug	No. of strains with MIC (mg/liter) of:										
		0.03	0.06	0.12	0.25	0.5	1	2	4	8	16	32
H. influenzae (n = 18)	Cefotiam					1	10	7				
	Cephalothin					1	2	8	3	1	3	
	Cefazolin							4	4	3	5	2
	Cefamandole			1	3	7	5	1	1			
	Cefuroxime			1	1	9	7					
	Cefoxitin						1	8	9			
N. gonorrhoeae (n = 7)	Cefotiam				1	2	4					
	Cephalothin						1	1	3	2		
	Cefazolin						1		4	1	1	
	Cefamandole									3	4	
	Cefuroxime	2	3	1	1							
	Cefoxitin					5	2					

We have also examined the effects of the inoculum and the differences between MICs and MBCs of cefotiam in 20 β-lactamase-negative strains of *H. influenzae* and 17 β-lactamase-producing strains. There was no difference in the behavior of the two groups of strains. We recorded an MIC (mean) of 1.69 mg/liter, whereas the MBC (mean) was 2.97 mg/liter.

The inoculum in the test had a significant effect at a concentration of 10^7 CFU/ml. The MIC (mean) of cefotiam for β-lactamase-negative strains was 1.37 mg/liter with an inoculum of 10^4 CFU/ml and 1.80 mg/liter with 10^6 CFU/ml. The MIC for β-lactamase-positive strains increased from 1.23 mg/liter with an inoculum of 10^4 CFU/ml to 2.82 mg/liter with an inoculum of 10^6 CFU/ml. With an inoculum of 10^7 CFU/ml, the MIC of cefotiam, however, was 20-fold greater than with an inoculum of 10^3 CFU/ml.

Cefuroxime and cefotiam were similar and had more activity against the *N. gonorrhoeae* β-lactamase-negative strains than did cephalothin or cefazolin; all strains were inhibited at a concentration of 0.5 mg/liter. The seven strains of β-lactamase-positive *N. gonorrhoeae* were inhibited by cefuroxime at the low concentration of 0.25 mg/liter and by cefotiam at a concentration of 0.5 mg/liter. Cefamandole, on the other hand, inhibited the β-lactamase-producing isolates only at the relatively high concentration of 16 mg/liter.

Against *N. meningitidis*, cefotiam was the most active agent; 0.06 mg/liter inhibited all strains. Cefuroxime and cefamandole had similar MICs and were more active than cefoxitin, cephalothin, and cefazolin. The increase of inoculum size from 10^4 to 10^7 CFU/ml did not alter the effect of cefotiam on *N. meningitidis*. The MBC, which was determined for 10 strains, was identical to the MIC.

In conclusion, we have found cefotiam, a new injectable cephalosporin, to be highly effective against both β-lactamase-positive and -negative strains of *H. influenzae* and *N. gonorrhoeae*. In vitro it was the most active cephalosporin against *N. meningitidis*. It now remains for clinical studies to show whether this cephalosporin is of value in the treatment of infections due to these organisms.

1. **Braveny, I.** 1979. In vitro activity of cefaclor against *H. influenzae* in comparison to other oral antibiotics. Infection 7(Suppl. 6):532–535.
2. **Nosaki, Y., A. Imada, and M. Yoneda.** 1979. SCE-963, a new potent cephalosporin with high activity for penicillin-binding proteins 1 and 3 of *Escherichia coli*. Antimicrob. Agents Chemother. 15:20–27.
3. **Tsuchiya, K., M. Kida, M. Kondo, S. Goto, M. Ogawa, A. Tsuji, and S. Kuwahara.** 1977. SCE-963, a new cephalosporin. II. In vitro and in vivo antibacterial activities. Program Abstr. Intersci. Conf. Antimicrob. Agents Chemother. 17th, New York, N.Y., abstr. no. 45.
4. **Zak, O., W. Tosch, E. A. Konopka, and F. Kradolfer.** 1978. In vitro characteristics of CGP 14221/E (SCE-963), a new injectable cephalosporin. Abstr. Annu. Meet. Am. Soc. Microbiol., A21, p. 4.

Pharmacokinetic Study of Cefmetazole in Healthy Volunteers

F. YAMASAKU,* Y. SUZUKI, K. SASAHARA, M. SEKINE, AND T. MORIOKA

Internal Medicine, Suibarago Hospital, Niigata, and Product Development Laboratories, Sankyo Co., Ltd., Tokyo, Japan

Cefmetazole is a new antibiotic of the cephamycin series that is resistant to the destructive activity of β-lactamase produced by gram-positive and gram-negative bacteria. It is, therefore, more active against gram-negative bacilli than are the cephalosporin antibiotics. To establish an appropriate dose regimen for infections due to gram-negative bacilli, we studied the pharmacokinetic behavior of cefmetazole in healthy volunteers.

The characteristics of four healthy volunteers employed for this study are shown in Table 1. Cefmetazole was infused continuously in accurate amounts by use of a Unita Perfusor at doses of 1, 2, and 4 g for 2 h and of 4 g for 4 h. All four treatments were conducted in crossover fashion by using four volunteers.

Bioassay of cefmetazole serum concentrations was carried out by the thin-layer cup method. *Bacillus subtilis* ATCC 6633 was used as the test organism when the serum level was more than 12.5 μg/ml, and *Micrococcus luteus* ATCC 9341 was used when the serum level was under 12.5 μg/ml. Standard curves of both methods are shown in Fig. 1. Urinary concentrations were determined by use of *B. subtilis* ATCC 6633.

Serum and urinary concentrations were also determined by the high-pressure liquid chromatography (HPLC) method. A Hitachi model 635A instrument and a μ Bond pack/C_{18} (Waters

Associates, Inc.) column were employed. Elution was with 10 mM phosphate buffer (pH 7.0)-methanol (4:1) and with the same phosphate buffer-acetonitrile (9:1) for serum and urinary samples, respectively. Detection was 254 nm for serum and 272 nm for urine. The standard curve was linear in the concentration range of 1 to 100 $\mu g/ml$. Good correlation between the bioassay and the HPLC method is shown in Fig. 1b.

Pharmacokinetic parameters were estimated by use of a curve-fitting computer program (BMDP-3R) for a one-compartment open model. Elimination rate constant, volume of distribution, elimination half-life, serum clearance, and renal clearance obtained from crossover trials for four volunteers are shown in Table 2. Urinary recoveries were good, and a mean value of 83.28 ± 8.13% (mean ± SD) was obtained for 16 trials.

After the 2-h continuous infusion of 0.5, 1.0, and 2.0 g of cefmetazole per h, the average ratio of cefmetazole concentrations at the termination of infusion was 1:2.1:4.0, indicating a good dose response in serum concentrations. Therefore, blood level profiles of specific dose regimens could be estimated from pharmacokinetic parameters. Blood levels for the 1-h infusion at doses of 0.5, 1.0, and 2.0 g were simulated by using pharmacokinetic parameters obtained from infusion experiments. The duration times of blood levels at the three doses were as follows: 1.0, 1.8, and 2.8 h for the level of 25 $\mu g/ml$; 1.9, 2.8, and 3.8 h for 12.5 $\mu g/ml$; 2.7, 3.5, and 4.7 h for 6.3 $\mu g/ml$; 3.5, 4.3, and 5.5 h for 3.1 $\mu g/ml$; and 4.2, 5.0, and 6.3 h for 1.6 $\mu g/ml$.

Cefmetazole was found to inhibit the growth of 90% of clinical isolates of *Escherichia coli* at a concentration of 6.25 $\mu g/ml$ and more than 80% at 3.12 $\mu g/ml$. It also inhibited the growth of more than 80% of *Klebsiella* isolates at a concentration of 6.25 $\mu g/ml$ and 70% at 3.12 $\mu g/ml$. For the *Proteus* group more than 70% of clinical isolates were inhibited in their growth at 12.5 $\mu g/ml$ (1).

For the treatment of diseases caused by cephalosporin- and penicillin-resistant pathogenic microbes, such as *Klebsiella* and indole-positive *Proteus* strains, administration of a dose three times a day that provides a blood level over 6.25 or 12.5 $\mu g/ml$ with a duration of more than 2 h is desirable.

Considering the growth-inhibiting concentra-

TABLE 1. *Characteristics of the four healthy volunteers*

Volunteer	Age (yr)	Height (cm)	Body wt (kg)	Body surface (m²)	Ccr[a] (ml/min)
1	20	175.5	66	1.81	106
2	19	167.3	66	1.74	118
3	20	162.5	51	1.53	116
4	19	161.0	61	1.64	118
Mean	19.5	166.0	61	1.68	114.5

[a] Creatinine clearance.

TABLE 2. *Mean pharmacokinetic parameters determined by bioassay[a]*

Expt	Infusion method	K_{el} (h⁻¹)	V_d (liters)	$T_{1/2}$ (h)	Serum clearance (ml/min)	Renal clearance (ml/min)
A	0.5 g/h for 2 h	1.02	7.9	0.68	132.8	120.3
B	1 g/h for 2 h	0.99	8.2	0.72	132.9	111.2
C	2 g/h for 2 h	0.85	9.3	0.82	132.4	113.2
D	1 g/h for 4 h	0.89	8.9	0.81	128.5	117.3
Mean ($n = 16$)		0.94	8.6	0.76	131.6	115.6
± SD		0.14	1.3	0.12	13.4	26.7

[a] K_{el}, elimination rate constant; V_d, total volume of distribution; $T_{1/2}$, apparent elimination half-life.

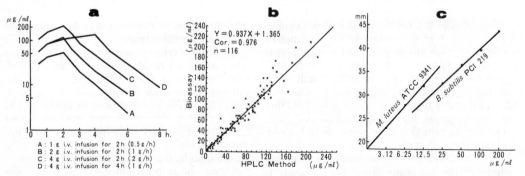

FIG. 1. *(a) Average serum levels of cefmetazole in four healthy adult volunteers after continuous intravenous infusions of the indicated doses. (b) Correlation of serum levels determined by bioassay and by the high-pressure liquid chromatography (HPLC) method. (c) Zone diameters of cefmetazole against Bacillus subtilis and Micrococcus luteus.*

tions for pathogenic microbes and the blood level simulation of cefmetazole, administration of 500 mg of cefmetazole is a rational dose for the aforementioned microbes. However, modifications of dose and of route of administration are necessary in accordance with factors such as

susceptibility of pathogenic microbes, location of the infection, severity of the infection, and dosing intervals.

1. **S. Goto.** 1979. Antibacterial activity of cefmetazole. J. J. A. Infect. Dis. **53**:52–65.

Pharmacokinetics of Cefmetazole in Normal Subjects and Patients with Impaired Renal Function

M. OHKAWA,* M. ORITO, T. SUGATA, M. SHIMAMURA, M. SAWAKI, E. NAKASHITA, K. KURODA, AND K. SASAHARA

Kanazawa University, Kanazawa and Sankyo, Tokyo, Japan

Cefmetazole is a new 7α-methoxycephalosporin derivative that has been shown to have marked resistance to inactivation by β-lactamase from gram-positive and gram-negative bacteria. Pharmacokinetics of cefmetazole were studied by single intravenous drip infusion employing 5 healthy volunteers and 16 patients with impaired renal functions. There were 16 males and 5 females, ranging from 25 to 84 years of age and from 41.0 to 68.5 kg of body weight. The subjects were divided into five groups according to creatinine clearance corrected to 1.73 m^2 of body surface area: group 1, five healthy volunteers with creatinine clearance of 95.6 to 155.6 ml/min; group 2, four patients with creatinine clearance of 65.5 to 86.8 ml/min; group 3, four patients with creatinine clearance of 35.2 to 52.7 ml/min; group 4, four patients with creatinine clearance of 10.2 to 24.8 ml/min; group 5, four patients with creatinine clearance of 0 to 9.7 ml/min.

One gram of the drug was diluted with 200 ml of 5% dextrose-water and administered intravenously by drip infusion over a period of 1 h Blood samples were obtained just prior to infusion and 1, 2, 4, and 6 h after the infusion was started. Urine specimens were collected from 0 to 2, 2 to 4, and 4 to 6 h.

The concentration of cefmetazole in serum and urine was determined by the thin-layer cup plate method, with *Micrococcus luteus* ATCC 9341 as the test organism and heart infusion agar as the medium. For the measurement of serum concentration, the standard solution series were prepared by using pooled serum of normal humans. The assay range was 200 to 0.78 μg/ml. For the measurement of urinary concentration, the standard solution series of 20 to 1.25 μg/ml were prepared with 1% phosphate buffer (pH

6.0). Pharmacokinetic parameters were estimated according to a one-compartment open model, using the BMDP-3R nonlinear regression program (2).

The mean serum concentration of each group at 1, 2, 4, and 6 h after beginning the 1-g dose infusion and mean cumulative urinary recoveries of cefmetazole are shown in Table 1. Pharmacokinetic parameters of cefmetazole after drip infusion of the 1-g dose to 5 normal subjects and 16 patients are shown in Table 2. Analysis shows that there was negative correlation between the serum concentration and the creatinine clearance ($P < 0.05$ at 1 h and $P < 0.001$ at 2, 4, and 6 h). The results demonstrated significant correlation between the cumulative urinary recovery and the creatinine clearance ($P < 0.001$ during 0 to 2, 0 to 4, and 0 to 6 h). A significant correlation ($P < 0.001$) and negative correlation ($P < 0.001$) were obtained, respectively, when elimination rate constants and the individual area under the serum concentration curves were plotted against creatinine clearance. Serum and renal clearance were corrected for 1.73 m^2 of body surface area. The results demonstrated significant correlations between the serum clearance and the creatinine clearance ($P < 0.001$), the renal clearance and the creatinine clearance ($P < 0.001$), and the serum clearance and the renal clearance ($P < 0.001$).

After administration of cefmetazole by 1-h intravenous drip infusion, peak serum concentrations were obtained at the end of the infusion in all subjects. As renal function decreased, the mean peak concentrations of cefmetazole increased. The mean serum half-life of cefmetazole in healthy volunteers, 0.81 h, was similar to that of cefoxitin (1, 3). The serum half-life of cefmetazole became more prolonged as renal function

TABLE 1. *Mean serum concentrations of cefmetazole and mean cumulative urinary recoveries*

Determination	Time (h)	Group 1	Group 2	Group 3	Group 4	Group 5
Serum concentration[a]	1	76.9 ± 33.0	92.0 ± 25.6	85.5 ± 10.7	113.3 ± 34.9	113.4 ± 35.5
	2	30.0 ± 13.0	59.5 ± 8.7	61.8 ± 4.6	78.8 ± 33.9	101.3 ± 32.7
	4	7.6 ± 4.1	23.0 ± 9.6	41.4 ± 14.3	62.0 ± 22.6	76.7 ± 24.5
	6	2.4 ± 1.7	9.0 ± 2.5	24.9 ± 12.3	47.8 ± 19.2	72.5 ± 17.1
Urinary recovery[b]	0~2	48.0 ± 15.0	38.4 ± 14.4	20.4 ± 11.0	7.9 ± 3.7	1.7 ± 3.3
	0~4	63.7 ± 16.8	51.7 ± 21.8	40.4 ± 11.8	13.6 ± 8.5	7.2 ± 14.2
	0~6	69.3 ± 17.2	59.7 ± 18.2	54.7 ± 22.2	20.0 ± 11.5	8.8 ± 16.2

[a] Micrograms per milliliter ± SD.
[b] Percent ± SD.

TABLE 2. *Pharmacokinetic parameters of cefmetazole after intravenous drip infusion of 1 g in 5 normal subjects and 16 patients with impaired renal function*[a]

Patient group	Creatinine clearance (ml/min per 1.73 m²)	Elimination rate constant (h⁻¹)	Half-life (h)	AUC[b] (µg/ml per h)	$V_d{}^c$ (% of total body wt)	Serum clearance (ml/min per 1.73 m²)	Renal clearance (ml/min per 1.73 m²)
1 (n = 5)	127.5 ± 23.3	0.91 ± 0.18	0.81 ± 0.19	139.5 ± 60.2	18.5 ± 6.0	164.0 ± 61.3	110.2 ± 40.4
2 (n = 4)	76.6 ± 10.7	0.44 ± 0.23	2.01 ± 1.30	238.0 ± 26.7	15.7 ± 2.5	67.3 ± 24.1	42.5 ± 14.7
3 (n = 4)	43.1 ± 8.3	0.26 ± 0.12	3.13 ± 1.60	285.9 ± 44.8	19.9 ± 3.9	35.0 ± 12.6	29.6 ± 14.8
4 (n = 4)	17.6 ± 6.2	0.13 ± 0.07	6.90 ± 3.87	403.2 ± 142.8	21.0 ± 6.3	25.5 ± 14.5	11.4 ± 7.2
5 (n = 4)	3.9 ± 4.8	0.07 ± 0.04	14.98 ± 9.42	491.1 ± 146.8	17.1 ± 5.3	14.0 ± 12.4	4.9 ± 9.0

[a] Results are given as the mean ± SD.
[b] Area under the serum concentration curve (0 to 6 h).
[c] Apparent volume of distribution.

decreased. A precipitous rise in serum half-life was observed when the creatinine clearance fell below 30 ml/min.

As renal function decreased, the area under the serum concentration curve increased. The mean apparent volume of distribution of cefmetazole in subjects with normal renal function was 18.5% of body weight and was not influenced by degree of renal impairment.

In subjects with normal renal function, cefmetazole was excreted primarily by the kidneys. Urinary excretion of cefmetazole decreased as renal function decreased; however, the mean urinary concentration of cefmetazole exceeded 200 µg/ml even in group 4 at 0 to 6 h after infusion. This concentration should be adequate to treat urinary tract infections caused by bacteria susceptible to cefmetazole.

The optimal dose and dosage interval for cefmetazole in patients with normal renal function depends largely on the susceptibility of various bacteria that cause infections, which must be determined in clinical trials. In patients with impaired renal function, the dose regimen could be estimated from the pharmacokinetic parameters of normal renal function. As a significant linear correlation was demonstrated between the elimination rate constant of cefmetazole and the creatinine clearance in this study, correct dosage adjustment of cefmetazole will be obtained by proper combination of prolongation of dosage interval and reduction of maintenance dose.

1. **Brumfitt, W., J. Kosmidis, J. M. T. Hamilton-Miller, and J. N. G. Gilchrist.** 1974. Cefoxitin and cephalothin: antimicrobial activity, human pharmacokinetics, and toxicology. Antimicrob. Agents Chemother. **6:**290–299.
2. **Dixon, W. J.** 1964. BMDP biological computer programs. Health Sciences Computing Facility, Los Angeles.
3. **Goodwin, C. S., E. B. Raftery, A. D. Goldberg, H. Skeggs, A. E. Till, and C. M. Martin.** 1974. Effects of rate of infusion and probenecid on serum levels, renal excretion, and tolerance of intravenous doses of cefoxitin in humans: comparison with cephalothin. Antimicrob. Agents Chemother. **6:**338–346.

Pharmacokinetic Studies on Cefmetazole, a New Cephamycin Derivative

Y. KAWADA

Gifu University School of Medicine, Gifu, Japan

The results of studies on absorption, distribution, excretion, and metabolism in humans of cefmetazole (CMZ), a new semisynthetic cephamycin derivative with a broad antibacterial spectrum, were accumulated from 34 research institutes in Japan.

Concentrations of CMZ in serum, urine, bile, sputum, or tissue were determined by either the cup plate or disk diffusion method, with *Micrococcus luteus* ATCC 9341 or *Bacillus subtilis* ATCC 6633 as the indicator strain. No differences were observed between results obtained with the two indicator strains.

For the purpose of comparison, concentrations of cefazolin (CEZ) were determined by the cup plate method with *B. subtilis* ATCC 6633 as the indicator strain.

Serum levels after intramuscular or intravenous injection of various single doses of CMZ are shown in Table 1. The half-life ranged from 1.1 to 1.4 h after intramuscular injection and was about 1 h after intravenous injection. When various doses of CMZ were administered by drip infusion, the half-life ranged from 1.1 to 1.4 h.

In a crossover study, serum levels achieved were found to be related to dosage for each route of administration.

No serum accumulation was observed when three healthy adults were given three 2-g doses of CMZ by drip infusion at 8-h intervals, or when a similar group was given three 0.5-g intramuscular doses at 8-h intervals.

Serum levels obtained after administration of 1 g of CMZ by drip infusion were slightly lower and the half-lives were shorter than those of CEZ when compared by a crossover method in three healthy adults. However, the situation was reversed if serum samples were diluted by buffer solution. This seemed to be due to a difference of protein-binding ratio between the two antibiotics.

Urinary excretion of CMZ was slightly quicker and urinary concentrations were slightly higher than those of CEZ when compared by a crossover method. Urinary recovery of CMZ within 6 h of administration of various doses by a variety of routes ranged from 74 to 92%. No metabolite of CMZ was detected in urine.

Biliary concentrations of CMZ after administration of a 2-g dose by drip infusion were compared to those of CEZ by a crossover method in six patients with T-tube drainage of the common bile duct. As shown in Fig. 1, biliary concentrations of CMZ were significantly higher than those of CEZ. Biliary recovery within 6 h ranged from 0.03 to 0.32% for CMZ and from 0 to 0.1% for CEZ. Even in the case in which the 6-h biliary recovery of CEZ was 0 and 0.001%, recovery of CMZ was 0.03 and 0.32%, respectively.

Tissue concentrations of CMZ and CEZ were studied in uterine tissue of patients undergoing operation for myoma uteri. The mean concentration of CMZ in 7 patients 30 to 60 min after a 1-g intravenous dose was 11.24 ± 0.96 µg/ml; this was significantly higher than the value obtained for CEZ (6.91 ± 0.63 µg/ml) when studied in the same way in 10 patients. However, when uterine tissue concentrations were estimated 1 to 2 h after administration of the dose, the mean concentration of CMZ was 4.82 ± 0.61 µg/ml (11 patients) and that of CEZ was 6.0 ± 0.90 µg/ml (8 patients). This difference is not significant.

The peak levels of CMZ achieved in sputa of

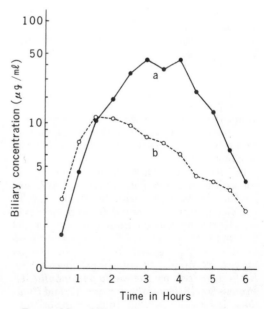

FIG. 1. *Mean biliary concentrations of (a) cefmetazole and (b) cefazolin after administration of a 2-g dose by drip infusion. Crossover study in six patients.*

TABLE 1. *Serum concentrations after administration of cefmetazole*

Route	Dose (g)	No. of pa-tients	Serum concn (µg/ml)						
			10 min	15 min	30 min	1 h	2 h	4 h	6 h
Intramuscular injection	0.5	17	—	29.5 ± 6.8	32.5 ± 10.1	26.2 ± 4.6	16.1 ± 2.7	5.8 ± 2.5	2.8 ± 2.2
	0.25	2	—	—	20.5 ± 3.5	12.3 ± 1.1	6.7 ± 1.0	2.5 ± 0.1	0.4
Intravenous injection	2	4	—	—	167 ± 20.2	99.8 ± 14.5	55.6 ± 5.1	13.5 ± 2.5	—
	1	19	183 ± 30.2	105.5 ± 19.5	82.1 ± 15.6	52.6 ± 11.2	24.8 ± 9.1	6.3 ± 2.5	1.9 ± 0.7
	0.5	5	85.3 ± 6.1	58.0 ± 6.7	37.1 ± 5.8	25.4 ± 6.1	12.6 ± 4.1	5.2 ± 1.7	0.9

8 patients, 2 to 5 h after administration of a 1-g intravenous dose, ranged from 2 to 4 µg/ml.

In conclusion, CMZ was rapidly absorbed to achieve a high serum level and was rapidly excreted into urine in active form. CMZ achieved higher concentrations than did CEZ in bile, sputa, and uterine tissue.

Clinical Use of Cefmetazole in Urinary Tract Infections Not Responding to Initial Treatment with β-Lactam Antibiotics

MASAAKI OHKOSHI,* SATOSHI KIMURA, KEISHI OKADA, AND NOBUO KAWAMURA

Department of Urology, Tokai University School of Medicine, Isehara, Japan

Recently, gram-negative bacteria rather than gram-positive bacteria have been increasing as the causative organisms of urinary tract infections, and organisms which were neglected as less toxigenic have become more important (1). In addition, the frequent use of β-lactam antibiotics has caused an increase in β-lactamase–producing bacteria (2).

Cefmetazole (CMZ), which has strong resistance against β-lactamase, was evaluated for clinical responses in patients in whom the β-lactam antibiotics commonly used were ineffective. Susceptibility of bacteria to CMZ in comparison with other antibiotics was also examined by the disk method.

In vitro study. Disk susceptibilities at one concentration of five antibiotics, i.e. CMZ, ampicillin (ABPC), carbenicillin (CBPC), cefazolin (CEZ), and cephaloridine (CER), were measured on 145 strains isolated from the urine of 134 patients with urinary tract infections during 6 months from December 1977 (*Staphylococcus aureus*, 22 strains, *Streptococcus faecalis*, 10; *Escherichia coli*, 58; *Klebsiella pneumoniae*, 14; *Proteus* spp., 9; *Enterobacter* spp., 12; and *Pseudomonas aeruginosa*, 20). In disk susceptibility tests organisms with a zone of inhibition over 16 mm were assessed to be susceptible and those with zones less than 16 mm were considered resistant.

The rates of susceptibility of each isolated organism to the five antibiotics are in Table 1. The rates of susceptibility to CMZ were 77.3% for *S. aureus*, 89.2% for *E. coli*, and 78.6% for *K. pneumoniae*. *E. coli* and *K. pneumoniae* were most highly susceptible to CMZ among the five antibiotics tested.

Table 2 shows the rates of susceptibility to CMZ for strains of *S. aureus*, *E. coli*, *K. pneumoniae*, and *Proteus* spp. resistant to ABPC, CBPC, CEZ, and CER. Many of the bacteria resistant to these four penicillins or cephalosporins, especially about 80% of *E. coli* and *K. pneumoniae*, were susceptible to CMZ.

We also determined the rates of susceptibility of CMZ-resistant strains to the other four antibiotics. Among five strains of *S. aureus*, 20% were susceptible to the two penicillins, 40% were susceptible to CEZ, and 60% were susceptible to CER. The results with eight CMZ-resistant *E. coli* strains showed 12.5% susceptible to the two penicillins, 37.5% susceptible to CEZ, and 25% susceptible to CER. None of three *K. pneumoniae* strains was susceptible to the penicillins, but 66.7% were susceptible to CEZ and CER. None of six strains of *Proteus* spp. was susceptible to CBPC, but 16.7% were susceptible to the other three drugs.

Clinical trial. Among 78 patients with complicated urinary tract infections hospitalized in the urological department during 6 months from December 1977, there were 45 cases in which the bacteria isolated were susceptible to the initial administered antibiotics. Of 35 patients to whom β-lactam antibiotics (CEZ, CEX [cephalexin], ABPC, CBPC) had been administered, 17 (48.6%) responded poorly both bacteriologically and clinically. The therapeutic effect of CMZ was evaluated in 8 of these 17 patients from whom the bacteria isolated were susceptible to CMZ (Table 3).

CMZ, 1.0 g twice a day, was administered successively for 5 days by one-shot intravenous injection. During the administration, the num-

bers of multinuclear leukocytes and bacteria in the urine were determined. To check side effects, we examined erythrocyte and leukocyte counts, glutamic oxalacetic and pyruvic transaminases, lactic dehydrogenase, blood urea nitrogen, etc., on peripheral blood before and after administration of CMZ.

The effects were assessed according to Criteria for Clinical Evaluation in Complicated Urinary Tract Infections (established in Japan) (3), by taking the number of bacteria and multinuclear leukocytes in urine as a parameter.

In this clinical trial, CMZ was administered to

TABLE 1. *Percentage of clinical isolates susceptible to five drugs[a]*

Organism (no. of strains)	CMZ	ABPC	CBPC	CEZ	CER
S. aureus (22)	77.3	63.6	63.6	86.4	86.4
E. coli (58)	86.2	41.4	29.3	75.9	39.7
K. pneumoniae (14) ...	78.6	0	0	64.3	35.7
Proteus spp. (9)	33.3	22.2	11.1	22.2	11.1
S. faecalis (10)	30.0	90.0	70.0	50.0	40.0
Enterobacter spp. (12)	0	0	0	0	0
P. aeruginosa (20)	5.0	0	0	5.0	0

[a] CMZ, Cefmetazole; ABPC, ampicillin; CBPC, carbenicillin; CEZ, cefazolin; CER, cephaloridine.

TABLE 2. *Percentage of strains resistant to other β-lactam antibiotics[a] that were susceptible to cefmetazole*

Organism	To-tal	Strains resistant to:			
		ABPC	CBPC	CEZ	CER
S. aureus	77.3	50.0	50.0	0	0
E. coli	86.2	79.4	82.9	64.3	82.9
K. pneumoniae	78.6	78.6	78.6	80.0	88.9
Proteus spp.	33.3	28.6	25.0	28.6	37.5
Total	78.6	69.8	71.8	51.7	74.1

[a] ABPC, Ampicillin; CBPC, carbenicillin; CEZ, cefazolin; CER, cephaloridine.

TABLE 3. *Clinical results with cefmetazole in complicated cystitis[a]*

Patient			Underlying disease	Treatment prior to CMZ	Causative organism (cells/ml)	WBC in the urine (cells/hpf)	MIC (µg/ml)			Clinical response
No.	Age (yr)	Sex					CMZ	CEZ	ABPC or CEX	
1	76	F	Bladder tumor	CEZ	K. pneumoniae 10⁶ ↓ (0)	10–15 ↓ 2–4	6.25	>100		Excellent
2	25	M	Neurogenic bladder	CEZ	Proteus spp. 10⁶ ↓ (0)	30–40 ↓ 0	1.56	25		Excellent
3	71	M	After TUR of BPH	ABPC	K. pneumoniae 10⁵ ↓ (0)	30 ↓ 1–2	6.25	>100	ABPC, >100	Excellent
4	81	M	After TUR of BPH	CEZ	E. coli 10⁶ ↓ E. coli 10⁶	>50 ↓ >50	1.56	25		Poor
5	74	M	After TUR of BPH	CEZ	K. pneumoniae 10⁶ ↓ (0)	40–50 ↓ 0	0.78	>100		Excellent
6	74	M	After TUR of BPH	CEX	K. pneumoniae 10⁶ ↓ (0)	>50 ↓ 10–29	1.56	>100	CEX, >100	Good
7	63	M	After TUR of BPH	CEX	E. coli 10⁶ ↓ (0)	>50 ↓ 0	0.78	6.25	CEX, >100	Excellent
8	63	M	Urethral stricture	CEZ	Proteus spp. 10⁶ ↓ (0)	50–60 ↓ 10–15	3.12	50		Good

[a] All patients received 1.0 g intravenously twice a day for 5 days. No side effects were observed in any of the eight patients. Abbreviations: CMZ, cefmetazole; CEZ, cefazolin; ABPC, ampicillin; CEX, cephalexin; WBC, leukocytes; hpf, high-power field; TUR, transurethral resection; BPH, benign prostatic hypertrophy.

eight patients with chronic complicated cystitis in whom CEZ, CEX, and ABPC had been ineffective both bacteriologically and clinically. The clinical response to CMZ was excellent in three, good in one, and poor in one (effective rate, 80%) of five patients in whom CEZ had been ineffective. With two patients in whom CEX had been ineffective, the clinical response to CMZ was excellent in one and good in one, and the clinical response to CMZ was excellent in one patient after ABPC was ineffective. The clinical response classified by causative organisms was excellent in two cases and good in one case for *K. pneumoniae*, excellent in one case and poor in one case for *E. coli*, and excellent in one case and good in one case for *Proteus* spp. As to the bacteriological effect, all seven strains except one strain of *E. coli* were eradicated in the patients who showed a clinical response to CMZ.

No side effects and no abnormal laboratory findings were observed.

Conclusion. Disk susceptibility of fresh clinically isolated strains to CMZ was examined, and also the correlation with susceptibility to ABPC, CBPC, CEZ, and CER was investigated. CMZ showed higher antibacterial activity against *E. coli*, *K. pneumoniae*, *S. aureus*, and *Proteus* spp. than those of ABPC, CBPC, CEZ, and CER, and many strains which were resistant to these four antibiotics displayed susceptibility to CMZ.

CMZ was used in patients with chronic complicated cystitis, including five patients with poor response to CEZ, two with poor response to CEX, and one with poor response to ABPC, and an effective rate of 87% was obtained.

From the above results, an excellent effect of CMZ can be expected in cases where a poor effect is observed after the treatment with other β-lactam antibiotics, if the isolated bacteria are susceptible to CMZ. Many strains of bacteria, especially *S. aureus*, *E. coli*, and *K. pneumoniae*, were found to be susceptible to CMZ even if they were resistant to other β-lactam antibiotics.

1. **Kumazawa, J.** 1975. The change of urinary tract infections. J. Jpn. Med. Assoc. **73**:650–654.
2. **Mitsuhashi, S., and S. Iyobe.** 1976. Distribution of strains resistant to antibiotics. Pharm. Mon. (Jpn.) **18**:2179–2184.
3. **Ohkoshi, M., et al.** Criteria for clinical evaluation in complicated urinary tract infections. Chemotherapy, in press.

Minimal Inhibitory Concentration of Cefmetazole for Clinical Isolates and Its Clinico-Bacteriological Effect: Comparison with Cefazolin

T. TSUJIMOTO,* K. YAMADA, AND H. YAMA

Hoshigaoka Koseinenkin Hospital, Osaka, Japan

The clinico-bacteriological effect of cefmetazole (CMZ), a new broad-spectrum antibiotic, was assessed in a controlled study designed to be quantitative, reproducible, and objective in its results. In this study cefazolin (CEZ) served as a control drug.

Selection of patients. In evaluating the effect of an antimicrobial agent exactly, the following conditions are desirable: (i) the disease studied is an intractable one for which spontaneous regression will not occur; (ii) the population of bacterial flora in pathological specimens is stable; and (iii) microorganisms from clinical specimens can be isolated quantitatively with the time course. As a disease which satisfies these conditions, chronic complicated urinary tract infection was chosen, and spinal cord injury patients with such infection were subjected to this approach on CMZ.

Dosage schedule of CMZ and CEZ. Four groups of patients were treated with 0.5 or 1.0 g of CMZ or CEZ twice daily intramuscularly for 7 days, as follows: group 1 (21 patients), 0.5 g of CMZ; group 2 (5 patients), 1.0 g of CMZ; group 3 (5 patients), 0.5 g of CEZ; group 4 (10 patients), 1.0 g of CEZ. Pretreatment was with 3 g of sulfamethizole per day orally for 1 to 2 weeks.

Bacteriological examination. Midstream clean-catch urines were submitted as clinical materials before and every morning after the start of CMZ or CEZ administration. A 0.1-ml sample from serial 10-fold saline dilutions of the urine was inoculated on the plate (quantitative culture). The isolation media were PEA blood agar for gram-positive bacteria, MacConkey agar and DHL agar for intestinal bacteria, NAC agar for *Pseudomonas aeruginosa*, EF agar for enterococci, etc. After quantitative culture on these media, identification of the microorganisms isolated was made by use of an APL analysis table for intestinal flora and the Yabuuchi method for glucose-nonfermenting gram-negative bacilli. The MIC was also determined for the strains detected before and after 7 days of treatment. Strains for which the viable count was 10^3 or more per ml before treatment were included in the analysis.

Effect of CMZ on the bacterial population in urine. Bacterial populations in urine showed quite the same tendency in all patients given CMZ. The bacterial pattern in urine was studied in terms of species and MIC. Illustrated in Table 1 is the time course of bacterial isolation for 60 strains detected in 21 patients given 0.5 g of CMZ twice daily (group 1). It is apparent that bacterial strains for which the MIC was 100 µg/ml or lower were undetectable in urine within 1 to 3 days of treatment (bactericidal zone of MIC), but those strains for which the MIC was 200 to 800 µg/ml were eradicated or reduced or persisted (minimum inhibitory zone of MIC). These antibacterial effects appear to be exhibited regardless of the bacterial species identified.

A different pattern was observed in 33 clinical isolates from 10 patients given 1.0 g of CEZ twice daily (group 4). The MIC for 17 strains was less than 100 µg/ml, and 14 of them were not detectable in urine within 1 to 4 days of the treatment. Although the remaining 3 showed a considerably lower MIC, they were seen to regrow on the 4th to 7th days of the treatment. Thus, the relationships of bacterial eradication, reduction, and persistence with MIC values seen with CMZ were not paralleled in the case of CEZ. *Streptococcus faecalis* was found to be the most fre-

TABLE 1. *Eradication and persistence of microorganisms after cefmetazole treatment (0.5 g twice daily intramuscularly) in relation to bacterial species and MICs*

Species	No. of strain	MIC µg/ml

Species	No. of strain	0.39	0.78	1.57	3.13	6.25	12.5	25	50	100	200	400	800 ≤
S. epidermidis	2				② ②								
S. faecalis	13										⍟⍟ ● ② ⍟ ● ● ⑦⍟ ● ② ③ ● ●		
A. faecalis	2										⑤ ⑦		⑦
Flavobacterium	1												
E. coli	1		②										
K. pneumoniae	1				②								
S. marcescens	12				① ①	② ②	② ③ ② ②	② ③	② ②				
P. mirabilis	1			①									
P. vulgaris	1				②								
P. morganii	7							③	②	② ③ ① ② ②			
P. rettgeri	16	②	① ②	① ① ① ①	① ② ② ② ②	② ③	③	②	Minimum Inhibitory Zone ● ● ●			
P. aeruginosa	3				Bactericidal Zone								

Note Ⓝ: Eradicated after N days treatment   ⍟: Suppressed (10^3 or over)   ●: Persisted after 7 days treatment

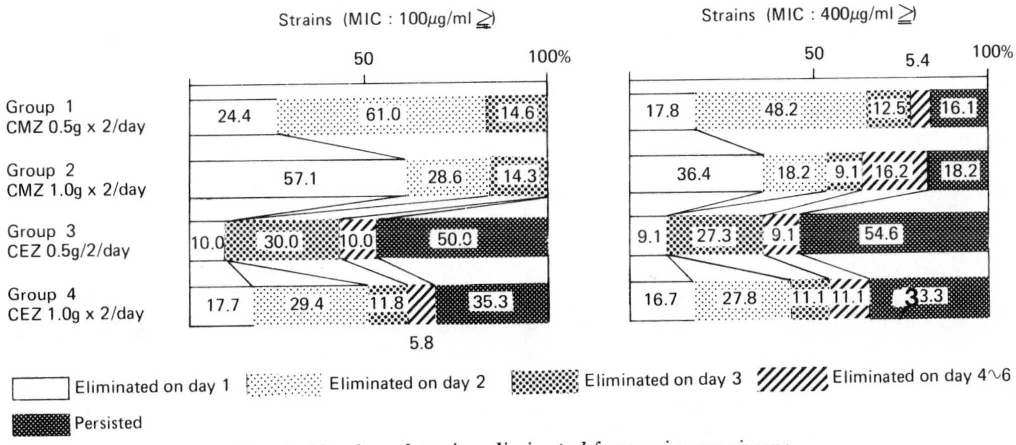

Strains (MIC : 100µg/ml ≥)   Strains (MIC : 400µg/ml ≥)

Group 1 CMZ 0.5g × 2/day	24.4 61.0 14.6	17.8 48.2 12.5 16.1
Group 2 CMZ 1.0g × 2/day	57.1 28.6 14.3	36.4 18.2 9.1 16.2 18.2
Group 3 CEZ 0.5g/2/day	10.0 30.0 10.0 50.0	9.1 27.3 9.1 54.6
Group 4 CEZ 1.0g × 2/day	17.7 29.4 11.8 35.3	16.7 27.8 11.1 11.1 33.3

☐ Eliminated on day 1   ▦ Eliminated on day 2   ▨ Eliminated on day 3   ⁄⁄⁄⁄ Eliminated on day 4∿6

■ Persisted

FIG. 1. *Number of strains eliminated from urine specimens.*

quently persistent species among the strains for which the MIC was less than 100 μg/ml, suggesting species specificity to CEZ.

Dose response to CMZ. The above effect of CMZ was investigated by group comparison based on day of eradication. As shown in Fig. 1, the bactericidal zone of the MIC was more than 100 μg/ml both for group 1 and group 2, and all bacterial strains were eradicated from urine within 1 to 3 days of CMZ treatment. Rate of eradicated to isolated strains at an MIC of 100 μg/ml on the 2nd day of treatment was 24.4% for group 1 and 57.1% for group 2, being significantly higher for the latter. Among strains for which MICs were more than 400 μg/ml, 17.8% and 36.4% were eradicated for group 1 and group 2, respectively. A clear dose-response relationship was thus recognized with CMZ.

A similar but unclear tendency was shown between group 3 and group 4 (CEZ). On the 2nd day of the treatment, few strains were eradicated, and many strains persisted. The rate of persisting strains in group 4 amounted to a considerable percentage, with 35.3% of the strains having an MIC of more than 100 μg/ml. In the case of clinical isolates showing MICs greater than 400 μg/ml, this value was as high as 33% in group 4, indicating a lesser antibacterial effect as compared to 16% in group 1. It can be said that CMZ is even more effective than CEZ under the present experimental condition.

Effect of CMZ and bacterial numbers. The effect of CMZ was estimated in terms of the bacterial count before treatment, on the day of bacterial eradication, and during persistence. Most of 60 strains isolated from patients given 0.5 g of CMZ twice daily (group 1) had a viable count of 10^4 to 10^8 per ml; however, the effect of CMZ was found to be exhibited regardless of the bacterial count.

Conclusion. CMZ was effective at an intramuscular dose of 0.5 g twice daily, without regard to the bacterial species and viable count before treatment. The clinical effect of CMZ was exactly related to the MIC. A significant dose-response relationship was noted between the groups given 0.5 and 1.0 g of CMZ twice daily. In contrast, the clinical effect of CEZ was not related to the MIC. It showed only a bacteriostatic effect even at a dose of 1.0 g twice daily.

Cefmetazole Concentration in Infected Tissues from Patients After Intravenous Administration and Clinical Effect for Patients with Cholecystitis and Peritonitis

TAKASHI NAKAMURA,* IKUO HASHIMOTO, YASUO SAWADA, JIROH MIKAMI, MASAMI NAKANISHI, YOICHI KASAI, AND YOSHIO SAHASHI

Department of Surgery, TENSHI General Hospital (Franciscan Missionaries of Mary), and 1st Surgical Department, School of Medicine, Hokkaido University, Sapporo, and Product Development Laboratory, Sankyo Co. Ltd., Tokyo, Japan*

Only a few of the studies on pharmacokinetics in patients treated with antibiotics have reported data on antibiotic concentrations in the tissues of patients (2). The few studies dealing with the concentrations of antibiotics in infected tissues have showed the concentration of antibiotics at a single point of time after administration of the drug (3, 4). Therefore, this study was performed to determine the concentration of cefmetazole in the infected tissue, plasma, and bile of patients as a function of time (1).

Cefmetazole (CS-1170, CMZ), supplied by Sankyo Co. Ltd., Tokyo, Japan, was given in a dose of 1 g by the intravenous route during operation on 33 patients with cholecystitis or peritonitis, of which 14 were female and 19 were male. During the operation, plasma, bile, and tissue specimens were taken and were sent to Sankyo Co. for determination of CMZ concentrations. The determination of CMZ concentration was carried out by the microbioassay with *Micrococcus luteus* ATCC 9341 as the test organism.

Infections due to gram-negative bacilli constitute a major problem among hospitalized patients. β-Lactamase is known to play an important role in the resistance of gram-negative bacteria to both penicillins and cephalosporins. CMZ is a newly developed cephamycin antibiotic which is not inactivated by β-lactamase. Since it is very important in chemotherapy to know the distribution of the drug in the infected target organ or tissues and the MIC of the drug for the pathogenic bacteria, this study was performed to determine the CMZ concentrations in infected tissues of patients. CMZ was also used

TABLE 1. *Clinical effect of cefmetazole after intravenous drip infusion for preoperative patients with cholecystitis and cholangitis (patients 1–6) and for postoperative patients with acute peritonitis (patients 7–11)[a]*

Patient	Age (yr)	Sex	Wt (kg)	Daily dose[b]	Dura-tion (days)	Organism in the operation	Clinical effect
1	76	F	45	4 g, 2 × 2	21	No growth	Good
2	58	M	49	4 g, 2 × 2	8	No growth	Good
3	50	F	52	4 g, 2 × 2	3	No growth	Good
				2 g, 2 × 1	7		
4	58	M	60	4 g, 2 × 2	17	E. coli (MIC, 1.56 μg/ml)	Good
5	34	M	84	4 g, 2 × 2	23	E. coli (MIC, 3.13 μg/ml)	Good
6	46	F	51	2 g, 1 × 2	16	No growth	Excellent
7	5	M	14.8	2 g, 0.5 × 4	1	E. coli (MIC, 3.13 μg/ml)	Excellent
				1.5 g, 0.5 × 3	5		
8	31	M	62	4 g, 2 × 2	5	No growth	Excellent
9	58	M	52.5	4 g, 2 × 2	11	No growth	Good
10	38	M	63	4 g, 2 × 2	6	E. coli (MIC, 3.13 μg/ml)	Good
11	10	M	25	2 g, 1 × 2	3	E. coli (MIC, 6.25 μg/ml)	Excellent
				1 g, 1 × 1	1		

[a] Patient 2 was diagnosed as having cholecyst-choledocholithiasis. In patients 3, 4, and 5, the cystic duct was obstructed. Patients 7 and 9 had complicated shock syndrome. Patient 7 was diagnosed as having panperitonitis with idiopathic cecal perforation and was administered 500 mg of cefmetazole intravenously. Patients 8, 9, 10, and 11 were diagnosed as having acute peritonitis with perforate appendicitis. No adverse effects of the drug treatment were observed in any of the 11 patients.

[b] A daily dose given in the table as "4 g, 2 × 2" means that the daily dose of 4 g was given as an intravenous drip infusion of 2 g twice daily.

TABLE 2. *Cefmetazole concentration in various body fluids and tissues during operation after intravenous administration of 1,000 mg to patients 1–6 in Table 1*

Patient	Cefmetazole concn at indicated time after injection				Inflammatory degree of gall bladder wall
	Plasma (μg/ml)	A-bile (μg/ml)	B-bile (μg/ml)	Gall bladder wall (μg/g)	
1	165.0 at 14 min 138.0 at 30 min 110.0 at 45 min 100.0 at 50 min	52.2 at 14 min	17.1 at 45 min	2.11 at 45 min	+
2	74.0 at 15 min 57.0 at 30 min	29.2 at 15 min 57.2 at 45 min	16.2 at 15 min	11.3 at 15 min	++
3	64.5 at 20 min			45.78[a] at 15 min	+++
4	43.5 at 50 min	46.8 at 20 min 40.8[c] at 30 min	ND[b] at 0 min ND[b] at 5 min 1.91 at 40 min	17.35 at 40 min	++
5	·71.0 at 15 min 48.5 at 30 min 47.0 at 45 min	48.5 at 30 min 27.0[c] at 40 min 59.5 at 45 min 8.8 at 90 min 4.4 at 105 min		20.22 at 15 min 13.71 at 30 min 11.13 at 45 min	+++
6	89.0 at 30 min	14.8 at 15 min 12.5[c] at 19 min	14.6 at 35 min	24.9 at 33 min	++

[a] Mucous membrane only; in the other parts of the gall bladder wall the concentration was 12.11 μg/g.
[b] White bile.
[c] Diluted by Biligrafin solution for cholangiography.

TABLE 3. *Cefmetazole concentration in various body fluids and tissues during operation after intravenous administration of 1,000 mg to patients 7-11 in Table 1*

Patient	Cefmetazole concn at indicated time after injection		
	Plasma (µg/ml)	Appendix (µg/g)	Ascites (µg/ml)
7		14.2 at 45 min	9.0 at 30 s 29.1 at 10 min 42.5 at 20 min 59.0 at 50 min
8	92.6 at 30 min	29.67, 28.26, and 25.00 at 30 min[a]	
9	43.5 at 50 min	49.67 at 7 min[b] 60.0 and 54.23 at 13 min[c] 44.75 at 15 min[d]	
10	55.0 at 25 min	12.27 at 5 min	20.2 at 5 min
11	113.0 at 20 min	18.5 at 20 min	49.5 at 10 min

[a] Concentrations in the mucous membrane, other parts of the appendix, and the mesoappendix, respectively.

[b] Concentration in the tip of the appendix.

[c] Concentration in the mucous membrane and other parts of the appendix, respectively.

[d] Concentration in the mesoappendix.

clinically in some patients with cholecystitis and peritonitis, whose tissues were taken and subjected to microbioassay for determination of CMZ.

The new knowledge obtained from this study on the CMZ concentration in infected tissues is as follows. (i) The CMZ concentration in purulent ascites increased gradually until 1 h after intravenous administration. (ii) The CMZ concentration in A-bile increased gradually until 30 min or 1 h, followed by a slow decline. (iii) The CMZ concentrations in white B-bile were very low. Further, CMZ was observed in white bile through the gall bladder wall 30 to 40 minutes after intravenous injection. (iv) In the case of cholecystitis, the CMZ concentration in the gall bladder wall reached a peak 15 min after intravenous injection, followed by a gradual decline. (v) The CMZ concentration in the infected mucous membranes was higher than that in other locations in patients with abdominal infection. (vi) CMZ concentrations in the inflammatory soft tissues reached a peak 10 to 15 min after intravenous injection, followed by a gradual decrease. (vii) CMZ concentrations in the gall bladder wall and appendix with infections were directly proportional to the degree of pathological changes of the inflammation. (viii) CMZ was distributed quickly in the seriously infected organs or tissues and stayed for a comparatively long time.

CMZ was used clinically in six patients with cholecystitis and five patients with acute peritonitis (Table 1). Tissue specimens were taken from these 11 patients and subjected to microbioassay as above for the CMZ determination (Tables 2 and 3). CMZ was given by drip infusion at a daily dose of 2 to 4 g. Clinical responses were excellent in four cases, good in seven cases, and fair or poor in none. No adverse effects were observed.

Cefmetazole therefore appears to be a very useful drug when used in the treatment of abdominal infections.

1. **Kasai Y., et al.** 1979. Clinical pharmacokinetics of intravenously administered Cefmetazole in the infected tissues. Chemotherapy (Tokyo) **27**:275–282. (In Japanese.)
2. **Kiss, J., et al.** 1978. Pharmacokinetic study of rifampicin in biliary surgery. Int. J. Clin. Pharmacol. **16**:105–109.
3. **Nakamura T., et al.** 1978. Debekacin concentration in various tissues of patients. Chemotherapy (Tokyo) **26**:377–378.
4. **Nakamura T., et al.** 1979. Bacampicillin concentration in various tissues of patients. Chemotherapy (Tokyo) **27**(S-4):202–205.

Clinical Experiences with Cefmetazole in Japan

KEIMEI MASHIMO

Director, Tokyo Koseinenkin Hospital, Tokyo, Japan

Cefmetazole is a new cephamycin antibiotic developed in 1973 by Sankyo Co., Ltd. (Japan). It is extremely stable for β-lactamase because it has a 7α-methoxy group. It displays better antibacterial potency against *Escherichia coli*, *Klebsiella*, etc., than conventional cephalosporin antibiotics such as cefazolin; in addition, it has excellent antibacterial activity against indole-positive *Proteus* strains and *Serratia*, against which conventional penicillin and cephalosporin antibiotics are ineffective.

Results of clinical examinations carried out on infections of middle and serious degree in departments of internal medicine, surgery, urology, and obstetrics and gynecology at university hospitals and public hospitals (total, 63 institutions) from December 1976 to October 1977 are summarized and reported.

A total of 1,049 patients were examined, but 97 were excluded because they were also receiving other antibacterial agents; thus 952 cases were analyzed. There were 492 men and 460 women, ranging in age from 15 to 89 years. The most frequent route of administration was intravenous drip infusion (495 patients), followed by intravenous and intramuscular injections. The most frequent daily dose was 2 g; 1 g was next

most frequent. The minimum and maximum daily doses were 0.5 and 6 g, respectively. In most patients, the drug was administered twice a day.

Clinical effects classified by each disease are shown in Table 1. There were 439 patients with urinary tract infections, and the effective rate of treatment was 71.1%. This is considered a satisfactory result because more than half of these were chronic complicated infections of the urinary tract. The effective rate in 243 cases of respiratory tract infection was 75.5%, and that in 63 cases of infections of the liver-bile duct was

TABLE 1. *Clinical effect of cefmetazole according to disease group*

Disease group	No. of cases	Clinical effect				Efficacy	
		Ex-cel-lent	Good	Poor	Un-known	No./total	Percent
Septicemia	16	2	10	1	3	12/16	75.0
Bacterial endocarditis	3		2		1	2/3	66.7
Soft tissue infection	29	6	14	3	6	20/29	69.0
Resiratory tract infection	243	60	124	22	37	184/243	75.7
Hepatobiliary tract infection	63	9	41	5	8	50/63	79.4
Peritonitis and intraperitoneal infection	55	9	37	5	4	46/55	83.6
Urinary tract infection	439	107	205	7	120	312/439	71.1
Prostatitis, epididymitis	5	2	3			5/5	100.0
Gynecological infection	85	21	57	1	6	78/85	91.8
Paranasal sinusitis, mumps	2	1			1	1/2	50.0
Prevention of postoperative infection	7		6		1	6/7	85.7
Other infections[a]	5		4		1	4/5	80.0
Total	952	217	503	44	188	720/952	75.6

[a] Enteritis, 2 cases; appendicitis, 2 cases; suppurative parotitis, 1 case.

TABLE 2. *Bacteriological effects of cefmetazole by main causative organisms*

Causative organism	No. of strains	Bacteriological effect			Percent eradicated
		Eradicated	Decreased	Persisted	
Staphylococcus	41	32	4	5	78.0
Streptococcus	31	24	2	5	77.4
Enterococcus	43	32	3	8	74.4
S. pneumoniae	11	10	1		90.9
Other gram-positive cocci	8	8			100.0
E. coli	218	192	14	12	88.1
Citrobacter	21	17	1	3	81.0
Klebsiella	112	92	6	14	82.1
Enterobacter	41	22	6	13	53.7
Serratia	79	64	1	14	81.0
Indole-positive *Proteus*	42	33	3	6	78.6
Indole-negative *Proteus*	28	24	3	1	85.7
Proteus sp.	5	4	1		80.0
Pseudomonas sp.	45	11	2	32	24.4
H. influenzae	21	17	2	2	81.0
H. parainfluenzae	4	4			100.0
Neisseria	1			1	0.0
Other gram-negative rods	23	14	2	7	60.9
Bacteroides	11	8	2	1	72.7
Others	5	4	1		80.0
Total	790	612	54	124	77.5

79.4%. The effective rate in 16 cases of septicemia and 3 cases of bacterial endocarditis, a total of 19 cases, was 73.7%. The effective rate in all 952 cases was 75.6%, which is an excellent result.

The bacteriological effect of cefmetazole is shown in Table 2. For 790 strains on which a bacteriological follow-up was possible, an eradication rate of 77.5% was obtained as a whole. The eradication rate for gram-positive cocci was 86.6%. For gram-negative bacilli, it was 88.1% for 218 strains of *E. coli* and 82.1% for 112 strains of *Klebsiella*. For 28 strains of *P. mirabilis* and 42 of indole-positive *Proteus*, the eradication rates were 85.7 and 78.6%, respectively. It is noteworthy that the eradication rate for 79 strains of *Serratia* was 81.0%. For 45 strains of *Pseudomonas*, the eradication rate remained at 24.4%. Among 55 patients in whom earlier chemotherapy (cefazolin, cephalothin, cefalexin, ampicillin,

carbenicillin, etc.) had failed to eradicate the bacteria, cefmetazole caused eradication in 46 patients (83.6%). These successful cases included eradication of 87.5% of 16 *E. coli* strains, 100% of 8 *Klebsiella* strains, 75.0% of 8 *Serratia* strains, and 100.0% in 5 strains of indole-positive *Proteus*.

Clinical side effects included eruption observed in 10 patients (1.0%) and 34 occurrences of such side effects as nausea, headache, etc., in 26 patients. Laboratory tests before and after administration revealed elevation of serum glutamic oxalacetic and pyruvic transaminases in 22 of 790 cases (2.8%) and 21 of 779 cases (2.7%), respectively, and eosinophilia in 8 of 433 cases (1.8%). However, no serious abnormality was observed.

The above results indicate that cefmetazole is widely effective and useful for infections due to gram-positive cocci and gram-negative bacilli.

Clinical Effects of Cefmetazole in Pediatric Patients

RYOCHI FUJII

Department of Pediatrics, Teikyo University School of Medicine, Tokyo, Japan

Cefmetazole (CMZ) is a cephamycin antibiotic with a broad spectrum, acting powerfully on many β-lactamase–producing resistant bacteria as well as on susceptible bacteria, because of its potent resistance against β-lactamase.

Since the high efficacy and safety of CMZ have been confirmed in adults, it was considered necessary to evaluate CMZ for future use in serious infections in children. Therefore, the departments of pediatrics of 14 institutions which were accustomed to cooperative study on clinical examinations in the Japan Society of Chemotherapy organized a study committee, and evaluation was made after administration of CMZ in various infections.

Blood level and urinary elimination. The mean blood levels achieved after a single intravenous (i.v.) injection of 15 mg/kg (six cases) and 30 mg/kg (three cases) in children were 46.8 and 97.0 μg/ml, respectively, at 15 min, and 1.2 and 3.2 μg/ml at 4 h. The biological half-lives were 0.81 and 0.75 h, respectively. Thus, a dose-response relationship was observed between these two dosage groups.

The mean blood levels of CMZ when administered by i.v. drip infusion over 60 min at doses of 15 mg/kg (two cases) and 30 mg/kg (two cases) were 45.0 and 69.5 μg/ml, respectively, as

a 60-min value at the time of completion of the i.v. drip infusion. The half-lives were 0.91 and 0.75 h, respectively. A dose-response relationship was observed as in the case of single i.v. injections.

The recovery rate in urine was examined after single i.v. injections of CMZ at doses of 15 mg/kg (five cases) and 30 mg/kg (six cases), and a high urinary recovery rate was observed. Within 6 h after administration the mean recovery rate was 89.6% in the group given 15 mg/kg and 91.9% in the group given 30 mg/kg.

Clinical results. The age distribution of patients examined was 77 infants, 65 young children, and 45 school children over 6 years old. There were 110 boys and 77 girls, a total of 187.

Daily dosage was usually 40 to 100 mg/kg administered as a single i.v. injection or as an i.v. drip infusion, by dividing the dose into two to four times a day.

As shown in Table 1, clinical efficacy according to each disease was 87.1% for pneumonia, 55.6% for pyothorax, 66.7% for septicemia, 62.5% for suppurative meningitis, 93.8% for bronchitis, 92.0% for urinary tract infections, and 100% for skin-soft tissue infection. The clinical response of a total of 187 patients to CMZ was excellent in 59, good in 95, fair in 10, poor in 15, and

TABLE 1. *Results of cefmetazole treatment classified by clinical diagnosis*

Diagnosis	Clinical effects						Efficacy (%)[a]
	Excellent	Good	Fair	Poor	Unknown	Total	
Upper respiratory tract infection	8	4				12	100
Bronchitis	6	9	1			16	93.8
Pneumonia	21	40	1	8	3	73	87.1
Pyothorax	1	4	1	3	1	10	55.6
Septicemia	3	3	2	1	1	10	66.7
Meningitis	1	4	2	1		8	62.5
Enteritis	1	3	1			5	80.0
Peritonitis		1	1			2	50.0
Urinary tract infection	10	13		2	3	28	92.0
Lymphadenitis	3	3	1			7	85.7
SSS syndrome	2	1				3	100
Pyoderma	3	10				13	100
Total	59	95	10	15	8	187	86.0

[a] Percent efficacy = (excellent + good)/(total number of patients − unknown) × 100.

TABLE 2. *Results of cefmetazole treatment classified by causative organisms*

Organism isolated	Bacteriological effects					Eradication rate (%)[a]
	Eradicated	Decreased	No change	Unknown	Total	
Staphylococcus aureus	17	3	2	5	27	91.0
S. epidermidis	3		1		4	75.0
Streptococcus haemolyticus	3		1		4	75.0
Gram-positive cocci	1			7	8	100
Subtotal	24	3	4	12	43	87.1
Haemophilus influenzae	8	1		2	11	100
Escherichia coli	18			3	21	100
Klebsiella	6	2	1		9	88.9
Proteus spp.	2				2	100
P. mirabilis	2				2	100
Salmonella C			1		1	0
Pseudomonas spp.			2	1	3	0
Subtotal	36	3	4	6	49	90.7
Haemophilus influenzae + *S. aureus*	1				1	100
H. influenzae + *Streptococcus pneumoniae*	1				1	100
E. coli + *Proteus* spp.	1				1	100
E. coli + enterococcus				1	1	
Subtotal	3			1	4	100
Total	63	6	8	19	96	89.6

[a] Percent eradication = (eradicated + decreased)/(total number of patients − unknown) × 100.

unknown in 8, for an effective rate (excellent plus good) of 86.0%.

Bacteriological effect classified by pathogenic bacteria. As shown in Table 2, the bacteriological eradication efficacy against pathogenic microorganisms was 91.0% for *Staphylococcus aureus* and 87.1% for gram-positive cocci as a whole. Against gram-negative bacilli, efficacy was 100% for *Haemophilus influenzae*, 100% for *Escherichia coli*, 88.9% for *Klebsiella*, and 100% for *Proteus mirabilis*. As a whole, the eradication efficacy was 90.7% for gram-negative bacilli.

Side effects and abnormal laboratory findings. The rate of appearance of subjective and objective symptoms was 5.3% (10 of 187 patients). These side effects included 2 cases of diarrhea (1.1%), 4 cases (2.1%) of urticaria-like eruption, 3 cases (1.6%) of vascular pain, and 1 case (0.5%) of dermal candidiasis.

Abnormal laboratory findings appeared in 9 of 187 cases (4.8%). Glutamic oxalacetic transaminase was elevated in one patient (0.5%), glutamic oxalacetic and pyruvic transaminases were elevated in three (1.6%), lactic dehydrogenase was elevated in three (1.6%), eosinophilia occurred in one (0.5%), and neutropenia occurred in one (0.5%). All of these abnormalities were light in degree and normal values returned upon discontinuation of CMZ.

No side effect considered serious was observed.

Conclusion. In the 187 cases of serious infections in infants, young children, and school children treated with single i.v. injections or i.v. drip infusion of CMZ at a daily dose of 40 to 100 mg/kg divided into two to four times, the bacteria isolated as pathogens were mostly *S. aureus*, *H. influenzae*, *E. coli*, *Klebsiella*, and *Proteus* spp.

The clinical efficacy rate as a whole was 86.0% (154 of 179 cases, excluding unknown cases), and 89.6% of the pathogenic bacteria were eradicated (69 of 77 cases, excluding unknown cases). No noteworthy serious side effect was observed. These results indicate a high efficacy and safety of CMZ for various bacterial infections in infancy and childhood.

Double-Blind Comparison of the Effects of Cefmetazole and Cefazolin in Respiratory Tract Infections

F. MIKI* AND K. SHIOTA

Osaka City University Medical School, Osaka, Japan

Cefmetazole (CMZ) is a new cephamycin antibiotic characterized by its more potent antibacterial activity against gram-negative bacteria than that of existing cephalosporins and also by its stability to numerous β-lactamases. To clarify the extent to which these characteristics are reflected in clinical practice, a double-blind comparative study on CMZ and cefazolin (CEZ) in respiratory tract infections was carried out in 38 institutions.

Patients and methods. Patients with chronic respiratory tract infections (infected pulmonary emphysema, infected pulmonary fibrosis, infected bronchial asthma, etc.) and patients with acute respiratory tract infections (pneumonia, lung abscess, etc.) who also had some underlying diseases such as lung cancer, pulmonary tuberculosis, pulmonary edema, chronic obstructive lung diseases, etc., were chosen as subjects. Only patients who were admitted to the hospitals were selected, regardless of sex. Patients omitted from the trial included children under 15 years of age, patients in whom the initial suspicion of infection was not confirmed, patients with extremely serious underlying diseases or complications, patients treated with CMZ or CEZ immediately before the present treatment was started, patients with infections due to *Pseudomonas aeruginosa*, *Streptococcus faecalis*, or *Enterobacter*, patients with a past history of hypersensitivity to cephalosporin preparations, women in gestation or lactation, and patients with renal disturbances and those requiring concomitant treatment with diuretics such as furosemide.

CMZ or CEZ was intravenously drip-infused twice daily for 14 days at a daily dose of 4 g.

For the purpose of evaluating efficacy and adverse reactions, body temperature, cough, sputum (volume and appearance), dyspnea, chest pain, rales, cyanosis, and other remarkable symptoms and signs were observed every day. Laboratory investigations including ESR, CRP, leukocyte count and leukocyte differentials, erythrocyte count, hemoglobin, hematocrit, platelet count, urine protein, urine sediment, serum glutamic oxalacetic and pyruvic transaminases, alkaline phosphatase, serum creatinine, blood urea nitrogen, arterial blood gas (P_{O_2}, P_{CO_2}), mycoplasmal antibody titer, cold hemagglutinin titer, X-ray examination of the chest, and bacteriological examination of sputum were performed before, during, and after treatment.

Evaluation and statistical analysis of results. A committee of 11 experienced doctors from seven institutions examined all the X-ray films and records of symptoms, signs, and laboratory data on each patient, and then clinical and bacteriological responses and adverse reactions were judged.

The clinical response was judged as excellent (in the case of rapid and complete remission), good (complete remission), fair (partial remission), or poor (no improvement).

The therapeutic effects were analyzed statistically for 176 patients (90 administered CMZ,

86 administered CEZ) after excluding those in whom the initial suspicion of infection was not confirmed or the medication was not performed in accordance with the rules of protocol. The side effects were also analyzed statistically in

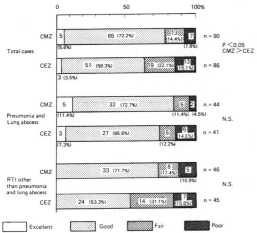

FIG. 1. *Clinical responses of 176 patients with respiratory tract infections (RTI) to treatment with cefmetazole (CMZ) or cefazolin (CEZ).*

231 patients (CMZ, 120; CEZ, 111) in whom the judgment was possible.

Results. No significant differences were observed between the two groups administered CMZ or CEZ concerning the background of patients, such as age, sex, body weight, and underlying diseases, or concerning symptoms, signs, chest X-ray findings, and laboratory findings before the treatment; therefore, it was confirmed that these antibiotics were administered to patient groups with little difference of background and severity. The causative bacteria isolated from sputum were *Staphylococcus aureus* in 8 patients treated with CMZ and in 1 patient treated with CEZ, *Streptococcus pneumoniae* in 9 and 4, *Escherichia coli* in 0 and 4, *K. pneumoniae* in 6 and 8, and *H. influenzae* in 9 and 6. In no patients treated with CMZ but in 2 treated with CEZ, mixed infection due to gram-positive and gram-negative bacteria was present. In the remaining 119 cases the causative bacteria were unclarified.

The clinical results in a total of 176 patients (90 administered CMZ, 86 administered CEZ) with pneumonia and lung abscess (85 patients) or respiratory tract infection other than pneu-

TABLE 1. *Side effects in 31 of 120 patients treated with cefmetazole and 25 of 111 patients treated with cefazolin*

Side effect[a]	Cefmetazole		Cefazolin	
	Administration continued	Administration discontinued	Administration continued	Administration discontinued
No. with side effects	26 (21.7)[b]	5 (4.2)	24(21.6)	1 (0.9)
Eruption	0	2 (1.7)	1 (0.9)	0
Fever	0	1 (0.8)	0	1 (0.9)
Itching	1 (0.8)	0	0	0
Diarrhea	0	1 (0.8)	0	0
Upper abdominal discomfort	0	0	1 (0.9)	0
Nausea	0	0	1 (0.9)	0
Nausea and anorexia	0	0	1 (0.9)	0
Tendency to hemorrage	0	0	1 (0.9)	0
GOT, GPT, Al-P elevation	2 (1.7)	0	2 (1.8)	0
GOT, GPT elevation	3 (2.5)	1 (0.8)	3 (2.7)	0
GOT, Al-P elevation	0	0	1 (0.9)	0
GOT elevation	1 (0.8)	0	4 (3.6)	0
GPT elevation	1 (0.8)	0	2 (1.8)	0
Al-P elevation	5 (4.2)	0	1 (0.9)	0
BUN S-creatinine elevation	1 (0.8)	0	0	0
BUN elevation	1 (0.8)	0	2 (1.8)	0
S-creatinine elevation	1 (0.8)	0	1 (0.9)	0
Decrease of Hb, Ht, RBC	1 (0.8)	0	2 (1.8)	0
Decrease of Hb, RBC	2 (1.7)	0	0	0
Decrease of Ht, RBC	1 (0.8)	0	0	0
Eosinophilia	10 (8.3)	0	3 (2.7)	0
Coombs test positive	1 (0.8)	0	0	0

[a] Abbreviations: GOT, glutamic oxalacetic transaminase; GPT, glutamic pyruvic transaminase; Al-P, alkaline phosphatase; BUN, blood urea nitrogen; S-creatinine, serum creatinine; Hb, hemoglobin; Ht, hematocrit; RBC, erythrocytes.

[b] Numbers in parentheses indicate percentages.

monia and lung abscess (91 patients) are shown in Fig. 1. In these 176 patients the therapeutic effects of CMZ were significantly superior to those of CEZ ($P < 0.05$). The efficacy rate in the patients treated with CMZ was higher than that with CEZ in the group with pneumonia and lung abscess as well as in the group with respiratory tract infections other than pneumonia and lung abscess; however, the differences between the two groups were not significant statistically.

By comparing symptoms, signs, chest X-ray findings, and laboratory findings on the 3rd, 7th, and 14th days after the beginning of the treatment with those before the treatment, differences between the CMZ group and the CEZ group concerning degrees of improvement in symptoms, signs, chest X-ray findings, leukocyte counts, ESR, and CRP were observed. CMZ gave a significantly better result in lowering body temperature on the 3rd day and in decreasing the volume of sputum on the 14th day than did CEZ in patients with pneumonia and those with lung abscess. As regards the decrease in cough on the 3rd day, CMZ was also significantly

more effective than CEZ in patients with respiratory tract infections other than pneumonia and lung abscess.

No significant differences in the bacteriological effects were observed between the two antibiotics.

As shown in Table 1, no serious adverse reactions were observed in any patient administered CMZ or CEZ. In five patients given CMZ and one given CEZ medication was discontinued because of side effects. No significant difference was noted between the two drugs in the occurrence of side effects.

Conclusion. CMZ was significantly more effective than CEZ in respiratory tract infections at a dose of 4 g daily. No significant difference was noted between the two drugs in the occurrence of side effects.

From these comparative results on therapeutic effects and side effects of these two drugs, it is thought that CMZ is more useful than CEZ in the treatment of acute and chronic respiratory tract infections.

Double-Blind Controlled Study Comparing Cefmetazole and Cefazolin in the Treatment of Chronic Complicated Urinary Tract Infections

J. KUMAZAWA,* S. NAKAMUTA, AND S. MOMOSE

Department of Urology, Faculty of Medicine, Kyushu University, Fukuoka, Japan

To confirm objectively the effectiveness, safety, and usefulness of cefmetazole (CMZ), a new cephamycin antibiotic, for treatment of chronic complicated urinary tract infections, it was compared in a double-blind study by using cefazolin (CEZ) as the standard treatment.

Subjects were male and female adults (above 16 years old) with chronic complicated urinary tract infections whose urine contained more than 10^4 bacteria/ml. The subjects were hospitalized and treated in the urological departments of 44 hospitals, mainly the urological departments of 8 university medical schools in the Kyushu district.

CMZ as well as CEZ was administered in the regimen of 1 g (potency) per dose and two doses per day (total, 2 g per day) for 5 consecutive days. The drugs were administered to a total of 248 patients (CMZ, 125; CEZ, 123).

A coordinating committee was organized to assess the efficacy of the drugs in accordance with Urinary Tract Infection Criteria for Clinical Evaluation of Antimicrobial Agent by using the

survey reports submitted by the institutions. In addition, the efficacy assessments made by the physicians in charge were evaluated by the committee.

The total number of cases assessed by the committee was 188 (CMZ, 94; CEZ, 94); the remaining cases were either excluded or dropped out of the study. Of the cases studied, cardiovascular diseases as systemic complications were found in 13.8% of the patients in the CMZ group and 3.2% in the CEZ group, the CMZ group being significantly higher in this respect. However, this is not considered to be directly related to the clinical efficacy as determined in the present study. No significant difference was observed between the two groups with respect to other background factors. The total number of cases assessed by the physicians in charge was 234 (CMZ, 120; CEZ, 114), with no significant difference in background factors found between the two groups.

Of the cases assessed by the committee, the overall rate of effectiveness was significantly higher in the CMZ group than in the CEZ group (Fig. 1). CMZ showed significantly higher efficacy against bacteriura. As to bacteriological response, the CMZ group showed a significantly higher rate of eradication and efficacy against *Serratia marcescens* as well as mixed infections due to *S. marcescens* and other bacteria.

In the cases of pyuria (+++), CMZ showed a significantly higher rate of efficacy; however, no significant difference between the two drug groups was noted in the correction of pyuria. Incidences of fever, pollakiuria, pain in urination, and lumbago were also investigated: no significant difference was observed between the two groups.

No significant difference in the overall clinical efficacy was noted between the two groups of patients subjected to assessments by the physicians in charge (Fig. 1).

CMZ and CEZ were challenged by the clinically isolated (from urines at the time of initial diagnoses) strains of *Escherichia coli, Klebsiella pneumoniae, S. marcescens,* and indole-positive *Proteus* (10^8 and 10^6 cells/ml each) to determine their MICs against these organisms. All of the strains showed higher susceptibilities to CMZ than to CEZ.

The relationship between the MIC for bacteria isolated from urine at the first diagnosis and the specific activity of β-lactamase showed values of less than one in all cases in which CMZ was used as substrate (Fig. 2). No correlation

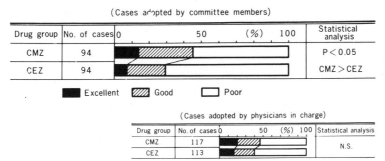

FIG. 1. *Overall clinical efficacy of cefmetazole (CMZ) and cefazolin (CEZ) in the patients analyzed by committee members and by the physicians in charge.*

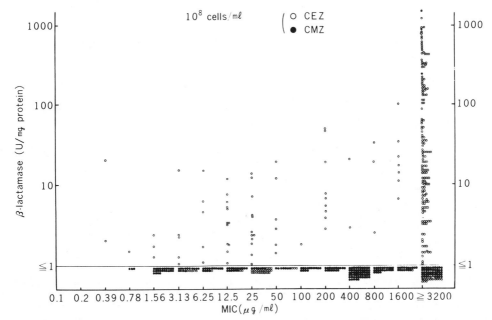

FIG. 2. *Relationship of β-lactamase activity and the MIC of cefmetazole (CMZ) and cefazolin (CEZ) for the organisms isolated from urines collected during the initial diagnosis (patients analyzed by committee members).*

was noted between specific activity of β-lactamase and the MIC for either antibiotic.

No significant difference was found between the two groups with respect to clinical usefulness of the drugs as determined by the physicians in charge.

No side effect was noted in the CMZ group, whereas three patients in the CEZ group required cessation of the drug. The rates of side effects in the two drug groups showed no significant variance.

In the laboratory findings, transient abnormal values of serum glutamic oxalacetic transaminase (SGOT) were found in three patients, serum glutamic pyruvic transaminase (SGPT) in two patients, and alkali phosphatase in one patient in the CMZ group; in the CEZ group transient abnormal values of blood urea nitrogen (one patient), serum creatinine (one patient), SGOT (four patients), and SGPT (two patients) were seen. However, there was no significant difference between the two groups in the rate of appearance of the side effects.

Based on the above findings, CMZ is considered to be a less toxic, safe, and clinically useful drug for the treatment of chronic complicated urinary tract infections.

Inhibition of the Type I β-Lactamase from *Enterobacter cloacae* by Cefonicid (SK&F 75073) and Related Compounds

DAVID J. NEWMAN,* RAJANIKANT J. MEHTA, BETTY ANNE BOWIE, CLAUDE H. NASH III,
AND PAUL ACTOR

*Microbiology Department, Research and Development Division, Smith Kline & French Laboratories,
Philadelphia, Pennsylvania 19101, U.S.A.*

Cefonicid (SK&F 75073) (1) was found to be resistant to hydrolysis by the type I β-lactamase from *Enterobacter cloacae* P99 (R. J. Mehta, D. J. Newman, B. A. Bowie, C. H. Nash III, and P. Actor, this volume), and further work indicated that cefonicid also inhibited the hydrolysis of the chromogenic cephalosporin, nitrocefin (Glaxo Ltd.). Since, to our knowledge, there were no good inhibitors of the type I β-lactamase from this organism (2), we decided to investigate further the inhibitory activities of cefonicid and related compounds when cephalothin was used as the enzyme substrate. The source of the organism and the method of isolation were reported by Mehta et al. (this volume). Reactions were performed in 100 mM potassium phosphate buffer, pH 7.0, in a total volume of 1 ml by use of a thermostatted cuvette assembly (30°C) and 10-mm cells. Substrates and inhibitors were added at suitable concentrations. After addition of suitable volumes of enzyme to initiate reaction, the time course was followed by observing the rate of decrease of absorbance at 260 nm in a recording Gilford 240 spectrophotometer. Control experiments were run with all compounds used as inhibitors to check that the *E. cloacae* enzyme did not hydrolyze the compound under the conditions of the assay.

The velocities of the reactions were calculated by tangential analysis of the progress curves, and apparent inhibition constants (K_{ia}) were obtained by drawing Dixon plots from regression lines calculated from the data. In all cases reported, the regression coefficients were at least 0.985. The initial Dixon plots were used in conjunction with Lineweaver-Burk plots to decide the type(s) of inhibition, and these were confirmed by a replotting of the inhibition data in the form "slope of Dixon plot versus the reciprocal of the substrate concentration." When this technique is used, the line from competitive inhibitors intersects the origin, whereas with noncompetitive inhibitors it intersects the abscissa in the negative quadrant.

The structures of the compounds tested are

TABLE 1. *Inhibition of the hydrolysis of cephalothin by the β-lactamase of E. cloacae P99*

Inhibitor	K_i (mol/liter)	Type of inhibition, comments
Cefonicid	800×10^{-9}	Noncompetitive
Cefamandole	$3,300 \times 10^{-9}$	Noncompetitive
SK&F 79433	92×10^{-9}	Noncompetitive
SK&F 80000	102×10^{-9}	Noncompetitive
SK&F 80303	45×10^{-9}	Noncompetitive
Clavulanic acid	—	No inhibition at 450 μM
CP45899	—	20% inhibition at 1,700 μM 80% inhibition at 17,000 μM
Tetrazoles		No inhibition at 100 μM
Oxime		No inhibition at 100 μM

shown in Fig. 1, and the kinetic constants for these compounds as inhibitors are given in Table 1. From inspection of our preliminary data, we thought that the substitution at the 3 position contributed significantly to the inhibition constants observed. Thus, with the substitution of an N-methylsulfonyl group for the N-methyl group on the tetrazole (see structures of cefonicid and cefamandole), the K_i was decreased fourfold and the type of inhibition remained the same. Further evidence for this idea was the approximately 20-fold decrease in K_i when SK&F 80303 was tested. However, this compound also had an altered 7 position when compared with the other two, as an α-hydroxyiminophenylacetic acid had been substituted for the mandelic acid in cefonicid and cefamandole. A check of the side-chain precursors (1-methyl-2-thiotetrazole, 1-methylsulfonyl-2-thiotetrazole, and α-hydroxyiminophenylacetic acid) did

not show any intrinsic inhibitory activity, nor did clavulanic acid or CP45899 (2), both potent β-lactamase inhibitors of all but type I enzymes. A search of our compound files was made for cephalosporins with a 7-α-hydroxyiminophenylacetyl substituent and with varied 3 substituents. Two such materials, SK&F 79433 and SK&F 80000, were identified and tested. Both of these compounds noncompetitively inhibited the hydrolysis of cephalothin with effectively identical kinetics. Since the 3 substituent of SK&F 79433 is the simple acetoxymethyl found in cephalothin and the K_i's of SK&F 79433 and 80000 are similar, we suggest that the noncompetitive inhibition of cephalothin hydrolysis by cephalosporins is effectively controlled by the substitution pattern of the 7 position and that it is possible that a 7-(2-thienyl-α-iminohydroxy) derivative of cephalothin might be an excellent inhibitor of the *E. cloacae* enzyme.

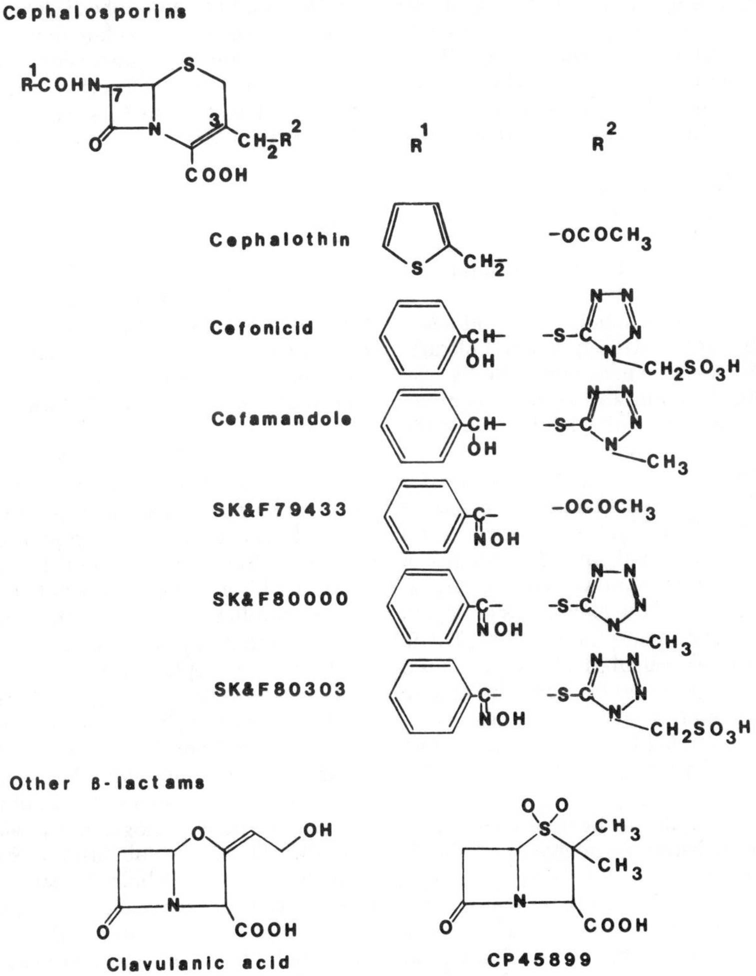

FIG. 1. *Compounds used.*

1. **Actor, P., J. V. Uri, I. Zajac, J. R. Guarini, L. Phillips, D. H. Pitkin, D. A. Berges, G. L. Dunn, J. R. E. Hoover, and J. Weisbach.** 1977. SK&F 75073, a new parenteral broad-spectrum cephalosporin with high and prolonged serum levels. Antimicrob. Agents Chemother. 13:784–790.

2. **English, A. R., J. A. Retsema, A. E. Girard, J. E. Lynch, and W. E. Barth.** 1978. CP-45899, a beta-lactamase inhibitor that extends the antibacterial spectrum of beta-lactams: initial bacteriological characterization. Antimicrob. Agents Chemother. 14:414–419.

Stability of Cefonicid (SK&F 75073) to β-Lactamases

RAJANIKANT J. MEHTA, DAVID J. NEWMAN, BETTY ANNE BOWIE,* CLAUDE H. NASH III,
AND PAUL ACTOR

*Microbiology Department, Research and Development Division, Smith Kline & French Laboratories,
Philadelphia, Pennsylvania 19101, U.S.A.*

The potency and antimicrobial spectrum of specific β-lactam compounds are the result of their stability toward inactivation by β-lactamase enzymes, their binding to cellular sites, and their rate of uptake by the cell. In this study we compared the β-lactamase stability of cefonicid (a new semisynthetic cephalosporin, SK&F 75073) (1) to that of cephalothin, cefamandole, and cefoxitin. In addition, we investigated the intrinsic permeability resistance of *Enterobacter cloacae* P99.

The β-lactamases used were isolated from *E. cloacae* P99, *Klebsiella aerogenes* K1, *Escherichia coli* RPI, and *Bacteroides fragilis* HH154 (2) by sonication, ultracentrifugation, and ultrafiltration, and from *Escherichia coli* strains TEM and RGN 238 by breakage in liquid nitrogen followed by ultracentrifugation and ultrafiltration. In the kinetic experiments, the hydrolysis of the cephalosporin antibiotics was monitored spectrophotometrically by following the rate of decrease of absorbance at 260 nm with a recording Gilford 240 spectrophotometer equipped with a constant-temperature (30°C) cuvette assembly. The reaction mixtures (total volume of 1 ml) contained suitable amounts of the enzyme preparations and various concentrations (50 to 200 μM) of the substrates dissolved in 100 mM potassium phosphate buffer, pH 7.0. The initial rates were calculated from tangential analysis of the progress curves. Apparent kinetic constants were determined by linear regression analysis of conventional Lineweaver-Burk plots (regression coefficients being equal to or greater than 0.985).

The kinetic constants for the isolated enzymes and the various substrates are given in Table 1. Cefoxitin was resistant to all the enzymes tested. Cefonicid and cefamandole were resistant to hydrolysis by the type I enzyme from *E. cloacae* under the conditions used. Further inspection showed that cefonicid and cefamandole differed significantly in their affinities (K_m's) and maximal velocities (V_{max}'s) for the type III A and III B enzymes, whereas with the type IV, the affinities differed but the maximal velocities were similar. With the anaerobe *B. fragilis*, cefonicid was not hydrolyzed; cefamandole exhibited a high affinity but a low intrinsic velocity with this preparation. Data from other sources (5) gave similar values for the K_m's with the type I and III A enzymes, but V_{max} data cannot easily be compared because neither absolute values nor the basis for the relative values were given in detail.

Since cefonicid was not hydrolyzed by the isolated enzyme from *E. cloacae* P99, it was surprising that the MIC for this strain (>200 μg/ml) was much higher than the MIC for other *E. cloacae* strains (1). We also had data showing that cefonicid was a noncompetitive inhibitor of the β-lactamase when cephalothin was used as the substrate (D. J. Newman, R. J. Mehta, B. A. Bowie, C. H. Nash III, and P. Actor, this volume). To determine whether membrane impermeability played a role in the intrinsic resistance of this strain, we attempted to study the rate of hydrolysis of cephalothin with cefonicid as an inhibitor, using both whole cells and cells whose membranes had been modified. Unfortunately, cephalothin and cefonicid could not be analyzed for cephalothin hydrolysis by the method of Mehta et al. (2) because of severe interference by cell metabolites on the high-pressure liquid chromatography columns used. Further experiments with the isolated enzyme indicated that cefonicid also inhibited the hydrolysis of the chromogenic cephalosporin, Nitrocefin. Thus, we substituted Nitrocefin for cephalothin in the whole-cell studies. The rate of hydrolysis of Nitrocefin was significantly accelerated when the outer cell membrane was disrupted either by pretreatment with polymyxin B at 1 μg/ml or by sonication. Under the

TABLE 1. *Comparative kinetic constants of various cephalosporins against five major gram-negative and one anaerobic β-lactamase*[a]

β-Lactamase[b]	Cephalothin		Cefonicid		Cefamandole	
	K_m[c]	V_{max}[d]	K_m	V_{max}	K_m	V_{max}
E. cloacae type I	60×10^{-6}	5.0×10^{-6}	NH[e]		NH	
E. coli TEM type III A	141×10^{-6}	9.8×10^{-6}	120×10^{-6}	3.7×10^{-6}	514×10^{-6}	26.6×10^{-6}
E. coli RPI type III B	166×10^{-6}	8.2×10^{-6}	66×10^{-6}	3.1×10^{-6}	236×10^{-6}	18.7×10^{-6}
K. aerogenes KI type IV	110×10^{-6}	11.5×10^{-6}	95×10^{-6}	11.3×10^{-6}	497×10^{-6}	10.0×10^{-6}
E. coli RGN238 type V	96×10^{-6}	8.3×10^{-6}	169×10^{-6}	8.5×10^{-6}	141×10^{-6}	5.9×10^{-6}
B. fragilis HH154 anaerobe	135×10^{-6}	14.1×10^{-6}	NH		18×10^{-6}	2.0×10^{-6}

[a] Cefoxitin was also tested but was found to be resistant to all the enzymes tested.
[b] Enzyme type according to references 3 and 4.
[c] Expressed in moles per liter.
[d] Expressed in moles per liter per minute.
[e] NH, No hydrolysis.

conditions of the experiment, vancomycin at 100 μg/ml had no accelerant effect.

From the experiments reported above, the following conclusions may be drawn. (i) Cefonicid is more stable than cefamandole with the preparations from *E. coli* TEM (III A), *E. coli* RPI (III B), and *B. fragilis*; it is equivalent with the preparations from *E. cloacae* P99 (I) and *K. aerogenes* K1 (IV) and is slightly less stable with the preparation from *E. coli* RGN 238 (V). (ii) Cefamandole is a substrate for the β-lactamase from the anaerobe *B. fragilis*. (iii) The high MIC of cefonicid against *E. cloacae* P99 may be due to the poor transport across the intact outer membrane.

1. Actor, P., J. V. Uri, I. Zajac, J. R. Guarini, L. Phillips, D. H. Pitkin, D. A. Berges, G. L. Dunn, J. R. E. Hoover, and J. A. Weisbach. 1977. SK&F 75073, a new parenteral broad-spectrum cephalosporin with high and prolonged serum levels. Antimicrob. Agents Chemother. 13:784–790.

2. Mehta, R. J., M. K. Fox, D. J. Newman, and C. H. Nash. 1977. An H.P.L.C. assay for cephalosporinase activity. J. Antibiot. 30:1132–1133.

3. Richmond, M. H., and N. A. Curtis. 1974. The interplay of β-lactamases and intrinsic factors in the resistance of Gram-negative bacteria to penicillins and cephalosporins. Ann. N.Y. Acad. Sci. 235:553–568.

4. Sykes, R. B., and M. Matthew. 1976. The β-lactamases of Gram-negative bacteria and their role in resistance to β-lactam antibiotics. J. Antimicrob. Chemother. 2: 115–157.

5. Vuye, A., and J. Pijck. 1978. Comparison of stabilities of cephalosporins against beta-lactamases from gram-negative organisms, p. 492–494. *In* Current chemotherapy, Proceedings of the 10th International Congress of Chemotherapy. American Society for Microbiology, Washington, D.C.

Comparison of Cefonicid with Cefamandole and Cefoxitin as Prophylactic Agents in Mouse Protection Tests

SARAH F. GRAPPEL,* LILLIAN PHILLIPS, PAUL ACTOR, AND JERRY A. WEISBACH

Smith Kline & French Laboratories, Philadelphia, Pennsylvania 19101, U.S.A.

Cefonicid (SK&F 75073) is a new cephalosporin with excellent activity against a broad spectrum of bacteria. Parenteral administration of cefonicid results in high and prolonged blood levels (1). The efficacy of cefonicid as a prophylactic antibiotic was, therefore, compared with that of cefamandole and cefoxitin in mouse protection tests.

Male albino Swiss mice, Webster-derived CD-1, weighing 18 to 20 g were used for these studies. Cultures of test organisms were diluted in 5.0% hog gastric mucin and injected intraperitoneally to produce uniformly lethal infections. The test antibiotics were administered subcutaneously in a single dose at the concentrations and time intervals before or after infection noted in the text. The final survival percentages for groups of 10 mice each were obtained after 3 days of observation. These percentages were used to estimate the LD_{50} for the inoculum as well as the ED_{50} of the antibiotics. The LD_{50} and the ED_{50} values were determined by the method of Litchfield and Wilcoxon (2).

A single subcutaneous dose of cefonicid at 40 mg/kg protected mice against lethal infections with *Staphylococcus aureus*, *Escherichia coli*,

TABLE 1. *Effect of a single subcutaneous dose of cefonicid and comparative compounds administered prior to infection in mouse protection tests*

Infecting organism	No. of LD$_{50}$'s	Cefonicid					Cefamandole					Cefoxitin				
		ED$_{50}^a$ (mg/kg)	Percent survivors^b				ED$_{50}^a$ (mg/kg)	Percent survivors^b				ED$_{50}^a$ (mg/kg)	Percent survivors^b			
			1 h	2 h	4 h	6 h		1 h	2 h	4 h	6 h		1 h	2 h	4 h	6 h
Staphylococcus aureus 674	3.2	3.7	100	80	70	60	4.8	0	0	0	0	32	0	0	0	0
Escherichia coli 12140	208	0.8	100	100	100	90	2.1	40	0	0	0	5.2	20	0	0	0
E. coli 1002	151	0.6	100	100	100	100	3.7	0	0	0	0	6.6	0	0	0	0
E. coli 801	10	11.5	80	60	60	50	1.4	20	20	0	0	6.8	10	20	0	0
Klebsiella pneumoniae 4200	480	0.6	100	100	90	100	0.6	0	0	0	0	33	0	0	0	0
Proteus mirabilis 442	4.6	0.3	100	100	100	100	9.6	0	0	0	0	5	10	0	0	0
P. mirabilis 416	10	0.6	100	100	100	100	4.3	0	0	0	0	5	0	0	0	0

^{a} Administered 1 h postinfection.
^{b} After administration of a single subcutaneous dose of 40 mg/kg at the indicated time preinfection.

TABLE 2. *Activity of cefonicid and comparative compounds administered subcutaneously 6 h preinfection or 1 h postinfection of mice*

Strain	No. of LD$_{50}$'s	ED$_{50}$ (mg/kg)					
		Cefonicid		Cefamandole		Cefoxitin	
		6 h pre-	1 h post-	6 h pre-	1 h post-	6 h pre-	1 h post-
S. aureus 674	3	65	8.1	. >100	15.5	>100	40
E. coli 12140	96	3.1	0.7	>100	0.6	>100	2.8
E. coli 1002	83	2.2	0.9	>100	2.7	>100	7.5
E. coli 801	8	33.0	10.5	>100	1.1	>100	5.7
K. pneumoniae 4200 ..	23	3.1	0.6	>100	1.3	>100	4.1
P. mirabilis 442	6	2.1	0.3	>100	8.4	>100	6.8
P. mirabilis 416	13	2.5	0.4	>100	4.8	>100	3.8

Klebsiella pneumoniae, and *Proteus mirabilis* when given as long as 6 h prior to infection (Table 1). No significant protection was obtained with cefamandole or cefoxitin when these compounds were administered 1, 2, 4, or 6 h prior to infection with the same strains. However, all of these compounds were effective when they were given 1 h postinfection in the same test. The ED$_{50}$'s obtained are shown in Table 1.

The ED$_{50}$'s for cefonicid administered 6 h prior to infection with each of the strains were determined (Table 2). No ED$_{50}$'s could be calculated for cefamandole or cefoxitin even when levels up to 100 mg/kg were used. However, all of the compounds were effective when adminis-

tered 1 h postinfection in the same test (Table 2).

Cefonicid's excellent activity against a broad spectrum of bacteria, even when administered several hours prior to infection, makes it a strong candidate for use in surgical prophylaxis.

1. **Actor, P., J. V. Uri, I. Zajac, J. R. Guarini, L. Phillips, D. H. Pitkin, D. A. Berges, G. L. Dunn, J. R. E. Hoover, and J. A. Weisbach.** 1978. SK&F 75073, new parenteral broad-spectrum cephalosporin with high and prolonged serum levels. Antimicrob. Agents Chemother. **13**:784–790.
2. **Litchfield, J. T., Jr., and F. Wilcoxon.** 1949. A simplified method of evaluating dose-effect experiments. J. Pharmacol. Exp. Ther. **96**:99–113.

Comparative In Vitro Activity of Cefonicid and Other Selected Cephalosporins Against *Neisseria gonorrhoeae*

IHOR ZAJAC,* HENRY BARTUS, PAUL ACTOR, AND JERRY WEISBACH

Smith Kline & French Laboratories, Philadelphia, Pennsylvania 19101, U.S.A.

Cefonicid, a new cephalosporin for parenteral administration, is currently under clinical investigation. This new cephalosporin has unique microbiological and pharmacokinetic properties

(1). We tested cefonicid against 60 strains of *Nesseria gonorrhoeae*, including five β-lactamase-producing strains, and found it to have excellent in vitro activity (Table 1). It was of interest to compare the activity of cefonicid and other selected cephalosporins under the conditions of low and high inoculum and in the presence of human serum against five strains of *N. gonorrhoeae* which produced β-lactamase. The presence of the enzyme was ascertained utilizing a unique property of nitrocefin which changes color with β-lactamase hydrolysis of the amide bond of the β-lactam ring (4).

All organisms were grown on supplemented Mueller-Hinton agar (1) at 37°C, 8% CO_2. The bacteria grown on slants were harvested by scraping the cells with a sterile cotton swab and resuspending by vigorous mixing on a Vortex mixer in a medium composed of Schaedler broth, yeast extract (0.025%), IsoVitaleX (10%), and glucose (1%), pH 7.1. The bacterial suspension was adjusted to 30% T and viability was determined. The MICs were determined by the agar dilution method (1). The surface of the agar was inoculated with the aid of a Steers replicator apparatus. After overnight incubation at 37°C, 8% CO_2, MICs were recorded as the lowest concentration of antibiotic completely inhibiting growth.

Concurrently, a duplicate set of inoculated plates was used for the determination of MBC. Areas inoculated with the Steers apparatus and showing no growth were removed and inoculated onto chocolate agar plates containing no antibiotics. The plates were incubated at 37°C, 8% CO_2, and were examined for growth at 24 and 48 h. The material transferred from the highest dilution and showing no growth on chocolate agar plates after 48 h of incubation was considered to be the MBC.

The results presented in Table 2 demonstrate that all low-inoculum MICs of cefonicid, cefamandole, cefuroxime, and cefoxitin were very similar, whereas cephapirin and penicillin were higher. Also there were negligible differences between MIC and MBC. Addition of human serum did not affect the MIC or MBC. Increasing the bacterial inoculum 100-fold resulted in no change of MIC for cefoxitin and cefuroxime. A slight increase in MIC of cefonicid and cefamandole and considerable increase for cephapirin and penicillin were observed when the inoculum was increased 100-fold.

A similar pattern was observed with these compounds when serum was incorporated into the medium. Cefoxitin and cefuroxime were not affected by the presence of serum, which is in agreement with the results reported in the lit-

TABLE 1. *Inhibitory effect of cefonicid and other selected cephalosporins on 60 strains of Neisseria gonorrhoeae*[a]

Compound tested	Cumulative % of organism inhibited (MIC, µg/ml)													
	0.003	0.006	0.012	0.025	0.05	0.1	0.2	0.4	0.8	1.6	3.1	6.2	12.5	25
Cefonicid	15	35	37	38	57	78	97	100						
Cefamandole ..		15	28	33	43	63	77	97	100					
Cefoxitin				8	12	27	38	82	95	100				
Cefazolin					15	33	45	72	98	100				
Cephapirin ...					15	32	38	52	80	98	100			
Penicillin G ...			3	22	35	43	53	67	87	92	93	93	98	100

[a] Fifty-five strains were non-β-lactamase producers and penicillin sensitive; five strains produced β-lactamase as determined by the chromophore method (4).

TABLE 2. *Effect of human serum on MIC and MBC of cefonicid and selected cephalosporins against five β-lactamase-producing strains of Neisseria gonorrhoeae at low and high inoculum*

Compound tested	Avg of two assays (µg/ml)							
	5×10^5 CFU/ml[a]				5×10^7 CFU/ml[a]			
	MIC	MIC/serum[b]	MBC	MBC/serum	MIC	MIC/serum	MBC	MBC/serum
Cefonicid	0.4	0.4	0.56	0.4	3.44	5.0	11.24	7.8
Cefamandole	0.96	0.56	1.42	1.04	5.6	12.0	31.24	40.0
Cefoxitin	0.6	0.68	1.28	0.8	0.64	0.96	1.42	1.42
Cephapirin	3.42	4.34	5.0	4.34	15.2	30.0	47.0	60.0
Cefuroxime	0.057	0.06	0.12	0.1	0.074	0.08	0.24	0.36
Penicillin G	2.26	1.72	5.14	3.44	220	1320	400	1600

[a] Average of five strains.
[b] Final serum concentration = 12.5%.

erature (2, 3). Cefonicid and cefamandole were only slightly affected; however, both the MIC and MBC of penicillin increased from 220 to 1,320 μg/ml and 400 to 1,600 μg/ml, respectively.

On the basis of these results, cefonicid shows considerable promise as an antigonococcal antibiotic. Its high and prolonged serum levels and effectiveness against β-lactamase-positive strains of *N. gonorrhoeae*, even in the presence of human serum in vitro, indicate the need for clinical trials to confirm and extend these in vitro observations.

1. Actor, P., J. V. Uri, I. Zajac, J. R. Guarini, L. Phillips,
D. H. Pitkin, D. A. Berges, G. L. Dunn, J. R. E. Hoover, and J. A. Weisbach. 1977. SK&F 75073, new parenteral broad-spectrum cephalosporin with high and prolonged serum levels. Antimicrob. Agents Chemother. 13:784–790.

2. Jorgenson, J. H., G. A. Alexander, and P. A. Grant. 1979. Comparison of three newer beta-lactam antibiotics against penicillinase-producing and non-penicillinase-producing *Neisseria gonorrhoeae*. Curr. Ther. Res. 25:74–78.

3. Phillips, I. 1978. The susceptibility of *Neisseria gonorrhoeae* to cefoxitin sodium. J. Antimicrob. Chemother. 4:61–64.

4. Uri, J. V., P. Actor, and J. A. Weisbach. 1978. A rapid and simple method for detection of β-lactamase inhibitors. J. Antibiot. 31:789–791.

Cefonicid (SK&F 75073) Serum Levels and Urinary Recovery After Intramuscular and Intravenous Administration

D. H. PITKIN,* P. ACTOR, F. ALEXANDER, J. DUBB, R. STOTE, AND J. A. WEISBACH

Smith Kline and French Laboratories, Philadelphia, Pennsylvania 19101, U.S.A.

Cefonicid (SK&F 75073) is a new parenterally active cephalosporin with broad-spectrum antimicrobial activity in vitro and in laboratory animals (1). The purpose of this study was to determine the safety, tolerance, serum levels, and urinary excretion of cefonicid in humans as compared to cefazolin and cefamandole.

Cefonicid was synthesized in the Smith Kline and French laboratories. Cefazolin was obtained as a commercial preparation from Smith Kline and French, and cefamandole was from Eli Lilly & Co. Antibiotics were dissolved in parenteral water and administered to human volunteers. None of the volunteers had a history of hypersensitivity towards penicillins or cephalosporins, a history of asthma, or had received antimicrobials or probenecid for 1 week before these studies (1 month in the case of benzathine penicillin G), or other medication for 48 h before or during these studies. A complete physical examination, a hematological and serum enzyme profile, and a urinalysis were obtained for each volunteer before and again 1 day after cephalosporin administration.

Subjects were randomized into equal groups and given cefonicid or one of the control cephalosporins. One week later, the groups were crossed over. Subjects were fasted for 8 h preceding dosing and were given 200 ml of water hourly for 6 h after dosing to insure adequate hydration. Blood and urine samples were obtained before and at selected intervals after dosing. Blood samples were permitted to clot in the cold, and the separated sera were stored at

−70°C for less than 2 weeks before assay. The voided urine was collected, the volume was measured, and a portion was stored at −70°C for assay. A disk agar diffusion assay employing penicillin seed agar buffered to pH 6.0 and seeded with *Bacillus subtilis* ATCC 6633 spores was used to determine the antibiotic content of each sample. Standards for assay of serum were prepared in pooled human serum devoid of background bioactivity, whereas standards for assay of urine were prepared in 1% phosphate buffer (pH 6.0).

Preliminary studies showed that single intramuscular (i.m.) or intravenous (i.v.) doses of 50 to 2,000 mg of cefonicid were safe and well tolerated in human volunteers. A single-dose pharmacokinetic study employing eight subjects in a crossover design was run using a 1-g i.m. dose of cefonicid in comparison to cefazolin, a cephalosporin known to produce high, long-lasting serum concentrations. The average peak serum concentration of cefonicid, 98 μg/ml, occurred 1 to 2 h after dosing, whereas the peak concentration of cefazolin, 70 μg/ml, was observed at 1 h (Fig. 1). Cefazolin was not detected in sera obtained 12 h after dosing, a time when more than 20 μg of cefonicid per ml was still present. Twenty-four hours after a single 1-g dose of cefonicid, the serum contained an average of 4.5 μg/ml. The apparent half-lives were 277 min for cefonicid and 126 min for cefazolin.

A study employing i.v.-administered drugs was carried out using the previously described procedures. The average 30-min serum concen-

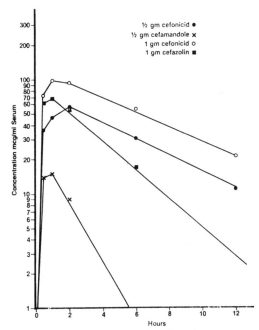

FIG. 1. *Serum concentration (in micrograms per milliliter) after i.m. dosing with selected cephalosporins.*

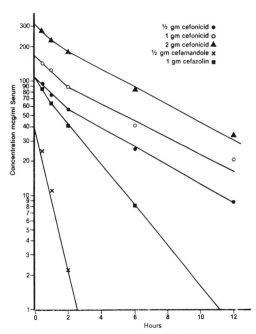

FIG. 2. *Serum concentrations (in micrograms per milliliter) after i.v. dosing with selected cephalosporins.*

trations of cefonicid and cefazolin were 148 and 88 µg/ml, respectively (Fig. 2). Twelve hours later, the subjects receiving cefonicid had a mean serum concentration of 15 µg/ml, whereas those receiving cefazolin were devoid of antibacterial activity. Twenty-four hours after the 1-g dose of cefonicid, an average of 2.6 µg/ml was still present. The half-lives of cefonicid and of cefazolin were 212 and 96 min, respectively.

A study comparing serum concentrations of cefonicid to those of cefamandole after an 0.5-g i.m. or i.v. dose was carried out. The peak cefonicid concentration, after the i.m. dose, was 58 µg/ml compared to 15 µg/ml for cefamandole (Fig. 1). The apparent half-lives were 270 and 60 min, respectively. A cefonicid concentration of 95 µg/ml was observed 30 min after the i.v. dose compared to 24 µg/ml for cefamandole. The half-lives were 222 and 30 min, respectively (Fig. 2).

Administration of a single 2-g i.v. dose of cefonicid to 10 volunteers for 10 consecutive days failed to produce any accumulation in the sera. This was evidenced by equivalent serum levels 24 h after each dose and by the ability to essentially superimpose day 1 and day 10 serum drug concentration profiles. Data for day 1 showed the presence of 282 µg of cefonicid per ml of serum 30 min after dosing. The half-life was 222 min.

TABLE 1. *Urinary recovery of cefonicid and cefazolin after a 1-g dose given i.m. or i.v.*

Drug	Route	Urinary recovery (%) at sampling intervals (h) of:						
		0/2	2/4	4/6	6/8	8/12	12/24	0/24
Cefonicid	i.m.	18	21	16	12	12	17	98
	i.v.	33	19	13	10	12	11	98
Cefazolin	i.m.	33	39	20	11	8	3	113
	i.v.	69	28	15	5	4	1	118

The urinary excretion patterns for cefonicid and cefazolin in volunteers receiving 1 g i.m. or i.v. are shown in Table 1. Essentially all of both drugs were recovered in urine samples collected within 24 h. Recovery of cefonicid remained nearly uniform at each sampling interval after an i.m. dose, whereas recovery of cefazolin was higher in the earlier hours. The front-end loading of the urinary excretion of cefazolin was more pronounced after an i.v. dose.

Serum concentrations of cefonicid were superior at all tested intervals to comparable doses of the commercially available cephalosporins tested. This compound does not appear to accumulate in the serum after repeated 2-g doses. All subjects tolerated cefonicid well without significant side effects. Cefonicid was excreted unchanged into the urine. Urinary concentrations of cefonicid were in excess of the MIC of susceptible urinary pathogens and were present for more than 24 h after a single i.m. or i.v. dose. The reported broad spectrum of in vitro activity and tissue penetration (2) in combination with the pharmacokinetics demonstrated in these studies suggest that cefonicid should be considered for additional clinical evaluation.

1. Actor, P., J. V. Uri, I. Zajac, J. R. Guarini, L. Phillips, D. H. Pitkin, D. A. Berges, G. L. Dunn, J. R. E. Hoover, and J. A. Weisbach. 1977. SK&F 75073, new parenteral broad-spectrum cephalosporin with high and prolonged serum levels. Antimicrob. Agents Chemother. 13:784–790.
2. Intoccia, A. P., S. S. Walkenstein, G. Joseph, R. Wittendorf, C. Girman, D. T. Walz, P. Actor, and J. A. Weisbach. 1978. Distribution in normal and inflammatory tissue of a new semisynthetic cephalosporin, SK&F 75073. J. Antibiot. 31:1188–1194.

Clinical Pharmacokinetics and Safety of FK 749 in Healthy Volunteers

MITSUYOSHI NAKASHIMA

Department of Pharmacology, Hamamatsu University, School of Medicine, Hamamatsu-shi, Shizuoka, 431-31, Japan

FK 749 is a new parenteral cephalosporin which exhibits the properties of broader antibacterial spectrum and more potent activities against gram-negative bacteria, and is more stable to β-lactamase than conventional cephalosporins.

The safety and pharmacokinetics of FK 749 in 38 healthy male volunteers were studied.

The dosage, number of volunteers, and observation items are shown in Table 1. Laboratory test items consisted of: erythrocyte, Hb, Ht, MCV, MCH, MCHC reticulocyte, heinz body, leukocyte, white blood picture, platelet count, serum iron, prothrombin time, partial thromboplastin time, fibrinogen volume, erythrocyte sedimentation rate, Coombs test, cyclic adenosine 5'-monophosphate receptor protein, serum glutamic oxalacetic transaminase, serum glutamic pyruvic transaminase, alkaline phosphatase, LDH, LAP, γ-guanosine 5'-triphosphate, total protein, serum protein fraction, total bilirubin, direct bilirubin, blood sugar, total cholesterol, CPK, blood urea nitrogen, serum creatinine, uric acid, serum electrolyte (Na, K, Ca, Cl, P), 24-h urine creatinine clearance, and urinalysis (specific gravity, pH, protein, glucose, urobilinogen, bilirubin, porphyrin, and urinary sediment).

The number of volunteers assigned to one dose schedule was six, except in the pilot study where the number was one to three. The dose was successively doubled after fully confirming the safety of each preceding dose.

FK 749 was well tolerated when given by intravenous (i.v.) or intramuscular (i.m.) injection. No abnormal findings attributable to the drug were observed in any of the items. Changes in laboratory test values encountered were within normal ranges and were considered to be

TABLE 1. *Outline of phase I study[a]*

Study	Administration route	Dose (mg)	No. of male volunteers	Age (yr)/body weight (kg)
Single dosing	i.v.	125	1	40/74.0
		250	1	36/54.5
		500	2	22, 33/63.0, 64.7
		1,000	2	32, 38/51.5, 73.5
	i.v.	500	6	24–38/54–67.5
		1,000	5	28–37/55–73
	d.i.	2,000	6	27–41/63–72
	i.m.	500	6	30–46/52–66
Repeated dosing	i.v.	1,000 b.i.d.[b] × 2 days	3	25–32/54.7–72.7
		1,000 b.i.d. × 5 days	6	35–40/53.5–70.0

[a] Observation items included clinical signs, laboratory tests (hematology, blood chemistry, urinalysis), physical tests (blood pressure, pulse rate, temperature, respiratory rate), polygraphy (blood pressure, pulse rate, deep body temperature, skin temperature, respiratory rate, ECG) and electrocardiogram. d.i., Drip infusion.

[b] b.i.d., Twice a day.

not meaningful from the safety point of view.

The serum and urinary concentrations, determined by the paper disk method using *Bacillus subtilis* ATCC 6633 as the test organism, are shown in Fig. 1. The serum concentrations after an i.v. bolus injection of 500 and 1,000 mg were as follows: 58.4 and 112.8 μg/ml, respectively, at 5 min; 17.1 and 31.0 μg/ml, respectively, at 1 h; and 2.9 and 4.9 μg/ml, respectively, at 4 h. The 24-h urinary excretion after 500- and 1,000-mg

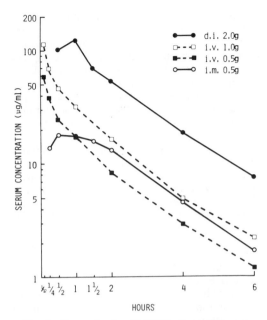

d.i. 2.0g
i.v. 1.0g
i.v. 0.5g
i.m. 0.5g

SERUM CONCENTRATION (µg/ml)

HOURS

FIG. 1. *Serum levels of FK 749 after a 500-mg i.m.* *(n = 6), 500-mg i.v. (n = 6), or 1,000-mg i.v. (n = 5)* *bolus injection and 2,000-mg i.v. drip infusion (n = 6)* *to healthy volunteers.*

doses was 88.1 and 88.6%, respectively, with the most being excreted during the first 6 h. The respective urinary concentrations after these doses were 602 and 1,599 µg/ml in the 0- to 2-h urine and 14 and 39 µg/ml in the 8- to 24-h urine.

The mean serum level after a 2,000-mg i.v. drip infusion reached a peak level of 123.7 µg/ml at the end of its 1-h infusion. After 6 h, 7.6 µg of FK 749 per ml still remained in the serum. Nearly 90% of the dose was recovered in 24-h urine. A urinary concentration of more than 1,000 µg/ml existed until 6 h after infusion.

The mean serum concentration after a 500-mg i.m. injection peaked at 30 min with the level of

18.1 µg/ml which, at 4 h, decreased to 4.6 µg/ml. The mean concentrations in the 2- to 4-h and 6- to 8-h urine were 1,018 and 154 µg/ml, respectively. Urinary excretion rate was 85.4% of the dose during 24 h.

The serum concentrations during a 5-day course of 1,000 mg twice a day was essentially the same as that obtained in the single-dosing study and showed no evidence of accumulation: the mean levels at 15 min and 6 h after a 1,000-mg injection during the 5-day course, determined on days 1, 3, and 5, were 61.6, 60.3, and 56.7 µg/ml and 3.4, 3.1, and 3.1 µg/ml, respectively.

Mathematical functions describing the time course of serum FK 749 concentrations were determined by a computer (FACOM 230-38), using weighted nonlinear least-squares regression analysis (NONLIN). Serum half-lives of FK 749 were 1.33, 1.30, 1.36, and 1.42 h after four different dosages, i.e., 500 mg i.m., 500 and 1,000 mg i.v. injection, and 2,000 mg i.v. drip infusion, respectively. The predicted serum levels were in excellent agreement with the actual concentrations in serum.

FK 749 exhibits marked intrinsic activities against gram-positive and gram-negative bacteria, including indole-positive *Proteus*, *Serratia*, *Enterobacter*, and *Bacteroides fragilis*. The 80% inhibiting concentration (IC_{80}) of FK 749 against clinically isolated strains of *Escherichia coli*, *Klebsiella*, *Proteus*, *Haemophilus influenzae*, and *Streptococcus pneumoniae* is as low as 0.1 µg/ml or less. The IC_{80}'s against *Serratia marcescens*, *B. fragilis*, and *Enterobacter* are 1.56, 3.12, and 6.25 µg/ml, respectively. The serum levels after an i.v. or i.m. injection of 500 mg exceeds these IC_{80} levels for 2 to 6 h or more. FK 749 was well tolerated when administered i.m. or i.v. Further clinical evaluation with 500- or 1,000-mg doses on various infectious diseases is well justified.

Ceftizoxime (FK 749), a New Parenteral Cephalosporin: In Vitro and In Vivo Antibacterial Activities

TAKAO TAKAYA, TOSHIAKI KAMIMURA, HITOSHI KOJO, YASUHIRO MINE, MINORU NISHIDA,* SACHIKO GOTO, AND SHOGO KUWAHARA

Fujisawa Pharmaceutical Co., Ltd., Osaka, and Toho University School of Medicine, Tokyo, Japan*

In the research for new cephalosporins with even greater antibacterial activity against a wide variety of gram-positive and gram-negative organisms, including the opportunistic pathogens,

ceftizoxime (FK 749), a distinctive new parenteral cephalosporin derivative, was recently developed (Fig. 1).

FK 749 is more potently active against various

gram-negative bacilli, including the opportunistic pathogens such as *Enterobacter, Citrobacter* species, and *Serratia marcescens*, than cephalosporins and cephamycins such as cefotiam, cefamandole, cefuroxime, cefotaxime, and cefmetazole. The antibiotic was also effective against anaerobic bacteria, and the activity of FK 749 against gram-negative anaerobes including species of *Bacteroides* was nearly the same as that of cefoxitin.

The inhibitory concentrations of FK 749 which were required to inhibit 80% of the test strains of *Staphylococcus aureus, Staphylococcus epidermidis,* and *Streptococcus pyogenes* were 3.13, 6.25, and ≤0.025 µg/ml, respectively (Table 1). The 80% inhibitory concentrations of FK 749 against the test strains of *Escherichia coli, Klebsiella pneumoniae, Proteus mirabilis,* and indole-positive *Proteus* species (except *Proteus morganii*) and *S. marcescens* were much lower, i.e., ≤0.025 to 1.56 µg/ml, than those of the other drugs tested. On the other hand, against *P. morganii, Citrobacter freundii, Enterobacter* species, *Haemophilus influenzae,*

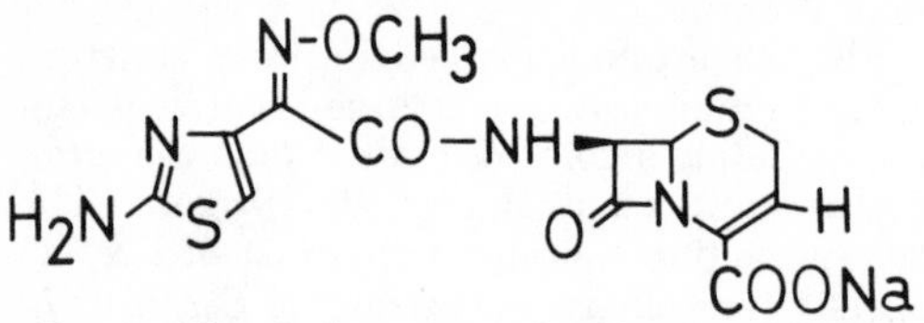

and *Bacteroides fragilis,* the 80% inhibitory concentrations of FK 749 (≤0.025 to 50 µg/ml) were almost the same as those of cefotaxime. However, the antibacterial activity of the drug was far more potent than that of the other drugs tested. The 50 and 80% inhibitory concentrations of FK 749 against 102 strains of *Pseudomonas aeruginosa* were higher than those of gentamicin and were almost the same as those of ticarcillin.

FK 749 was extremely stable to various types of β-lactamases and was highly effective against other cephalosporin- and cephamycin-resistant strains of *E. coli, K. pneumoniae,* and *P. mirabilis.* These resistant strains showed no cross-resistance between FK 749 and cefotiam, cefamandole, cefuroxime, and cefmetazole.

The effect of the test antibiotics on the viable cell count of *E. coli* no. 5 was investigated with an inoculum of 10^6 colony-forming units per ml in both heart infusion broth and 90% defibrinated rabbit blood. The bactericidal activity of FK 749 and cefotaxime at 5 µg/ml was more potent than that of the other antibiotics tested, and the viable cell counts were decreased markedly in 1 h by both drugs. The other drugs showed almost the same bactericidal activity as that of FK 749 when tests were carried out for 3 h. In the presence of 90% defibrinated rabbit blood, the bactericidal activity of FK 749 did not decrease and, in fact, was superior to its activity in heart infusion broth. The activity of cefotax-

FIG. 1. *Chemical structure of ceftizoxime (FK 749).*

TABLE 1. *Comparative antibacterial activity against clinical isolates[a]*

Organism		MIC (µg/ml) required for 80% of strains					
		FK 749	Cefotiam	Cefamandole	Cefuroxime	Cefotaxime	Cefmetazole
S. aureus	(207)[b]	3.13	0.78	0.78	1.56	3.13	1.56
S. pyogenes[c]	(42)	≤0.025	0.1	0.1	≤0.025	≤0.025	0.78
E. coli	(499)	0.1	0.39	3.13	6.25	0.2	1.56
K. pneumoniae	(302)	≤0.025	0.39	6.25	3.13	0.1	1.56
P. mirabilis	(253)	≤0.025	0.78	3.13	6.25	0.05	6.25
H. influenzae[c]	(42)	≤0.025	0.78	0.78	1.56	≤0.025	6.25
P. vulgaris	(63)	0.1	400	400	>400	3.13	3.13
P. morganii	(56)	6.25	100	50	100	6.25	12.5
P. rettgeri	(42)	≤0.025	25	50	50	0.2	50
P. inconstans B	(42)	0.05	3.13	12.5	12.5	0.39	12.5
C. freundii	(63)	50	100	200	100	25	200
E. cloacae	(68)	6.25	400	400	400	12.5	>400
E. aerogenes	(42)	6.25	25	100	100	6.25	400
S. marcescens	(89)	1.56	>400	>400	>400	6.25	200
B. fragilis[d]	(41)	3.13	100	400	50	6.25	25
P. aeruginosa	(102)	FK749	TIPC	CBPC	GM	HR-756	
50%		50	50	100	3.13	50	
80%		200	>400	400	25	100	

[a] HI agar, stamp method, 37°C, 20 h, 10^6 colony-forming units per ml.
[b] Number in parentheses indicates number of strains.
[c] Supplemented with 5% horse blood.
[d] GAM agar, GasPak method.

TABLE 2. *Protective effect on infection in mice*[a]

Organism	MLD[b]	ED$_{50}$ (mg/kg)			
		FK 749	Cefotiam	Cefotaxime	Cefmetazole
S. aureus 47	1	1.44	3.03	1.42	1.98
E. coli 54	1	1.78	4.92	1.33	25.7
K. pneumoniae 38	1	<0.24	7.70	0.75	20.3
P. mirabilis 73	1	<0.24	1.65	<0.24	3.90
P. vulgaris 63	1	<0.24	7.81	0.24	2.57
	100	5.11	—[c]	64.5	—
E. cloacae 63	1	3.68	57.5	2.83	>62.5
C. freundii 13	1	4.50	109	18.0	—
S. marcescens 32	1	16.1	>244	53.1	>244

		FK 749	CBPC	HR-756	T-1220	TIPC
P. aeruginosa 93	1	30.5	48.3	45.3	37.6	31.3

[a] ICR strain mice, 4 weeks old. Subcutaneous therapy at 1 h after intraperitoneal infection. Infection via 5% mucin suspension, 0.5 ml/mouse.

[b] MLD, Minimum lethal dose.

[c] —, Not tested.

ime, however, decreased in the presence of the blood.

The mean MBC of FK 749 for *E. coli* (eight strains) was almost the same as that of cefotaxime, but was lower for the other organisms than any other antibiotics tested. The bactericidal activity of FK 749 was 8 (cefotiam) to 138 (cefamandole) times higher for *E. coli* than the other test drugs except for cefotaxime, was about 4 (cefotaxime) to 134 (cefamandole) times higher for *K. pneumoniae* (eight strains) than any other test antibiotics, and was about 4.6 (cefotaxime) to >111 (cefamandole) times higher for *P. mirabilis* (five strains) than any other antibiotics tested.

The therapeutic effect of subcutaneous FK 749 in mice infected with various kinds of organisms was compared with that of the other an-

tibiotics (Table 2). The ED$_{50}$ value of FK 749 for *S. aureus* 47 infection was 1.44 mg/kg and was about the same as that of cefotaxime and cefamandole. The effect of FK 749 on infections due to *E. coli*, *K. pneumoniae*, indole-negative and -positive *Proteus* species, and *Enterobacter cloacae* 63 was almost the same as that of cefotaxime and was by far superior to that of the other test drugs. In contrast, FK 749 was more effective than cefotaxime against infections due to *C. freundii* 13 and *S. marcescens* 32 and was equal to ticarcillin and piperacillin in effect against infections due to *P. aeruginosa* 93.

In view of the finding that the antibacterial activity of FK 749 is more potent than related antibiotics in various in vitro and in vivo tests, it is concluded that the antibiotic has a considerable potential for clinical application.

Pharmacokinetics of Ceftizoxime (FK 749) in Animals After Parenteral Dosing

TAKEO MURAKAWA, HIROSHI SAKAMOTO, SHIGEMI FUKADA, SHOJI NAKAMOTO, TOSHIHARU HIROSE, NORIKAZU ITO, AND MINORU NISHIDA*

Research Laboratories, Fujisawa Pharmaceutical Co., Ltd., Osaka, Japan

The in vitro and in vivo antibacterial activities of FK 749, a new parenteral cephalosporin derivative, were reported previously. In the present study the pharmacokinetics, metabolism in animals, serum protein binding, and stability of FK 749 were evaluated and compared with those of cefotiam (SCE 963), cefamandole, cefotaxime (HR 756), and cefmetazole.

Serum concentration. The serum concentrations of FK 749 in different species of animals are shown in Table 1. FK 749 showed favorable serum levels in each species of animals. The elimination rate of FK 749 from the serum differed according to species and was the fastest in mice, followed in descending order by rats, monkeys, and dogs. The antibiotic concentration in the serum was undetectable in mice 1.5 h after a single subcutaneous (s.c.) and intravenous (i.v.) dose of 20 mg/kg, but was 1.4 and 1.7 μg/ml in dogs 6 h after an i.v. and an intramuscular (i.m.) dose, respectively. The pharmacokinetic parameters are shown in Table 2. The biological half-life of FK 749 was 0.267 h for mice, 0.333 h for rats, 0.738 h for monkeys, and 1.06 h for dogs. When the body clearance rates of FK 749 were compared among these animals, the drug clearance was faster in small animals such as mice and rats than in large animals such as dogs and monkeys. The serum concentration of FK 749 was compared with those of cefotiam, cefamandole, cefotaxime, and cefmetazole in mice, rats, dogs, and monkeys. In dogs the serum concentration of FK 749 was the highest of all the antibiotics tested. In monkeys the serum concentration of FK 749 was also the highest of the test drugs except cefmetazole.

Tissue concentration. The tissue concentrations of FK 749 and the related antibiotics were determined in rats after a single i.m. dose of 20

mg/kg. FK 749 was well distributed to all the tissues tested. The tissue concentrations 15 min after injection were the highest in the kidneys, i.e., 68.6 μg/g, followed by the liver (12.6 μg/g), the lungs (7.0 μg/g), and the heart (3.2 μg/g). The tissue concentrations of FK 749 were higher than those of cefotiam except in the liver. Although the serum concentration of cefotaxime was the highest in rats, the liver and kidney concentrations of this antibiotic were the lowest. These results were evinced by the instability of cefotaxime in the tissue homogenates and suggest the formation of a desacetyl metabolite of cefotaxime in the body.

Urinary excretion in dogs and monkeys. Urinary recovery in dogs and monkeys after an i.m. dose of 20 mg/kg is shown in Table 3. In dogs, the 24-h urinary recovery of FK 749 was 93.8% and was the highest of all the antibiotics tested. In monkeys, 71.5% of the given dose was excreted in the 4-h urine and 80.3% was excreted in the 24-h urine. More than 80% of given FK 749 was excreted in the 24-h urine in both species

TABLE 1. *Serum concentrations of FK 749 in animals after parenteral dosing*

Animal	Route	Serum concn (mean ± SE [μg/ml])								
		3^a	5	7	10	15	30	45	60	90
Mouse	i.v. (n = 16)	23.0 ± 1.1	ND^b	14.8 ± 1.2	ND	6.6 ± 0.5	2.0 ± 0.2	0.7 ± 0.1	0.4 ± 0.1	$—^c$
	s.c. (n = 20)	ND	ND	ND	ND	22.3 ± 0.8	10.6 ± 0.6	1.8 ± 0.2	0.2 ± 0.1	—
Rat	i.v. (n = 10)	ND	41.4 ± 0.8	ND	28.0 ± 1.3	18.2 ± 0.8	9.9 ± 1.3	ND	3.3 ± 0.7	1.0 ± 0.1
	i.m. (n = 10)	ND	ND	ND	ND	22.4 ± 1.5	14.0 ± 0.7	ND	4.4 ± 0.2	1.0 ± 0.1
		0.25^d	0.5		1.0	2.0	3.0	4.0		6.0
Dog	i.v. (n = 5)	69.3 ± 2.4	47.9 ± 1.2		31.8 ± 2.0	15.2 ± 0.9	ND	4.1 ± 0.6		1.4 ± 0.4
	i.m. (n = 5)	51.2 ± 6.2	46.5 ± 2.3		41.5 ± 1.0	23.6 ± 1.2	10.7 ± 1.2	5.8 ± 1.2		1.7 ± 0.5
Monkey	i.v. (n = 5)	51.8 ± 2.9	30.9 ± 1.5		14.7 ± 1.1	6.2 ± 0.5	ND	0.9 ± 0.2		—
	i.m. (n = 5)	36.9 ± 2.3	36.6 ± 0.9		28.8 ± 1.9	13.2 ± 1.3	ND	2.1 ± 0.6		—

[a] Time after injection (in minutes).
[b] ND, Not determined.
[c] —, Not detected.
[d] Time after injection (in hours).

TABLE 2. *Pharmacokinetic parameters^a*

Animal	A (μg/ml)	α (h^{-1}) ($T_{1/2\beta}$ [h])	B (μg/ml)	β (h^{-1}) ($T_{1/2\beta}$ [h])	K_{12} (h^{-1})	K_{21} (h^{-1})	K_e (h^{-1})	V_c (ml/kg)	V_t (ml/kg)	CL-body (ml/h per kg)	AUC (μg·h/ml)
Mouse	27.6	7.44 (0.093)	4.52	2.60 (0.267)	0.863	3.28	5.90	624	164	3,670	5.45
Rat	48.6	11.0 (0.063)	26.8	2.08 (0.333)	3.47	5.25	4.38	265	175	1,160	17.3
Dog	61.9	4.57 (0.152)	58.1	0.653 (1.06)	1.50	2.55	1.17	167	98.3	195	100
Monkey	78.0	5.09 (0.136)	38.4	0.939 (0.738)	1.65	2.31	2.07	172	123	356	56.2

[a] The parameters were obtained by analysis of serum data in animals after a single i.v. injection. AUC, Area under the curve; CL-body, body clearance. V_c and V_t, Volume of distribution in central and tissue compartment; K_e, elimination constant; K_{12} and K_{21}, transfer rate constant between V_c and V_t. A and B, Drug concentration at zero time in α and β phases. α and β, Elimination rate constant in α and β phases.

TABLE 3. *Urinary recovery of FK 749 and related antibiotics in dogs and monkeys after a single i.m. injection of 20 mg/kg*

Antibiotic	Recovery (%)					
	Dog (n = 5)			Monkey (n = 5)		
	0–6 h	6–24 h	Total	0–6 h	6–24 h	Total
FK 749	91.9	1.9	93.8	78.0	2.3	80.3
Cefotiam	57.0	1.1	58.1	51.0	0.3	51.3
Cefamandole	68.9	1.8	70.7	77.8	0.2	78.0
Cefotaxime	61.0	1.2	62.2	68.1	0.8	68.9
Cefmetazole	50.6	3.9	54.5	80.0	0.2	80.2

tested. The 24-h urinary excretion was 51.3% for cefotiam, 78.0% for cefamandole, 68.9% for cefotaxime, and 80.2% for cefmetazole.

Biliary excretion in rats. The 24-h biliary recovery was 3.7% for FK 749, 35.7% for cefotiam, 24.6% for cefamandole, 1.0% for cefotaxime, and 79.1% for cefmetazole. FK 749 was mainly excreted in the urine.

Serum protein binding. The human serum protein binding of FK 749 was 31% and was similar to that of cefotaxime (37%), but was lower than that of cefotiam (53%), cefamandole (75%), and cefmetazole (66%). The serum protein binding of FK 749 was also the lowest of the test drugs, i.e., 13% in mice, 32% in rats, 25% in rabbits, and 17% in dogs.

Stability in biological fluids. FK 749 was more stable than cefotiam and cefotaxime in human serum and urine, and in rat tissue homogenate at 37°C. The half-lives were 93 to 170 h for FK 749, 16 to 30 h for cefotiam, and 55 to 59 h for cefotaxime in the test samples. Cefotaxime was very unstable in rat tissue homogenate; i.e., the half-lives were 0.1 h for cefotaxime, 16 h for cefotiam, and 120 to 170 h for FK 749. FK 749 was the most stable of the three antibiotics tested in the buffers at pH 5.0, 7.0, and 9.2. The half-lives at pH 7.0 were 148 h for FK 749, 44 h for cefotaxime, and 17 h for cefotiam.

It is of interest to note that the species of animal which most closely resembles humans in the pharmacokinetic profile of FK 749 is the monkey (unpublished data on phase I study). In conclusion, the results of this study suggest that FK 749, with its excellent antibacterial activity, has high promise for clinical application.

Ceftizoxime (FK 749), Its Affinity to Penicillin-Binding Proteins and β-Lactamases and Its Antibacterial Activity

TAKESHI YOKOTA,* REIKO SEKIGUCHI, EIKO AZUMA, AND MINORU NISHIDA

Department of Bacteriology, School of Medicine, Juntendo University, Tokyo 113, and *Research Laboratories, Fujisawa Pharmaceutical Co. Ltd. Osaka 532, Japan*

Ceftizoxime (FK 749) is a novel cephalosporin, devised by Fujisawa Pharmaceutical Co., Ltd. (Osaka, Japan), that possesses the methoxy-imino radical on the 7-Z(2) position and no side chain on the 3 position. The drug exhibits marked antibacterial activities, especially on gram-negative rods and including opportunistic pathogens, i.e., *Enterobacter* species, *Citrobacter* species, *Serratia marcescens*, *Proteus* species, and *Pseudomonas aeruginosa*, although the effect on the last species is moderate (2). Since FK 749 shows strong activities even for β-lactamase-producing bacteria and its bactericidal activity is more prominent than other newly developed cephalosporins (2, 3), it is of interest to investigate the stability to various β-lactamases and the affinity to murein-transpeptidases that have been known to be the target enzyme group of β-lactams and as the penicillin-binding proteins (PBPs) of bacteria.

Affinity of FK 749 to PBPs of *Escherichia coli* and *Vibrio cholerae.* The affinity of FK 749 to PBPs was examined by the competitive binding of the drug against [14C]penicillin G by the method of Spratt (4). The membrane fractions of *E. coli* NIHJ JC2 and of *V. cholerae* E2 were prepared from the sonic lysates by successive ultracentrifugations. Thirty-microliter volumes of membrane suspension were preincubated at 30°C for 10 min with 0.1 volume of FK 749 solution to make the final concentrations of 0.5, 1.0, 5.0, and 25 µg/ml before the addition of 3 µl of [14C]penicillin G (1 µmol/50 µCi per ml) followed by further incubation at 30°C for 10 min. The reaction was terminated by cooling and the addition of 3 µl of a mixture of 20% Sarkosyl and 60 mg of cold penicillin G per ml. After dissolving the inner membrane by letting it stand at room temperature, the outer membrane component was eliminated by centrifugation. The resulting clear supernatants were subjected to 10% acrylamide slab gel electrophore-

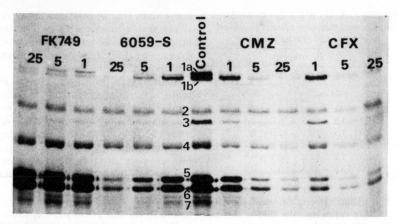

FIG. 1. *Competition of various cephalosporin derivatives for PBPs of E. coli NIHJ JC2. Indicated amounts of drugs (in micrograms per milliliter) were preincubated with membrane fractions at 30°C for 10 min before the addition of [^{14}C]penicillin G.*

sis. The radioactive bands of PBPs were identified by a fluorographic method (1).

It was revealed that FK 749 manifests a strong binding affinity to the 1b and 3 fractions of PBPs of both *E. coli* and *V. cholerae* followed by that to the 1a fraction. Other cephalosporin derivatives showed high binding affinities to the 1a and 3 fractions followed by that to the 1b fraction (Fig. 1). Since the 1b fraction of PBPs has been elucidated as an essential cross-linking enzyme of the murein biosynthesis required for cell elongation (5), it is tenable to assume that β-lactam drugs showing a high affinity to the 1b fraction are predominant in bactericidal activity. In fact, FK 749 was confirmed to exhibit a stronger bactericidal effect on *E. coli* cells than cefmetazole, cefamandole, cefotiam, cefuroxime, and cefotaxime (HR 756) (2). Furthermore, when the cells of *E. coli* NIHJ JC2 were incubated in L broth supplemented with 20% human serum and 2% of the complement of guinea pigs, the bacteria were more rapidly killed in the presence of a 50% growth inhibitory concentration of FK 749 than in the absence of it. In that case, the 50% inhibitory dose was determined spectrophotometrically by growing the microbe in L broth containing serially increasing concentrations of the drug. Although enhancement of bactericidal effect of the complement by subinhibitory doses of drugs was common in 7-Z(2)-methoxyimino derivatives of cephalosporins, the effect of FK 749 was more prominent than cefuroxime and HR 756.

Stability of FK 749 to various β-lactamases. The 105,000 × *g* supernatants of sonic extracts of *Enterobacter cloacae* Nek39, *Proteus vulgaris* 33, *Proteus mirabilis* JY10, *E. coli*

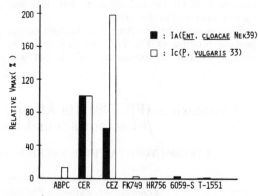

FIG. 2. *Stabilities of ceftizoxime (FK 749) and other cephalosporins against type Ia and Ic β-lactamases.*

CSH2 carrying the RK1 plasmid, *Klebsiella* 42, and *E. coli* CSH2 carrying RE45 were employed as crude enzymes of the types Ia, Ic, II, III(TEM), IV, and V β-lactamases, respectively. The V_{max} values of the enzymes were measured by the macroiodometric method for each drug and expressed as relative to those for ampicillin and cephaloridine, taken as 100 in the case of penicillinases and that of cephalosporinases, respectively. Although cephaloridine and cefazolin were well hydrolyzed by type Ia and Ic cephalosporinases, FK 749, HR-756, 6059-S, and cefoperazone (T-1551) were not destroyed by them (Fig. 2). In the case of penicillinase-type enzymes, the TEM-type(III) β-lactamase specified by the majority of R(*b1a*) plasmids hydrolyzed ampicillin and cephaloridine effectively, cefazolin and T-1551 moderately, and HR-756 slightly, but not FK 749 or 6059-S. The oxacillin-hydrolyzing enzyme (V) encoded by the minority of R(b1a) plasmids destroyed all of the drugs except 6059-S.

Since we previously reported that gram-negative rods producing β-lactamases as perienzymes become resistant to β-lactams not only due to hydrolysis by the enzymes but also depending on an unknown barrier directed by β-lactamase itself (which does not hydrolyze the drugs but binds them and prevents their passing through the periplasmic space to the sensitive site [6]), the affinity of FK 749 to β-lactamases was examined as K_i values by the modified acidimetric method. It may be noteworthy that FK 749 is not only quite stable to the TEM-type β-lactamase but also possesses a high K_i value, indicating that the drug is indifferent to R(b1a) plasmids. This enzymological characteristic correctly reflected the MIC of FK 749 which showed that the transfer of 51 different R(b1a) plasmids encoding the TEM-type β-lactamase to E. coli CSH2 resulted in no change of the drug susceptibilities from the R⁻ parent strain. On the other hand, MICs of 6059-S, which possessed 100-fold-higher affinity (1/100 the K_i of FK 749), and of CFX, which had 20-fold-higher affinity to the enzyme, were elevated to 10 and 2 times, respectively, by inheriting the R plasmids.

Although some clinical isolates of E. cloacae resistant to more than 50 μg of CFX were also slightly resistant to FK 749 because of its high affinity to the type Ic β-lactamase, more than 70% of the strains were inhibited in growth by less than 6.35 μg of FK 749 per ml. It may be noteworthy that FK 749 is not only effective on various β-lactamase-producing bacteria but is also expected to have a better therapeutic effect in vivo because of its strong bactericidal activity.

1. **Bonner, M., and R. A. Laskey.** 1974. A film detection method for tritium-labelled proteins and nucleic acids in polyacrylamide gels. Eur. J. Biochem. **46**:83–88.
2. **Kamimura, T., Y. Matsumoto, N. Okada, Y. Mine, M. Nishida, S. Goto, and S. Kuwahara.** 1979. Ceftizoxime (FK 749), a new parenteral cephalosporin: in vitro and in vivo antibacterial activities. Antimicrob. Agents Chemother. **16**:540–548.
3. **Kojo, H., M. Nishida, S. Goto, and S. Kuwahara.** 1979. Antibacterial activity of ceftizoxime (FK 749), a new cephalosporin, against cephalosporin-resistant bacteria, and its stability to β-lactamase. Antimicrob. Agents Chemother. **16**:549–553.
4. **Spratt, B. G.** 1975. Distinct penicillin-binding proteins involved in the division, elongation and shape of Escherichia coli K12. Proc. Natl. Acad. Sci. U.S.A. **72**:2999–3003.
5. **Tamaki, S., S. Nakajima, and M. Matsuhashi.** 1977. Thermosensitive mutation in Escherichia coli simultaneously causing defects in penicillin-binding protein-1Bs and in enzyme activity for peptidoglycan synthesis in vitro. Proc. Natl. Acad. Sci. U.S.A. **74**:5472–5476.
6. **Yamamoto, T., and T. Yokota.** 1977. Beta-lactamase-directed barrier for penicillins of Escherichia coli carrying R plasmids. Antimicrob. Agents Chemother. **11**:936–940.

Antibacterial Activity and β-Lactamase Stability of a New Semisynthetic Cephalosporin, Ceftizoxime (FK 749)

HAROLD C. NEU* AND KWUNG P. FU

Departments of Medicine and Pharmacology, College of Physicians and Surgeons, Columbia University, New York, New York 10032, U.S.A.

Although chemical modifications of the cephalosporin nucleus have enlarged the antibacterial spectrum of compounds in this class, many gram-negative species have remained resistant and there have been decreases in the activity against gram-positive organisms. FK 749 is a new cephalosporin with the structure (6R,7R)-[(z)-2-(2-imino-4-thiazolin-4-yl)-2methoxyimino acetamino]-8-oxo-5-thia-1-azabicyclo[4.2.0]oct-2-ene-2-carboxylate. The structural similarities to recently developed compounds such as cefotaxime and cefoxitin caused us to compare its in vitro activity with that of other β-lactam compounds and to determine specifically its activity against multiply resistant isolates.

FK 749 was obtained from Fujisawa Pharmaceuticals, and other agents were obtained from their respective manufacturers. Susceptibility tests were performed in either broth or agar, with the use of Mueller-Hinton medium and a final inoculum of 10^5 colony-forming units (CFU). β-Lactamase stability was determined by the spectrophotometric assay.

FK 749 inhibited the majority of Staphylococcus aureus and S. epidermidis isolates at concentrations of 3.1 μg/ml. In contrast, it inhibited streptococcal species, with the exception of S. faecalis and S. faecium, at concentrations of 0.2 μg/ml or lower. Most Haemophilus influenzae and Neisseria meningitidis strains were in-

TABLE 1. *Comparative activity of FK 749 and other β-lactam antibiotics*

Organism (no. of strains)	Drug	MIC (μg/ml)	
		For 50% of isolates	For 90% of isolates
Staphylococcus aureus (16)	FK 749	1.6	3.1
	Cefotaxime	1.6	3.1
	Cefoxitin	1.6	3.1
	Cephalothin	0.1	0.4
Streptococcus pyogenes (10)	FK 749	0.1	0.2
Haemophilus influenzae (5)	FK 749	0.05	0.1
Neisseria gonorrhoeae (5)	FK 749	0.05	0.1
Enterococci (33)	FK 749	1.6	>100
Escherichia coli (40)	FK 749	0.02	0.04
	Cefotaxime	0.05	0.4
	Cefoxitin	1.6	6.3
	Cefoperazone	0.4	25
Klebsiella pneumoniae (32)	FK 749	0.02	0.05
	Cefotaxime	0.02	0.2
	Cefoxitin	3.1	25
	Cefoperazone	3.1	50
Enterobacter (36)	FK 749	0.1	0.8
	Cefotaxime	0.04	3.1
	Cefamandole	1.3	6.3
	Cefoperazone	0.2	0.5
Citrobacter (32)	FK 749	0.05	0.2
	Cefotaxime	0.05	0.2
	Cefamandole	0.8	200
	Cefoperazone	0.4	12.5
Serratia (32)	FK 749	6.3	12.5
	Cefotaxime	25	50
	Cefoxitin	50	>100
	Cefamandole	>100	>100
	Cefoperazone	50	>100
	Carbenicillin	50	>100
Proteus mirabilis (20)	KF 749	<0.0063	<0.0063
	Cefotaxime	<0.0063	<0.025
	Cefoxitin	1.6	12.5
Proteus, indole-positive (27)	FK 749	0.02	6.3
	Cefotaxime	0.05	1.6
	Cefoxitin	1.3	12.5
	Cefoperazone	1.3	25
	Cefamandole	25	200
	Carbenicillin	12.5	100
Providencia (16)	FK 749	0.01	0.05
	Cefotaxime	0.4	1.3
	Cefoxitin	3.1	12.5
	Carbenicillin	100	>400
Pseudomonas aeruginosa (80)	FK 749	12.5	100
	Cefotaxime	12.5	50
	Cefoperazone	3.1	12.5
	Carbenicillin	50	>200
Bacteroides fragilis (30)	FK 749	25	50
	Cefotaxime	25	100
	Cefoxitin	6.3	25
	Carbenicillin	50	>100

hibited at concentrations below 0.1 μg/ml. The activity of FK 749 against the aforementioned species was comparable to that of cefotaxime and cefoperazone. It was more active than cefoxitin against streptococci, but less active than cephalothin, cefamandole, or cefuroxime.

FK 749 showed remarkable activity against gram-negative enteric bacteria. It inhibited the majority of isolates of *Escherichia coli, Klebsiella pneumoniae, Enterobacter cloacae, E. aerogenes, E. hafniae, E. agglomerans, Proteus mirabilis, P. morganii, P. rettgeri, P. vulgaris, Providencia, Citrobacter diversus,* and *C. freundii* at concentrations below 0.2 μg/ml. It had activity similar to that of cefotaxime against most of these isolates, but was more active at lower concentrations against *Enterobacter, Citrobacter,* and *Proteus.* It was manyfold (8- to 256-fold) more active than cefamandole and cefoxitin against the aforementioned species (Table 1).

FK 749 inhibited the majority of multiresistant isolates of *Serratia marcescens* at concentrations of 12.5 μg/ml. At this concentration only 31% were inhibited by cefotaxime, 13% by cefoperazone, and 3% by carbenicillin.

FK 749 was less active than cefoperazone and cefotaxime against *Pseudomonas aeruginosa.* At 12.5 μg/ml 84% of isolates were inhibited by cefoperazone, 61% by cefotaxime, 36% by FK 749, and 2% by carbenicillin. FK 749 was not active against most other species of *Pseudomonas* tested (*P. cepacia, P. maltophilia,* and *P. diminuta*).

FK 749 inhibited many strains of *Bacteroides fragilis.* It was slightly less active than cefoxitin against *B. fragilis* subsp. *fragilis,* but was more active than carbenicillin or cefoperazone. Other anaerobic species which were inhibited at concentrations below 12 μg/ml were *Clostridium perfringens,* peptococci, peptostreptococci, and *Fusobacterium,* but FK 749 was less active than penicillin against most of these anaerobic species.

Varying the growth conditions did not appreciably alter the MICs of FK 749 when assays were run in different media (Mueller-Hinton, brain heart infusion, tryptic soy) or at pH 6, 7, and 8. The effect of varying the inoculum size from 10^3 to 10^7 CFU did increase both the MICs and MBCs, but the actual increase in inhibitory level was minimal. For example, the MIC for an *E. coli* isolate was 0.0063 μg/ml at 10^3 CFU and 0.2 μg/ml at 10^7 CFU. MBCs were within a twofold dilution of the MICs for most of the isolates at inocula of 10^3 and 10^5 CFU, but at 10^7 CFU the MBCs of *Serratia* were appreciably increased.

FK 749 inhibited isolates resistant to cephalothin and carbenicillin, with the exception of *P. aeruginosa* and *Acinetobacter,* at concentrations below 1 μg/ml (Table 2). It also inhibited isolates resistant to gentamicin and tobramycin at similar concentrations.

There was no effect of the presence of a detectable β-lactamase in a bacterial isolate upon the MICs. For example, against two *P. morganii* isolates with β-lactamase detected by nitrocefin, the MICs were 0.2 and 6.3 μg/ml. FK 749 was not hydrolyzed by β-lactamases of *E. coli, Klebsiella, Shigella, P. morganii, P. mirabilis, S. aureus, Citrobacter,* and *P. aeruginosa.* It had a β-lactamase stability similar to that of cefuroxime and cefoxitin.

Combinations of FK 749 and gentamicin or carbenicillin, when tested against 64 isolates of *P. aeruginosa, K. pneumoniae, S. marcescens, P. mirabilis, E. coli,* and indole-positive *Pro-*

TABLE 2. *Activity of FK 749 against bacteria resistant to cephalothin and carbenicillin (MIC > 200 μg/ml)*

Organism	MIC (μg/ml)			
	FK 749	Cefotaxime	Cefoxitin	Cefamandole
E. coli	0.012	0.05	3.2	100
E. coli	0.05	0.05	12.5	3.1
K. pneumoniae	0.0063	0.025	12.5	6.3
K. pneumoniae[a]	0.025	0.1	25	50
S. marcescens	0.4	25	>400	>400
S. marcescens[a]	3.1	25	>400	>400
P. mirabilis	0.0063	0.1	>400	>400
P. rettgeri[a]	0.0063	0.05	1.6	0.8
P. morganii	6.3	3.1	12.5	25
E. cloacae	0.0063	0.05	>400	6.3
P. aeruginosa	25	12.5	>400	>400
P. aeruginosa	6.3	3.1	200	>400
P. stuartii[a]	0.05	1.6	>400	>400

[a] Also resistant to gentamicin and tobramycin, MIC ≥ 25 μg/ml.

teus, rarely demonstrated synergy (4 of 64 isolates). However, a fourfold decrease in MIC of one agent, partial synergy, was found for 30 of 64 isolates.

These studies demonstrate that FK 749 is an extremely active cephalosporin with a spectrum of activity similar to that of cefotaxime and superior to that of cefoxitin and cefamandole. It significantly enlarges the cephalosporin spectrum, inhibiting gram-negative aerobic and anaerobic species resistant to β-lactam compounds and to the aminoglycosides.

SCE 1365, a New Cephalosporin: In Vitro Antibacterial Activities

S. GOTO,* M. OGAWA, A. TSUJI, S. KUWAHARA, K. TSUCHIYA, M. KONDO, AND M. KIDA

*School of Medicine, Toho University, Tokyo, and Takeda Chemical Industries, Ltd., Osaka, Japan**

In previous reports (3, 4), cefotiam, i.e., 7β-[2-(2-aminothiazol-4-yl)acetamido]-3-[[[1-(2-dimethylaminoethyl)-1H-tetrazol-5-yl]thio]-methyl]ceph-3-em-4-carboxylic acid, having excellent antibacterial and pharmacokinetic properties, was presented. Although cefotiam has high and broad antibacterial activities, some of the gram-negative bacteria still remained resistant. Therefore, further chemical modifications of the cefotiam molecule were conducted in Takeda Chemical Industries, Ltd., and SCE 1365, i.e., 7β-[2-(2-aminothiazol-4-yl)-[z]-2-methoxyiminoacetamido]-3-[(1-methyl-1H-tetrazol-5-yl)-thiomethyl]-ceph-3-em-4-carboxylic acid, was finally selected based on the broad spectrum of antibacterial activity, the resistance to hydrolysis by β-lactamases, and some physicochemical properties (2).

The test strains were gram-positive and gram-negative bacteria from laboratory stocks and recent clinical isolates. Strains of *Escherichia coli* and *Klebsiella pneumoniae* not inhibited by cefazolin at 50 μg/ml or higher concentration and strains of *Serratia marcescens* not inhibited by gentamicin at 25 μg/ml or higher concentration were classified arbitrarily as resistant. MIC and MBC values were determined by the serial twofold dilution method using Trypticase soy agar (BBL Microbiology Systems, Cockeysville, Md.) or Trypticase soy broth (BBL Microbiology Systems). MIC was defined as the lowest concentration of cephalosporin that prevented visible growth after overnight cultivation at 37°C. MBC was defined as the lowest concentration of cephalosporin that inhibited visible growth on the subculture plate. Bactericidal effect was evaluated by the method of time-kill curve in Trypticase soy broth. After the addition of cephalosporins to a suspension of test bacteria, the number of colony-forming units was determined at various intervals by plating out samples. Bacteriolytic effect was followed by measuring the absorbance in an automated continuously recording photometer. Morphological changes of bacteria were observed by a scanning electron microscope and by a transmission electron microscope. β-Lactamase activity was determined by the UV method (for cephalosporins) and microiodometric method (for penicillins) using 200 μmol of each substrate.

SCE 1365 exhibited a super-broad spectrum of antibacterial activity against various pathogenic bacterial species, including *Haemophilus influenzae,* indole-positive *Proteus, S. marcescens, Citrobacter freundii,* and *Enterobacter cloacae.* The spectrum and activity of SCE 1365 were similar to those of cefotaxime (1) against a wide variety of bacterial species tested. In the activities against clinical isolates of *Staphylococcus aureus* and *Staphylococcus epidermidis,* SCE 1365 resembled cefotiam but was less active than cefazolin. Against *Streptococcus pyogenes,* SCE 1365 was more potent than cefotiam and cefazolin. The activity of SCE 1365 against several gram-negative bacteria was excellent. SCE 1365 inhibited the most strains of *H. influenzae* at 0.025 μg/ml or below, and it was about 60 times and 500 to 1,000 times as active as cefotiam and cefazolin, respectively. SCE 1365 inhibited the most strains of cefazolin-susceptible *E. coli* and *K. pneumoniae, Proteus mirabilis, Proteus vulgaris, Proteus morganii,* and *Proteus rettgeri* at 0.2 μg/ml or below, and it was about 2 to 100 times and about 10 to 1,000 times more active than cefotiam and cefazolin, respectively. Furthermore, SCE 1365 inhibited the most strains of cefazolin-resistant *E. coli* and *K. pneumoniae, Proteus inconstans,* gentamicin-susceptible *S. marcescens,* and *E. cloacae* at 0.78 μg/ml or below, and it was about 2 to 4 times and 10 to 100 times more potent than cefotiam and cefazolin, respectively. The activity of SCE 1365 against gentamicin-resistant strains of *S. marcescens* was inferior to that against gentamicin-susceptible strains, and all the strains tested were inhibited at less than 6.25 µg of SCE 1365 per ml. Inhibition of the growth of most strains of *Pseudomonas aeruginosa*, *Pseudomonas cepacia*, and *Pseudomonas maltophilia* required 25 µg of SCE 1365 per ml, and the activity of SCE 1365 against *P. aeruginosa* was about two times and one-fourth to one-eighth times the activities of carbenicillin and cefsulodin (5), respectively. SCE 1365 inhibited most strains of *Acinetobacter calcoaceticus* at 50 µg/ml or below (Table 1).

SCE 1365 also showed bactericidal activity. The MBCs of SCE 1365 against *E. coli* (10 strains), *K. pneumoniae* (10 strains), and *S. marcescens* (7 strains) were close to the MICs determined by the tube dilution assay. Kill-curve analysis of SCE 1365 against *S. aureus* FDA 209 P, *E. coli* NIHJ JC-2, and *S. marcescens* IFO 12648 was compared with that of cefotaxime. A definite decrease in number of colony-forming units was observed at a concentration of 0.78 µg/ml for *S. aureus*, 0.39 µg/ml for *E. coli*, and 0.2 µg/ml for *S. marcescens*, which were the MICs determined by the broth dilution assay. Bacteriolysis of *S. aureus* and *E. coli* was observed at concentrations higher than 0.78 µg/ml and 0.2 µg/ml, respectively, when SCE 1365 was added

at early exponential growth phase (opacity, 20%). For *S. marcescens*, however, no bacteriolysis was observed, but the increase of opacity of the culture was dose-dependently inhibited. Although SCE 1365 and cefotaxime had a similar MIC against *S. marcescens* IFO 12648, cefotaxime did not prevent the increase of opacity of the culture of *S. marcescens*.

SCE 1365 was markedly resistant to hydrolysis by penicillinases and cephalosporinases except for the cephalosporinase of *P. vulgaris*. Although SCE 1365 was slightly hydrolyzed by the *P. vulgaris* enzyme, the K_m value for SCE 1365 was of the order of 10^{-4} M, and this means that the enzyme had relatively low affinity to SCE 1365. Moreover, SCE 1365 was a potent competitive inhibitor of cephalosporinases of *E. cloacae*, *C. freundii*, and *P. aeruginosa* (Table 2). The high stability of SCE 1365 to β-lactamase may be one of the factors for its potent antibacterial activity, especially against cefazolin-resistant strains.

SCE 1365 showed a high affinity to penicillin-binding proteins 1A and 3 and to a less extent to penicillin-binding proteins 1B and 2. The gram-negative rods became filaments when treated with SCE 1365 of a wide range of concentrations. This may reflect the preferential high affinity of

TABLE 1. *Comparative activities of SCE 1365, cefotaxime, cefotiam, and cefazolin against clinical isolates*[a]

| Organism[b] | MIC which inhibited the following cumulative % of isolates: | | | | | | | |
| | SCE 1365 | | Cefotaxime | | Cefotiam | | Cefazolin | |
	50%	80%	50%	80%	50%	80%	50%	80%
S. aureus (105)	1.56	1.56	3.13	3.13	0.78	0.78	0.39	0.78
S. epidermidis (52)	0.78	1.56	0.78	1.56	0.39	0.78	0.2	0.39
S. pyogenes (37)	0.013	0.013	0.013	0.013	0.05	0.05	0.1	0.1
E. coli (CEZ[s]) (104)	0.1	0.2	0.1	0.1	0.2	0.2	1.56	3.13
E. coli (CEZ[r]) (31)	0.2	0.39	0.2	0.2	0.78	1.56	25	50
K. pneumoniae (CEZ[s]) (75)	0.1	0.1	0.05	0.1	0.2	0.39	3.13	3.13
K. pneumoniae (CEZ[r]) (100)	0.2	0.78	0.2	0.78	1.56	12.5	25	100
H. influenzae (69)	0.013	0.025	0.025	0.025	0.78	1.56	25	50
P. mirabilis (110)	0.05	0.1	0.025	0.05	0.78	0.39	6.25	6.25
P. vulgaris (116)	0.1	0.2	0.1	0.39	25	50	>100	>100
P. morganii (124)	0.05	0.1	0.05	0.2	0.78	3.13	>100	>100
P. rettgeri (81)	0.013	0.1	0.013	0.025	0.2	0.78	12.5	50
P. inconstans (37)	0.1	0.39	0.1	0.78	0.2	3.13	50	>100
S. marcescens (GM[s]) (105)	0.2	0.78	0.39	1.56	6.25	>100	>100	>100
S. marcescens (GM[r]) (39)	3.13	6.25	6.25	12.5	>100	>100	>100	>100
C. freundii (82)	0.39	12.5	0.39	25	1.56	100	>100	>100
E. cloacae (78)	0.39	0.78	0.39	0.78	3.13	25	>100	>100
P. aeruginosa (157)	12.5	25	12.5	25	>100	>100	>100	>100
P. cepacia (32)	6.25	12.5	6.25	6.25	>100	>100	>100	>100
P. maltophilia (21)	6.25	12.5	50	100	>100	>100	>100	>100
A. calcoaceticus (45)	25	50	12.5	25	50	100	>100	>100

[a] Inoculum size: one loopful of bacterial suspension (10^6 colony-forming units per ml). Medium: Trypticase soy agar (TSA), blood-TSA, chocolate agar.

[b] Abbreviations: CEZ[s] and CEZ[r], cefazolin sensitive and resistant, respectively; GM[s] and GM[r], gentamicin sensitive and resistant, respectively. Number in parentheses indicates number of strains.

TABLE 2. *Apparent affinity constants of SCE 1365 and other cephalosporins for β-lactamase*

Type of enzyme	Source of enzyme	Apparent affinity constants (M)[a]							
		SCE 1365		Cefotaxime		Cefuroxime		Cefoxitin	
		K_m	K_i	K_m	K_i	K_m	K_i	K_m	K_i
Penicillinase	S. aureus 1840		$>10^{-4}$		$>10^{-4}$		$>10^{-4}$		1.1×10^{-5}
	E. coli TN713		$>10^{-4}$		$>10^{-4}$		$>10^{-4}$		$>10^{-4}$
	K. pneumoniae TN1698		$>10^{-4}$		$>10^{-4}$		4.6×10^{-4}		2.0×10^{-5}
	P. aeruginosa GN3407		6.9×10^{-5}		$>10^{-4}$		9.3×10^{-5}		$>10^{-4}$
Cephalosporinase	E. cloacae TN1282		9.8×10^{-8}		7.6×10^{-8}		5.2×10^{-8}	1.4×10^{-6}	1.3×10^{-6}
	C. freundii GN1706		9.8×10^{-9}		5.3×10^{-9}		7.1×10^{-9}		7.6×10^{-7}
	P. aeruginosa U31		3.0×10^{-7}		2.2×10^{-7}		4.9×10^{-8}		3.5×10^{-7}
	S. marcescens TN81		1.8×10^{-6}		7.7×10^{-6}		1.6×10^{-6}		3.8×10^{-7}
	P. vulgaris GN4413	2.9×10^{-4}	$>10^{-4}$	5.6×10^{-4}	$>10^{-4}$	4.2×10^{-4}	$>10^{-4}$		2.3×10^{-7}

[a] Inhibition constants (K_i) were determined by assessing the ability of antibiotics to inhibit the hydrolysis of ampicillin (penicillinase) or cephalothin (cephalosporinase).

the cephalosporin to penicillin-binding protein 3. By the electron microscopy study on the ultrathin sections, the filamentous cells of *S. marcescens* IFO 12648 treated with SCE 1365 showed several morphological changes such as expansion of nucleoid area, vacuole formation, and plasmolysis.

1. Heymes, R., A. Lutz, and E. Schrinner. 1978. Experimental evaluation of HR-756, a new cephalosporin derivative: pre-clinical study. Infection 5:259–260.
2. Ochiai, M., O. Aki, A. Morimoto, T. Okada, and Y. Matsushita. 1977. New cephalosporin derivatives with high antibacterial activities. Chem. Pharm. Bull. 25: 3115–3117.
3. Tsuchiya, K., M. Kida, M. Kondo, H. Ono, M. Takeuchi, and T. Nishi. 1978. SCE-963, a new broad-spectrum cephalosporin: in vitro and in vivo antibacterial activities. Antimicrob. Agents Chemother. 14:551–568.
4. Tsuchiya, K., M. Kondo, Y. Kita, Y. Noji, M. Takeuchi, and T. Fugono. 1978. Absorption, distribution and excretion of SCE-963, a new broad-spectrum cephalosporin, in mice, rats, rabbits and dogs. J. Antibiot. 31: 1272–1282.
5. Tsuchiya, K., M. Kondo, and H. Nagatomo. 1978. SCE-129, antipseudomonal cephalosporin: in vitro and in vivo antibacterial activities. Antimicrob. Agents Chemother. 13:137–145.

SCE 1365, a New Cephalosporin: In Vivo Antibacterial Activities and Fates in Experimental Animals

K. TSUCHIYA, M. KONDO,* Y. KITA, I. YAMAZAKI, T. FUGONO, S. GOTO, M. OGAWA, A. TSUJI, AND K. KUWAHARA

Takeda Chemical Industries, Ltd., Osaka,* and School of Medicine, Toho University, Tokyo, Japan

SCE 1365 is a new cephalosporin which shows excellent in vitro antibacterial activity against gram-negative bacteria including *Haemophilus influenzae*, indole-positive *Proteus*, *Serratia marcescens*, *Citrobacter freundii*, and *Enterobacter cloacae*. Its activity is comparable with that of cefotaxime but more potent than those of cefotiam and cefazolin. Cefotaxime, however, has the acetoxymethyl moiety at the 3 position of the cephalosporin. Usually, the cephalosporins having the acetoxymethyl moiety at the 3 position are metabolized to the deacetyl form in the body, and the deacetylcephalosporins are less active than the parent compounds. Therefore, it is imperative to conduct a comparative study on in vivo antibacterial activities of SCE 1365, cefotaxime, cefotiam, and cefazolin and on the fate in experimental animals of SCE 1365 and cefotaxime.

The protective effect against systemic infection was tested in Slc:ICR mice infected with various strains of gram-positive and gram-negative bacteria. Mice were infected intraperitoneally with the bacteria in 0.5 ml of 5% mucin except *Streptococcus pneumoniae* type I, which was suspended in Trypticase soy broth. Groups of five mice at each dose level were given subcutaneously 0.2 ml of the cephalosporin solutions per mouse at 0 and 4 h after infection with *S. pneumoniae*, at 0, 2, and 4 h after infection with *Pseudomonas aeruginosa*, and at 0 h after infections with other bacteria. All experiments were repeated five times. The ED_{50} values were calculated by probit analysis from the number of animals surviving 5 days after infection (2). The therapeutic effects against pneumonia caused by *Klebsiella pneumoniae* and pyelonephritis caused by *Proteus mirabilis* in mice were tested. *Klebsiella* pneumonia was induced by the method of Nishi and Tsuchiya (submitted for publication). Slc:ICR mice were infected with *K. pneumoniae* DT-S by the aerosol method, resulting in a deposition of about 10^4 colony-forming units (CFU) of bacteria per lung. The number of bacteria in the lung increased to about 10^8 CFU per tissue at the time of start of chemotherapy. Pyelonephritis due to *P. mirabilis* was produced by the method of Iwahi and Tsuchiya (1). CF 1/b (Takeda) mice were infected with *P. mirabilis* IFO 3849 by ascending route. This treatment resulted in a deposition of about 10 CFU of the organism per kidney, and the number of bacteria in the kidney reached about 10^4 CFU per tissue at the time of start of chemotherapy. Cephalosporins were administered subcutaneously to groups of 10 mice at each dose level in two dosing series a day, each of which consisted of four doses at 30-min intervals. The treatments with cephalosporins

started at 30 h after infection and continued for 10 days for mice with *Klebsiella* pneumonia, and the treatment started at 3 days after infection and continued for 5 days for mice with pyelonephritis caused by *P. mirabilis*. The concentrations of SCE 1365 in the body fluids and tissues were assayed by the cylinder plate diffusion method using *P. mirabilis* ATCC 21100 as the test organism and DST agar. The cefotaxime concentrations in the plasma, urine, and bile specimens were assayed by the same method as that for SCE 1365 assay, and its concentrations in the tissues were assayed by the paper disk method after homogenation with methanol.

The protective activity of SCE 1365 in mice infected with *S. aureus* resembled those of cefotaxime and cefotiam and was inferior to that of cefazolin (Table 1). In mice infected with *S. pyogenes* and *S. pneumoniae*, SCE 1365 and cefotaxime, however, were more potent than cefotiam and cefazolin. The activities of SCE 1365 and cefotaxime in mice infected with gram-negative bacteria were 30 to 3,000 times more potent than those of cefotiam and cefazolin, especially in mice infected with *K. pneumoniae*, *S. marcescens*, and *Proteus* species. Moreover, in mice infected with *Proteus vulgaris* GN 4721,

TABLE 1. *Protective effects of SCE 1365 and other cephalosporins against experimental intraperitoneal infection in mice*

Organism (CFU/ mouse)	Cephalosporin	ED_{50} (mg/kg)	MIC (10^6 CFU/ml)	Organism (CFU/ mouse)	Cephalosporin	ED_{50} (mg/kg)	MIC (10^6 CFU/ml)
S. aureus 308 A-1 (10^8)	SCE 1365	2.72	0.78	*S. marcescens* TN 66 (10^3)	SCE 1365	0.163	0.2
	Cefotaxime	4.13	1.56		Cefotaxime	0.241	0.2
	Cefotiam	2.01	0.39		Cefotiam	6.12	0.39
	Cefazolin	1.23	0.2		Cefazolin	186	>100
S. pyogenes E-14 (10^4)	SCE 1365	0.040	0.013	*C. freundii* TN 549 (10^5)	SCE 1365	0.272	0.2
	Cefotaxime	0.025	0.013		Cefotaxime	0.278	0.2
	Cefotiam	0.103	0.05		Cefotiam	1.34	0.78
	Cefazolin	0.318	0.2		Cefazolin	80.7	100
S. pneumoniae type I (10^2)	SCE 1365	0.665	0.006	*E. cloacae* TN 618 (10^4)	SCE 1365	0.064	0.2
	Cefotaxime	0.913	0.013		Cefotaxime	0.064	0.2
	Cefotiam	5.07	0.05		Cefotiam	0.126	0.39
	Cefazolin	0.854	0.1		Cefazolin	3.95	6.25
E. coli O-111 (10^6)	SCE 1365	0.020	0.013	*P. mirabilis* GN 4336 (10^6)	SCE 1365	0.053	0.1
	Cefotaxime	0.017	0.013		Cefotaxime	0.079	0.05
	Cefotiam	0.066	0.025		Cefotiam	3.61	0.78
	Cefazolin	1.84	0.78		Cefazolin	10.6	6.25
E. coli T-7 (10^3)	SCE 1365	0.435	0.2	*P. vulgaris* GN 4712 (10^2)	SCE 1365	0.165	0.1
	Cefotaxime	0.259	0.2		Cefotaxime	0.534	0.05
	Cefotiam	0.952	0.39		Cefotiam	51.9	6.25
	Cefazolin	31.7	12.5		Cefazolin	89.3	>100
K. pneumoniae DT (10^3)	SCE 1365	0.233	0.025	*P. morganii* TN 373 (10^6)	SCE 1365	0.093	0.025
	Cefotaxime	0.445	0.025		Cefotaxime	1.17	0.025
	Cefotiam	5.25	0.1		Cefotiam	58.8	0.39
	Cefazolin	10.0	1.56		Cefazolin	167	>100
K. pneumoniae S 22 (10^6)	SCE 1365	0.447	0.1	*P. rettgeri* TN 338 (10^7)	SCE 1365	0.256	0.006
	Cefotaxime	0.349	0.1		Cefotaxime	1.43	0.006
	Cefotiam	5.62	0.78		Cefotiam	9.72	0.025
	Cefazolin	48.1	12.5		Cefazolin	42.5	0.39

TABLE 2. *Tissue levels and excretions of SCE 1365 and cefotaxime after a single dose of 20 mg/kg in experimental animals*

Animal	Cephalo-sporin	Tissue	Mean concn (μg/ml or g)							Mean % excretion (0–24 h)[a]	
			1/12 h	1/4 h	1/2 h	1 h	2 h	4 h	6 h	Urine	Bile
Mice (n = 5)	SCE-1365	Plasma	20.3	22.9	15.1	5.1	0.4	0[b]	NT	65.8	NT[c]
		Lung	7.1	7.6	5.9	2.3	0.5	0	NT		
		Liver	6.7	14.1	10.7	3.6	0.3	0	NT		
		Spleen	2.2	2.5	1.8	0.6	0	0	NT		
		Kidney	41.0	63.3	49.2	12.4	4.9	0.9	NT		
		Brain	0.2	0.3	0.2	0	0	0	NT		
	Cefotaxime	Plasma	19.5	28.7	25.5	7.7	0.8	0	NT	36.0	NT
		Lung	3.2	4.0	3.7	0.7	0	0	NT		
		Liver	0.3	1.2	1.6	0	0	0	NT		
		Spleen	0.9	1.3	1.5	0.3	0	0	NT		
		Kidney	3.3	10.8	8.8	2.6	0	0	NT		
		Brain	0	0	0	0	0	0	NT		
Rats (n = 6)	SCE-1365	Plasma	30.3	66.7	49.1	27.4	6.7	0.3	0.1	52.5	32.6
		Lung	6.6	13.4	9.6	5.7	1.2	0	0		
		Liver	13.0	27.3	19.4	10.9	2.3	0	0		
		Spleen	1.9	3.7	2.8	1.6	0.4	0	0		
		Kidney	35.8	122	96.1	42.7	11.7	0.8	0.4		
		Brain	0.3	0.5	0.5	0	0	0	0		
	Cefotaxime	Plasma	36.2	43.4	32.6	17.3	2.5	0.1	0	48.7	1.27
		Lung	1.9	3.0	2.6	1.5	0.3	0	0		
		Liver	0.6	1.6	1.2	0.8	0	0	0		
		Spleen	0.5	1.0	0.8	0.5	0	0	0		
		Kidney	4.5	17.4	14.1	4.6	1.3	0	0		
		Brain	0	0	0	0	0	0	0		
Rabbits (n = 3)	SCE 1365	Plasma	NT	28.5	40.3	17.9	12.4	4.8	1.6	81.4	0.27
		Lung	NT	5.6	7.3	4.3	2.0	1.2	0.3		
		Liver	NT	3.6	5.5	2.7	1.5	0.8	0		
		Spleen	NT	1.6	2.7	1.3	1.0	0.7	0		
		Kidney	NT	63.8	90.3	65.0	29.3	12.2	4.7		
		Brain	NT	0.2	0.3	0	0	0	0		
	Cefotaxime	Plasma	NT	55.0	34.0	24.6	9.7	3.5	1.4	72.2	0.21
		Lung	NT	3.1	2.3	1.8	0.4	0	0		
		Liver	NT	1.4	0.7	0	0	0	0		
		Spleen	NT	0.9	0.4	0	0	0	0		
		Kidney	NT	59.1	36.3	20.6	5.6	2.3	0.7		
		Brain	NT	0	0	0	0	0	0		
Dogs (n = 3)	SCE 1365	Plasma	NT	NT	22.7	13.3	4.5	0.5	0	64.5	9.9
		Lung	NT	NT	7.9	5.5	2.2	0.4	0		
		Liver	NT	NT	63.6	52.8	28.4	0.4	0		
		Spleen	NT	NT	2.5	1.7	0.5	0	0		
		Kidney	NT	NT	281	180	61.0	24.3	1.9		
		Brain	NT	NT	0.2	0	0	0	0		
	Cefotaxime	Plasma	NT	NT	34.0	25.3	6.3	2.1	0	55.5	0.54
		Lung	NT	NT	8.4	6.1	1.3	0	0		
		Liver	NT	NT	4.6	3.0	0.8	0	0		
		Spleen	NT	NT	2.7	1.1	0	0	0		
		Kidney	NT	NT	76.8	95.3	10.9	6.7	0.2		
		Brain	NT	NT	0	0	0	0	0		

[a] The mean values of percent excretion in dogs were estimated on the 0- to 6-h urine and bile.
[b] 0, Not detected.
[c] NT, Not tested.

Proteus morganii TN 373, and *Proteus rettgeri* TN 338, SCE 1365 was about 3 to 13 times more potent than cefotaxime, although both cephalosporins had the same MICs. In mice infected with *P. aeruginosa* and *Acinetobacter calcoaceticus*, SCE 1365 and cefotaxime showed more potent activity than cefotiam and cefazolin, whereas the activities of both SCE 1365 and cefotaxime were much inferior to those in mice infected with the strains of other bacterial species. The therapeutic effect of SCE 1365 on *Klebsiella* pneumonia in mice was about 2 times more than cefotaxime, 4 times more than cefotiam, and 64 times more than cefazolin. The MICs of SCE 1365, cefotaxime, cefotiam, and cefazolin against *K. pneumoniae* DT-S were 0.025, 0.025, 0.1, and 1.56 μg/ml, respectively. The therapeutic activity of SCE 1365 on pyelonephritis caused by *P. mirabilis* in mice was close to that of cefotaxime, although the in vitro activity of SCE 1365 against the organism used was 4 times less than that of cefotaxime (MIC of SCE 1365 = 0.78 μg/ml, MIC of cefotaxime = 0.2 μg/ml). In this model infection, SCE 1365 was more potent than cefotiam and cefazolin.

Since SCE 1365 has potent in vivo antibacterial activity, its fate in experimental animals was compared with that of cefotaxime (Table 2). The peak levels of SCE 1365 and cefotaxime in the plasma and tissue were reached 15 min after administration in mice and rats and 30 min after administration in rabbits and dogs. Although the SCE 1365 level in plasma was similar to that

of cefotaxime, the tissue levels of SCE 1365 were several times higher than those of cefotaxime. In mice and rats, SCE 1365 showed distribution at high concentrations in various tissues with the descending order in the kidneys, plasma, liver, lung, spleen, and brain; in rabbits—kidneys, plasma, lung, liver, spleen, and brain; and in dogs—kidneys, liver, plasma, lung, spleen, and brain. The plasma and tissue levels of SCE 1365 lasted much longer than those of cefotaxime. Both cephalosporins were principally excreted in the urine. The high biliary excretions of SCE 1365 in rats and dogs may reflect high hepatic levels, and the biliary excretion of cefotaxime was much lower. Like the cephalosporins which have the acetoxymethyl moiety at the 3 position, cefotaxime was metabolized to deacetylcefotaxime in the body, whereas no active metabolites were observed in the specimens from animals given SCE 1365.

The results of these experiments indicate that SCE 1365 is a potentially useful parenteral cephalosporin.

1. **Iwahi, T., and K. Tsuchiya.** 1979. Establishment of experimental urinary tract infection with *Proteus mirabilis* in mice and therapeutic effect of cefotiam on the infection model. Antimicrob. Agents Chemother. Submitted for publication.

2. **Tsuchiya, K., M. Kida, M. Kondo, H. Ono, M. Takeuchi, and T. Nishi.** 1978. SCE 963, a new broad spectrum cephalosporin: in vitro and in vivo antibacterial activities. Antimicrob. Agents Chemother. **14**:551–568.

In Vitro Properties of GR 20263—a Highly Active Broad-Spectrum Cephalosporin with Antipseudomonal Activity

P. B. HARPER,* SUSAN M. KIRBY, AND CYNTHIA H. O'CALLAGHAN

Glaxo Group Research Ltd., Greenford, Middlesex UB6 0HE, England

A high level of broad-spectrum antibacterial activity, coupled with good activity against relatively resistant *Pseudomonas* species, has until now been mainly associated with aminoglycoside antibiotics. GR 20263 (Fig. 1) is one of a new generation of parenteral β-lactam antibiotics which has a breadth of spectrum and a level of activity at least as good as gentamicin.

GR 20263 is a new parenteral aminothiazolyl cephalosporin which combines exceptionally high broad-spectrum antibacterial activity, particularly against strains of *Pseudomonas aeruginosa*, with high stability to a wide range of β-lactamases.

GR 20263 was highly active against a wide range of gram-negative organisms, showing little change in MIC when the challenge inoculum was increased from 10^5 colony-forming units (CFU)/ml to 10^7 CFU/ml (Table 1). Strains of *Escherichia coli*, *Klebsiella pneumoniae*, *Enterobacter cloacae*, *Serratia*, *Providence*, *Citrobacter*, *Proteus* (indole positive and negative), *Salmonella*, *Shigella*, and *Haemophilus influenzae* were all susceptible over the range <0.06 to 2 mg/liter. Geometric mean MICs ranged from 0.13 to 1.11 mg/liter, indicating that the majority of isolates tested were exquisitely susceptible to this antibiotic. The very small inoculum effect seen against all of these organisms is further evidence of the high intrinsic activity of the compound. Activity against gram-positive organisms was more modest, the majority of isolates of *Staphylococcus aureus* falling within the range of 4 to 8 mg/liter, whereas the geometric mean MIC against nonfecal *Streptococcus* sp. was 1.0 mg/liter.

The compound was especially active against isolates of *P. aeruginosa*. When compared with antipseudomonal compounds presently available, or shortly to be made available, GR 20263 was the most active (Table 2). More than 90% of the isolates tested were susceptible to 4 mg of GR 20263 per liter, whereas four times this concentration of cefotaxime or gentamicin was required to achieve the same standard.

GR 20263 was stable to the β-lactamases from

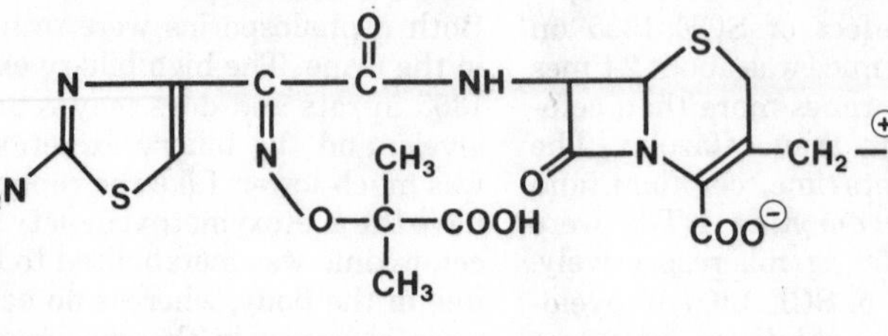

(6R, 7R) - 7 - [(Z) - 2 - (2 - AMINOTHIAZOL - 4 - YL) - 2 -
(2 - CARBOXYPROP - 2 - YLOXYIMINO) ACETAMIDO] - 3 -
(PYRIDINIUM - 1 - YLMETHYL) CEPH - 3 - EM - 4 - CARBOXYLIC ACID

FIG. 1. *GR 20263.*

TABLE 1. *GR 20263—geometric mean MICs and range*

Organism	MIC range (mg/liter)										Geometric mean MIC (mg/liter)	
	≤0.06	0.1	0.2	0.5	1	2	4	8	16	≥32	10^5 CFU/ml	10^7 CFU/ml
S. aureus (25)[a]							11	12	1	1	6.8	9.7
Streptococcus sp., nonfecal (12)		1	2	1	4	2				2	1.0	5.0
E. coli (24)	3	13	1	5	2						0.19	0.31
K. pneumoniae (25)			2	3	10	10					1.1	2.0
E. cloacae (22)	1	12	8		1						0.14	0.37
Serratia sp. (14)	1	9		2	2						0.19	0.43
P. vulgaris (14)	5	6	2			1					0.13	1.2
Citrobacter/Providencia (23)	1	6	4	2	4	1	2			3	0.71	3.8
S. typhimurium (24)		3	20		1						0.20	0.22
H. influenzae (21)	19	2									0.04	0.13
B. fragilis (22)							5	10	3	4	10.9	23.0

[a] Number of strains tested.

TABLE 2. *P. aeruginosa—cumulative percentage sensitivity to antipseudomonal β-lactams*

Antibiotic	Cumulative % MIC[a] (10^5 CFU/ml)								Geometric mean[a] MIC (mg/liter)	
	<0.5[b]	0.5	1	2	4	8	16	32	10^5 CFU/ml	10^7 CFU/ml
GR 20263	4	8	40	88	92	96	100		1.6	2.5
Piperacillin			20	72	84	96		100	2.5	11.3
Azlocillin	4			20	60	92	96	100	4.2	160.3
Gentamicin	4		8	20	24	88	92		6.7	10
Amikacin	4		8	12		72	88	92	9.3	21.5
Cefotaxime	4			8		36	92	96	11	22
Carbenicillin	4			8			12	32	38.5	71.0

[a] Twenty-five isolates.
[b] Milligrams per liter.

a wide range of gram-positive and gram-negative organisms. The use of partially purified enzymes in the UV spectrophotometer proved to be insufficiently sensitive to measure hydrolytic breakdown. A procedure requiring incubation with a heavy inoculum of an enzyme producer, followed by microbiological assay of residual compound, was developed to measure stability. The compound proved to be remarkably stable. Little or no breakdown of GR 20263 was seen after incubation for 4 h, with a heavy inoculum (10^8 to 10^{10} CFU/ml) of organisms mediating a wide range of chromosomally and plasmid-borne β-lactamases.

GR 20263 was rapidly bactericidal, judged by both viable count and turbidimetric (Abbot MS2) measurements, at or close to the MIC. The compound has an affinity for penicillin-binding proteins 3 and 1a, producing longforms as a transient step to lysis of the damaged cell. The MIC and MBC values were generally the same, and in only a few cases was the MBC one doubling dilution higher than the MIC. Since the compound is stable in human serum ($t_{1/2} >$ 6 h) and shows a low order of binding to serum proteins (17%), the activity of GR 20263 was unimpaired in the presence of human serum. We found no evidence of antagonism, and there were several examples in which the activity of the compound was enhanced by as much as 10-fold in the presence of serum. The presence of up to 50% of human serum in growth medium had no adverse effect on the rate of kill of the compound.

The high level of activity seen in vitro was sustained in vivo (see P. Acred, D. M. Ryan, and P. W. Muggleton, this volume) where metabolic stability, low serum binding, and high stability in the presence of serum are coupled with good pharmacokinetics to give a high order of protection in experimental animals.

GR 20263 is at least as active as gentamicin in vitro against gram-negative pathogens. It was the most potent antipseudomonal compound tested, being eightfold more active than cefotaxime. By the agar dilution method, which does give less favorable MICs for aminoglycosides, GR 20263 was, on the average, four times more active than gentamicin against the strains of *P. aeruginosa* tested. Because of its high activity against the gram-negative organisms, GR 20263 should be of considerable value in the treatment of the seriously ill patient.

In Vivo Properties of GR 20263

P. ACRED,* D. M. RYAN, S. M. HARDING, AND P. W. MUGGLETON

Glaxo Group Research Ltd., Greenford, Middlesex UB6 OHE, England

GR 20263, (6R,7R)-7-[(Z)-2(2-aminothiazol-4-yl)-2-(2-carboxyprop-2-yloxyimino) acetamido]-3-(pyridinium-1-ylmethyl) ceph-3-em-4-carboxylic acid, is a new parenteral aminothiazolyl cephalosporin with exceptionally high broad-spectrum antibacterial activity combined with high stability to a wide range of bacterial β-lactamase enzymes. An outstanding characteristic of this new cephalosporin is activity comparable to that of the aminoglycoside antibiotics against *Pseudomonas aeruginosa*. The in vitro properties of GR 20263 have been described by Harper et al. (P. B. Harper, S. M. Kirby, and C. H. O'Callahan, this volume). The present paper describes some of the in vivo characteristics of this new cephalosporin.

The chemotherapeutic efficacy of GR 20263, the related aminothiazolyl cephalosporin cefotaxime (HR-756), and the aminoglycoside antibiotic gentamicin was compared in mice infected with a range of gram-positive and gram-negative bacteria. The mice received an intraperitoneal challenge of 10- to 100-fold the LD_{50} of the infecting organisms. Groups of 10 mice were treated subcutaneously with serial fourfold dilutions of the antibiotics, the doses being administered at 1 and 5 h postinfection. In the *P. aeruginosa*-infected mice the antibiotics were administered at 1, 3, and 5 h postinjection. The ED_{50} values (milligrams per kilogram per dose) were calculated by probit analysis of the numbers of mice surviving on the 5th day of the experiment. GR 20263 proved more active than cefotaxime (Table 1) in protecting animals against infections with 7 of 10 strains of indole-positive *Proteus* spp., *Enterobacter cloacae,* and *Serratia* spp.; the activity of GR 20263 was similar to that of gentamicin against most of the test strains. Activity of the three antibiotics was similar against infections due to *Proteus mirabilis* and *Klebsiella* spp. GR 20263 and cefotaxime were equally effective against infections due to *Escherichia coli,* and both cephalosporins were more active than gentamicin. The two aminothiazolyl antibiotics were less active than gentamicin against *Staphylococcus aureus.* The therapeutic efficacy of GR 20263 was equal to that of gentamicin against three of the four experimental infections due to *P. aeruginosa* (Table 2), and it was significantly more active in these tests than cefotaxime and the antipseudomonal penicillins azlocillin and carbenicillin.

In general, the results in vivo reflected the in vitro susceptibility of the various gram-negative and gram-positive strains used in the experimental infections.

GR 20263 has low affinity for serum proteins. The extent of binding, as determined by the Centriflo cone filtration technique (Amicon Ltd.), when added to the serum of various animal species at a concentration of 25 mg/liter, was as follows: mouse, 13%; rat, 19%; rabbit, 11%;

TABLE 1. *Activity of GR 20263 against a range of gram-positive and gram-negative bacterial infections in mice*

Infecting organism and strain	GR 20263		Cefotaxime		Gentamicin	
	$ED_{50}{}^a$	MIC^b	ED_{50}	MIC	ED_{50}	MIC
Staphylococcus aureus						
853	34.0	8	15.5	0.5	1.4	1
630	90.0	8	15.2	1	2.2	2
Escherichia coli						
851	0.3	0.2	0.1	0.06	1.2	8
573	0.5	0.2	0.2	0.06	1.5	4
2023	0.3	0.5	0.1	0.06	2.4	4
2025	0.3	0.2	0.1	0.06	1.0	4
Proteus mirabilis						
1126	3.0	4	0.9	0.1	3.1	16
1315	3.1	4	1.2	0.5	6.3	16
P. morganii						
1375	3.0	2	2.6	8	0.9	1
1901	0.5	2	2.3	31	1.2	4
265	5.3	0.5	25.0	8	1.8	1
519	2.8	8	5.4	16	0.5	2
P. vulgaris						
1356	3.5	8	23.0	>62	1.2	4
Enterobacter cloacae						
2010	0.1	0.5	0.6	0.5	0.4	1
781	2.7	2	14.0	2	2.7	2
800	9.6	0.5	55.8	0.5	0.6	2
Klebsiella spp.						
2011	0.6	2	0.8	16	0.6	1
Curtis	1.9	2	5.4	4	2.2	16
43403	16.0	1	22.0	0.2	1.2	2
Serratia spp.						
1131	10.0	0.25	74.0	8	1.0	4
3999	0.8	0.1	5.0	0.25	1.0	4

[a] Doses (milligrams per kilogram) administered subcutaneously at 1 and 5 h after intraperitoneal challenge with the infecting organisms.
[b] Expressed in milligrams per liter. Inoculum, 10^7 colony-forming units/ml.

TABLE 2. *Activity of GR 20263 against acute, fatal Pseudomonas aeruginosa infections in mice*

Infecting strain	GR 20263		Cefotaxime		Gentamicin		Azlocillin		Carbenicillin	
	$ED_{50}{}^a$	MIC^b	ED_{50}	MIC	ED_{50}	MIC	ED_{50}	MIC	ED_{50}	MIC
SM2	1.6	1	33.0	16	3.6	2	18.3	4	102.0	31
SM5	4.7	2	100.0	16	6.3	8	73.0	31	>200.0	62
23	4.5	1	>200.0	16	6.3	2	25.0	8	>200.0	125
24	25.0	2	73.0	16	2.6	8	73.0	8	100.0	125

[a] Doses (milligrams per kilogram) administered subcutaneously at 1, 3, and 5 h after intraperitoneal challenge with the infecting organisms.
[b] Expressed in milligrams per liter. Inoculum, 10^7 colony-forming units per ml.

dog, 20%; cynomolgus monkey, 8%; and human, 17%. The new cephalosporin was also stable in serum from the various species.

Serum concentrations of GR 20263 achieved in various animal species after parenteral administration of a dose of 25 mg/kg (monkeys, 10 mg/kg) were species dependent, as were the serum half-life values. In all species, peak serum concentrations occurred within 15 to 30 min after dosing and were as follows: mice, 26 mg/liter; rats, 45 mg/liter; rabbits, 63 mg/liter; dogs, 41 mg/liter, and cynomolgus monkeys, 31 mg/liter. The corresponding serum half-lives in these species were 21, 23, 48, 60, and 58 min, respectively.

GR 20263 is similar to cefuroxime in its pattern of distribution into the peritoneal, pericardial, and pleural fluids of rabbits (1). In common with other β-lactam antibiotics, GR 20263 penetrates the cerebrospinal fluid and aqueous humor of normal uninfected rabbits to only a limited extent.

GR 20263 was recovered unchanged and in high concentrations in the urine of various animal species, the percentage of the parenterally administered cephalosporin recovered being 53% in mice, 62% in rats, 52% in rabbits, 71% in dogs, and 45% in cynomolgus monkeys. Experiments in rodents indicated that less than 5% of parenterally administered GR 20263 was excreted in bile.

Preliminary results in human volunteers showed peak serum concentrations of 10, 23, and 27 mg/liter after intramuscular administration of doses of 250, 500, and 750 mg, with half-lives of 1.4, 1.6, and 1.8 h for the respective doses. Serum concentrations exceeded 8 mg/liter for periods of 1.5, 4.2, and 6.1 h after each of the three intramuscular doses. Urinary recovery of GR 20263 ranged from 48 to 88% in the volunteers. Preliminary studies indicated that the rate of excretion is not affected by administration of probenecid, and it is therefore assumed there is no net tubular secretion.

GR 20263 is a new outstandingly active parenteral cephalosporin that has high antibacterial activity both in vitro and in vivo and good pharmacokinetic properties. These characteristics, together with the high activity of GR 20263 against *P. aeruginosa,* indicate that this cephalosporin is a potential replacement for the more toxic aminoglycoside antibiotics.

1. **Ryan, D. M., C. H. O'Callaghan, and P. W. Muggleton.** 1976. Cefuroxime, a new cephalosporin antibiotic: activity in vivo. Antimicrob. Agents Chemother. **9:**520–525.

Pharmacological Studies on YM09330, a New Parenteral Cephamycin Derivative

A. TACHIBANA,* M. KOMIYA, Y. KIKUCHI, K. YANO, AND K. MASHIMO

Central Research Laboratories, Yamanouchi Pharmaceutical Co., Ltd., Tokyo 174, and *Tokyo Kosei Nenkin Hospital, Tokyo, Japan*

YM09330 is a new injectable cephamycin derivative which is characterized by high activity against gram-negative bacteria including β-lactamase-producing bacteria. Its activity against gram-negative bacteria is much higher than those of cefmetazole and cefoxitin. The present communication describes pharmacological properties of YM09330 in comparison with cefmetazole and cefazolin as well as a tautomerism of YM09330 observed in body fluids.

Concentration in plasma. Concentrations of these cephalosporins in plasma, tissue, urine, and bile were determined by the paper disk method on nutrient agar with *Escherichia coli* NIHJ for YM09330 and with *Bacillus subtilis* ATCC 6633 for cefazolin and cefmetazole as the test organisms.

YM09330 was administered intravenously in a dose of 20 mg/kg to experimental animals. The plasma concentration curves of YM09330 in animals tested are shown in Fig. 1. The average concentrations at 30 min after administration were 5.5 μg/ml, 16.1 μg/ml, 23.9 μg/ml, 42.6 μg/ml, and 75.7 μg/ml for mice, rats, rabbits, dogs, and monkeys, respectively. The persistence of plasma levels was observed in monkeys, dogs, and rabbits, in that order. These plasma concentration curves were analyzed by applying the one-compartment model for mice and the two-compartment model for the others with a first-order rate constant (1). The pharmacokinetic parameters of YM09330 in several species are shown in Table 1. The concentration in the central compartment at time zero and the area under plasma concentration curve for YM09330 were highest in monkeys (177 μg/ml and 168.3 h ·

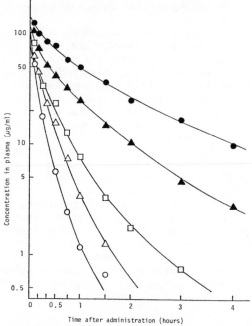

Time after administration (hours)

FIG. 1. *Plasma levels of YM09330 after intrave-nous injection of 20 mg/kg into mice (○), rats (△), rabbits (□), dogs (▲), and monkeys (●).*

TABLE 1. *Pharmacokinetic parameters of YM09330 after intravenous administration of 20 mg/kg to experimental animals*

Animal	$C_p^{0\,a}$	$t_{1/2}\,\beta$ (min)	AUC^b (h·µg per ml)	$K_{el}^{\ c}$ (h^{-1})	$V_p^{\ d}$ (ml/kg)
Mouse[e]	66	13.0	20.6	3.20	303
Rat	111	15.9	26.0	4.26	180
Rabbit	134	30.5	42.0	3.19	150
Dog	164	55.5	83.3	1.97	122
Monkey	177	75.5	168.3	1.05	113

[a] Drug concentration in the plasma immediately after intravenous injection.

[b] Total area under the drug concentration in the plasma versus time curve.

[c] Apparent first-order elimination rate constant.

[d] Apparent volume of distribution of central compartment.

[e] Based on one-compartment model.

µg per ml, respectively) after intravenous administration of 20 mg/kg, followed by dogs, rabbits, rats, and mice, in that order. A similar result was observed in the value of biological half-life, it being longest in monkeys (75.5 min).

In comparison with cefmetazole and cefazolin, the values for area under concentration curve and biological half-life in YM09330 were much higher than those in cefmetazole but lower than those in cefazolin, except for the half-life value in dogs.

Concentrations in tissue. The concentrations of YM09330 in the tissue of mice and rats were highest in the kidneys, followed by those in the plasma, liver, lung, heart, and spleen (in that order). YM09330 showed similar distribution to cefazolin, whereas those of cefmetazole in mice and rats were highest in the liver followed by the kidneys. In dogs, YM09330 was also distributed in various tissues after an intravenous injection, with a pattern similar to that in rat tissue. YM09330 was administered intravenously in 20-mg/kg, 50-mg/kg, and 100-mg/kg dosages. The increasing dose of YM09330 resulted in a corresponding increase in the concentrations not only in plasma but also in all the tissues examined.

Urinary and biliary excretion. The recoveries in urine during 48 h of treatment were 67.2, 52.0, 74.3, 52.8, and 59.7% of the dose for mice, rats, rabbits, dogs, and monkeys, respectively. The major part of the amounts recovered in the urine was excreted within the first 6 h after administration. The biliary excretion of the drug in rats was also as much as 47% within the first 3 h but only 1% in the succeeding hours. Altogether 99% of the intravenously given dose was recovered both from the urine and from the bile in rats.

Metabolism and tautomerism. Metabolism of YM09330 in rats was examined by thin-layer chromatography, bioautography, and high-performance liquid chromatography. Almost no metabolite of YM09330 was detected in the urine or bile. It was found, however, that a small part of the given YM09330 was recovered in the urine and bile of rats as a biological active tautomer of YM09330. The tautomer has a 3-hydroxy-4-carboxy isothiazole ring at the 7-β-position of β-lactam skeleton, showed a lower R_f value and a longer retention time than YM09330 on thin-layer chromatography and high-performance liquid chromatography, respectively, and possessed quite a similar antibacterial activity compared with YM09330. In the investigation of the equilibrium reaction between YM09330 and the tautomer, it was concluded that YM09330 was easily converted to the tautomer by the high alkaline pH (over pH 9) and the high concentration of Mg^{2+} (about 20 mM).

YM09330 excreted into urine was found mostly unchanged in mice, rats, and dogs (Table 2), only 3 to 8% of the dose being changed to the tautomer. In rabbits and monkeys, on the other hand, a large amount of the tautomer was recovered in urine because of the high concentra-

TABLE 2. *Excretion of YM09330 and its tautomer in urine and bile after administration of 20 mg/kg to animals*

Sample	Animal	Administration route[a]	Recovery[b] (% of the dose)			
			Bioassay[c]	HPLC[d]		
				YM09330 (A)	Tautomer (B)	Total (A + B)
Urine	Mouse	i.v.	64.6	56.2	8.07	64.3
	Rat	i.v.	50.1	45.3	2.95	48.3
		i.m.	41.8	34.6	6.66	41.2
	Rabbit	i.v.	73.7	17.7	58.7	76.3
	Dog[e]	i.v.	52.8	49.2	5.89	55.1
		i.m.	52.4	47.3	4.35	51.6
	Monkey	i.v.	58.1	42.7	23.5	66.2
Bile	Rat	i.v.	48.0	41.7	3.13	44.1
		i.m.	51.8	47.4	5.54	52.9
	Rabbit	i.v.	4.42	4.42	1.40	5.82

[a] i.v., Intravenous; i.m., intramuscular.
[b] During 6 h of administration.
[c] Expressed as YM09330.
[d] HPLC, High-performance liquid chromatography.
[e] During 24 h of administration.

tion of Mg^{2+} (about 20 mM) in rabbit urine and the high pH value (about pH 9) of monkey urine. However, the recoveries by biological assay method were the same as those by high-performance liquid chromatography, in spite of differences in the extent of the tautomer formation.

Binding to serum protein. Protein binding of YM09330, cefmetazole, and cefazolin was determined by the ultracentrifugation method. YM09330 was highly bound to the serum protein in humans (91% bound) and monkeys (87% bound), whereas it was bound relatively lower to serum in dogs (39% bound), rabbits (51% bound), and rats (30% bound). The extent of binding of

YM09330 to human serum was similar to that of cefazolin (87% bound) and cefmetazole (85% bound).

The LD_{50} value of YM09330 in mice and rats was ≥5 g/kg intravenously, and no nephrotoxicity was observed in the acute toxicological studies in rats and rabbits, indicating that YM09330 is one of the low-toxic cephalosporin derivatives like cefmetazole and cefazolin.

1. **Gibaldi, M., and D. Perrier.** 1975. Multicompartment models, p. 45–96. *In* J. Swarbrick (ed.), Drugs and pharmaceutical sciences, vol. 1. Pharmacokinetics. Marcel Dekker, New York.

SM-1652, a New Parenterally Active Cephalosporin: Microbiological Studies

TOSHIAKI KOMATSU,* TAKAO OKUDA, HIROSHI NOGUCHI, MASATOMO FUKASAWA, KUNIICHIRO YANO, MASUHIRO KATO, AND SUSUMU MITSUHASHI

Pharmaceuticals Division, Sumitomo Chemical Co., Ltd., Osaka, Central Research Laboratories, Yamanouchi Pharmaceutical Co., Ltd., Tokyo, and Department of Microbiology, School of Medicine, Gunma University, Maebashi, Japan*

SM-1652, sodium 7-[D(−)-α-(4-hydroxy-6-methylpyridine-3-carboxamido)-α-(4-hydroxyphenyl)acetamido]-3-[(1-methyl-1H-tetrazol-5-yl)thiomethyl]-3-cephem-4-carboxylate, is a new antipseudomonal cephalosporin derivative with broad-spectrum activity.

Antibacterial activities were generally deter-

mined with heart infusion agar as the test medium by the standard method of Japan Society of Chemotherapy (1).

The activity of SM-1652 against gram-positive bacteria was generally comparable to that of cefazolin (CEZ). Against gram-negative bacteria SM-1652 exceeded CEZ in potency and broad-ness. It displayed very potent activity against *Pseudomonas aeruginosa*, *P. cepacia*, indole-positive *Proteus*, *Enterobacter*, *Vibrio parahaemolyticus*, and *Haemophilus influenzae*, as well as *Enterobacteriaceae* such as *Escherichia coli*, *Klebsiella pneumoniae*, *P. mirabilis*, etc. SM-1652 also showed fair activity against *Serratia* and *Acinetobacter*. It was more active than CEZ against *Bacteroides*, but almost equivalent to CEZ against other anaerobes.

The above-mentioned activities were confirmed against 1,746 clinical isolates (Table 1). At a concentration of 3.13 µg/ml, SM-1652 inhibited *Staphylococcus aureus* almost completely (95%). It inhibited 100% of strains of *Streptococcus* groups A, B, C, and G, *S. pneumoniae*, and *H. influenzae*, and it inhibited 92% of *V. parahaemolyticus* strains. In contrast, CEZ inhibited only 20% of *H. influenzae* and 15% of *V. parahaemolyticus* strains at this concentration.

At 12.5 µg/ml, SM-1652 inhibited coagulase-negative *Staphylococcus* (93%), *E. coli* (85%), *Salmonella* (96%), *Klebsiella* (93%), and *P. mirabilis* (95%) to the same extent as CEZ. The most characteristic findings were that the majority of *Streptococcus* group D (77%), indole-positive *Proteus* (74%), *E. cloacae* (84%), *P. aeruginosa* (87%), and *P. cepacia* (81%) isolates were inhibited by SM-1652 at 12.5 µg/ml, whereas this concentration of CEZ inhibited the growth of the strains by only 36, 27, 8, 0, and 0%,

respectively. SM-1652 also inhibited *Serratia* spp. (36%), *P. maltophilia* (48%) and *Acinetobacter* (42%) isolates to a considerable extent at 12.5 µg/ml.

The concentrations of SM-1652 which inhibited 50% and 75% of clinical isolates (MIC_{50} and MIC_{75}) are also shown in Table 1. The MIC_{75} of SM-1652 for *H. influenzae* (0.16 µg/ml), indole-positive *Proteus* (14 µg/ml), *E. cloacae* (5.8 µg/ml), *P. aeruginosa* (6.3 µg/ml), *P. cepacia* (8.8 µg/ml), and *V. parahaemolyticus* (1.5 µg/ml) was very low compared with that of CEZ (10, >200, >200, >200, >200, and 6.3 µg/ml, respectively). The MIC_{75} of SM-1652 for *Serratia* spp., *P. maltophilia*, and *Acinetobacter* was 60, 44, and 48 µg/ml, whereas that of CEZ was more than 200 µg/ml. In species other than those mentioned above, the MIC_{75} of SM-1652 was generally almost the same as that of CEZ.

Effects of different culture media (heart infusion agar, tryptic soy agar, nutrient agar, and Mueller-Hinton agar) and pH values (5, 6, 7, 8, and 9) on the MICs of SM-1652 were not great compared with CEZ. The addition of human serum (Moni-Trol I) at 20 to 50% slightly increased the MICs when an agar dilution method was used.

The MBC was determined with a loop transfer method after determination of the MIC by a broth dilution method in which *E. coli* and *P. aeruginosa* were used. Peaks of MBC distribution were no more than one twofold dilution

TABLE 1. *Antibacterial activity of SM-1652 compared with that of cefazolin (CEZ) against clinical isolates*

Organism (no. of strains)	Percentage of strains inhibited at:				MIC_{50} (µg/ml)		MIC_{75} (µg/ml)	
	3.13 µg/ml		12.5 µg/ml					
	SM-1652	CEZ	SM-1652	CEZ	SM-1652	CEZ	SM-1652	CEZ
Staphylococcus aureus (100)	95	97	100	99	1.8	0.3	2.4	0.5
Coagulase-negative *Staphylococcus* (144)	65	78	93	90	1.2	0.4	2.4	0.9
Streptococcus group A, B, C, G (104)	100	100	100	100	0.1	0.06	0.2	0.08
Streptococcus group D (104)	2	0	77	36	8.6	15	12	21
S. pneumoniae (17)	100	100	100	100	≦0.01	0.02	0.03	0.04
Haemophilus influenzae (25)	100	20	100	88	0.09	6.6	0.16	10
Escherichia coli (200)	71	85	85	98	1.1	1.1	4.6	1.6
Salmonella spp. (50)	36	96	96	100	3.8	1.4	5.2	2.0
Klebsiella pneumoniae (200)	73	86	93	99	1.6	1.3	3.8	2.1
Proteus mirabilis (100)	15	21	95	96	5.1	4.4	8.0	6.0
Indole-positive *Proteus* (77)	8	18	74	27	7.2	110	14	>200
Citrobacter freundii (22)	0	5	32	23	>200	>200	>200	>200
Enterobacter cloacae (50)	44	4	84	8	3.4	>200	5.8	>200
Serratia spp. (130)	1	0	36	0	18	>200	60	>200
Pseudomonas aeruginosa (200)	54	0	87	0	2.9	>200	6.3	>200
P. maltophilia (82)	20	0	48	0	14	>200	44	>200
P. cepacia (26)	42	0	81	8	3.8	>200	8.8	>200
Acinetobacter (102)	8	1	42	1	18	>200	48	>200
Vibrio parahaemolyticus (13)	92	15	100	100	1.0	4.6	1.5	6.3

TABLE 2. *Protective effects of SM-1652 against experimental infection in mice*

Organism[a]	Challenge dose (cells/mouse)	Drug[b]	Route[c]	MIC (μg/ml)	ED$_{50}$ (mg/kg)
Streptococcus pyogenes S-23	10^4	SM-1652	s.c.	0.1	0.44
		CEZ	s.c.	0.2	0.75
Pseudomonas aeruginosa KB29	2×10^5	SM-1652	s.c.	3.13	7.8
		Cefsulodin	s.c.	3.13	3.8
		SBPC	s.c.	50	192
P. aeruginosa KB15	10^5	SM-1652	s.c.	6.25	3.8
		CBPC	s.c.	200	140
Escherichia coli No. 34	10^4	SM-1652	s.c.	3.13	1.6
		CEZ	s.c.	1.56	8.6
	10^4	SM-1652	i.v.	3.13	2.4
		CEZ	i.v.	1.56	10.4
Klebsiella pneumoniae KB14	5×10^4	SM-1652	s.c.	1.56	2.3
		CEZ	s.c.	1.56	2.3
Proteus vulgaris No. 125	10^6	SM-1652	s.c.	12.5	15
		CEZ	s.c.	>200	200
Serratia KB1	8×10^6	SM-1652	s.c.	25	15
		SBPC	s.c.	12.5	26.5
		CEZ	s.c.	>200	>1,200
Enterobacter cloacae No. 65	10^6	SM-1652	s.c.	1.56	0.87
		CEZ	s.c.	50	10.2

[a] Challenge, with 5% mucin except for *S. pyogenes*, intraperitoneally.
[b] Medication, 1 and 3 h after infection. CEZ, cefazolin; SBPC, sulbenicillin; CBPC, carbenicillin.
[c] Subcutaneous (s.c.) or intravenous (i.v.).

higher than the MIC peaks at the inoculum size of 10^4 and 10^6 colony-forming units/ml, except for 10^6 colony-forming units/ml with *P. aeruginosa*. The bactericidal action was also confirmed by the viable-cell counting method.

Stability of SM-1652 to β-lactamases was determined by the macroiodometric method described by Perret (2). SM-1652 was more resistant than cephaloridine and was as stable as cephalothin and CEZ to hydrolysis by penicillinase type I (TEM type). It was very stable to penicillinases II and III (oxacillin-hydrolyzing enzymes) and penicillinase IV (carbenicillin-hydrolyzing enzyme). To cephalosporinase originated from *E. freundii* GN346, *P. vulgaris* GN76, *P. morganii* GN926, *E. coli* GN5482, and *P. aeruginosa* GN918, SM-1652 was much more resistant than cephalothin, cephaloridine, and CEZ. With the hydrolysis rate of cephaloridine assumed to be 100%, those of SM-1652, cephalothin, CEZ, and penicillin G were 1 to 4%, 15 to 95%, 74 to 265%, and 4 to 25%, respectively.

Protective effects of SM-1652 against experimental systemic infections in mice are illustrated in Table 2. Male ICR mice were challenged intraperitoneally with test organisms suspended in 5% mucin and were treated with test materials subcutaneously or intravenously 1 and 3 h after challenge. SM-1652 showed protective effect comparable to that of CEZ against gram-positive bacteria such as *S. pyogenes*. Potent in vitro activity of SM-1652 against gram-negative bacilli was confirmed by the in vivo experiment. Against *P. aeruginosa*, the protective effect of SM-1652 was about 25 and 40 times that of sulbenicillin and carbenicillin, respectively, and was comparable to that of cefsulodin (SCE-129). SM-1652 was several times as effective as CEZ against *E. coli* and was equivalent to CEZ against *K. pneumoniae*. It showed, furthermore, in vivo activity against *P. vulgaris*, *Serratia*, and *Enterobacter*, whereas CEZ was inactive or much less potent against these organisms.

Influence of the challenge dose on the ED$_{50}$ of SM-1652 was slight, as was the case with CEZ, against both *E. coli* and *K. pneumoniae*. In *P. aeruginosa* the ED$_{50}$ of SM-1652 was increased to some extent, as was also observed with sulbenicillin.

Total ED$_{50}$ values of SM-1652 on divided dosing were not greatly influenced, as was the case with those of CEZ, against both *E. coli* and *K. pneumoniae*, but they were somewhat decreased against *P. aeruginosa*.

In conclusion, SM-1652 is a novel antipseudomonal cephalosporin derivative with broad-spectrum activity that exhibits a potent protective effect in vivo upon parenteral administration.

1. **Japan Society of Chemotherapy.** 1974. Determination method of MIC. Chemotherapy (Tokyo) **22**:1126–1128. (In Japanese).
2. **Perret, C. J.** 1954. Iodometric assay of penicillinase. Nature (London) **174**:1012–1013.

SM-1652, a New Parenterally Active Cephalosporin: Pharmacological Studies

HIDEFUMI MATSUI,* KUNIICHIRO YANO, HIROSHI NAKATANI, AND KEIMEI MASHIMO

Central Research Laboratories, Yamanouchi Pharmaceutical Co., Ltd., Tokyo, Pharmaceuticals Division, Sumitomo Chemical Co., Ltd., Osaka, and Tokyo Kosei Nenkin Hospital, Tokyo, Japan*

SM-1652, sodium 7-[D(−)-α-(4-hydroxy-6-methylpyridine-3-carboxamido)-α-(4-hydroxyphenyl)acetamido]-3-[(1-methyl-1H-tetrazol-5-yl)thiomethyl]-3-cephem-4-carboxylate, is a novel semisynthetic cephalosporin antibiotic. It is a compound developed as a result of collaborative research between Yamanouchi Pharmaceutical Co. and Sumitomo Chemical Co. The compound has a broad spectrum of activity against both gram-positive and -negative microorganisms, including *Pseudomonas*, in vitro and in vivo (see T. Komatsu, T. Okuda, H. Noguchi, M. Fukazawa, K. Yano, M. Kato, and S. Mitsuhashi, this volume). The experiments described below were undertaken to determine and compare the pharmacokinetics of SM-1652 and cefazolin (CEZ) in laboratory animals after intravenous (i.v.) administration and to gain information on the tolerability of SM-1652.

Male ddY mice weighing approximately 30 g, male SD rats weighing approximately 200 g, male albino rabbits weighing approximately 3 kg, rhesus monkeys of both sexes weighing approximately 5 kg, and female beagle dogs weighing approximately 10 kg were used for the pharmacokinetic studies. In the measurements of the concentrations of SM-1652 or CEZ in plasma of mice and rats, a group of three animals was sacrificed at each indicated time. In rabbits, monkeys, and dogs, blood samples were consecutively withdrawn from each of the animals in the usual manner. SM-1652 levels in biological materials were determined by a disk agar diffusion assay, with *Bacillus subtilis* ATCC 6633 or *Escherichia coli* NIHJ as test organism.

Pharmacokinetics. Figure 1 shows SM-1652 concentrations in plasma of mice, rats, rabbits, monkeys, and dogs after i.v. injection of the drug in a dose of 20 mg/kg. As the body size of the animal species increased from mice to monkeys, SM-1652 levels in plasma became higher. Plasma concentrations of SM-1652 in dogs were similar to those in rats in the early period after dosing, although the body size of dogs was greatest of the five species studied.

It is pertinent to consider plasma levels of a drug in terms of their height and duration. C^0 (calculated drug level in plasma immediately after i.v. administration) as a parameter indicating the height of the drug level and $T_{1/2}$ (plasma half-life) as a parameter reflecting the duration of the antibiotic concentrations are listed in Ta-

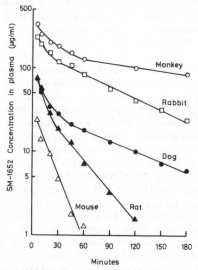

FIG. 1. *SM-1652 concentrations in plasma after intravenous administration of 20 mg/kg to mice, rats, rabbits, monkeys, and dogs.*

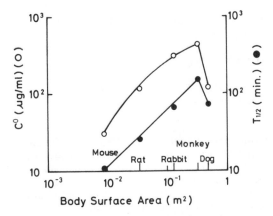

FIG. 2. *Relationship between body surface area and C^0 (calculated drug level in plasma immediately after i.v. administration) or $T_{1/2}$ (plasma half-life).*

TABLE 1. *Calculated drug level immediately after intravenous injection (C^0) and plasma half-life ($T_{1/2}$) of SM-1652 and cefazolin (CEZ).*

Species	C^0 (µg/ml)		$T_{1/2}$ (min.)	
	SM-1652	CEZ	SM-1652	CEZ
Mouse	30.3[a]	86.6[a]	11.0[a]	11.2[a]
Rat	114.9	89.0[a]	26.0	21.6[a]
Rabbit	307.7±35.3[b]	493.7±94.3	65.8± 4.8	24.7± 0.9
Monkey	428.4±37.2	211.8±17.8	150.9±16.7	42.3± 3.7
Dog	118.2±13.8	169.0±16.6	72.6± 3.1	43.9± 3.7

[a] Based on single-compartment model
[b] Mean±SE

ble 1. C^0 values of SM-1652 were 1.3- and 2-fold higher than those of CEZ in rats and monkeys, respectively, but they were 35, 60, and 70% of those of CEZ in mice, rabbits, and dogs, respectively. In mice and rats, $T_{1/2}$ values of SM-1652 were similar to those of CEZ, whereas the values were 2.7, 3.5, and 1.7 times those of CEZ in rabbits, monkeys, and dogs, respectively. These observations demonstrate that SM-1652 is a novel cephalosporin derivative that yields high and prolonged blood levels.

Species difference in C^0 and $T_{1/2}$. Body surface area was employed as an index of the body size of the species. The relationship between body surface area and C^0 or $T_{1/2}$ is illustrated in Fig. 2. From mice to monkeys, both C^0 and $T_{1/2}$ increased as body surface area increased. However, the curves rapidly declined from monkeys to dogs. These findings indicate that SM-1652 disposition in dogs is considerably different from what is expected from the general trend of drug disposition in animal bodies, i.e., that drug levels in plasma become higher and more prolonged in proportion to the increase of the body size of the animal species (1).

Urinary and biliary excretion. The urinary recoveries of SM-1652 were 31.7 ± 1.8 (mean ± SE), 35.2 ± 2.2, 74.1± 5.5, 44.6 ± 0.7, and 70.6 ± 2.7% of the doses in mice, rats, rabbits, mon-

keys, and dogs, respectively, over a period of 24 h after i.v. administration. During the 24-h collection period, 59.6 ± 5.5 and 19.1 ± 4.5% of the SM-1652 administered were excreted into bile in rats and rabbits, respectively, and the corresponding figures in dogs were 19.1 ± 1.5% over 9 h after drug administration. Therefore, 90 to 95% of SM-1652 doses were recovered in urine and bile in an unchanged form in rats, rabbits, and dogs. On bioautogram, no active metabolite was detected in the species examined.

Binding to serum. The percentages of SM-1652 binding to serum determined by the ultrafiltration method were 44, 46, 90, 93, 30, and 96 in mice, rats, rabbits, monkeys, dogs, and humans, respectively.

Acute toxicity. The LD$_{50}$ values of SM-1652 against 5-week-old ICR mice were 4.4 and 4.3 g/kg i.v. for males and females, respectively. Those for 5-week-old SD rats were 5.85 and 6.10 g/kg i.v. for males and females, respectively.

These studies demonstrate that SM-1652 is a well-tolerated antibiotic yielding high and prolonged blood levels upon i.v. administration to laboratory animals. SM-1652 is, therefore, a promising cephalosporin derivative for the treatment of infections due to gram-positive and -negative microorganisms, including *Pseudomonas*, in clinical practice.

1. **Dedrick, R. L., K. B. Bischoff, and D. S. Zaharko.** 1970. Interspecies correlation of plasma concentration history of methotrexate. Cancer Chemother. Rep. (Part 1) **54:**95–101.

In Vitro and In Vivo Antibacterial Activities of YM09330, a New Cephamycin Derivative

M. TODA,* T. SAITO, K. YANO, K. SUZAKI, M. SAITO, AND S. MITSUHASHI

Central Research Laboratories, Yamanouchi Pharmaceutical Co., Tokyo, 174, and Department of
Microbiology, School of Medicine, Gunma University, Maebashi, Japan*

YM09330, disodium 7-β-[4-(carbamoyl carboxylatomethylene)-1,3-dithietan-2-yl]carboxamido-7-α-methoxy-3-(1-methyltetrazol-5-yl)-thiomethyl-Δ3-cephem-4-carboxylate, is a new cephamycin-type antibiotic with a broad spectrum of antibacterial activity.

The susceptibility distribution of YM09330 was examined against about 1,500 clinical isolates of gram-positive and -negative bacteria at an inoculum size of 10^6 colony-forming units per ml (Table 1). Against both *Staphylococcus aureus* and *Streptococcus pyogenes*, YM09330 was slightly less active than cefoxitin and cefazolin. Against gram-negative bacteria, YM09330 showed the highest activity, being 3.5- to over 100-fold more potent than cefazolin. The MIC for 70% of clinical isolates (MIC_{70}) of *Escherichia coli*, *Klebsiella pneumoniae*, *Haemophilus influenzae*, *Proteus mirabilis*, indole-positive *Proteus* spp., and *Serratia marcescens* was 0.17 to 4.5 μg of YM09330/ml, indicating that YM09330 is one of the most active cephamycin derivatives. YM09330 was shown to be more active than any of the above cephalosporins against *Pseudomonas cepacia* strains which were shown to produce a strong β-lactamase that hydrolyzed cefuroxime and cefamandole. The MIC_{70} of YM09330 against *P. cepacia*

strains was found to be 12.5 μg/ml. Further, YM09330 was more active than the above two cephalosporins against *Enterobacter cloacae* and *Citrobacter freundii*, but its activity was rather weak; the MIC_{70} against clinical isolates was 30 and 17.5 μg/ml, respectively.

The MICs of YM09330 against gram-negative organisms were compared under various conditions. Changes in inoculum size had no significant effect on MICs for *E. coli* NIH JC-2 and *S. marcescens* IMAI 184. No significant difference in the MICs of YM09330 was observed when growth media were changed. Heart infusion agar, Mueller-Hinton agar, tryptic soy agar, and nutrient agar were the media used.

The bactericidal activity of YM09330 against *E. coli* GN6370 was examined in antibiotic medium 3 (Difco Penassay broth) containing serial twofold dilutions of the antibiotic. A clear decrease in viable bacteria was observed at 0.1 μg/ml, which was the same concentration of YM09330 as the MIC determined by the agar dilution method. At a concentration of 0.1 μg/ml, regrowth was not observed during an incubation time of 24 h.

The dose-response curve of YM09330 showed a steep gradient and gave ID_{50} values (1) of 0.023 μg/ml against *E. coli* NY-17, 0.041 μg/ml against

TABLE 1. *Susceptibility of clinical isolates to YM09330, cefoxitin (CFX), cefmetazole (CMZ), and cefazolin (CEZ)*[a]

Organism (no. of strains)	YM09330		CFX		CMZ		CEZ	
	MIC_{50}	MIC_{70}	MIC_{50}	MIC_{70}	MIC_{50}	MIC_{70}	MIC_{50}	MIC_{70}
Staphylococcus aureus (200)	3.84	5.10	1.28	1.54	0.56	0.68	0.19	0.28
Streptococcus pyogenes (175)	0.96	1.28	0.32	0.48	0.22	0.32	0.01	0.15
Escherichia coli (160)	0.32	0.38	5.32	6.88	1.21	1.44	1.87	2.81
Klebsiella pneumoniae (200)	0.13	0.17	4.38	5.79	1.17	1.40	3.60	5.16
Haemophilus influenzae (58)	0.52	0.66	1.28	1.48	1.71	2.50	7.04	10.2
Proteus mirabilis (100)	0.18	0.25	5.01	5.95	2.65	3.75	5.95	9.40
Proteus vulgaris (54)	0.21	0.30	4.22	5.47	2.18	2.70	>100	>100
Proteus rettgeri (31)	0.18	0.86	5.63	30.0	3.91	21.25	80.0	>100
Proteus morganii (54)	2.96	4.22	10.31	12.50	7.18	10.60	>100	>100
Enterobacter cloacae (81)	3.13	30.0	84.5	>100	62.5	>100	>100	>100
Citrobacter freundii (65)	0.34	17.5	45.0	95.0	20.0	45	11.5	>100
Serratia marcescens (241)	1.36	4.53	25.0	65.0	13.8	45	>100	>100
Pseudomonas cepacia (79)	5.90	12.5	60.0	80.0	35.0	50	>100	>100

[a] The inoculum was one loopful of 10^6 colony-forming units/ml. The MIC_{50} and MIC_{70} were the concentrations (micrograms per milliliter) of a drug required to inhibit 50 and 70%, respectively, of the tested strains.

TABLE 2. *Substrate profiles of β-lactamase produced by various gram-negative bacteria*

Cephalosporinase producer	Relative rate of hydrolysis[a] of						
	CEZ	CET	CEX	CTM	CMD	CXM	YM09330
Escherichia coli GN5482	70	370	54	42	<0.1	<0.1	<0.1
Enterobacter cloacae GN7471	52	420	56	76	<0.1	<0.1	<0.1
Citrobacter freundii GN346	116	125	80	8	<0.1	<0.1	<0.1
Serratia marcescens 48	457	389	30	60	<0.1	<0.1	<0.1
Proteus vulgaris GN7919	555	190	48	150	225	219	<0.1
P. morganii GN5407	68	232	28	36	4	<0.1	<0.1
P. rettgeri GN4425	36	44	<0.1	22	4	<0.1	<0.1
Pseudomonas aeruginosa GN98	131	495	33	33	<0.1	<0.1	<0.1
P. cepacia GN11164	115	176	60	69	147	85	<0.1

[a] β-Lactamase activity was assayed by the method of Samuni (2). The rate of hydrolysis of cephaloridine was taken as 100. Other drugs were cefazolin (CEZ), cephalothin (CET), cephalexin (CEX), cefotiam (CTM), cefamandole (CMD), and cefuroxime (CXM).

K. pneumoniae ATCC 10031, 0.074 μg/ml against *P. mirabilis* 1278, 0.044 μg/ml against *P. vulgaris* IID 874, 0.16 μg/ml against *P. morganii* Kono, and 0.045 μg/ml against *S. marcescens* IID 620.

Enzymatic studies using a spectrophotometric assay (2) were carried out on the resistance of YM09330 to β-lactamases obtained from various bacteria which were shown to produce cephalosporinase. The results in Table 2 indicate that YM09330 has strong resistance to all types of β-lactamase. It was not hydrolyzed by any of the β-lactamases tested, whereas cefamandole and cefuroxime were hydrolyzed by *P. vulgaris*-type and *P. cepacia*-type β-lactamases.

Inner membrane protein fractions were prepared from *E. coli* JE 1011, *S. marcescens* GN7403, and *P. aeruginosa* NCTC 10490 by the method of Spratt (3). The affinity of YM09330 for penicillin-binding proteins (PBPs) was detected by measuring the competition for the binding of ^{14}C-labeled penicillin G to the PBPs and by the direct binding of ^{14}C-labeled YM09330 to them. YM09330 showed a high affinity for almost all PBPs, with a stronger affinity for PBP 3, a strong affinity for PBPs 1A, 1Bs, 4, and 5/6, and little affinity for PBP 2. In the course of our experiments, new binding proteins were found in the inner membrane fraction of *E. coli* JE 1011. Through the direct binding of ^{14}C-YM09330, four new binding proteins were detected: Y-1 (molecular weight, 75,000), Y-2 (68,000), Y-3 (57,000), and Y-4 (53,000). But their functions are not yet known. In addition to the above four proteins, several bands of proteins

were observed at a molecular weight of about 30,000.

The ED$_{50}$ of YM09330 was 0.12 mg/kg in mice infected with *E. coli* NY-17. Mice were challenged intraperitoneally with 8 LD$_{50}$, and the drug was given subcutaneously 2 h after infection. YM09330 was shown to have a protective effect about 40 times greater than that of cefoxitin. On the other hand, the ED$_{50}$ of YM09330 was 0.18 mg/kg in mice infected with *S. marcescens* IID 620. Thus, YM09330 was shown to have a protective effect about 90 times greater than that of cefoxitin.

The effect of YM09330 on the morphology of *E. coli* NY-17 and *S. marcescens* IID 625 was examined by phase-contrast and scanning electron microscopy. On exposure to serial dilutions of YM09330 in Mueller-Hinton broth, both strains showed long filamentous shapes at concentrations near the MIC after 2 h of incubation; then lysis proceeded in the long filaments down to the MIC, to give only elongated filaments attached to spheroplast-like structures at the MIC after 18 h. Cefoxitin and cefazolin did not show such a lytic change under corresponding conditions.

1. **Kato, T., S. Kurashige, Y. A. Chabbert, and S. Mitsuhashi.** 1978. Determination of the ID$_{50}$ values of antibacterial agent in agar. J. Antibiot. **31:**1299–1303.
2. **Samuni, A.** 1975. A direct spectrophotometric assay and determination of Michaelis constants for β-lactamase reaction. Anal. Biochem. **63:**17–26.
3. **Spratt, B. G.** 1977. Properties of the penicillin binding proteins of *Escherichia coli* K 12. Eur. J. Biochem. **72:** 341–352.

Diastereomeric 7-α-Ureidoacetyl Cephalosporins: Preparation and Antibacterial Activity In Vitro of 7-(α-Ureido-2-Amino-4-Thiazolylacetyl) Cephalosporins

H. BREUER, K. R. LINDNER, AND U. D. TREUNER*

Squibb International Research Center, von Heyden GmbH, D-8400 Regensburg, Federal Republic of Germany

In a previous paper (1) we reported that the L-diastereomers of 7-acyl-α-ureido cephalosporins show antimicrobial activity superior to that of their corresponding D-diastereomers. This contradicts the general studies made so far with penicillins and cephalosporins. From a series of derivatives, the L-diastereomeric 2-furyl-α-ureido cephalosporin (compound 1, SQ 69,613) proved to be the most potent (Fig. 1).

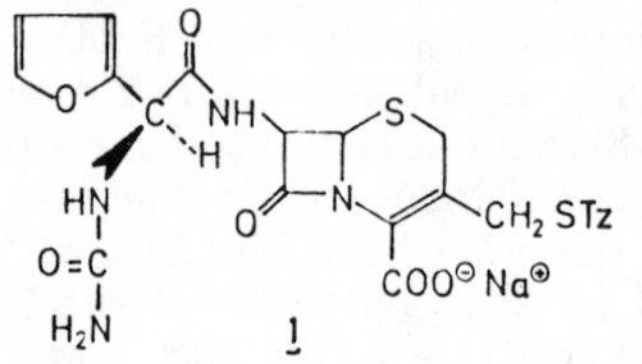

FIG. 1. *Structure of compound 1 (SQ 69,613).*

These findings and reports on the activity-enhancing influence of the 2-amino-4-thiazolyl substituent in 7-acyl side chains of cephalosporins (HR-756 [cefotaxime; 2, 3] and SCE-963 [K. Tsuchiya et al., Program Abstr. Intersci. Conf. Antimicrob. Agents Chemother. 17th, New York, N.Y., abstr. no. 45, 1977) prompted us to synthesize compounds of the type 2 and to investigate the antimicrobial activity of the separated L- and D-diastereomers together with their D,L-mixtures.

Chemistry. The scheme in Fig. 2 shows the synthetic routes used. The reactions were carried out according to known methods.

Separation of the diastereomers. The mixture (1:1) of diastereomers 2, as obtained by both synthetic routes, was separated into D- and L-isomers by means of preparative high-perform-

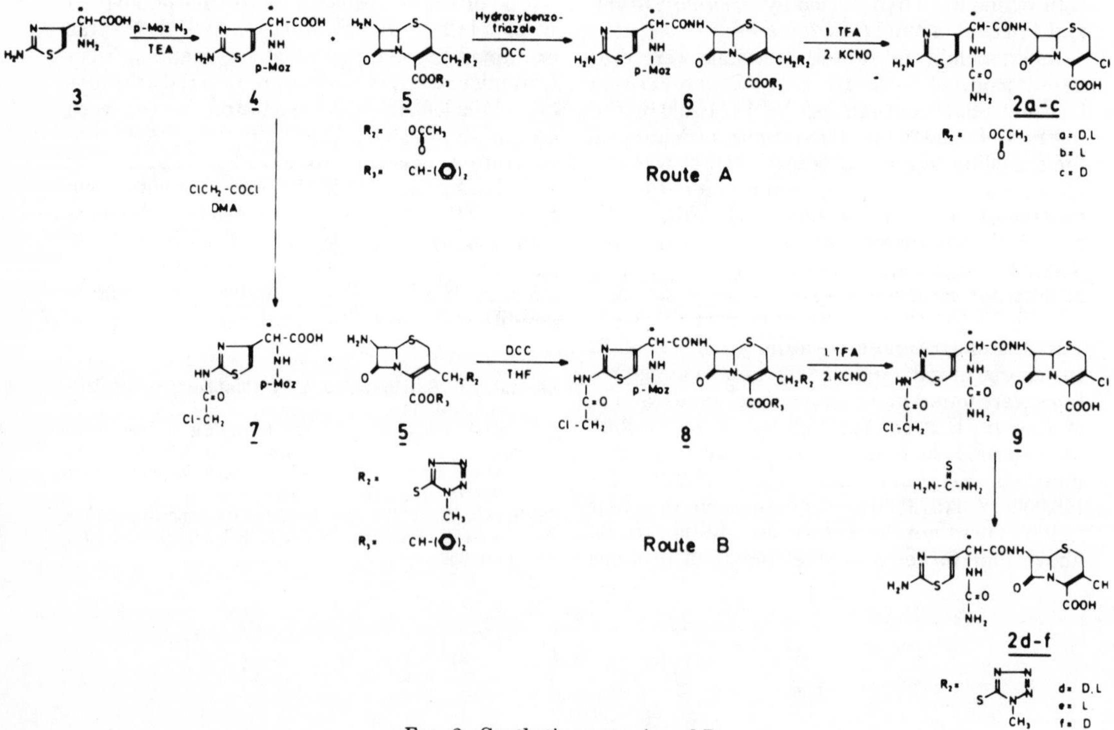

FIG. 2. *Synthetic routes A and B.*

TABLE 1. *In vitro MICs of aminothiazolylureido cephalosporins, SQ 69,613, and cefoxitin (plate dilution test; inoculum, 10^4 and 10^5 colony-forming units)*

mpound No. / R_2		4a D,L / STz		4b L / STz		4c D / STz		3 SQ 69,613 L / STz		4d D,L / OCCH₃		4e L / OCCH₃		4f D / OCCH₃		Cefoxitin		HR-756 Cefotaxime	
ganism	SC-No.	10⁴CFU	10⁵CFU	10⁴CFU	10⁵CFU	10⁴CFU	10⁵CFU	10⁴CFU	10⁵CFU	10⁴CFU	10⁵CFU	10⁴CFU	10⁵CFU	10⁴CFU	10⁵CFU	10⁴CFU	10⁵CFU	10⁴CFU	10⁵CFU
aureus	2400	3.1	6.3	3.1	6.3	6.3	12.5	6.3	12.5	6.3	6.3	6.3	6.3	6.3	25	3.1	3.1	1.6	1.6
aureus	2399	3.1	3.1	3.1	6.3	3.1	3.1	3.1	6.3	6.3	6.3	6.3	6.3	6.3	6.3	1.6	3.1	0.8	1.6
coli TEM+	10404	<0.2	<0.2	<0.2	<0.2	<0.2	0.8	1.6	>50	<0.2	<0.2	<0.2	<0.2	0.4	1.6	3.1	6.3	<0.2	<0.2
coli TEM-	10439	<0.2	<0.2	<0.2	<0.2	<0.2	<0.2	0.4	0.8	<0.2	<0.2	<0.2	<0.2	<0.2	0.4	6.3	6.3	<0.2	<0.2
coli RGN 238	10854	<0.2	<0.2	<0.2	<0.2	<0.2	0.4	1.6	3.1	<0.2	<0.2	<0.2	<0.2	0.4	0.8	6.3	12.5	<0.2	0.8
tr. freundii	10204	<0.2	1.6	<0.2	<0.2	<0.2	3.1	0.8	12.5	<0.2	25	<0.2	3.1	0.8	50	>50	>50	<0.2	6.3
ig. sonnei	10944	<0.2	0.8	<0.2	0.4	<0.2	3.1	1.6	25	0.4	6.3	<0.2	3.1	3.1	25	25	50	0.8	6.3
:t typhimur.	10943	<0.2	<0.2	<0.2	<0.2	<0.2	<0.2	1.6	0.8	<0.2	<0.2	<0.2	<0.2	<0.2	0.4	3.1	12.5	<0.2	<0.2
t. cloac. P99+	10435	50	>50	25	50	>50	>50	>50	>50	>50	>50	>50	>50	>50	>50	>50	>50	50	>50
it cloac. P99-	10441	<0.2	<0.2	<0.2	0.4	<0.2	0.4	0.8	1.6	<0.2	<0.2	<0.2	<0.2	<0.2	0.4	12.5	25	<0.2	<0.2
.t. cloacae	8415	<0.2	6.3	<0.2	0.8	<0.2	6.3	0.8	1.6	<0.2	1.6	<0.2	0.4	0.8	25	1.6	6.3	<0.2	3.1
aerog. KI+	10436	0.4	>50	0.8	>50	6.3	>50	>50	>50	0.8	50	0.8	50	12.5	>50	1.6	6.3	0.8	>50
aerog. KI-	10440	<0.2	<0.2	<0.2	<0.2	<0.2	0.8	0.4	0.8	<0.2	<0.2	<0.2	<0.2	<0.2	0.4	3.1	6.3	<0.2	<0.2
pneumoniae	8340	<0.2	<0.2	<0.2	<0.2	<0.2	1.5	0.4	0.8	<0.2	<0.2	<0.2	<0.2	<0.2	0.4	1.6	6.3	<0.2	<0.2
pneumoniae	11 056	<0.2	1.6	<0.2	<0.2	<0.2	3.1	3.1	50	<0.2	0.4	<0.2	0.2	0.4	3.1	6.3	12.5	<0.2	0.8
ot. rettgeri	8217	<0.2	0.4	<0.2	<0.2	<0.2	1.6	0.8	50	<0.2	<0.2	<0.2	<0.2	<0.2	1.6	12.5	50	<0.2	1.6
ot. vulgaris	10 950	<0.2	>50	<0.2	>50	<0.2	>50	>50	>50	<0.2	>50	<0.2	>50	1.6	>50	3.1	6.3	<0.2	>50
ot. vulgaris	10 951 B	<0.2	>50	<0.2	>50	0.4	>50	>50	>50	<0.2	>50	<0.2	>50	1.6	>50	3.1	12.5	<0.2	>50
c: mirabilis	9574	<0.2	<0.2	<0.2	<0.2	<0.2	0.8	1.6	1.6	<0.2	<0.2	<0.2	<0.2	0.4	0.8	3.1	6.3	<0.2	<0.2
aeruginosa	9545	1.6	25	3.1	6.3	25	25	>50	>50	>50	>50	25	>50	>50	>50	50	>50	0.8	6.3
aeruginosa	8329	>50	>50	50	>50	>50	>50	>50	>50	>50	>50	50	>50	>50	>50	>50	>50	12.5	50
r. marcescens	9782	<0.2	1.6	<0.2	1.6	<0.2	>50	25	>50	0.4	25	<0.2	3.1	6.3	>50	6.3	25	<0.2	1.6

ance liquid chromatography, using a 7-μm, reversed-phase C-8 column (25-mm inside diameter by 250 mm). The eluent used was a mixture of methanol and 0.01 M phosphate buffer. The subsequent removal of the inorganic matter, introduced by the solvent system, was accomplished by high-performance liquid chromatography on an RP-8 column (16-mm inside diameter by 250 mm; 25 to 40 μm) using MeOH-water as the solvent.

The configurational assignment of the separated isomers is based on the analogous retention times experienced with stereospecific D- and L-ureido cephalosporins previously synthesized by us (1). Compounds 2b and 2e, thus assigned to have the L-configuration, show the greater antimicrobial activity. These results are in agreement with earlier findings (1).

Microbiology. The MICs of the compounds prepared are given in Table 1. Cefoxitin, as well as SQ 69,613 (compound 1) and HR-756 are included for comparison.

The following conclusions can be made from the data in Table 1. (i) The 2-amino-4-thiazolylureido cephalosporins 2a–f are broad-spectrum antibiotics with outstanding antimicrobial activity. They show the great activity-enhancing

influence of the 2-amino-4-thiazolyl substituent. (ii) The compounds having the L-configuration at C-2 of the 7-acyl side chain, 2b and 2e, are distinctly more active than the corresponding D-diastereomers 2c and 2f. (iii) Compound 2e, having $R_2 = $ STz (SQ 81,015), is the most potent compound of the series. Its antimicrobial spectrum is comparable to that of the glycoside antibiotics, except for the low activity against *Staphylococcus aureus* and *Pseudomonas aeruginosa* strains. (iv) The inoculum effect shown by these compounds is small, especially that of the L-isomers. This may be due to greater β-lactamase stability of the L-compounds. (v) The ureido cephalosporins 2a–f are distinctly superior in activity to cefoxitin.

1. Breuer, H., U. D. Treuner, H. J. Schneider, M. G. Young, and H. I. Basch. 1978. Diastereomeric 7-ureidoacetyl cephalosporins. I. Superiority of 7α-H-L-isomers over D-isomers. J. Antibiot. 31:546–560.
2. Bucourt, R., R. Heymes, A. Lutz, L. Penasse, and J. Perromet. 1978. Cephalosporines à chaines amino-2-thiazolyl-4-acetyles. Tetrahedron 34:2233–2243.
3. Ochiai, M., O. Aki, A. Morimoto, T. Okada, and Y. Matsushita. 1977. New cephalosporin derivatives with high antibacterial activities. Chem. Pharm. Bull. 25:3115–3117.

Comparison of D and L Isomers in 7-Substituted Cephalosporins

NAFSIKA H. GEORGOPAPADAKOU,* FUNG Y. LIU, AND MIGUEL A. ONDETTI

The Squibb Institute for Medical Research, Princeton, New Jersey 08540, U.S.A.

7-Ureidoacetyl cephalosporins are potent broad-spectrum β-lactam antibiotics active against β-lactamase–producing members of the *Enterobacteriaceae* (2). Unlike most β-lactam antibiotics, their L side chain isomers are better antibiotics than the corresponding D side chain isomers (Table 1). Also, in the 7-methoxy series, the L isomer acts synergistically with the D isomer. It has been suggested that the apparent superiority of the L isomer and its synergistic activity may not reflect differences in intrinsic activity but rather β-lactamase inhibition by the L series (3).

In the present study the intrinsic activities of the most representative compounds of the series were compared on the basis of their ability to

bind to specific enterobacterial membrane proteins. These proteins bind penicillin (penicillin-binding proteins, PBPs) and are presumably involved in cell wall biosynthesis (7). The same compounds were also compared on the basis of their ability to inhibit *Streptomyces* R61 DD-carboxypeptidase activity (5).

PBP assay. Solubilized (2% Triton X-100) membranes of sonicated *Escherichia coli* (SC 8,294) and *Enterobacter cloacae* (SC 8,415) were incubated (~100 μg of protein) at 30°C with the appropriate cephalosporin for 10 min in a total volume of 50 μl. Then 10 nmol of ^{14}C-penicillin G (Amersham-Searle; specific activity, 54 μCi/μmol) was added, and the incubation was continued for another 10 min. Protein was precipitated with four volumes of cold acetone and subjected to sodium dodecyl sulfate-polyacrylamide gel electrophoresis (4), followed by fluorography (1). Protein-bound ^{14}C-penicillin was determined by visual examination of the X-ray film.

DD-Carboxypeptidase assay. Partially purified *Streptomyces* R61 DD-carboxypeptidase (5) was incubated at 30°C with the appropriate cephalosporin for 0 or 30 min in a total volume of 20 μl. Two nanomoles of ^{14}C-diacetyl-L-Lys-D-Ala-D-Ala (6) was added, and the incubation was continued for 30 min. Reaction was stopped by the addition of 5 μl of 0.25 M HCl, and the hydrolysis product (^{14}C-diacetyl-L-Lys-D-Ala) was separated from the substrate by high-voltage paper electrophoresis at pH 3.5 (8). Percentage hydrolysis was determined from liquid scintillation counting of the two radioactive spots.

The results, summarized in Table 2, were identical for both *E. coli* and *E. cloacae* PBP systems. In the aminoacetyl pair (SQ 68,112 and

TABLE 1. *Antibiotic activity of D and L isomers of substituted ureidoacetyl and aminoacetyl cephalosporins (3)*

SQ no.	R	R	MIC (μg/ml)	
			E. coli SC 8,294	*E. cloacae* SC 8,415
68,112 (D*)	H–	–H	1.6	9.4
68,806 (L*)	H–	–H	9.4	>100
68,381 (D*)	NH$_2$CO–	–H	1.2	75.0
68,653 (L*)	NH$_2$CO–	–H	0.4	1.6
14,359 (D*)	NH$_2$CO–	–OCH$_3$	0.4	1.2
14,526 (L*)	NH$_2$CO–	–OCH$_3$	3.1	6.2

TABLE 2. *Binding of D and L isomers of substituted ureidoacetyl and aminoacetyl cephalosporins to enterobacterial PBPs and inhibition of DD-carboxypeptidase activity by these compounds*

SQ no.	Amt (μg/ml) to inhibit penicillin G binding completely					I$_{50}^a$ for DD-carboxypeptidase (M)	
	PBP 1	PBP 2	PBP 3	PBP 4	PBP 5/6	0 min^b	30 min
68,112	10	>30	0.2	2.0	>30	5×10^{-6}	2.5×10^{-5}
68,806	$\geq$30	>30	2.0	30	>30	3×10^{-5}	10^{-4}
68,381	2.0	30	0.5	2.0	>30	6×10^{-5}	10^{-4}
68,653	$\geq$30	>30	0.5	10	>30	2.7×10^{-5}	10^{-4}
14,359	2.0	>30	0.1	0.1	2.0	2×10^{-6}	7×10^{-6}
14,526	$\geq$30	>30	10	2.0	30	10^{-5}	4×10^{-6}

^{a} Amount to cause 50% inhibition.
^{b} Preincubation time.

SQ 68,806) the L isomer was an order of magnitude less active than the D isomer (binding to PBPs 1, 3, 4, and inhibition of DD-carboxypeptidase activity). In the ureidoacetyl pair (SQ 68,381 and SQ 68,653), the L isomer was also less active than the D-isomer, although the difference was less pronounced (an order of magnitude for PBPs 1 and 4, none for PBP 3, and twofold for DD-carboxypeptidase). Finally, in the ureidoacetyl-7-methoxy pair (SQ 14,339 and SQ 14,526), the L isomer was less active than the D isomer by the same magnitude as in the aminoacetyl pair. None of the compounds bound to PBP 2 to any significant extent, and only the D isomer of the ureidoacetyl-7-methoxy pair bound to PBP 5/6.

On the basis of these results one would expect in the ureidoacetyl pair the L isomer to be a poorer antibiotic than the D isomer and in the ureidoacetyl-7-methoxy pair the L isomer not to enhance the activity of the D isomer since it did not bind to any additional PBP. Therefore, the observed in vitro superiority of the L isomer in the ureidoacetyl pair and the synergism with the D isomer in the ureidoacetyl-7-methoxy pair do not reflect increased intrinsic activity of the L isomer.

1. **Bonner, W. M., and R. A. Laskey.** 1974. A film detection method for tritium labelled proteins and nucleic acids in polyacrylamide gels. Eur. J. Biochem. **46:**83–88.
2. **Breuer, H., U. D. Treuner, H. G. Schneider, M. G. Young, and H. I. Basch.** 1978. Diasteromeric 7-ureidoacetyl cephalosporins. I. Superiority of 7α-H-L-isomers over D-isomers. J. Antiobiot. **31:**546–560.
3. **Gadebusch, H. H., H. I. Basch, P. Lukaszow, B. Remsburg and R. Schwind.** 1978. Diastereomeric 7-ureidoacetyl cephalosporins. III. Contributions of D- and L-isomers to the growth-inhibiting activities of 7α-H and 7α-OCH₃ derivatives for gram-positive and gram-negative bacteria. J. Antibiot. **31:**570–579.
4. **Laemmli, U. K.** 1970. Cleavage of structural proteins during the assembly of the head of bacteriophage T4. Nature (London) **227:**680–685.
5. **Leyh-Bouille, M., J. Coyette, J. M. Ghuysen, J. Idczak, H. R. Perkins, and M. Nieto.** 1971. Penicillin-sensitive DD-carboxypeptidase from *Streptomyces* strain R61. Biochemistry **10:**2163–2170.
6. **Perkins, H. R., M. Nieto, J. M. Frere, M. Leyh-Bouille, and J. M. Ghuysen.** 1973. *Streptomyces* DD-carboxypeptidase as transpeptidases. The specificity for amino compounds acting as carboxyl acceptors. Biochem. J. **131:**707–708.
7. **Spratt, B. G.** 1975. Distinct penicillin-binding proteins involved in the division, elongation and shape of *Escherichia coli* K12. Proc. Natl. Acad. Sci. U.S.A. **72:**2999–3003.
8. **Tamura, T., Y. Imae, and J. L. Strominger.** 1976. Purification to homogeneity and properties of two D-alanine carboxypeptidases from *Escherichia coli.* J. Biol. Chem. **251:**414–423.

Piperacillin in the Treatment of Severe Infections: Clinical Evaluation and Pharmacokinetics in Serum, Wound Fluid, and Subcutaneous Tissue

THOMAS O. LINGLÖF,* OTTO CARS, AND FOLKE NORDBRING

Departments of Infectious Diseases and *Clinical Microbiology, University Hospital, S-750 14 Uppsala, Sweden*

Clinical study. The safety and efficacy of piperacillin, a new semisynthetic injectable penicillin, were studied. The bacterial spectrum of piperacillin is similar to that of carbenicillin, but the drug is distinctly more active (2, 4).

Herein we report our experience with piperacillin in the treatment of severe infections in 53 patients admitted to our care. The study was carried out from October 1978 to July 1979. The patients ranged in age from 8 months to 96 years (mean 60.7 years) and consisted of 36 males and 17 females including 2 children. Piperacillin was administered by a slow intravenous bolus injection (5 min) in a dose of 2 g every 8 h in most of the cases. In children and in patients with impaired renal function, the dose was reduced. Treatment duration ranged from 4 to 29 days, excluding four cases who died during the first 3 days from the severity of their conditions or underlying disease. Each patient was examined, and routine cultures and standard laboratory tests were performed before, during, and after the treatment.

In those cases where it has been our normal practice, mainly urinary tract infections, a follow-up course of an appropriate oral antibiotic was given. Of the 53 patients, 3 were considered not to be suffering from bacterial infection. Fifty patients were thus evaluated. The clinical diagnoses are shown in Table 1. Organisms considered to be of etiological importance were cultured from all but 6 of the 50 cases. The organism isolated included 25 *Escherichia coli*, 12 *Pseudomonas*, 6 *Klebsiella*, 8 *Enterobacter*, 4 *Proteus*, 4 *Bacteroides fragilis*, 2 *Enterococcus*, and 7 other various species. Susceptibility tests were performed with the disk diffusion method (3).

The clinical and bacteriological results of the

study are summarized in Table 1. Clinical cure or improvement (4 cases) occurred in 38 out of 41 evaluable cases. Three patients (7.3%) failed to respond to piperacillin. These patients responded well to other antibiotics. In nine cases a valid clinical judgment could not be made either because of the patients' early death or because culture revealed additional nonsusceptible organisms which required further antimicrobial therapy.

The bacteriological outcome was considered successful in 32 cases. Twenty-eight of these showed eradication, and five showed marked reduction. In three cases (8.6%) bacteriological failure occurred. Fourteen cases could not be judged bacteriologically, including the four deaths and six cases where culture was negative. In the remainder, evaluation was not possible because follow-up cultures were not feasible to obtain. Five cases relapsed bacteriologically posttreatment, and in three of these further treatment was considered unnecessary. Two relapsed significantly, and both of these patients responded well to a second course of piperacillin and were thus considered as cures.

Adverse reactions were very few. Two cases of local thrombophlebitis were noticed, and four cases showed mild and clinically insignificant elevation of liver transaminases.

Pharmacokinetic study. Serum concentrations of piperacillin were measured using an agar diffusion method with *Bacillus stearothermophilus* as the test organism. Samples were assayed in triplicate, and standards were prepared in pooled human serum. The coefficient of variation was 6%. From 18 patients with normal serum creatinine, blood samples were drawn at 5 min, 10 min, 30 min, 1 h, 2 h, 4 h, and 6 h after a 2-g intravenous dose. The serum concentrations (mean ± SD) were 150 ± 39, 110 ± 33, 63 ± 19, 38 ± 16, 15 ± 7.3, 7.0 ± 3.7, and 4.0 ± 3.2, respectively. The mean elimination half-life in these patients was 122 ± 46 min, which contrasts

with a serum half-life of approximately 60 min previously reported in volunteers (5). Our findings thus seem to be at variance with the results of pharmacokinetic studies in healthy volunteers and indicate that patients who are ill and confined to bed may be expected to excrete the drug more slowly.

One important factor in the treatment of bacterial diseases is the ability of antibiotics to achieve active concentrations at the site of the infection. Tissue concentrations in humans have in most cases been measured by different homogenizing or extraction techniques that require large tissue samples. This imposes limitations on pharmacokinetic studies in tissues. To meet the need of serial measurements in each patient, we developed an agar diffusion technique utilizing very small pieces of tissue. Specimens of the subcutaneous tissue were obtained from patients with infected wounds by means of scissors and forceps. The samples were then rapidly cleaned of any visible blood and sealed in small preweighed plastic tubes to prevent evaporation. The wet weight of each biopsy was usually 10 to 20 mg, and it was often possible to obtain two biopsies at each time point. Without previous homogenization, the samples were then sealed into wells in agar plates preinoculated with the test strain. After prediffusion at room temperature for 1 h, the plates were incubated overnight. Round and distinct zones of inhibition formed around tissue pieces.

Standards for the tissue assay were prepared in phosphate-buffered saline. This would result in a degree of underestimation of the tissue levels if piperacillin were bound to proteins or other constituents of the tissues. However, serum protein binding of piperacillin is low (1), and in preliminary experiments we could not demonstrate binding of piperacillin to homogenates of human subcutaneous tissue. The coefficient of variation in the tissue assay was 13 to 20%.

TABLE 1. *Result of clinical and bacteriological outcome in 50 patients treated with piperacillin*

Infections	Clinical				Bacteriological		
	No. of patients	No. cured or improved	Failure	No. not evaluable	No. eradicated or showing marked reduction	Failure	No. not evaluable
UTI[a]	19	18	0	1	17	0	2
Septicemia	12	10	0	2	8	0	4
Soft tissue	12	7	0	5	7	2	3
Abdominal	5	3	1	1	0	1	4
Pneumonia	2	0	2	0	0	0	2

[a] UTI, Urinary tract infection.

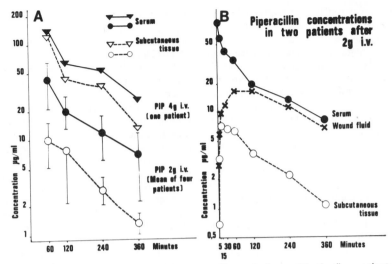

FIG. 1. (A) Serum and subcutaneous tissue concentrations of piperacillin in five patients with wound infections. (B) Serum, wound fluid, and subcutaneous tissue concentrations of piperacillin in two patients with wound infections.

Figure 1A shows the serum and subcutaneous concentrations obtained from five patients with wound infections. At 1 h after injection, serum and tissue levels decreased fairly parallel to one another. In two of the patients (Fig. 1B), measurements were also made at 5, 15, and 30 min after injection to concentrations in wound fluid which was sampled using small glass capillaries holding 10 μl. Maximum concentrations in wound fluid and tissue were found within 1 h. The wound fluid concentrations almost reached the same level as in serum. The mean ratio of subcutaneous to serum levels during elimination in all the patients was 0.47. Evidently, within the tissue samples there is a substantial proportion of fat into which piperacillin does not pass, and therefore the true values for levels in the interstitial fluid of the tissue might be higher. Piperacillin thus seems to pass rapidly into subcutaneous tissue and wound fluid and is eliminated at approximately the same rate in serum and tissue.

1. **American Cyanamid Co.** 1978. Piperacillin sodium injectable antibiotic. Clinical investigators brochure. American Cyanamid Co., Lederle Laboratories Division, Pearl River, N.Y.

2. **Dicksson, G. M., T. J. Cleary, and T. A. Hoffman.** 1978. Comparative evaluation of piperacillin in vitro. Antimicrob. Agents Chemother. 14:919–921.

3. **Ericsson, H. M., and J. C. Sherris.** 1971. Antibiotic sensitivity testings. Report of an international collaborative report. Acta Pathol. Microbiol. Scand. Suppl. 217:1–90.

4. **Renkonen, O.-V.** 1978. Susceptibility of 500 clinical isolates to piperacillin, p. 601–603. *In* Current Chemotherapy, Proceedings of the 10th International Congress of Chemotherapy. American Society for Microbiology, Washington, D.C.

5. **Tjandramaga, T. B., A. Mullie, R. Verbesselt, P. J. De Schepper, and L. Verbist.** 1978. Piperacillin: human pharmacokinetics after intravenous and intramuscular administration. Antimicrob. Agents Chemother. 14:829–837.

Use of Piperacillin as Initial or Supplanting Therapy in Serious Bacterial Infections

JOSÉ IGNACIO SANTOS,* GAY WENERSTROM, BARBARA J. SAXON, AND JOHN M. MATSEN

University of Utah, College of Medicine, Salt Lake City, Utah, U.S.A.

Piperacillin is a new semisynthetic penicillin derivative with broad-spectrum activity against *Pseudomonas aeruginosa*, *Enterobacteriaceae* including *Klebsiella pneumoniae*, and anaerobes (2–5). Its wider spectrum of activity is an improvement over other existing available beta-lactam antibiotics; in addition, it has the added advantage of being less toxic than the aminoglycoside drugs. Currently, aminoglycosides in combination with semisynthetic penicillins or cephalosporins provide the mainstay of therapy for serious gram-negative bacillary infections in most hospitals. No antibiotic alone or in combination has been entirely satisfactory for the treatment of these infections. Piperacillin may provide a single-drug alternative to these regimens, possibly resulting in equally effective and less toxic therapy.

To explore this possibility, we evaluated the clinical and bacteriological efficacy, patient tolerance, and toxicity of piperacillin in an open, noncomparative study in 35 hospitalized adult patients with documented serious bacterial infections.

Materials and methods. Consenting hospitalized adult patients with serious infections caused by susceptible bacteria were eligible for the study. Patients were excluded if they had a history of hypersensitivity to penicillin or had received presumably effective antibiotics. Exception was made in five cases where said therapy failed and organism eradication and clinical cure could, therefore, be evaluated with piperacillin. Additionally, seven patients, where piperacillin was used as initial therapy, also received a second and in one case a third antibiotic. Combined therapy was initiated in most instances despite an initial clinical response at the discretion of the attending physician because of concern for the severity of the underlying illness.

Piperacillin was administered either by intravenous drip or intramuscularly in the gluteal region. Dosage ranged from 200 to 300 mg/kg per day depending on the severity of infection. The drug was given in divided doses at 4- to 6-h intervals. The intravenous preparation was infused over 3 to 5 min. The patients were examined daily by one of the investigators throughout the study to determine clinical response and possible clinical adverse effects.

In addition to routine hospital admission laboratory determinations and the related clinical studies concerned with the patient's illness, laboratory tests were used to monitor hepatic, renal, and hematopoietic function on each patient pretreatment, at least every 4 days during treatment, and 2 to 3 days posttreatment.

Etiological diagnosis was sought in all patients with multiple blood cultures and, when appropriate, cultures of urine, sputum, or aspirates from infected sites before the initiation of therapy.

Pathogens recovered from patients were tested for susceptibility to piperacillin and carbenicillin by the Bauer-Kirby disk diffusion method and by the microbroth dilution MIC method (1). Where feasible, a biological assay of piperacillin in the serum and the appropriate body fluids was determined by the *Sarcina lutea* (ATCC 9341) assay.

The overall assessment of response was based on both clinical and bacteriological criteria and designated as either cure or failure. The severity of infection was evaluated by one of the investigators before the start of antibiotic therapy and included parameters such as age of the patient, pretreatment signs and symptoms, presence of concurrent disease, site and duration of infection, and the nature of the pathogen.

Results. Thirty-five patients between the ages of 17 and 85 years were studied. Twenty-nine were male. Table 1 is a case tabulation giving the number and nature of infections treated and the final clinical and bacteriological outcome. Causative organisms listed were recovered from pre-piperacillin therapy cultures. A specific bacterial etiology was identified in all patients. Aerobic gram-negative bacilli accounted for the most common etiological agent occurring singly or as a polymicrobial infection in 27 of 35 (77%) patients. The most common causative organisms included *Escherichia coli* and *P. aeruginosa* which were cultured as single or predominant pathogens in 13 (37%) and 11 (31%) of the patients, respectively.

Twenty-three infections were considered severe, five were moderate, and seven were mild. In all but 4 cases there was a clinical cure, and all of the 23 classified as severe had a bacteriological cure.

The results of piperacillin therapy according to category of etiological agent included a clinical cure for 25 of 27 (93%) patients infected with aerobic gram-negative bacilli. Of the five patients with gram positive cocci, only three had a clinical cure; the two failures were staphylococci. The two failures from gram-negative aerobic rods included one *P. aeruginosa* and one *K. pneumoniae*.

TABLE 1. *Outcome of 35 patients treated with piperacillin*

Diagnosis	No. of patients	Bacteriological		Clinical	
		Cure	Failure	Cure	Failure
Sepsis	9	9	0	8	1
UTI[a]	8	5	3	7	1
Peritonitis	7	7	0	7	0
Soft tissue infection	7	5	2	5	2
Pneumonia	1	1	0	1	0
Miscellaneous	3	3	0	3	0

[a] UTI, Urinary tract infection.

TABLE 2. *Comparative susceptibility of 109 bacterial isolates recovered from 35 study patients*

Organism	No. tested	Piperacillin MIC (μg/ml)		Carbenicillin MIC (μg/ml)	
		Range	Mean	Range	Mean
P. aeruginosa	40	0.25–64	22.18	2–256	86.0
E. coli	24	0.5–256	27.5	0.5–256	180.3
Serratia	13	1–256	32.8	8–256	172.3
S. aureus	2	0.5–8	4.25	0.5–2	1.25
S. epidermidis	5	4–32	12	2–64	35.6
Enterococcus	10	1–8	2.9	4–64	28.4
Klebsiella	8	4–256	66.5	16–256	74.5
P. mirabilis	7	0.5–2	1.07	0.5–32	5.71

Overall study results included 31 of 35 (89%) patients with a clinical cure and 30 of 35 (86%) with a bacteriological cure.

Only one potential toxic complication occurred in one patient who sustained a transient pancytopenia while on piperacillin; however, the patient was concomitantly being administered three other drugs well associated with hematopoietic dyscrasias, making a cause and effect association difficult to define.

During the course of the study, 109 bacterial isolates were obtained from the 35 patients. Table 2 depicts the range and mean MIC of piperacillin and carbenicillin for these clinical isolates. In all cases except for *Staphylococcus aureus*, the mean MIC of piperacillin was significantly less than that of carbenicillin; the differences are most significant for the *Pseudomonas*, *E. coli*, and *Serratia* groups.

Discussion. In this open noncomparative therapeutic study in a medical and surgical patient population, piperacillin performed very well both in efficacy and patient tolerance.

The clinical and bacteriological response in almost 90% of the patients was excellent and rapid. Serious clinical adverse effects were not observed. Only the one clinically significant laboratory abnormality previously noted was encountered in a study patient, and circumstances surrounding the case made a cause and effect relationship unevaluable.

The organisms isolated were in general very susceptible to piperacillin. MIC data on the clinical isolates indicate that piperacillin is appreciably more active against *P. aeruginosa*, *E. coli*, and *Serratia* than carbenicillin.

If we chose not to evaluate the 7 patients who received concomitant antibiotics and whose organisms were either susceptible to the added antibiotic alone or where synergy with piperacillin could be demonstrated in vitro (4/7), we would end up with 31 evaluable cases and the overall cure rate for piperacillin would be 29 of 31 (96%). It should also be pointed out that, in the four cases where the added antibiotic was effective against the pathogen(s) in question, in vitro synergy could not be demonstrated.

Based on this limited, open, noncomparative study, piperacillin appears to be a safe, effective, and well-tolerated antibiotic when used in patients with infections due to susceptible bacteria. Potential advantages over carbenicillin and ticarcillin warrant further comparative studies to determine the role of this antimicrobial.

1. **Bauer, A. W., W. M. M. Kirby, J. C. Sherris, and M. Turck.** 1966. Antibiotic susceptibility testing by a standard single-disc method. Am. J. Clin. Pathol. **45:**493–496.
2. **Bodey, G. P., and B. LeBlanc.** 1978. Piperacillin: in vitro evaluation. Antimicrob. Agents Chemother. **14:**78–87.
3. **Fu, K. P., and H. C. Neu.** 1978. Piperacillin, a new penicillin active against many bacteria resistant to other penicillins. Antimicrob. Agents Chemother. **13:**358–367.
4. **Verbist, L.** 1978. In vitro activity of piperacillin, a new semisynthetic penicillin with an unusually broad spectrum of activity. Antimicrob. Agents Chemother. **13:** 349–357.
5. **Winston, D. J., D. Want, L. S. Young, W. J. Martin, and W. L. Hewitt.** 1978. In vitro studies of piperacillin, a new semisynthetic penicillin. Antimicrob. Agents Chemother. **13:**944–950.

Clinical Effectiveness of Piperacillin Sodium in Serious Gram-Negative and Anaerobic Infections

R. M. KLUGE,* AND R. B. GAINER

West Virginia University Medical Center, Morgantown, West Virginia 26506, U.S.A.

Piperacillin sodium is an investigational semisynthetic penicillin which has in vitro activity against most gram-positive and gram-negative organisms, including anaerobes (3, 4). Of particular interest is its activity against *Pseudomonas aeruginosa*, indole-positive *Proteus* species, and *Bacteroides fragilis*. Piperacillin exhibits much greater inhibitory activity than carbenicillin and ticarcillin against these organisms. Its pharmacokinetics are such that the inhibitory index of piperacillin for most organisms is much greater than carbenicillin or ticarcillin, i.e., the ratio between the mean peak serum level of piperacillin and the MIC required to inhibit the majority of organisms is several-fold higher than for carbenicillin (2).

The study was designed as an open noncomparative evaluation of the efficacy, safety, and tolerance of piperacillin sodium in the parenteral therapy of hospitalized adult patients with infections caused by susceptible strains of aerobic and/or anaerobic organisms. Patients were eligible for inclusion if they had strong presumptive evidence of infection or documented bacteriological evidence of infection. Disease categories considered for inclusion were genitourinary tract, respiratory tract, skin and soft tissue, bone and joint, gastrointestinal, and bacteremia.

Appropriate specimens for culture were obtained before piperacillin therapy as were basic hematology and chemistry studies and urinalysis. Direct and indirect Coombs tests were also performed. All laboratory tests were repeated at 4-day intervals during treatment and 2 to 3 days after treatment. Cultures were repeated during treatment as indicated and 2 to 3 days after treatment. Patients with urinary tract infections had additional cultures obtained 8 to 10 days and 4 to 6 weeks posttherapy. Standard isolation and identification procedures were employed by the hospital diagnostic microbiology laboratories. Routine antimicrobial sensitivity testing was performed using the Bauer-Kirby and standard MIC techniques.

All patients with serious infections received intravenous piperacillin sodium in doses ranging between 200 and 300 mg/kg per day, given in divided doses every 4 or 6 h. Those with less serious genitourinary tract infections received 150 to 200 mg/kg per day. Therapy was to be administered for at least 5 days. Patients were monitored daily for any evidence of allergic reactions and for local tolerance.

Results. Twenty-two patients were entered into the study. Four were found subsequently to have sterile cultures and are therefore not included in the analysis. One patient had infection in the perinephric space caused by *Staphylococcus aureus* and was dropped from the study. Two patients were eliminated from the study because of a break in protocol, i.e., antibiotics were added or changed. That left 15 patients with documented bacterial infections who received piperacillin therapy.

The sites of infection included: genitourinary tract, five (two with pyelonephritis, one with prostatitis); bacteremia, three; peritonitis, two; osteomyelitis two; and one patient each with pneumonia, enterocutaneous fistula, chronic rectal cryptitis, perineal wound, and pelvic cellulitis. Two patients had two separate but coexisting infections which explains the 17 sites in 15 patients.

A variety of organisms were isolated, and in seven patients two or more organisms were recovered. There were six *Escherichia coli* isolates; three each of *Proteus mirabilis*, *Klebsiella pneumoniae*, and *Streptococcus pyogenes*; two each of *Clostridium perfringens*, *Streptococcus faecalis*, *P. aeruginosa*, and *Pseudomonas fluorescens*; and one each of *Enterobacter cloacae*, *Serratia marcescens*, and *B. fragilis*.

All of the aerobic organisms were susceptible to piperacillin: MICs ranged between 0.0078 and 32 μg/ml. Anaerobes recovered in this study were not tested, but other investigators report that 85 to 95% of *Bacteroides* and *Clostridium* species are susceptible to 25 μg or less of piperacillin per ml (1, 4).

Four patients with rapidly or ultimately fatal underlying disease and marked neutropenia at the time antibiotic therapy was initiated died. Three of these patients died before completing 5 days of piperacillin. The remaining 12 patients had adequate courses of piperacillin. The average duration of antibiotic treatment was 14.6 days; the average dose was 15 g/day. These patients had excellent clinical and bacteriological responses.

In general, side effects were of a mild and

transient nature. Three patients had increased serum bilirubin, serum glutamic oxalacetic transaminase, serum lactate dehydrogenase, or alkaline phosphatase; one patient had a transient elevation of blood urea nitrogen; one developed a 10% eosinophilia during therapy without other allergic manifestations; and one patient had decreased serum potassium levels. A very serious adverse reaction occurred in one patient who developed a suprainfection with a piperacillin-resistant organism. No local reactions or chemical thrombophlebitis were noted.

Summary. Piperacillin sodium was administered to 15 patients with documented bacterial infections. Three patients died before completing 5 days of therapy. The 12 patients who completed treatment had excellent clinical and bacteriological responses. Side effects were generally of a mild and transient nature. A suprainfection due to a piperacillin-resistant organism developed in one neutropenic patient. Piperacil-

lin appears to be a safe and effective antimicrobial for the treatment of serious gram-negative and anaerobic infections.

1. **Bach, V., H. Thadepalli, and I. Roy.** 1977. Antimicrobial activity of piperacillin against anaerobic bacteria in vitro. *In* Program Abstr. Intersci. Conf. Antimicrob. Agents Chemother. 17th, New York, N.Y., abstr. no. 321.
2. **Evans, M., P. Wilson and T. Leung.** Pharmacokinetics of piperacillin: comparison of bolus and slow intravenous infusion. *In* Program Tenth International Congress of Chemotherapy, September 1977, Zurich, Switzerland, abstr. no. 76.
3. **Shah, P. P., D. J. Briedis, H. G. Robson, and J. P. Conterato.** 1979. In vitro activity of piperacillin compared with that of carbenicillin, ticarcillin, ampicillin, cephalothin, and cephamandole against *Pseudomonas aeruginosa* and *Enterobacteriaceae*. Antimicrob. Agents Chemother. **15**:346–350.
4. **Winston, D. J., D. Wang, L. S. Young, W. J. Martin, and L. W. Hewitt.** 1978. In vitro studies of piperacillin, a new semisynthetic penicillin. Antimicrob. Agents Chemother. **13**:944–950.

Efficacy, Safety, and Tolerance of Piperacillin Sodium in Patients with Urinary Tract Infections

P. J. P. VAN BLERK, C. S. BLOCK,* E. YOURASSOWSKY, E. SCHOUTENS, S. SANDER, AND T. BERGAN

Johannesburg Hospital and South African Institute for Medical Research, Johannesburg, South Africa; Hopital Brugmann, Brussels, Belgium; Aker Hospital, Oslo, Norway

The efficacy, safety, and tolerance of intramuscular (i.m.) piperacillin sodium in the treatment of uncomplicated urinary tract infections (UTI) caused by susceptible bacteria were assessed in an open, noncomparative, multiclinic trial. The study incorporated 64 patients including 50 nonpregnant females and 14 males, ranging in age from 21 to 87 years (mean 67.2), and 20 to 88 years (mean 61.8), respectively. Seven had upper tract infections, 41 had lower tract infections, and infections were unlocalized in 16. The illness was of less than 10 days' duration before treatment in 46 patients, 10 to 20 days in 9 patients, and more than 20 days in 9 patients. Forty patients had acute disease, 11 had chronic disease, and 13 had recurrent or unspecified disease. There were six asymptomatic patients. Of the remaining 58, 22 were febrile, 16 had chills, 50 had dysuria, 46 had frequent micturition, 40 had urgent voidance, and 17 had costovertebral angle tenderness. Fifty-five patients had one or more associated diseases, usually cardiovascular disorders.

Piperacillin was administered in a total daily

dose of 4 g, as two 12-hourly (46 patients) or four 6-hourly (18 patients) i.m. injections. No concurrent antimicrobial treatment was allowed. Duration of therapy ranged from 5 to 10 days (mean 7.4 days) and was determined by clinical assessment of response. The one exception was a patient who underwent a gastrectomy for bleeding and died with acute cardiorespiratory insufficiency, unrelated to piperacillin therapy, on the third postoperative day. His UTI was diagnosed before surgery and he was treated with 2 g of piperacillin every 12 h for 4 days without adverse reactions. In most cases, concurrently administered non-antimicrobial drugs were cardiovascular agents. Piperacillin was reconstituted with either sterile distilled water (19 patients) or 0.25 to 0.5% lidocaine (44 patients). In one case 1% lidocaine was used as the diluent.

Efficacy was evaluated by clinical and bacteriological criteria. Clinical response was judged, at the end of therapy, from the time course of signs and symptoms (fever, chills, frequency of micturition, urgency, dysuria, and costovertebral angle tenderness) and graded as cure, improvement, or failure. Bacteriological response was defined from the results of urine cultures done before, during, and after therapy. Posttherapy cultures were done 8 to 10 days after completion of treatment. From these short-term results, the response was interpreted as elimination (negative culture), failure (original organism recovered), or superinfection (one or more new organisms isolated). If this culture was negative, a long-term specimen was taken at 4 to 6 weeks, with results being judged as cure (elimination maintained), relapse (original organism re-isolated), or reinfection (due to new organism).

Sixty-three patients had positive urine cultures (at least 10^5 colony-forming units per ml). A single organism was isolated in 61 instances, and two were isolated in two cases. *Escherichia coli* was the most frequent isolate (40), followed by *Proteus mirabilis* (14), enterococci (3), *Klebsiella* spp. (3), *Pseudomonas aeruginosa* (2), and *Proteus morganii*, *Providencia* spp., and *Staphylococcus epidermidis* (one each). The susceptibilities of these organisms are shown in Table 1.

Fifty-seven patients could be assessed clinically. The seven exclusions comprised six asymptomatic patients and one with an incorrect diagnosis. Thirty-nine (68%) were considered cured, 15 (26%) were improved, and 3 (6%) were clinical failures. Eight patients were excluded from the bacteriological assessment. Three had resistant urinary isolates, two did not have UTI, and one each had other antibacterial therapy, indwelling bladder catheter, or died before completion of therapy. Six of the 56 patients evaluated (11%) were bacteriological failures, with elimination of original organisms being achieved at short-term follow-up in 50 (89%). Of these 50,

TABLE 1. *Susceptibilities of urinary isolates to piperacillin*[a]

Organisms	MIC (µg/ml)			
	<1	<8	<50	≥50
E. coli (39)[b]	22	34	36	39
Proteus spp. (13)	13			
Klebsiella spp. (3)	1	2	2	3
S. faecalis (3)	2	3		
P. aeruginosa (2)	1	2		
Providencia spp. (1)				1
S. epidermidis (1)	1			
Total	40 (65%)	55 (89%)	57 (92%)	62 (100%)

[a] Four organisms were not tested by serial dilution.
[b] Number of organisms is indicated in parentheses.

TABLE 2. *Comparison between clinical and bacteriological responses*

Clinical response	Bacteriological response					
	Cure	Rein-fec-tion	Re-lapse	Super-infec-tion	Fail-ure	Total
Cure	28	3	2	2	3	38
Improvement	8	1			2	11
Failure		1			1	2
Total	36	5	2	2	6	51[a]

[a] Excluded for combined clinical and bacteriological assessment were six asymptomatic patients, three with resistant microbes, and one each with indwelling catheter, other antimicrobial therapy, wrong diagnosis, and unrelated death.

TABLE 3. *Effect of dosage regimen and duration of treatment*

Response	Dosage regimen		Duration of treatment (days)			
	2 g, 12 hourly	4 g, 6 hourly	6	7–8	9–10	Total
Clinical						
Cure	27	12	10	19	10	39
Improvement	10	5	3	9	3	15
Failure	2	1	1	1	1	3
Total	39	18	14	29	14	57
Bacteriological						
Cure	27	14	10	22	9	41
Re-infection	5		1	3	1	5
Relapse	2		1	1		2
Superinfection	1	1	1	1		2
Failure	5	1	3		3	6
Total	40	16	16	27	13	56

41 (82%) were cured, 2 (4%) suffered relapses, 5 (10%) became reinfected, and 2 (4%) had superinfections. Clinical and bacteriological responses are compared in Table 2. The different dosing regimens used and the duration of therapy did not appear to affect the outcome of treatment (Table 3).

Systemic tolerability of piperacillin was assessed by clinical observation and laboratory tests performed before, during, and after therapy. These included hematology, blood chemistry, and urinalysis. No significant adverse systemic reactions could be ascribed to piperacillin treatment.

Significant hematological findings were the development of mild leukopenia (less than $3,000/mm^3$) in three patients and eosinophilia in five. One patient demonstrated a thrombocytopenia during therapy. In none of these patients did the changes require therapeutic intervention or discontinuation of treatment. Important blood chemical findings included small increases in serum creatinine concentrations in two patients, but no significant alteration in creatinine clearances was demonstrated in any patient. Minor temporary elevations in alkaline phosphatase levels occurred in two instances. Local tolerance was assessed daily. Treatment was considered well tolerated in 57 cases (including 14 with mild or sporadic discomfort), moderately well in 6, and poorly tolerated in one due to pain, erythema, and induration which disappeared when 1% lidocaine was used as drug diluent. An apparent tendency to better tolerance of the injections when lidocaine was used as the diluent was not statistically significant (93% tolerated well with and 80% without anesthetic, and 7 and 15% tolerated the injections moderately well with and without, respectively).

Studies in healthy volunteers have shown that 1 g of piperacillin i.m. yields a mean peak serum level of 22 mg/ml and urine levels above 50 mg/ml (chosen here as resistance breakpoint) for at least 6 h.

This study indicates that i.m. piperacillin sodium was safe, reasonably effective, and well tolerated in the treatment of UTI caused by susceptible pathogens.

Mezlocillin and Piperacillin: a Comparative Clinical Evaluation

JONATHAN R. SPICEHANDLER,* LEON BERNHARDT, MICHAEL S. SIMBERKOFF, AND JAMES J. RAHAL, JR.

Department of Infectious Diseases, New York Veterans Administration Hospital and New York University School of Medicine, New York, New York 10010, U.S.A.

Mezlocillin and piperacillin are new antibiotics of the acylureido-penicillin group which have a wide spectrum of antimicrobial activity encompassing those of the cephalosporins and the penicillins. These antibiotics also present significantly less sodium load to the patient contrasted to carbenicillin, and thus fluid overload, electrolyte disorders, and bleeding may be limited. Because of these potential clinical benefits, clinical trials were undertaken to compare mezlocillin and piperacillin with respect to efficacy and toxicity.

An open, prospective, randomized, comparative study was conducted on patients hospitalized at the Manhattan Veteran's Administration Hospital, New York. All patients entered in the study were evaluated by the Infectious Disease staff both for microbiological and clinical evidence of infection and response to therapy. Bacterial cultures were obtained before, during, and after completion of therapy. A quantitative in vitro evaluation was performed on all isolates utilizing the tube dilution assay.

When a patient with an infection likely caused by pathogens susceptible to either antibiotic was found, he was randomly allocated to receive either piperacillin or mezlocillin intravenously (3 g every 4 h) for a total daily dose of 18 g. Informed consent was obtained from all patients. Antibiotic serum concentrations were determined at 1 and 4 h posttherapy, and dosage was adjusted. Other body fluid concentrations were determined when available.

Patients were included for evaluation if there was clinical evidence of serious systemic infection, a bacteriological diagnosis and in vitro sensitivity were confirmed, and the patient received antibiotic therapy for a minimum of 5 days.

A total of 29 patients was included in the trial: 15 in the mezlocillin group and 14 in the piperacillin group. Age range was comparable in both groups, and all patients were male.

In the piperacillin group, the infectious diagnosis was pneumonia in seven patients, including four pneumococcal, two aspiration pneumonias with mixed flora, and one *Escherichia coli* pneumonia. Four patients had septicemia including *Streptococcus pneumoniae* (pneumonia), *Bacteroides fragilis* (empyema), *Streptococcus salivarius* and *Streptococcus mitior* (cellulitis), and *Providencia alcalifaciens* (source unknown). Three patients had soft tissue infections including a mixed gram-negative (*Proteus mirabilis*, *Morganella morganii*, and *E. coli*), *S. salivarius* and *S. mitior*, and a third patient with cellulitis but no bacteriological isolate. Two patients had empyema—both were mixed infections (*B. fragilis*, *Peptostreptococcus*, and *Proteus mirablis*, and *Bacteroides melaninogenicus* and *Fusobacterium* sp.). One patient had a *Pseudomonas cepacia* endocarditis.

In the mezlocillin group the infectious diagnosis was pneumonia in five patients, including two pneumococcal, and one each of *Haemophilus influenzae*, *Haemophilus aphrophilus*, and *Klebsiella pneumoniae*. Two patients had mixed purulent bronchitis with fever and leukocytosis. Two patients had septicemia including *E. coli* (cellulitis) and *S. pneumoniae* (pneumonia). Three patients had soft tissue infections including *E. coli* (cellulitis), *Pseudomonas aeruginosa* (epididymitis), and a third patient with clinical cellulitis but no bacteriological isolate. Four patients had urinary tract infections, all nosocomially acquired acute infections with systemic signs of fever and leukocytosis. The bacterial isolates included three *P. aeruginosa* and one *K. pneumoniae*. One patient had empyema (*P. aeruginosa*) and one patient had osteomyelitis (*P. aeruginosa*).

Antibiotic susceptibility was defined as an MIC less than or equal to 62 μg/ml. For piperacillin, MICs ranged between <0.1 and 15.6 μg/ml and MBCs ranged between <0.1 and 125 μg/ml. One isolate, *P. cepacia*, exhibited a disparity between the MIC and MBC, and that patient failed on therapy. For mezlocillin, MICs ranged between <0.9 and 125 μg/ml and MBCs ranged between 0.9 and >500 μg/ml. Four isolates, one *K. pneumoniae* and three *P. aeruginosa*, exhibited a disparity between MIC and MBC, and two of those patients failed on therapy.

Antibiotic serum concentrations were determined at 1 and 4 h posttherapy during days 1, 3, and 5 of therapy employing a microbiological assay. Mean serum concentrations for piperacillin and mezlocillin were comparable at 1 and 4 h, 126 to 54 μg/ml and 127 to 43 μg/ml, respectively. Urinary concentrations of mezlocillin were excellent. Pleural fluid concentrations were excellent with both agents except for one patient in the piperacillin group.

Clinical cure was obtained in 11 of 14 patients with piperacillin (78%). Bacteriological eradication was obtained in 8 of 11 patients (72%). One failure was in a diabetic with severe peripheral vascular disease who had been treated for extensive mixed gram-negative cellulitis of the lower extremity. Although in vitro testing confirmed antibiotic susceptibility, the infection progressed, requiring surgical amputation. Operative cultures revealed persistence of the pathogens despite continued antibiotic susceptibility. Failure was probably due to the patient's underlying disease and lack of effective surgical drainage. The second failure was in an active drug addict who developed prosthetic valve endocarditis due to *P. cepacia*. The patient initially did well with surgical valve replacement and piperacillin therapy. Extensive myocardial abscesses were observed at surgery. Two weeks into antibiotic therapy, the patient relapsed with fever and positive blood cultures. Although initially

the organism was susceptible to piperacillin, follow-up blood isolates were resistant to all antimicrobials except trimethoprim-sulfamethoxazole. Resistance soon developed to this agent as well as numerous investigational antibiotics, and the patient expired. The third failure was in a patient with recurrent empyema after a previous thoracotomy. All isolates demonstrated in vitro sensitivity. Despite good serum concentrations, virtually no piperacillin was detected in pleural fluid. Although local inactivation of the antibiotic was considered, no evidence to support this was demonstrated. The patient improved on chloramphenicol therapy.

Clinical cure was obtained in 12 of 15 patients with mezlocillin (80%), with one unevaluable case (early discontinuation of antibiotic). Bacteriological eradication was obtained in 9 of 12 patients (75%). The first failure was in a patient with severe peripheral vascular disease and osteomyelitis. Although the MIC was 31 μg/ml, the subsequent MBC was 500 μg/ml. Clinically the associated cellulitis improved, but the drainage and original pathogen persisted despite the addition of an aminoglycoside. The second failure occurred in a patient with a urinary catheter that developed a *P. aeruginosa* infection. The patient initially responded, manifested by diminished pyuria and sterilization of the urine. In vitro testing revealed an MIC of 62 μg/ml and an MBC of 125 μg/ml. Because of clinical improvement and high urinary mezlocillin concentrations, therapy was continued. The catheter could not be removed, and the organism was reisolated while on therapy.

The only adverse reactions were noted with mezlocillin and consisted of three patients who developed significant eosinophilia, one patient with a generalized urticarial reaction, and one patient with moderate diarrhea. The antibiotic was discontinued in three of the five patients. No patient in either group developed fluid overload, significant electrolyte disturbance, or clinical bleeding.

In summary, a randomized, comparative clinical trial revealed equal efficacy with piperacillin and mezlocillin. Both antibiotics were highly effective in the therapy of serious infections. Adverse reactions were limited to mezlocillin and required the discontinuance of therapy in three patients (20%).

Piperacillin and mezlocillin appear to be promising new antibiotics in the parenteral therapy of serious infections. Their broad range of antimicrobial activity and possibly diminished toxicity make them attractive alternatives to currently available semisynthetic penicillins.

Efficacy of Piperacillin in the Therapy of Serious Infections

ALICE S. PRINCE, STEPHEN J. PANCOAST, AND HAROLD C. NEU*

Departments of Medicine and Pharmacology, College of Physicians and Surgeons, Columbia University, New York, New York 10032, U.S.A.

Piperacillin is a new semisynthetic piperazine derivative of ampicillin. It has a broad spectrum of activity against many gram-positive and -negative aerobic and anaerobic bacteria, including many *Klebsiella*, *Pseudomonas*, and *Bacteroides*, which are frequently resistant to carbenicillin (1). Since piperacillin is a β-lactam compound that would not have the nephrotoxicity and ototoxicity associated with use of aminoglycosides and since it may have fewer side effects than carbenicillin, we studied its efficacy and safety in the therapy of serious infections.

The patients were all hospitalized at The Columbia Presbyterian Medical Center. All patients included in the study had clinical evidence of infection. Patients with pneumonia had chest X-ray evidence of pneumonitis in addition to white cells and bacteria in the sputum. Patients with cystic fibrosis had exacerbations of their underlying pulmonary disease as manifested by fever, increased sputum production, and deterioration in pulmonary function. Patients with urinary tract infection had fever, urinary symptoms, and $>10^5$ organisms per ml of urine. Bacterial cultures were taken before therapy and identified by standard methods. Piperacillin MICs were determined for all organisms. Piperacillin serum levels were determined by an agar well diffusion technique. Laboratory studies included evaluation of hematological, hepatic, and renal function. Patients were observed daily for adverse reactions.

Patients were considered cured if there was both clinical improvement and bacteriological eradication of the infecting organism. Patients were considered improved if there was clinical improvement but the infecting organism was not eradicated. Patients were classified as failed if the infection did not clear clinically and the pathogen was not eradicated.

Intravenous therapy was given in doses ranging from 100 to 500 mg/kg per day and intramuscularly with 60 to 90 mg/kg per day. Doses were adjusted for the patient's renal function and the severity of the infection. The lower doses were used to treat urinary tract infections, and high (300 to 500 mg/kg per day) doses were used to treat pulmonary infections in patients with cystic fibrosis.

There were 32 patients treated with piperacillin. They ranged in age from 12 to 78 years. The underlying diseases included cystic fibrosis, diabetes mellitus, chronic renal disease, alcoholism, chronic pulmonary disease, malignancy, chronic neurological disease, and cirrhosis. Twenty-one patients had ultimately fatal underlying disease, and six had rapidly fatal underlying disease. There were 39 sites of infection in the patients.

Fifty bacterial isolates obtained before initiation of treatment included the following: *Pseudomonas aeruginosa* (29), *Klebsiella* (5), *Proteus* (3), *Escherichia coli* (2), *Achromobacter xyloxidans* (2), *Serratia* (2), and one each of *Salmonella*, *Pseudomonas multophilia*, *Enterobacter aerogenes*, *Streptococcus pneumoniae*, *Haemophilus influenzae*, *Haemophilus parainfluenzae*, and *Bacteroides fragilis*. Twenty-two (45%) of these organisms were not susceptible to carbenicillin; eight isolates (16%) had MICs to piperacillin >50 μg/ml, including four *P. aeruginosa* from the cystic fibrosis patients, and 11 (65%) were not susceptible to carbenicillin. Four (23%) strains had piperacillin MIC values >50 μg/ml. The mean carbenicillin and piperacillin MICs for these patients are shown in Table 1. Piperacillin was two- to threefold more active than carbenicillin.

Piperacillin concentrations were measured in serum and urine. Intravenous doses of 250 to 500 mg/kg per day gave mean peak levels of 190 μg/ml and trough levels of 0 to 40 μg/ml. Intramuscular doses of 60 to 90 mg/kg per day gave peak serum levels of 10 to 14 μg/ml. Urine levels were all $>1,000$ μg/ml in the absence of renal failure. There was no evidence of drug accumulation after multiple dosing. Patients with cystic fibrosis in general required higher doses to achieve

TABLE 1. *Mean MIC values of pretreatment cultures*

Organism (no.)	Mean MIC (μg/ml)	
	Carbenicillin	Piperacillin
P. aeruginosa (29)	184	59
Klebsiella (5)	360	108
Proteus (3)	4.6	1.2
E. coli (2)	3.9	1.9
Serratia (2)	206	28

TABLE 2. *Response to piperacillin therapy*

| Infection | No. | Cure | | Side effect[a] |
		Clinical	Bacterio-logical	
Bacteremia	7	6	7	2
Pneumonitis	5	4	4	1
Exacerbation of cystic fibrosis	12	10	1	2
Urinary tract	12	10	9	1
Soft tissue	1	1	1	
Peritonitis	2	2	2	
Total	39[b]	33 (85%)	23 (59%)	6 (19%)[c]

[a] Side effects were: phlebitis, 3; rash, 1; fever, 1.
[b] Several patients had infection at more than one site.
[c] Percent calculated on 32 patients.

the same serum levels as were achieved in the other patients.

The infections treated included seven episodes of bacteremia, 17 pulmonary infections (12 in patients with cystic fibrosis), 12 urinary tract infections, two episodes of peritonitis, and one soft tissue infection.

Overall there were 39 infections in the 32 patients which were evaluable for clinical efficacy. Clinical cure or improvement occurred in 88% (Table 2). Bacteremias due to *Klebsiella*, *P. aeruginosa*, *Enterobacter*, *Serratia*, *Proteus*, *E. coli*, and *Arizona* were all cleared. The six patients who completed therapy were both clinical and bacteriological cures. One of the patients with *P. aeruginosa* sepsis had disseminated carcinoma. One patient had sepsis due to *E. aerogenes* and *K. pneumoniae* from a small bowel obstruction.

Pulmonary infections were treated in 17 patients, 12 of whom had cystic fibrosis. There was clinical improvement in 14 patients and complete eradication of pathogens from the sputum in four patients who did not have cystic fibrosis. The patients with cystic fibrosis did show a decrease in volume of sputum and marked improvement in well-being. However, in 11 of 12 patients with cystic fibrosis, the suspected pathogens could be cultured in the sputum, although in decreased numbers. Three patients failed to improve during piperacillin therapy. These patients had at least one organism in the sputum with piperacillin MIC value >400 µg/ml at the time when they were considered to be a clinical failure. For example, one patient had a *Klebsiella* with an MIC >400 µg/ml.

Urinary tract infections were cured clinically and bacteriologically in 75% of the patients including six with *Pseudomonas*. The other organisms for which there was complete cure were *Serratia*, *Klebsiella*, and *Proteus*. Two patients with staghorn calculi improved clinically, but continued to have asymptomatic bacteriuria after piperacillin had been discontinued.

The other infections included one patient with a large sacral decubitus ulcer infected with *B. fragilis*, *E. coli*, and *P. mirabilis*. The wound healed. Two patients with peritonitis both showed marked improvement and ultimate cure.

Side effects of piperacillin therapy were observed in six patients (19%). Three patients developed phlebitis; two patients developed urticarial rashes. One patient who was given oxacillin in addition to piperacillin for a suspected but undocumented staphylococcal infection developed drug fever after 11 days of therapy, but was able to tolerate oxacillin subsequently without reaction. Therapy was stopped in the patients with rash and fever. There was no evidence of renal, hematological, or hepatic toxicity in any patient treated with piperacillin.

Piperacillin was shown in this study to be a safe and effective antibiotic to treat serious infections due to gram-negative bacteria. It seems particularly useful against *P. aeruginosa*, many of which were carbenicillin resistant. Development of resistant organisms was not a major problem in this study although larger studies certainly will be needed to determine the extent to which this may occur.

1. **Fu, K. P., and H. C. Neu.** 1978. Piperacillin, a new penicillin active against many bacteria resistant to other penicillins. Antimicrob. Agents Chemother. **13:**358–367.

Piperacillin in the Treatment of Bacteremia and Bacterial Endocarditis

BENJAMIN M. LIMSON,* RODRIGO F. GUANLAO, AND LUCITA Z. DEPAKAKIBO

Department of Biological Research, Philippine Heart Center for Asia, Quezon City, Philippines

Piperacillin sodium (T-1220), a new semisynthetic penicillin derivative, has been studied in Japan and the United States for the past 4 years, and its unusually broad spectrum against aerobic and anaerobic bacteria has been documented (2–6). Compared to other β-lactam antibiotics of similar chemical structure such as carbenicillin, ticarcillin, ampicillin, and cephalosporin agents, piperacillin showed superior potency against *Pseudomonas* species, the *Klebsiella-Enterobacter-Serratia* group, *Proteus* species, *Acinetobacter* species, and *Citrobacter* species. Furthermore, it showed remarkable activity against anaerobic bacteria, particularly *Bacteroides* species, peptostreptococci, peptococci, and enterococci.

Perhaps the more significant role of piperacillin was its use in serious blood stream infections. Early trials in which large doses of piperacillin were used in the treatment of septicemia gave a high cure rate (1).

This report evaluates the efficacy of moderate doses of piperacillin in the treatment of bacteremia and infective endocarditis caused by aerobic and anaerobic bacteria.

Recent clinical isolates of gram-positive and gram-negative bacteria were routinely tested for susceptibility to piperacillin by the disk diffusion method. Blood and other appropriate specimens from infected sites were cultured under aerobic and anaerobic conditions. In patients with confirmed bacterial endocarditis, the serum bactericidal activity of piperacillin (as a test of adequate dosage) was verified when a 1:8 or greater dilution of serum was bactericidal against the patient's causative pathogen. Serum samples were obtained midway between doses of the drug on the second or third day of treatment.

Piperacillin sodium, in 2-g vials, was supplied by Lederle Laboratories Division, American Cyanamid Co., Pearl River, N.Y. The daily dose was 200 to 300 mg/kg, administered in divided portions every 4 to 6 h by intermittent intravenous drip over 20 to 30 min. Duration of treatment was 10 to 14 days for bacteremia and 14 days for bacterial endocarditis. After obtaining specimens for cultures and other laboratory tests, treatment was started on strong clinical presumptive evidence and was continued upon bacteriological confirmation of in vitro susceptibility of the pathogen to piperacillin.

Routine in vitro disk susceptibility tests on recent clinical isolates of *P. aeruginosa, Proteus* species, *K. pneumoniae, E. aerogenes, S. marcescens, Escherichia coli, C. freundii, A. calcoaceticus, B. fragilis,* and streptococci showed that 76.8% of 200 strains were susceptible.

A total of 20 patients with confirmed blood stream infection were entered into the study, but two patients were dropped because of chills and generalized itching with the first two doses of piperacillin. The rest completed a 10- to 14-day course of treatment without side reactions. There were 18 evaluable patients, of whom 13 were females and 5 were males, aged 16 to 67 years. There were 11 cases of bacteremia related to primary foci of infection in various sites and 7 cases of bacterial endocarditis associated with chronic rheumatic valve disease.

As shown in Table 1, 10 of 11 patients with bacteremia were clinically cured, and the pathogen was eradicated. The associated conditions included septic shock, pyelonephritis, pneumonia, catheter-induced phlebitis, pelvic inflammatory disease, post-partum complications, diabetes mellitus, cerebral thrombosis, coronary artery disease, and mitral stenosis. Of the etiological microorganisms, seven were aerobic gram-negative bacilli, two were anaerobic, and one was streptococcal. The fever subsided on the fourth to the seventh day of piperacillin treatment. There were four patients with septic shock who received in addition two or three massive intravenous doses of hydrocortisone or methylprednisolone. Cultures of blood and other specimens were negative in 48 to 72 h.

One patient with multi-organ infection and pneumococcal bacteremia responded partially to piperacillin. This patient was in coma with bacteremia, pneumonia, meningitis, and hepatitis. The pneumonia and bacteremia cleared up, but the meningitis and hepatitis persisted, together with low-grade fever.

Also shown in Table 1 are the results of piperacillin treatment in seven patients with bacterial endocarditis caused by aerobic and anaerobic streptococci. All had a background of inactive chronic rheumatic mitral and/or aortic valve disease with congestive heart failure. The duration of fever prior to piperacillin treatment ranged from 2 to 9 weeks, and four patients had failed to respond to earlier treatment with pen-

TABLE 1. *Piperacillin treatment in bacteremia and bacterial endocarditis*[a]

Age	Sex	Disease and associated conditions	Causative pathogen	Dose every 6 h (g)	Daily dose (mg/kg)	Duration (days)	Clinical outcome
					Treatment		
		BACTEREMIA					
30	F	Septic shock, postpartum pyelonephritis	*Enterobacter aerogenes*	3	210	14	Cure
46	F	Pelvic inflammatory disease, coronary insufficiency	*Peptostreptococcus*	2	200	10	Cure
60	F	Septic shock, pyelonephritis, diabetes mellitus	*Escherichia coli*	3	206	10	Cure
65	F	Pyelonephritis, coronary insufficiency	*Citrobacter freundii*	3	230	10	Cure
67	F	Septic shock, pyelonephritis, diabetes mellitus	*Pseudomonas aeruginosa*	3	230	14	Cure
23	F	Septic shock, postpartum, pneumonia	*Klebsiella pneumoniae*	3	218	10	Cure
48	M	Pneumonia, myocardial infarct	*P. aeruginosa*	3	218	10	Cure
62	M	Pneumonia, cerebral thrombosis	*Bacteroides fragilis*	3	262	10	Cure
48	F	Phlebitis, postcardiac catheter, mitral stenosis	*Streptococcus faecalis*	3	235	10	Cure
50	F	Phlebitis, cardiovascular pump catheter, myocardial infarct	*Acinetobacter calcoaceticus*	3	250	10	Cure
30	F	Meningitis, pneumonia, hepatitis	*S. pneumoniae*	3	214	14	Improved
		BACTERIAL ENDOCARDITIS					
42	F	Rheumatic mitral regurgitation	Microaerophilic streptococcus	3	222	14	Cure
16	F	Rheumatic mitral stenosis and regurgitation	*S. faecalis*	2	200	14	Cure
17	M	Rheumatic mitral regurgitation	*S. faecalis*	2.5	228	14	Cure
29	M	Rheumatic mitral stenosis	Viridans streptococcus	3	214	14	Cure
47	F	Rheumatic mitral stenosis, aortic regurgitation	Microaerophilic streptococcus	3	250	14	Cure
24	M	Rheumatic aortic regurgitation	*S. faecalis*	3	226	14	Cure
23	F	Acute endometritis, post-partum, rheumatic mitral stenosis/regurgitation	*Peptostreptococcus*	4	300	14	Cure

[a] The bacteriological outcome in all patients was eradication of the causative organism.

icillin/streptomycin, ampicillin, or other broad-spectrum antibiotics. With piperacillin treatment the fever subsided in 4 to 7 days, and blood cultures were negative in 2 to 3 days. Follow-up laboratory tests every 2 weeks posttreatment up to 2 months showed no recurrence of infection. All seven patients with streptococcal endocarditis were considered cured clinically, and the causative pathogen was eradicated.

These results with intravenously administered piperacillin sodium in patients with life-threatening bacteremia and bacterial endocarditis caused by aerobic and anaerobic bacteria, against which the choices of antimicrobial agents are generally limited, were achieved with significantly lower doses than those previously employed. Earlier investigators have administered piperacillin doses of 12 to 24 g/day in six divided portions for bacterial septicemia and have achieved a high cure rate (1). In our series the dose range of piperacillin was 8 to 12 g/day, and our results show that the lower dosage of piperacillin is just as effective as the higher dosages previously employed in serious blood stream infections. The use of lower dosages may have the advantages of economy and fewer side reactions.

1. **Gooding, P. G.** 1978. Results of U.S. phase II studies of piperacillin, observations in 109 patients, p. 1–72. Medical Research Division, American Cyanamid Co., Pearl River, N.Y.
2. **Jones, R. N., C. Thornsberry, A. L. Barry, P. C. Fuchs, T. L. Gavan, and E. H. Gerlach.** 1977. Piper-

acillin (T-1220), a new semisynthetic penicillin: in vitro antimicrobial activity comparison with carbenicillin, ticarcillin, ampicillin, cephalothin, cefamandole and cefoxitin. J. Antibiot. **30**:1107–114.

3. **Kuck, N. A., and G. S. Redin.** 1978. In vitro and in vivo activity of piperacillin, a new broad spectrum semisynthetic penicillin. J. Antibiot. **31**:1175–1182.

4. **Monif, G. R. G., P. R. Clark, J. J. Shuster, and H. Baer.** 1978. Susceptibility of the anaerobic bacteria, group D streptococci, *Enterobacteriaceae*, and *Pseudomonas* to semisynthetic penicillins: carbenicillin, pi-

peracillin, and ticarcillin. Antimicrob. Agents Chemother. **14**:643–649.

5. **Ueo, K., Y. Fukuoka, T. Hayashi, T. Yasuda, H. Taki, M. Tai, Y. Watanabe, I. Saikawa, and S. Mitsuhashi.** 1977. In vitro and in vivo antimicrobial activity of T-1220, a new semisynthetic penicillin. Antimicrob. Agents Chemother. **12**:455–460.

6. **Winston, D. J., D. Wang, L. S. Young, W. J. Martin, and W. L. Hewitt.** 1978. In vitro studies of piperacillin, a new semisynthetic penicillin. Antimicrob. Agents Chemother. **13**:944–950.

Clinical Evaluation of Intravenous Piperacillin

BHAVANI S. RAO, DANIEL W. WHITE, VINH T. BACH, AND HARAGOPAL THADEPALLI*

Division of Infectious Diseases, Department of Medicine, Charles R. Drew Postgraduate Medical School, Martin Luther King, Jr., General Hospital and U.C.L.A. School of Medicine, Los Angeles, California 90059, U.S.A.

Piperacillin, a new semisynthetic penicillin, at 25 µg/ml is more effective than carbenicillin and ticarcillin against *Pseudomonas, Proteus, Klebsiella, Serratia,* and *Bacteroides fragilis* (1, 3). We report the clinical evaluation of piperacillin in 28 patients. Seven of them had pure aerobic infections, 7 had anaerobic infections, and 14 others had mixed infections. The diagnoses were lung abscess in four patients, empyema in one, osteomyelitis of the mandible in seven, necrotizing fasciitis in four, oropharyngeal, ischiorectal, or intraabdominal abscess in seven, urinary tract infection in three, and suppurative arthritis in two.

Cultures were obtained by transtracheal aspiration, thoracentesis, surgically drained pus, or "clean-catch" urine, and processed for aerobic and anaerobic bacteria (Table 1). MIC of the anaerobic bacteria was determined by agar dilution method (1). The serum antibiotic levels were determined by agar well diffusion method (2) against *Bacillus subtilis* (ATCC 6633). The piperacillin dose was 5 g every 6 h, diluted with 5% dextrose water given intravenously. The clinical responses were graded as "cure," "recurrence," or "failure" based on microbiological, clinical, and roentgenographic evaluation.

Results. The clinical results are summarized in Table 2. Twelve out of 14 patients with mixed aerobic/anaerobic infections were cured. In one patient with *B. capillosus* infection, the infection recurred; he needed surgical drainage and a second course of piperacillin therapy. The infection also recurred in another patient with *B. corrodens* infection. He underwent lobectomy and needed a second course of piperacillin therapy. He was considered as a failure since the

bacteria were still present in the abscess cavity at the time of surgery. The bacterial isolates in these two patients were susceptible to piperacillin at 8 µg/ml. All seven patients that had exclusively anaerobic infections and seven patients with pure aerobic infections promptly responded and were cured with the piperacillin therapy.

Six patients in this study had *Pseudomonas aeruginosa* (MIC ≤ 32 µg/ml) infections. Four of these had earlier failed on gentamicin (MIC > 5 µg/ml) alone or with carbenicillin (MIC > 100 µg/ml). All six patients with *Pseudomonas* infections were cured with piperacillin therapy.

TABLE 1. *Aerobic and anaerobic bacterial isolates derived from the initial pretherapy cultures*

Isolates	No.	MIC (µg/ml)
Aerobic		
Streptococcus	10	2–64
Enterococcus	3	4
S. aureus	4	32–128
E. coli	3	4
Proteus	3	4–8
Pseudomonas	6	4–32
Klebsiella	1	8
Enterobacter	1	8
Citrobacter	1	8
Serratia	1	8
Anaerobic		
Peptococcus	1	4
Peptostreptococcus	13	2–16
Bacteroides	20	2–128
Fusobacterium	2	2–16
Acidaminococcus	1	0.5
Lactobacillus	1	8
Eubacterium	4	0.5–2
Veillonella	1	2

TABLE 2. *Summary of clinical results*

Diagnosis	No. of patients	Cure	Recurrence	Failure
Lung abscess	4	3		1
Osteomyelitis of the mandible	7	6	1	
Necrotizing fasciitis	4	4		
Oropharyngeal abscess	3	3		
Intraabdominal abscess	3	3		
Urinary tract infection	3	3		
Chronic suppurative arthritis	2	2		
Rectal abscess	1	1		
Empyema	1	1		

Fourteen patients had *Bacteroides* infections, of which two had *B. fragilis* (MIC ≤ 4 µg/ml). All but two patients, as mentioned earlier, responded to piperacillin therapy. Both patients that had *B. fragilis* infection were cured.

The average serum piperacillin levels were 266 ± 158.5, 96 ± 41, 59 ± 37.5, 32 ± 23, and 16 µg/ml at the end of 1, 2, 3, 4, and 5 h, respectively, after a single intravenous infusion of 5 g of piperacillin in 5% dextrose water given within 15 min.

The adverse effects were minor: two had pruritus, one had lactate dehydrogenase elevation, and another eosinophilia, but none required discontinuation of therapy.

It was not known at the time of initiation of therapy that four patients treated with piperacillin had *Staphylococcus aureus* infections. One of these isolates was resistant (MIC = 128 µg/ml) to piperacillin. But all four patients responded to therapy. Gentamicin was added in two of these patients to achieve cure.

Discussion. Carbenicillin (4), ticarcillin (6), and mezlocillin (5) are effective in the treatment of aerobic and anaerobic infections. Piperacillin in vitro is known to be effective in the treatment of aerobic and anaerobic infections (1, 3). In our study, 21 patients had anaerobic infections: 19 of them were cured on the initial course and 2 others were cured on the second course of piperacillin. Both patients with *B. fragilis* infections were also cured with piperacillin. Piperacillin is not indicated for penicillinase-producing *S. aureus* infections, although four of our patients with *S. aureus* infections were cured.

Piperacillin, in our study, was found to be safe and effective in the treatment of aerobic, anaerobic, and mixed infections. Further trials are needed to compare its efficacy with carbenicillin or ticarcillin, which are proven to be effective in such infections.

1. **Bach, V. T., I. Roy, and H. Thadepalli.** 1977. *In vitro* activity of piperacillin against anaerobic bacteria in comparison with carbenicillin and ticarcillin. Curr. Ther. Res. **22:**583–587.
2. **Bennett, J. V., J. L. Brodie, E. J. Benner, and W. M. M. Kirby.** 1966. Simplified accurate method for antibiotic assay of clinical specimens. Appl. Microbiol. **14:** 170–177.
3. **Roy, I., W. M. Abernathy, V. T. Bach, and H. Thadepalli.** 1978. *In vitro* activity of piperacillin against aerobic bacteria. Curr. Ther. Res. **23:**200–205.
4. **Thadepalli, H.** 1976. Treatment of anaerobic infections with carbenicillin. Curr. Ther. Res. **20:**589–603.
5. **Thadepalli, H., and B. Rao.** 1979. Clinical evaluation of mezlocillin. Antimicrob. Agents Chemother. **16:**605–610.
6. **Webb, D., H. Thadepalli, I. Roy, and V. T. Bach.** 1978. Ticarcillin disodium in anaerobic infections. Arch. Intern. Med. **138:**1618–1620.

Complications of the Treatment of Bacterial Infections with Piperacillin

EMILIO BOUZA,* LUIS BUZÓN, JESÚS MARTINEZ-BELTRAN, MARTA RODRIGUEZ, IGNACIO MONEO, AND CARMEN BURGALETA

Infectious Disease Unit and Microbiology,* Immunology, and Hematology Services of the Centro Especial "Ramón y Cajal," Madrid, Spain

Piperacillin (Pp) is a new piperazine penicillin derivative with a wide spectrum of in vitro activity against gram-positive and gram-negative bacteria, including *Pseudomonas* (2, 11). There is a scarcity of clinical studies testing such efficacy and the possible incidence of complications, which would supposedly be similar to those caused by other penicillins (W. L. Hewitt, W. Murphy, D. Wang, and D. J. Winston, Program Abstr. Intersci. Conf. Antimicrob. Agents Chemother. 18th, Atlanta, Ga., Abstr. no. 167, 1978; E. Schrinner, N. Klesel, M. Limbert, and A. Lutz, 18th ICAAC, abstr. no. 80).

We treated 19 patients with 80 to 240 mg (mean 187.6) of intravenous sodium Pp per kg per day over periods of time varying from 10 to 42 days (mean 16.7), with the exception of one patient whose treatment was discontinued on day 3 of therapy. The diseases, microorganisms, methods of specimen collection, possible complications of therapy, and the final fates of the patients are summarized in Table 1. All aerobic microorganisms proved to have an MIC to Pp ≤64 μg/ml. Anaerobic bacteria were all susceptible to a disk of 100 μg of the said drug. The patients were examined daily by one of the authors, and routine blood, urine, sera, and specimens for bacterial cultures were taken before and after treatment and at least once a week during the treatment period. In 10 cases, serum levels of Pp were run, showing an oscillation from 60 to 140 μg/ml in the "peak" and from 7 to 29.9 μg/ml in the "valley." Bone marrow aspirates, in vitro cultures of granulocytic precursors, and detection of leukolytic antibodies were determined in some of the patients who had developed neutropenia. Neutropenia was defined as a total neutrophil count ≤2,000/μl and considered severe if absolute count was ≤500/μl.

We divided our patients into two groups (Table 1). Group 1 included the 9 patients who showed adverse effects directly or indirectly attributable to Pp. Group 2 consisted of the 10 patients who recovered without such effects. Complications are summarized in Table 1. In case 2, Pp was discontinued on day 3 of therapy due to a clinical setting of spiking fevers and shock, and treatment was switched to ampicillin plus gentamicin. Blood cultures taken during the episode proved later to be sterile. Two patients (cases 1 and 4) with pneumonia caused by *Streptococcus pneumoniae* developed pulmonary cavitation. Case 1 died with an *Escherichia coli* pulmonary abscess while on treatment with carbenicillin and gentamicin. This patient was also a diabetic. Case 4 also developed a lung cavity during therapy and required surgery for definitive cure. On two occasions thrombophlebitis appeared, interfering at certain points with the administration of further intravenous therapy. Neutropenia was the most noteworthy adverse effect in our cases (Table 2). In case 5, it appeared at the end of therapy, on day 10. All of the four remaining cases started the neutropenia during week 4 of therapy. The neutrophil nadir in the five cases was ≤1.750/μl and in two cases was inferior to 500/μl. Absolute eosinophilia was found in one patient only. After withdrawal of the drug, the recovery time to a normal neutro-

TABLE 1. *Patients treated with piperacillin*[a]

Case	Age	Sex	Diagnosis	Microorganism	Sample origin	Dose (mg/kg per day)	Days on treatment	Complications	Evolution
1	71	F	Pneumonia	*Streptococcus pneumoniae*	TTA	80	14	Superinfection (lung abscess)	D
2	27	M	Osteomyelitis	*Streptococcus faecalis*	BS	185	3	Septic episode	C + Surgery
3	23	M	Osteomyelitis	*Pseudomonas aeruginosa*	BS	171	26	Neutropenia (day + 26)	C + Surgery
4	42	M	Pneumonia	*S. pneumoniae*	TTA	185	30	Neutropenia (day + 28); lung abscess	C + Surgery
5	62	F	Erysipelas	*Streptococcus*, group A	NA	133	10	Neutropenia (day + 10)	C
6	42	M	Osteomyelitis	*Proteus mirabilis* *Streptococcus* Anaerobes	BS	225	25	Neutropenia (day + 25)	I + Surgery
7	82	F	Pneumonia	*S. pneumoniae*	TTA	200	10	Thrombophlebitis	C
8	57	M	Pneumonia	*S. pneumoniae*	TTA	197	11	Thrombophlebitis	C
9	63	M	Lung abscess	Anaerobes	TPA	182	22	Neutropenia (day + 22)	C
10	67	M	Pneumonia	*S. pneumoniae*	TTA	218	10	None	C
11	41	F	Lung abscess	*Serratia marcescens* Anaerobes	TTA	207	42	None	C + Surgery
12	17	F	Pneumonia		Sputum	240	12	None	C
13	62	M	Osteomyelitis	*Escherichia coli*	BS	200	28	None	C + Surgery
14	73	F	Pneumonia	*S. pneumoniae*	TTA	130	12	None	C
15	36	M	Pneumonia	*S. pneumoniae*	TTA	235	10	None	C
16	40	M	Pneumonia	*S. pneumoniae*	TPA	209	14	None	C
17	60	M	Pneumonia	*S. pneumoniae*	TPA	190	14	None	C
18	46	M	Pneumonia	*S. pneumoniae*	TTA	185	11	None	C
19	54	M	Pneumonia	*S. pneumoniae*	TTA	194	11	None	C

[a] Abbreviations: C, cured; D, died; I, improved; TTA, translaryngeal aspirate; TPA, transpulmonary aspirate; BS, bone sample; NA, needle aspiration.

TABLE 2. *Patients with neutropenia*

Case	Age (yr)	Sex	Dose (mg/kg per day)	Initial leuko-cyte count[a]	Neu-tro-phils (%)	Eosino-phils (%)	Neutro-penia (day 1)	Nadir leuko-cyte count[a]	Nadir neu-tro-phils[a]	Zenit eosin-ophils[a]	Days to re-cover	Bone marrow	Leuko-lytic anti-bodies
3	23	M	171	10.3	41	1	26	3.2	0.7	0.6	7	Maturation arrest	+
4	42	M	185	14.5	78	0	28	4.4	1.7	0.2	5	ND[b]	ND
5	62	F	133	4.7	50	0	10	3.2	1.4	0.1	7	Granulocytic hyperpla-sia	+
6	42	M	225	10.7	59	0	23	2.8	0.1	0.0	4	ND	ND
9	63	M	182	9.1	74	0	22	1.0	0.0	0.0	7	ND	+

[a] $\times 10^9$ per liter.
[b] ND, Not done.

phil count was 4 to 7 days. No complications were found during the neutropenic period.

Examination of bone marrow aspirate in case 3 showed a maturation arrest at the myelocytic stage, and in case 5 showed granulocytic hyperplasia without arrest. Incubation in semisolid media of bone marrow aspirates of both patients with progressive amounts of Pp (2 to 20 µg/ml) failed to show toxic effects of Pp on granulocytic precursors. Sera from three patients, after recovery from neutropenia, showed the presence of a "leukolytic factor" for patient and control leukocytes previously incubated with Pp. The effect was complement dependent, decreased with serum dilution, and disappeared when immunoglobulins were removed.

Clinical assays with sodium Pp are lacking, especially those devoted to long-term treatment of bacterial infections such as osteomyelitis, lung abscesses, endocarditis, and arthritis. In our series, nine patients received sodium Pp during 14 days or more.

Neutropenia is a well-known side effect of all β-lactam antibiotics in general, especially to semisynthetic penicillins (4, 7, 8). Information in literature is usually provided on a case report basis, and the total incidence is difficult to evaluate. Yow et al. reviewed the side effects of methicillin in 3,000 patients during a 10-year period (12). Total incidence of neutropenia was 0.5%, and the figure increased to 16% when only cases treated for 10 or more days were considered. In a recent review of neutropenia induced by β-lactam antibiotics, the incidence was higher when dosages greater than 150 mg/kg per day were administered, and the duration of treatment was prolonged 2 or more weeks (4).

We only found three previously reported cases of neutropenia related to Pp (G. M. Dickinson, D. G. Droller, R. L. Greenman, and T. A. Hoffman, 18th ICAAC, abstr. no. 166; 10). Therefore,

it was remarkable that 5 out of 19 patients treated by us with this drug developed neutropenia. Case 5 developed neutropenia on day 10 of therapy. This complication appeared in four of the six patients who received therapy for 3 weeks or more, which implies a much higher incidence than that reported previously for all other β-lactam drugs (3–5, 7, 8).

Information is incomplete on the possible mechanisms of β-lactam drug-induced neutropenia. The two major theories are: a simple toxicity mechanism (1, 4, 8) and an immunologically mediated reaction (5, 9). Our data suggest that there is a serum factor, which is leukolytic in vitro for Pp-coated leukocytes. The effect is complement dependent and probably immunologically mediated. The drug does not seem directly toxic for granulocytic precursors. We excluded the possibility of other medications, administered concomitantly with the antibiotic as offending agents, since they were continued during the episode of leukopenia.

Thrombophlebitis and superinfection are two well-reported complications of antibiotic therapy.

Thirteen of the 19 patients were considered cured at the end of the initially planned treatment with sodium Pp. Ten of the 12 cases presenting pneumonia were cured without major problems, but only 1 of the 4 cases of osteomyelitis completed treatment with this antibiotic.

Piperacillin should be added to the list of drugs that may induce neutropenia and should be administered with careful leukocyte monitoring, especially when the administration period exceeds 2 weeks.

1. **Chu, J. Y., D. M. O'Connor, and R. R. Schmidt.** 1977. The mechanism of oxacillin induced neutropenia. J. Pediatr. **90:**668.
2. **Fu, K. P., and H. C. Neu.** 1978. Piperacillin, a new

penicillin active against many bacteria resistant to other penicillins. Antimicrob. Agents. Chemother. **13**:358–367.

3. **Ghosh, J. S.** 1979. Oxacillin induced granulocytopenia. Acta Haematol. **61**:59.

4. **Homayouni, H., T. A. Gross, U. Setia, and T. J. Lynch.** 1979. Leukopenia due to penicillin and cephalosporin homologues. Arch. Intern. Med. **139**:827–828.

5. **Markowitz, S. M., M. Rothkopf, F. D. Holden, D. M. Stith, and R. J. Duma.** 1975. Nafcillin induced agranulocytosis. J. Am. Med. Assoc. **232**:1150–1152.

6. **Price, T. H., and D. C. Dale.** 1978. The selective neutropenias. Clin. Haematol. **7**:501–521.

7. **Rahal, J. J., and N. S. Simberkoff.** 1978. Adverse reactions to anti-infective agents. Dis. Mon. Oct.: 1–67.

8. **Reyes, M. P., M. Palutke, and A. M. Lerner.** 1973. Granulocytopenia associated with carbenicillin. Am. J. Med. **54**:413–418.

9. **Weitzman, S. A., T. P. Stossell, and M. Desmond.** 1978. Drug induced immunological neutropenia. Lancet **1**:1068–1071.

10. **Wilson, C., G. Greenhood, J. S. Remington, and K. L. Vosti.** 1979. Neutropenia after consecutive treatment courses with nafcillin and piperacillin. Lancet **1**:1150.

11. **Winston, D. J., D. Wang, L. S. Young, W. J. Martin, and W. L. Hewitt.** 1978. In vitro studies of piperacillin, a new semisynthetic penicillin. Antimicrob. Agents Chemother. **13**:944–950.

12. **Yow, M. D., L. H. Taber, F. F. Barret, A. A. Mintz, G. R. Balnkinship, E. Clark, and D. J. Clark.** 1976. A ten year assessment of methicillin associated side-effects. Pediatrics **58**:329–334.

Piperacillin: In Vitro Activity on 3,500 Bacterial Isolates

JESÚS MARTÍNEZ-BELTRÁN,* EMILIO BOUZA, ELENA LOZA, AND FERNANDO BAQUERO

Microbiology Service and Infectious Disease Unit, Centro Especial "Ramón y Cajal," Madrid, Spain

Piperacillin is a new semisynthetic piperazine penicillin derivative with a wide spectrum of activity, including gram-positive aerobic cocci, *Enterobacteriaceae*, nonfermentative gram-negative bacilli, and anaerobic bacteria (1, 3, 5–7). This spectrum of activity and its inferior toxicity, compared with aminoglycosides, arouse clinical interest in this drug.

We report the pattern of in vitro susceptibility to piperacillin in 3,500 nonselected, recent clinical isolates, including 2,331 *Enterobacteriaceae*, 434 nonfermentative gram-negative bacilli, and 735 gram-positive aerobic cocci. In 2,500 of them we have compared the activity of piperacillin with that of ampicillin, carbenicillin, cefazolin, cefamandole, cefoxitin, gentamicin, tobramycin, and amikacin. Against 50 strains of *Pseudomonas aeruginosa* and 20 isolates of *Streptococcus faecalis*, the MBC/MIC ratio was compared for piperacillin, carbenicillin, and ampicillin.

Identification of microorganisms and MIC and MBC determinations were performed by well-established routines (2, 4). The standard reference strains *Escherichia coli* ATCC 25922, *P. aeruginosa* ATCC 27853, and *Staphylococcus aureus* ATCC 25923 were always tested as internal controls. In agar dilution tests, antibiotic final concentrations varied from 256 to 8 µg/ml for piperacillin, 256 to 64 µg/ml for carbenicillin, and 16 to 4 µg/ml for the remaining drugs in a twofold dilution. For broth dilution studies, the range of concentrations was from 512 to 0.125 µg/ml for piperacillin, carbenicillin, and ampicillin.

Standard powders of antibiotics were supplied by manufacturers. Piperacillin was a gift of Lederle Laboratories. Isolates were considered susceptible if they were inhibited at 64 µg/ml for piperacillin and carbenicillin, 8 µg/ml for ampicillin, cefazolin, cefamandole, cefoxitin, and amikacin, and 4 µg/ml for gentamicin and tobramycin.

We found that the standard reference organisms were inhibited by 8 µg of piperacillin per ml. The results of the in vitro susceptibility tests on 3,500 isolates to piperacillin are summarized in Table 1. At a concentration of 64 µg/ml, piperacillin was active against more than 60% of *E. coli* and *Enterobacter* and 50% of *Klebsiella* and *Serratia*, whereas 8 µg/ml was only active for 31 and 35% of *Klebsiella* and *Serratia*, respectively, the most resistant *Enterobacteriaceae* to piperacillin. With the exception of a strain of *Salmonella mendoza* (MIC > 256), all *Salmonella* and *Yersinia enterocolitica* isolates were very susceptible to piperacillin. Against indole-positive and indole-negative *Proteus*, piperacillin showed similar activity. It inhibited 85 and 80%, respectively, at 64 µg/ml. The activity of piperacillin for *P. aeruginosa* was remarkable: 8 µg/ml inhibited 75% and 64 µg/ml inhibited 98% of isolates. Only two isolates were resistant to 256 µg of the drug per ml. Nine of nine isolates of *Pseudomonas cepacia* were susceptible to 8 µg of piperacillin per ml. All isolates of *S. faecalis* were inhibited by 32 µg/ml.

The comparative activity of piperacillin with other antibiotics is summarized in Table 2. At critical concentrations, piperacillin appeared superior to carbenicillin against *E. coli*, *Klebsiella*,

TABLE 1. *In vitro activity of piperacillin against gram-positive and -negative organisms*

Organism	No. tested	Cumulative % susceptible to indicated MIC (µg/ml)						
		≤8	16	32	64	128	256	>256
E. coli	870	48	53	59	65	69	74	100
Klebsiella sp.	510	31	38	45	51	56	61	100
Enterobacter sp.	170	50	55	59	61	70	74	100
S. marcescens	165	35	39	45	50	52	54	100
Citrobacter sp.	48	58	60	63	63	77	85	100
Salmonella sp.	68	94	99	99	99	99	99	100
Y. enterocolitica	10	70	80	90	100			
P. mirabilis	340	63	69	76	85	88	90	100
Proteus indole-positive	150	65	69	74	80	85	90	100
P. aeruginosa	386	75	85	93	98	99	99	100
P. cepacia	9	100						
Pseudomonas sp.	8	38	38	50	50	62	62	100
A. calcoaceticus	31	32	68	81	93	100		
S. aureus	350	53	64	75	85	91	97	100
S. epidermidis	195	71	78	84	88	94	98	100
S. faecalis	190	96	98	100				

TABLE 2. *Comparative activity of piperacillin with other β-lactam and aminoglycoside antibiotics*

Organism	Percent inhibited at critical concn[a]								
	PP (64 µg/ ml)	CB (64 µg/ ml)	AMP (8 µg/ ml)	CFZ (8 µg/ ml)	CFM (8 µg/ ml)	CFX (8 µg/ ml)	GTA (4 µg/ ml)	TOB (4 µg/ ml)	AK (8 µg/ ml)
E. coli (600)[b]	65	45	36	76	74	89	93	92	99
Klebsiella sp. (355)	51	8	1	48	55	88	66	68	100
Enterobacter sp. (111)	61	58	10	23	72	24	77	78	100
S. marcescens (115)	50	22	2	3	6	15	44	48	100
Citrobacter sp. (26)	63	58	19	31	88	27	96	96	100
Salmonella sp. (34)	99	97	97	100	100	100	100	100	100
Y. enterocolitica (10)	100	0	0	0	100	100	100	100	100
P. mirabilis (220)	85	64	48	62	74	87	95	95	99
Proteus indole-positive (107)	80	73	2	0	39	49	93	98	100
P. aeruginosa (253)	98	79	0	0	0	0	71	85	86
P. cepacia (9)	100	0	0	0	0	0	0	0	0
Pseudomonas sp. (8)	50	62	0	0	0	0	75	75	75
A. calcoaceticus (31)	93	81	16	6	6	10	84	90	87
S. aureus (340)	85	95	62	97	98	97	98	98	100
S. epidermidis (162)	88	91	72	98	99	75	83	89	100
S. faecalis (119)	100	97	100	5	3	2	6	4	3

[a] Abbreviations: PP, piperacillin; CB, carbenicillin; AMP, ampicillin; CFZ, cefazolin; CFM, cefamandole; CFX, cefoxitin; GTA, gentamicin; TOB, tobramycin; AK, amikacin.
[b] Total number tested.

and *Serratia* and similar to carbenicillin for *Enterobacter* and *Citrobacter*. Cefoxitin was the most active β-lactam antibiotic for *Klebsiella*, cefamandole for *Enterobacter* and *Citrobacter*, and piperacillin for *Serratia*. For *Klebsiella*, *Enterobacter*, and *Serratia*, we already have a β-lactam drug that equals the activity of gentamicin and tobramycin. Ten isolates of *Yersinia enterocolitica*, resistant to clinical concentrations of ampicillin, carbenicillin, and cefazolin, were susceptible to 64 µg of piperacillin per ml and 8 µg each of cefamandole and cefoxitin per ml. Against all *Enterobacteriaceae*, amikacin

was the most active drug. Piperacillin was the most active drug of the β-lactam drugs and aminoglycosides tested against *P. aeruginosa*. For *P. cepacia*, piperacillin had a noteworthy activity, especially important as all isolates were resistant to aminoglycosides, including amikacin. Against *S. aureus* and *Staphylococcus epidermidis*, piperacillin proved to be inferior to other β-lactam drugs, as was expected. For *S. faecalis*, piperacillin, ampicillin, and carbenicillin had a similar activity at critical concentrations.

The MBC/MIC ratio was obtained to compare the bactericidal activity of piperacillin and carbenicillin against 50 strains of *P. aeruginosa*. Carbenicillin was more bactericidal than piperacillin, even when MICs for piperacillin were 16 times less. For carbenicillin, 49 of the 50 strains showed a MBC/MIC ratio less than 4. Such a ratio for piperacillin was 32 for 18 strains and 64 for 21 strains of *P. aeruginosa*. For *S. faecalis*, MIC and MBC values were very similar, and the MBC/MIC ratio was always equal or less than 2 for piperacillin, carbenicillin, and ampicillin.

The results of this study with 3,500 isolates emphasizes the broad spectrum of activity of piperacillin against gram-negative bacilli and *S. faecalis*, combining ampicillin and carbenicillin activities. At critical concentrations, piperacillin was more active than carbenicillin against *Klebsiella*, *Serratia*, *Yersinia*, *P. aeruginosa*, and *P. cepacia* and had a similar activity to gentamicin and tobramycin against *Serratia*, *Salmonella*, and *Yersinia*. We did not find the high activity of piperacillin against *Klebsiella*, *Enterobacter*, and *Serratia* reported by other authors (3, 6, 7). Piperacillin was the most active antibiotic against *P. aeruginosa* and *P. cepacia*. Its activity against *S. aureus* and *S. epidermidis* was as to be expected for this group, and was clearly inferior to the cephalosporins. The activity against *S. faecalis* was excellent, as previously reported (3, 6, 8).

Piperacillin had a very high inhibitory rate against *P. aeruginosa*. Nevertheless, it was less bactericidal as the ratio of MBC/MIC shows, although the clinical significance of this fact is unknown. Clinical studies to test efficacy, and to rule out undesirable side effects, are required to assess the role of this drug in the treatment of human infections.

1. **Bodey, G. P., and B. Leblanc.** 1978. Piperacillin: in vitro evaluation. Antimicrob. Agents Chemother. **14**:78–87.
2. **Eriksson, H. M., and J. C. Sherris.** 1971. Antibiotic sensitivity testing. Report of an international collaborative study. Acta Pathol. Microbiol. Scand. Sect. B Suppl. **217**:1–90.
3. **Fu, K. P., and H. C. Neu.** 1978. Piperacillin, a new penicillin active against many bacteria resistant to other penicillins. Antimicrob. Agents Chemother. **13**:358–367.
4. **Lennette, E. H., E. H. Spaulding, and J. P. Truant (ed.).** 1974. Manual of clinical microbiology, 2nd ed. American Society for Microbiology, Washington, D.C.
5. **Ueo, K., Y. Fukuoka, T. Hayashi, T. Yasuda, H. Taki, H. Tai, M. Tai, Y. Watanabe, Y. Saikawa, and S. Mitsuhashi.** 1977. In vitro and in vivo antibacterial activity of T-1220, a new semisynthetic penicillin. Antimicrob. Agents Chemother. **12**:455–460.
6. **Verbist, L.** 1978. In vitro activity of piperacillin, a new semisynthetic penicillin with an unusually broad spectrum of activity. Antimicrob. Agents Chemother. **13**:349–357.
7. **Winston, D. J., D. Wang, L. S. Young, W. J. Martin, and W. L. Hewitt.** 1978. In vitro studies of piperacillin, a new semisynthetic penicillin. Antimicrob. Agents Chemother. **13**:944–950.

Diffusion and Pharmacokinetics of Piperacillin in Prostatic Tissue

ULF TUNN* AND DIETER ADAM

Urological Clinic of the Ruhruniversitat, Marien Hospital, Herne, and The Hospital for Children of the University of Munich, Munich, Federal Republic of Germany*

Piperacillin is a new semisynthetic penicillin and has a broad spectrum against gram-positive and gram-negative bacteria, including *Pseudomonas aeruginosa*, *Escherichia coli*, *Klebsiella pneumoniae*, and *Proteus* and other microorganisms, which are often involved in infections of the genitourinary tract.

The present study was undertaken to determine blood and prostatic tissue concentrations of piperacillin after bolus injection of 4.0 g. This method allows it to prove, firstly, the extent of diffusion of piperacillin into the prostatic tissue and, secondly, the time course of drug elimination.

Materials and methods. In 21 patients (mean age ± SEM, 69.6 ± 2.9 years; range, 62 to 82 years) suffering from benign prostatic hyperplasia (BPH) and undergoing transurethral resection of the prostate, piperacillin concentrations were determined simultaneously in serum and prostatic tissue after a bolus injection over 3 min of 4.0 g.

Prostatic tissue. Prostatic tissue was removed by transurethral resection of the prostate with continuous irrigation, simultaneous suction, and low intravesical pressure. This procedure ensures that no contamination of prostatic tissue with urine occurs. BPH tissue was resected at different intervals 15, 30, 45, 60, 120, and 135 min after bolus injection of piperacillin. Tissue samples were washed with isotonic glycocoll solution to eliminate residual blood. The tissue was blotted dry with sterile filter paper and stored at −40°C.

TABLE 1. *Concentrations of piperacillin in serum (A)[a] and in prostatic tissue (B)[b] after a single intravenous dose of 4.0 g*

Determi-nation[c]	Piperacillin concn at:																	
	15[d]			30			45			60			120			135		
	A	B	B/A	A	B	B/A	A	B	B/A	A	B	B/A	A	B	B/A	A	B	B/A
X̄	328.7	55.4	0.26	211.8	52.7	0.49	185.0	71.5	0.41	119.1	70.7	0.6	35.3	27.5	0.78	31.4	14.7	0.52
SEM	84.5	5.9	0.05	52.5	5.9	0.12	17.4	4.9	0.06	16.4	10.4	0.05	6.2	7.3	0.12	6.0	2.9	0.14
n	8			11			5			4			6			5		

[a] In micrograms per milliliter.
[b] In micrograms per gram.
[c] X̄, Mean; SEM, standard error of the mean; n, number of samples.
[d] Minutes after injection.

Assay. The assay of piperacillin in the serum and homogenized tissue was performed by a standard agar diffusion method using the inhibition of *E. coli* on agar (Oxoid Ltd.) by the method of Adam et al. (1).

Data processing. Calculation of data was done with an Olivetti Programma 101 disk-computer. Means, SD, SEMs, regression lines, and correlation coefficients of Pearson-Bravais were evaluated.

Results. Serum and prostatic tissue levels of piperacillin after bolus injection of 4.0 g are shown in Table 1, including mean serum concentrations and the regression line of the values. The average serum drug concentrations (mean ± SEM) ranged from 328.7 µg/ml (±84.5) 15 min after injection to 31.4 µg/ml (±6.0) 135 min after injection. The average biological half-life was 42 min.

The corresponding concentrations in the prostatic tissue after bolus injection of 4.0 g of piperacillin are also shown in Table 1. Peak concentrations were measured 45 min after administration. At this time the average piperacillin concentration was 71.5 µg/g of BPH tissue. Plateau levels were obtained between 45 and 60 min after application. Thereafter, the average prostatic tissue drug level decreased continuously. After 135 min, the concentration in the BPH tissue was 14.7 µg/g.

The ratio (R) of prostatic tissue to serum concentration of piperacillin at different intervals after application of prostatic tissue is delayed compared to the decline of serum levels,

TABLE 2. *Regression equations of piperacillin concentrations[a]*

Concn	Y	R	No. of samples
Serum concn, X = 15–135 min	323.6 − 2.386·X	0.6101	38
Tissue concn, X = 0–135 min	68.1 − 0.33·X	0.61	39
X = 0–45 min	43.37 + 0.45·X	0.30	25
X = 60–135 min	115.26 − 0.74·X	0.86	14

[a] X, Minutes after injection; Y, regression equation of piperacillin concentration; R, correlation coefficient.

the distribution ratio increases until 120 min after drug injection.

Statistical data are shown in Table 2.

Conclusions. (i) The mean serum concentrations of piperacillin after bolus injection of 4.0 g are several times higher than MICs of the drug within 120 min after injection. (ii) The mean levels of piperacillin in tissue of BPH increases within 45 min after injection and decreases continuously after 60 min. (iii) The BPH tissue drug value indicates good tissue penetration and delayed tissue elimination. (iv) The estimated concentrations of piperacillin in serum and BPH tissue are suited for the treatment of infections caused by piperacillin-susceptible microorganisms.

1. **Adam, D., et al.** 1976. Studies on the diffusion of cephradine and cephalothin into human tissue. Infection **4:** 105.

Diffusion of Piperacillin into Human Heart Muscle

DIETER ADAM,* BRUNO REICHART, AND BERNHARD ROTHENFUSSER

Kinderklinik der Universität, D-8000 Munich 2, and Herzchirurgische Klinik im Klinikum Grosshadern der Universität, D-8000 Munich 70, Federal Republic of Germany*

Infection after open-heart surgery is a serious complication since eradication of infection in these cases is difficult even with appropriate antibiotic therapy. This fact has encouraged many surgeons to administer antibiotics prophylactically. Although most observations supporting such usage have been uncontrolled (1, 2), some recent randomized double-blind trials give hope that chemoprophylaxis in open-heart surgery may be of some value (3, 4).

To provide protection during an operation, an antibiotic theoretically should reach concentrations in tissue that are greater than the MIC of the antibiotic for the suspected pathogen. An approach that may reduce the frequency of postoperative (wound) infections is to use chemoprophylaxis for only a short period, starting with the first dose 30 to 60 min preoperatively, continuing the administration during the operation, and discontinuing the chemoprophylaxis with the end of the operation.

This report examines the characteristics of the penetration of piperacillin into the heart muscle tissue (HMT) of patients who underwent open-heart surgery and provides data concerning the most appropriate time to administer the drug to ensure adequate intraoperative levels.

Fifty patients who underwent cardiac surgery with cardiopulmonary bypass were the subjects of this study. Their ages ranged from 19 to 60 years. All of the patients who participated in the study had normal clinical and laboratory values. Twenty-eight patients received a single dose of 100 mg/kg and 22 patients a single dose of 50 mg/kg by rapid intravenous (i.v.) (<5 min) injection at various times (5 to 70 min) before the removal of the heart muscle material. Heart muscle was removed after an ischemia of 5 min, so that the blood portion in the tissue was low. Before treating the material in a Stomacher no. 80 (A. J. Seward Co., Ltd., London), the tissue samples were freed from visible blood with a dry sterile swab and dipped into a sterile glucose solution. Serum samples were collected before the administration of the antibiotic as control (in no case was antimicrobial activity detectable) and at precisely the time of tissue removal. The centrifuged serum and the tissue samples were stored at −30°C until analyzed. Antibiotic concentrations were determined by the agar diffu-

sion method using punched holes, with *Escherichia coli* 6311/65 as the test organism. Excess drug concentration due to contamination with blood was found to be <5% of the measured total drug levels in tissue. Correction of this amount of contamination was thought to be insignificant.

As shown in Fig. 1, at 10 to 20 min after a 100-mg/kg i.v. dose of piperacillin, the mean concentrations in serum were about 500 µg/ml, ranging from 462.5 to 594.5 (SD, ±57.3) µg/ml. At 60 min after that dose, the serum concentrations ranged from 142.8 to 262.5 µg/ml, with a mean of 199.0 (SD, ±45.7) µg/ml. The corresponding HMT concentrations ranged at 10 to 20 min after the administration of the drug from 104.1 to 120.5, with a mean of 113.5 (SD, ±6.5) µg/g, and at 60 min from 30.6 to 101.0, with a mean of 60.0 (SD, ±26.3). The ratio varied from 0.23 to 0.30.

As shown in Fig. 2, 5 min after a 50-mg/kg i.v. dose of piperacillin, the mean concentrations in serum were 232.0 µg/ml, ranging from 184.0 to 242.0 (SD, ±43.8) µg/ml. At 70 to 75 min after that dose, the serum concentrations ranged from 19.2 to 66.7, with a mean of 49.2 (SD, ±26.1) µg/ml. The corresponding HMT concentrations

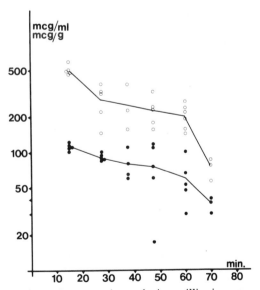

FIG. 1. *Concentrations of piperacillin in serum* (○) *and in heart muscle tissue* (●) *after a 100-mg/kg i.v. bolus injection.*

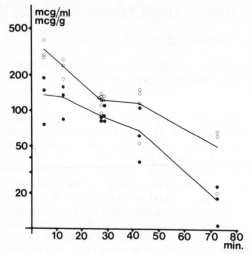

FIG. 2. *Concentrations of piperacillin in serum* (O) *and in heart muscle tissue* (●) *after a 50-mg/kg i.v. bolus injection.*

ranged at 5 min after the administration of the drug from 77.4 to 190.1, with a mean of 137.6 (SD, ±56.8) μg/ml, and at 70 to 75 min after the injection from 10.9 to 23.3, with a mean of 17.4 (SD, ±6.2) μg/ml. The ratio varies from 0.42 to 0.35.

Conclusions. Piperacillin, a low-protein-bound new penicillin, shows an excellent diffusibility into the HMT. It is of interest to note that the ratios are markedly higher after a 50-mg/kg dose compared to a 100-mg/kg dose. There may be a saturation effect if a high dose was given, and the penetration of the drug into the HMT may be limited depending on the concentration of the drug in the serum at a given time. However, the concentrations in the HMT

are high after a 100-mg/kg dose as well as after a 50-mg/kg dose. The peak values are reached also in the HMT very soon after the administration of the drug. The results of the study indicate that a single 50-mg/kg dose of piperacillin should be administered no more than 60 to 75 min before removal of the heart muscle to ensure an adequate antibiotic concentration in this tissue if the reason for the administration is to carry out a perioperative chemoprophylaxis. To meet this requirement the antibiotic should be given in the operating room, probably by the anesthesiologist at the start of the surgical procedure. If the lag time between the onset of the operation and the entry of the antibiotic into the HMT is longer, an intraoperative dose must be given. A prospective double-blind study with cefamandole done by Stone and co-workers (4) emphasized the importance of adequate pre- and intraoperative levels of antibiotics in patients who underwent colon, gastric, and biliary surgery; it was found that the rate of wound infections was about 15% when the drug was administered after the operation or when no antibiotic was given. The infection rate dropped down to 4% when the drug was administered preoperatively.

1. **Carey, J. S., and R. K. Hughes.** 1970. Control of infection after thoracic and cardiovascular surgery. Ann. Surg. **172**:916–926.
2. **Nelson, R. M., C. B. Jenson, and C. A. Peterson.** 1965. Effective use of prophylactic antibiotics in open heart surgery. Arch. Surg. **90**:731–736.
3. **Perdue, G. D., Jr.** 1975. Antibiotic as an aid in the prevention of infection after peripheral arterial surgery. Ann. Surg. **41**:296–300.
4. **Stone, H. H., C. A. Hooper, L. D. Kolb, C. E. Geheber, and E. J. Dawkins.** 1976. Antibiotic prophylaxis in gastric, biliary and colonic surgery. Ann. Surg. **184**:443–452.

Pharmacokinetics of Intravenous Piperacillin in Patients Undergoing Chronic Hemodialysis and in Patients with Cystic Fibrosis

ELLIOT F. FRANCKE, ALICE S. PRINCE, STEPHEN J. PANCOAST, AND HAROLD C. NEU*

Departments of Medicine* and Pharmacology, College of Physicians and Surgeons, Columbia University, New York, New York 10032, U.S.A.

Piperacillin, a piperazine penicillin, has a broad in vitro activity against many gram-positive and gram-negative bacteria, including streptococci, true enterococci, *Listeria, Escherichia coli,* indole-positive and -negative *Proteus, En-* *terobacter,* and *Pseudomonas aeruginosa.* It also inhibits anaerobic species such as *Bacteroides fragilis* (1). Infections with these organisms occur frequently in patients with diminished renal function, in whom treatment with carbenicillin is difficult since the drug accumulates in the presence of renal failure, and in whom aminoglycoside therapy carries a higher risk of toxicity than in patients with normal renal function. Another population in which infections with *Pseudomonas*, often resistant to other antibiotics, occur is patients with cystic fibrosis (3). Therefore, we studied the pharmacokinetics of piperacillin in patients with creatinine clearances of <7 ml/min and in patients with cystic fibrosis.

Seven volunteers, four female and three male, with creatinine clearances of <7 ml/min and undergoing chronic hemodialysis were given a bolus injection of 1 g of piperacillin at the start of a 4-h dialysis with a Travenol RSP apparatus. Ages ranged from 32 to 75 years, and weight ranged from 44.1 to 70.4 kg. Three of the patients received an additional bolus of 2 g of piperacillin during an interdialysis period.

Six patients with cystic fibrosis and acute, infectious, pulmonary exacerbations were given doses ranging from 350 to 500 mg of piperacillin per kg per day in a 60-min intravenous infusion. Blood samples were drawn at the end of infusion at 15, 30, 60, 120, 180, and 240 min. During dialysis, samples of dialysis fluid were obtained at 30, 60, 120, 180, and 240 min. Bioassay of samples was performed using an agar well diffusion method with *P. aeruginosa* as the assay organism. Each sample was assayed in quadruplicate against standards prepared in serum. Dialysis samples were assayed with samples prepared in potassium phosphate buffer. Linear regression analysis was used to determine actual serum and dialysis concentrations. Kinetic data were then computed using a two-compartment linear model (2).

In the volunteers undergoing dialysis, serum levels after a 1-g bolus injection ranged from 98.5 to 229.8 µg/ml, with a mean of 153.1 ± 16.6 µg/ml. Mean level at 30 min was 60.4 ± 3.9 µg/ml, and that at 4 h was 8.4 ± 1.9 µg/ml. Kinetic parameters are given in Table 1. Mean elimination half-life during dialysis was 1.26 ± 0.14 h during dialysis and 2.12 h off dialysis. Mean clearance was 0.094 ± 0.012 liter/kg of body weight on dialysis and 0.060 liter/kg off dialysis. Dialysis removed 48% of a dose in 4 h.

Since the mean serum half-life of piperacillin in patients undergoing dialysis was not significantly different from the half-life off dialysis, and since 48% of a 1-g bolus injection of piperacillin could be recovered in the dialysate fluid, there may be differences in the metabolism and nonrenal excretion of piperacillin patients while they are undergoing dialysis. Based on peak

TABLE 1. *Pharmacokinetic data of piperacillin in patients requiring hemodialysis*

Parameter[a]	Mean ± SE
During dialysis	
K_{12} (h^{-1})	0.5004 ± 0.134
K_{21} (h^{-1})	1.2678 ± 0.078
K_e (h^{-1})	0.9543 ± 0.080
V_1 (liters/kg)	0.100 ± 0.011
V_D (liters/kg)	0.164 ± 0.017
Cl (liters/h per kg)	0.094 ± 0.012
$t_{1/2\alpha}$ (h)	0.349 ± 0.042
$t_{1/2\beta}$ (h)	1.261 ± 0.138
Between dialysis	
$t_{1/2\beta}$ (h)	2.12
Cl (liters/h per kg)	0.0602

[a] K_{12} and K_{21}, First-order tissue distribution rate constants; K_e, elimination rate constant; V_1, apparent volume of distribution of central compartment; V_D, total volume of distribution; Cl, clearance; $t_{1/2\alpha}$, α-phase half-life; $t_{1/2\beta}$, β-phase half-life.

TABLE 2. *Pharmacokinetic parameters of piperacillin in patients with cystic fibrosis*

Parameter[a]	Mean ± SE
$t_{1/2\beta}$ (h)	0.617 ± 0.08
V_D (liters/1.73 m^2)	8.27 ± 3.63
Cl (liters/h)	9.51 ± 5.14
Cl (ml/min per 1.73 m^2)	96.7 ± 22.0

[a] For explanations of parameter abbreviations, see Table 1, footnote a.

levels and a 35 to 45% reduction in serum level per hour, patients with creatinine clearances less than 10 ml/min should receive a dose of 0.5 to 1.0 g of piperacillin every 6 h, regardless of dialysis status, to treat most susceptible streptococci, *Haemophilus influenzae*, and *Neisseria*. A dose of 2 g every 6 h should treat most susceptible *Enterobacteriaceae*, *Bacteroides*, and *P. aeruginosa*.

In patients with cystic fibrosis, peak serum levels after 60 min of infusion ranged from 85 to 387 µg/ml, with trough levels less than 5 µg/ml. Urine levels ranged from 1,139 to 7,640 µg/ml (mean, 3,414). Mean elimination half-life was 0.617 ± 0.08 h; mean clearance was 9.51 ± 5.1 liters/h, and mean volume of distribution was 8.27 ± 3.6 liters/1.73 m^2 (Table 2).

In patients with cystic fibrosis the reduced half-life of 0.617 h versus 1.02 h in normals, and the smaller volume of distribution of 8.27 liters/1.73 m^2 versus 15 to 24 liters/1.73 m^2 in normals, combine to result in serum levels comparable to those in normal individuals. Thus, for susceptible *P. aeruginosa* a dose of 300 mg/kg per day divided into 4- or 6-h doses would provide adequate levels of piperacillin.

1. **Fu, K. P., and H. C. Neu.** 1978. Piperacillin, a new penicillin active against many bacteria resistant to other penicillins. Antimicrob. Agents Chemother. 13:358–367.
2. **Greenblatt, D. J., and J. Koch-Weser.** 1975. Clinical pharmacokinetics (first of two parts). N. Engl. J. Med.

293:704–705.
3. **Parry, M. F., and H. C. Neu.** 1976. Tobramycin and ticarcillin therapy for acute exacerbations of pulmonary disease in patients with cystic fibrosis. J. Infect. Dis. 134(Suppl.):194–197.

Correlation of In Vivo and In Vitro Synergistic Responses of *Enterobacteriaceae* to Mecillinam Combined with Ampicillin, Carbenicillin, and Cephalothin

ROY CLEELAND,* WILLIAM DeLORENZO, GEORGE BESKID, EDITH TITSWORTH, JAMES CHRISTENSON, AND E. GRUNBERG

Hoffmann-La Roche, Inc., Nutley, New Jersey 07110, U.S.A.

Mecillinam is an amidino β-lactam antibiotic with a mode of action different from that of other β-lactam compounds. It has been demonstrated that, when mecillinam is combined with other β-lactam compounds, marked synergy occurs both in vitro (3, 4) and in vivo (1, 2) against members of the *Enterobacteriaceae*. However, before the results of an in vitro test of the synergistic effect of mecillinam with other β-lactam compounds can be used to predict a successful clinical outcome, extensive clinical testing is required. Unfortunately, with new agents such as mecillinam this is difficult until a sufficient base of clinical results has been obtained.

In the present studies, two in vitro tests, the broth dilution method and the disk susceptibility test (Kirby-Bauer procedure), were used to predict in vivo activity. For the determination of the synergistic potential of mecillinam by the broth dilution method when combined with the three class β-lactam compounds ampicillin, carbenicillin, and cephalothin, the MICs of mecillinam and other β-lactam components were compared with the MIC of each compound combined with mecillinam in a 10:1 ratio. Synergy in vitro was considered to have occurred if the fractional inhibitory concentration (FIC) index was equal to or less than 0.50. The FIC index was calculated by dividing the MIC value obtained for each of the components in the combination by the MIC value for each component alone and adding the two quotients. For determination of synergy by diffusion assay, combination disks were developed containing 10 μg of ampicillin plus 1 μg of mecillinam, 50 μg of carbenicillin plus 1 μg of mecillinam, and 2.5 μg of cephalothin plus 0.25 μg of mecillinam. These ratios were determined through extensive testing to be quite suitable for detection of synergy. It was found that an increase of 2 mm in the size

of the zone produced by the combination disk over the larger zone produced by either component disk was a reliable in vitro measure of synergy.

The correlation of synergy as determined by disk susceptibility testing to clinical synergy would, as mentioned above, require extensive clinical testing. Since an adequate number of clinical cases is not yet available, as an alternative the synergistic responses obtained in vitro were compared with the synergistic responses seen in vivo when the three class β-lactam antibiotics were combined with mecillinam and tested against strains of *Enterobacteriaceae* in lethal mouse infections.

To determine synergy in vivo, groups of 10 mice were infected with 100 to 1,000 minimal lethal doses of properly diluted overnight cultures and treated with graded doses of mecillinam, the other β-lactam antibiotics, and a 10:1 combination of β-lactam compound and mecillinam immediately after infection. Survival of the animals was determined 14 days after infection, and, based on survival, the 50% protective dose (PD_{50}) in milligrams per kilogram was determined. Synergy in vivo was considered to have occurred if the FIC index was equal to or less than 0.60. The FIC index was calculated by dividing the PD_{50} value obtained for each of the components in the combination by the PD_{50} value for each component alone and adding the two quotients.

In Table 1 are summarized the results of in vivo tests performed with 73 to 84 strains of *Enterobacteriaceae* to determine the synergistic response of ampicillin, carbenicillin, and cephalothin when combined with mecillinam. The synergistic response ranged from 61 to 73% depending on the combination. The highest response rates overall were seen with *Escherichia coli, Klebsiella pneumoniae*, and *Enterobacter*;

TABLE 1. *In vivo synergistic responses of members of the Enterobacteriaceae to mecillinam combined in 1:10 ratios with ampicillin, carbenicillin, and cephalothin*

Organism	Mecillinam plus		
	Ampicillin	Carbenicillin	Cephalothin
E. coli	12/20[a] (60)[b]	11/13 (85)	14/16 (88)
K. pneumoniae	24/28 (85)	21/26 (77)	21/28 (75)
Enterobacter	8/9 (89)	9/9 (100)	4/9 (44)
Serratia	4/12 (33)	6/10 (60)	3/9 (33)
Proteus-Providencia	3/15 (20)	7/15 (47)	6/15 (40)
Total	51/84 (61)	54/73 (74)	48/77 (62)
Synergistic effect of combination on resistant organisms[c]	9/29 (31)	9/19 (47)	3/19 (16)

[a] Number of strains responding synergistically/number of strains tested. Criterion for synergy: a fractional inhibitory concentration index ≤0.6.
[b] Number in parentheses indicates percentage of strains responding.
[c] Number of strains sensitive to the combination/number resistant to both single agents.

TABLE 2. *Correlation of the synergistic responses of members of the Enterobacteriaceae seen by disk susceptibility tests[a] with those seen in vivo*

Organism	Mecillinam plus		
	Ampicillin (1:10)[b]	Carbenicillin (1:50)	Cephalothin (1:10)
E. coli	18/20[c] (90)[d]	11/13 (83)	8/16 (50)
K. pneumoniae	13/28 (46)	18/26 (69)	19/28 (68)
Enterobacter	3/9 (33)	3/9 (33)	6/9 (67)
Serratia	9/12 (88)	4/10 (40)	6/9 (67)
Proteus-Providencia	14/15 (93)	11/15 (75)	11/15 (73)
Total	57/84 (68)	47/73 (64)	50/77 (65)
False-positive results[e]	2/33 (6)	1/19 (5)	1/29 (3)
False-negative results[f]	28/51 (55)	27/54 (50)	25/48 (52)

[a] Kirby-Bauer technique, Mueller-Hinton agar. Synergy by disk test indicated by a ≥2-mm increase in zone size of the combination disk compared to that of the larger zone of either of the component disks.
[b] Ratios of mecillinam to each compound.
[c] Number of strains showing agreement between disk and in vivo tests in terms of synergy or no synergy/number of strains tested.
[d] Number in parentheses indicates percentage of strains in agreement.
[e] False-positive result: synergy demonstrated by disk test but not in vivo.
[f] False-negative result: synergy not demonstrated by disk test but demonstrated in vivo.

lower rates of synergy were seen with *Serratia* and *Proteus-Providencia*. Of interest is the fact that strains resistant to mecillinam as well as the other individual β-lactam compounds (PD_{50} > 250 mg/kg) were susceptible to the combination; 31, 47, and 16% responded to mecillinam-ampicillin, mecillinam-carbenicillin, and mecillinam-cephalothin combinations, respectively.

Having determined the extent of in vivo synergy that could be expected, we next undertook studies to ascertain the reliability of the disk susceptibility tests in correctly predicting a synergistic response. The results of these tests, summarized in Table 2, show that there was an overall total agreement of 68% with the ampicillin-mecillinam combinations. For the carbenicil-lin-mecillinam combination the overall agreement rate was 64%, and for the cephalothin-mecillinam combination the overall rate of agreement was 65%. The false-positive rates (i.e., synergy by disk test without corresponding synergy in vivo) were very low, between 3 and 6%. The major discrepancies were in the category of false-negative results; that is, the disk failed to correctly predict the synergy seen in the in vivo mouse protection test.

A similar analysis of the reliability of MIC tests in correctly predicting in vivo synergy was carried out in the preferred broth medium for demonstration of mecillinam in vitro activity (NIH broth) and in the medium most frequently used for determination of MICs of antibiotics

(Mueller-Hinton broth). The overall correlation was less than that seen by disk assay (48 to 66%). More significant was the fact that there was a false-positive rate of 18 to 30%, which was much higher than the 3 to 6% rate seen with the disk test.

From these results, it is apparent that comparison of the MIC of the combination with the MICs of the individual components is not as reliable a means for predicting in vivo synergy as is the disk diffusion assay utilizing combination disks.

The usefulness of the disk diffusion assay for predicting synergy in humans can be assessed only after extensive clinical trials. However, the initial clinical findings with the disk test have been quite encouraging. For example, based on the synergistic response of isolates to either the ampicillin-mecillinam or cephalothin-mecillinam disks, nine patients with serious gram-negative infections were treated with mecillinam in combination with ampicillin or cephapirin. The pathogens were completely eradicated in six patients. Clear-cut synergy, as defined by the disk test system, was present in all cases. Three patients whose organisms also exhibited a clear-

cut synergistic response responded partially, as measured by a reduction of the organisms in the clinical specimen, but complete eradication was not achieved.

On the basis of extensive experimental data and a limited number of clinical cases, we consider the disk diffusion assay to be useful in predicting the effect of mecillinam in combination with other β-lactam antibiotics.

1. **Grunberg, E., and R. Cleeland.** 1977. *In vivo* activity of the 6β-amidinopenicillanic acid derivative, mecillinam, chemically linked or combined in varying ratios with 6-aminopenicillanic acid derivatives. J. Antimicrob. Chemother. 3(Suppl. B):59–70.
2. **Grunberg, E., R. Cleeland, G. Beskid, and W. F. DeLorenzo.** 1976. In vivo synergy between 6β-amidinopenicillanic acid derivatives and other antibiotics. Antimicrob. Agents Chemother. 9:589–594.
3. **Neu, H. C.** 1976. Synergy of mecillinam, a beta-amidinopenicillanic acid derivative, combined with beta-lactam antibiotics. Antimicrob. Agents Chemother. 10:535–542.
4. **Tybring, L., and N. H. Melchior.** 1975. Mecillinam (FL 1060) a 6β-amidinopenicillanic acid derivative: bactericidal action and synergy in vitro. Antimicrob. Agents Chemother. 8:271–276.

Scanning Electron Microscopy of the Morphological Effects on *Escherichia coli* of Mecillinam and Other β-Lactam Antibiotics When Used as Single Agents and in Combination

MICHAEL J. KRAMER* AND YOLANDA R. MAURIZ

Department of Chemotherapy, Hoffmann-La Roche, Inc., Nutley, New Jersey 07110 U.S.A.

Mecillinam, a 6β-amidinopenicillanic acid derivative, has been shown to be more active in vitro and in vivo against certain gram-negative bacteria (particularly *Enterobacteriaceae*) than against gram-positive organisms (4). It was further shown that mecillinam was synergistic, both in vitro and in vivo, when combined with other penicillins and cephalosporins (1, 3).

Morphological studies have revealed a striking difference between the structural modifications produced in susceptible bacteria by mecillinam and other penicillins and cephalosporins. Whereas, in general, penicillins caused the formation of filaments at subinhibitory concentrations and spheroplasts at concentrations greater than or equal to the MIC, and cephalosporins primarily caused filament formation (3), mecillinam produced large stable spherical forms at concentrations of drug ranging from 1 to 1,000

MICs (5). Furthermore, it was demonstrated (6) that, whereas mecillinam bound preferentially with penicillin-binding protein (PBP) 2 of *Escherichia coli*, which is involved in the maintenance of cell shape, other penicillins bound to at least two different PBPs and not exclusively with PBP 2.

In view of the demonstrated synergy of mecillinam with other β-lactam antibiotics and the difference in morphological effects produced by mecillinam as compared with these agents, the morphological changes induced in three isolates of *E. coli* treated in vitro with mecillinam in combination with penicillins and cephalosporins were evaluated by scanning electron microscopy. The combination effect was compared with that seen with the individual antibiotics.

The procedure for the in vitro morphological studies included the incorporation of the peni-

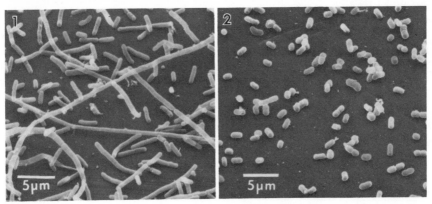

FIG. 1 and 2. *Scanning electron microscopy of the effect of (1) cephalothin (one MIC) and (2) mecillinam (one-fourth MIC) against Escherichia coli 736 after 4 h at 37°C.*

cillins and cephalosporins into Mueller-Hinton agar either alone or in combination with mecillinam, placement of antibiotic-containing agar in the central area of a glass microscope slide, inoculation of the agar slide with the test organism, and incubation at 37°C for 4 h. An Amicon SEP 15 ultrafilter was then lightly touched to the area of bacterial growth, fixed in 2.5% buffered glutaraldehyde, and further processed for scanning electron microscopy by standard procedures. Doses of the individual antibiotics used in combination were selected on the basis of discernible morphological changes produced in the test organism over a 4-h period.

In the case of *E. coli* 257 the penicillins ampicillin, amoxicillin, and carbenicillin and the cephalosporins cephalothin, cephalexin, cefazolin, cefamandole, and cefoxitin were tested as single agents and in combination with mecillinam. *E. coli* isolates 736 and 503-79 were tested only against a single cephalosporin (cephalothin) and against two penicillins (ampicillin and carbenicillin) as single agents and in combination with mecillinam.

When tested against the *E. coli* isolates at doses ranging from one-fourth to one MIC, mecillinam caused the conversion from the normal rod shape to a cocco-bacillary form. Varying degrees of filament formation resulted from single testing of the other penicillins and cephalosporins. There was no indication of lysis with any of the single agents at the doses tested. In contrast, when mecillinam was combined with penicillins and cephalosporins, extensive lysis and cell destruction were observed. Scanning electron micrographs of *E. coli* 736 treated in vitro with cephalothin, mecillinam, or a combination of cephalothin with mecillinam are shown in Fig. 1, 2, and 3, respectively. If, however,

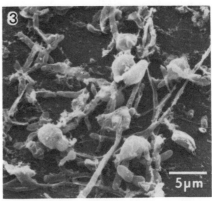

FIG. 3. *Scanning electron microscopy of the combination effect of cephalothin (one MIC) and mecillinam (one-fourth MIC) against Escherichia coli 736.*

another β-lactam antibiotic such as carbenicillin was substituted for mecillinam in the mecillinam-cephalexin combination, the morphological changes seen with the carbenicillin-cephalexin combination were not significantly different from those caused by carbenicillin or cephalexin when tested as single agents.

These studies further substantiate the potential usefulness of mecillinam as a synergistic agent with other β-lactam antibiotics.

1. **Baltimore, R. S., J. O. Klein, C. Wilcox, and M. Finland.** 1976. Synergy of mecillinam (FL1060) with penicillins and cephalosporins against *Proteus* and *Klebsiella*, with observations on combinations with other antibiotics and against other bacterial species. Antimicrob. Agents Chemother. **9:**701–705.
2. **Greenwood, D., and F. O'Grady.** 1973. Comparison of the response of *Escherichia coli* and *Proteus mirabilis* to seven β-lactam antibiotics. J. Infect. Dis. **128:**211–222.

3. **Grunberg, E., R. Cleeland, G. Beskid, and W. F. DeLorenzo.** 1976. In vivo synergy between 6-β-amidinopenicillanic acid derivatives and other antibiotics. Antimicrob. Agents Chemother. **9:**589–594.

4. **Lund, F., and L. Tybring.** 1972. 6-β-Amidinopenicillanic acids—a new group of antibiotics. Nature (London) New Biol. **236:**135–137.

5. **Melchior, N. H., J. Blom, L. Tybring, and A. Birch-Andersen.** 1973. Light and electron microscopy of the early response of *Escherichia coli* to a 6β-amidinopenicillanic acid (FL1060). Acta Pathol. Microbiol. Scand. Sect. B **81:**393–407.

6. **Spratt, B. G.** 1977. The mechanism of action of mecillinam. J. Antimicrob. Chemother. **3**(Suppl. B):13–19.

Comparative Clinical Pharmacology of Bacmecillinam Alone or in Combination with Bacampicillin and of Pivmecillinam

JOHN-OLOF LERNESTEDT,* BRIAN G. PRING, AND DOUGLAS WESTERLUND

Medical Department and Research and Development Laboratories, Astra Läkemedel AB, S-151 85 Södertälje, Sweden

The 6β-amidinopenicillanic acid mecillinam, which is remarkable because of its enhanced activity against the *Enterobacteriaceae*, is very poorly absorbed upon oral administration. Therefore pro-drugs of mecillinam such as pivmecillinam have been developed in order to provide mecillinam in an orally absorbable form. Bacmecillinam, the 1'-ethoxycarbonyloxyethyl ester of mecillinam, is a new pro-drug of mecillinam containing a carbonate group in the ester moiety. The hydrolysis of bacmecillinam is catalyzed by esterases present in blood and tissues, the products of hydrolysis being mecillinam, ethanol, acetaldehyde, and carbon dioxide. In experimental studies in mice and dogs, bacmecillinam has shown superior oral absorption compared to pivmecillinam, giving rise to higher initial serum levels of mecillinam.

On combining mecillinam with other β-lactam antibiotics such as ampicillin, a synergistic effect is shown against many strains of gram-negative bacteria both in vitro and in vivo. Synergy is obtained within a wide range of ratios of the two components but appears to be optimal when the ratio is close to 1:1. Moreover, the development of resistance in vitro by several gram-negative strains to the combination of mecillinam and ampicillin has been found to be less than to mecillinam alone (1). Therefore, a pharmaceutical preparation containing mecillinam and ampicillin or their pro-drugs is of potential clinical value. Such a preparation is an equimolar mixture of bacmecillinam and bacampicillin, which is a pro-drug of ampicillin containing the same ester group as bacmecillinam. This combination has been assigned the code number A 2382.

The present study was undertaken to compare the absorption and excretion of equimolar doses of bacmecillinam and pivmecillinam in fasting volunteers. Furthermore, the purpose was to elucidate the absorption and excretion of mecillinam when given combined with ampicillin as the esters bacmecillinam and bacampicillin in the equimolar mixture A 2382 and to determine the ratios of the two antibiotics in serum and urine. Eleven normal male volunteers, aged from 21 to 35 years, participated in the study, which was performed in triple crossover fashion. The subjects received at 1-week intervals in a randomized order tablets containing 200 mg of bacmecillinam, 200 mg of pivmecillinam (Selexidin), or 500 mg of A 2382, i.e., 244 mg of bacmecillinam and 256 mg of bacampicillin. These doses correspond to 137 mg of mecillinam, or 166 mg of mecillinam plus 178 mg of ampicillin, respectively. No food was allowed from midnight until 2 h after administration of the test dose.

Blood samples were drawn from the cubital vein just before, and 0.25, 0.5, 0.75, 1.0, 1.5, 3.0, 6.0, and 8.0 h after administration. Urine was voided immediately before drug intake and thereafter was collected at 2-h intervals during 8 h. To minimize breakdown of mecillinam in the specimens, blood samples were immediately centrifuged, and the plasma was rapidly frozen in an ethanol-Dry Ice bath (−70°C) and stored at this temperature until analyzed. Urine specimens were frozen and stored in the same way. The concentrations of ampicillin and mecillinam in plasma and urine were determined by reversed-phase liquid chromatography followed by post-column derivatization as described by Westerlund et al. (2). The areas under the serum concentration curves (AUC) were calculated by the trapezoidal method and the plasma half-lives were calculated by the formula $0.693/K_{el}$, K_{el} being the overall elimination rate constant. The Student t test was used in assessing significant differences between drugs with regard to different pharmacokinetic parameters.

The mean plasma concentrations of mecillinam after administration of pivmecillinam and bacmecillinam and of mecillinam and ampicillin after administration of the combination A 2382 are shown in Fig. 1. The peak of the mean plasma curve was 2.59 µg/ml after bacmecillinam and 1.40 µg/ml after pivmecillinam, both peaks being reached 0.75 h after administration. This difference is statistically significant ($P < 0.001$). The individual mean peak plasma concentrations were 2.73 µg/ml and 1.63 µg/ml after bacmecillinam and pivmecillinam, respectively, which also gave a statistically significant difference at $P < 0.001$. The median time to reach the individual peak was 0.75 h after bacmecillinam and 1.0 h after pivmecillinam. After administration of the combination A 2382, the peaks of the mean plasma curves were 2.62 µg/ml for mecillinam and 3.69 µg/ml for ampicillin, and the corresponding individual mean peaks were 2.80 and 4.29 µg/ml. The median time to reach the individual mean peak was 0.75 h for mecillinam and 0.5 h for ampicillin. The mean AUC was 4.30 µg·h·ml^{-1} after bacmecillinam and 3.14 µg·h·ml^{-1} after pivmecillinam, this difference being

TABLE 1. *Mean molar ratios of ampicillin to mecillinam in plasma and urine after oral administration of 500 mg of an equimolar combination of bacampicillin and bacmecillinam, A 2382, to volunteers*

Fluid	Sampling time (h)	Molar ratio of ampicillin to mecillinam (mean ± SD)
Plasma	0.25	2.39 ± 0.59
	0.5	1.59 ± 0.25
	0.75	1.30 ± 0.21
	1.0	1.14 ± 0.21
	1.5	1.09 ± 0.16
	3.0	1.29 ± 0.25
	6.0	1.68 ± 0.35
	8.0	2.32 ± 0.80
Urine	0–2	1.35 ± 0.14
	2–4	1.33 ± 0.28
	4–6	1.47 ± 0.19
	6–8	1.50 ± 0.20

significant at $P < 0.001$. Thus, the mean AUC after bacmecillinam exceeds that after pivmecillinam by 37%. After A 2382, the mean AUCs for mecillinam and ampicillin were 4.82 and 6.67 µg·h·ml^{-1}, respectively. The mean plasma half-life of mecillinam was 0.92 h after bacmecillinam and 0.96 h after pivmecillinam; the corresponding times after A 2382 were 0.94 h and 1.08 h for mecillinam and ampicillin, respectively.

During the 8-h sampling interval, the mean urinary recovery of mecillinam was 43.8% after bacmecillinam and 34.6% after pivmecillinam. This difference is significant at $0.05 > P > 0.01$. After administration of the combination A 2382, the urinary recoveries of mecillinam and ampicillin during 8 h were 44.0% and 55.9%, respectively.

Since optimal synergistic activity between ampicillin and mecillinam against gram-negative bacteria has been observed when the molar ratio of the antibiotics is in the region of 1:1, it was of interest to determine the molar ratio of the two antibiotics in plasma and urine at different times after administration of A 2382. In Table 1 the mean molar ratios of ampicillin to mecillinam in plasma and urine at the different sampling times are presented. The mean molar ratios of ampicillin to mecillinam in plasma were below 2:1 except for the first and last sampling times. In urine, the mean molar ratios at the different sampling times were more uniform and lay in the range of 1.3 to 1.5.

In conclusion, the oral absorption of bacmecillinam is superior to that of pivmecillinam in fasting normal volunteers with the tablet formulations used. Plasma concentrations of mecillinam were significantly higher after bacmecilli-

µg/ml

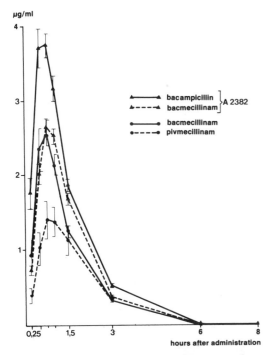

FIG. 1. *Mean plasma concentration curves of mecillinam after administration of 200 mg of bacmecillinam or pivmecillinam and of ampicillin and mecillinam after administration of 500 mg of an equimolar combination of bacampicillin and bacmecillinam, A 2382, to 11 volunteers.*

nam, as were the AUC and cumulative urinary recovery. The equimolar combination of bacmecillinam and bacampicillin, A 2382, gave ratios of ampicillin and mecillinam in plasma and urine within the limits usually regarded as optimal for synergy in vitro against strains belonging to the *Enterobacteriaceae* and appears suitable from a pharmacokinetic point of view for synergy in vivo.

1. Sjöberg, B., P. Bamberg, B. Ekström, U. Forsgren, L. Magni, and B. G. Pring. 1978. Synergistic action in vitro between amidinopenicillanic acids and penicillins or cephalosporins, p. 432–434. *In* Current chemotherapy, Proceedings of the 10th International Congress of Chemotherapy. American Society for Microbiology, Washington, D.C.

2. Westerlund, D., J. Carlqvist, and A. Theodorsen. 1979. Analysis of penicillins in biological material by reversed phase liquid chromatography and post-column derivatization. Acta Pharm. Suec. **16:**187–214.

Mecillinam, a New Amidino-Penicillin Derivative in the Treatment of Serious Gram-Negative Infections

SESSINE NAJJAR,* JEAN MESSIHI, AND LEON G. SMITH

Department of Infectious Diseases, Saint Michael's Medical Center, Newark, New Jersey 07102, U.S.A.

Mecillinam is a new β-lactam antibiotic which is more stable than the semisynthetic penicillins to the action of penicillinase. The purpose of our study was to evaluate the efficacy and safety of mecillinam when administered parenterally to patients with serious gram-negative infections.

Fifteen hospitalized patients with gram-negative infections were studied. Appropriate laboratory data were obtained before, during, and at termination of therapy. Patients were entered in the study after informed written consent was obtained. Ten patients received mecillinam as a single agent, and five received combination therapy.

Bacteriology studies. Susceptibility studies were carried out on all isolates by using Kirby-Bauer techniques. MICs were also obtained. The following disk concentrations were used: mecillinam, 10, 1, and 0.25 μg; mecillinam, 0.25 μg, in combination with cephalothin, 2.5 μg; and mecillinam, 1 μg, in combination with ampicillin, 10 μg, or carbenicillin, 50 μg. Synergistic effect was present when disk susceptibility of mecillinam in combination with the β-lactam antibiotic showed an inhibition zone of growth that was $\geq$2 mm greater than that of each antibiotic alone.

Dosage, route of administration, and duration of therapy. When mecillinam was given alone, the dose was 60 mg/kg per 24 h in six equally divided doses. When used in combination with either ampicillin or carbenicillin, the dose was dropped to 40 mg/kg per 24 h in four equally divided doses. All the patients received the treatment intravenously, and the duration of therapy ranged from 4 to 20 days.

Mecillinam given as a single agent. Ten patients were treated with mecillinam alone (Table 1). Two patients had bacteremia secondary to pyelonephritis, seven patients had urinary tract infection, and one patient had a recurrent abdominal wall infection.

In the first group of patients, the organisms were resistant to ampicillin and carbenicillin and susceptible to mecillinam (*Escherichia coli*). The clinical response to mecillinam therapy was good in both cases. In the second group of patients, we isolated five *E. coli*, one ampicillin–carbenicillin-resistant *Enterobacter aerogenes*, and one *Klebsiella pneumoniae*. Six of the isolates were mecillinam susceptible, and one ampicillin-resistant *E. coli* was also resistant to mecillinam. The clinical response in all cases was excellent.

The abdominal wall drainage yielded three organisms: *Enterobacter cloacae*, ampicillin-resistant *Citrobacter freundii*, and ampicillin-resistant *Klebsiella oxytoca*. All three organisms were susceptible to mecillinam. The bacteriological response was good, but the clinical response was poor, and self-induced wound infection was suspected in this case.

Mecillinam given in combination with a β-lactam antibiotic. Five patients were included in this group (Table 2). One patient had pyelonephritis with bacteremia (*Proteus mirabilis*); another one had bronchopneumonia (*K. pneumoniae*); the third patient had cholangitis with bacteremia (*E. coli*); the fourth patient had pyelonephritis (*E. coli*); and the last patient had chronic osteomyelitis of the tibia (*Proteus mirabilis*). Synergistic effect of combination therapy was noted with all isolates except with the *P. mirabilis* bacteremia. Despite this in vitro

TABLE 1. *Clinical evaluation of mecillinam*

Patient	Age (yrs)	Sex	Diagnosis	Underlying disease	Bacteriology	Daily mecillinam dosage (mg)	Associated antibiotics (amt)	Results Clinical	Results Bacteriological
1	80	F	Hydronephrosis, bacteremia	Polycystic kidney, atrial fibrillation	*Proteus* and *E. coli* in urine	720	Ampicillin (8 g)	Poor	Blood and urine sterile
2	28	F	Pyelonephritis, bacteremia	Kidney stones, gout	*E. coli* in blood and urine	2,200		Recovered	Recovered
3	63	F	UTI[a]	Renal failure, diabetes mellitus, congestive heart failure, hypertension	*E. coli* in urine	1,600		Fair	Urine sterile
4	42	F	UTI	Pelvic inflammatory disease	*E. coli* in urine	2,000		Recovered	Recovered
5	88	M	Bronchopneumonia	Chronic obstructive pulmonary disease, congestive heart failure	*K. pneumoniae*	2,200	Ampicillin (4 g)	Fair	No *Klebsiella* in sputum
6	63	M	Cholangitis, bacteremia	Congestive heart failure	*E. coli*	3,080	Ampicillin (4 g)	Cholecystectomy	Recovered
7	52	F	Postoperative wound infection	Obesity, psychiatric disorder	*E. cloacae, C. freundii, K. oxytoca*	4,200	None	Poor	*Staphylococcus aureus* isolated from wound
8	68	M	Pyelonephritis	Epididymitis, seizures, chronic alcoholism	*E. coli*	2,480	Ampicillin (8 g)	Recovered	Recovered
9	44	F	Pyelonephritis, bacteremia	Diabetes mellitus, hypertension	*E. coli*	5,460	None	Recovered	Recovered
10	33	F	Chronic osteomyelitis	Obesity	*P. mirabilis*	3,440	Carbenicillin (20 g)	Less sinus drainage, improvement on X-ray	
11	77	M	UTI	Chronic obstructive lung disease, latent syphilis, renal insufficiency	*E. aerogenes*	2,760	None	Good	Good
12	78	M	UTI	Diabetes mellitus, hypertension	*K. pneumoniae*	4,080	None	Recovered	Recovered
13	42	F	Recurrent UTI	None	*E. coli*	4,020	None	Recovered	Recovered
14	51	M	UTI	Benign prostatic hypertrophy	*E. coli*	3,000	None	Good	Good
15	67	F	UTI	Felty's syndrome	*E. coli*	3,000	None	Good	Good

[a] UTI, Urinary tract infection.

TABLE 2. *Synergistic study of mecillinam dose and duration of therapy*

Patient	Bacteria	Source	Daily mecillinam dose (mg)	β-Lactam antibiotic (amt)	MIC (μg/ml)	Duration of treatment (days)
1	*P. mirabilis*	Blood	720	Ampicillin (8 g)	64	8
	E. coli	Urine			0.25	
2	*K. pneumoniae*	Sputum	2,200	Ampicillin (4 g)		12
3	*E. coli*	Blood, cholangitis	3,080	Ampicillin (4 g)		12
4	*E. coli*	Urine	2,480	Ampicillin (8 g)	2	
5	*P. mirabilis*	Osteomyelitis	3,440	Carbenicillin (20 g)	64	20

result, all five cases responded well to the combination of mecillinam-ampicillin (first four cases) or mecillinam-carbenicillin.

This discrepancy between the in vitro resistance and the in vivo response has no explanation at the present time. This sort of discrepancy was also noted in one case of urinary tract infection with mecillinam-resistant and ampicillin-resistant *E. coli*.

Toxicity. No sign of serious side effects or toxicity was noted in the 15 patients. Side effects were limited to transient elevations of alkaline phosphatase and transaminase in three patients.

Pharmacokinetics. Mecillinam serum levels were determined in eight patients. Seven patients who received 60 mg of mecillinam per kg per day intravenously had a mean peak level of 12.05 μg/ml (range, 5.65 to 19.37) and a mean trough level of 4.06 μg/ml (range, 3.33 to 5.73). One patient received 40 mg of mecillinam per kg per day intravenously with a mean peak level of 5.23 μg/ml and a mean trough level of 0.31 μg/ml (range, 0.19 to 0.43).

Conclusions. Infection was eradicated in 9 of 10 patients (7 with urinary tract infection) treated with mecillinam alone and in all 5 patients given combination therapy. In five instances the isolate was susceptible to mecillinam and resistant to the β-lactam antibiotics tested. No serious side effects were noted, and this drug was well tolerated.

On the basis of these data, mecillinam, when given alone, offers a certain advantage in the treatment of gram-negative infection resistant to currently available β-lactam antibiotics. Because of inadequate numbers, the clinical impact of in vitro synergism is still uncertain. Since the major indication of mecillinam would be combination therapy, further synergistic studies are needed in the future.

1. **Greenwood, D., and F. O'Grady.** 1973. A new beta-lactam antibiotic with novel properties. J. Clin. Pathol. **26**:1–6.
2. **Neu, H. C.** 1977. Mecillinam, an amidino penicillin which acts synergistically with other β-lactam compounds. J. Antimicrob. Chemother. **3**(Suppl. B):45–52.

Mecillinam in Urinary Tract Infections

JEROME A. ERNST* AND VICTOR LORIAN

Bronx-Lebanon Hospital Center, Bronx, New York 10456, U.S.A.

Mecillinam, a new derivative of G-aminopenicillanic acid with a substituted amidino group in the 6 position (1), was administered to 14 patients with symptoms of urinary tract infections consisting of flank pain, dysuria, fever, leukocytosis, pyuria, and bacteriuria. When used alone, the drug was given in a daily dose of 60 mg/kg intravenously in six divided doses. When used with another β-lactam antibiotic—either ampicillin or cephalothin—mecillinam was given in a daily dose of 40 mg/kg intravenously in four divided doses. Against all of the organisms

treated, the MICs were 4 μg/ml or lower. Dosage of mecillinam in both the single and combined drug groups was reduced according to the patient's creatinine clearance. However, the initial loading dose of 10 mg/kg was not changed. Sterile urine upon completion of therapy was considered a successful response.

Ten patients received mecillinam as a single agent. The mean dose of mecillinam given daily was 3,310 mg, and the mean duration of therapy was 7 days. The MICs for the organisms isolated from our patients ranged from 0.097 to 0.390 μg/

ml, with a mean of 0.2 μg/ml. All patients had sterile urines within 24 h after beginning treatment.

Eight of nine patients had sterile urines and were discharged from the hospital after therapy was completed, a success rate of 89%. Of those eight patients, four had repeat urine cultures after 1 to 2 months, and two of those four had bacteriuria. One patient who originally was infected with *Escherichia coli* again had *E. coli* which again was susceptible to mecillinam.

One patient had a rise in eosinophil count while on therapy which returned to the pretreatment value when the therapy was finished. Therapy was stopped in one patient who, immediately after receiving the first dose of mecillinam, developed urticaria. This resolved with no complications, but she was withdrawn from the study.

Four of our patients received mecillinam together with either ampicillin or cephalothin. All had urinary tract infections due to *E. coli*, and two also had septicemia. MIC levels for the organisms ranged from 0.097 to 3.125 μg/ml, with a mean of 0.9 μg/ml. Three of these four patients had a successful response. The fourth developed a *Pseudomonas* infection after her *E. coli* infection was eradicated. She had originally been treated with mecillinam and ampicillin, had chronic renal failure with a creatinine clearance of 12 ml/min, and eventually died in the hospital from other causes.

We have shown mecillinam to be an effective agent in the treatment of urinary tract infections. The efficacy of the oral form, pivmecillinam, has been shown before. Wise et al. (2) treated 35 patients with the oral form and had a cure rate of 83%. Ishigami (in press) conducted a double-blind trial in 243 patients with acute cystitis and found pivmecillinam to be significantly more effective than amoxycillin on both clinical and bacteriological grounds, primarily as a result of its efficacy in infections due to ampicillin-resistant *E. coli*.

We had some trouble with the assay of mecillinam levels in blood. At 4°C 10% of activity has been shown to be lost every day. Once we began storing our samples at −70°C, the levels we obtained on assay were much higher and more compatible with the results reported in the literature, as well as with the good clinical results we obtained.

It is our impression that mecillinam compares favorably with other currently used antibiotics in the treatment of urinary tract infections, and we consider it a very promising drug.

1. **Lund, F., and L. Tybring.** 1972. 6 β-Amidinopenicillanic acids—a new group of antibiotics. Nature (London) New Biol. **236:**135–137.
2. **Wise, R., D. S. Reeves, J. M. Symonds, and P. J. L. Wilkinson.** 1976. A clinical investigation of pivmecillinam: a novel β-lactam antibiotic in the treatment of urinary tract infections. Chemotherapy (Basel) **22:**335–339.

Mecillinam in the Treatment of Patients with Severely Impaired Renal Function

PER L. SVARVA,* TERJE WESSEL-AAS, AND JOHAN A. MAELAND

University Clinic of Trondheim, 7000 Trondheim, Norway

Mecillinam is an amidinopenicillanic acid that is particularly active against members of the *Enterobacteriaceae.* Thus, mecillinam has been used successfully in the treatment of patients with urinary tract infections.

Special problems are encountered when patients with renal insufficiency require antimicrobial therapy because of the risk of accumulation of a potentially toxic antibiotic. Our study was designed to evaluate mecillinam in the treatment of such patients in terms of its clinical usefulness, the serum levels achieved, and any signs of toxicity.

Twelve patients with severe renal insuffi-

ciency were included in the study. The serum creatinine levels ranged from 245 to 872 μmol/ liter (median, 555 μmol/liter). All the patients had a bacteriologically verified urinary tract infection caused by gram-negative bacilli. The patients received 400 mg of mecillinam intravenously every 6 h, which is the normally recommended dose for this antibiotic. No adjustment of the dose was made for renal function. All the patients recovered from the infection, and neither clinical nor laboratory data indicated side effects possibly caused by the antibiotic. The treatment period averaged 8 days.

Serum levels of mecillinam were determined

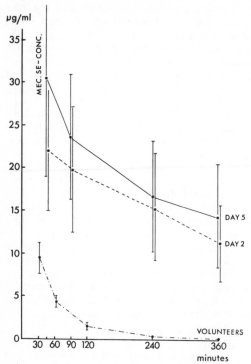

FIG. 1. *Serum concentrations of mecillinam in patients with severe renal insufficiency, determined on day 2 (----) and day 5 (———) of the treatment period, and in healthy volunteers (—·—·—).*

on days 2 and 5 of the treatment period by the paper-disk diffusion method. Blood for the testing was drawn at 45, 90, 240, and 360 min after the morning dose. As shown in Fig. 1, very high concentrations of mecillinam were recorded in the patients, and the half-life of the antibiotic was estimated to be five to six times that in healthy individuals. In the patients the concentrations of mecillinam continued to be very high throughout the observation period. Slightly higher concentrations were observed on day 5 than on day 2, but there was no significant difference in the trough levels of the antibiotic. This indicates that a steady-state situation was reached within the first 2 days of the treatment period and that no accumulation took place within the observation period. No correlation was observed between serum creatinine levels and mecillinam concentrations.

In conclusion, we have shown that in patients with renal insufficiency serum levels and the half-life of mecillinam were greatly increased. In spite of this, no definite accumulation or side effects of the antibiotic were observed. We think that this antibiotic can be given safely and in normal doses for short-term treatment of patients with renal insufficiency. Nevertheless, we believe that a dosage schedule adjusted to the renal function of this group of patients would be preferable.

Treatment of Systemic Infections with Mecillinam Alone or Combined with Other β-Lactam Antibiotics

STEPHEN J. PANCOAST, ELLIOT L. FRANCKE, AND HAROLD C. NEU*

Departments of Medicine and Pharmacology, College of Physicians and Surgeons, Columbia University, New York, New York 10032, U.S.A.

Mecillinam is an amidino penicillin with an unusual degree of activity against gram-negative bacilli, even though it is hydrolyzed by gram-negative β-lactamases (1, 4). It appears to bind specifically to the protein involved in cell shape in gram-negative species (3). Mecillinam also acts synergistically with other β-lactam antibiotics to inhibit members of the *Enterobacteriaceae* and *Pseudomonas* resistant to it and to other penicillins or cephalosporins (2). We have evaluated the clinical efficacy and safety of mecillinam alone and in combination with other β-lactam antibiotics when used to treat serious gram-negative infections.

Mecillinam was used as the sole agent to treat

five males and three females aged 21 to 79 years. One patient received 1 day of treatment with penicillin G. Mecillinam was used in combination with cefazolin in one male (age, 63 years) and one female (age, 73 years) and in combination with ampicillin in two males and one female (ages, 27 to 77 years). Mecillinam was given as an intravenous infusion of 15 mg/kg of body weight every 4 to 6 h when used alone and 10 mg/kg of body weight when combined with another agent. The MICs were determined for all organisms, and the degree of synergy was determined by checkerboard agar dilution. Laboratory studies evaluating hematological, hepatic, and renal function were performed before, during, and after therapy. Patients were considered cured if all signs of infection resolved and cultures became negative. Patients were classified as failures of therapy if they did not become afebrile and cultures remained positive.

Treatment with mecillinam alone. The eight patients treated with mecillinam alone ranged in age from 21 to 79 years (Table 1). Four of the patients had bacteremia, one had meningitis, one had osteomyelitis, and one, suspected of having sepsis, had a urinary tract infection due to *Escherichia coli*. Only one patient could be considered a failure of therapy. A 78-year-old man with widely metastatic carcinoma of the colon and diabetes mellitus developed septicemia due to *E. coli* and *Klebsiella pneumoniae*. Both organisms were resistant to ampicillin and cephalothin but susceptible to mecillinam. In spite of 3 days of therapy with adequate serum levels, he died, and both organisms, still susceptible to mecillinam, were cultured from his blood, although the urine was negative.

Successful cases included a patient with osteomyelitis of the femur due to a strain of *Aeromonas hydrophila* resistant to ampicillin and cephalothin. Previous therapy for 2 weeks with gentamicin had been unsuccessful. The patient received mecillinam for 55 days without side effects.

The most impressive success with mecillinam was the therapy of meningitis due to *E. coli* in a 77-year-old man with squamous cell carcinoma of the maxillary antrum that developed after surgery which produced a dural tear and cerebrospinal fluid leak. The *E. coli* strain was resistant to ampicillin (MIC > 400 µg) and chloramphenicol (MIC > 100 µg). The patient was treated with mecillinam at 12 g/day for 21 days. The cerebrospinal fluid cultures were negative after 72 h of treatment. The only side effect of

therapy was slight diarrhea. Sepsis and pneumonia due to an ampicillin-resistant *E. coli* strain responded to therapy, as did sepsis due to *Salmonella typhimurium* and *S. typhi*. No significant adverse reactions occurred in any of the patients.

Mecillinam combined with other agents. The patients treated with mecillinam and another agent ranged in age from 27 to 77 years (Table 2). Addition of mecillinam to the ampicillin therapy of *E. coli* sepsis in a patient with Hodgkin's disease resulted in a fall in temperature, clinical improvement, and eradication of the organism from the blood. Mecillinam and cefazolin were used to treat a patient with multiple liver abscesses and sepsis due to *K. pneumoniae*. Surgery was required and, although the patient was clinically improved and blood became sterile, the organism, susceptible to both agents, could be cultured from the biliary drainage tube. One patient received ampicillin and mecillinam for only 1 day. He had sepsis due to multiple organisms: *Klebsiella*, susceptible to mecillinam with synergy with ampicillin; *Enterobacter*, resistant to both agents; and *S. faecalis*, resistant to mecillinam. Therapy was changed to gentamicin and ampicillin, but he died with positive blood cultures. One 27-year-old male with Wiskott-Aldrich syndrome and *Salmonella enteritidis* sepsis remained febrile after mecillinam treatment although his blood cultures were negative. At 5 days ampicillin was also given, and he became afebrile. Whether the addition of ampicillin was helpful was unclear. One 63-year-old man with Waldenstrom's macroglobulinemia and metastatic carcinoma of the lung was cured of his *E. coli* sepsis, but he developed a urinary infection due to a *Serratia marcescens* strain resistant to mecillinam and cephalothin. This group of patients treated with mecilli-

TABLE 1. *Treatment of eight patients with mecillinam alone*

Age	Sex	Source of infection	Pathogen	Underlying disease[a]	Treatment (days)	Outcome	
						Clinical	Bacterial
70	M	Osteomyelitis	*Aeromonas hydrophila*	Hip prothesis, NF	55	Cure	Cure
77	M	Meningitis	*Escherichia coli*	Carcinoma, UF	21	Cure	Cure
78	M	Sepsis	*E. coli* *Klebsiella pneumoniae*	Carcinoma, RF	3	Failure	Failure
62	M	Sepsis, pneumonia	*E. coli*	Alcoholism, UF	11	Cure	Cure
36	M	Pyelonephritis	*E. coli*	End-stage renal disease, UF	9	Cure	Cure
67	F	Sepsis	*Salmonella typhimurium*	Diabetes, UF	17	Cure	Cure
21	F	Sepsis	*S. typhi*	None	17	Cure	Cure
79	F[b]	Sepsis	*E. coli*	Diabetes, UF	10	Cure	Cure

[a] NF, Nonfatal; RF, rapidly fatal; UF, ultimately fatal.

[b] Received 1 day of penicillin G.

TABLE 2. *Treatment of five patients with mecillinam and another agent*

Age	Sex	Source of infection	Pathogen	Underlying disease[a]	Treatment		Outcome	
					Agent	Dura-tion (days)	Clinical	Bacte-rial
67	M	Sepsis, urinary	*Escherichia coli*	Hodgkin's, RF	Mecillinam	6	Cure	Cure
					Ampicillin	12		
77	M	Sepsis, abdominal	*Klebsiella pneumoniae*	Colon reaction, shock, UF	Mecillinam	1	—[b]	—
			Enterobacter cloacae		Ampicillin	1		
			Streptococcus faecalis					
73	F	Sepsis, liver abscesses	*K. pneumoniae*	Diabetes, UF	Mecillinam	16	Cure	Cure
					Cefazolin	18	Cure	Failure
63	M	Sepsis	*E. coli*	Macroglobulinemia, carcinoma, RF	Mecillinam	7	Cure	Cure
					Cephalothin	5		
					Ticarcillin	1		
27	M	Sepsis	*Salmonella enteritidis*	Wiskott-Aldrich, UF	Mecillinam	10	Cure	Cure
					Ampicillin	6		

[a] NF, Nonfatal; RF, rapidly fatal; UF, ultimately fatal.
[b] Not able to be evaluated.

nam, although small, illustrates that in selected situations mecillinam therapy alone or in combination with another agent is effective in eradicating serious infection such as sepsis and meningitis due to gram-negative bacteria resistant to ampicillin and cephalothin. The MICs of mecillinam ranged from 0.04 to 5 μg/ml, whereas the mean MICs of ampicillin were >400 μg/ml. Further studies of the combination of mecillinam with other antibiotics are needed to determine whether the in vitro synergy and the synergy shown in treating animal infections will be beneficial in humans. The high penetration of mecillinam into the cerebrospinal fluid suggests that it would be an excellent agent for treatment of meningitis due to *E. coli*. It is hoped that studies of this aspect of its use will be possible in the future.

1. **Neu, H. C.** 1975. Mecillinam, a novel penicillanic acid derivative with unusual activity against gram-negative bacteria. Antimicrob. Agents Chemother. **9**:793–799.
2. **Neu, H. C.** 1976. Synergy of mecillinam, a beta-amidino penicillanic acid derivative, combined with beta-lactam antibiotics. Antimicrob. Agents Chemother. **10**:535–542.
3. **Spratt, B. G.** 1975. Distinct penicillin binding proteins involved in the division, elongation and shape of *Escherichia coli* K12. Proc. Natl. Acad. Sci. U.S.A. **72**:2999–3003.
4. **Tybring, L.** 1975. Mecillinam (FL 1060), a 6β-amidino penicillanic acid derivative: in vitro evaluation. Antimicrob. Agents Chemother. **8**:266–270.

Pharmacokinetics of Clavulanic Acid in Patients with Normal and Impaired Renal Function

DIETRICH HÖFFLER AND AXEL DALHOFF*

Städtische Kliniken, Darmstadt, and Beecham-Wülfing, Neuss, Federal Republic of Germany*

Clavulanic acid is a fused β-lactam microbial metabolite produced by *Streptomyces clavuligerus*. It inhibits a wide range of β-lactamases progressively and irreversibly, but its own intrinsic antibacterial activity, although of broad spectrum, is relatively low. Clavulanic acid protects other β-lactam antibiotics from inactivation by many β-lactamases produced by gram-positive and gram-negative bacteria, thus allowing the intrinsic activity of compounds such as amoxycillin against these organisms to be manifested.

The purpose of this study was to determine the pharmacokinetics of clavulanic acid in patients with normal and impaired renal function.

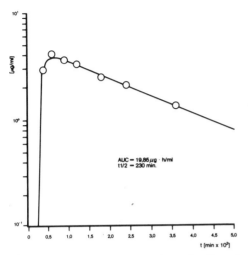

FIG. 1. *Mean serum concentrations of sodium clavulanate in patients with impaired renal function.*

$$Y(t) = P_1 P_3 \{\exp[-P_2(t - t_0)]$$
$$- \exp[-P_3(t - t_0)]\}/(P_3 - P_2)$$

By adopting this equation for all sampling times, serum concentrations of sodium clavulanate declined linearly with a half-life of approximately 90 min, but an optimal fit of the serum concentration versus time curve was not obtained by this procedure. The mean values deviated from the regression line, indicating a more rapid distribution in the early phase of disposition but a slower distribution in the late phase. A better fit was obtained if the 6-h value was omitted. These observations indicate a biphasic elimination of sodium clavulanate with a half-time of approximately 72 min for the first phase and approximately 172 min for the second phase. It can be assumed that in the early phase sodium clavulanate undergoes a rapid distribution from plasma into tissues and simultaneous excretion. In patients with different degrees of renal insufficiency, serum concentrations declined with a half-time of 230 min (Fig. 1). This indicates that sodium clavulanate is renally excreted at least to some extend and that the excretion rate is dependent on renal function.

In summary, the pharmacokinetic parameters of sodium clavulanate are in the same range as the values for amoxycillin—if administered orally—with which sodium clavulanate will be administered simultaneously in clinical use. Further studies need to be undertaken to confirm the distribution pattern of sodium clavulanate in healthy volunteers and to enable us to give dosage recommendations for patients with different degrees of renal insufficiency.

Sodium clavulanate was administered to fasting subjects, and food intake was allowed 90 min after dosing. Each patient received a single dose of 250 mg.

In six patients with normal renal function peak drug concentrations were obtained 60 min after dosing (range, 40 to 90 min). Considerable intersubject variations were observed in this panel of patients. The maximal concentrations ranged from 1.35 to 4.5 µg/ml, thereafter declining to 0.3 µg/ml at 6 h.

The serum concentration versus time curves were calculated by use of the equation:

Inhibitory Activity of Clavulanic Acid Against 16 β-Lactamases Produced by Gram-Negative Bacteria

JEAN-CLAUDE PECHERE, ROBERT LETARTE,* AND ROGER GUAY

Department of Microbiology, School of Medicine, Laval University, Quebec, Quebec, Canada

One of the important mechanisms of bacterial resistance to penicillins and cephalosporins is the production of β-lactamases that hydrolyze the antibiotic molecule (2). Clavulanic acid, a β-lactam analog from *Streptomyces clavuligerus* (4), has been shown to bind irreversibly to the β-lactamase and to inhibit to differing extents its hydrolyzing activity. Investigations of the effect of clavulanic acid on the MICs of penicillins and cephalosporins suggested that Richmond types II, III, IV, and V β-lactamases were

inhibited by clavulanic acid (0.5 to 2.0 µg/ml), whereas type I cephalosporinases remained unaffected (3). We have evaluated the inhibitory properties of clavulanic acid by checking the variation of the β-lactamase itself extracted from 16 strains of gram-negative rods, including 12 members of the *Enterobacteriaceae*.

The inhibitory effect of clavulanic acid was assessed on *Escherichia coli* MULB-127, *Enterobacter cloacae* P-99 and MULB-260, *E. aerogenes* MULB-250, *Serratia marcescens* MDA-

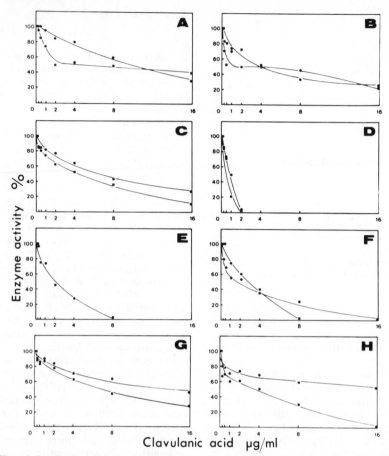

FIG. 1. *Effect of clavulanic acid on eight chromosomally mediated β-lactamases of Enterobacteriaceae (A, Enterobacter cloacae P-99; B, E. aerogenes MULB-250; C, E. cloacae MULB-260; D, Klebsiella pneumoniae; E, Serratia marcescens N-12; F, S. marcescens MDA-761; G, Citrobacter freundii MULB-601; H, Proteus vulgaris Ro-104). Activity (%) on penicillin G (●) and cephalothin (■) was measured with various concentrations of clavulanic acid.*

761, *Acinetobacter calcoaceticus* MULB-811, *Proteus vulgaris* Ro-104, and *Citrobacter freundii* MULB-601, the presumably chromosome-dependent cephalosporinases of *A. xylosoxidans* MULB-901, *S. marcescens* N-12, *Bacteroides fragilis* MULB-1008, and *Klebsiella pneumoniae*, and the four plasmid-mediated β-lactamases of *Escherichia coli* strains R-TEM, 1573 E (R-1818), and JC-6310 (pUB5451), and *Haemophilus* (TEM-like). Each strain was grown to late logarithmic phase in tryptic soy broth at 37°C in the presence of cephalothin (100 μg/ml), except for *B. fragilis* and *H. influenzae*, which were grown in supplemented *Brucella* broth with cephalothin (100 μg/ml) under anaerobic and aerobic conditions, respectively. Bacterial cells were harvested by centrifugation, washed twice, suspended in 0.1 M NaCl, sonicated, and centrifuged (40,000 × g) to give a clear super-

natant which was the source of enzyme. The hydrolyzing velocity (V_0) was measured with 10 U of penicillin G or cephalothin, depending on the preferential substrate of the β-lactamase. The inhibitory effect was evaluated by comparing the V_0 values of the enzyme before and after incubation (37°C, 1 h) with various concentrations (0.25 to 20 μg/ml) of clavulanic acid. All enzymatic assays were performed by use of a computerized microacidimetric method (1).

Figures 1 and 2 show that in 15 out of 16 strains tested complete or partial inhibition of the β-lactamases was obtained with increasing concentrations of clavulanic acid. The four plasmid-mediated β-lactamases and *H. influenzae* β-lactamase were totally inhibited by clavulanic acid at less than 2 μg/ml when penicillin was used as substrate (Fig. 2A, B, C, G, and H), confirming the close substrate-inhibitor-enzyme

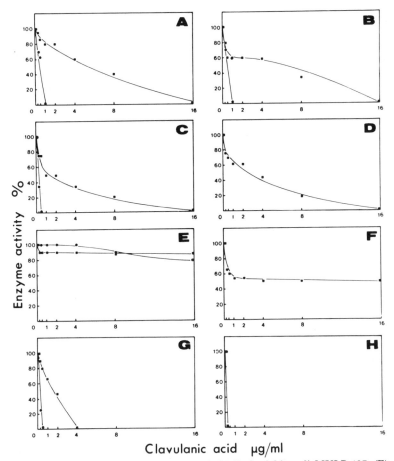

FIG. 2. *Effect of clavulanic acid on β-lactamases of (D) Escherichia coli MULB-127, (E) Acinetobacter xylosoxydans MULB-901, (F) A. calcoaceticus MULB-812, and (H) Bacteroides fragilis MULB-1008, and on the four plasmid-mediated β-lactamases of E. coli strains (A) R-TEM, (B) 1573 E, and (C) JC-6310, and of (G) Haemophilus influenzae. Activity (%) on penicillin G (●) and cephalothin (■) was measured with various concentrations of clavulanic acid.*

structural relationships. Activity of Richmond type I cephalosporinases of strains P-99, MULB-250, and MULB-260 (Fig. 1A–C) was decreased to a lesser extent (50 to 90%) by a clavulanic acid concentration of 16 μg/ml, as evaluated with its preferential substrate, cephalothin.

The present work clearly demonstrated that type I cephalosporinase activity can be lowered by increasing both inhibitor concentration and preincubation time. For example, MICs of cephalothin for reference P-99 and MULB-250 β-lactamase–producing strains were over 5,120 μg/ml, even with a clavulanic concentration of 16 μg/ml. Similar observations have already been reported, and the assumption has been made that type I cephalosporinases could not be inhibited by clavulanic acid. Measurement of enzyme activity proved to be more reliable in inhibition studies than evaluation of MIC values

because residual enzyme activity could eventually lead to a constant high MIC.

B. fragilis β-lactamase appeared very sensitive to a very low level of clavulanic acid, 0.25 μg/ml (Fig. 2H). This observation was in good correlation with the MIC reduction observed in that species (5) because of the synergistic effect of clavulanic acid used with other β-lactam drugs. On the other hand, there are cases in which clavulanic acid has acted as a poor inhibitor of the β-lactamase (4), namely, *Pseudomonas aeruginosa* A Sabath type. *A. xylosoxidans* MULB 901 (Fig. 2E) should be classified in that category.

1. **Letarte, R., M. Devaud-Felix, J. C. Pechere, and D. Allard-Leprohon.** 1977. Enzymatic and immunological characterization of a new cephalosporinase from

Enterobacter aerogenes. Antimicrob. Agents Chemother. **12**:201–205.

2. **Neu, H. C.** 1974. The role of beta-lactamases in the resistance of Gram-negative bacteria to penicillin and cephalosporin derivates. Infect. Dis. Rev. **11**:133–149.

3. **Neu, H. C., and K. P. Fu.** 1978. Clavulanic acid, a novel inhibitor of β-lactamases. Antimicrob. Agents Chemother. **14**:650–655.

4. **Reading, C., and M. Cole.** 1977. Clavulanic acid: a beta-lactamase inhibiting beta-lactam from *Streptomyces clavuligerus.* Antimicrob. Agents Chemother. **11**:852–857.

5. **Wust, J., and T. D. Wilkins.** 1978. Effect of clavulanic acid on anaerobic bacteria resistant to beta-lactam antibiotics. Antimicrob. Agents Chemother. **13**:130–133.

Response of Staphylococcal Renal Infection in Mice to Treatment with Clavulanic Acid and Penicillin

M. S. HEEREMA,* D. M. MUSHER, AND T. W. WILLIAMS, JR.

Department of Medicine, Baylor College of Medicine, Houston, Texas 77030, U.S.A.

The ability of clavulanic acid to inhibit the β-lactamases of *Staphylococcus aureus* and many gram-negative bacteria has been demonstrated in vitro (2), but very little in vivo work with clavulanic acid has been reported (3). We evaluated the effect of benzylpenicillin and clavulanic acid in experimental *S. aureus* infections in mice.

Female CBA mice were injected intravenously (i.v.) with approximately 10^7 colony-forming units (CFU) of β-lactamase–producing *S. aureus.* The subsequent renal infection produced approximately 10^8 CFU of *S. aureus* per kidney at 1 week, declining to 10^7 CFU at 2 weeks (1). The individual kidneys from sacrificed animals were homogenized aseptically, and 10-fold serial dilutions of the homogenates were cultured to determine the CFU of *S. aureus* per kidney. Penicillin, clavulanic acid, or saline was administered subcutaneously in 0.1-ml amounts every 4 h.

The effect of antibiotic therapy when begun immediately prior to i.v. challenge of 25-g mice with 10^7 CFU of *S. aureus* was examined. There were four treatment groups: penicillin, 5,000 U/kg per dose; clavulanic acid, 1 mg/kg per dose; penicillin plus clavulanic acid; and saline. Treatment was administered every 4 h for 24 h. After an additional 24 h without treatment, the kidneys were cultured. As shown in Table 1, prophylactic treatment with penicillin or clavulanic acid alone did not reduce the bacterial counts per kidney, but a highly significant decrease in the mean number of *S. aureus* cells per kidney was observed when penicillin and clavulanic acid were given together.

In a series of experiments on established infections, mice were inoculated i.v. with about 10^7 CFU of *S. aureus*, and 24 h later the mice were randomized into treatment groups to receive various doses of penicillin and/or clavulanic acid for 24 to 120 h. In a representative experiment, 25-g mice were treated for 120 h with penicillin (5,000 U/kg per dose), clavulanic acid (1 mg/kg per dose), penicillin plus clavulanic acid, or saline beginning 24 h after i.v. inoculation of 7.5×10^6 CFU of *S. aureus.* The results in Table 1 show that either drug alone reduced the CFU of *S. aureus* by about 90%; these values were not statistically significant ($P > 0.05$). However, the drug combination produced a 99.9% decline in *S. aureus*; this difference was highly significant when compared to any of the other three groups ($P < 0.01$). The effect of doubling the doses of penicillin or clavulanic acid was no greater than that observed with either of these drugs given

TABLE 1. *Colony-forming units (CFU) of Staphylococcus aureus from kidneys of mice treated with clavulanic acid and penicillin singly and in combination[a]*

Treatment	Mean log CFU of *S. aureus* per kidney ± SD	
	Prophylaxis	Established infection
Penicillin	6.5 ± 1.2	7.4 ± 0.5
Clavulanic acid	7.3 ± 0.6	7.1 ± 0.8
Penicillin plus clavulanic acid	1.7 ± 1.4	4.9 ± 0.8
Saline	6.9 ± 0.6	8.2 ± 1.2

[a] Penicillin (5,000 U/kg), clavulanic acid (1 mg/kg), penicillin (5,000 U/kg) plus clavulanic acid (1 mg/kg), or saline was administered immediately prior to intravenous challenge with 7.5×10^6 CFU of *S. aureus* in the prophylaxis experiment and 24 h after intravenous inoculation of 10^7 CFU of *S. aureus* in the established infection experiment. There were 8 to 10 kidneys in each group.

alone at the concentrations used in the above experiment.

Mice weighing 15 g were inoculated with 2.0×10^7 CFU of *S. aureus*, and 24 h later survivors were randomly divided into treatment groups: penicillin, 25,000 U/kg per dose; clavulanic acid, 2 mg/kg per dose; penicillin plus clavulanic acid; and saline. Injections were given for 72 h, and the number of survivors was recorded. There were no deaths among mice treated with the drug combination, compared to 80% mortality in the control group. Mice treated with either drug alone succumbed less rapidly, but by 72 h none of the penicillin-treated animals and only 20% of the clavulanic acid-treated animals were still alive.

In the three examples of experimental infection described, penicillin and clavulanic acid given together were markedly more effective than either drug alone. These findings extend the in vitro experiments in which small quantities of clavulanic acid were found to potentiate the activity of various β-lactam antibiotics against β-lactamase–producing bacteria. If clavulanic acid proves to be relatively nontoxic, it may play a unique role in the therapy of bacterial infections.

1. **Musher, D. M., R. E. Baughn, G. B. Templeton, and J. N. Minuth.** 1977. Emergence of variant forms of *Staphylococcus aureus* after exposure to gentamicin and infectivity of the variants in experimental animals. J. Infect. Dis. **136**:360–368.
2. **Neu, H. C., and K. P. Fu.** 1978. Clavulanic acid, a novel inhibitor of β-lactamases. Antimicrob. Agents Chemother. **14**:650–655.
3. **Ninane, G., J. Joly, M. Kraytman, and P. Pilot.** 1978. Bronchopulmonary infection due to β-lactamase-producing *Branhamella catarrhalis* treated with amoxicillin/clavulanic acid. Lancet **1**:257.

Synergy of Clavulanic Acid with Penicillins Against Ampicillin and Carbenicillin-Resistant Gram-Negative Organisms, Related to Their Type of Beta-Lactamase

A. M. PHILIPPON,* G. C. PAUL AND P. A. NEVOT

Service de Bactériologie, C.H.U. Cochin, 75014 Paris, France

Resistance to β-lactam antibiotics is mainly related to β-lactamase biosynthesis in gram-negative bacilli. One way of achieving effective antibiotherapy is the use of β-lactamase competitive inhibitors such as clavulanic acid (CA). This potent irreversible inhibitor reduces markedly the antibiotic MIC of clinical isolates of different bacterial species, including *Bacteroides fragilis*. The characterization of β-lactamase was exceptional (2, 4).

This study was undertaken to examine the effect of CA on in vitro potentiation with ampicillin or carbenicillin against ampicillin- and carbenicillin-resistant gram-negative bacilli producing at least one β-lactamase without induction.

Clinical strains were isolated from patients hospitalized in different units at Cochin between January 1977 and December 1978. All strains had β-lactamase activity, revealed by the iodometric method in crude extracts of uninduced cultures broken by ultrasound. The MICs were measured by using a replicating device on Mueller-Hinton medium, inoculated with approximately 10^4 colony-forming units. Organisms were tested for growth inhibition with various concentrations of ampicillin or carbenicillin with or without CA in a final concentration of 1 or 10 μg/ml. Control plates with CA (1 or 10 μg/ml) were included in each assay.

The MIC was defined as the lowest amount of antibiotic inhibiting visible growth after incubation at 37°C for 18 h.

No inhibitory effect was noted when CA was acting alone.

The β-lactamases can most readily be differentiated and identified by analytical isoelectric focusing (1). All the β-lactamases were isolated from crude broken-cell preparations of uninduced cultures and compared with the following reference β-lactamases: *Escherichia coli* K-12 R111 (TEM1), K-12 RP4 (TEM2), K-12 P453 (Pitton type 2), K-12 RGN238 (OXA1), K-12 R46 (OXA2), and K-12 R55 (OXA3); *Pseudomonas aeruginosa* PU21 RPL11 (PSE1), PU R151 (PSE2), PU Rms149 (PSE3), and strain Dalgleish (PSE4) (1). Some unusual enzymes were examined by determination of substrate profile and molecular weight.

The influence of CA on resistance of clinical isolates of *E. coli*, *Proteus mirabilis*, *Klebsiella pneumoniae*, and *Citrobacter diversus* biotypes a and b to ampicillin was studied according to the isoelectric point (pI) of the β-lactamase (Table 1). There was a progressive decrease in ampicillin MIC with increasing amounts of CA. *E. coli* and *P. mirabilis* strains were highly resistant to ampicillin, but the CA potentiation (1.0 and 10 µg/ml) was significant for strains producing β-lactamase of pI 5.4 or 5.6 (TEM1- and TEM2-like β-lactamases). Nevertheless, six *E. coli* strains biosynthesizing a β-lactamase (pI = 7.4) were only significantly inhibited at a CA concentration of 10 µg/ml. This enzyme appeared unusual; the substrate profile indicated an oxacillin-hydrolyzing β-lactamase, active against methicillin and identified as OXA1 (1).

There was a bimodal distribution of ampicillin susceptibilities in *K. pneumoniae* isolates tested, reflecting the types of β-lactamases. Strains producing only one β-lactamase (pI = 7.7) had a low level of resistance (mean agar dilution MIC of ampicillin, 40.3 µg/ml). The CA synergy was marked not only with 1 µg/ml but also with 10 µg/ml. Nine isolates with two β-lactamases (pI = 7.7 plus 5.4) were highly resistant (mean agar dilution MIC of ampicillin, 4,096 µg/ml), but the synergy was also significant with 1 µg of CA per ml, although the geometric mean MIC was higher than that obtained with low-resistance strains. The predominant β-lactamase (pI = 7.7) appeared similar to the one of Pitton type 2 (3).

The behavior of *C. diversus* strains, biotype b (*Levinea malonatica*), appeared similar to that of *K. pneumoniae*: low ampicillin resistance with the biosynthesis of one β-lactamase (pI = 4.8), higher for two enzymes (pI = 4.8 plus 5.4). In any case, the clavulanate potentiation (1 and 10 µg/ml) was marked and significant. It is important to note that all tested strains produced an unknown β-lactamase, a narrow-spectrum penicillinase, probably chromosomally mediated (unpublished data). We also observed a low resistance level for all strains of *C. diversus*, biotype a (*L. amalonatica*), producing only one penicillinase with a different pI from one strain to another. The potentiation effect was somewhat less marked.

The β-lactamase-inhibiting activity of CA was also investigated with carbenicillin against species (usually producing an inducible and chromosomally mediated cephalosporinase inactive against carbenicillin). We analyzed the CA synergy for carbenicillin-resistant clinical isolates producing a noninducible β-lactamase (see Table 2). The potentiation effect of CA appeared variable, as a function of resistance levels, species, and types of β-lactamase. CA synergy was more effective with increasing concentrations (except some strains of *P. aeruginosa*). CA (1 µg/ml) failed to potentiate appreciably carbenicillin activity against *C. freundii* and *Enterobacter cloacae* producing a TEM2-like β-lactamase (pI = 5.6). Nevertheless, the CA synergy was significant with 10 µg/ml for these isolates and

TABLE 1. *Summary of clavulanic acid (CA) potentiation of ampicillin*

Species	No. of isolates	pI of β-lactamase	MIC (µg/ml)[a]		
			Ampicillin	Ampicillin + clavulanate	
				1 µg/ml	10 µg/ml
E. coli	12	5.4	966	21.3	3.0
	1	5.6	>8,192	512	16
	1	5.4 + 5.6	8,192	256	16
	6	7.4	1,024	256	4.0
P. mirabilis	10	5.4	4,096	45.2	3.0
	9	5.6	1,895	13.7	1.8
	1	5.4 + 5.6	4,096	32	2.0
K. pneumoniae	9	7.7	40.3	2.0	0.6
	9	7.7 + 5.4	4,096	54.8	1.8
	1	5.4	64	2.0	0.5
	1	7.1	32	1.0	0.5
C. diversus					
Biotype b	10	4.8	39.4	1.5	0.3
	2	4.8 + 5.4	4,096	90.5	0.7
Biotype a	3	6.05	80.6	32.0	2.5
	3	7.0	64	12.7	1.6
	3	7.85	32	6.3	1.0

[a] Geometric mean.

TABLE 2. *Summary of clavulanic acid (CA) potentiation of carbenicillin*

Species	No. of isolates	pI of β-lactamase	MIC (μg/ml)[a]		
			Carbenicillin	Carbenicillin + clavulanate	
				1 μg/ml	10 μg/ml
C. freundii	8	5.4	>8,192	332.0	20.7
	7	5.6	>8,192	3,042	70.6
	5	5.4 + 5.6	>8,192	675.6	42.2
E. cloacae	9	5.4	>8,192	752.2	74.6
	5	5.6	>8,192	4,705	147.0
S. marcescens	10	5.4	>8,192	3,104	315.2
	4	5.6	>8,192	>8,192	1,217.7
Proteus (indole positive)	9	5.4	1,289	23.5	5.0
	8	5.6	2,656	38.0	14.7
	1	5.4 + 5.6	4,096	64.0	32.0
P. inconstans	2	5.4	1,024	11.3	2.8
	5	5.6	1,552	24.2	4.6
Acinetobacter	19	5.4	4,096	1,705	38.4
P. aeruginosa	24	5.4	1,084	497.3	76.1
	4	5.3	4,870	724.1	107.6
	56	5.70	>8,192	1,786	237.5
	2	5.75	5,792	512	64.0
	3	7.4	256	256	203.1
	8	7.0	608.8	469.5	394.8

[a] Geometric mean.

with 1 and 10 μg/ml for *C. freundii* and *E. cloacae*, producing a TEM1-like enzyme. *Serratia marcescens* appeared to be less susceptible.

The notable CA synergy, even with 1 μg/ml, was explained by the moderate resistance level for indole-positive *Proteus* and *P. inconstans*. A significant potentiation was also seen, but was less marked, against *Acinetobacter* spp., biosynthesizing only TEM1-like enzyme.

The behavior of *P. aeruginosa* appeared to be markedly affected with 10 μg of CA per ml for isolates producing TEM1-like β-lactamase. Nevertheless, a majority of strains produced a carbenicillin-hydrolyzing enzyme (PSE), individualized by isoelectric point: 5.3, 5.70, and 5.75. These enzymes were found only in *P. aeruginosa* and appeared similar to PSE1 and PSE4 (1). The carbenicillin resistance was high, but we observed a marked effect of CA (1 and 10 μg/ml). Nevertheless, 13 of 62 isolates had carbenicillin MICs of 64 μg/ml. No appreciable lowering of the carbenicillin MIC was noted for strains producing oxacillin-hydrolyzing β-lactamase with pI's of 7.0 (OXA3) and 7.4 (OXA1).

The CA effect on the synergistic potential of ampicillin or carbenicillin appeared variable, depending on resistance levels, bacterial species, and types of β-lactamases. Although CA has a marked effect, it was sometimes incompatible with clinically attainable levels.

1. **Matthew, M.** 1979. Plasmid-mediated β-lactamases of Gram-negative bacteria: properties and distribution. J. Antimicrob. Chemother. **5**:349–358.
2. **Neu, H. C., and K. P. Fu.** 1978. Clavulanic acid, a novel inhibitor of β-lactamases. Antimicrob. Agents Chemother. **14**:650–655.
3. **Pitton, J. S.** 1972. Mechanisms of bacterial resistance to antibiotics. Rev. Physiol. **65**:15–93.
4. **Reading, C., and M. Cole.** 1977. Clavulanic acid: a beta-lactamase-inhibiting beta-lactam from *Streptomyces clavuligerus*. Antimicrob. Agents Chemother. **11**:852–857.

Augmentin (Amoxicillin Plus Sodium Clavulanate, a Beta-Lactamase Inhibitor) Is Active in Amoxicillin-Resistant Infections

J. KOSMIDIS,* A. ANYFANTIS, C. STATHAKIS, K. MANTOPOULOS, AND G. K. DAIKOS

First Department of Propedeutic Medicine, Athens University School of Medicine, King Paul's Hospital, Athens 609, Greece

A recent approach to overcome the increasing rate of bacterial resistance to β-lactam antibiotics, when due to β-lactamase production, is the concomitant use of a β-lactamase inhibitor. This approach has been used in the past with stable β-lactams which can inhibit β-lactamases and thus potentiate the action of a second, β-lactamase-susceptible compound. This inhibition, however, is of the competitive and reversible type, and protection of a labile agent requires a high concentration of the inhibitor, which is often pharmacokinetically impossible to achieve.

Clavulanic acid (1, 2) is a β-lactam with a structure resembling the penicillins and is produced by *Streptomyces clavuligerus*. It has a weak intrinsic antibacterial activity but is a potent inhibitor of the β-lactamases of Richmond types II, III, IV, and V, produced by a wide range of bacteria. Inhibition is progressive and irreversible and effected even at low concentrations of clavulanic acid. A marked in vitro synergy between this compound and various labile β-lactam antibiotics against a variety of β-lactamase-producing bacteria has been shown (1–3).

We investigated the efficacy and safety of a combination of amoxicillin and clavulanate sodium in the treatment of infections due to amoxicillin-resistant organisms. This combination has been given the trade name Augmentin. Thirty-eight patients were treated. Twenty-four were males and 14 were females. Their ages ranged from 18 to 76 years, with a majority above 60. They were suffering from a variety of infections (Table 1) often in the presence of one or more factors usually associated with antibiotic treatment failure such as renal stone (8 patients), other anatomical abnormalities (6), malignancy (6), diabetes (3), and other functional abnormalities (6). A total of 22 patients had one or more aggravating factors. In 21 cases previous antibiotic courses had failed including ampicillin or its analogs (3 patients), mezlocillin (1), cephapirin/cephalexin (4), gentamicin (5), co-trimoxazole (7), nalidixic acid (5), nitrofurantoin (3), colistin (1), and erythromycin (1). All pathogens were resistant to amoxicillin by standard disk sensitivity techniques and included: *Escherichia coli* (6 strains), *Citrobacter freundii* (2), *Kleb-*

siella pneumoniae (6), *Enterobacter aerogenes* (3), *Proteus mirabilis* (9), other *Proteus* spp. (4), *Providencia* spp. (2), *Acinetobacter calcoaceticus* var. *anitratus* (1), and *Staphylococcus aureus* (5). Augmentin was given by mouth as tablets containing 250 mg of amoxicillin and 125 mg of clavulanate sodium. Patients suffering from lower urinary tract infection or soft-tissue infection received one tablet three times daily; those with upper urinary tract infection and respiratory infections were given two tablets three times daily. In the vast majority of patients treatment lasted 8 days. The patients were observed carefully for evaluation of efficacy and occurrence of side effects, and the following laboratory tests were performed before, during, and after treatment: full blood count, platelet count, SGPT, serum bilirubin, alkaline phosphatase, urea, creatinine, clotting parameters (activated partial thromboplastin time and partial thromboplastin time), and complete urinalysis.

In addition to the above clinical trial, penetration in sputum of the ingredients of Augmentin was studied in three patients with exacerbation of chronic bronchitis. They were given two tablets three times a day, and sputum and serum were collected every 2 h for 6 h after the first dose and again after a dose on day 4 of treatment. Concentrations of clavulanate were assayed by using a technique developed by P. Hunter (Beecham Research Laboratories, data on file) which measures β-lactamase inhibitory activity, whereas levels of amoxicillin were measured by a conventional agar well plate technique with *Sarcina lutea* as the indicator organism.

Finally, 134 consecutive clinical isolates were tested for susceptibility to amoxicillin alone and to Augmentin. Disks containing 20 μg of amoxicillin plus 10 μg of clavulanic acid or 20 μg of amoxicillin alone were used.

Results of treatment are shown in Table 1. Twenty-six of 34 patients with symptoms (76.5%) were clinically cured, four improved, and four failed. Twenty-eight of the 38 pathogens (73.7%) were eradicated and 10 persisted. The latter included *E. coli* (1), *K. pneumoniae* (3), *P. mirabilis* (3), *P. vulgaris* (1), *A. calcoaceticus* var. *anitratus* (1), and *S. aureus* (1). There was no appreciable difference in the success rate

TABLE 1. *Results of treatment with Augmentin of 38 infections due to amoxicillin-resistant bacteria*

Infection	No. of patients	Clinical results				Bacteriological results	
		Cure	Improvement	Failure	NA[a]	Eradication	Persistence
Acute cystitis	7	7				7	
Recurrent cystitis	3	2		1		1	2
Acute/recurrent cystitis on chronic active pyelonephritis	10	6	3	1		5	5
Acute pyelonephritis	3	2		1		3	
Recurrent pyelonephritis	2	2				2	
Chronic active pyelonephritis	4				4	3	1
Chronic urethritis	1	1				1	
Osteomyelitis	1		1				1
Cellulitis/carbuncle/infected acne	4	4				4	
Chronic otitis media	1			1			1
Pneumonia	1	1				1	
Exacerbated chronic bronchitis	1	1				1	

[a] NA, Nonevaluable (asymptomatic).

TABLE 2. *Penetration in sputum*[a]

Treatment day	Collection period (h)	Clavulanic acid level (μg/ml)	Amoxicillin level (μg/ml)
1	Before	0	0
	0–1	1.21	0.53
	1–2	0.22	0.19
	2–4	0.18	0.04
	4–6	0.08	0.03
4	Before	0.03	0
	0–2	0.25	0.03
	2–4	0.22	0.04
	4–6	0.01	0

[a] Mean values in three patients with chronic bronchitis given two tablets three times a day.

between the two dosage groups. Clinical or bacteriological failure was always associated with one or more aggravating factors.

Side effects included mild to moderate diarrhea in four cases, nausea and vomiting in one case, and a maculopapular rash in one case. In only one patient with diarrhea was the side effect severe enough to cause discontinuation of treatment. Gastrointestinal side effects were observed in 2 of 13 patients receiving two tablets three times a day. No toxicity on the liver, kidneys, or bone marrow was caused by treatment in any of the 38 patients. In only one case a transient elevation of alkaline phosphatase up

to 8.3 units (upper normal, 8.0), quickly reverting to normal, was observed.

Levels of both components of Augmentin in sputum are shown in Table 2. It can be seen that penetration into sputum was more effective on day 1, when sputum was more purulent.

Of the 134 isolates studied 84 were resistant to amoxicillin, and of these only 33 were also resistant to the combined Augmentin disk.

Our results of treatment with Augmentin are very satisfactory. Success in infections due to amoxicillin-resistant organisms, often in the presence of aggravating factors, was about 75%. Gastrointestinal side effects were the only problem, but in all except one case treatment was not discontinued. The advent of clavulanic acid has opened new prospects for the β-lactam group of antibiotics by resensitizing the bacteria that have become resistant by virtue of β-lactamase production.

1. **Neu, H. C., and K. P. Fu.** 1978. Clavulanic acid, a novel inhibitor of β-lactamases. Antimicrob. Agents Chemother. **14**:650–655.
2. **Reading, C., and M. Cole.** 1977. Clavulanic acid: a beta-lactamase-inhibiting beta-lactam from *Streptomyces clavuligerus*. Antimicrob. Agents Chemother. **11**:852–857.
3. **Wise, R., J. M. Andrews, and K. A. Bedford.** 1978. In vitro study of clavulanic acid in combination with penicillin, amoxycillin, and carbenicillin. Antimicrob. Agents Chemother. **13**:389–393.

Amoxicillin/Clavulanic Acid (Augmentin) Therapy in Complicated Urinary Tract Infection

DONALD A. LEIGH* AND KATHERINE BRADNOCK

Department of Microbiology, Wycombe General Hospital, High Wycombe, Buckinghamshire, England

Over the past decade, there has been a marked increase in the number of bacteria which produce β-lactamases, and this has limited the value of the β-lactam antibiotics in chemotherapy. The introduction of cephalosporins and cephamycins with marked resistance to the action of β-lactamases, such as cefuroxime, cefamandole, cefotaxime, and cefoxitin, has extended the spectrum of antibacterial compounds active against these strains, but there is still a need for an effective oral antibiotic.

Clavulanic acid (BRL 14151), Z-(2R.5R)-3-(hydroxyethylidene)-7-oxo-4-oxa-1 azabicyclo-(3.2.0.) heptane-2-carboxylic acid, is a new compound produced by *Streptomyces clavuligerus* which has a chemical structure with similarities to those of the β-lactam antibiotics. It has intrinsic antibacterial activity, but this approaches therapeutic levels for only a few species of bacteria, and its main property is the irreversible progressive inhibition of β-lactamase formation (1, 4). It is active against most β-lactamases, with the greatest inhibition occurring with types II, III, IV, and V. The activity against type I enzymes is confined to that produced by *Bacteroides fragilis*. When prescribed with a β-lactam antibiotic, it potentiates the antibacterial effect by inactivation of β-lactamase and increases the susceptibility of highly resistant strains of bacteria to therapeutically attainable antibiotic concentrations. This action has been reported with many β-lactam antibiotics (2, 3, 6). In the case of bacteria that do not produce β-lactamase, the presence of clavulanic acid does not interfere with the action of the β-lactam antibiotic. Augmentin (BRL 25000) is a new formulation of clavulanic acid (125 mg) and amoxicillin (250 mg). The pharmacokinetic properties of the two compounds, i.e., peak serum concentration, serum half-life, and excretion, are similar. Augmentin was used in the treatment of chronic urinary tract infections caused by bacteria with multiple antibiotic resistance.

Clinical trial. Ages of the 75 patients included in the study are shown in Table 1. Most patients were over 70 years of age. Serious complications were present in the majority of these patients, and 47 (63%) had indwelling urinary catheters during part or all of the treatment period. Although 18 patients had asymptomatic infection, 29 (39%) had chronic recurrent infections, and 11 (15%) had neurogenic bladders and paraplegia. Seven patients (9%) developed their infection after prostatectomy, five had cerebral thrombosis, and three suffered from retention. All patients had reduced renal or bladder function, and most had received previous courses of parenteral antibiotic therapy. The infections were due to strains of *Enterobacteriaceae*, 39 (52%) being *Klebsiella* spp., 21 (28%) *Escherichia coli*, and 9 (11%) *Proteus* species; the remaining infections were due to either *Enterobacter* or *Citrobacter* species or were mixed infections (Table 1). The strains were generally susceptible only to nalidixic acid, colistin, gentamicin, amikacin, and the β-lactamase–resistant cephalosporins and cephamycins. The inhibitory concentration of amoxicillin was always in excess of 125 mg/liter and frequently exceeded 8,000 mg/liter. However, in the presence of clavulanic acid, the MICs fell to between 0.8 and 31 mg/liter.

Augmentin was prescribed, after informed consent, in a dose of 375 mg three times a day for 10 days, and urine specimens were examined during treatment and between 2 and 3 weeks after treatment. When possible, biochemical and hematological parameters were assessed, although the coexistence of underlying disease resulted in there being considerable abnormalities present in most patients before treatment was started. Urine culture was carried out by

TABLE 1. *Ages and infecting organisms of the 75 patients treated with Augmentin*

Age and organism	Women	Men	Total
Age (yr)[a]			
<39	2	1	3
40–59	7	3	10
60–69	2	4	6
70–79	7 (19%)	15 (38%)	22 (29%)
80–89	16 (44%)	15 (38%)	31 (41%)
>90	2	1	3
Total	36	39	75
Infecting organism			
Escherichia coli	16 (44%)	5	21 (28%)
Klebsiella spp.	11	28 (72%)	39 (52%)
Proteus spp.	6	2	8 (11%)
Citrobacter spp.	1	1	2
Enterobacter spp.	—	2	2
Mixed growth	2	1	3

[a] Ages ranged from 18 to 96 years.

TABLE 2. *Reasons for failure of Augmentin therapy*

No.	Sex	Age (yr)	Infection	Infecting organism	Complicating features
4	F	81	Simple	*Proteus*	—
9	M	90	Simple	*Klebsiella*	Retention, catheter
14	M	84	Chronic	*Klebsiella*	Catheter
17	M	78	Chronic	*Klebsiella*	Retention, catheter
20	F	82	Chronic	*Escherichia coli*	Catheter (permanent), senility
21	F	82	Chronic	*E. coli*	Catheter, Parkinsonism
22	M	80	Simple	*Klebsiella*	Catheter, cerebral thrombosis
24	F	82	Simple	*Klebsiella*	—
27	F	86	Simple	*Klebsiella*	—
30	M	76	Simple	*Klebsiella*	Carcinoma of prostate, catheter
34	M	77	Chronic	*Klebsiella*	Catheter
36	M	78	Chronic	*Klebsiella*	Catheter
38	F	82	Chronic	*E. coli*	Catheter (permanent), senility
41	F	46	Chronic	*Proteus*	Catheter (permanent), paraplegia
44	M	19	Chronic	*Proteus*	Catheter (permanent), paraplegia
46	M	79	Postoperative	*Klebsiella*	Catheter, prostatectomy
49	F	78	Chronic	*Klebsiella*	Catheter, diabetes
50	M	86	Chronic	*E. coli*	Catheter, diabetes
55	F	83	Chronic	*Proteus, Klebsiella*	Catheter
56	M	89	Postoperative	*Klebsiella*	Catheter, prostatectomy
59	M	75	Simple	*Klebsiella*	—
60	M	78	Chronic	*Klebsiella*	Catheter, amputation
71	F	76	Simple	*Klebsiella*	—
74	M	60	Postoperative	*Klebsiella*	Catheter, prostatectomy

conventional laboratory methods, and cure resulting from treatment was assessed as the eradication of the original infecting strain. In 74 patients whose urine was cultured while they were receiving treatment, 90% had a sterile specimen but in 4% reinfection due to a different strain had occurred. The overall cure rate after treatment was 64%, but 18 patients showed reinfection, in 9 cases due to *Pseudomonas aeruginosa*. Nine patients died during the follow-up period as a result of their underlying disease. The cure rate was higher in infections due to *E. coli*, but these were generally less complicated than those caused by *Klebsiella*. The activity of the potassium salt was marginally greater than that of the sodium salt. The majority of treatment failures (Table 2) showed severe abnormalities and had indwelling catheters.

Augmentin was generally well tolerated in a dose of 375 mg, but in four patients in whom the dose was increased to 750 mg, severe nausea and vomiting occurred which precluded completion of therapy. Six patients (8%) complained of side effects, and four of these (5%) had significant diarrhea. The other two patients had a single loose stool and urethral irritation. No significant changes were seen in the biochemical and hematological parameters.

Discussion. The introduction of Augmentin represents a significant and important advance in chemotherapy. Clavulanic acid potentiates the action of amoxicillin against most β-lactam-ase–producing strains of *Enterobacteriaceae*. In addition, the activity against *B. fragilis*, also reported by Wise (5), with penicillin is so great as to merit its use in the treatment of anaerobic infections and suggests that it may be of value in preoperative prophylaxis in gastrointestinal surgery. The broad spectrum of activity shown by the combination of clavulanic acid and amoxicillin makes it an appropriate alternative therapy to parenteral antibiotics in the prophylaxis of patients with leukemia, and febrile and infective episodes have been successfully treated in two patients (D. A. Leigh, unpublished data). Soft tissue infections such as diabetic leg ulcers and postoperative amputation wounds have also responded to Augmentin treatment. Although the administration of 250 mg of clavulanic acid caused marked gastrointestinal irritation in the patients treated in this study, a dose of 125 mg was well tolerated, and only 5% of patients developed diarrhea. It is possible that calibration of the dose is necessary, as the cure rate in this group of patients with very complicated infections was low and might have been improved by an increased dose of 175 mg. Urinary infections due to strains of *Enterobacteriaceae* are usually treated with aminoglycosides, but in geriatric patients with reduced and variable renal function it is difficult to control the dose by serum assay, and toxic effects may occur. This study has shown that Augmentin is effective in severe complicated infections and is a treatment acceptable to and well tolerated by elderly patients.

This study was supported by a grant from Beecham Pharmaceuticals Ltd. (England).

1. **Brown, A. G., D. Butterworth, M. Cole, G. Hanscomb, G. D. Hood, C. Reading, and G. N. Rolinson.** 1976. Naturally occurring β-lactamase inhibitors with antibacterial activity. J. Antibiot. **29**:668–669.
2. **Neu, H. C., and K. P. Fu.** 1978. Clavulanic acid, a novel inhibitor of β-lactamases. Antimicrob. Agents Chemother. **14**:650–655.
3. **Paisley, J. W., and J. A. Washington.** 1978. Combined activity of clavulanic acid and ticarcillin against ticarcillin-resistant gram-negative bacilli. Antimicrob. Agents Chemother. **14**:224–227.
4. **Reading, C., and M. Cole.** 1977. Clavulanic acid: a beta-lactamase-inhibiting beta-lactam from *Streptomyces clavuligerus.* Antimicrob. Agents Chemother. **11**:852–857.
5. **Wise, R.** 1977. Clavulanic acid and susceptibility of *Bacteroides fragilis* to penicillin. Lancet **2**:145.
6. **Wise, R., J. M. Andrews, and K. A. Bedford.** 1978. In vitro study of clavulanic acid in combination with penicillin, amoxycillin, and carbenicillin. Antimicrob. Agents Chemother. **13**:389–393.

Comparative Activity of BRL 25000 with Amoxicillin Against Resistant Clinical Isolates

HERMAN W. VAN LANDUYT* AND ANNEMIE LAMBERT

Department of Microbiology, A. Z. St. Jan, B-8000 Brugge, Belgium

Clavulanic acid is a β-lactam antibiotic isolated from *Streptomyces clavuligerus.* Although the compound has only poor antibiotic properties, it is a potent inhibitor of many β-lactamases found in clinical isolates (2). In combination with other antibiotics it can protect them against the inactivation by many bacterial β-lactamases and render the bacteria susceptible to them (1).

BRL 25000 (Augmentin) is a mixture of amoxicillin trihydrate and potassium clavulanate in a proportion of 2:1. The in vitro activity of this formulation was compared with that of amoxicillin against 570 clinical isolates, including 428 strains of *Enterobacteriaceae,* 102 of *Staphylococcus aureus,* and 40 of *Haemophilus* (see Table 2). All the isolates were resistant to ampicillin, as determined by the Kirby-Bauer technique, and all were β-lactamase producers, as determined by the rapid chromogenic cephalosporin method.

The MICs for the strains were determined by an agar dilution technique with the use of an automatic multipoint inoculator (Denley, Great Britain). The test medium was Mueller-Hinton medium (Difco), and the final inoculation spot contained 2×10^5 to 4×10^5 colony-forming units. For the *Haemophilus* strains the medium was supplemented with 1% hemoglobin (Oxoid) and 1% IsoVitaleX (BBL Microbiology Systems). The incubation time at 37°C was 18 h for the *Enterobacteriaceae* and *S. aureus* strains and 24 h for the *Haemophilus* strains. The activity of the two compounds was checked by comparing the geometric mean MICs, the concentrations required to inhibit 90% of the strains (MIC$_{90}$), and the percentage of strains inhibited at a given concentration of 2 μg/ml for the *S. aureus* and *Haemophilus* strains and 8 μg/ml for the *Enterobacteriaceae* strains (Tables 1 and 2).

The geometric mean MICs of BRL 25000 were less than 2 μg/ml for the *S. aureus* and *Haemophilus* strains, and more than 90% of these strains were inhibited at this concentration. Among the *Enterobacteriaceae* isolates, the geometric mean MICs of BRL 25000 were below 8 μg/ml for the *Klebsiella, P. mirabilis,* and *P. vulgaris* strains, 73%, 80%, and 100% of the strains, respectively, being inhibited at this concentration. The MIC$_{90}$ for each of the above five groups was at least four twofold dilutions lower for BRL 25000 than for amoxicillin.

Only 27% of the *E. coli* strains and 38% of the *Citrobacter* strains were inhibited by BRL 25000 at a concentration of 8 μg/ml. The MIC$_{90}$ of BRL 25000 for these strains was two twofold dilutions lower than that of amoxicillin. There was also a lowering in geometric mean MICs of BRL 25000 against these strains, but none fell below the level of 8 μg/ml.

The differences between BRL 25000 and amoxicillin were minimal for the other *Enterobacteriaceae* isolates. Only 3% of the *Enterobacter* strains were inhibited at a BRL 25000 concentration of 8 μg/ml. The MIC$_{90}$ for the *Enterobacter* and *P. morganii* strains was only

TABLE 1. *In vitro activity of ampicillin (AMP), amoxicillin (AMX), and BRL 25000 (AUG) against β-lactamase-producing bacteria*[a]

Organism (no. of strains tested)	Drug	MIC range	MIC_{50}	MIC_{90}	Geometric mean MIC
Staphylococcus aureus (102)	AMP	2->128	32	>128	24.88
	AMX	2->128	16	128	16.10
	AUG	0.5-64	2	2	1.63
Escherichia coli (163)	AMP	32->128	>128	>128	227.26
	AMX	64->128	>128	>128	224.55
	AUG	4-128	16	64	19.12
Klebsiella (117)	AMP	16->128	64	>128	75.54
	AMX	32->128	128	>128	151.09
	AUG	2-64	4	16	6.23
Enterobacter (29)	AMP	16->128	64	>128	63.99
	AMX	16->128	>128	>128	162.55
	AUG	4-128	64	128	68.75
Citrobacter (8)	AMP	16->128	32	>128	69.79
	AMX	64->128	>128	>128	181.01
	AUG	4-128	16	128	24.67
Serratia (15)	AMP	64->128	>128	>128	185.25
	AMX	128->128	>128	>128	212.79
	AUG	128->128	>128	>128	203.18
Proteus mirabilis (20)	AMP	16->128	>128	>128	207.93
	AMX	32->128	>128	>128	222.86
	AUG	1-16	8	16	5.65
P. vulgaris (26)	AMP	32->128	128	>128	142.40
	AMX	64->128	>128	>128	201.38
	AUG	2-8	4	8	3.69
P. morganii (44)	AMP	32->128	64	>128	97.92
	AMX	64->128	128	>128	149.83
	AUG	64-128	128	128	104.29
P. rettgeri (1)	AMP	>128	>128	>128	256
	AMX	>128	>128	>128	256
	AUG	32	32	32	32
Providencia (5)	AMP	>128	>128	>128	256
	AMX	>128	>128	>128	256
	AUG	64->128	128	>128	127.99
Haemophilus (40)	AMP	2->128	8	16	8.28
	AMX	2->128	8	32	11.51
	AUG	0.5-8	1	2	1.14

[a] All MICs are given in micrograms per milliliter of medium. The MIC_{50} and MIC_{90} were the concentrations that inhibited 50 and 90% of the strains, respectively.

TABLE 2. *Inhibition of β-lactamase-producing bacteria by fixed concentrations of ampicillin (AMP), amoxicillin (AMX), and BRL 25000 (AUG)*[a]

Organism	No. tested	Percentage of strains inhibited		
		AMP	AMX	AUG
Staphylococcus aureus	102	8	9	93
Haemophilus	40	12.5	7.5	95
Escherichia coli	163	0	0	27
Klebsiella pneumoniae	117	0	0	73
Enterobacter	29[b]	0	0	3
Citrobacter	8[c]	0	0	38
Serratia marcescens	15	0	0	0
Proteus mirabilis	20	0	0	80
P. vulgaris	26	0	0	100
P. morganii	44	0	0	0
P. rettgeri	1	0	0	0
Providencia stuartii	5	0	0	0

[a] Each drug was tested at a concentration of 2 µg/ml against *S. aureus* and *Haemophilus* isolates and 8 µg/ml against the *Enterobacteriaceae* isolates.

[b] *E. cloacae*, 14; *E. aerogenes*, 7; *E. hafniae*, 1; *E. agglomerans*, 4; *E. liquefaciens*, 3.

[c] *C. freundii*, 5; *C. diversus*, 3.

one twofold dilution lower for BRL 25000 than for amoxicillin. There was no difference between BRL 25000 and amoxicillin in the MIC_{90} for the *Serratia* and *Providencia* strains.

In conclusion, it can be stated from this study that the addition of clavulanic acid to amoxicillin in a ratio of 1:2 to form BRL 25000 (Augmentin) enlarges the spectrum of this compound toward certain groups of β-lactamase–producing bacteria which have become more and more resistant to amoxicillin. Furthermore, this combination is active against the *Haemophilus* strains for which amoxicillin was one of the first-choice drugs before the emergence of β-lactamase–producing strains. Further clinical studies are needed to support these in vitro observations.

1. **Neu, H. C., and K. P. Fu.** 1978. Clavulanic acid, a novel inhibitor of β-lactamases. Antimicrob. Agents Chemother. **14:**650–655.
2. **Reading, C., and M. Cole.** 1977. Clavulanic acid: a beta-lactamase-inhibiting beta-lactam from *Streptomyces clavuligerus*. Antimicrob. Agents Chemother. **11:**852–857.

Clinical and Pharmacokinetic Studies with Clavulanic Acid

A. P. BALL,* I. D. FARRELL, A. M. GEDDES, P. DAVEY, AND G. R. BROOKES

East Birmingham Hospital, Birmingham B9 5ST, England

Clavulanic acid is a naturally occurring compound derived from *Streptomyces clavuligerus*, which, although it has little intrinsic antibacterial activity, is a potent β-lactamase inhibitor. It is active against staphylococcal β-lactamase and class II to V plasmid-mediated enzymes produced by members of the *Enterobacteriaceae*, but has little activity against class I β-lactamases. In vitro studies (1, 2; I. D. Farrell, G. R. Brooks, A. P. Ball, and A. M. Geddes, this volume) have shown synergy between clavulanic acid and penicillins against β-lactamase–producing *Staphylococcus aureus* and *Enterobacteriaceae* isolates. Some β-lactamase–producing gram-negative species, e.g., *Klebsiella aerogenes*, are predictably inhibited by amoxicillin (AMX) plus a small concentration of clavulanic acid (<1 mg/liter), but others, including some *Escherichia coli* strains, require the addition of higher concentrations of clavulanic acid (5 to 10 mg/liter) (Farrell et al., this volume). In the present study, we investigated the efficacy, safety, and tolerance of sodium and potassium clavulanate in combination with AMX at three dose levels, in adult patients with AMX-resist-

ant urinary tract infections. The disposition characteristics of the individual components were studied simultaneously.

All patients included entered the trial after confirmation of significant bacteriuria in at least two midstream urine specimens. Patients were excluded only if one or more of the following criteria were present: age < 12 years, pregnancy, penicillin allergy, severe gastrointestinal disease, significant renal impairment, or bladder catheterization.

Three series of 20 patients received oral therapy for 7 days as follows: series I, 250 mg of AMX and 125 mg of sodium clavulanate every 8 h; series II, 500 mg of AMX and 125 mg of potassium clavulanate every 8 h; series III, 500 mg of AMX and 250 mg of potassium clavulanate every 8 h.

Safety and tolerance were monitored by routine complete blood count, biochemistry, and urinalysis on days 0 and 7 and by frequent assessment of subjective patient response.

The causative organisms isolated were *E. coli* (susceptible to AMX, treated during initial assessment in series I) in 10 patients, *E. coli* (resistant to AMX) in 31, *K. aerogenes* (resistant to AMX) in 10, and other resistant organisms in 9 (*Proteus* spp., 3; *S. aureus*, 3; *Serratia marcescens*, 1; mixed infection due to *Citrobacter* sp. and *K. aerogenes*, 1; mixed infection due to *E. coli* and *K. oxytoca*, 1). The MICs of combinations of AMX and clavulanic acid for these organisms are reported by Farrell et al. (this volume).

The results of treatment of the 60 patients related to anatomic diagnosis and infecting organism are shown in Table 1.

No intolerance was detected in patients in series I and II, but in series III, in which the dose of potassium clavulanate was doubled (to 250 mg every 8 h), eight patients complained of nausea and two of these were withdrawn from the study after the onset of vomiting. In the other six patients, nausea was tolerated during continued therapy. No patient developed diarrhea during or after treatment. Adverse reactions were infrequent. One patient developed a penicillin rash and candidal vulvo-vaginitis, and another developed a slight rise in serum glutamic pyruvic transaminase and blood urea (due to accelerated hypertension and its treatment). Slight, transient eosinophilia occurred in four patients.

Single-dose pharmacokinetic studies were undertaken in six fasting volunteers. Four were given 250 mg of AMX and 125 mg of sodium clavulanate orally, and two were given 500 mg of AMX and 250 mg of potassium clavulanate. Blood samples were obtained at time zero, at 15, 30, 45, 60, 75, and 90 min, and at 2, 3, 4, 5, and 6 h. Urine specimens were obtained between 0 and 2 h, 2 and 4 h, and 4 and 6 h. All assays were performed on the day of study. AMX was assayed by a standard large-plate agar well technique with *Sarcina lutea* NCTC 8340 as the assay organism. Clavulanic acid was assayed by use of a spore suspension of *K. aerogenes* (BRL 1003) in agar containing 60 mg of benzylpenicillin per liter. Inactivation of β-lactamase by clavulanic acid resulted in inhibition zones due to benzylpenicillin around the wells, allowing comparison with zones produced by known clavulanic acid concentrations.

After oral dosage of 250 mg of AMX and 125 mg of sodium clavulanate, peak serum concentrations of 4.0 ± 1.75 (SD) mg of AMX and 2.55 ± 0.97 mg of clavulanic acid per liter were found at 75 and 60 min, respectively. After twice this dose (500 mg/250 mg) the peak serum concentrations were 7.0 mg of AMX and 5.9 mg of clavulanic acid per liter, both at 75 min. The corresponding serum elimination half-lives were 70.7 min (250 mg) and 63.2 min (500 mg) for AMX and 69.0 min (125 mg) and 61.2 min (250 mg) for clavulanic acid.

Urine recoveries after administration of the two doses are shown in Table 2. The increased drug concentrations in the 2- to 4-h urines from the volunteers given the higher dose pos-

TABLE 1. *Results of therapy with three dose regimens related to underlying diagnosis and to causative organism*

Diagnosis or organism	No of successes/total no. of patients			
	Series I	Series II	Series III	Overall
DIAGNOSIS				
ASB[a]/cystitis	4/9 (44%)	6/10 (60%)	7/12 (58%)	17/31 (55%)
Cystitis following surgery, tumor, or catheter	3/6 (50%)	5/7 (71%)	4/5 (80%)	12/18 (66%)
Cystitis with prostatitis	1/1 (LT Co-T)[b]	1/1 (LT Co-T)[b]	1/1	3/3
Cystitis with epididymitis	0/1	—	—	0/1
Acute pyelonephritis	1/3	2/2	2/2	5/7 (71%)
Overall result	9/20 (45%)	14/20 (70%)	14/20 (70%)	37/60 (62%)
ORGANISM[c]				
E. coli (S)	6/10 (60%)	—	—	—
E. coli (R)	2/6 (33%)	9/12 (75%)	9/13 (69%)	18/25 (72%)[d]
K. aerogenes (R)	—	4/6 (66%)	3/4 (75%)	7/10 (70%)[d]
Other species (R)	1/4	1/2	2/3	—
Overall result	9/20 (45%)	14/20 (70%)	14/20 (70%)	

[a] Asymptomatic bacteriuria.

[b] Two negative posttreatment midstream urine specimens, followed by long-term co-trimoxazole (two tablets at night).

[c] S and R indicate susceptibility and resistance to AMX.

[d] Series II and III combined.

TABLE 2. *Urinary recovery of amoxicillin (AMX) and clavulinic acid (CLV) after oral administration of single doses to healthy volunteers*

Treatment[a]	Time (h)	Percent recovered		Concn in urine (mg/liter)	
		AMX	CLV	AMX	CLV
AMX, 250 mg;	0–2	52	24	475	131
NaCLV, 125 mg	2–4	24	9	162	32
	4–6	8	2	170	22.8
	Total	84	36.5		
AMX, 500; KCLV,	0–2	32.5	28	282	117
250 mg	2–4	18.5	13	855	310
	4–6	4	3	106	45
	Total	55	44		

[a] NaCLV and KCLV are sodium and potassium clavulanate.

sibly reflect higher urine flow rates in the first 2 h.

The disposition characteristics of the two agents indicate rapid absorption from the gut and fairly rapid clearance from the serum, predominantly by renal elimination. Serum levels after low dosage, especially of clavulanic acid, may be inadequate for invasive infection, and this is reflected by therapeutic failure in two of three patients with pyelonephritis in series I (250 mg/125 mg). However, at higher dosage, peak serum concentrations sufficient to inhibit most susceptible organisms were obtained, and at these dosage levels all four patients with pyelonephritis were cured (Table 1). Although urine elimination had fallen to minimal levels by 4 to 6 h, drug concentrations were adequate for eradication of most infections. Notably, less than 50% of the administered dose of clavulanic acid was recovered from the urine in 6 h, suggesting a significant nonrenal elimination route.

The results of the clinical study revealed no significant adverse reactions, but they did indicate that high dosage of the combination (series III) is likely to be associated with gastrointestinal intolerance. This appeared to be an effect of the high dose (250 mg every 8 h) of clavulanic acid and did not occur with doses of 125 mg every 8 h. However, the satisfactory comparable results in series II (AMX, 500 mg; potassium clavulanate, 125 mg) and series III (AMX, 500 mg; potassium clavulanate, 250 mg) suggest that acceptable results may be obtained without the use of doses of clavulanic acid likely to produce intolerance. Both *E. coli* and *K. aerogenes* infections were eradicated in over two-thirds of patients in series II, results which are comparable to those expected with other agents in hospital infections. Of the 12 treatment failures in series II and III, 5 were due to inadequate β-lactamase inhibition by clavulanic acid and 5, including 2 withdrawn because of intolerance, failed as a result of clinical factors. Only 2 failures are unexplained.

It is concluded that combinations of clavulanic acid and AMX are effective in urinary infections due to AMX-resistant pathogens and that a combination of AMX (500 mg) and potassium clavulanate (125 mg) administered every 8 h for 7 days produces a satisfactory cure rate while avoiding intolerance.

We are grateful to Beecham Pharmaceuticals, United Kingdom Division, for the combination clavulanic acid/amoxicillin (Augmentin) tablets used in this study.

1. **Neu, H. C., and K. P. Fu.** 1978. Clavulanic acid, a novel inhibitor of β-lactamases. Antimicrob. Agents Chemother. **14**:650–655.
2. **Reading, C., and M. Cole.** 1977. Clavulanic acid: a beta-lactamase-inhibiting beta-lactam from *Streptomyces clavuligerus*. Antimicrob. Agents Chemother. **11**:852–857.

Evaluation of Amoxicillin With and Without BRL 14151 in the Treatment of Urinary Tract Infections

DANIEL STAMBOULIAN,* BEATRIZ SARACHIAN, EDUARDO ARGÜELLO, AND BEATRIZ BELFORTE

British Hospital of Buenos Aires, Buenos Aires, Argentina

BRL 14151 is a new β-lactam derivative produced by *Streptomyces clavuligerus* and named clavulanic acid (3). This compound, isolated as the sodium salt, resembles the nucleus of penicillin but differs in having no acylamino side chain, having oxygen instead of sulfur, and containing a β-hydroxyethylidine substituent in the oxozolidine ring (4). Sodium clavulanate is a potent irreversible inhibitor of many β-lactamases at very low concentrations. It inhibits the β-lactamases from resistant *Staphylococcus aureus*, *Haemophilus influenzae*, *Bacteroides*, and *Proteus* strains and plasmid-carrying strains of *Escherichia coli*, *Klebsiella*, *Salmonella*, *Shigella*, and *Neisseria*. The chromosomally mediated β-lactamases of *E. coli* and *Klebsiella*, and the cephalosporinase type found in *Pseudomonas aeruginosa* and *Enterobacter cloacae*, are less well inhibited (1). BRL 14151 alone has a broad spectrum but weak antibacterial activity. The addition of this compound to ampicillin or amoxicillin (AMX) produces a synergistic effect against many gram-negative β-lactamase–producing organisms.

In the present study we determined the safety and efficacy of a combination of sodium clavulanate (BRL 14151) with AMX after oral administration in patients with uncomplicated urinary tract infections due to organisms resistant to AMX but susceptible to AMX plus BRL 14151. Doses of 250 mg of AMX or 250 mg of AMX plus 50 or 125 mg of BRL 14151 were administered orally three times daily to 31 patients aged 20 to 69 years for up to 9 days according to a randomized double-blind comparative protocol. Patients were assigned to treatment groups in the sequence that they entered the trial.

In all cases the patients were clinically evaluated before, during, and after therapy, and standard laboratory measurements were obtained to check response, side effects, and appearance of any allergic reactions. All microorganisms isolated from the urine were resistant to ampicillin (10 μg) by the Kirby-Bauer disk method. In addition, these organisms were tested subsequently by the broth dilution method for their susceptibility to AMX alone and AMX plus BRL 14151.

Urine cultures with colony counts were carried out before therapy, on days 3 and 6 of therapy, less than 7 days after treatment, and 10 days after treatment. Those patients who failed to respond favorably within 2 days were withdrawn from the study. The bacteriological response to therapy was defined by the urine culture results as follows: success or cure, negative culture less than 7 days after treatment and during the long-term follow-up; relapse or persistence, reemergence of the initial pathogen or persistence during treatment or follow-up period; reinfection, appearance of a new pathogen.

The two treatment groups were well matched as regards age, sex, and diagnosis and were comparable in terms of the distribution of causative organisms. Cystitis and asymptomatic bacteriuria were observed in the majority of patients (27 of 31).

E. coli was the predominant pathogen isolated, infecting 8 of 11 patients (73%) in the AMX group and 13 of 18 (65%) in the AMX + BRL 14151 group. The other microorganisms were *Klebsiella pneumoniae* (3 and 6) and *Citrobacter freundii* in 1 patient in the second group.

In the AMX group negative urine cultures during treatment were found in 4 of 11 patients (36%) versus 17 of 18 (94%) in the AMX + BRL 14151 group. This difference was statistically highly significant (Fischer's test, $P < 0.01$). The four cases in the AMX group in which the organisms were eradicated from urine despite their resistance could be considered as spontaneous cure. This occurs frequently in uncomplicated urinary tract infections (2). The patient with persistent organisms in the clavulanic acid group turned out to be infected with *Klebsiella* strain resistant to AMX + BRL 14151 (MIC, 160 μg/ml).

Success and cure after therapy on short-term and long-term follow-up were obtained in 67% and 56%, respectively, in the AMX + BRL 14151 group (Table 1). When considering the percentage of therapeutic failure, we should bear in mind that 3 (17%) were reinfections. This fact is related to the host rather than to drug failure. Additionally, in our series we had many cases of asymptomatic bacteriurias and history of recurrent infections despite the treatments. Side effects were observed in four patients in the AMX + BRL 14151 group and none in the AMX group. Two had vomitings severe enough that treatment was discontinued, one patient had mild nausea, and one had mild diarrhea. No evidence of hepatic, renal, or hematopoietic toxicity was ever noted in any patient in either group. No allergic reactions were observed.

BRL 14151 in concentrations of 10 μg/ml combined with AMX (0.15 to 320 μg/ml) showed marked synergy (MIC ≤ 10 μg) against 90% of *E. coli* and 80% of *Klebsiella* strains (Table 2). The two strains of *Klebsiella* with little or no change in their susceptibility to AMX + BRL 14151 were reidentified as *Enterobacter aerogenes* by use of the API 20E system. It is known

TABLE 1. *Bacteriological results of amoxicillin plus BRL 14151 after therapy*

Time of culture after therapy	Negative culture	Relapse or persistence	Reinfection
Short-term follow-up (less than 7 days)	12 (67%)	3 (17%)	3 (17%)
Long-term follow-up (more than 7 days)	10 (56%)	5 (28%)	3 (17%)

TABLE 2. *Synergism of amoxicillin + BRL 14151 against gram-negative bacilli resistant to amoxicillin*[a]

Organism	Cumulative % inhibition by a concn (μg/ml)[b] of:											
	0.15	0.30	0.60	1.2	2.5	5	10	20	40	80	160	320
Escherichia coli (20 strains)	25	25	35	50	75	85	90	95	100			
Klebsiella pneumoniae (10 strains)	40	40	50	50	60	60	80	80	80	80	90	100
Citrobacter freundii (1 strain)										100		

[a] An amoxicillin concentration of 100 μl/ml or higher was required for inhibition of all strains.
[b] The concentrations shown are those of amoxicillin; in all cases they were combined with BRL 14151 at a concentration of 10 μg/ml.

that the addition of BRL 14151 to ampicillin or AMX has no effect on organisms such as *Citrobacter* and *Enterobacter*, as occurred in our patients. This is due to the production of chromosomally mediated β-lactamase by these organisms (1, 3).

In summary, the data obtained in this clinical study indicate, despite the small number of cases, that BRL 14151 added to AMX was safe and highly efficacious for the treatment of uncomplicated urinary tract infections caused by gram-negative organisms resistant to AMX. Side effects were related to the gastrointestinal tract but were not a serious problem. The in vitro study shows that BRL 14151 (10 μg/ml) combined with AMX had marked synergy against the majority of the responsible organisms isolated.

1. Brown, A. G., D. Butterworth, M. Cole, G. Hanscomb, J. D. Hood, and C. Reading. 1976. Naturally-occurring β-lactamase inhibitors with antibacterial activity. J. Antibiot. 20:668–669.
2. Kunin, C. M. 1974. Detection, prevention and management of urinary tract infections, 2nd ed. Lea & Febiger, Philadelphia.
3. Reading, C., and M. Cole. May 1977. Clavulanic acid: a beta-lactamase-inhibiting beta-lactam from *Streptomyces clavuligerus*. Antimicrob. Agents Chemother. 11:852–857.
4. Spratt, B. G., V. Jobanputra, and W. Zimmermann. 1977. Binding of thienamycin and clavulanic acid to the penicillin-binding proteins of *Escherichia coli* K-12. Antimicrob. Agents Chemother. 12:406–409.

Comparative In Vivo and In Vitro Activity of Two Novel β-Lactamase Inhibitors—Clavulanic Acid and CP-45,899

PAMELA A. HUNTER* AND JANE R. WEBB

Beecham Pharmaceuticals, Betchworth, England

CP-45,899, penicillanic acid sulfone (3), a semisynthetic β-lactamase inhibitor, was compared with clavulanic acid as a synergist with various labile β-lactam antibiotics in several in vitro and in vivo systems against a range of organisms.

The spectrum of inhibition of CP-45,899 against isolated β-lactamases has been shown by English et al. (3) to be similar to that of clavulanic acid (5). These findings have been confirmed in these laboratories by C. Reading (unpublished data). As with clavulanic acid (4), these β-lactamase–inhibitory properties result in a synergistic effect when CP-45,899 is used in conjunction with various labile β-lactam antibiotics (1, 3), but we have found these effects to be less marked than those seen with clavulanic acid both in vivo and in vitro.

In vitro activity against organisms producing R_{TEM}. A particular weakness, in spite of good activity against the isolated enzyme, was against organisms producing a plasmid-mediated β-lactamase of the R_{TEM} type. *Escherichia coli* (R_{TEM}) and *Klebsiella aerogenes* (R_{TEM}) strains were not rendered fully susceptible to ampicillin (Table 1), cefazolin, or cephaloridine, even in the presence of 10 μg of CP-45,899 per ml, whereas 2 to 5 μg of clavulanic acid per ml rendered such organisms fully susceptible to cefazolin and cephaloridine. Other organisms which can produce the R_{TEM} β-lactamase are *Haemophilus influenzae* and *Neisseria gonorrhoeae*. Against these organisms we found CP-45,899 to be less potent than clavulanic acid as a synergist with ampicillin, carbenicillin, and benzylpenicillin, particularly when heavy inocula were used.

Stability in the presence of R_{TEM} β-lactamase. The reason for this lower activity against organisms producing R_{TEM} is most probably the reduced stability of CP-45,899 in the

TABLE 1. *In vitro activity of ampicillin alone and in the presence of CP-45,899 or clavulanic acid against β-lactamase–producing organisms* [a]

Organism (no. of strains)	Method[b]	Geometric mean MIC (µg/ml) of ampicillin									
		Alone	+ CP-45,899 at a concn (µg/ml) of:					+ Clavulanic acid at a concn (µg/ml) of:			
			0.5	1.0	2.5	5	10	0.5	1.0	2.5	5
B. fragilis (8)	A	>80	80	61.7	18.3	—	—	10	5.45	2.5	—
B. fragilis (12)	A	37.8	1.67	1.13	0.79	—	—	0.94	0.83	0.83	—
E. coli[c] (6)	B	>2,000	—	>500	—	500	201	—	69	—	12
H. influenzae (15)	C	>320	—	>40	30.3	3.5		—	1.81	0.72	0.31
K. aerogenes (6)	B	500	—	27	—	7.0	2.7	—	2.3	—	1.7
K. aerogenes[c] (6)	B	>2,000	—	>500	—	>500	315	—	55.7	—	15.6
N. gonorrhoeae (6)	D	>40	2.24	—	—	—	—	0.22	—	—	—
P. mirabilis (3)	B	>2,000	—	125	—	11	4	—	27	—	2.8
P. vulgaris (3)	B	2,000	—	31	—	7.8	4.9	—	4.9	—	2.4
S. aureus (9)	E	296	23	10	3.4	1.25	—	1.6	0.92	0.43	0.06

[a] MICs of CP-45,899 and clavulanic acid alone were >40 µg/ml and >20 µg/ml, respectively (except against *N. gonorrhoeae*).

[b] (A) Serial dilution in DST agar plus 5% horse blood. Inoculum heavy (undiluted 48-h broth culture). Incubation in H_2/CO_2 (GasPak BBL Microbiology Systems). (B) Microtiter technique. Medium: tryptic soy broth. Inoculum heavy (final dilution 1:500 of overnight broth culture). (C) Serial dilution in "chocolate" agar (DST plus 5% horse blood) plus 1% Difco supplement B. Inoculum moderate (ca. 10^5 colony-forming units/ml). Incubation in 10% CO_2. (D) Serial dilution in "chocolate" agar plus 1% Difco supplement B. Inoculum heavy (ca. 10^6 colony forming units/ml). Incubation in 10% CO_2. (E) Microtiter technique. Medium: brain heart infusion. Inoculum heavy (final dilution 1:500 of overnight broth culture).

[c] Strains producing plasmid-mediated β-lactamase.

presence of this enzyme, and not lack of penetration as has been suggested by English et al. (5) and Aswapokee and Neu (1). Using a 6-h culture of a strain of *E. coli* producing the R_{TEM} β-lactamase, we found 50 µg of CP-45,899 per ml to be degraded rapidly; 30 min after addition of CP-45,899 to the culture, only 33% remained, and by 1 h less than 10% was detected. Under the same conditions, >75% of clavulanic acid remained after 6 h (Table 2). The compounds were assayed by a β-lactamase-inhibition microbiological assay technique described previously (2).

Activity against other organisms in vitro. Both CP-45,899 and clavulanic acid lack good inhibitory activity against β-lactamases which are predominantly active against cephalosporins (3, 5). Consequently, both compounds have little effect on the activity of ampicillin and cephaloridine against organisms producing such enzymes, e.g., *Enterobacter* spp., *Citrobacter freundii*, *Serratia marcescens*, *Proteus morganii*, *P. rettgeri*, and *E. coli* (non-plasmid-carrying strains). *Bacteroides fragilis* strains show a bimodal distribution in their resistance to ampicillin, some strains having a high degree of resistance. Against these highly resistant strains CP-45,899 at <2.5 µg/ml had little effect on the activity of ampicillin (Table 1), whereas even 1 µg of clavulanic acid per ml did have an effect. However, against the less resistant

TABLE 2. *Comparative stability of CP-45,899 and clavulanic acid in the presence of an E. coli R_{TEM} broth culture*

Time (h)	Percent remaining[a]			
	Clavulanic acid		CP-45,899	
	+ R_{TEM}[b]	− R_{TEM}[c]	+ R_{TEM}	− R_{TEM}
0.5	98	89	33	100
1	87	90	≈5	97
2	80	95	<5	91
6	78	97	<5	100

[a] Starting concentration, 50 µg/ml.
[b] Tryptone soy broth culture containing *E. coli* R_{TEM}.
[c] Sterile tryptone soy broth control.

strains, CP-45,899 was more effective, although still not equal to clavulanic acid in activity. Against *Klebsiella aerogenes* (non-plasmid-carrying strains) and *Staphylococcus aureus*, when used in conjunction with ampicillin, levels of CP-45,899 below 5 µg/ml had a poor effect, and even 5 µg/ml did not equal the effect seen with 1 µg of clavulanic acid per ml. Only against *P. mirabilis* and *P. vulgaris* strains did CP-45,899 plus ampicillin approach clavulanic acid plus ampicillin in activity (Table 1).

Activity with ticarcillin in vitro. When CP-45,899 was used with ticarcillin, synergistic effects were seen only at high concentrations (5 to 10 μg/ml) against ticarcillin-resistant strains of *Providencia alcalifaciens, Pseudomonas aeruginosa*, and *S. marcescens*. However, these synergistic effects were less than the effects seen with lower concentrations of clavulanic acid (e.g., in the presence of 10 μg of CP-45,899 per ml MICs of ticarcillin ranged from 62 μg/ml against *P. alcalifaciens* to 2,000 μg/ml against *P. aeruginosa* Dalgleish, whereas in the presence of 5 μg of clavulanic acid per ml the corresponding values were 8 and 125 μg/ml).

Activity against *S. aureus* determined with a biophotometer. The comparative effects of CP-45,899 and clavulanic acid on the activity of ampicillin against a log-phase culture of a β-lactamase–producing strain of *S. aureus* were studied by use of a biophotometer. Ampicillin alone at 1 μg/ml had little effect, only delaying the development of turbidity by 1.5 h. When clavulanic acid at 0.5 μg/ml was added to the ampicillin, no growth occurred over a 24-h period. However, the addition of CP-45,899 at 0.5 μg/ml had only a marginal effect, allowing turbidity to develop by 3 h, and even 1 μg/ml allowed growth after 18 h. With concentrations of ampicillin below 1 μg/ml, the levels of CP-45,899 required to prevent the development of turbidity were in excess of the ampicillin concentration, whereas clavulanic acid was still effective at lower concentrations.

In vivo activity—acute intraperitoneal infections. In vivo experiments with acute intraperitoneal mouse infections confirmed the in vitro findings. Using various infecting organisms, we determined the 50% curative dose (CD_{50}, milligrams per kilogram) of ampicillin alone and in the presence of CP-45,899 or clavulanic acid. The compounds were administered by the subcutaneous route at 1 and 5 h postinfection. Against a strain of *S. aureus* the CD_{50} of ampicillin alone was >1,000 mg/kg. In the presence of 5 mg of clavulanic acid per kg the CD_{50} of amoxicillin was reduced to 1.1 mg/kg, whereas 5 mg of CP-45,899 per kg only reduced the CD_{50} of ampicillin to 100 mg/kg. Against a *K. aerogenes* infection the difference between the compounds, although less, was still significant. Ampicillin alone had a slight effect, with a CD_{50} of 440 mg/kg; at a dose of 2 mg/kg, CP-45,899 reduced this figure to 120 mg/kg while clavulanic acid reduced it to 36 mg/kg. When the inhibitor dosage was increased to 10 mg/kg, CP-45,899

reduced the ampicillin CD_{50} to 38 mg/kg and clavulanic acid reduced it to 20 mg/kg. When the infecting organism was a strain of *E. coli* producing the R_{TEM} β-lactamase, as would be anticipated from the in vitro results, no effect was seen with CP-45,899, whereas clavulanic acid had a marked effect even at doses as low as 1 mg/kg. Only against a *Proteus vulgaris* infection did CP-45,899 plus ampicillin show activity that almost equalled that of clavulanic acid plus ampicillin. Inhibitor doses of 5 mg/kg reduced the CD_{50} of ampicillin from >1,000 mg/kg alone to 35 mg/kg with CP-45,899 and 29 mg/kg with clavulanic acid.

In vivo activity—subacute infections. Further studies were made with the use of a *S. aureus* localized mouse thigh lesion model. Compounds were administered subcutaneously at 1, 3, and 5 h postinfection, and the infected thighs were measured over a period of 6 days. By comparing the average thigh sizes of treated groups with an infected control group and a noninfected control group, percent protection was calculated. Ampicillin alone at 25 mg/kg had a negligible effect, as did the inhibitors alone. When ampicillin was administered with CP-45,899, even at equal doses (each at 25 mg/kg), the protective effect was less than complete (72%). Lowering the dose of inhibitor produced a corresponding reduction in the protective effect of the ampicillin. Clavulanic acid was considerably more effective, since a dose of only 6.25 mg/kg plus ampicillin at 25 mg/kg produced 82% protection.

1. **Aswapokee, N., and H. C. Neu.** 1978. A sulfone β-lactam compound which acts as a β-lactamase inhibitor. J. Antibiot. **31**:1238–1244.
2. **Brown, A. G., D. Butterworth, M. Cole, G. Hanscomb, J. D. Hood, C. Reading, and G. N. Rolinson.** 1976. Naturally-occurring β-lactamase inhibitors with antibacterial activity. J. Antibiot. **29**:668–669.
3. **English, A. R., J. A. Retsema, A. E. Girard, J. E. Lynch, and W. E. Barth.** 1978. CP-45,899, a beta-lactamase inhibitor that extends the antibacterial spectrum of beta-lactams: initial bacteriological characterization. Antimicrob. Agents Chemother. **14**:414–419.
4. **Hunter, P. A., K. Coleman, J. Fisher, D. Taylor, and E. Taylor.** 1979. Clavulanic acid, a novel β-lactam with broad spectrum β-lactamase inhibitory properties. Synergistic activity with ampicillin and amoxycillin. Drugs Under Exp. Clin. Res. **5**:1–6.
5. **Reading, C., and M. Cole.** 1977. Clavulanic acid: a beta-lactamase-inhibiting beta-lactam from *Streptomyces clavuligerus*. Antimicrob. Agents Chemother. **11**:852–857.

Activity of Amoxicillin/Clavulanic Acid (2:1) [BRL 25000, Augmentin] In Vitro and In Vivo

K. R. COMBER, R. HORTON, LINDA MIZEN, A. R. WHITE, AND R. SUTHERLAND*

Beecham Pharmaceuticals Research Division, Betchworth, Surrey, England

Clavulanic acid is a progressive inhibitor of β-lactamases produced by many strains of gram-negative and gram-positive bacteria (1, 3) and is capable of protecting β-lactam antibiotics from inactivation by these bacteria (2, 3). Bioavailability studies in animals and in human volunteers have shown that clavulanic acid is well absorbed by the oral route and that its pharmacokinetics are comparable with those of amoxicillin (AMX). For instance, after oral administration to human volunteers serum concentrations of clavulanic acid are similar to the antibiotic levels produced by equivalent doses of AMX (Beecham Research Laboratories, unpublished data). This paper describes the properties of an AMX/clavulanic acid formulation containing two parts of AMX to one part of clavulanic acid (BRL 25000, Augmentin).

In vitro activity. The results in Table 1 show typical MICs of BRL 25000 (AMX/clavulanic acid, 2:1), AMX, and clavulanic acid against a range of AMX-susceptible and AMX-resistant strains of gram-negative and gram-positive bacteria. MICs were determined after 18 h at 37°C by serial dilution of the compounds in Mueller-Hinton agar. The inoculum, 0.001 ml of an undiluted overnight broth culture of the test organism (approximately 5×10^5 cells), was applied to the agar by use of a multipoint inoculator (Denley, Billingshurst, England).

In general, the formulation showed the activity that would be expected from its AMX content against bacteria susceptible to AMX, and there was no evidence of antagonism between AMX and clavulanic acid against these bacteria. Clavulanic acid showed a low, relatively uniform order of activity against most of these AMX-susceptible organisms, with the exception of the gonococcus, which was relatively susceptible, and was unlikely to have contributed to the antibacterial activity of the formulation. A significant number of β-lactamase–producing bacteria resistant to AMX were susceptible to AMX plus clavulanic acid as a result of the β-lactamase–inhibitory activity of clavulanic acid. These bacteria included strains of *Escherichia coli*, *Klebsiella aerogenes*, *Proteus mirabilis*, *P. vulgaris*, *Haemophilus influenzae*, *Neisseria gonorrhoeae*, *Staphylococcus aureus*, and *Bacteroides fragilis*. On the other hand, against

AMX-resistant bacteria producing β-lactamases not inhibited by clavulanic acid, the formulation was no more active than would be expected from the activities of the individual constituents. These bacteria included strains of *Enterobacter* sp., *Providencia* sp., *Proteus morganii*, *P. rettgeri*, *Pseudomonas aeruginosa*, and *Serratia marcescens*.

There was good correlation ($r = 0.94$) between MICs and inhibition zone diameters produced by a susceptibility disk containing 30 μg of BRL 25000 (AMX, 20 μg; clavulanic acid, 10 μg) against 145 strains of gram-negative and gram-positive bacteria in the FDA/NCCLS standardized susceptibility test.

Antibacterial activity in vivo. AMX/clavulanic acid was shown to be effective in the treatment of experimental infections resistant to treatment with AMX. The results in Table 2 compare the median protective doses (PD_{50}) of BRL 25000, AMX, and clavulanic acid against AMX-susceptible and AMX-resistant bacteria.

TABLE 1. *Antibacterial spectrum of BRL 25000 (amoxicillin/clavulanic acid [2:1]), amoxicillin, and clavulanic acid*

Organism	MIC (μg/ml)		
	BRL 25000	Amoxicillin	Clavulanic acid
Escherichia coli	5.0	5.0	50
E. coli[a]	25	>500	50
Klebsiella aerogenes	2.5	125	50
Proteus mirabilis	1.25	1.25	125
P. mirabilis[a]	12.5	>500	125
P. morganii	250	500	125
P. vulgaris	5.0	>500	125
Pseudomonas aeruginosa	250	>500	125
Enterobacter cloacae	125	500	125
Serratia marcescens	125	125	125
Bacteroides fragilis	1.25	25	50
Haemophilus influenzae	0.25	0.25	12.5
H. influenzae[a]	1.25	>50	>50
Neisseria gonorrhoeae	0.01	0.005	1.25
N. gonorrhoeae[a]	1.25	>10	5.0
Staphylococcus aureus	0.1	0.05	25
S. aureus[a]	2.5	125	25
Streptococcus pyogenes	0.01	0.01	25
S. pneumoniae	0.02	0.02	12.5
S. faecalis	0.5	0.5	250

[a] β-Lactamase-producing strain.

TABLE 2. *Activity of BRL 25000 (amoxicillin/clavulanic acid [2:1]), amoxicillin, and clavulanic acid against intraperitoneal infections in mice*

Organism	PD$_{50}$ (mg/kg)		
	BRL 25000	Amoxicillin	Clavu-lanic acid
Staphylococcus aureus Smith	0.35	0.23	96
Escherichia coli 8	25	25	>200
E. coli JT39	114	>1,000	340
Klebsiella aerogenes T767	84	>2,000	>2,000
K. pneumoniae 62	400	>3,200	>3,200
Proteus mirabilis 889	280	>1,000	>1,000
P. vulgaris E	120	>1,000	>1,000

In these tests, the mice were infected intraperitoneally with an infective inoculum (10 to 100 median lethal doses) of the bacteria suspended in hog gastric mucin, the compounds were administered by the oral route 1 and 5 h after infection, and the PD$_{50}$ values were calculated after 4 days.

As was the case in vitro, clavulanic acid alone showed little activity, and the formulation showed the activity to be expected from its AMX content against infections due to the AMX-susceptible strains, *S. aureus* Smith and *E. coli* 8. However, the formulation of AMX plus clavulanic acid was significantly more effective than AMX against the infections due to the β-lactamase–producing bacteria which had failed to respond to AMX therapy. BRL 25000 was also efficacious against various other mouse experimental infection models. For instance, the formulation was as effective as cephalexin in the treatment of a pyelonephritis due to an amoxicillin-resistant strain of *E. coli* and as effective as cefazolin against a respiratory infection caused by *K. pneumoniae*. Also, BRL 25000 was active against a localized groin infection produced by subcutaneous injection of *B. fragilis* (4) and was more effective than cefoxitin in reducing the bacterial counts in groin tissue.

Bioavailability and tissue distribution in animals. In bioavailability studies with the formulation of AMX plus clavulanic acid in rats, mice, dogs, and squirrel monkeys, clavulanic acid was absorbed by the oral route to the same extent as AMX. There was no evidence of interaction between the two compounds, and the serum levels and urinary excretion values obtained in dogs after administration of BRL 25000 were similar to those measured after administration of the individual constituents.

After oral administration of BRL 25000 to rats, clavulanic acid and AMX were distributed in a similar fashion throughout body tissues. At 1 h after dosing, the ratio of AMX to clavulanic acid ranged from 1.5 to 4.0 in serum and tissues. Clavulanic acid penetrated more rapidly than AMX into silastic tissue cages implanted subcutaneously in rats, and proportionally higher concentrations of clavulanic acid were found in tissue cage fluid up to 2 h after dosing. Serum and tissue cage fluid levels of clavulanic acid and AMX were similar after administration of BRL 25000 to those found when the compounds were administered separately.

Conclusion. This specific formulation of AMX and clavulanic acid has been undergoing limited clinical trials, and the results of treatment of urinary tract and respiratory tract infections have been encouraging. As expected from the experimental data described briefly here, the clinical results with AMX/clavulanic acid show it to be effective in the treatment of various infections due to β-lactamase–producing bacteria.

1. **Brown, A. G., D. Butterworth, M. Cole, G. Hanscomb, J. D. Hood, C. Reading, and G. N. Rolinson.** 1976. Naturally occurring β-lactamase inhibitors with antibacterial activity. J. Antibiot. **29**:668–669.
2. **Hunter, P. A., C. Reading, and D. A. Witting.** 1978. In vitro and in vivo properties of BRL 14151, a novel β-lactam with β-lactamase-inhibiting properties, p. 478–480. *In* Current chemotherapy, Proceedings of the 10th International Congress of Chemotherapy. American Society for Microbiology, Washington, D.C.
3. **Reading, C., and M. Cole.** 1977. Clavulanic acid: a beta-lactamase-inhibiting beta-lactam from *Streptomyces clavuligerus.* Antimicrob. Agents Chemother. **11**:852–857.
4. **Walker, C. B., and T. D. Wilkins.** 1976. Use of semisolid agar for initiation of pure *Bacteroides fragilis* infection in mice. Infect. Immun. **14**:721–725.

Clavulanic Acid: Human Pharmacokinetics and Penetration into Cerebrospinal Fluid

REINER MÜNCH,* RUEDI LÜTHY, JÜRG BLASER, AND WALTER SIEGENTHALER

Department of Medicine, University of Zürich,* Institute for Biomedical Engineering, University of Zürich, and Federal Institute of Technology, CH-8091 Zürich, Switzerland

Clavulanic acid, a product of *Streptomyces clavuligerus*, acts as an irreversible inhibitor of many clinically important β-lactamases of Richmond types II, III, IV, and V (3, 4). Few data are available on human pharmacokinetics after oral administration of clavulanic acid, and there are no data on its penetration into human cerebrospinal fluid (CSF). The aim of our study was (i) to report on pharmacokinetics after oral administration of 250 mg of clavulanic acid, (ii) to study its entry into CSF of human adults without meningeal inflammation, and (iii) to obtain some information on its in vitro stability.

Of the 22 patients (7 females, 15 males) who took part in our investigations, 18 were studied for CSF penetration of clavulanic acid; 15 of the 18 received a diagnostic lumbar puncture and 3 had a continuous CSF drainage after a neurosurgical procedure. In the remaining 4 patients, only serum and urine concentrations were measured. All subjects fasted for at least 4 h before and up to 1 h after ingestion of clavulanic acid.

A single dose of 250 mg of clavulanic acid was given to 21 subjects, and 1 subject received five doses of 250 mg at 6-h intervals. Blood samples were drawn before and 20, 40, 60, and 90 min after administration and at the time of CSF collection. If possible, further samples were drawn 120, 180, 240, and 360 min after administration of the drug. CSF samples obtained by a lumbar puncture were drawn at various time intervals after oral administration of clavulanic acid (Fig. 1, upper panel). Sampling schedules of blood and CSF in the neurosurgical patient studied on a multiple-dose regimen are indicated in Fig. 2. Three of 15 patients who underwent a lumbar puncture showed elevated CSF protein concentrations, with 40, 61, and >100 mg/100 ml (normal range, ≤34 mg/100 ml), whereas all cell counts were within the normal range (≤5/mm³).

In two of three neurosurgical patients with continuous CSF drainage, routine CSF analyses were done. In both cases, CSF protein concentrations were elevated (198 and 310 mg/100 ml). In one of these two patients the CSF cell count was 167/mm³, whereas it was normal in the other. Specimens were stored at −196°C and assayed within 1 week by a slightly modified

large agar plate method, using a β-lactamase-producing strain of *Klebsiella aerogenes*.

The results of the degradation studies showed a time-dependent loss of activity of clavulanic acid which was best described by an exponential function and which seemed to be related to temperature and pH. In pooled human serum a loss of activity of 4.2 ± 1.0%/h could be observed at room temperature, while at 37°C the mean degradation rate was 11.2 ± 0.1%/h. At 37°C the loss of activity of clavulanic acid averaged 6.5 ± 0.8%/h and 10.9 ± 1.9%/h in phosphate buffer of pH 7 and 5, respectively.

The mean serum concentration time course after ingestion of clavulanic acid is shown in Fig. 1 (lower panel). The serum level averaged 4.3 ± 2.2 μg/ml (range, 0.1 to 9.5 μg) after 60 min. Individual peak serum concentrations were reached between 40 and 60 min. The observed wide range in peak serum concentrations may be due to an interindividual variability in gastrointestinal absorption and/or in vivo degra-

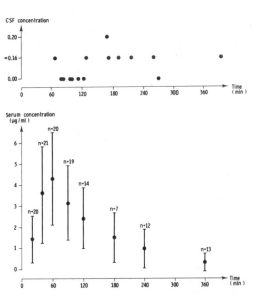

FIG. 1. *Serum concentrations ($\bar{x}$ ± SD) and CSF concentrations obtained by lumbar puncture after oral administration of 250 mg of clavulanic acid to the indicated number of patients.*

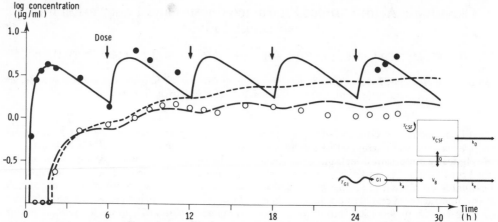

FIG. 2. *Measured serum (●) and CSF (○) concentration time courses in one patient with a continuous CSF drainage studied in a multiple-dose regimen. Measured clavulanic acid concentrations in serum and CSF during the first 6 h were analyzed with a linear multicompartment model with two constant parameters (volume of CSF, V_{CSF} = 0.135 liter; CSF degradation rate, k_D = 10%/h) and six variable parameters (τ_{GI} = gastrointestinal absorption lag time; τ_{CSF} = CSF lag time; V_B = volume of distribution minus V_{CSF} (liters); Q = transfer constant (liters/h), k_a = absorption rate constant; k_e = elimination rate constant). Curves: ——————, fitted serum concentration time course; -----, fitted CSF concentration time course (no CSF degradation of clavulanic acid); – – –, fitted CSF concentration time course incorporating an hourly degradation rate of 10%.*

dation. Urinary excretion after 300 to 400 min ranged from 0.8 to 54.3% of the administered dose. The three patients with peak serum concentrations of <2 µg/ml had a urinary recovery during the first 6 h of <5% of the administered dose, indicating a very poor absorption in these three patients.

Data on 14 patients were sufficient (more than five measurable serum concentrations) for pharmacokinetic analysis with a one-compartment open model. The pharmacokinetic parameters of the model were adapted to the experimental serum concentration time course with a nonlinear fitting program (C. M. Metzler, G. L. Elfring, and A. J. McEwen, A Users Manual for NONLIN and Associated Programs, Research Biostatistics, The Upjohn Co., Kalamazoo, Mich., 1974). The terminal serum half-life averaged 52 ± 28 min (range, 35 to 151 min), which is comparable to most penicillins (1). The absorption rate constant (k_a) averaged 2.6 ± 1.1 h^{-1} (range, 1.2 to 4.7 h^{-1}), and the lag time between ingestion and appearance of the drug in serum (τ_{GI}) was 16 ± 9 min (range, 9 to 34 min). No remarkable differences in drug absorption velocity were observed regardless of the form of administration (capsules or dissolved drug).

Penetration of clavulanic acid into CSF in patients with noninflamed meninges was only minimal (Fig. 1, upper panel). In only 1 of 15 patients was the measured CSF concentration of clavulanic acid, 0.2 µg/ml, within the range of

the standards. In 7 of 15 patients no clavulanic acid was detected in CSF, and in 7 clavulanic acid was detectable but was below the lowest standard concentration (0.16 µg/ml) and had to be extrapolated.

In contrast to these findings, CSF concentrations of clavulanic acid were considerably higher in neurosurgical patients with a continuous CSF drainage. In both patients who received a single dose, equalization between the serum and CSF concentration time course was attained after approximately 220 min. Peak CSF concentrations were measured 240 min after administration of clavulanic acid. At that time CSF concentrations were 2.42 µg/ml for one patient and 0.38 µg/ml for the other; the corresponding serum levels were 2.27 µg/ml and 0.32 µg/ml, respectively. In contrast to these patients, no such equalization was observed during the first 6 h in the multiple-dose study (Fig. 2). This may be attributed to a lower drug penetration into CSF. The higher penetration of clavulanic acid into the CSF of the neurosurgical patients may be due to a difference in permeability of the blood-brain barrier in the postsurgical period, a hypothesis which is supported by elevated CSF protein levels in two patients (2).

Another interesting result of the multiple-dose trial was that modelling of CSF concentrations appeared improved when the in vitro degradation rate of clavulanic acid was incorporated as one route of elimination into the pharmacokinetic model (Fig. 2). According to the measured loss of activity at 37°C in pooled human serum, a degradation in CSF of 10%/h was assumed for the model. This procedure is capable of predicting accurately CSF concentration time courses. Without considering any degradation of clavulanic acid in CSF, equalization between serum and CSF would occur after approximately 12 h. The differences between measured and predicted serum concentrations in the multiple-dose study probably reflect an intraindividual variability of gastrointestinal absorption of clavulanic acid (Fig. 2). In conclusion, oral absorption of clavulanic acid shows remarkable inter- and intraindividual variability. The serum half-life of clavulanic acid is comparable to that of other penicillins and, as with other β-lactam antibiotics, penetration through intact meninges is poor. Disturbance of the blood-brain barrier,

as shown in the neurosurgical patients, results in better drug penetration. The present observations need to be confirmed by CSF measurements of clavulanic acid concentrations in patients with meningeal inflammation.

1. **Barza, M., and L. Weinstein.** 1976. Pharmacokinetics of the penicillins in man. Clin. Pharmacokinetics 1:297–308.
2. **Davson, H.** 1967. Blood-brain and blood-CSF barriers: further considerations, p. 224–315. *In* H. Davson (ed.), Physiology of the cerebrospinal fluid. J. and A. Churchill Ltd., London.
3. **Neu, H. C., and K. P. Fu.** 1978. Clavulanic acid, a novel inhibitor of β-lactamases. Antimicrob. Agents Chemother. 14:650–655.
4. **Reading, C., and M. Cole.** 1977. Clavulanic acid: a beta-lactamase-inhibiting beta-lactam from *Streptomyces clavuligerus.* Antimicrob. Agents Chemother. 11:852–857.

Clinical Trial of Clavulanic Acid/Amoxicillin Formulation in Urinary Tract Infections

D. S. REEVES,* P. J. ELLIOTT, H. A. HOLT, Z. MOJADDEDI, AND S. T. CHAPMAN

Department of Medical Microbiology, Southmead Hospital, Bristol BS10 5NB, England

Broad-spectrum penicillins have for many years been used successfully for the treatment of urinary infections due to coliforms. Since their introduction, an increasing number of strains of otherwise susceptible species, such as *Escherichia coli*, have been resistant to these penicillins, usually as a result of the production of β-lactamase. Clavulanic acid is a potent, irreversible inhibitor of β-lactamases and thus is of potential interest as an agent to combine with β-lactamase–unstable β-lactam antibiotics. It is a particularly efficient inhibitor of TEM-type β-lactamases, which are the ones most frequently found in *E. coli, Haemophilus influenzae,* and *Neisseria gonorrhoeae* (3). Clavulanic acid is a naturally occurring β-lactam compound (1) with only weak intrinsic antibacterial activity and is absorbed after oral administration as the potassium or sodium salt.

The aims of our study were to assess the efficacy of a clavulanic acid/amoxicillin (AMX) formulation (Augmentin, BRL 25000) as treatment for urinary infections in hospitalized patients, its tolerability, any toxic effects, and its pharmacology. The overall study design was open and noncomparative. The patients came from various services of the hospital. Many of the infections were asymptomatic, being discov-

ered on routine examination of the urine. All the patients were admitted for conditions other than urinary infection, and most had serious underlying disease or had recently undergone surgery, sometimes of the urinary tract. The criterion for commencing treatment was the finding of a significant bacteriuria ($\geq 10^5$ colony-forming units/ml), the isolated bacteria being susceptible to clavulanic acid/AMX on disk testing. Disks contained 10 μg of clavulanic acid plus 20 μg of AMX. The criterion of infection for determining efficacy was significant bacteriuria with the same bacterial species in two successive midstream urines. A single isolate was accepted from catheter specimens and from patients with symptoms referable to the urinary tract. Patients were not included in the study if they were less than 16 years of age, were hypersensitive to β-lactam drugs, or were pregnant or possibly pregnant.

The first 18 patients were treated with a dosage of one tablet of clavulanic acid/AMX every 8 h for 5 days; each tablet contained 125 mg of sodium clavulanate plus 250 mg of AMX trihydrate. Later, a formulation with the potassium salt became available which appeared to give better absorption. The dosage for the remaining 12 patients was increased to two tablets every 8 h to see whether an improvement in efficacy followed and whether tolerability was as good as at the lower dose.

Assessment of tolerability and any side effects was by a physician questioning the patient before, during, and after therapy. Hematological and biochemical screening tests were done before and after therapy.

To assess the pharmacokinetics of clavulanic acid/AMX under more controlled conditions than its administration to patients would allow, we administered two tablets of clavulanic acid (potassium salt)/AMX to four healthy volunteers in a fasting state. Blood and urine samples were collected at the times indicated below.

Quantitation and identification of bacterial isolates were performed by standard laboratory techniques. Isolates were subcultured, saved, and used for confirmation of species (and type, when necessary) and of susceptibility to antimicrobials. Toxicological screening tests were done by standard automated methods. Clavulanic acid was assayed microbiologically by a large-plate method. The indicator strain was a multiresistant *Klebsiella aerogenes* surface inoculated to give a confluent growth on Oxoid DST agar containing penicillin (60 mg/liter). The ranges of standards were 0.5 to 8 mg/liter for serum and 1 to 16 mg/liter for urine, which was usually diluted in buffer. Preincubation was for 1 h at 4°C, followed by incubation at 37°C for 18 h. AMX was assayed microbiologically by a large-plate method with the use of *Bacillus subtilis* (NCTC 10,400) incorporated into Difco Penassay seed agar.

Of the 30 patients so far entered into the study, 25 were female (mean age, 66 years; range, 26 to 89 years) and 5 were male (55 years; 28 to 65 years). Because of the difficulties of collecting high-quality midstream urines from ill patients, in only 21 of the 30 patients was the infection confirmed on the second midstream urine, and only these patients were included in assessing efficacy. Their infecting bacteria were *E. coli* in 11 (6 AMX-resistant), *Proteus mirabilis* in 5 (1 resistant), *Streptococcus faecalis* in 1, *Staphylococcus aureus* in 1, group B streptococcus in 1, and *E. coli* plus *S. faecalis* in 2 (coliforms both resistant).

Bacteriological cure (Table 1) was taken as the eradication (or $<10^3$ colony-forming units/ml) of the original infecting organism; a reinfection with a different strain was not taken as a failure. Although the numbers were small, there was a trend for greater efficacy with the larger dose of clavulanic acid/AMX. Ten of 30 patients had symptoms referable to the urinary tract before therapy; in 8 (80%) they resolved.

Of 18 patients taking one tablet every 8 h, 1 had mild indigestion, 1 had a slight skin rash, and 1 vomited once, dubiously related to the drug. On the high dosage (12 patients), 2 had nausea (1 with vomiting which improved on lowering doses to one tablet), 1 patient had diarrhea, and 1 had a slight skin rash. In no patient was treatment discontinued. On the lower dose, of 13 patients with pairs of samples, 4 had mild rises in liver enzymes, 2 being attributable to primary illness; on the higher dose (9 pairs), the figures were 3 and 2, respectively. No patients showed hematological abnormalities not readily explainable by underlying disease.

Blood concentrations of clavulanic acid in 14

TABLE 1. *Bacteriological results of treatment with clavulanic acid/amoxicillin*

| Group | No. of patients cured | | | |
| | 2 weeks after entry | | 6 weeks after entry | |
	Assessable	Cured	Assessable	Cured
Patients on doses of one tablet	14	9 (64%)	13	8 (62%)
Patients on doses of two tablets	6	5 (83%)	4	3 (75%)
Patients with amoxicillin-resistant bacteria	9	6 (67%)	7	3 (43%)
Patients with urethral catheter	9	7 (78%)	8	6 (75%)
All patients	20	14 (70%)	17	11 (65%)

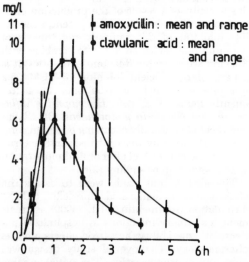

FIG. 1. *Blood concentrations of clavulanic acid and amoxicillin in four fasting volunteers taking 250 mg of potassium clavulanate/500 mg of amoxicillin.*

patients were, after dosing with the initial one tablet: at 0.5 h, 0.3 (range 0 to 1.3) mg/liter; at 1 h, 1.2 (0 to 2.7) mg/liter; at 2 h, 2.0 (0.6 to 5.1) mg/liter; at 4 h, 1.3 (0 to 3.9) mg/liter; and at 8 h, 0.4 (0 to 1.0) mg/liter. The mean urine concentration of clavulanic acid in 52 collections of 8-h duration taken during the first 48 h of treatment was 34 mg/liter (range, 0 to 141 mg/liter). Mean excretion was 17 mg (0 to 81 mg), 14% of the dose given. These figures are undoubtedly low because of the instability of clavulanic acid at room temperature and difficulties in ensuring that urines arrived promptly in the laboratory. In volunteers the mean peak concentration of clavulanic acid (6.1 mg/liter) was more than twice that in the patients (2.0 mg/liter) who received half the dose (Fig. 1). The urinary recovery (28%) was also significantly higher; that for AMX was 71%.

In an on-going trial we have found clavulanic acid/AMX to be efficacious in curing urinary infections in a difficult group of patients, comparing well with other therapies investigated by us (2, 5). Future patients will be treated with two tablets every 8 h since the results so far suggest that this could be a better treatment than the lower dose. The relatively high cure rate in patients with infecting bacteria resistant to AMX is encouraging. Although a group treated with AMX alone would be desirable as a comparison, ethical considerations made this difficult. The treatment was well tolerated, particularly at the lower dosage, with which side effects were no more frequent than might have been expected with any broad-spectrum penicillin. In our experience, unexplained mild rises in liver enzymes are not uncommon in ill patients.

The results of the toxicity screening tests were therefore unremarkable.

Blood concentrations of clavulanic acid in patients on the smaller dose were low, but urine concentrations were sufficient to potentiate the activity of AMX to inhibitory levels against most strains of coliforms (4). There were technical reasons why the urinary concentrations may have been higher. In volunteers we demonstrated a greater urinary recovery of clavulanic acid and significantly higher blood concentrations. Certainly, for tissue infections due to coliforms, we believe that the two-tablet dose at least would be necessary for giving potentiation against coliforms. This dose would probably also be necessary for infections in sites where access of antibiotics is difficult, such as bronchial infections, even though respiratory pathogens may be inhibited in vitro by lower concentrations of clavulanic acid with AMX.

1. Howarth, T. T. A., A. G. Brown, and T. J. King. 1976. Clavulanic acid, a novel β-lactam isolated from Streptomyces clavuligerus. J. Chem. Soc. Chem. Commun., p. 266–267.
2. Leigh, D. A., D. S. Reeves, K. Simmons, A. L. Thomas, and P. J. Wilkinson. 1976. Talampicillin: a new derivative of ampicillin. Br. Med. J. 3:1378–1380.
3. Reading, C., and M. Cole. 1977. Clavulanic acid: a beta-lactamase-inhibiting beta-lactam from Streptomyces clavuligerus. Antimicrob. Agents Chemother. 11:852–857.
4. Reeves, D. S., M. J. Bywater, and H. A. Holt. 1978. Antibacterial synergism between beta-lactam antibiotics: results using clavulanic acid (BRL 14151) with amoxicillin, carbenicillin or cephaloridine. Infection 6(Suppl. 1):9–15.
5. Wise, R., D. S. Reeves, J. M. Symonds, and P. J. Wilkinson. 1976. A clinical investigation of pivmecillinam. Chemotherapy (Basel) 22:335–339.

Clinical Evaluation of the Formulation Clavulanic Acid plus Amoxicillin in the Treatment of Urinary Tract Infections due to β-Lactamase-Producing Bacteria

F. W. GOLDSTEIN,* M. D. KITZIS, C. MALHURET, P. BOURQUELOT, AND J. F. ACAR

Hôpital Saint Joseph, Université Pierre et Marie Curie, Paris, France

Clavulanic acid, a β-lactamase inhibitor, was shown, when tested in vitro, to protect amoxicillin (AMX) from inactivation by β-lactamase-producing bacteria, rendering these bacteria susceptible to AMX (3).

A previous study in six patients with urinary tract infections due to β-lactamase–producing bacteria demonstrated that, after a single dose of clavulanic acid plus AMX, the urine level of

AMX achieved a normal range and the bacterial count dramatically decreased (1).

The purpose of this study was to assess the clinical effectiveness of the formulation clavulanic acid plus AMX.

Eleven patients, aged 27 to 79 years, with severe urinary tract infections entered the study. The patients received 500 mg of AMX and 250 mg of clavulanic acid three times a day for 10

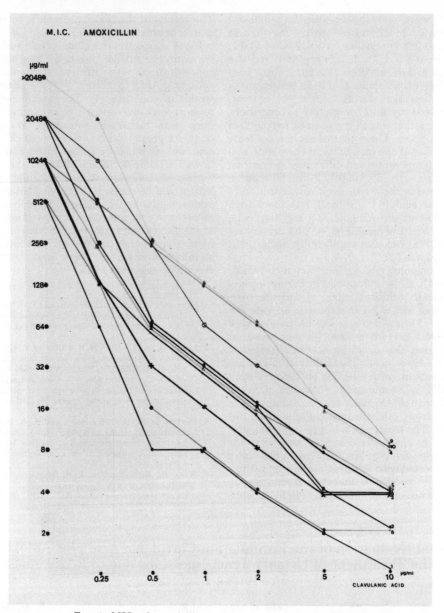

FIG. 1. *MICs of amoxicillin in the presence of clavulanic acid.*

days or more. A clinical, bacteriological, and biological follow-up lasted for at least 1 month. Urine cultures with exact bacterial and leukocyte counts were taken before treatment, after 48 h, 5 days, and 10 days of treatment, and at 48 h, 7 days, 2 weeks, and 1 month after the end of the treatment.

Routine susceptibility testing and determinations of MICS of AMX and clavulanic acid were performed on Mueller-Hinton agar (inoculum, 10^5 bacteria/ml). Inhibition of β-lactamase was demonstrated by the paper-strip method as previously described (1). Antibiotic assays in the urine were performed by a microbiological method (2). The protective effect of clavulanic acid could be demonstrated in vitro (Fig. 1) by the decrease of the MICs of AMX and in vivo by the urinary level of AMX which, in presence of clavulanic acid, reached a normal range in spite of the β-lactamase–producing infecting organism.

Of the 11 patients with urinary tract infections, cure was not expected in two cases for anatomical reasons. All the urines were cleared by 48 h after initiation of therapy except for one of the above two patients. Six of eight patients were cured; the two others relapsed within the week following the end of treatment. One patient had two episodes of treatment at a 1-month interval. Another patient was given gentamicin 3 days after sterilization of the urine and clinical improvement. Tolerance was good except for one patient in whom treatment had to be discontinued for intolerance (nausea, vomiting). No laboratory abnormalities attributable to the treatment have been observed.

The formulation of clavulanic acid and AMX appears to be an effective treatment of urinary tract infections due to β-lactamase–producing bacteria. Further clinical studies are, however, necessary to confirm these observations.

1. Acar, J. F., F. W. Goldstein, and Y. A. Chabbert. 1973. Synergistic activity of trimethoprim-sulfamethoxazole on Gram-negative bacilli: observations in vitro and in vivo. J. Infect. Dis. 128(Suppl.):470–477.
2. Goldstein, F. W., M. D. Kitzis, and J. F. Acar. 1979. Effect of clavulanic acid and amoxicillin formulation against β-lactamase producing Gram-negative bacteria in urinary tract infections. J. Antimicrob. Chemother. 5:705–709.
3. Wise, R., J. M. Andrews, and K. A. Bedford. 1978. In vitro studies of clavulanic acid in combination with penicillin, amoxicillin, and carbenicillin. Antimicrob. Agents Chemother. 13:389–393.

Laboratory Efficacy of Amoxicillin and Clavulanic Acid Combinations and Its Correlation with the Clinical Response to Treatment

I. D. FARRELL,* G. R. BROOKES, A. P. BALL, AND A. M. GEDDES

Public Health Laboratory, East Birmingham Hospital, Birmingham, B9 5ST, England

Clavulanic acid is a naturally occurring β-lactam compound produced by *Streptomyces clavuligerus* which is a potent inhibitor of bacterial β-lactamases, although it has little intrinsic antibacterial activity. It readily penetrates bacterial cell walls, and it progressively and irreversibly inhibits most of the clinically important β-lactamases. It has been shown that clavulanic acid has little activity against class I β-lactamases (1), which are cephalosporinases usually mediated by chromosomal mechanisms.

The degree of potentiation achieved when increasing concentrations of clavulanic acid were combined with amoxicillin (AMX) against recent isolates of AMX-resistant organisms has been investigated.

The MIC of AMX alone against these isolates was compared with the results of MIC titrations of AMX in the presence of clavulanic acid at concentrations of 0.5, 2.5, and 10 mg/liter. Clavulanic acid had a marked effect on the susceptibility of AMX-resistant strains of *Haemophilus influenzae*, *Bacteroides fragilis*, and *Staphylococcus aureus*, even at a concentration of 0.5 mg/liter. The MICs of AMX were substantially reduced in the presence of clavulanic acid for most strains of *Klebsiella aerogenes* and *K. ozaenae*.

The effect of clavulanic acid was not as pronounced with strains of *Escherichia coli* in that some strains remained relatively resistant. The susceptibility of some strains of indole-positive *Proteus* spp. was unaffected by the addition of clavulanic acid; these strains were identified as *P. morganii*.

An AMX plus clavulanic formulation is available for clinical trial from Beecham Research Laboratories. The antibiotic combination is taken orally every 8 h for 7 days and contains AMX trihydrate (250 mg) and potassium clavulanate (125 mg). Volunteer studies (A. P. Ball, I. D. Farrell, A. M. Geddes, P. G. Davey, and G. R. Brookes, this volume) have confirmed that peak serum concentrations after a single dose are approximately in the ratio of 2:1, AMX to clavulanic acid. The mean peak serum concentrations of AMX (4.0 mg/liter) were seen at 75 min and those of clavulanic acid (2.55 mg/liter) were seen at 60 min.

The MIC of AMX against recent AMX-resistant clinical isolates is compared with the MIC of the 2:1 combination of AMX and clavulanic acid in Table 1. The MIC of the 2:1 combination of AMX and clavulanic acid is expressed in terms of the AMX content and is the concentration of AMX in the lowest 2:1 combination of AMX and clavulanic acid to give complete or almost complete inhibition.

Sixty patients with urinary tract infections were treated with a combination of AMX and either sodium or potassium clavulanate as described by Ball et al. (this volume). The causa-

TABLE 1. *MICs of amoxicillin (AMX) alone and combined with clavulanic acid (AMX/CA) against recent AMX-resistant clinical isolates*[a]

Organism (no. of strains)	Drug	No. of strains susceptible to AMX at a concn (mg/liter) of:												
		0.13	0.25	0.5	1	2	4	8	16	32	64	128	256	≥512
Staphylococcus aureus (20)	AMX				1	2	6	9	2					
	AMX/CA			9	11									
Bacteroides (20)	AMX						5	3	1	4	6	1		
	AMX/CA	1	6	5	4	4								
Haemophilus influenzae, β-lactamase producing (9)	AMX					2		4	3					
	AMX/CA			2	7									
H. influenzae, non-β-lactamase producing (11)	AMX		1	3	3	1	1	2						
	AMX/CA		1	3	3	2	2							
Escherichia coli (25)	AMX													25
	AMX/CA							1	7	15	1	1		
Klebsiella aerogenes (39)	AMX								3	2	14	2	2	16
	AMX/CA				3	15	6	7	7	1				
K. ozaenae (20)	AMX							1	1	2	4	7	5	
	AMX/CA			4	10	5				1				
Proteus spp., indole positive (19)	AMX											1	5	13
	AMX/CA		1	2	3	2	1					6	4	

[a] All MICs of the combination are expressed in terms of the AMX concentration. The drugs were combined in a 2:1 ratio of AMX to clavulanic acid.

tive organisms were *E. coli* (AMX susceptible) in 10, *E. coli* (AMX resistant) in 31, *K. aerogenes* (AMX resistant) in 10, other resistant organisms in 7 (*Proteus* spp., 3; *S. aureus*, 3; *Serratia marcescens*, 1), and mixed resistant infections in 2. The 10 AMX-susceptible *E. coli* isolates were included during the initial assessment of tolerance and safety.

The bacterial synergy studies showed that the MICs of AMX for resistant *E. coli* isolates (mode MIC ≥ 512 mg/liter) when titrated against a 2:1 combination of AMX and clavulanic acid fell into two groups. Isolates which were considered susceptible to the combination (range, <0.12 to 16 mg/liter) had a mode MIC of 8 mg/liter, and resistant isolates (≥32 mg/liter) had a mode MIC of 64 mg/liter. All 10 *K. aerogenes* isolates (mode MIC of AMX alone, 256 mg/liter) became

susceptible to AMX (mode MIC, 2 mg/liter) in the presence of clavulanic acid, as did the three *S. aureus* isolates. All other isolates were susceptible to the combination except for two of the three strains of *Proteus* spp., against which the MIC of AMX was unaffected by clavulanic acid. Overall, 40 of the 50 resistant isolates (80%) were susceptible to AMX (MIC < 32 mg/liter) in the presence of clavulanic acid.

Seven of the 10 patients with infections caused by bacteria which remained resistant to AMX in the presence of clavulanic acid failed to respond to treatment with a combination of AMX and clavulanic acid.

1. **Neu, H. C., and K. P. Fu.** 1978. Clavulanic acid, a novel inhibitor of β-lactamases. Antimicrob. Agents Chemother. **14:**650–655.

Pharmacokinetics of CP-45,899 and Pro-Drug CP-47,904 in Animals and Humans

G. FOULDS,* W. E. BARTH, J. R. BIANCHINE, A. R. ENGLISH, D. GIRARD, S. L. HAYES, M. M. O'BRIEN, AND P. SOMANI

Pfizer, Inc., Groton, Connecticut 06340; Ohio State University, Columbus, Ohio 43210; and University of Miami, Miami, Florida 33152, U.S.A.*

CP-45,899 (Fig. 1) is a new β-lactamase inhibitor currently undergoing clinical investigation. When administered parenterally to dogs and rats, its pharmacokinetic characteristics are similar to those of ampicillin and amoxicillin. The intravenous (i.v.) data are consistent with a two-compartment pharmacokinetic model. Elimination half-lives of CP-45,899 in beagle dogs (0.85 h) are similar to those of ampicillin (0.65 h) and amoxicillin (1.1 h). The principal pathway of elimination is excretion in the urine, with up to 90% of a dose being recovered in the urine of beagle dogs. Biliary excretion of CP-45,899 is insignificant in the rat; only 1.5% of a parenteral dose of CP-45,899 appears in bile within 6 h.

CP-45,899 was administered i.v. and intramuscularly (i.m.) in single doses of up to 1,000 mg to 10 human subjects. The drug was well tolerated by all subjects and caused no significant side effects except for some pain on i.m. injection. Serum levels 10 min after completion of a 30-min i.v. infusion of 1,000 mg of CP-45,899 were approximately 43 µg/ml. Peak serum levels after i.m. injection of 1,000 mg were approximately 30 µg/ml. The half-life for elimination of drug was approximately 1 h. Areas under the serum level versus time curves and urinary recoveries were the same after i.v. and i.m. administration, indicating that the i.m. dose was completely bioavailable. Approximately 75% of the dose was recovered in urine. The data after i.v. infusion were consistent with a two-compartment model with kinetic parameters very similar to those of amoxicillin and ampicillin.

In a further study, designed to reveal the possible pharmacokinetic interaction of CP-45,899 with ampicillin or penicillin G, 500 mg of CP-45,899 was administered alone and in combination with 500 mg of ampicillin (i.m.) or penicillin G (i.v. bolus and infusion). No major changes in serum concentrations, volumes of distribution, distribution rate kinetics, or urinary recoveries of CP-45,899, penicillin G, or ampicillin were observed due to co-administration. Oral absorption studies showed that CP-45,899 is well

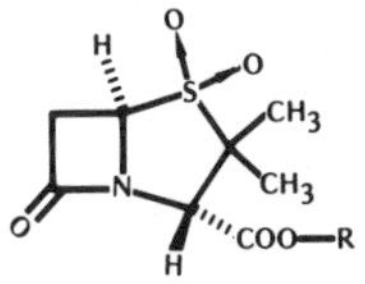

FIG. 1. *Structures of CP-45,899 and CP-47,904.*

absorbed by beagle dogs and mice, but poorly absorbed by rats and rhesus monkeys. In humans, single oral doses of 500 mg produced peak serum concentrations of approximately 1.4 µg/ml. However, pro-drug CP-47,904 (Fig. 1), the pivaloyloxymethyl ester of CP-45,899, gave serum concentrations of CP-45,899 in all four animal species equal to or better than those following administration of oral CP-45,899.

Studies in the rat have shown that CP-47,904 is hydrolyzed during its passage through the intestinal wall. At doses as high as 100 mg/kg, essentially no (<0.01 µg/ml) intact CP-47,904 reached the portal blood.

In humans, oral CP-47,904 efficiently delivered CP-45,899 to serum. A tablet equivalent to 250 mg of CP-45,899 produced mean peak serum concentrations of 4.9 µg of CP-45,899 per ml. Comparison of areas under the serum concentration versus time curves and urinary recoveries of CP-45,899, after oral administration of CP-47,904 and parenteral administration of CP-45,899, suggested that greater than 85% of a dose of CP-47,904 is absorbed and delivered as CP-45,899 to the peripheral circulation. Studies using both CP-47,904 and ampicillin have indicated the absence of any major pharmacokinetic interaction between these drugs. CP-45,899 serum concentrations, urinary recoveries, and areas under the curves after administration of CP-47,904 were not markedly affected by co-administration of 500 mg of oral ampicillin. Likewise, ampicillin serum concentrations, urinary recoveries, and areas under the curves were not affected by co-administration of 125 or 250 mg of CP-47,904.

Laboratory Evaluation of FR 31564, a Phosphonic Acid-Containing Antibiotic: In Vitro and In Vivo Antibacterial Activities and Pharmacokinetics in Animals

HITOSHI KOJO, TOSHIAKI KAMIMURA, SHIGEO NONOYAMA, YASUHIRO MINE, MINORU NISHIDA,* SACHIKO GOTO, AND SHOGO KUWAHARA

Fujisawa Pharmaceutical Co., Ltd., Osaka,* and Toho University School of Medicine, Tokyo, Japan

FR 31564 is a novel phosphonic acid-containing antibiotic developed for parenteral and oral use. This antibiotic was devised by chemical modification (2) to improve the antibacterial activity of its parent compound FR 900098, which was isolated from culture filtrates of *Streptomyces rubellomurinus* (1). This report describes a laboratory evaluation of the in vitro and in vivo antibacterial activities of FR 31564 and its pharmacokinetics in animals.

FR 31564 exerted antibacterial activity against most gram-negative bacteria except *Serratia marcescens* and glucose-nonfermenting gram-negative rods excluding *Pseudomonas aeruginosa*, and also against *P. aeruginosa*, *Citrobacter freundii*, and *Enterobacter* species which are relatively resistant to β-lactam antibiotics. Unlike fosfomycin, FR 31564 was inactive against gram-positive bacteria. The antibacterial activity of FR 31564 against several organisms including *Escherichia coli* and *Klebsiella pneumoniae* was enhanced several times by adding either 10% rabbit blood or glucose-6-phosphate to the test medium. The mean MICs of FR 31564 against clinical isolates were compared to those of fosfomycin and other antibiotics (Table 1). The mean MICs of FR 31564 against 100 strains each of *Escherichia coli* and *Klebsiella pneumoniae* were 5.79 and 3.82 µg/ml, respectively, much lower than those of fosfomycin, ampicillin, and piperacillin. FR 31564 was almost as active as fosfomycin and was less active than cefazolin and amikacin against 50 strains each of *Proteus mirabilis*, *P. vulgaris*, and *P. rettgeri*, with mean MICs of 5.22, 4.42, and 8.78 µg/ml, respectively. The mean MICs of FR 31564 for 50 strains of *Enterobacter aerogenes* and 100 strains each of *E. cloacae* and *C. freundii* were 6.70, 1.80, and 2.92 µg/ml, respectively. FR 31564 was more active than fosfomycin against *Enterobacter* species and almost as active as fosfomycin against *Citrobacter*. FR 31564 was more active than fosfomycin against 50 strains of *P. aeruginosa*, with a mean MIC of 9.74 µg/ml. FR 31564 was also active against gram-negative bacteria resistant to β-lactam antibiotics as well as gentamicin-resistant *P. aeruginosa* strains.

FR 31564, like fosfomycin, was incorporated into bacterial cells by the active transport system for α-glycerophosphate and also by that for hexose phosphates when glucose-6-phosphate

TABLE 1. *Antibacterial activity of FR 31564 and other antibiotics against clinical isolates*

Organism (no. of strains)	Antibiotic	Mean MIC[a] (µg/ml)
Escherichia coli (100)	FR 31564	5.79
	Fosfomycin	15.3
	Ampicillin	19.9
	Cefazolin	1.83
Klebsiella pneumoniae (100)	FR 31564	3.82
	Fosfomycin	38.2
	Cefazolin	2.54
Proteus mirabilis (50)	FR 31564	5.22
	Fosfomycin	3.21
	Ampicillin	0.443
	Cefazolin	1.29
P. vulgaris (50)	FR 31564	4.42
	Fosfomycin	2.72
	Piperacillin	0.523
P. rettgeri (50)	FR 31564	8.78
	Fosfomycin	9.03
	Piperacillin	2.44
Enterobacter cloacae (100)	FR 31564	1.80
	Fosfomycin	64.6
	Piperacillin	8.13
	Gentamicin	1.97
Citrobacter freundii (100)	FR 31564	2.72
	Fosfomycin	3.00
	Piperacillin	9.41
	Gentamicin	2.61
Pseudomonas aeruginosa (50)	FR 31564	9.74
	Fosfomycin	18.4
	Ticarcillin	25.3
	Piperacillin	4.67
	Gentamicin	16.0

[a] Nutrient agar (Difco), 10^{-3} dilution, stamp method, 37°C, 20 h.

TABLE 2. *Comparative efficacy of subcutaneous doses of FR 31564 and other drugs for infection in mice*[a]

Organism	ED$_{50}$ (mg/kg)					
	FR 31564	Fosfomycin	Ampicillin	Cefazolin	Piperacillin	Gentamicin
Escherichia coli 23	1.89	15.4[b]	3.85	1.74		
Klebsiella pneumoniae 74	0.59	26[b]		1.87[b]	7.21[b]	
Proteus mirabilis 8	4.59	3.48	<0.87[c]	6.06	1.52[c]	
P. vulgaris 8	0.73	2.76[b]			0.90	
Enterobacter aerogenes 9	7.68	12.7			9.11	0.36[c]
E. cloacae 63	8.14	>217[b]			1.29[c]	0.42[c]
Citrobacter freundii 13	0.92	6.07[b]			14.5[b]	0.84
Pseudomonas aeruginosa 26 ...	1.85	92.5[b]			75.0[b]	10.2[b]

[a] Mice: JCL ICR strain males 4 weeks old weighing 23.5 ± 1.5 g, 10 mice/group. Challenge: one minimal lethal dose, mucin suspension, intraperitoneally. Therapy: 1 and 3 h after challenge, subcutaneously.

[b] Significant (FR 31564 superior to other drug).

[c] Significant (FR 31564 inferior to other drug).

was added to the test medium. But the incorporation rate of FR 31564 was higher than that of fosfomycin. FR 31564 was scarcely inactivated in the bacterial culture fluids.

The therapeutic effect of FR 31564 after subcutaneous and oral administration was studied in experimental infections in mice. After either type of dosing, FR 31564 was much superior to fosfomycin against most gram-negative bacteria, excluding *P. mirabilis* and *E. aerogenes* (Table 2). The protective effect of FR 31564 against *P. aeruginosa* was the most potent among the five drugs including fosfomycin, piperacillin, gentamicin, and cefazolin. The therapeutic activity of FR 31564 was substantially more potent than expected from the results of the in vitro studies.

The results of the pharmacokinetic study in animals indicated that FR 31564, given parenterally and orally, was well absorbed, was distributed rapidly into the body fluids and tissues, and was excreted unchanged, mainly in the urine. After intramuscular injection of 20 mg/kg, the mean serum concentrations of FR 31564 peaked at 33.3 μg/ml for rats and 41.4 μg/ml for dogs, each at 15 min, and at 33.5 μg/ml for monkeys at 30 min. The mean peak serum concentrations after intravenous injection of the same dose were 33.0 μg/ml for rats, 54.8 μg/ml

for dogs, and 48.4 μg/ml for monkeys, each at 15 min. The 24-h urinary recovery of FR 31564 when administered parenterally ranged from 85 to 95% in rats, dogs, and monkeys. The serum concentrations of FR 31564 peaked at 0.5 to 2 h in mice and rats given a single oral dose of 100 mg/kg and in dogs given a single dose of 40 mg/kg. The mean serum concentrations of FR 31564 peaked at 8.99 μg/ml (half-life, 4.5 h) in mice, 8.10 μg/ml (4.1 h) in rats, and 16.6 μg/ml (3.4 h) in dogs. The 24-h urinary recovery after oral dosing was 45.8% in rats and 37.8% in dogs. The binding of FR 31564 to serum proteins of different kinds of animals and to rat tissues was extremely low.

The results presented here indicate that FR 31564 is a very promising parenteral and oral antibiotic for the treatment of infections due to a wide range of gram-negative bacteria.

1. Imanaka, H., M. Okuhara, Y. Kuroda, T. Goto, M. Okamoto, H. Terano, E. Iguchi, J. Hosoda, M. Kohsaka, and H. Aoki. 1979. Studies on new phosphonic acid-containing antibiotics. I. FR 900098. Isolation and characterization. J. Antibiot. (in press).
2. Kamiya, T., K. Henmi, H. Takeno, and M. Hashimoto. 1979. Studies on new phosphonic acid-containing antibiotics. II. Synthesis of FR 31564 and related antibiotics. J. Antibiot. (in press).

Studies on New Phosphonic Acid-Containing Antibiotics: Synthesis of FR-31564 and Related Antibiotics

TAKASHI KAMIYA,* KEIJI HEMMI, HIDEKAZU TAKENO, AND MASASHI HASHIMOTO

Research Laboratories, Fujisawa Pharmaceutical Company, Ltd., Osaka, Japan

Recently, a great deal of attention has been given to the production of new chemotherapeutic substances by chemical modification of antibiotics produced by microorganisms. During a search for modification of the new phosphonic acid-containing antibiotics FR-900098 (Ia) and

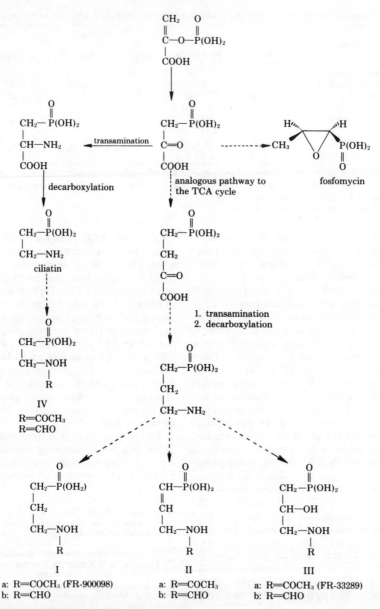

FIG. 1. *Biogenesis of FR-900098 and other congeners. TCA, Tricarboxylic acid.*

FR-33289 (IIIa), which were isolated from the fermentation broth of *Streptomyces rebellomurinus* by Imanaka et al. (2), we have obtained 3-(N-formyl-N-hydroxyamino)-propylphosphonic acid (FR-31564) (Ib), a promising new antibiotic, as the most potent antibiotic among the derivatives. This report relates the synthesis of FR-31564 and related antibiotics.

The structures of Ia and IIIa were determined as 3-(N-acetyl-N-hydroxyamino)-propylphos-

phonic acid and 3-(N-acetyl-N-hydroxyamino)-2(R)-hydroxypropylphosphonic acid on the basis of spectroscopic and chemical evidence, respectively. For confirmation of these antibiotics, Ia and IIIa were synthesized.

Ia and IIIa are active against gram-negative organisms, but their activities are relatively low. Consequently, we have started a program of chemical modification which enhances their activities.

TABLE 1. *Antimicrobial activity*

Structure	MIC (μg/ml)[a]				
	S. aureus 209P	B. subtilis ATCC 6633	P. vulgaris IAM 1025	E. coli NIHJ JC2	P. aeruginosa IAM 1095
OH OH O $\mid$ $\mid$ $\parallel$ R—NCH$_2$CHCH$_2$P(OH)$_2$					
R=COCH$_3$	>400	400	400	50	400
R=CHO	>100	100	50	25	25
OH O $\mid$ $\parallel$ R—NCH$_2$CH=CHP(OH)$_2$					
R=COCH$_3$	>1,000	2.5	600	10	600
R=CHO	>100	6.25	3.13	12.5	1.56
OH O $\mid$ $\parallel$ R—NCH$_2$CH$_2$CH$_2$P(OH)$_2$					
R=COCH$_3$	>1,000	200	125	400	250
R=CHO	>100	6.25	3.13	12.5	0.78
R=CF$_3$CO	>100	>100	>100	>100	40
R=ClCH$_2$CO	>100	>100	>100	>100	>100
R=HOCH$_2$CO	>100	>100	>100	>100	>100
R=CH$_3$(CH$_2$)$_2$CO	>100	>100	>100	>100	>100
R=C$_6$H$_5$CO	>100	>100	>100	>100	>100
R=⟨thienyl⟩—CH$_2$CO	>100	>100	>100	>100	>100

[a] Agar dilution assay.

The structures of these antibiotics, when considered with those of biogenesis, suggested that there exist some congeners in nature. We anticipated that these antibiotics are derived from 3-phosphonopyruvate in connection with the biosyntheses of ciliatin (4), fosfomycin (1), and hadacidin (5), as shown in Fig. 1. It is, therefore, reasonable to presume that congeners such as II and IV are produced in the culture broth. This possibility is of interest in connection with their chemical modification.

These congeners were synthesized by the method described above. It is of interest that IIa was later found to be produced as a minor product in the culture broth. This result is in accord with our expectation based on biogenesis of these new antibiotics. IIa was found to have activity similar to that of FR-900098, but IV did not show any activity against gram-negative and -positive organisms.

It was subsequently realized that major changes in activity would result from appropriate change in the N-acetyl side chain of these antibiotics. In particular, we were interested in N-formyl derivatives in connection with the biosynthesis of hadacidin (5), N-formyl-N-hydroxyaminoacetic acid. A number of N-acyl deriva-

tives common in penicillins and cephalosporins were synthesized. However, none of the N-acyl derivatives proved to have significant antibacterial activity, except N-formyl derivatives (see Table 1). It is of interest that these formyl derivatives, Ia, IIa, and IIIa, were found to be more active than the parent antibiotics (see Table 1). Although some other related derivatives were synthesized, it was found that they did not show any improved activity.

FR-31564 proved to have the highest activity against gram-negative organisms among all of the derivatives and was effective orally (3). It was later found to be produced as a minor product in culture broth (2).

1. **Horiguchi, M., J. S. Kittredge, and E. Roberts.** 1968. Biosynthesis of 2-aminoethylphosphonic acid in tetrahymena. Biochim. Biophys. Acta **165**:164–166.
2. **Imanaka, H., M. Okuhara, Y. Kuroda, T. Goto, M. Okamoto, H. Terano, E. Iguchi, J. Hosoda, M. Kohsaka, and H. Aoki.** 1979. Studies on new phosphonic acid-containing antibiotics. I. FR 900098. Isolation and characterization. J. Antibiot., in press.
3. **Mine, Y., T. Kamimura, S. Noyama, M. Nishida, S. Goto, and S. Kuwahara.** 1979. In vitro and in vivo antibacterial activities of FR31564, a new phosphonic acid-containing antibiotic. J. Antibiot., in press.

4. **Rogers, T. O., and J. Bunbaum.** 1974. Biosynthesis of fosfomycin by *Streptomyces fradiae*. Antimicrob. Agents Chemother. **5:**121-132.

5. **Stevens, R. L., and F. E. Thomas.** 1966. The biosynthesis of hadacidin. Biochemistry **5:**74-81.

Discovery, Isolation, and Characterization of New Phosphonic Acid Antibiotics

MASAKUNI OKUHARA,* YOSHIO KURODA, TOSHIO GOTO, MASANORI OKAMOTO, HIROSHI TERANO, EIKO IGUCHI, JUNJI HOSODA, MASANOBU KOHSAKA, HATSUO AOKI, AND HIROSHI IMANAKA

Research Laboratories, Fujisawa Pharmaceutical Co., Ltd., Osaka, Japan

Discovery of nocardicin A by the use of an *Escherichia coli* mutant strain which is supersensitive to penicillin proved the usefulness of such a screening system (1). We undertook, therefore, another screening program using a mutant strain of *Pseudomonas aeruginosa* NCTC 10490 supersensitive to nocardicin C, which has only weak antibacterial activity (2). Using this system, we isolated a strain of *Streptomyces* from a soil sample and identified it as *Streptomyces rubellomurinus* sp. nov., which produces a new antibiotic FR-900098.

FR-900098 was produced by cultivating *S. rubellomurinus* under submerged, aerobic conditions in aqueous medium containing 5% soluble starch, 0.5% cotton seed meal, 2.5% gluten meal, 0.5% dried yeast, 1% $MgSO_4 \cdot 7H_2O$, 1% KH_2PO_4, and 0.7% $Na_2HPO_4 \cdot 12H_2O$. Production of the antibiotic reached a maximum after 3 days of incubation at 30°C on a rotary shaker at 220 rpm. The clear filtrate obtained after separation of the mycelial cake was passed through a column of activated charcoal. The effluent and the wash were combined and adjusted to pH 2.0 with a cation-exchange resin (Duolite C-20, H^+ cycle). The acidified solution was passed through a column of anion-exchange resin (Duolite A-6, OH^- cycle). The resin was washed with water, and the antibiotic activity was eluted with 0.1 N sodium hydroxide solution. The active fractions were adjusted to pH 2.0 with Duolite C-20 (H^+ cycle) and again adsorbed onto a column of activated charcoal. The active fractions eluted by 60% aqueous acetone were evaporated to dryness after adjustment of the pH to 6.5. The residue was applied to a column packed with cellulose powder. The column was washed with 80% propanol and eluted with 75% propanol. The white powder obtained by evaporating the active fraction under reduced pressure was dissolved in a small volume of methanol, and 10 volumes of acetone were added to the solution. Colorless crystal of FR-900098 was obtained as the monosodium salt.

FR-900098 (mp, 193 to 194°C) is soluble in water, methanol, and dimethylsulfoxide, slightly soluble in ethanol, and substantially insoluble in acetone, ethyl acetate, and hexane. The observed specific rotation $[\alpha]_D^{25}$ is 0 (c = 1.0, H_2O). It moves toward the anode with phosphate buffer, pH 6.5, at 300 V upon paper electrophoresis for 2 h. Potentiometric titration of the monosodium salt showed an equivalent weight of 240, with a pK'_a of 2.0, 7.2, 9.4. Elemental analysis gave C 27.74%, H 5.02%, N 6.66%, P 12.35%, and Na 10.31%, values consistent with $C_5H_{11}NO_5PNa$. Color reactions were as follows: positive in $FeCl_3$, I_2, and $KMnO_4$ tests, and negative in ninhydrin, Ehrlich, Dragendorff, and Molisch tests. The UV absorption spectrum in 0.1 N sodium hydroxide solution showed an absorption, λ_{max}, at 230 nm ($E_{1cm}^{1\%}$, 325) and end absorption in acidic and neutral solution. Elemental analysis, titration, and color tests suggested the existence of phosphonic acid. The infrared spectrum in KBr (Fig. 1) showed maxima at: 3,600 to 2,600, 1,615 (—CO—N—), 1,160 (P—O), 1,040, and 885 cm^{-1}. The nuclear magnetic resonance spectrum, shown in Fig. 1, had the following characteristics: acetyl protons at δ 1.95 (3H, s), two protons at δ 1.35 (2H, m), two protons at δ 1.75 (2H, m), and two protons at δ 3.50 (2H, t, J = 7 Hz). Irradiation of the signals at δ 1.75 changed the triplet signals at δ 3.80 into a singlet. The fact that two methylene protons were observed at δ 3.50 indicated the existence of —CH_2—N— (or O). The above-mentioned information suggests the partial structure of this antibiotic as CH_3—, —CO—, —N(OH)—, —N—CH_2—, and —CH_2—PO_3H. Studies by chemists in our laboratories have shown that the chemical structure is 3-(*N*-acetyl-*N*-hydroxy)aminopropylphosphonic acid.

FR-900098 showed unique antibacterial activ-

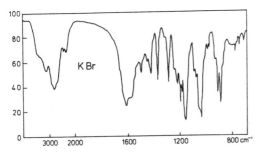

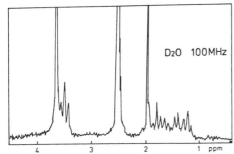

FIG. 1. *Infrared and nuclear magnetic resonance spectra of FR-900098.*

TABLE 1. *Antibacterial spectra of FR-900098, FR-33289, FR-31564, and FR-32863*

Organism	MIC (μg/ml)[a]			
	FR-900098	FR-33289	FR-31564	FR-32863
Staphylococcus aureus 209P	>800	>400	>100	>100
Bacillus subtilis ATCC 6633	200	400	6.25	6.25
Sarcina lutea PCI-1001	8	400	0.1	0.2
Klebsiella pneumoniae NCTC-418	800	400	50	100
Shigella flexneri 1a EW 8	8	200	6.25	50
Salmonella typhi O-901	2	200	0.39	0.78
Proteus vulgaris IAM 1025	125	400	3.13	3.13
Pseudomonas aeruginosa IAM 1095	250	400	0.78	1.56
Escherichia coli NIHJ JC 2	400	50	12.5	12.5
Pseudomonas III	1.6	25	0.05	0.1
Pseudomonas III[r][b]	>100	>100	>100	>100
Saccharomyces cerevisiae	>250	>250	>250	>250
Penicillium chrysogenum	>250	>250	>250	>250

[a] MIC by agar dilution assay with nutrient agar plates.

[b] Strain of *Pseudomonas* III highly resistant to FR-900098.

ity against a wide spectrum of gram-negative bacteria and no inhibitory effect on gram-positive bacteria, yeast, and fungi (Table 1). When susceptible cells were treated with the antibiotic in a hypertonic medium, all cells were transformed into protoplasts. Thus, it seems likely that the antibiotic inhibits bacterial cell wall synthesis. Each of five ICR mice was given a single intravenous dose of 100 mg of FR-900098 (4 to 5 g/kg); all survived.

Our continued efforts to isolate new cell wall-inhibitory antibiotics from culture broths of *Streptomyces* have yielded three phosphonic acid antibiotics which were distinct from, but resembled, FR-900098. FR-31564 and FR-32863 (FR-900136) were produced by strain No. 8006, which has been identified as *S. lavendulae*. The strain designated *S. rubellomurinus* subsp. *indigoferus* was found to produce FR-33289. Fermentation and isolation procedures of these antibiotics were essentially the same as those described for FR-900098. From the physical and biological properties, the chemical structure of FR-31564 ($C_4H_9NO_5PNa$) is considered to be equivalent to 3-(*N*-formyl-*N*-hydroxy)aminopropylphosphonic acid, which has been synthesized by the chemists in our laboratories. FR-32863 ($C_4H_7NO_5PK$) and FR-33289 ($C_5H_{11}NO_6PNa$) were determined as 3-(*N*-formyl-*N*-hydroxy)amino-1-*trans*-propenylphosphonic acid and 3-(*N*-acetyl-*N*-hydroxy)amino-2-hydroxypropylphosphonic acid, respectively.

The antibacterial spectra of these compounds are compared with that of FR-900098 in Table 1. All of them showed activity against gram-negative bacteria but not against gram-positive bacteria. FR-31564 and FR-32863 exhibited a similar range of potencies, whereas FR-900098 and FR-33289 appeared to have much weaker antibacterial activity. Cross-resistance shown in Table 1 suggests a close resemblance of these antibiotics to FR-900098 in their biological activity.

In summary, FR-900098 and its derivatives are interesting new antibiotics containing phosphorus in their structure. Their activity against gram-negative bacteria and their low toxicity in experimental animals suggest that they have potential as effective chemotherapeutic agents.

1. **Aoki, H., H. Sakai, M. Kohsaka, T. Konomi, J. Hosoda, T. Kubochi, E. Iguchi, and H. Imanaka.** 1976. Nocardicin A, a new monocyclic β-lactam antibiotic. I. Discovery, isolation and characterization. J. Antibiot. **29:**492–500.
2. **Hosoda, J., T. Konomi, N. Tani, H. Aoki, and H. Imanaka.** 1977. Isolation of new nocardicins from *Nocardia uniformis* subsp. *tsuyamanensis*. Agric. Biol. Chem. **41:**2013–2020.

Interactions Between Alafosfalin and Other Inhibitors of Bacterial Cell Wall Synthesis

DAVID GREENWOOD* AND RUTH VINCENT

Department of Microbiology, University Hospital, Queen's Medical Centre, Nottingham NG7 2UH, England

Alafosfalin is a novel antibacterial agent with a broad spectrum of activity (1, 2). Structurally, alafosfalin is L-alanyl-L-1-aminoethylphosphonic acid; susceptible bacteria actively transport the compound, which is cleaved intracellulary to yield L-alanine and the antibacterially active L-1-aminoethylphosphonic acid (1, 3). The primary site of action of this active metabolite of alafosfalin is in the bacterial cell wall, where it competitively inhibits alanine racemase (1, 3), the enzyme responsible for generating D-alanine residues which terminate the pentapeptide side chain of N-acetylmuramic acid and which are engaged in the final cross-linking reaction which is believed to give the bacterial cell wall its rigidity.

Since alafosfalin owes its antibacterial activity to interference with bacterial cell wall synthesis, it is possible that it may interact synergically with other cell wall-active agents in much the same way that trimethoprim and sulfonamides interact by blocking sequential steps in a metabolic pathway. Preliminary results suggest that such synergy does indeed occur (2).

The largest group of cell wall-active compounds—penicillins and cephalosporins—generally attack multiple sites within the bacterial cell wall (4), but certain members of the β-lactam family, notably mecillinam and cephalexin (and the closely related cephradine), act at separate, single sites (5, 8). The unrelated compound fosfomycin acts by interfering with the formation of the lactyl moiety which converts N-acetylglucosamine to N-acetylmuramic acid (9). These three compounds, mecillinam, cephalexin, and fosfomycin, seemed the most likely candidates for synergic interaction with alafosfalin and were selected for investigation. Since one potential clinical application of alafosfalin is in the treatment of urinary tract infection, the action and interaction of these drugs was examined in an in vitro model which simulates some of the conditions of exposure to drug which exist in the treatment of bacterial cystitis, and *Escherichia coli*, the most common urinary pathogen, was chosen for intensive study.

Interactions in static culture. In preliminary studies, dense broth cultures of *E. coli* were exposed to alafosfalin, alone and in combination with mecillinam, cephalexin, and fosfomycin, in a simple static system. When such experiments were continuously monitored turbidimetrically, it was found that mixtures of alafosfalin with mecillinam or cephalexin were able to cause a dramatic fall in opacity of *E. coli* cultures at drug concentrations at which the individual components merely inhibited growth (Fig. 1). Mixtures of alafosfalin and fosfomycin showed little or no synergy when tested in this way.

Microscopic examination of cultures exposed to antibiotic showed the typical conversion of the rod-shaped bacteria to long filaments by cephalexin, and to spherical forms by mecillinam (5). The very low concentration of alafosfalin used (0.015 µg/ml) had little effect on bacterial morphology. In combination, alafosfalin plus either cephalexin or mecillinam caused rapid and complete lysis of the great majority of the bacteria.

Bactericidal synergy between alafosfalin and cephalexin or mecillinam was also demonstrated by performing sequential viable counts over a 6-h period on cultures exposed to these compounds.

Bladder model. The design and use of the bladder model have been described elsewhere (6, 7). In the model, 20 ml of an overnight broth culture of bacteria was diluted at 1 ml per min with fresh broth; at hourly intervals a pump emptied the system (simulating micturition), leaving behind a residual volume of 20 ml. After 4 h of such dilution and "micturition," cultures were exposed to 12.5 mg of alafosfalin (alone and in the presence of 12.5 mg of mecillinam, cephalexin, or fosfomycin) in one of two ways: (i) the whole "dose" was introduced as a single pulse achieving an instantaneous peak level of 625 µg/ml, which subsequently declined because of the washout effect; (ii) the "dose" was introduced over a 12-h period by use of a gradient-forming device which arranged for a peak level of 50 µg/ml to be achieved after 2 h and for the concentration subsequently to decline exponentially over a further 10 h. The opacity of the culture was continuously recorded, and the results were expressed as the time taken from the commencement of drug exposure for the opacity of the culture to reattain a level of 50% of maximum.

Two strains of *E. coli* and one of *Proteus mirabilis* were tested in the single-pulse experi-

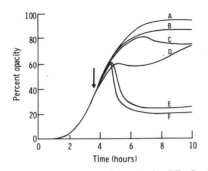

FIG. 1. *Continuous opacity records of Escherichia coli ECSA 1. Drug(s) added at arrow to achieve the following concentrations (μg/ml): (A) no drug; (B) alafosfalin, 0.015; (C) cephalexin, 16; (D) mecillinam, 2; (E) alafosfalin, 0.015, plus cephalexin, 16; (F) alafosfalin, 0.015, plus mecillinam, 2.*

TABLE 1. *Suppression of bacterial growth in the bladder model by alafosfalin alone, and in combination with cephalexin, mecillinam, and fosfomycin*

Bacterial strain	Time (h) to recovery[a] after exposure to 12.5 mg of						
	ALA	CEX	ALA + CEX	MEC	ALA + MEC	FOS	ALA + FOS
12.5-mg pulse *Escherichia coli*							
ECSA 1	16	8	9.5	11.5	21	12	14.5
E. coli ECSA 11	19	11	16	15	23	14	15
Proteus mirabilis							
RU	6.5	10	8	NE	10	NT	NT
12.5 mg over 12 h							
E. coli ECSA 1	22	18.5	25	26	29	NT	NT

[a] Time taken from commencement of exposure to drug(s) for the opacity of the culture to reattain a level of 50% of maximum. ALA, alafosfalin; CEX, cephalexin; MEC, mecillinam; FOS, fosfomycin. NE, no effect; NT, not tested.

ments (Table 1). The period of suppression of growth of *E. coli* by alafosfalin was found to be shorter in the presence of cephalexin than in its absence, whereas with mecillinam growth was suppressed for longer by the mixture than by either component. In the therapeutically more realistic conditions of prolonged exposure, however, enhancement of growth suppression was observed with combinations of alafosfalin and both mecillinam and cephalexin (Table 1).

These results indicate that the combination of

alafosfalin and mecillinam exhibits bactericidal synergy against *E. coli* in conventional static culture and that the combination also enhances suppression of bacterial growth in dynamic conditions similar to those which exist in the infected urinary bladder during treatment. Alafosfalin and cephalexin can also be shown to be strikingly synergic in terms of the early bactericidal effect, but in certain test conditions suppression of bacterial growth by alafosfalin may be paradoxically reduced by the presence of cephalexin. This reduced effect was not found in experiments in which the bacteria were exposed to concentrations of drugs which rose and fell as they do during treatment, and is unlikely to have therapeutic significance. However, since the combination with mecillinam was found to be consistently superior in the bladder model system, the present results suggest that mecillinam may have some advantages as a partner to alafosfalin if combination therapy is contemplated.

1. **Allen, J. G., F. R. Atherton, M. J. Hall, C. H. Hassall, S. W. Holmes, R. W. Lambert, L. J. Nisbet, and P. S. Ringrose.** 1978. Phosphonopeptides, a new class of synthetic antibacterial agents. Nature (London) **272:**56–58.
2. **Allen, J. G., F. R. Atherton, M. J. Hall, C. H. Hassall, S. W. Holmes, R. W. Lambert, L. J. Nisbet, and P. S. Ringrose.** 1979. Phosphonopeptides as antibacterial agents: alaphosphin and related phosphonopeptides. Antimicrob. Agents Chemother. **15:**684–695.
3. **Atherton, F. R., M. J. Hall, C. H. Hassall, R. W. Lambert, W. J. Lloyd, and P. S. Ringrose.** 1979. Phosphonopeptides as antibacterial agents: mechanism of action of alaphosphin. Antimicrob. Agents Chemother. **15:**696–705.
4. **Blumberg, P. M., and J. L. Strominger.** 1974. Interaction of penicillin with the bacterial cell: penicillin-binding proteins and penicillin-sensitive enzymes. Bacteriol. Rev. **38:**291–335.
5. **Greenwood, D., and F. O'Grady.** 1973. The two sites of penicillin action in *Escherichia coli.* J. Infect. Dis. **128:**791–794.
6. **Greenwood, D., and F. O'Grady.** 1977. Is your dosage really necessary? Antibiotic dosage in urinary infection. Br. Med. J. **2:**665–667.
7. **Greenwood, D., and F. O'Grady.** 1978. An *in vitro* model of the urinary bladder. J. Antimicrob. Chemother. **4:**113–120.
8. **Spratt, B. G.** 1975. Distinct penicillin-binding proteins involved in the division, elongation, and shape of *Escherichia coli* K12. Proc. Natl. Acad. Sci. U.S.A. **72:**2999–3003.
9. **Strominger, J. L.** 1973. The actions of penicillin and other antibiotics on bacterial cell wall synthesis. Johns Hopkins Med. J. **133:**63–81.

In Vitro and In Vivo Antibacterial Activity of TA-058, a New Broad-Spectrum Semisynthetic Penicillin

TAKESHI NISHINO,* NOBUO ISHII, TERUO TANINO, SATOSHI OHSHIMA, AND TOTARO YAMAGUCHI

Department of Microbiology, Kyoto College of Pharmacy, Kyoto, and Microbiological Research Laboratory, Tanabe Seiyaku Co., Ltd., Toda, Saitama, Japan*

TA-058, 6[D-2-(D-2-amino-3-N-methylcarbamoyl propionamido)-2-p-hydroxy-phenylacetamido] penicillanic acid, is a new semisynthetic penicillin derived from aminobenzylpenicillin. This compound is characterized by a very low toxicity (its LD_{50} intravenously in mice is greater than 10 g/kg) and a high solubility in water. TA-058 showed an antibacterial spectrum broader than those of ampicillin and carbenicillin against aerobic and anaerobic bacteria. We report herein the in vitro and in vivo activities of TA-058 compared with those of ampicillin (ABPC), carbenicillin (CBPC), piperacillin (PIPC), and apalcillin (APPC) against gram-positive and gram-negative bacteria.

TA-058 was as active as CBPC, PIPC, and APPC but less active than ABPC against gram-positive bacteria. The MICs of TA-058 were lower than those of ABPC and CBPC against gram-negative bacteria. TA-058 was particularly active against *Escherichia coli, Salmonella typhi, Shigella flexneri, Proteus mirabilis,* and *Haemophilus influenzae.*

The activity of TA-058 against *E. coli* which possess β-lactamase was similar to those of the other penicillins tested. At lower concentrations TA-058 was twice as active as CBPC but less active than APPC and PIPC. TA-058 was about two times more active than the other penicillins against *P. mirabilis*, but less active than the others against *P. vulgaris.* Against *P. aeruginosa*, TA-058 and CBPC were equally inhibitory, but less so than APPC and PIPC. TA-058 inhibited a majority of *H. influenzae* strains at concentrations below 0.1 µg/ml. Against *H. influenzae*, TA-058 was less active than PIPC but more active than APPC and CBPC.

The bactericidal activity against *E. coli* KC-

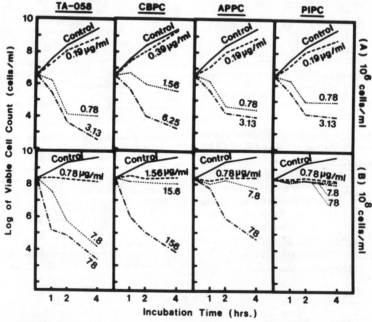

FIG. 1. *Bactericidal activities of TA-058, carbenicillin (CBPC), apalcillin (APPC), and piperacillin (PIPC) against Escherichia coli KC-14 (A) after a small inoculum of 10^6 cells per ml and (B) after a large inoculum of 10^8 cells per ml. The number of viable cells at the appropriate times after addition of antibiotics was counted on antibiotic-free agar.*

TABLE 1. *Chemotherapeutic effects of TA-058 (subcutaneously) and other penicillins on experimental infection in mice[a]*

Test organism	Challenge dose[b]		Injection[c]		ED$_{50}$ (mg/kg)[d]			
	Cells/mouse	No. of LD$_{50}$	No. of times	Time (h) after infection	TA-058	APPC	PIPC	CBPC
Escherichia coli KC-14	7.8×10^3	50	1	2	1.2	3.8	4.5	11.5
	2.5×10^4	85	1	2	1.8	6.5	6.5	18.0
	2.5×10^6	8,500	1	2	6.0	24.5	55.5	46.0
	2.5×10^7	85,000	1	2	25.5	325.0	875.0	240.0
					$(0.78)^e$	(0.39)	(0.78)	(1.56)
Klebsiella pneumoniae	1.2×10^3	300	1	2	8.5	65.0	86.5	460.0
					(0.39)	(0.39)	(0.39)	1.56)
Pseudomonas aeruginosa E-2	2.2×10^3	150	1	2	175.0	50.0	390.0	375.0
					(50)	(1.56)	(6.25)	(50)
P. aeruginosa E-2	1.3×10^3	125	1	2	750.0	79.0	295.0	375.0
			2	2, 3	175.0	19.5	72.5	250.0
			4	2, 3, 4, 5	66.0	12.0	31.5	69.5
			5	2, 3, 4, 5, 6	107.5	12.5	28.5	115.0
					(50)	(6.25)	(6.25)	(50)

[a] Ten male mice of ddY(s) strains weighing 18 to 20 g were used at each dose level.

[b] Cells were suspended in 3% mucin solution and injected intraperitoneally.

[c] Test compounds were administered subcutaneously in a single dose 2 h after infection or repeatedly 2, 3, 4, 5, and 6 h after infection.

[d] ED$_{50}$ was calculated from the survival rate 1 week after infection. APPC, apalcillin; PIPC, piperacillin; CBPC, carbenicillin.

[e] Numbers in parentheses are MICs (micrograms per milliliter) determined by the usual twofold dilution method with heart infusion agar.

14 of TA-058 was compared with those of CBPC, APPC, and PIPC as shown in Fig. 1. Logarithmically growing cells in heart infusion broth were exposed to various concentrations of TA-058, CBPC, PIPC, and APPC. When the inoculum size was 2×10^6 cells per ml, the killing rates were similar for all four penicillins. However, when the inoculum size was 10^8 cells per ml, TA-058 was more potent than the other three.

Chemotherapeutic effects of TA-058 in mice experimentally infected with *E. coli* KC-14, *K. pneumoniae*, and *P. aeruginosa* E-2 are shown in Table 1. Against the infections due to *E. coli* KC-14 and *K. pneumoniae*, TA-058 was much more effective than APPC, PIPC, and CBPC. Against *P. aeruginosa*, TA-058 was also more effective than PIPC and CBPC, but less so than APPC. The in vivo activities of TA-058 were not significantly influenced by the inoculum size. These properties support the view that the in vitro determination of antibacterial activity has an excellent predictive value for in vivo responses.

Comparative In Vitro Activity of CI-867, a New Semisynthetic Penicillin, with Ticarcillin and Piperacillin

JULIO V. CARDENAS,* DONALD POHLOD, LOUIS D. SARAVOLATZ, RAMON DEL BUSTO, KEITH H. BURCH, TOM MADHAVAN, EVELYN J. FISHER, AND EDWARD L. QUINN

Henry Ford Hospital, Detroit, Michigan 48202, U.S.A.

With the introduction of carbenicillin (1) a new group of semisynthetic penicillins have evolved which have attracted attention because of their antimicrobial activity against *Pseudomonas aeruginosa* and other gram-negative bacilli. Similar antibiotics with greater antibacterial activity against these organisms have been introduced, such as ticarcillin and piperacillin. The purpose of this study was to compare the in vitro activity of a new semisynthetic penicillin, CI-867, against recent isolates from Henry Ford Hospital. Preliminary studies with this compound, prepared from amoxicillin, showed that it has a prolonged half-life of 2 h compared to the other antipseudomonal β-lactam penicillins.

The bacteria studied were 24 strains of cephalothin-susceptible and 24 cephalothin-resistant E. coli, 24 Enterobacter sp., 13 indole-positive Proteus, 24 Proteus mirabilis, 24 Klebsiella sp., 16 Klebsiella sp. resistant to cephalothin, gentamicin, and tobramycin, 24 Pseudomonas aeruginosa, 21 Serratia sp., 24 penicillin-resistant and 24 penicillin-susceptible Staphylococcus aureus, 11 group A streptococci, 15 group B streptococci, 23 Streptococcus faecalis, 24 S. pneumoniae, 4 penicillinase-producing Neisseria gonorrhoeae (PPNG), and 15 strains of Legionella pneumophila. All 334 isolates were recovered from human sources with the exception of 2 environmental isolates of L. pneumophila. Eleven strains of L. pneumophila and the 4 PPNG were provided by the Center for Disease Control, Atlanta, Ga.

The activities of CI-867, ticarcillin, and piperacillin were determined simultaneously by the agar dilution method, utilizing Mueller-Hinton agar (BBL Microbiology Systems). In the case of the streptococci, sheep blood (Cleveland Scientific) was added; for PPNG chocolatized blood and IsoVitaleX (BBL) was used. For L. pneumophila a medium containing Mueller-Hinton agar, 1% hemoglobin (Difco), and 1% IsoVitaleX was used. Prepared plates were used within 24 h. All plates containing twofold dilutions of the antibiotics were inoculated with a Steers applicator with a inoculum containing 10^5 organisms. The antibiotic concentration that prevented visible growth after 18 h (48 h for L. pneumophila) of incubation at 37°C was recorded as the MIC. CI-867 was supplied by Warner-Lambert/Parke-Davis as a dry powder, piperacillin was supplied by Cyanamide USA, and ticarcillin was supplied by Beecham Pharmaceuticals; all were stored at 4°C, prepared each day in a sterile medium, and used within 24 h.

Table 1 shows the mean geometric MIC for each antibiotic against the 334 isolates. Results of tests with gram-negative bacteria showed that CI-867 was more active than ticarcillin against cephalothin-resistant E. coli, Klebsiella sp., Serratia sp., PPNG, and, of particular interest, P. aeruginosa. They were similarly active, within one dilution, against cephalothin-susceptible E. coli, indole-positive Proteus, Enterobacter sp., and L. pneumophila; CI-867 was less active than ticarcillin against P. mirabilis. In comparison with piperacillin, CI-867 was equally active against both types of E. coli, Enterobacter sp., P. aeruginosa, and Serratia sp. It was also active against two of four PPNG that piperacillin was not active against. CI-867 was less active against both types of Proteus and Klebsiella. All three antibiotics were ineffective against the resistant strain of Klebsiella sp.

With gram-positive organisms, CI-867 was more active than ticarcillin against group B streptococci, S. faecalis, and S. pneumoniae. In comparison with piperacillin, CI-867 was equally

TABLE 1. Comparative in vitro activities of CI-867, ticarcillin, and piperacillin

Organism (no. of strains)	Geometric mean MIC (µg/ml)		
	Ticarcillin	Piperacillin	CI-867
Penicillin-resistant S. aureus (24)	6.01	10.1	>21
Penicillin-susceptible S. aureus (24)	0.79	0.51	0.87
Group A streptococci (11)	<0.41		<0.02
Group B streptococci (15)	1.15	<0.24	0.15
S. faecalis (23)	31	1.89	1.71
S. pneumoniae (24)	0.73	<0.45	<0.05
Cephalothin-susceptible E. coli (24)	1.3	<0.41	0.82
Cephalothin-resistant E. coli (24)[a]	<17	>8.02	>4.17
Enterobacter sp. (24)	11.4	6.56	>6.07
Indole-positive Proteus (13)	4.43	>0.52	>6.2
P. mirabilis (24)	0.91	0.54	3.1
Klebsiella sp. (21)	>145	>8.76	>25
Resistant Klebsiella sp. (16)	>500	>282.5	>50
P. aeruginosa (24)	34.1	7.58	4.29
Serratia sp. (21)	>94.1	>16.6	>22.9
PPNG (4)	>50	500	14.9
L. pneumophila (15)	1.24	4.7	2.58

[a] MIC range, 12.5 (11 strains) to >50.0 (2 strains) µg/ml.

TABLE 2. *Summary of in vitro activity of CI-867*

Organism	% Inhibited at CI-867 concn of (µg/ml):										
	0.05	0.1	0.2	0.4	0.8	1.6	3.1	6.3	12.5	25	50
Cephalothin-susceptible *E. coli*	—[a]	—	—	8.3	83.3	100					
Cephalothin-resistant *E. coli*	—	—	—	4.1	16.6	62.5	66.6	66.6	70.8	70.8	70
Enterobacter sp.	—	—	—	—	—	16.6	54.16	66.6	83.3	83.3	83
Indole-positive *Proteus*	—	—	—	—	—	30.7	61.4	69.2	69.2	69.2	84
P. mirabilis	—	—	—	—	—	—	100				
Klebsiella sp.	—	—	—	—	—	—	—	—	25.0	75.0	79.10
Resistant *Klebsiella* sp.	—	—	—	—	—	—	—	—	—	—	—
P. aeruginosa	—	—	—	—	—	8.2	54.1	91.6	100		
Serratia sp.	—	—	—	—	—	—	9.1	22.7	36.4	45.4	50
Penicillin-resistant *S. aureus*	—	—	—	—	—	—	—	25	37.5	62.5	62
Penicillin-susceptible *S. aureus*	—	—	—	83.3	100						
Group A streptococci	100										
Group B streptococci	—	55.5	88.8	88.8	100						
S. faecalis	—	—	—	—	—	86.9	100				
S. pneumoniae	66.6	75	91.6	100							
PPNG	—	—	—	—	—	—	25	50	50	50	100
L. pneumophila	—	—	—	—	20	46.6	60	100			

[a] — = 0%.

active against the same organisms. It was somewhat less effective than the other two antibiotics against penicillin-resistant *S. aureus*.

Table 2 gives the cumulative percentage inhibited at different concentrations of CI-867. At a concentration of 50 µg/ml (single intramuscular injection of 30 mg/kg in dogs produces a peak of 83 µg/ml in 0.5 h and at 2 h level is 48 µg/ml), CI-867 inhibits against all isolates of cephalothin-susceptible *E. coli*, *P. mirabilis*, and *P. aeruginosa* and penicillin-susceptible *S. aureus*, group A and B streptococci, *S. faecalis*, *S. pneumoniae*, PPNG, and *L. pneumophila*, as well as against most strains of cephalothin-resistant *E. coli* (70%), *Enterobacter* sp. (83%), indole-posi-

tive *Proteus* (84%), *Klebsiella* sp. (79%), penicillin-resistant *S. aureus* (62.5%), and *Serratia* sp. (50%).

The results presented here show that CI-867 has a spectrum of antibacterial activity greater than that of ticarcillin and comparable to that of piperacillin. Further laboratory and clinical studies appear warranted because CI-867 has the advantages of a prolonged half-life and enhanced activity against *P. aeruginosa* and *S. faecalis*.

1. **Neu, H. C., and H. Swarz.** 1969. Carbenicillin: use in serious infections caused by Pseudomonas. Clin. Res. **17**:372.

Synthesis and Structure-Activity Relationships of a Series of Sulfonamidophenylpyridone Derivatives of Ampicillin and Amoxicillin

J. S. KALTENBRONN,* T. H. HASKELL, L. DOUB, J. KNOBLE, C. BAIRD, D. DeJOHN, U. KROLLS, N. JENESEL, G. G. HUANG, AND C. HEIFETZ

Warner-Lambert Pharmaceutical Research Division, Ann Arbor, Michigan 48105, U.S.A.

Among the more serious infections encountered in hospitals are those found among the species of *Klebsiella*, *Enterobacter*, and *Pseudomonas*. A synthetic program at the Warner-Lambert Research Laboratories in Ann Arbor, Mich., undertaken to find penicillins capable of combating these infections has led to a series of sulfonamidophenylpyridone derivatives of ampicillin and amoxicillin which show high activity

against these species. Table 1 shows the generic structure for this series and the in vitro activities against the above-named species. Included for comparison are the activities of piperacillin (PIP) and ticarcillin (TIC). From Table 1 it can be seen that the activities of these compounds compare favorably with those of PIP and are much more potent than TIC. No obvious trends in structure-activity relationships seem to be

TABLE 1. *In vitro activities in micrograms per milliliter (MIC)*

x	y	Klebsiella Pneumoniae MGH2	Enterobacter Cloacae IMM 11	Pseudomonas Aeruginosa #28	Pseudomonas Aeruginosa CB–CS
H_2N	H	6.3	6.3	6.3	6.3
CH_3NH	H	3.1	3.1	3.1	6.3
$(CH_3)_2N$	H	0.8	1.6	1.6	1.6
$(CH_3)_2N$	OH	6.3	6.3	1.6	3.1
$(C_2H_5)_2N$	H	1.6	1.6	1.6	0.8
$(HOCH_2CH_2)_2N$	H	1.6	3.1	3.1	3.1
$(HOCH_2CH_2)_2N$	OH	6.3	3.1	1.6	6.3
$HOCH_2CH_2NH$	H	6.3	6.3	6.3	3.1
⟨pyrrolidine⟩N	H	3.1	3.1	6.3	6.3
⟨piperidine⟩N	H	1.6	3.1	3.1	6.3
⟨piperidine-CH_2OH⟩N	H	6.3	3.1	12.5	3.1
$(CH_3)_2NCH_2CH_2NH$	H	12.5	6.3	6.3	3.1
$(CH_3)_2NCH_2CH_2NH$	OH	3.1	1.6	0.8	—
⟨pyridyl⟩-NH	H	6.3	6.3	6.3	6.3
⟨pyridyl⟩-NH	H	3.1	3.1	6.3	3.1
PIP	—	1.6	0.8	3.1	—
TIC	—	>200	3.1	12.5	12.5

TABLE 2. *In vivo activities in mice[a]*

x	y	Pseudomonas aeruginosa UI-18	Pseudomonas aeruginosa BRK-12-4-4	Enterobacter cloacae IMM-11	Klebsiella pneumoniae MGH2
$(CH_3)_2N$	H	310	268	84	—[b]
$(CH_3)_2N$	OH	132	200	44	—
$(HOCH_2CH_2)_2N$	H	300	140	64	—
$(HOCH_2CH_2)_2N$	OH	70	62	42	90
$(CH_3)_2NCH_2CH_2NH$	H	138	220	70	—
$(CH_3)_2NCH_2CH_2NH$	OH	92	54	12	96
PIP		150	100	20	38
TIC		240	286	12	3200

[a] Generic structure as in Table 1. Values are 50% protective doses in mice, expressed in milligrams per kilogram. Numbers are the total of two doses given by the subcutaneous route.
[b] —, Not done.

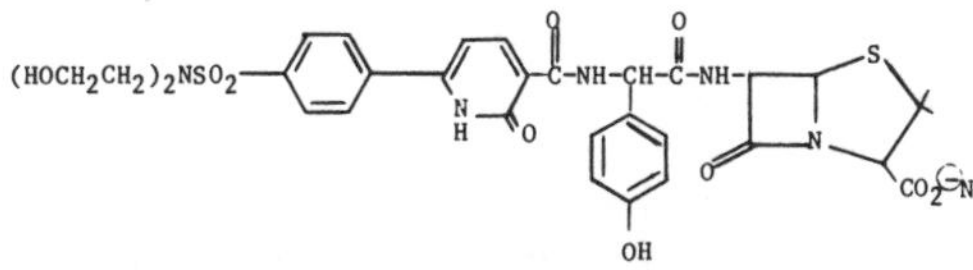

FIG. 1. *CI-867*.

present in this series. Good MIC values are obtained when x is either an aliphatic or aromatic amine. There is no striking difference in MIC values when x is a primary, secondary, or cyclic amine.

Although the in vitro MIC values of ampicillin and amoxicillin derivatives bearing identical side chains are similar, when tested in vivo in mice the amoxicillin derivatives show a definite superiority. Table 2 compares three sets of derivatives against two strains of *Pseudomonas* and one each of *Enterobacter* and *Klebsiella*. The in vivo activities of PIP and TIC are included for comparison.

Based on these and other data, one compound, CI-867, was selected for further evaluation (Fig. 1).

When tested in vitro against the expanded array of gram-positive and gram-negative species that we use in our early evaluation process, CI-867 had an activity profile similar to PIP and was clearly superior to TIC, especially against *Pseudomonas* and *Klebsiella* spp. In addition to the data listed in Table 1, this expanded in vitro evaluation showed the following MIC values for CI-867, PIP, and TIC, respectively: *Staphylococcus aureus* UC-76: 0.8, 0.4, 0.4; *Streptococcus*

faecalis MGH-2: 0.2, 1.6, 25; *Serratia marcescens* IMM-16: 6.3, 0.8, 3.1; *Pseudomonas aeruginosa* BRK-12-4-4: 3.1, 3.1, 25; *Pseudomonas aeruginosa* UI-18: 1.6, 1.6, 25; *Escherichia coli* Vogel: 0.4, 0.8, 1.6; *E. coli* Brig: 0.8, 0.8, 3.1; and *Proteus vulgaris* 1810: 3.1, 0.2, 0.8.

The in vivo results versus *Pseudomonas* sp. (Table 2) show the advantage of CI-867 compared to both PIP and TIC.

When tested in vitro against reference standard bacteria in both agar dilution and broth dilution tests, CI-867 again showed activity similar to PIP and was approximately four times more potent than TIC. MIC values are as follows for CI-867 agar/broth, PIP agar/broth, and TIC agar/broth, respectively: *S. aureus* ATCC 25923: 0.8/0.8, 0.8/1.6, 0.8/3.1; *E. coli* ATCC 25922: 3.1/ 3.1, 1.6/3.1, 12.5/12.5; *P. aeruginosa* ATCC 27853: 3.1/3.1, 1.6/3.1, 12.5/25.

Blood level studies in dogs and mice showed higher peak blood levels than either PIP or TIC, with a longer half-life, particularly in dogs. Values of peak blood levels (μg/ml)/half-life (h) obtained from a 30-mg/kg intramuscular dose in dogs were as follows: CI-867, 83/2.3; PIP, 40/0.7; TIC, 62/0.8. A 300-mg/kg subcutaneous dose in mice gave values (peak blood level [μg/ml]/half-life [h]) of: CI-867, 92/1.0; PIP, 47/0.3; TIC, 89/ 0.7.

Single intravenous doses as high as 4,000 mg/ kg showed no toxic manifestations in mice. Like PIP and TIC, CI-867 is not active by the oral route of administration.

CI-867 has been scheduled for clinical trial.

CI-867, a Novel Penicillin Derivative Active Against Gram-Negative Pathogens

C. L. HEIFETZ* AND J. A. SESNIE

Warner-Lambert Pharmaceutical Research Division, Detroit, Michigan 48232, U.S.A.

Pseudomonas aeruginosa and species of *Klebsiella* and *Enterobacter* continue to contribute a high incidence of infections, attended by significant morbidity and mortality, in people in immunologically compromised conditions. Drugs currently available for treatment of gram-negative infections are either toxic at doses close to therapeutic levels or of low potency and limited spectrum. Increasing occurrence of aminoglycoside resistance has added to the problem. These factors have stimulated the search for new highly potent, nontoxic, broad-spectrum antibacterial agents.

In an effort to produce a suitable therapeutic agent, a series of sulfonamidophenyl-substituted pyridone semisynthetic penicillins were synthesized for antibacterial evaluation (J. S. Kaltenbronn et al., this volume). The evaluations emphasized the therapeutic potencies of the novel derivatives against clinically important and relatively intransigent gram-negative bacteria in experimental infections of laboratory mice. In vitro data were obtained to help indicate the breadth of spectrum. This process led to the selection of CI-867 as a candidate for further development (2). Herein are described the antibacterial attributes of this new agent along with data obtained simultaneously with ticarcillin and piperacillin.

Therapeutic activities of the three semisynthetic penicillins were compared in acute mouse protection tests in which 18- to 22-g female Charles River CD-1 mice were used. (1). Subcutaneous doses in twofold rising incremental series were administered concurrently with bacterial challenge, and were repeated in 2 h in some cases, as indicated. Challenges were accomplished by the intraperitoneal injection of an estimated 100 median lethal doses in 0.5-ml volumes of 5% hog gastric mucin or tryptic soy broth. Generally, >90% of the untreated controls died within 48 to 72 h. Final survival percent-

TABLE 1. *Relative activity of CI-867 in mouse therapy tests, compared with ticarcillin and piperacillin*

Organism	No. of doses[a]	PD$_{50}$ (mg/kg, total dose)		
		CI-867	Ticarcillin	Piperacillin
Pseudomonas aeruginosa				
UI-18	2	70 (1.6)[b]	240 (12.5)	150 (1.6)
BRK 12-4-4	2	62 (3.1)	186 (25)	100 (3.1)
Homma IID 1117	2	100 (3.1)	310 (25)	250 (3.1)
PA86	2	92 (1.6)	192 (12.5)	168 (1.6)
PA220	2	75 (3.1)	. 140 (25)	90 (3.1)
Bold 6-22	2	128 (3.1)	2,000 (25)	1,080 (6.3)
Enterobacter cloacae				
IMM-11	2	42 (3.1)	21 (3.1)	20 (0.8)
IMM-50	1	80 (3.1)	75 (1.6)	45 (1.6)
HFH-5	1	22 (3.1)	16 (1.6)	9 (1.6)
HFH-18	1	13 (1.6)	6 (3.1)	5 (1.6)
Klebsiella pneumoniae				
MGH-2[c]	2	90 (6.3)	3,200 (>50)	38 (1.6)
AD[c]	2	10 (0.4)	3 (0.8)	10 (0.2)
IMM-40	2	132 (6.3)	>400 (>50)	132 (6.3)
HFH-50	2	240 (6.3)	>1,600 (200)	430 (1.6)
HFH-67	2	220 (6.3)	>400 (200)	100 (3.1)
Proteus mirabilis				
MGH-1	2	34 (3.1)	70 (0.8)	25 (0.2)
658	1	26 (3.1)	22 (0.4)	5 (0.4)
P. morganii				
RC-2362	2	74 (3.1)	23 (0.8)	6 (0.4)
37-2	1	118 (3.1)	50 (0.4)	21 (0.8)
P. rettgeri				
M1771	2	30 (1.6)	7 (0.2)	34 (0.1)
M1050	1	28 (1.6)	11 (0.1)	6 (0.8)
P. vulgaris				
1810	2	74 (3.1)	40 (0.8)	22 (0.2)
50	1	32 (3.1)	13 (0.4)	6 (0.1)
277	1	110 (6.3)	180 (1.6)	10 (0.4)
Providencia stuartii				
B2328	1	161 (25)	5 (0.8)	30 (3.1)
120	1	80 (12.5)	10 (0.8)	22 (1.6)
Escherichia coli				
Vogel	1	14 (0.4)	12 (1.6)	12 (0.8)
07D	1	6 (0.8)	11 (1.6)	11 (1.6)
Brig	1	16 (0.8)	6 (3.1)	5 (0.8)
04	1	12 (0.8)	10 (1.6)	7 (0.8)
MGH-1	1	11 (0.8)	12 (3.1)	7 (0.4)
MGH-2	1	12 (0.8)	14 (1.6)	6 (0.8)
Serratia marcescens				
IMM-16	2	136 (6.3)	44 (3.1)	14 (0.8)
Berman	2	100 (6.3)	18 (6.3)	20 (1.6)
01	1	37 (6.3)	17 (3.1)	22 (0.4)
06	1	100 (6.3)	19 (12.5)	11 (0.8)

[a] Administered subcutaneously.

[b] MICs (micrograms per milliliter) are given in parentheses.

[c] Challenge administered in tryptic soy broth; all others administered in 5% hog gastric mucin.

TABLE 2. *Relative activity of CI-867 in vitro, compared with ticarcillin and piperacillin*

Organism (no. of strains)	Drug	Cumulative percent inhibited by a concn (µg/ml) of:										
		<0.2	0.2	0.4	0.8	1.6	3.1	6.3	12.5	25	50	>50
Pseudomonas spp. (90)[a]	CI-867			1	2	24	64	91	96	97	98	100
	Ticarcillin							2	17	44	84	100
	Piperacillin			1	11	43	80	93	97	98		100
Klebsiella spp. (78)[b]	CI-867	3		4	6	9	21	55	73	90	91	100
	Ticarcillin			1	3						4	100
	Piperacillin	4	5	9	15	41	76	87	91	92	94	100
Enterobacter spp. (43)[c]	CI-867				7	30	77		86			100
	Ticarcillin				7	26	63	74	81		84	100
	Piperacillin			2	16	44	77	86				100
Serratia spp. (30)[d]	CI-867				3		7	43	63	73		100
	Ticarcillin			3	13	23	33	57	63	67	77	100
	Piperacillin	3	7	37	57	67	73	80	87	93	100	
Escherichia coli (16)	CI-867				6	38	56	75				100
	Ticarcillin					31	56	69	75			100
	Piperacillin				6	38	69	75			81	100
Proteus, indole negative (13)	CI-867				8	15	77	92				100
	Ticarcillin		15	39	77	85	92					100
	Piperacillin	15		77	92				100			
Proteus spp., indole positive (39)[e]	CI-867						23	51	64	80	85	100
	Ticarcillin	3	5	23	54	77	80	82	90			100
	Piperacillin	8	15	54	69	80	85		90	92	97	100
Providencia spp. (16)[f]	CI-867							6	13	56	88	100
	Ticarcillin			25	63	81			88			100
	Piperacillin			6	19	69	88	94				100
Salmonella spp. (7)[g]	CI-867							43	100			
	Ticarcillin						14	71	86	100		
	Piperacillin					43	100					
Shigella spp. (5)[h]	CI-867		40	60		80	100					
	Ticarcillin				40	60	80	100				
	Piperacillin	40			80	100						

[a] *P. aeruginosa,* 83 strains; non-*P. aeruginosa,* 7 strains.
[b] *K. pneumoniae,* 67 strains; *K. oxytoca,* 11 strains.
[c] *E. cloacae,* 34 strains; *E. aerogenes,* 7 strains; *E. sakazakii,* 2 strains.
[d] *S. marcescens,* 29 strains; *S. liquefaciens,* 1 strain.
[e] *P. morganii,* 15 strains; *P. rettgeri,* 13 strains; *P. vulgaris,* 11 strains.
[f] *P. alcalifaciens,* 2 strains; *P. stuartii,* 14 strains.
[g] *S. enteritidis,* 2 strains; *S. typhimurium,* 2 strains; *S. typhi,* 2 strains; *S. paratyphi,* 1 strain.
[h] *S. dysenteriae,* 2 strains; *S. flexneri,* 1 strain; *S. sonnei,* 2 strains.

ages, obtained after 4 to 7 days of observation among groups of 8 to 16 mice, were pooled and used to estimate median protective doses (PD$_{50}$) by the log-probit method (4). MICs were determined by microtitration dilution in tryptic soy broth in 100-µl final volumes (1, 3). Inocula contained 1,000 colony-forming units of bacteria derived from overnight cultures. All incubations were at 37°C for 16 to 18 h. The MIC was the lowest concentration of compound, in twofold dilution series, inhibiting visible growth. Bacteria tested included fresh clinical isolates and strains from our culture collection, which include a high proportion of antibiotic-resistant strains.

In acute mouse protection tests (Table 1) against 36 gram-negative isolates, the geometric mean PD$_{50}$ values (total dose, milligrams per kilogram) were 85 against six *P. aeruginosa* strains, 31 against four *E. cloacae* strains, 91 against five *K. pneumoniae* strains, 66 against nine indole-positive *Proteus* strains, 30 against two *P. mirabilis* strains, 11 against six *Escherichia coli* strains, and 84 against four *Serratia marcescens* strains. CI-867 was markedly more effective in mice than ticarcillin against *P. aeruginosa* and *K. pneumoniae* and more than twice as effective as piperacillin against the former. Thus, to include *P. aeruginosa* in their therapeutic ranges, piperacillin and ticarcillin required severalfold higher doses than CI-867.

The in vitro data (Table 2) indicate that CI-867 possesses a broad spectrum of action against gram-negative bacteria, including those for which new agents are required. In broth dilution tests, median MICs ranged from 1.6 μg/ml (*E. coli* and *P. mirabilis*) through 3.1 μg/ml (*Pseudomonas, Enterobacter*, indole-positive *Proteus, Salmonella-Shigella*) and 6.3 μg/ml (*Klebsiella*) to 12.5 μg/ml (*Serratia* and *Providencia*). Ticarcillin was virtually inactive against *Klebsiella* and was markedly less effective than CI-867 against *P. aeruginosa*. Although against *P.*

aeruginosa, piperacillin and CI-867 were roughly equivalent in vitro, the latter was markedly more effective in mouse therapy tests.

These studies indicate that CI-867 has potential usefulness as a therapeutic agent against clinically important and relatively intransigent gram-negative bacteria and merits further study.

1. **Heifetz, C. L., J. A. Chodubski, I. A. Pearson, C. A. Silverman, and M. W. Fisher.** 1974. Butirosin compared with gentamicin in vitro and in vivo. Antimicrob. Agents Chemother. **6:**124–135.
2. **Kaltenbronn, J. S., T. H. Haskell, L. Doub, J. Knoble, D. de John, U. Krolls, N. Jenesel, G. Huang, C. L. Heifetz, and M. W. Fisher.** 1979. CI-867, a new broad-spectrum semi-synthetic penicillin. J. Antibiot. **32:**621–625.
3. **Marymont, J. H., Jr., and R. M. Wentz.** 1966. Serial dilution antibiotic sensitivity testing with the microtitrator system. Am. J. Clin. Pathol. **45:**548–551.
4. **Miller, L. C., and M. L. Tainter.** 1944. Estimation of the ED_{50} and its error by means of logarithmic-probit graph paper. Proc. Soc. Exp. Biol. Med. **57:**261–274.

Gas Chromatographic-Mass Spectrometric Characteristics of a Group of β-Lactam Compounds Determined by Use of a Desk-Top Quadrupole Mass Spectrometer

THOMAS F. BRODASKY

Research Laboratories, The Upjohn Co., Kalamazoo, Michigan 49001, U.S.A.

Pursuant to the goals of a program designed to investigate various analytical procedures for a number of antibiotic families, a comprehensive study of the gas chromatographic-mass spectrometric (GC-MS) properties of a selected group of penicillins, cephalosporins, and azetidinones was undertaken. In addition to the generation of analytical data, this study presented an opportunity to evaluate a newly acquired desk-top quadrupole GC-MS unit.

The instrument used in this investigation was a Hewlett-Packard model 5992A GC-MS unit (Hewlett-Packard Co., Avondale, Calif.). The mass analyzer is a quadrupole unit with a range from 10 to 800 atomic mass units. The electron source is operated at 70 eV with electron multiplier voltages between 2,200 and 2,800 V. The columns used were either 45 or 80 cm long, 2.0 mm in inner diameter, glass, and were packed with UCW 982 on high-efficiency Chromosorb W.

With all penicillins investigated, the side-chain groups were responsible for the appearance of strong ions in the low mass region,

whereas molecular ions varied in intensity depending on the compound. Aside from these features, the penicillins generally gave a group of peaks related to the formation and subsequent fragmentation of a thiazolidine ring (114, 142, 160, 174, and 232 m/z [ratio of the ionic mass to the ionic charge]) (2). The spectrum of 6-aminopenicillanic acid (6APA) · trimethylsilyl derivative (TMS) exemplifies these fragmentations, although it contains only an amine as a substituent on the lactam ring. The chromatogram of the TMS derivative is a single peak, with the mass spectrum shown in Fig. 1. The molecular ion at 360 m/z and thiazolidine ions at 114 and 232 m/z are apparent. The loss of thioacetone (74 m/z) as assigned in this fragmentation is unique to this compound among those lactam compounds giving the thiazolidine ions.

In view of the reproducible fragmentations of the penicillins and 6APA, SIM (selected ion monitoring) experiments were carried out monitoring various ions from the thiazolidine ring. Retention times and selected ions allow recognition of individual members in mixtures. The

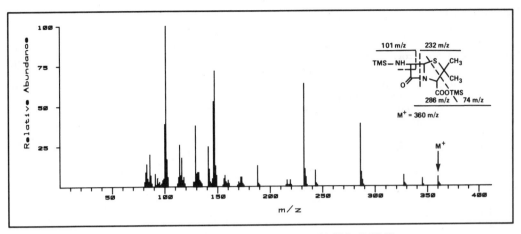

FIG. 1. *Electron impact mass spectrum of 6APA·di-TMS.*

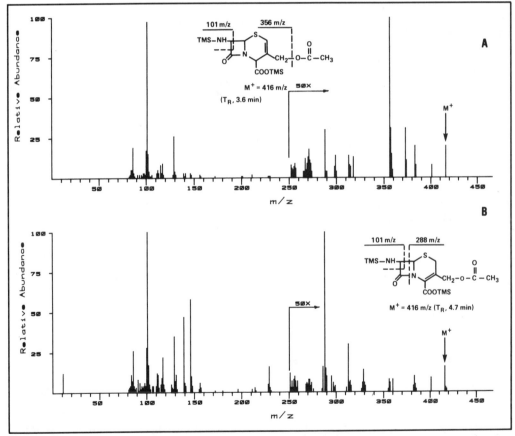

FIG. 2. *Composite electron impact mass spectrum of (A) 7ACA·di-TMS Δ² isomer and (B) 7ACA·di-TMS Δ³ isomer.*

three ions (232, 174, and 114 m/z) gave the best results, but the program allows monitoring of up to six ions. It would be profitable, in cases where the presence of specific compounds was sus-pected, to include ions representative of the side-chain fragments.

As with the penicillins, our purpose in study-ing the cephalosporins was the establishment of reproducible fragmentation patterns suitable for generation of a mass spectral library. A computer search of the literature failed to reveal any work, other than pyrolysis gas chromatography (3, 5) and a study of cephalexin (4), which dealt with gas chromatography of this group of β-lactam compounds. Numerous experiments with cephalothin and cephaloglycin failed to produce any gas chromatographic peaks giving spectra consistent with the structures. These results prompted us to investigate model compounds, such as 7-aminocephalosporanic acid (7ACA), containing all the functionality of the cephalosporins except for the side chain on the lactam ring. The total ion abundance chromatogram of the TMS derivative of 7ACA contained two well-resolved peaks of nearly equal intensity. The mass spectra of these peaks (Fig. 2) revealed that the compound having the lower gas chromatographic retention time preferentially loses a 60 m/z fragment (CH₃COOH). This anomaly is not due to a second component in the sample but to a transformation occurring during derivatization or chromatography. Cocker described the isomerization of the double bond in cephalosporin acids under the influence of pyridine and indicated that this isomerization is facilitated when the carboxylic group is esterified (1). Based on these studies, it would appear that the doublet is due to the Δ^2,Δ^3 isomers.

The Hewlett-Packard 5992 GC-MS unit is not equipped with a means of introducing samples directly into the source chamber. Such a system could be of value in examining the cephalosporins in view of their unsatisfactory gas chromatographic characteristics. A device (T. F. Brodasky, patent pending) was constructed which allows evacuation of a small chamber containing a melting-point capillary holding the sample.

After evacuation by the roughing pump, the isolation valve is opened and the gas chromatograph oven is programmed from 80 to 300°C in an attempt to volatilize sufficient of the sample to obtain its mass spectrum. A sample of the methyl ester of cephalothin, which had failed to give a peak when the GC-MS mode of operation was used, was examined by use of this direct inlet system. Monitoring the total ion abundance led to the appearance of a peak at approximately 250°C. The mass spectrum of this peak is nearly identical to one obtained by probe on an Atlas CH5.

Among the compounds examined, representing the nonclassical β-lactam antibiotics, were the azetidinones with various substituents on the ring. Although only two compounds representing the unsubstituted lactam nitrogen group were run, it appears that the loss of 115 m/z (TMSN=C=O|⁺) may be a characteristic fragmentation pathway and could be useful in identifying this group.

1. **Cocker, J. D., S. Eardley, G. I. Gregory, M. E. Hall, and A. G. Long.** 1966. Cephalosporanic acids. IV. 7-Acylamidoceph-2-en-4-carboxylic acids. J. Chem. Soc., p. 1142–1151.

2. **Flynn, E. H. (ed.).** 1972. Cephalosporins and penicillins—chemistry and biology, p. 312–369. Academic Press Inc., New York.

3. **Müller, M., J. Seibl, and W. Simon.** 1978. Characterization of some penicillins and cephalosporins by pyrolysis mass spectroscopy. Anal. Chim. Acta **100:**263–269.

4. **Nakagawa, T., J. Haginaka, M. Masada, and T. Uno.** 1978. Gas chromatographic and gas chromatographic-mass spectrometric analysis of cephalexin. J. Chromatogr. **154:**264–266.

5. **Roy, T. A., and S. S. Szinai.** 1976. Pyrolysis GLC identification of food and drug ingredients. II. Qualitative and quantitative analysis of penicillins and cephalosporins. J. Chromatogr. Sci. **14:**580–584.

Immunological Cross-Reactivity of Penicillins and Cephalosporins Related to Side-Chain Configuration

DEBRA K. ALLEMENOS,* RICHARD S. GRIFFITH, AND BRUCE H. PETERSEN

Lilly Laboratory for Clinical Research, Wishard Memorial Hospital, Indianapolis, Indiana 46202, U.S.A.

Immunological cross-reactivity between compounds of similar chemical configuration frequently occurs. When the compounds are drugs, this reactivity can have clinical significance. Because of their frequent use, immunological cross-reactivity between the penicillins and cephalosporins has received a great deal of attention (1).

In these studies several cephalosporins of differing chemical composition were evaluated for cross-reactivity with antibodies to penicillin G, cephalexin, cefamandole, and cephalothin. The methods and procedures used in this study have been described (1).

Antibody to penicillin G appears to be directed to the benzylpenicilloyl determinant, with the acyl side chain determining the role of its immunogenicity: 6-aminopenicillanic acid (6-APA) did not effectively inhibit the anti-penicillin G antibody. Similarities of the acyl side chains have been shown to be responsible for the cross-reactivity of antibody to penicillin G and the cephalosporins (2). The phenyl group of the penicillin G side chain does not seem to be readily distinguishable immunologically from the thiophene ring of the cephalothin side chain. Penicillin V and cephalothin effectively inhibited antibody to penicillin G. Cephalexin, which has a similar acyl side chain but with a substituted α-amino group, failed to cause inhibition. Ampicillin, also with this same amino-substituted side chain, poorly inhibited antibodies to penicillin G. From these experiments, it became apparent that the addition of the amino group altered the antigenic specificity of the side chain. Cephalosporins that do not have an acyl side chain similar to that of penicillin G failed to inhibit the antibody.

On the other hand, antibody to cephalothin appears to recognize both the 7-aminocephalosporanic acid (7-ACA) nucleus and the thiophene side chain substituted at the R_1 position. Two cephalosporin nuclei, 7-ACA and 7-aminodeacetoxycephalosporanic acid (7-ADCA), inhibited the antibody to cephalothin, supporting the supposition that some antibody specificity is directed toward the 7-ACA nucleus. Cefamandole, which has a 7-ACA nucleus and phenyl side chain, and penicillin G were effective inhibitors of the anticephalothin antibody, presumably because of the immunologically similar groups at R_1 (Table 1). Cephalexin, which has a 7-ADCA nucleus and an amino-substituted phenyl side chain, was as effective an inhibitor of the antibody as 7-ACA or 7-ADCA. The failure of cephalexin, with its substituted phenyl side chain, to inhibit the antibody as well as cefamandole gives further support to the observation that the addition of an amino group to the acyl side chain alters immunological reactivity.

Antibody to cephalexin appears to be strongly influenced by the 7-ACA nucleus. 7-ACA and 7-

TABLE 2. *Immunological cross-reactivity of cephalosporins as determined by haptene inhibition* [a]

Antibiotic inhibitor	Concn (mM) inhibiting antibody to	
	Cephalexin	Cefamandole
Cephalexin	0.38	25
Cefamandole	50	<0.38
Cephalothin	25	50
Cefazolin	50	6.25
Cefoxitin	200	25
Cefuroxime	200	100
Cefotaxime	200	25
7-ACA	25	>100
7-ADCA	25	>100

[a] Results are expressed as the lowest concentration of antibiotic giving inhibition of agglutination.

ADCA were effective inhibitors of antibody to cephalexin (Table 2). The acetyl side chain of 7-ACA appears to have little effect on antibody binding. Most penicillin derivatives did not effectively inhibit antibody to cephalexin. Ampicillin, however, with an acyl side chain similar to that of cephalexin, gave partial inhibition of anti-cephalexin antibodies at concentrations of 200 and 400 mM. Complex side chains substituted at the R_1 and R_2 positions on the cephalosporin molecule did affect antibody specificity. The side chain at the R_1 position of cephapirin and cephalothin made the molecule a more effective inhibitor of antibody to cephalexin than was 7-ACA. Substitution of an amino group to the side chain at the R_2 position appeared to alter antigen recognition strongly, as is evidenced by the failure of cefuroxime and cefoxitin to inhibit anti-cephalexin antibody.

Antibody specificity to cefamandole, on the other hand, appears to be primarily affected by side chains substituted at the R_1 and R_2 positions of the nucleus. 7-ACA and 7-ADCA did not inhibit antibody to cefamandole, whereas cefazolin, which has a similar chain at the R_2 position, effectively inhibited the antibody (Table 2). The nitrogen constituents in the cefazolin ring at the R_1 position apparently do not affect antibody binding. Penicillin G, which has a phenyl side chain, inhibited antibody to cefamandole at a concentration of 100 mM, whereas the free penicillin nucleus 6-APA did not inhibit at concentrations of 200 mM. The complex ring structure of cefotaxime makes its antigenic reactivity more difficult to explain. Possibly the most reasonable explanation is that the side chain at the R_1 position of cefotaxime is compatible with antibody to cefamandole because of similarities to the R_2 position side chain of cefamandole. We have already shown that the acetyl side chain is

TABLE 1. *Immunological reactivity of human anti-cephalothin antibody for other antibiotics*

Inhibitor	Concn (mM) [a]
Cephalothin	0.39
Penicillin G	12.5
Cephalexin	25
Cefamandole	2.6
7-ACA	25
7-ADCA	25

[a] The lowest concentration of antibiotic which inhibited agglutination.

not involved in the inhibition of antibody to cefamandole.

Although there was limited cross-reactivity between the cephalosporins, it appeared to be largely determined by the group substituted at the R_1 and R_2 position rather than reactivity of antibody to the nucleus. Cross-reactivity of anti-cephalexin antibody, specific for the 7-ADCA nucleus, with other cephalosporins was largely eliminated by substitutions of complex groups at the R_2 position. There appear to be different degrees of cross-reactivity between penicillins and the different cephalosporins, apparently more related to the side-chain substitution than to the nucleus. The clinical relevance of these results cannot be determined, possibly because the sensitivity of in vitro immunological tests for cross-reactivity far exceeds the level of clinical relevance.

1. **Petersen, B. H., and J. Graham.** 1974. Immunologic cross-reactivity of cephalexin and penicillin. J. Lab. Clin. Med. **83**:860–870.
2. **Petz, L. D.** 1978. Immunologic cross-reactivity between penicillins and the cephalosporins. A review. J. Infect. Dis. **13**:S74–S79.

Immunogenic Derivatives of Cephalosporins: In Vitro Assay of Spontaneous Cephalosporylation of Model Compounds

NEWTON E. HYSLOP, JR.,* ANNE L. BUCHINSKI, AND NORA LIU

Medical Service (Infectious Disease Unit), Massachusetts General Hospital, and Department of Medicine, Harvard Medical School, Boston, Massachusetts 02114, U.S.A.*

The spontaneous immunogenicity of drugs is closely related to their ability to react chemically with functional groups on biological substrates to form covalent linkages and to do so under physiological conditions and at concentrations used in therapy. This principle is best exempli-

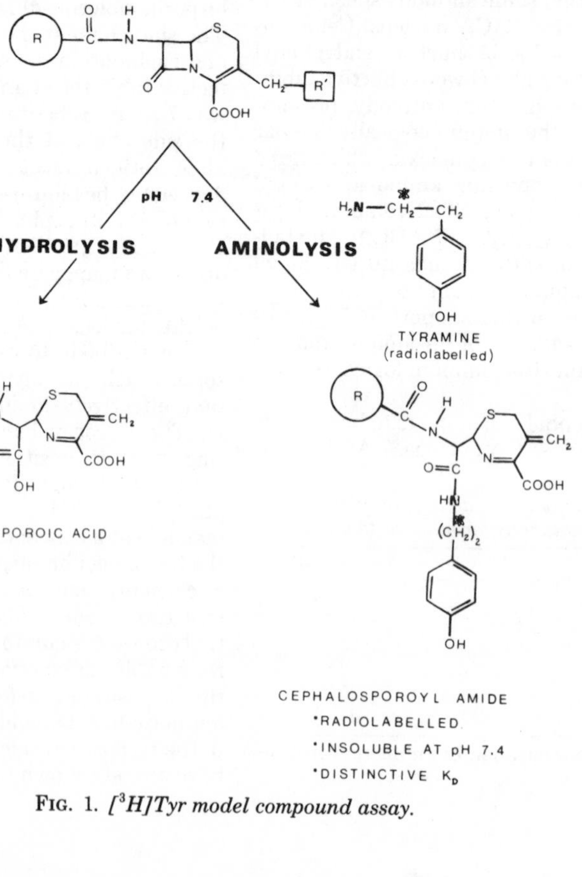

FIG. 1. *[³H]Tyr model compound assay.*

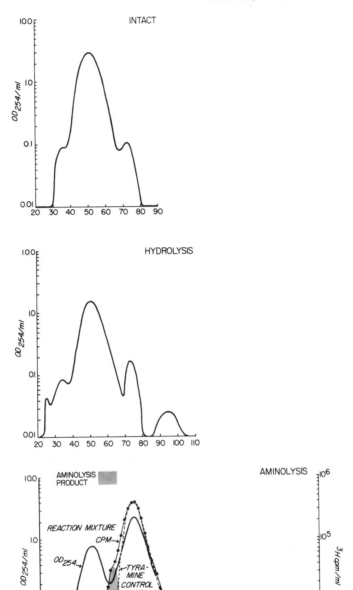

FIG. 2. *Sephadex G-10 chromatography of cephaloridine. (Top) Intact; (middle) products formed under hydrolysis conditions (0.1 M PO$_4$ buffer, pH 7.4; 18 h, 37°C); (bottom) products formed under aminolysis conditions (5 × 10^{-2} M Tyr, 0.1 M PO$_4$ buffer, pH 7.4; 18 h, 37°C).*

fied by the in vivo immunogenicity of penicillins.

While penicillins are capable of several degradative reactions resulting in products able to react with proteins, membranes, or other carriers, the penicilloylation reaction is the principal in vivo route to haptenic substitution and is the most common object of the immune response. In this reaction an amide linkage of side chain and thiazolidine ring to carrier results when the β-lactam ring undergoes aminolysis by the free NH_2 groups of the carrier to form the penicilloyl determinant.

Cephalosporins also undergo immunochemically significant degradative in vivo reactions. A cephalosporyl haptenic analog of the penicilloyl determinant is thought to result from aminolysis of the β-lactam ring of cephalosporins, although model compound aminolysis studies conducted with concentrated solutions suggest that this reaction is accompanied by cleavage of large R' side chains, as indicated in Fig. 1. Knowledge about rates of cephalosporylation and accessory reactions under physiological conditions is limited, however, due to lack of any assay for detecting reactions of the β-lactam ring of cephalosporins which is comparable in sensitivity to the penamaldate assay for the penicilloates and penicilloylamides of penicillins.

Previous studies of immunochemically significant cephalosporin degradation reactions have used spectroscopic analysis of concentrated solutions to identify aminolysis products and high-pressure liquid chromatography to identify hydrolysis products in dilute solutions (1, 2, 4). The objective of our studies was to determine if a direct assay of β-lactam aminolysis by model amines could be based on the ability of highly cross-linked dextran gels to separate the products of β-lactam aminolysis from the intact and hydrolyzed cephalosporin in the mixture (3).

Selected cephalosporins at 5×10^{-3} M were subjected to hydrolysis and aminolysis under physiological conditions (pH 7.4, 37°C, 0.1 M PO_4 buffer) for varying lengths of time up to 18 h. Samples (1.0 ml) of reaction solutions and of intact cephalosporins were chromatographed on Sephadex G-10 and eluted over 2 h with phosphate-buffered saline at pH 7.4 or 9.5. Eluates were monitored for absorbancy at 254 nm (A_{254}) on an ISCO UA-5 monitor with a scale expander. Aminolysis was conducted with amine in 10-fold

molar excess; epsilon-aminocaproic acid and γ-aminobutyric acid were compared with tyramine (Tyr) as model amines.

As substrates for detection of aminolysis of the β-lactam ring by alteration of chromatographic elution position, both epsilon-aminocaproic and γ-aminobutyric acids had the advantage of insignificant A_{254}. However, the resultant elution positions of their cephalosporoylamides and the respective cephalosporoates overlapped too closely to be distinctive. While Tyr as a substrate had the disadvantages of significant A_{254} (see Fig. 1) and of the insolubility of its cephalosporylamide derivatives at pH 7.4, the latter were soluble at pH 9.5 and had distinctive chromatographic elution positions.

Results of a typical experiment are shown in Fig. 2, where elution profiles of reaction samples eluted with pH 9.5 phosphate-buffered saline are shown for intact cephaloridine (top), for cephaloridine hydrolyzed for 18 h (middle), and for cephaloridine reacted for 18 h with excess [³H]Tyr. Integration of the difference between the position of prechromatographed [³H]Tyr (dashed line) and the counts per minute (dots) of the fractions is indicated by the shaded areas; A_{254} is shown as a solid line. Note that polymers were not detected.

These results indicate that direct measurement of aminolysis of the β-lactam of cephalosporins in dilute solutions is possible with suitable model compound substrates. The unique characteristics of the Tyr aminolysis product suggest that the Tyr assay may be useful for studies on the effect of side chain structures on rates of β-lactam aminolysis under physiological conditions.

1. **Bundgaard, H.** 1975. Chemical studies related to cephalosporin allergy. 1. Kinetics of aminolysis of cephalosporins and effect of C-3 substituents on β-lactam reactivity. Arch. Pharm. Chem. Sci. Ed. **3**:94–123.

2. **Hamilton-Miller, J. M. T., G. G. F. Newton, and E. P. Abraham.** 1970. Products of aminolysis and enzymatic hydrolysis of the cephalosporins. Biochem. J. **116**:371–384.

3. **Hyslop, N. E., Jr., and R. J. Milligan.** 1974. Chromatography of penicillins, penicilloates, and penicilloylamides on dextran gels. Antimicrob. Agents Chemother. **5**:617–629.

4. **Yamana, T., and A. Tsuji.** 1976. Comparative stability of cephalosporins in aqueous solution: kinetics and mechanisms of degradation. J. Pharm. Sci. **65**:1563–1574.

Clinical Experience with Netilmicin

J. FALISEVAC, S. SCHONWALD,* V. CAR, B. GMAJNICKI, AND M. STRITOF

University Hospital of Infectious Diseases, Zagreb, Yugoslavia

Netilmicin, a new semisynthetic aminoglycoside derived from sisomicin, has been shown to have good in vitro activity against a wide variety of gram-negative bacteria and *Staphylococcus aureus* (3). Some investigators have also demonstrated that netilmicin has good activity against strains of bacteria resistant to other aminoglycosides (2, 5).

Clinically, netilmicin has been shown to be effective in the treatment of many serious and life-threatening infections, including septicemia and urinary tract, pulmonary, and soft-tissue infections (1, 4).

A total of 69 patients, participating in three separate clinical trials, were treated with netilmicin. Forty of the patients had infections due to *S. aureus* and were treated at a dosage of 6 mg/kg per day given in three equal doses. Ten patients, with systemic infections due to gram-negative organisms, received netilmicin at a dosage of 200 mg twice a day. The remaining 19 patients had infections due to gram-negative or gram-positive organisms and received netilmicin at a dosage of 150 mg three times a day.

Infections treated with netilmicin included pneumonia, endometritis, biliary tract infections, cellulitis, mastitis, pyelonephritis, carbuncles, and furuncles. Causative organisms included *Escherichia coli*, *Klebsiella pneumoniae*, *Proteus mirabilis*, *S. aureus*, *Streptococcus pneumoniae*, and *Enterococcus*.

All patients had documented infection or fever with or without septicemia. In addition, all patients had normal renal function before inclusion in the studies. Before therapy, all patients underwent complete physical examination, including extensive laboratory testing as well as puretone audiometry and electronystagmography. Auditory and vestibular functions were normal in all patients before receiving netilmicin.

Overall, the outcome of therapy was very favorable. Combining the results for all three studies, 85.6% of the patients (59 patients) were completely cured of their infections, 7.2% experienced clinical improvement (5 patients), 4.3% failed to respond to therapy (3 patients), and the outcome was indeterminate in 2.9% (2 patients). Therefore, 92.8% of the patients had favorable clinical responses to netilmicin therapy.

The overall bacteriological outcome of netilmicin therapy was also very favorable. Eradication of the causative organism was observed in 94.3% of the cases (65 isolates), and persistence was observed in only 2.9% (2 isolates). Results were indeterminate in 1.4% and not specified in 1.4% (one isolate each). None of our patients experienced ototoxicity, nephrotoxicity, or other adverse reactions, and local tolerance was good in all patients.

Based on our experience, it can be said that netilmicin, whether administered on a milligram-per-kilogram basis or as a simplified dosage, is effective and safe in the treatment of a wide variety of both local and systemic infections caused by gram-negative and gram-positive organisms.

1. Chadwick, P., A. W. Bruce, T. D. V. Cooke, and G. J. Marty. 1978. Therapeutic experience with netilmicin. GMA J. 119:1189–1193.
2. Devaud, M., F. H. Kayser, and U. Huber. 1977. Resistance of bacteria to the newer aminoglycoside antibiotics: an epidemiological and enzymatic study. J. Antibiot. 30:655–664.
3. Digranes, A., B. Ostervold, S. T. Madsen, C. O. Solberg, and K. Haeger. 1978. Susceptibility of 327 clinical isolates to netilmicin. J. Intern. Med. Res. 6:409–413.
4. Panwalker, A. P., J. B. Malow, V. M. Zimelis, and G. G. Jackson. 1978. Netilmicin: clinical efficacy, tolerance, and toxicity. Antimicrob. Agents Chemother. 13:170–176.
5. Watanakunakorn, C., and C. A. Kauffman. 1978. In vitro susceptibility of gentamicin and/or tobramycin resistant gram-negative bacilli to seven aminoglycosides. Infection 6:111–115.

High-Dose Netilmicin Therapy of Patients with Septicemia and Pyelonephritis

C. O. SOLBERG,* S. TSCHUDI MADSEN, A. DIGRANES, S. STOKSTAD, K. B. HELLUM, F. J. HALVORSEN, AND K. BAKKE

Medical Department B, Departments of Microbiology and Otolaryngology, School of Medicine, University of Bergen, Bergen, Norway

Netilmicin has an antibacterial spectrum similar to that of gentamicin (1). Results of animal experiments and clinical studies indicate that the drug may be less nephrotoxic and ototoxic than gentamicin (3–6). The purpose of the present study was, therefore, to examine the efficacy and tolerance of high-dose netilmicin therapy in patients with severe or chronic (or both) infections. The penetration of the drug into skin blister fluid was also examined.

The study included 32 patients, 18 males and 14 females aged 19 to 65 years (mean, 46.5 years). Sixteen patients had septicemia and 16 had recurrent pyelonephritis, 14 with abnormal pyelograms. Eighteen patients either had failed to respond to treatment with β-lactam antibiotics for 2 to 6 days or had shown only minor improvement. Each patient was given 200 mg (2.2 to 3.3 mg/kg; mean, 2.8 mg/kg) of netilmicin intramuscularly every 8 h for 7 to 10 days (mean, 8.8 days). The MICs of netilmicin and gentamicin were determined by an agar dilution method, and the antibiotic concentrations in patient sera and skin blister fluid were determined by an agar well diffusion method as previously described (6). In addition to physical examination and urinalysis, the following laboratory blood studies were performed before, during, and after therapy: hemoglobin, erythrocytes, leukocytes with differential count, ESR, serum electrolytes, creatinine and liver function tests, including serum glutamic oxaloacetic transaminase, bilirubin, and alkaline phosphatase. At least one creatinine clearance was obtained during the course of treatment. Nephrotoxicity was defined as an increase in serum creatinine of 30 μmol/liter or more. Otoneurological examination including pure-tone audiograms and caloric nystagmography was performed immediately before treatment or within 32 h of treatment in all patients and again after treatment in 31 patients, and 3 months later in 21 patients. Ototoxicity was defined as a mean decrease in auditory acuity of greater than 10 decibels in the range of 250 to 8,000 Hz or a decrease of at least 15 decibels in two or more frequencies in either ear, or both.

Sixteen infections were caused by *Escherichia coli*, 5 by *Pseudomonas aeruginosa*, 4 by *Sal-* *monella* sp., 4 by *Proteus mirabilis*, 2 by *Klebsiella* sp., and 1 by *Enterobacter* sp. All bacteria except 1 *P. aeruginosa* strain were inhibited by 2.0 mg of netilmicin per liter or less. The MICs of netilmicin and gentamicin closely paralleled each other.

Twenty-six patients were cured, i.e., the clinical symptoms disappeared and the infecting organism was not isolated from appropriate specimens after treatment. Two patients with pyelonephritis were not cured. Each had bladder stones and the pyelonephritis was caused by *P. aeruginosa* or *Klebsiella* sp. Two patients with septicemia, 1 infection caused by *P. mirabilis* and the other by *E. coli*, seemed to have been cured when netilmicin treatment was discontinued after 8 and 10 days, respectively, but 3 to 5 days later clinical symptoms reappeared and blood cultures became positive. Combined treatment with ampicillin and gentamicin for 2 weeks was successful. One of the patients who failed to respond to therapy had acute leukemia, granulocytopenia, and *E. coli* septicemia. Later, he also failed to respond to combined treatment with carbenicillin and gentamicin even in the presence of granulocyte transfusions. The other patient who did not respond to therapy had salmonella septicemia and spondylitis with spastic paraparesis. For the last 6 years he had been treated for Weber-Christian's disease with 15 to 50 mg of prednisone per day. Surgery to remove the osteomyelitic focus and long-term treatment with other aminoglycosides, co-trimoxazole, and penicillins were also unsuccessful.

Netilmicin and creatinine serum level determinations were performed on treatment day 5 or 6. In the 27 patients with normal serum creatinine levels (<120 μmol/liter), the mean netilmicin concentrations and range at 1 (peak values) and 8 (trough values) h after intramuscular injection were 12.6 (8.8 to 18.5) and 2.0 (0.5 to 5.0) mg/liter, respectively (Fig. 1). In the five patients with elevated serum creatinine levels (125 to 162 μmol/liter), the corresponding netilmicin concentrations were 21.5 (18.5 to 26.0) and 5.8 (4.0 to 8.5) mg/liter.

Skin blisters were produced as previously described (2) by tightly strapping a perspex block with eight bores (diameter, 8 mm) to the mid-volar area of the forearm and applying a controlled suction (-0.3 kg/cm^2) to each bore. After 2 h, a half-spherical blister containing 0.15 ml of serous fluid had developed at each bore through dermoepidermal separation. After blister production, four patients each received 200 mg of netilmicin intramuscularly, and antibiotic serum and blister fluid concentrations were measured at serial intervals; i.e., fluid from one blister was harvested each time a serum sample was obtained. The mean netilmicin peak level in serum was 10.6 mg/liter after 0.5 h (Fig. 2). In the blister fluid a delayed entry and elimination of the antibiotic was demonstrated. At 2 h serum and blister fluid concentrations were equal. Later, blister fluid levels were a little higher than the serum levels.

Netilmicin was well tolerated. Only two patients showed impairment of renal function, the serum creatinine levels increasing from 84 to 117 and 132 to 179 µmol/liter, respectively. However, 3 to 4 months later serum creatinine clearance values had returned to pretreatment levels.

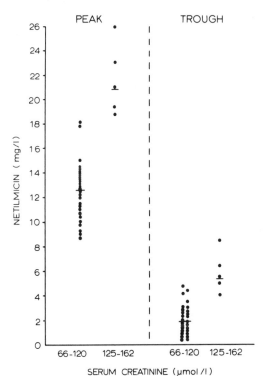

FIG. 1. *Peak and trough serum levels in patients with normal (<120 µmol/liter) and slightly elevated (125 to 162 µmol/liter) serum creatinine receiving 200 mg (2.2 to 3.3; mean, 2.8 mg/kg) of netilmicin intramuscularly every 8 h for 7 to 10 days (mean, 8.8 days). Bars = median serum levels.*

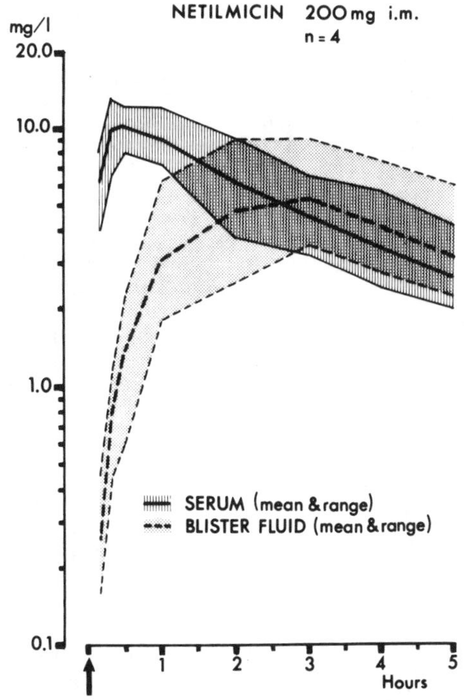

FIG. 2. *Antibiotic concentrations in serum and dermal suction blisters in four patients after intramuscular (i.m.) injection of 200 mg (2.4 to 2.6 mg/kg) of netilmicin; mean and individual observations.*

Eight patients had presbyacusis and five complained about uncharacteristic dizziness before or during therapy. No deterioration of audiometric and vestibular functions was demonstrated in any patient during and after therapy.

In the present study, patients with septicemia or chronic/recurrent pyelonephritis received high doses of netilmicin for short treatment periods. The efficacy of the drug seemed comparable to that of gentamicin. Despite high netilmicin doses and serum levels nephrotoxicity occurred in only 2 of 32 patients (6%) and ototoxicity was not demonstrated.

1. **Eickhoff, T. C., and J. M. Ehret.** 1977. In vitro activity of netilmicin compared with gentamicin, tobramycin, amikacin, and kanamycin. Antimicrob. Agents Chemother. **11:**791–796.
2. **Hellum, K. B., A. Schreiner, A. Digranes, and I. Bergman.** 1978. Skin blister produced by suction: a new model for studies of penetration of antibiotics in humans, p. 620–622. *In* Current chemotherapy, Proceedings of the 10th International Congress of Chemotherapy. American Society for Microbiology, Washington, D.C.
3. **Jonsson, M., I. Julander, G. Tunevall, and K. Haeger.** 1978. Netilmicin treatment of serious infections in pa-

tients with renal insufficiency. J. Int. Med. Res. **6**:226–234.

4. **Luft, F. C., M. N. Yum, and S. A. Kleit.** 1976. Comparative nephrotoxicities of netilmicin and gentamicin in rats. Antimicrob. Agents Chemother. **10**:845–849.

5. **Panwalker, A. P., J. B. Malow, V. M. Zimelis, and G. G. Jackson.** 1978. Netilmicin: clinical efficacy, toler-

ance, and toxicity. Antimicrob. Agents Chemother. **13**:170–176.

6. **Solberg, C. O., S. Tschudi Madsen, A. Digranes, S. Stokstad, K. B. Hellum, F. J. Halvorsen, and K. Bakke.** High dose netilmicin therapy: efficacy, tolerance and tissue penetration. J. Antimicrob. Chemother., in press.

Comparative Efficacy and Toxicity of Netilmicin and Gentamicin in Serious Gram-Negative Infections

MITCHELL V. BRODEY,* ROBERT W. BUNDTZEN, AND WILLIAM A. CRAIG

Department of Medicine, William S. Middleton Memorial Veterans Hospital, Madison, Wisconsin 53705, U.S.A.

Netilmicin is a new semisynthetic aminoglycoside derived by ethylation of the 1-*N*-position of the deoxystreptamine ring of sisomicin. It has been shown to possess in vitro activity against a number of enterobacteriaceae and *Pseudomonas aeruginosa* resistant to gentamicin (3, 6). Several uncontrolled clinical studies have shown netilmicin to be effective in the treatment of serious gram-negative infections (2, 3). In addition, animal studies have suggested that netilmicin may be less nephrotoxic (4) and ototoxic (1) than gentamicin.

This report presents the results of a prospective randomized study designed to determine the relative efficacy and toxicity of netilmicin and gentamicin in the therapy of serious gram-negative infections.

Seventy-one patients with known or suspected serious gram-negative infections were prospectively randomized to receive either netilmicin or gentamicin. All subjects were adult male in-patients at the William S. Middleton Memorial Veterans Hospital. Netilmicin was given initially at a dose of 2.5 mg/kg per 8 h, and gentamicin was given at 1.7 mg/kg per 8 h. At 72 h doses were reduced to netilmicin, 2 mg/kg per 8 h and gentamicin, 1 mg/kg per 8 h. Maintenance doses were adjusted for renal function according to the following formula: Normal maintenance dose/serum creatinine = adjusted maintenance dose.

Of the 71 patients entered into the study, 42 were considered evaluable for efficacy (Table 1). The others were excluded because a gram-negative pathogen was not identified, they did not receive the drug for 72 h, or they received another antibiotic effective against the suspected pathogen. All deaths are included despite the fact that the patient may have received the antibiotic for less than 72 h. Twenty-two patients received netilmicin, and 20 patients received gentamicin. The mean age was similar in both groups, as was duration of therapy and the use of concomitant antibiotics. There was no significant difference in initial leukocyte count between the two groups, and no patient was neutropenic. One patient in the gentamicin group was in shock at the initiation of therapy. Patients were categorized as to their underlying disease according to the classification of McCabe and Jackson (5), and no significant difference was noted. *Escherichia coli* was responsible for 30% of the infections in the netilmicin group and 29% in those treated with gentamicin, including

TABLE 1. *Demographic characteristics of patients evaluated for efficacy of netilmicin and gentamicin*

Characteristic	Netilmicin	Gentamicin
No. of patients	22	20
Mean age (yrs)	64 (24–87)[a]	63 (20–80)[a]
Underlying disease (no. of patients)		
Nonfatal	14	15
Ultimately fatal	8	5
Rapidly fatal	0	2
Duration of therapy (days)	9.5 (4–18)[a]	10.5 (2–32)[a]
Concomitant antibiotics (no. of patients)	14	12
Leukocyte count (thousands)	14.7 (5.4–45)[a]	13.6 (5.2–44)[a]
Patients with:		
Shock	0	1
Bacteremia	5	4
Organism		
E. coli	9 (2)[b]	8(2)[b]
Pseudomonas	8 (1)[b]	7
Klebsiella	8 (2)[b]	5 (1)[b]
Proteus	1	5 (1)[b]
Other	4	3
Anatomic site		
Urinary tract	6	8
Pneumonia	6	7
Soft tissue	5	4
Bone	2	0
Intraabdominal	3	1

[a] Range.
[b] Bacteremia.

TABLE 2. *Demographic characteristics of patients evaluated for nephrotoxicity*

Characteristic	Netilmicin	Gentamicin
No. of patients	31	31
Mean age (yrs)	59 (21–87)[a]	61 (20–83)
Mean creatinine before therapy	2.1 (0.6–14.1)	2.0 (0.7–14)
Mean days of therapy	8.7 (3–14)	9.6 (3–33)
Previous renal disease	7	8
Shock	0	0
Renal impairment		
Doubtful	2	2
Possible or probable	5 (16%)	6 (15%)

[a] Parentheses indicate range.

two bacteremias in each group. *Pseudomonas aeruginosa* accounted for 27% of the infections in those receiving netilmicin, including one bacteremia, and in 25% of the gentamicin group. The remainder of the infections were caused by *Klebsiella, Proteus, Enterobacter, Serratia,* and *Moraxella.*

Of the patients with documented serious gram-negative infections, 95% treated with netilmicin and 85% treated with gentamicin had favorable responses (Table 1). All patients with genitourinary (14), soft-tissue (9), bone (2), and intraabdominal (4) infections were cured or improved. Five patients in the netilmicin group and four in the gentamicin group had bacteremias, all of which cleared on therapy. Failures were confined to pulmonary infections. Of the six patients with pulmonary infections treated with netilmicin, one patient died of his *E. coli* pneumonia. Three of the seven patients with gentamicin died; two had lung infections with *Pseudomonas,* and one had a lung infection with *E. coli.*

The mean peak level obtained for netilmicin was 6.7 µg/ml, and that for gentamicin was 5.8 µg/ml. None of the 20 patients receiving netilmicin who had mean peak serum levels ≥4 µg/ml failed, whereas one of the two who had levels <4 µg/ml died. Of the patients treated with gentamicin who failed, two had mean peak serum levels ≥4 µg/ml, and one had a level <4 µg/ml. The only other patient treated with gentamicin with a mean peak serum level <4 µg/ml was cured of *Pseudomonas* soft-tissue infection.

Of the 62 patients considered evaluable for nephrotoxicity, 31 received netilmicin and 31 received gentamicin (Table 2). The other nine patients were not evaluated because they had not received the designated aminoglycoside for at least 72 h. No significant differences between the two groups were noted with respect to age, mean creatinine at the start of therapy, preexisting renal impairment or shock, and duration of therapy. Five patients receiving netilmicin and six patients receiving gentamicin exhibited changes in renal function that were considered possibly or probably due to the administered aminoglycosides. Two patients in each group had rises in creatinine for which the relationship to the study drug was considered doubtful.

Serial audiograms could be obtained in 24 patients receiving netilmicin and 26 patients receiving gentamicin. One patient receiving gentamicin sustained a moderate but permanent decrease in auditory function. This patient had received prior aminoglycosides and had a preexisting hearing deficit. He received a 5-day course of gentamicin with a mean peak serum level of 6.6 µg/ml and a mean trough serum level of 1.9 µg/ml.

Superinfections occurred in two patients in each of the study groups. All four patients responded to appropriate chemotherapy.

In conclusion, netilmicin and gentamicin appear to be equally effective in the therapy of serious gram-negative infections with no significant differences in toxicity.

1. **Brummett, R. E., K. E. Fox, R. T. Brown, and D. L. Himes.** 1978. Comparative ototoxic liability of netilmicin and gentamicin. Arch. Otolaryngol. **104:**579–584.
2. **Jahre, J. A., K. P. Fu, and H. C. Neu.** 1979. Clinical evaluation of netilmicin therapy in serious infections. Am. J. Med. **66:**67–73.
3. **Klastersky, J. D., F. Meunier-Carpentier, C. Coppens-Kahan, D. Daneau, and J. M. Prevost.** 1977. Clinical and bacteriological evaluation of netilmicin in gram-negative infections. Antimicrob. Agents Chemother. **12:**503–509.
4. **Luft, F. C., R. Block, R. S. Sloan, M. N. Yum, R. Costello, and D. R. Maxwell.** 1978. Comparative nephrotoxicity of aminoglycoside antibiotics in rats. J. Infect. Dis. **138:**541–545.
5. **McCabe, W. R., and G. G. Jackson.** 1962. Gram negative bacteremia. I. Etiology and ecology. Arch. Intern. Med. **110:**847–855.
6. **Meyers, B. R., and S. Z. Hirschman.** 1977. Antimicrobial activity in vitro of netilmicin and comparison with sisomicin, gentamicin, and tobramycin. Antimicrob. Agents Chemother. **11:**118–121.

Comparative Efficacy and Toxicity of Netilmicin and Gentamicin in Serious Systemic Infections

P. LEAL DEL ROSAL,* J. J. GAMEZ, AND L. LEAL DEL ROSAL

Hospital Clinica del Parque, Calle 12 y de la Llave, Chihuahua, Chihuahua, Mexico

Netilmicin is active in vitro against a wide variety of gram-negative bacteria, including certain gentamicin-resistant isolates, and *Staphylococcus aureus* (3). Clinical trials have confirmed the in vivo activity of netilmicin in several different types of infection (1, 2). The objective of this study was to compare the safety and efficacy of netilmicin and gentamicin in patients with serious systemic infections.

Forty-three male and 35 female patients aged 14 to 93 years who had documented infections were impaneled. All infections were severe; all intraabdominal infections were complicated by perforated viscus and leakage of infected material or by abscesses. Virtually all patients required corrective surgery before or during antibiotic therapy. Treatment was assigned randomly such that 40 patients received netilmicin and 38 received gentamicin. The dosage regimen was 2 mg of netilmicin or 1.5 mg of gentamicin per kg intramuscularly or by intravenous infusion every 8 h; in a few patients, dosages were adjusted downward to avoid excessive serum levels. Serum aminoglycoside levels 1 h after administration averaged 6 to 10 µg/ml in the netilmicin group and 4 to 8 µg/ml in the gentamicin group. Trough levels were generally 2.5 µg/ml or less in both groups. Most patients were treated for 7 to 10 days. Thirteen netilmicin and 16 gentamicin patients received concomitant antimicrobials, mainly clindamycin. One patient in the netilmicin group and two in the gentamicin group received ethacrynic acid. During the study, a "blind" observer evaluated the responses to treatment and assessed adverse reactions. The results were compared between the groups via Fisher's exact test (two-tailed, α = 0.10).

Data from 63 patients were evaluable for efficacy: the infections were caused by organisms susceptible in vitro to the two study drugs; the patients were treated for at least 72 h; and no one received another antimicrobial potentially effective against the pathogens being treated with aminoglycosides. Sixty-eight sites of infection were identified: 40 were intraabdominal, primarily peritonitis or cholecystitis; 20 were skin or soft-tissue sites, mainly involving surgical or traumatic wounds and cellulitis; six were in the lower respiratory tract; and two were in the genitourinary tract. The most common pathogens were *Escherichia coli* (34), *Pseudomonas aeruginosa* (12), and *Klebsiella pneumoniae* (11); isolated less frequently were species of *Enterobacter, Proteus, Serratia,* and *Staphylococcus.* Table 1 shows the good clinical and bacteriological responses. The two drugs produced comparable clinical results, but netilmicin was associated with a greater bacterial elimination rate. Two strains each of *E. coli, P. aeruginosa,* and *K. pneumoniae* persisted after treatment with gentamicin, as did one each of *Enterobacter agglomerans, Proteus mirabilis,* and *Staphylococcus aureus.* One *S. aureus* persisted in the netilmicin group. Clinical and bacteriological re-

TABLE 1. *Clinical and bacteriological responses at all 68 sites*

Response	Treatment group	
	Netilmicin (n = 38)	Gentamicin (n = 30)
Clinical		
Resolution	29[a]	20
Improvement	6	4
Failure	3	6
	(P = 0.40)	
Indeterminate	0	0
Bacteriological		
Elimination	34	21
Reduction	1	0
Persistence	1	9
	(P = 0.004)	
Indeterminate	2	0

[a] Number of sites.

TABLE 2. *Nephrotoxic and ototoxic reactions observed and relationship to therapy[a]*

Reaction	Netilmicin (N)		Gentamicin (G)		N vs G (Pr/Pos)
	Pr/Pos	Doubt	Pr/Pos	Doubt	
Renal	2[b]	4	5	4	P = 0.26
Auditory[c]	2	0	1	0	P = 1.0
Vestibular	2	0	0	0	P = 0.49

[a] Pr/Pos = probably and possibly related, combined; doubt = doubtfully related.
[b] Number of patients.
[c] Hearing loss of at least 15 dB at two or more of six test frequencies from 250 to 8,000 Hz.

sponses for the 40 intraabdominal sites were almost identical to those just described for all sites.

Safety data were collected from all 78 patients. Table 2 summarizes the results on nephrotoxicity and ototoxicity. Renal reactions were indicated in six netilmicin and eight gentamicin patients by increases in serum creatinine levels of $\geq 25\%$ above base line (increment, at least 0.5 mg/dl) to values of 1.3 mg/dl or more and in a ninth gentamicin patient by granular casts in the urine. None of these 15 patients received ethacrynic acid. When the incidences of reactions considered probably or possibly drug related were compared, there was no significant difference between the drug groups. Hearing loss was observed in 2 of 36 netilmicin patients and 1 of 33 gentamicin patients who had serial audiograms. Vestibular disturbance, indicated by transient dizziness or vertigo, was detected in two netilmicin patients. The differences between the groups in auditory and vestibular reactions were not statistically significant.

In addition to these renal and eighth-cranial-nerve reactions, five netilmicin and eight gentamicin patients had appreciable increases in platelet counts and a few in each group had increases in serum glutamic oxalacetic transaminase (SGOT), alkaline phosphatase, and bilirubin levels that were considered possibly or probably related to treatment.

Netilmicin was at least as safe and effective as gentamicin in this group of patients with serious systemic infections caused by organisms susceptible to both study drugs.

1. Chadwick, P., A. W. Bruce, T. D. V. Cooke, and G. J. Hardy. 1978. Therapeutic experience with netilmicin. Can. Med. Assoc. J. 119:1189–1193.
2. Maigaard, S., N. Frimodt-Möller, and P. O. Madsen. 1978. Comparison of netilmicin and amikacin in treatment of complicated urinary tract infections. Antimicrob. Agents Chemother. 14:544–548.
3. Schering Corporation. 1976. Informational material for the investigational drug SCH 20569. Schering Corp., Bloomfield, N.J.

Antibacterial Activity and Enzyme Stability of UK 31214, a Kanamycin B Derivative

RONALD R. CUTLER,* WENDY FARRELL, AND FIONA A. DRASAR

The London Hospital Medical College, London EI 2AD, England

The increasing emergence of bacteria resistant to aminoglycosides causes problems in the treatment of many serious infections. Gram-negative rods and *Staphylococcus aureus* resistant to gentamicin may cause particular difficulties (2, 3).

Resistance to these antibiotics may be due to impaired transport of the antibiotic across the membrane, but the majority of strains possess one or more plasmid-mediated enzymes capable of modifying aminoglycosides by acetylation, adenylylation, or phosphorylation. Because of these and other problems related to the nephro- and ototoxicity of aminoglycosides in current use, it is necessary to develop new enzyme-stable aminoglycosides of low toxicity.

UK 31214 is a semisynthetic aminoglycoside derived from kanamycin B. The following work is related to the comparative susceptibility of a number of strains of gram-negative and gram-positive organisms to UK 31214 and other aminoglycosides, as measured by MIC determinations, and to the stability of UK 31214 to inactivation by aminoglycoside-modifying enzymes.

MIC determinations. The activity of UK 31214 was compared with those of gentamicin, tobramycin, amikacin, and kanamycin A and B by using a range of gram-negative rods and *S. aureus* strains, either resistant (MIC ≥ 8 μg/ml) or susceptible to gentamicin. An agar dilution method was used which incorporated twofold dilutions of antibiotic into DST (Oxoid) agar, and an inoculum of 10^3 colony-forming units was applied to the surface of the agar by using a multipoint inoculator (Denley Instruments Ltd.). The recorded MIC was the minimum concentration of antibiotic required to reduce growth of the organisms to one colony or no growth.

The results of MIC determinations for gentamicin-susceptible and -resistant organisms for UK 31214, amikacin, and tobramycin are given in Fig. 1. It was found that 89% of gentamicin-susceptible, gram-negative rods were susceptible (MIC ≤ 8 μg/ml) to UK 31214. The most susceptible groups of gentamicin-resistant bacilli were *Enterobacter* and *Citrobacter* spp. and *Escherichia coli*, *Klebsiella*, and *Serratia* spp.

Thirty-one percent of gentamicin-resistant *Pseudomonas aeruginosa* were susceptible to UK 31214, but all gentamicin-resistant strains of *Providencia* spp., *Proteus* spp., *Acinetobacter* spp., and *Alcaligenes* spp. were resistant (MIC ≥ 16 μg/ml).

Susceptibilities to UK 31214 and to tobramycin (MIC of tobramycin ≤ 4 μg/ml) were similar for gentamicin-susceptible, gram-negative rods (Fig. 1). However, UK 31214 showed increased activity over tobramycin for gentamicin-resistant *E. coli*, *Enterobacter* spp., *Citrobacter* spp., *Klebsiella*, and *Serratia* spp. The majority of gentamicin-resistant, gram-negative bacilli, with the exception of *Acinetobacter* and *Alcaligenes* spp., were susceptible to amikacin.

Ninety-seven percent of gentamicin-susceptible and 34% of gentamicin-resistant *S. aureus* were susceptible to UK 31214. Amikacin was the most active antibiotic against resistant *S. aureus*. For all gentamicin-susceptible and -resistant organisms, UK 31214 was more active than either kanamycin A or B. For resistant organisms, 22% were susceptible to kanamycin A and 15% were susceptible to kanamycin B; for gentamicin-susceptible strains, 59% and 63%, respectively, were susceptible (MIC ≤ 8 μg/ml).

Enzyme detection by aminoglycoside modification. Gram-negative bacilli and *S. aureus* were investigated for their ability to produce aminoglycoside-modifying enzymes. Using single-enzyme preparations, the stability of UK 31214 to enzymatic modification was compared with that of other aminoglycosides (Table 1). Enzymes were detected by the radioactive technique of Benveniste and Davies (1). To obtain cell-free enzyme preparations, gram-negative rods were disrupted by sonication. Lysostaphin (50 μg/ml, 37°C, 1 h; Dickinson & Co. Ltd.) was used to disrupt the *S. aureus* strains. Modification was detected in a suitably buffered system containing enzyme, aminoglycoside, and the radiolabeled compound to be transferred to the aminoglycoside.

When the stability of UK 31214 to selected single-enzyme preparations was compared with that of gentamicin, it was found to be more stable to modification by gram-negative-derived AAC3-1, AAC3-2, and AAC2′ (see Table 1). UK 31214 was 50 to 100 times more stable to modification by AAC3-1 and AAC3-2 and 4 to 5 times more stable to modification by AAC2′. The stability to ANT2″ was more variable; with two preparations, the modification of UK 31214 was roughly comparable with that of gentamicin, but with two other preparations tested it was only half as stable as gentamicin.

The activity of 12 preparations of APH2″ was measured; in 7 cases the stability of UK 31214 was two to six times greater than that of gentamicin. Acetylases produced by *S. aureus* showed a high degree of modification for each of the aminoglycosides tested.

Aminoglycoside-modifying enzymes were detected in 83% of the gentamicin-resistant gram-negative rods and in all but 1 of the 32 strains of *S. aureus* tested.

The relationship between the MIC of UK 31214 and the ability of various enzymes to modify this antibiotic was not consistent. A high MIC was frequently connected with substantial modification of UK 31214 (compared with gentamicin) when acetylases from *S. aureus* were studied, but no such relationship was found between the MIC and APH2″ from *S. aureus* or AAC2′ and ANT2″ from gram-negative rods.

UK 31214 is active against most gentamicin-susceptible *S. aureus* and gram-negative rods

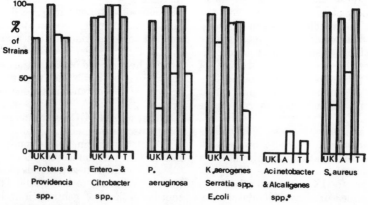

FIG. 1. *Susceptibility of gentamicin-resistant (open bars) and -susceptible (lined bars) organisms to UK 31214 (UK), amikacin (A), and tobramycin (T).* *, No gentamicin-susceptible strains tested.

TABLE 1. *Stability of UK 31214 and other aminoglycosides to enzymatic modification*

Organism	Enzyme[a]	No. of strains	No. of single-enzyme preparations with stability to enzymatic modification less than gentamicin[b]						
			UK	A	T	Ka	Kb	B	L
Gram-negative rods	ANT2″	4	2	—[c]	2	—	—	—	—
	AAC2′	2	0	0	1	—	—	—	—
	AAC3-1	2	0	0	0	0	0	—	—
	AAC3-2	1	0	0	0	0	0	—	—
S. aureus	AAC3-1 AAC6′	11	11	10	10	11	10	—	—
	APH2″	12	5	—	—	—	—	5	5

[a] ANT[2″], Aminoglycoside 2″-nucleotidyltransferase; AAC[2′], aminoglycoside 2′-acetyltransferase; AAC3-1, aminoglycoside 3-acetyltransferase-1; AAC3-2, aminoglycoside 3-acetyltransferase-2; AAC6′, aminoglycoside 6′-acetyltransferase; APH2″, aminoglycoside 2″-phosphotransferase.

[b] UK, UK 31214; A, amikacin; T, tobramycin; Ka, kanamycin A; Kb, kanamycin B; B, butirosin; L, lividomicin.

[c] —, Not tested.

and many gentamicin-resistant organisms. Its stability to modification by a number of enzymes compares favorably with the stability of other aminoglycosides.

1. **Benveniste, R., and J. Davies.** 1971. R-factor mediated gentamicin resistance: a new enzyme which modifies aminoglycoside antibiotics. FEBS Lett. **14**:293–296.

2. **Murray, B. E., and R. C. Moellering, Jr.** 1979. Aminoglycoside-modifying enzymes among clinical isolates of *Acinetobacter calcoaceticus* subsp. *anitratus*: explanation for high-level aminoglycoside resistance. Antimicrob. Agents Chemother. **15**:190–199.

3. **Speller, D. C. E., D. Raghunath, M. Stephens, A. C. Viant, D. S. Reeves, P. J. Wilkinson, J. M. Broughall, and H. A. Holt.** 1976. Epidemic infection by a gentamicin-resistant *Staphylococcus aureus* in three hospitals. Lancet **i**:464–466.

UK-31,214, a New Aminoglycoside: In Vitro Study

RICHARD WISE,* JENNIFER M. ANDREWS, KEITH A. BEDFORD, AND ADRIAN P. GILLETT

Department of Medical Microbiology, Dudley Road Hospital, Birmingham, England

The emergence of organisms resistant to gentamicin and the appreciation of the problems of aminoglycoside toxicity have stimulated research for new compounds which may show activity against such resistant strains and less toxicity. UK-31,214, 1-*N*-dihydroxy isopropyl kanamycin B, is a novel compound and was compared with other clinically available aminoglycosides against recent isolates.

Susceptibility testing was by a routine agar plate dilution procedure using Isosensitest agar and broth, pH 7.2 (Oxoid, Basingstoke, U.K.), throughout. Two inocula of 10^3 and 10^6 colony-forming units (CFU) were used. The plates were incubated overnight in air at 37°C, and the MIC was defined as that microgram of antibiotic per milliliter of agar which gave an estimated (by counting) 99% reduction in the initial inoculum.

The minimum bactericidal concentrations (MBC) of UK-31,214, gentamicin, and amikacin against 20 selected strains were determined in Isosensitest broth.

The rate of killing of three strains of *Pseudom-* onas aeruginosa by gentamicin and UK-31,214 alone and in combination with carbenicillin was studied. The aminoglycosides were added to broth in a final concentration equivalent to the MIC. Carbenicillin was added to give a final concentration of 100 μg/ml. The strains of *P. aeruginosa* were added to give an initial viable count of about 10^4 to 10^5 CFU/ml. Samples were removed at 1, 2, 4, 6, and 24 h.

The protein binding of UK-31,214 and gentamicin in 100% human serum was determined by an Amicon Centriflo cone ultrafiltration technique.

The activity of the four aminoglycosides are compared in Table 1. Against *Escherichia coli*, *Klebsiella pneumoniae*, indole-positive *Proteus* spp., and *Enterobacter* spp., UK-31,214 and amikacin had similar activity and gentamicin was about fourfold more active. *E. coli* W677/ R5, a known 6′-acetylating strain, was susceptible to UK at 32 μg/ml, to amikacin at 16 μg/ml, to gentamicin at 0.5 μg/ml, and to tobramycin at 16 μg/ml. *Proteus mirabilis* was fourfold more

TABLE 1. *MICs required to inhibit cumulative percentage of isolates*

Organism (no. tested)	Antibiotic (inoculum, 10^3 CFU)	50%	75%	90%
E. coli (34)	UK-31,214	1	2	2
	Amikacin	1	1	2
	Gentamicin	0.25	0.25	1
	Tobramycin	0.5	1	1
Klebsiella pneumoniae (25)	UK-31,214	1	1	2
	Amikacin	1	1	2
	Gentamicin	0.25	0.5	0.5
	Tobramycin	0.5	0.5	0.5
Proteus mirabilis (24)	UK-31,214	2	4	8
	Amikacin	0.5	2	2
	Gentamicin	0.25	0.5	0.5
	Tobramycin	0.25	0.5	1
Indole-positive *Proteus* (10)	UK-31,214	1	1	1
	Amikacin	1	1	2
	Gentamicin	≤0.12	0.25	0.25
	Tobramycin	≤0.25	≤0.25	≤0.25
Enterobacter spp. (20)	UK-31,214	1	1	1
	Amikacin	1	1	2
	Gentamicin	0.25	0.25	0.5
	Tobramycin	0.5	0.5	0.5
P. aeruginosa (all strains) (54)	UK-31,214	2	8	32
	Amikacin	2	8	32
	Gentamicin	1	2	16
	Tobramycin	0.25	1	4
P. aeruginosa (gentamicin R) (12)	UK-31,214	32	64	>128
	Amikacin	16	64	>128
	Gentamicin	16	64	>128
	Tobramycin	4	8	>128
Providencia stuartii (27)	UK-31,214	4	4	8
	Amikacin	0.5	0.5	1
	Gentamicin	4	8	16
	Tobramycin	4	4	8
S. aureus (30)	UK-31,214	1	1	8
	Amikacin	1	1	4
	Gentamicin	0.12	0.25	32
	Tobramycin	0.12	0.25	16

susceptible to amikacin than to UK-31,214. The activities of UK-31,214 and amikacin against *P. aeruginosa* were similar. Twelve strains of *P. aeruginosa* resistant to gentamicin (MIC ≥8 µg/ml) were equally susceptible to UK and amikacin. None of the gentamicin-resistant strains were susceptible to 8 µg or less of UK or amikacin per ml. Seven of these 12 strains were moderately susceptible (MIC ≤32 µg/ml) to amikacin and UK-31,214, the remaining 5 being more resistant.

All 27 strains of *Providencia stuartii* were eightfold more susceptible to amikacin (the most active aminoglycoside tested) than to UK-31,214. A previous study (1) showed that many of these strains produced a phosphorylating enzyme, confirming kanamycin resistance, and when such strains were resistant, showing MIC ≥8 µg/ml (as were 44% of these isolates), they also possessed an acetylating enzyme.

Five strains of *Citrobacter* spp. were tested and were found to be equally susceptible to UK-31,214 and amikacin (mode MIC 1 µg/ml), and nine strains of *Serratia* spp. were twice as sus-

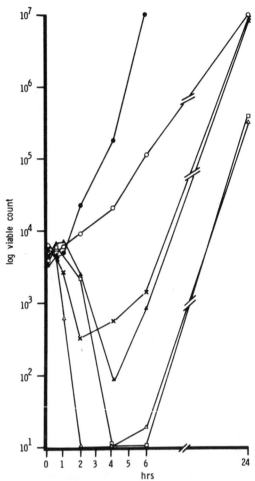

FIG. 1. *Comparative bactericidal activity of gentamicin and UK-31,214 (both at the MIC) alone and combined with carbenicillin (at 100 μg/ml). Symbols: ●, control; ○, carbenicillin (100 μg/ml); ×, gentamicin (0.5 μg/ml); ▲, UK-31,214 (1 μg/ml); △, gentamicin (0.5 μg/ml) plus carbenicillin (100 μg/ml); □, UK-31,214 (1 μg/ml) plus carbenicillin (100 μg/ml).*

ceptible to amikacin (mode MIC 2 μg/ml) as to UK (mode MIC 4 μg/ml).

Amikacin and UK-31,214 were equally active against *Staphylococcus aureus*. In five gentamicin-resistant strains (MICs in all cases 32 μg/ml), the MICs of amikacin were 1, 2, 4, 4, and 4 μg/ml and the UK-31,214 MICs were 2, 8, 8, 8, and 8 μg/ml.

On increasing the inoculum to 10^6 CFU, the MICs of all four antibiotics against the majority of strains tested was doubled. The MBCs of amikacin, UK-31,214 and gentamicin were usually the same or twofold higher than the MIC. The protein binding of gentamicin and UK-31,214 was 25% and 12%, respectively.

The viable count study of UK-31,214 or gentamicin in combination with carbenicillin for one of the strains tested is shown in Fig. 1. When combined with carbenicillin at 100 μg/ml, no viable cells could be demonstrated by 2 h in the case of gentamicin and by 4 h in UK-31,214. Regrowth was observed with the gentamicin/carbenicillin combination at 6 h, but not with UK-31,214 carbenicillin. Both showed regrowth after overnight incubation. Similar results were obtained from the other two strains tested.

UK-31,214 appears to share many of the properties of amikacin, being a broad-spectrum bactericidal aminoglycoside exhibiting little inoculum effect. The spectrum of activity includes all the common gram-negative pathogens and *S. aureus*. Although less active than gentamicin or tobramycin against *P. aeruginosa*, it could be expected that if, like amikacin, UK-31,214 can be administered in proportionally higher doses, that it would be clinically effective against these pathogens.

1. **McHale, P., L. English, A. Speekenbrink, C. Keane, and R. Wise.** 1978. Kanamycin resistance in *Providencia stuartii*. J. Antimicrob. Chemother. **4:**273–278.

UK-31,214, a New Semisynthetic Aminoglycoside: Pharmacological Profile

JAMES R. C. BAIRD,* ANTHONY J. CARTER, DAVID M. COWLEY, AND JOHN T. HENDERSON

Pfizer Central Research, Sandwich, Kent, England

Aminoglycoside antibiotics have been reported to cause adverse effects in man. Ototoxicity and nephrotoxicity are the major hazards in their clinical use, but neuromuscular blocking and cardiovascular depressant activities have also been observed. In a new aminoglycoside, reduction or elimination of one or more of these effects, particularly ototoxicity and nephrotoxicity, would represent a substantial advantage over existing compounds.

UK-31,214 is a new and potentially useful aminoglycoside antibiotic in terms of antibacterial potency and spectrum. As part of its development, it was subjected to screening in animals to determine its side-effect profile. In all experiments, established aminoglycosides—one or more of amikacin, kanamycin A, netilmicin, and gentamicin—were included for comparison.

Ototoxicity was assessed using Preyer's reflex in newborn guinea pigs. Test compounds were administered subcutaneously to groups of animals each day for the duration of the experiment immediately following measurement of the threshold sound intensity at a frequency of 12 KHz for Preyer's reflex. In a 21-day experiment, UK-31,214, at 150 mg base per kg/day, had little effect on the mean threshold sound intensity, the thresholds closely resembling those of the control group. In contrast, with amikacin at 100 and 150 mg base per kg/day, the mean threshold sound intensities began to rise after 14 and 10 days of treatment, respectively. Thereafter, they continued to rise steadily so that, by the end of the experiment, both doses had produced some degree of hearing loss. On increasing the treatment period to 31 days in another experiment, UK-31,214 at 150 mg base per kg/day again had little effect until towards the end of the experiment when the mean threshold sound intensities were slightly elevated. At 225 mg base per kg/day, the compound also had little effect until day 26, when the mean threshold sound intensity began to increase slowly over the remaining 5 days of the experiment. In the same experiment, gentamicin produced dose-related increases in the mean threshold sound intensity at 33.3 and 50 mg base per kg/day, although 25 mg base per kg/day was without effect. Thus, UK-31,214 produced only slight auditory toxicity in newborn guinea pigs and was less audiotoxic than gentamicin and amikacin.

Nephrotoxicity was assessed using the urinary excretion of lactate dehydrogenase (LDH), glutamate-oxalacetate transaminase (GOT), and exfoliated tubular cells in the rat. The animals were subjected to an initial acclimatization period of 3 days, a treatment period of 5 days, and a posttreatment period of 3 days. Throughout the experiment, 17-h urine samples were collected (4°C) over each night from the animals individually housed in metabolism cages. LDH and GOT were measured on an LKB-8600 series reaction rate analyzer using Boehringer test kit assays and tubular cell counts made, following

staining with "Sedicolor" (Ortho Diagnostics), by using a Neubauer hemocytometer and a light microscope at a magnification of ×150. The compounds were administered subcutaneously daily during the treatment period just before the animals were placed in the metabolism cages.

UK-31,214, at 90 mg base per kg/day, significantly increased urinary LDH and tubular cell counts on the first day of treatment. The levels remained significantly elevated for the remainder of the treatment period. Thereafter, during the posttreatment period, they fell towards control levels. In contrast, gentamicin and netilmicin, both at 30 mg base per kg/day, produced progressively rapid increases in urinary LDH and tubular cell counts during the treatment period, with the levels either continuing to rise or remaining elevated during the posttreatment period. UK-31,214, at 90 mg base per kg/day, and gentamicin and netilmicin, both at 30 mg base per kg/day, had less effect on the urinary excretion of GOT, but the respective patterns of such effects as did occur resembled those observed with LDH and tubular cells. These results suggest that UK-31,214 had a slight nephrotoxic potential in the rat which overall resembled those of gentamicin and netilmicin. However, UK-31,214 was less active in this test and its effects declined when treatment stopped, whereas the effects of gentamicin and netilmicin continued after cessation of treatment.

Neuromuscular blocking activity was assessed using the rat phrenic nerve-diaphragm preparation in vitro. Contractions of the diaphragm were produced by electrical stimulation (0.2 Hz, 1 m·sec, supramaximal voltage) of the phrenic nerve and recorded as changes in tension. In this test, UK-31,214, at concentrations much higher than those required for antibacterial activity in vitro, displayed neuromuscular blocking activity. It was less active than gentamicin and more active than kanamycin A.

Cardiac depressant activity was assessed using the cat papillary muscle preparation in vitro. The muscles were stimulated electrically (0.5 Hz, 1 m·sec, 2 to 3 V above threshold) and the resulting contractions were recorded as changes in tension. In this test, UK-31,214, at concentrations much higher than those required for antibacterial activity in vitro, displayed cardiac depressant activity. It was less active than both kanamycin A and gentamicin.

The results obtained from these studies indicate that, compared to established aminoglycosides and taking antibacterial potency into account, UK-31,214 has an improved, though characteristic, aminoglycoside side-effect profile.

UK-31,214, a New Semisynthetic Aminoglycoside: Activity Against Bacterial Clinical Isolates and Pharmacokinetic Properties

KEITH W. BRAMMER,* SIDNEY JEVONS, AND KENNETH RICHARDSON

Pfizer Central Research, Pfizer Limited, Sandwich, Kent, England

UK-31,214 is a new semisynthetic derivative of kanamycin B, 1-N(1,3-dihydroxy-2-propyl) kanamycin B. Preliminary evaluation of its antibacterial properties and of its potential for ototoxicity and nephrotoxicity in laboratory animals (J. R. C. Baird, A. J. Carter, D. M. Cowley, and J. T. Henderson, this volume; K. Richardson, K. W. Brammer, and S. Jevons, this volume) indicated that UK-31,214 merited further study as a possible candidate for evaluation in man. This paper summarizes the results of an extensive evaluation of the antibacterial properties of UK-31,214, both in vitro and in vivo, and of a comparative pharmacokinetic study with amikacin in dogs.

Antibacterial activity in vitro. Antibacterial activity of UK-31,214 was determined against over 600 unselected clinical bacterial isolates of the genera and species most relevant to aminoglycoside therapy in man, i.e., *Escherichia coli*, *Klebsiella* spp., *Pseudomonas* spp., *Proteus* spp., (indole-negative and indole-positive), *Enterobacter* spp., *Serratia* spp., *Providencia* spp., and *Staphylococcus aureus*. Approximately half of these isolates were aminoglycoside-resistant as evidenced principally by resistance to gentamicin. The isolates were obtained from hospitals in Europe and the United States.

The antibacterial potency of UK-31,214 in vitro was determined on the basis of MIC using a standard agar plate technique and Diagnostic Sensitivity Test Agar medium (Oxoid Ltd., England). The agar surface was inoculated with 1 × 10⁴ to 5 × 10⁴ cells of each organism, and the presence or absence of bacterial growth was recorded after incubation at 37°C for 18 h. The recorded MIC was the minimum antibiotic concentration which, when incorporated in the medium, reduced growth of the organism to five colonies or less. UK-31,214 exhibited potent antibacterial activity against essentially all the aminoglycoside-susceptible isolates, with MICs against more than 99% of the isolates of 12.5 μg/ml or less. In general, the potency of UK-31,214 against these isolates was similar to that of amikacin and about one-third that of gentamicin. UK-31,214 also exhibited potent activity against the aminoglycoside-resistant isolates, 87% of them being inhibited by UK-31,214 at a concentration of 12.5 μg/ml or less. At this same con-

centration, amikacin inhibited the growth of 89% of the isolates and gentamicin inhibited the growth of only 21%. Overall, therefore, UK-31,214 was shown to have an antibacterial potency and spectrum similar to that of amikacin. Its spectrum of activity against aminoglycoside-resistant bacteria was far superior to that of gentamicin.

Activity against bacterial infections in mice. Antibacterial activity in vivo was demonstrated with UK-31,214 against acute systemic infections in mice. Infections which caused the deaths of all untreated mice within 48 h were established by intraperitoneal inoculation of standardized suspensions of selected bacteria in 5% hog gastric mucin. One aminoglycoside-susceptible strain and one aminoglycoside-resistant strain of each of the five species, *E. coli*, *Proteus mirabilis*, *Klebsiella pneumoniae*, *Pseudomonas aeruginosa*, and *S. aureus*, were used to infect the mice. The aminoglycoside-resistant strains possessed the aminoglycoside-inactivating enzymes indicated in Table 1. Kanamycin B, the antibiotic from which UK-31,214 was derived and which was known to be inactivated by the enzymes present in the resistant strains, was evaluated in parallel with UK-31,214. Kanamycin B or UK-31,214 was administered subcutaneously to groups of infected mice at 0.5 and 4 h postinfection at a range of dose levels, increasing in twofold steps, up to 50 mg/kg. The dose level of antibiotic which gave 50% survival of the mice at 72 h (the PD$_{50}$) was calculated in each case. The results are summarized in Table 1. UK-31,214 was effective against both aminoglycoside-susceptible and aminoglycoside-resistant bacterial infections, whereas kanamycin B was effective only against the aminoglycoside-susceptible infections. Kanamycin B was generally more potent than UK-31,214 against the aminoglycoside-susceptible bacterial infections, with the exception of that due to *Pseudomonas* 48. This is consistent with its known in vitro antibacterial potency and spectrum. The results with UK-31,214 indicate that the antibacterial properties demonstrated against bacteria in vitro translate to an in vivo situation.

Pharmacokinetic properties in dogs. A study of the pharmacokinetic properties of UK-31,214 after both intravenous and intramuscular

TABLE 1. *Activity of UK-31,214 against acute bacterial infections in mice*

Organism	Enzyme content	PD$_{50}$ (mg antibiotic/kg of mouse body wt)	
		UK-31,214	Kanamycin B
(a) Using bacterial strains without detectable aminoglycoside-inactivating activity			
E. coli 172		2.6	1.9
P. mirabilis 8		3.6	1.4
K. pneumoniae 33		1.5	0.4
P. aeruginosa 48		7.8	31.9
S. aureus 223		4.0	0.7
(b) Using bacterial strains known to possess the aminoglycoside-inactivating enzymes indicated			
E. coli 174	APH(3')	6.2	>50
P. mirabilis 318	APH(3'), AAC(3)	9.3	>50
K. pneumoniae 62	APH(3', 5"), AAD(2")	2.9	>50
P. aeruginosa 399	AAD(2")	16.8	>50
S. aureus 246	APH(3', 5")	8.6	>50

TABLE 2. *Pharmacokinetic characteristics of UK-31,214 and amikacin in dogs*

Pharmacokinetic parameter	Antibiotic	
	UK-31,214	Amikacin
Serum half-life (h)	0.80	0.97
Volume of distribution (% body wt)	24.2	25.1
Renal clearance value (ml/min)	32.0	32.1

administration was undertaken. The dog was selected for this evaluation as experience had shown that results with aminoglycosides in this species provided a reliable indication of the corresponding properties in man. Amikacin, an aminoglycoside of similar antibacterial potency and spectrum, was evaluated in parallel; the experimental design by each route of administration being a crossover in two beagle dogs. After administration of either UK-31,214 or amikacin at 5 mg/kg, blood samples were taken from the saphenous vein at appropriate intervals up to 6 h after dosing, and serum was separated. Total bladder urine was collected via a catheter

at appropriate intervals up to 24 h after dosing. All serum and urine samples were assayed for UK-31,214 or amikacin concentration, as appropriate. A standard agar plate bioassay procedure using *Bacillus subtilis* ATCC 6633 as indicator organism was used for both compounds. The serum concentration/time profile by each route of administration was similar for the two compounds, and in each case more than 80% of the dose was excreted unchanged in the urine. The serum concentration and urinary excretion data from the intravenously dosed dogs were used to calculate the pharmacokinetic parameters listed in Table 2. It is apparent that UK-31,214 behaves very similarly to amikacin when administered parenterally to dogs. A distribution volume of about 25% of body weight, consistent with antibiotic localization in the extracellular body water, is commonly reported for aminoglycoside antibiotics in man (1).

1. **Mawer, G. E.** 1979. Aminoglycoside pharmacology, p. 121–135. *In* D. Reeves and A. Geddes (ed.), Recent advances in infection, No. 1. Churchill Livingstone, London.

UK-31,214, a New Semisynthetic Aminoglycoside: Structure, Synthesis, and In Vitro Evaluation

KENNETH RICHARDSON,* KEITH W. BRAMMER, AND SIDNEY JEVONS

Pfizer Central Research, Pfizer Limited, Sandwich, England

The clinical usefulness of aminoglycoside antibiotics is limited by two main factors: (i) their susceptibility to modification (resulting in activation) by enzymes present in many resistant bacteria, and (ii) their potential for toxicity to the animal host, especially ototoxicity and nephrotoxicity. We undertook a program of 1-N-alkyl modifications of kanamycin B in an attempt to minimize these limitations, and this paper describes the synthesis of these compounds and the antibacterial properties of one of the derivatives prepared during this study, namely UK-31,214 [1-*N*-(1,3-dihydroxy-2-propyl)kanamycin B, Fig. 1].

The 1-*N*-alkyl substituted compounds were prepared using a derivative of kanamycin B protected on all amino groups except the 1-amine. Thus, 2′,3,3″,6′-tetra-*N*-formylkanamycin B (Takeda Chemical Industries, Ltd., Belgian patent 817,546, 13 January 1975) was reductively alkylated at the 1-position, using the appropriate carbonyl compound (2 to 5 equivalents) and sodium cyano borohydride (3 equivalents) in dimethylsulfoxide containing a catalytic amount of 2 N hydrochloric acid. Yields were 80 to 90%. The formyl protecting groups were removed by treatment with 1 N sodium hydroxide solution at 55°C for 4 h, and the 1-*N*-alkyl derivatives were isolated by ion-exchange chromatography on a column of Sephadex CM-25 in yields of approximately 60%. In this manner glyceraldehyde was used to produce the 2,3-dihydroxypropyl derivative, erythrose gave the trihydroxybutyl analog, ribose gave the tetrahydroxypentyl compound, and 1-hydroxyacetone yielded the 1-hydroxy-2-propyl derivative. The most interesting compound produced in this manner was UK-31,214, the 1,3-dihydroxyisopropyl analog which was prepared by reductive alkylation using 1,3-dihydroxyacetone as the carbonyl compound.

UK-31,214 was evaluated against a panel of aminoglycoside-susceptible bacterial isolates in comparison with gentamicin and kanamycin B. All of the isolates of *Escherichia coli* were inhibited by UK-31,214 at 3.1 µg/ml or less, *Proteus* spp., *Staphylococcus aureus*, and *Pseudomonas aeruginosa* at 6.2 µg/ml or less, and *Klebsiella* spp. at 1.6 µg/ml or less. Against this group of organisms, gentamicin was approximately three times more potent while kanamycin B was twice as potent as UK-31,214, except for *P. aeruginosa* where it was eight times less potent.

UK-31,214 was also evaluated against 12 aminoglycoside-resistant bacterial isolates which have been proven to possess aminoglycoside-modifying enzymes, as shown in Table 1. Amikacin was used as a comparative agent since it is known to be resistant to the most commonly encountered aminoglycoside-inactivating enzymes (2). Good activity was demonstrated by UK-31,214 against isolates possessing enzymes capable of 3′-phosphorylation, 3-acetylation, and 2″-adenylylation, and this activity was similar to that shown by amikacin. UK-31,214 was only

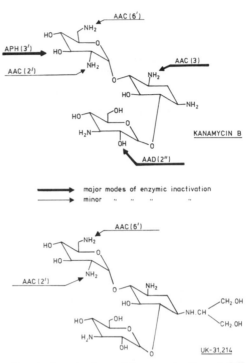

FIG. 1. *Inactivation of kanamycin B and UK-31,214*

TABLE 1. *Activity of UK-31,214 against bacterial isolates possessing proven inactivating enzymes*[a]

Organism	Enzyme(s) present	UK-31,214 (MIC in µg/ml)	Amikacin (MIC in µg/ml)
E. coli 174	APH(3′)	6.2	3.1
E. coli 175	APH(3′), AAD(2″)	12.5	12.5
E. coli 176	AAC(6′)	50	50
E. coli 271	AAC(3)	3.1	3.1
E. coli 272	AAC(3)	3.1	3.1
E. coli 273	AAD(2″)	3.1	3.1
P. aeruginosa 53	AAC(3)	3.1	1.6
P. aeruginosa 54	AAC(3), APH(3′)	3.1	1.6
P. aeruginosa 238	AAC(3), APH(3′)	1.6	1.6
Enterobacter 21	AAD(2″), APH(3′)	3.1	1.6
Providencia 17	AAC(2′)	25	12.5
Klebsiella pneumoniae 62	AAD(2″), APH(3′)	3.1	3.1

[a] MICs were determined by a standard agar plate technique using Diagnostic Sensitivity Test Agar (Oxoid Ltd., England). 1×10^4 to 5×10^4 cells of each organism were inoculated onto the agar surface and incubated at 37°C for 18 h. The recorded MIC was the minimum concentration of antibiotic which reduced growth of the organism to five or fewer colonies.

moderately active against isolates of *E. coli* 176 and *Providencia* 17, which are known to possess enzymes capable of 6′-acetylation and 2′-acetylation, respectively.

These data suggest that substitution on the 1-position with a 1,3-dihydroxyisopropyl group prevents inactivation by 3′-phosphorylation, 2″-adenylylation, or 3-acetylation, which are the most frequently encountered modes of aminoglycoside inactivation according to data generated by Andrews et al. (1). It appears likely, however, that 1-*N*-substitution by the 1,3-dihydroxyisopropyl group does not prevent suscep-

tibility to the relatively uncommon 2′- and 6′-acetylating enzymes (see Fig. 1).

1. **Andrews, R. J., K. W. Brammer, H. E. Cheeseman, and S. Jevons.** 1978. UK-18,892: resistance to modification by aminoglycoside-inactivating enzymes. Antimicrob. Agents Chemother. **14**:846–850.
2. **Price, K. E., T. A. Pursiano, M. D. De Furia, and G. E. Wright.** 1974. Activity of BB-K8 (amikacin) against clinical isolates resistant to one or more aminoglycoside antibiotics. Antimicrob. Agents Chemother. **5**:143–152.

Pharmacokinetics and Toxicological Screening of Intramuscular and Intravenous UK 31214 in Human Volunteers

PETER WILSON* AND BARRY D. COOKSON

The London Hospital Medical College, London, England

UK 31214 is a new aminoglycoside derived from kanamycin B which is active against gentamicin-susceptible and -resistant bacteria. Animal studies of the toxicity of UK 31214 show it to have considerably less nephrotoxic and ototoxic potential than currently available aminoglycosides. This study was designed to establish the pharmacokinetics and to assess the safety of the drug in humans.

Ten normal healthy male volunteers with normal hearing and vestibular function were given UK 31214 in three dosage regimes. Two subjects were assigned to the 1.25-mg/kg regimen, two subjects to the 2.5-mg/kg regimen, and six subjects to the 5-mg/kg regimen. Each subject received his dose of UK 31214 intramuscularly (i.m.), followed some 6 weeks later by the same dose administered as an intravenous (i.v.) bolus. To establish pharmacokinetic data from serum concentrations, blood samples were taken at various intervals (Fig. 1 and 2). Urine samples were taken at 0 to 2, 2 to 4, 4 to 8, 8 to 12, and 12 to 24 h to establish urinary excretion of the drug.

Before the study, all volunteers had their hematology and plasma biochemistry monitored. Pure tone audiometry and caloric irrigation at 30 and 44°C were also carried out. All the prestudy screening as above was repeated at 24 h and at 4 to 8 weeks postdose. Prestudy urinary enzymology consisted of *N*-acetyl-β-glucosaminidase, lactate dehydrogenase, gamma-glutamyl transpeptidase, and alanine aminopeptidase. These enzymes were monitored for two 24-h periods prestudy, on the study day, and then by continuous 12-hourly urine collections for the following 6 days.

After i.m. injection, peak serum levels obtained at 1.25 h were 3.9 ± 0.1, 8.2 ± 1.1, and

13.9 ± 1.8 mg/liter for the 1.25-, 2.5-, and 5-mg/kg regimens, respectively (see Fig. 1). These data produced a mean half-life of 2.0 h, with a mean area under the curve of 37 mg/liter per h (5 mg/kg) (computer derived).

After i.v. injection of UK 31214 at 1.25 mg/kg, serum concentrations failed to reach 10 µg/ml; at 2.5 mg/kg, serum concentrations exceeded 20 µg/ml for 5 min; at 5 mg/kg, they exceeded 20 µg/ml for 25 min (see Fig. 2). These data produced a mean half-life of 1.3 h, with a mean area under the curve of 35 mg/liter per h (5 mg/kg).

Over 80% of the administered dose could be recovered in the urine over the 24-h period. The greatest percentage recovery occurred in the lowest-dosage group, and within each subject urinary recovery was greatest after i.v. injection.

Urinary enzyme excretion, expressed as enzyme excretion per 24 h, showed changes with subject-to-subject variation. No changes were, however, observed with the *N*-acetyl-β-glucosaminidase monitoring. Minimal changes could be seen in three subjects with lactate dehydrogen-

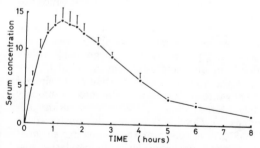

FIG. 1. *Serum concentrations (milligrams per liter) of UK 31214 in six subjects after i.m. administration of 5 mg/kg (mean values ± SD).*

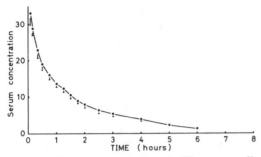

FIG. 2. *Serum concentrations (milligrams per liter) of UK 31214 in five subjects after i.v. administration of 5 mg/kg (mean values ± SD).*

ase excretion (5-mg/kg group), centered around day 3 to 5 postdose. Alanine aminopeptidase excretion in response to the UK 31214 challenge was inconsistent: some subjects showed an apparent increase in enzyme excretion after either i.m. or i.v. administration, but no subject showed an increase on both occasions in the 5-mg/kg group, and both routes of administration were equally likely to produce an increased alanine aminopeptidase enzymuria. In the 2.5-mg/kg group, one subject showed an increase in alanine

aminopeptidase and gamma-glutamyl transpeptidase excretion after both i.m. and i.v. administration which reached its maximum after 3 to 4 days. Gamma-glutamyl transpeptidase excretion showed the greatest changes after the second UK 31214 challenge (i.v.) in five of the six subjects in the 5-mg/kg group. In only one subject did this increased enzymuria not return to normal limits at 7 days postdose. All subjects had agreed to abstain from alcohol during the period of the trial, and a note was made of any sexual activity.

No significant changes were observed in the auditory or vestibular functions. There was negligible pain at the site of i.m. injection, and no phlebitis was observed related to i.v. administration. No eosinophilia was noted.

In conclusion, the pharmacokinetics of UK 31214 would appear to be comparable to that of amikacin, showing a similar half-life and rapid, high urinary excretion. Urinary toxicology based on enzyme excretion is difficult to interpret out of context, but comparable studies based on a double-blind, randomized, crossover design involving other aminoglycoside antibiotics are in progress.

In Vitro Evaluation of Fortimicin A: a Six-Center Collaborative Study

HERBERT M. SOMMERS,* ARTHUR L. BARRY, PETER C. FUCHS, THOMAS L. GAVAN, E. HUGH GERLACH, RONALD N. JONES, AND CLYDE THORNSBERRY

Northwestern Memorial Hospital Chicago, Illinois 60611, U.S.A.; University of California-Davis, Sacramento, California, 95817, U.S.A.; St. Vincent Hospital, Portland, Oregon 97225, U.S.A.; The Cleveland Clinic Foundation, Cleveland, Ohio 44106, U.S.A.; St. Francis Hospital, Wichita, Kansas 67214, U.S.A.; Clinical Microbiology Laboratories, of Kaiser Foundation Hospitals, Clackamas, Oregon 97015, U.S.A.; and Clinical Bacteriology Section, Center for Disease Control, Atlanta, Georgia 33033 U.S.A.

Fortimicin A (test drug no. ABBOTT-44747) is the most active member of the fortimicin complex, a group of aminoglycoside antibiotics derived from *Micromonospora olivoastrospora* as described by Nara et al. (2). The compound was first synthesized by the Tokyo Research Laboratory of Kyowa Hakko Kogyo Co., Ltd., Tokyo, Japan, and is under development for medical application in the United States by Abbott Laboratories, North Chicago, Ill. Early investigations demonstrated that fortimicin A has a wide spectrum of antimicrobial activity similar to that of amikacin, although demonstrating relatively weak activity against *Pseudomonas aeruginosa* (1). To confirm these reports of in vitro activity, a six-center collaborative evaluation of fortimicin A was designed, using large,

high-volume clinical microbiology laboratories in five widely separated geographic areas of this country (California, Illinois, Kansas, Ohio, and Oregon).

During a 60-day interval in late 1978 and early 1979, the MIC of fortimicin A was determined on over 11,000 recently isolated bacteria. Amikacin and gentamicin MICs were determined concurrently with that of fortimicin A (tested as the sulfate) using either broth microdilution or agar dilution procedures as recommended by the International Collaborative Study. Bacteria tested included those responsible for clinical infection of the urinary tract, surgical wounds, respiratory tract, meninges, blood, skin, and throat (Table 1).

Approximately 60% of all organisms tested

were members of the *Enterobacteriaceae*. With a 90% endpoint for the MIC, fortimicin A and amikacin were comparable against most species of *Enterobacteriaceae* except *Serratia marcescens*, against which fortimicin A was fourfold more effective than amikacin. On a weight basis, gentamicin was more effective against the *Enterobacteriaceae* in vitro than either fortimicin A or amikacin. Against *Staphylococcus aureus*, gentamicin was more active than either fortimicin A or amikacin at ≤0.5 μg/ml. All three agents were effective against 90% or more isolates of *S. aureus* at 2.0 μg/ml. Fortimicin A, amikacin, and gentamicin were all ineffective against *Streptococcus faecalis*, requiring 16 μg/ml or greater for inhibition of 60% or more of the isolates.

Fortimicin A was slightly less active against most nonenteric gram-negative bacteria than amikacin and gentamicin, including *P. aeruginosa* (Table 2). Whereas amikacin and gentamicin were able to inhibit 57 and 74% of *P. aeruginosa* isolates at 4 μg/ml, respectively, fortimicin A required 32 μg/ml for inhibition of 60% of the isolates, due in part to endemic resistance at one of the participating medical centers. At 16 μg/ml, fortimicin A inhibited between 16 and 75% of *P. aeruginosa* strains, depending upon participating hospital, whereas gentamicin at 4 μg/ml inhibited 62 to 90%.

TABLE 1. *Modal MICs and the MICs inhibiting 90% of Enterobacteriaceae*[a]

Organism (no.)	Modal MIC (μg/ml)			90% MIC[b]		
	Fort	Amik	Gent	Fort	Amik	Gent
Citrobacter diversus (127)	≤0.5	≤0.5	≤0.5	2	2	4
C. freundii (130)	≤0.5	≤0.5	≤0.5	4	2	≤0.5
Escherichia coli (3,759)	2	2	2	4	4	2
Enterobacter aerogenes (352)	2	2	≤0.5	4	2	≤0.5
E. agglomerans (83)	4	4	2	8	8	4
E. cloacae (406)	2	2	≤0.5	4	2	2
Klebsiella oxytoca (199)	2	2	≤0.5	2	2	2
K. pneumoniae (1,010)	2	2	≤0.5	4	2	2
Morganella morganii (159)	2	2	≤0.5	4	4	2
Proteus mirabilis (791)	2	2	≤0.5	8	4	2
P. vulgaris (99)	2	2	≤0.5	4	2	2
Providencia rettgeri (58)	2	2	≤0.5	4	2	2
P. stuartii (35)	2	≤0.5	2	4	4	8
Salmonella enteritidis (95)	2	2	2	4	2	4
Serratia marcescens (438)	2	2	≤0.5	4	16	128[c]

[a] Abbreviations: Fort, fortimicin A; amik, Amikacin; gent, gentamicin.
[b] Calculated to closest $\log_2$ dilution step.
[c] High MIC values skewed by endemic hospital organism populations.

TABLE 2. *Antimicrobial activity of fortimicin A (fort), amikacin (amik), and gentamicin (gent) tested on 1,173 isolates of nonenteric gram-negative bacteria*

Organism (no.)	Antibiotic tested	Cumulative % inhibited at MIC (μg/ml) of:						
		<0.5	2.0	4.0	8.0	16	32	128
Acinetobacter calcoaceticus var. *anitratus* (123)	Fort	3	44[a]	72	80	85	88	93
	Amik	19	68	86	91	93	98	98
	Gent	41	84	87	91	94	97	100
A. calcoaceticus var. *lwoffi* (13)	Fort		85	92	100			
	Amik	23	23	100				
	Gent	85	92	92	92	100		
Pseudomonas aeruginosa (881)	Fort	1	3	7	14	33	60	84
	Amik	6	24	57	78	88	94	99
	Gent	9	33	74	86	93	95	97
Pseudomonas species (126)	Fort	2	14	16	17	35	44	67
	Amik	10	29	37	50	56	63	93
	Gent	17	31	47	58	72	87	95
Other gram-negative bacilli (30)	Fort	13	37	40	43	50	60	67
	Amik	13	37	43	60		63	77
	Gent	33	47	57	60	67	70	77

[a] Underlined percentage is modal MIC value.

Fortimicin A, like amikacin, gentamicin, netilmicin, sisomicin, and tobramycin showed a distinct rise in the MIC as the number of organisms in the inoculum was increased. Fortimicin A performed somewhat less well to a large inoculum (10^7) of bacteria than did the other aminoglycoside agents tested.

Fortimicin A showed activity similar to that of amikacin in resistance to bacterial strains known to have specific inactivating enzymes. Enteric organisms containing aminoglycoside-6'-N-acetyltransferase I were fourfold more susceptible to fortimicin A than amikacin, as were three strains of *Staphylococcus aureus* known to contain 3'-O-phosphotransferase. Fortimicin A was effective against a strain of *S. aureus* containing aminoglycoside - 4' - O - nucleotidyltransferase, whereas amikacin required four times the same amount of drug for inhibition of this strain. Isolates of *P. aeruginosa* known to have a wide variety of aminoglycoside-inactivating enzymes were all resistant to fortimicin A. Bacterial permeability mutants were not susceptible to fortimicin A, amikacin, gentamicin, netilmicin, sisomicin, or tobramycin.

The minimal lethal concentration of fortimicin A was the same as the MIC in most bacterial strains tested. Fortimicin was similar to amikacin, gentamicin, netilmicin, sisomicin, and tobramycin in exerting a bactericidal effect on most enteric bacteria. Both amikacin and fortimicin A required a fourfold increase in concentration to kill two of ten strains of *S. aureus*.

Papers presented at this meeting have shown that fortimicin A is considerably less nephrotoxic and ototoxic than gentamicin (C. L. Yang, B. Buratto, S. B. Lehrer, I. A. Heyman, and J. L. Emerson, this volume; E. T. Kimura, S. Tekeli, J. P. Lewkowski, K. R. Majors, and J. W. Kesterson, this volume; R. E. Brummett, K. E. Fox, T. Bendrick, D. Himes, and R. Davis, Proc. 10th Int. Congr. Chemother., abstr. no. 776, 1979). This would suggest that fortimicin A should be further investigated as an antibiotic to use against susceptible bacteria causing infections in patients who require long-term administration in preference to gentamicin or other nephro- and ototoxic aminoglycosides.

1. **Girolami, R. L., and J. M. Stamm.** 1977. Fortimicins A and B, new aminoglycoside antibiotics. IV. In vitro study of fortimicin A compared with other aminoglycosides. J. Antibiot. **30**:564-570.
2. **Nara, T., M. Yamamoto, I. Kawamoto, K. Takyama, R. Okachi, S. Takawasa, T. Sata, and S. Sato.** 1977. Fortimicins A and B, new aminoglycoside antibiotics. I. Producing organism, fermentation and biological properties of fortimicins. J. Antibiot. **30**:533-540.

Vestibular Toxicity Study with Fortimicin A Sulfate (ABBOTT-44747) in Cats

CHRISTINE L. YANG,* BRUNO BURATTO, STEPHEN B. LEHRER, IRWIN A. HEYMAN, AND JAMES L. EMERSON[1]

Division of Drug Safety Evaluation, Abbott Laboratories, North Chicago, Illinois 60064, U.S.A.

Fortimicin A sulfate (test drug no. ABBOTT-44747) is a unique aminoglycoside antibiotic with particular activity against gram-negative pathogens and *Staphylococcus*. Many aminoglycoside antibiotics are known to induce vestibular toxicity and nephrotoxicity in experimental animals as well as humans. The present study was designed to determine the potential of fortimicin A to produce vestibular toxicity and nephrotoxicity in cats after subchronic administration and to compare the relative vestibular toxicity and nephrotoxicity of gentamicin with fortimicin A.

This study was conducted in minimal-disease cats weighing 2.5 to 4.0 kg at the initiation of treatment. Sixty selected cats (30 males and 30

females) were divided into six groups, each consisting of five males and five females. Three of the groups received fortimicin A in base dosages of 12, 35, or 105 mg/kg per day, and two groups received gentamicin, 7 or 20 mg/kg per day, for 3 months. The remaining group received normal saline, the vehicle for both drugs. Daily doses were administered subcutaneously at a volume of approximately 0.5 ml per kg of body weight. Animals were weighed once a week. Gait, stance, and righting reflex were evaluated daily. Postrotatory vestibular nystagmus (PRN) was monitored twice each week. Blood was collected from each animal once before the initiation of treatment and before necropsy. Serum urea nitrogen and creatinine were measured from each blood sample. Kidneys and middle ears were examined

[1] Present address: The Coca Cola Co., Atlanta, GA 30301.

grossly at necropsy. Representative sections from kidneys were submitted for histological examination.

Signs of vestibular toxicity included the appearance of unsteady gait and stance, impaired righting reflex, abnormally diminished PRN. The occurrence of these signs is summarized in Table 1. The onset of vestibular toxicity in gentamicin-treated animals appeared to be dose and sex related. Vestibulotoxic effects induced by gentamicin were irreversible and, once present, persisted to study termination. One male cat in the fortimicin A-treated group (base dosage of 105 mg/kg per day) exhibited slightly unsteady gait and stance and impaired righting reflex only from days 28 through 36. However, abnormally decreased PRN in this animal persisted from day 28 throughout the study. Mean duration of PRN in the vehicle control group varied from 14.3 to 20.5 s during the treatment period. PRN values of less than 8.5 s were considered abnormal. A relatively gradual diminution of abnormal PRN was observed in most of the affected animals. However, some affected animals in the high-dose gentamicin group demonstrated a relatively abrupt change from normal response to loss of all PRN response.

Fortimicin A at base dosages of 12, 35, or 105 mg/kg per day did not affect serum creatinine or urea nitrogen values. Gentamicin at base dosages of 7 and 20 mg/kg per day in males and 20 mg/kg per day in females caused significant elevations of these parameters. Gross renal findings in cats treated with fortimicin A at base dosages of 35 or 105 mg/kg per day and genta-

micin at 7 or 20 mg/kg per day were primarily color changes (diffusely pale green-tan or tan cortex–red medulla). The incidence of renal microscopic lesions is given in Table 2. No treatment-related changes were observed in cats treated with fortimicin A at 12 mg/kg per day. Histopathological lesions observed in the kidneys of cats given gentamicin at 7 or 20 mg/kg per day and fortimicin A at 35 or 105 mg/kg per day were, for the most part, characterized by degenerative changes in cortical tubular epithelium, cortical tubular cell necrosis, and regeneration and peritubular connective tissue changes. These renal tubular changes in cats given fortimicin A at 35 or 105 mg/kg per day were predominantly focal, minimal, and reversible. Renal lesions observed in cats given gentamicin (7 or 20 mg/kg per day) were more severe and diffuse than those observed in cats given the highest base dosage of fortimicin A (105 mg/kg per day). One male cat given gentamicin (base dosage of 20 mg/kg per day) was found dead on day 36. Death was attributed to renal toxicity. In addition, three male and three female cats in the gentamicin high-dose group (20 mg/kg per day) and one male cat in the gentamicin low-dose group (7 mg/kg per day) were killed in a moribund condition between study days 22 and 79. Renal toxicity was present in moribund animals. No gross pathological abnormalities were observed in the middle ears of cats given gentamicin or fortimicin A. Histopathological evaluation of the middle ears was not performed.

In conclusion, the relative vestibular toxicity and nephrotoxicity of fortimicin A were signifi-

TABLE 1. *Occurrence of vestibular toxicity in cats given subcutaneous doses of fortimicin A (ABBOTT-44747) or gentamicin*

Test substance	Base dosage (mg/kg per day)	Sex	Incidence[a]	No. showing given symptom at first day of onset[a]		
				Unsteady gait and stance	Impaired righting reflex	Abnormality of PRN
0.9% saline	0	M	0	—[b]	—	—
		F	0	—	—	—
Fortimicin A	12	M	0	—	—	—
		F	0	—	—	—
Fortimicin A	35	M	0	—	—	—
		F	0	—	—	—
Fortimicin A	105	M	1	28[c]	28[c]	28
		F	0	—	—	—
Gentamicin	7	M	3	56[d]	56	49
		F	0	—	—	—
Gentamicin	20	M	5	17	18	21
		F	5	28	28	25

[a] There were five animals in each test group.
[b] —, Not present.
[c] Effects were transient and reversible and occurred only from days 28 through 36.
[d] Effects induced by gentamicin were irreversible and, once present, persisted to study termination.

TABLE 2. *Incidence of microscopic renal lesions in cats given subcutaneous doses of fortimicin A (ABBOTT-44747) or gentamicin*

Test substance	Base dosage (mg/kg per day)	Degeneration of cortical tubular epithelium		Cortical tubular cell basophilia		Cortical tubular necrosis		Peritubular fibrosis	
		Focal	Diffuse	Focal	Diffuse	Focal	Diffuse	Focal	Diffuse
0.9% saline	0	1	0	1	0	1	0	2	0
Fortimicin A	12	0	0	1	0	2	0	2	0
Fortimicin A	35	2	0	7	0	3	0	6	0
Fortimicin A	105	8	0	6	0	5	0	5	0
Gentamicin	7	3	5	8	0	6	2	6	2
Gentamicin	20	1	3	7	3	4	6	3	7

[a] There were 10 animals in each test group.

cantly less than those of gentamicin for the following reasons. (i) Gentamicin at a base dosage level of 20 mg/kg per day produced severe vestibular toxicity in all 10 treated cats, whereas fortimicin A at 105 mg/kg per day gave only an equivocal response, since only one cat exhibited transient, reversible alterations in righting reflex, stance, and gait and a persistent decreased PRN. The remaining nine cats treated with this dosage were free of any adverse vestibular effects during the 3-month treatment period. (ii) No

signs of vestibular toxicity were observed in cats treated with fortimicin A at 12 or 35 mg/kg per day. Gentamicin at 7 mg/kg per day produced vestibular toxicity in three treated cats. (iii) Fortimicin A at base dosage levels of 35 and 105 mg/kg per day produced minimal renal morphological changes, whereas gentamicin at 7 and 20 mg/kg per day produced more severe and widespread renal pathological changes which resulted in several moribund animals or death.

Some Structure-Activity Relationships of Fortimicins at C-1 and C-2

RONALD E. CARNEY* AND JAMES B. McALPINE

Division of Antibiotics and Natural Products, Abbott Laboratories, North Chicago, Illinois 60064 U.S.A.

Fortimicin A 1 (Fig. 1) differs structurally from previously known aminoglycosides mainly in certain aspects of the cyclitol, and it is possible to draw a structural analogy with gentamicin C2 in which C-2, C-1, C-6, and C-5 of fortimicin are seen as the counterparts of C-2, C-3, C-4, and C-5 of gentamicins. The only apparent differences in large segments of these molecules is that the purpurosamine B in fortimicin A is epimeric at C-6' to that present in gentamicin C2. The analogy is strengthened by the observation that the only aminoglycoside-inactivating enzyme known to act upon fortimicin A is aminoglycoside-3-N-acetyltransferase [AAC(3)]-I, which acetylates the C-1 and C-3 amino groups of fortimicin A and the gentamicins, respectively (6). Enthusiasm for this analogy must be tempered by the knowledge that fortimicin A exists, at physiological pH, predominantly with its cyclitol in the alternate chair conformation to that shown in the structures depicted here. Nonetheless, struc-

ture-activity relationships of the gentamicins suggested certain key compounds as the targets of a fortimicin modification program.

2-Hydroxygentamicin C1 was reported by Daum et al. (2) to be less potent than gentamicin C1, and this fact suggested that 2-deoxyfortimicin A may be more potent than the parent.

The four primary amino groups of fortimicin A were protected as benzoxycarbonyl derivatives, and the procedure of Barton and McCombie (1) was used to deoxygenate. The C-2 hydroxyl group was found to be much more reactive than that at C-5, and the 2-O-thiocarbonylimidazolide was isolated in 60% yield from treatment of the tetra-N-benzyloxycarbonyl fortimicin A with N,N'-thiocarbonyldiimidazole in ethyl acetate. Reduction with tri-n-butylstannane and subsequent deprotection in methanolic hydrogen chloride gave 2-deoxyfortimicin A 2 as the tetrahydrochloride. The position of deoxygenation was evidenced by the β-shift ($\Delta\delta = 3.7$

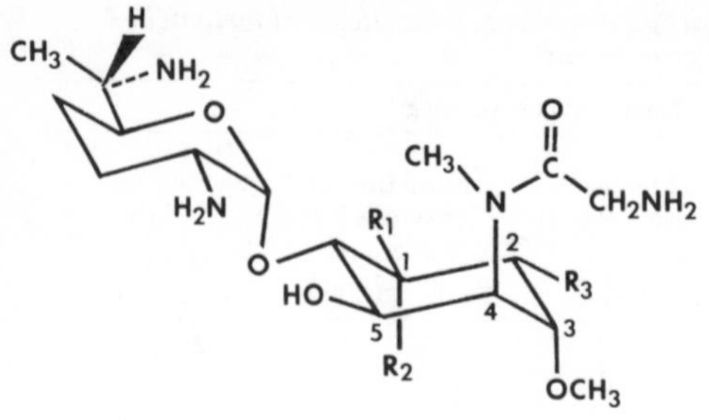

	R_1	R_2	R_3
1	NH_2	H	OH
2	NH_2	H	H
3	H	NH_2	OH
4	H	NH_2	H

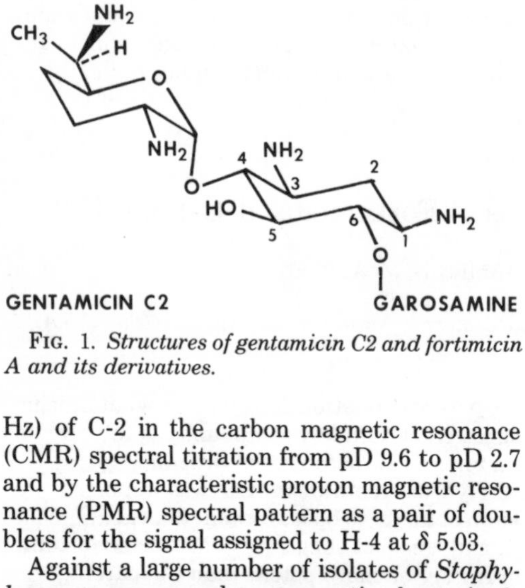

GENTAMICIN C2   GAROSAMINE

FIG. 1. *Structures of gentamicin C2 and fortimicin A and its derivatives.*

Hz) of C-2 in the carbon magnetic resonance (CMR) spectral titration from pD 9.6 to pD 2.7 and by the characteristic proton magnetic resonance (PMR) spectral pattern as a pair of doublets for the signal assigned to H-4 at δ 5.03.

Against a large number of isolates of *Staphylococcus aureus* and gram-negative bacteria, 2-deoxyfortimicin A was slightly more potent (1.35-fold) than fortimicin A, with no change in antibacterial spectrum or in activity against resistant strains. The acute toxicity of 2-deoxyfortimicin A as measured in male mice after an intravenous injection was twice that of fortimicin A. Thus, the effects of a hydroxyl group at C-2 in the fortimicins on antibacterial activity and acute toxicity resemble closely those of an analogous substitution in the gentamicins.

Mild oxidation of tetra-*N*-benzyloxycarbonyl-fortimicin A with either Jones reagent or Goldman-Albright reagent gave as the major product

a monoketone, reduction of which with sodium borohydride in methanol gave a single product isomeric with the starting material. After deprotection, a diastereomer of fortimicin A was obtained with a PMR spectrum which, measured at 270 MHz, showed the only large coupling constant for the cyclitol protons to be $J_{3,4}$, indicating that the cyclitol was in the fortimicin A-type conformation and that epimerization could have occurred at C-1 or C-6. These possibilities are the likely consequences of oxidation of the secondary alcohols at C-2 and C-5, respectively. The reaction sequence was repeated, using sodium borodeuteride as the reductant. The noise-decoupled CMR spectrum of the product differed from a similar spectrum of the undeuterated product by the loss of one carbon signal, which was assigned to C-2 by the β-shift (4.6 ppm) that it exhibited on titration. Thus, C-1 was the position of epimerization.

1-*epi*-Fortimicin A 3 was almost indistinguishable from fortimicin A in its biological activity. It displayed similar potency and antimicrobial spectrum, with no change in activity against resistant strains bearing the AAC(3)-I enzyme despite the fact that this enzyme acetylates fortimicin at the C-1 amine.

Deoxygenation of 1-*epi*-fortimicin A after the reaction sequence used earlier led to 5-deoxy-1-*epi*-fortimicin A. *N,N'*-thiocarbonyldiimidazole reacted preferentially with the hydroxyl group at C-5. Presumably, the cyclitol ring of tetra-*N*-benzyloxycarbonyl-1-*epi*-fortimicin A adopts the chair conformation, with the C-2 hydroxyl group axial and sterically shielded by two equatorial adjacent bulky groups and a 1,3-diaxial interaction with the C-6 oxygen. Since no trace of a di-*O*-substituted derivative could be detected in the reaction with *N,N'*-thiocarbonyldiimidazole, 2-deoxy-1-*epi*-fortimicin A was sought via tetra-*N*-benzyloxycarbonyl-1,2-di-*epi*-fortimicin A. This was detected as a minor product of reduction of the 2-oxo compound under certain reduction conditions, sodium borohydride in chloroform being the most favorable.

Barton deoxygenation of tetra-*N*-benzyloxycarbonyl-1,2-di-*epi*-fortimicin A led smoothly to 2-deoxy-1-*epi*-fortimicin A 4 which was identical to sporaricin A (3). This identity confirms the structural assignment of 1-*epi*-fortimicin A.

2-Deoxy-1-*epi*-fortimicin A incorporates the two structural variations previously described, and the biological activity of this molecule is as would have been predicted from the consideration of those seen for 2-deoxyfortimicin A and 1-*epi*-fortimicin A. 2-Deoxy-1-*epi*-fortimicin A was approximately 1.5 times as active as fortimicin A in vitro against a selection of gram-negative bacteria, with no change in antibacterial spectrum or in activity against resistant strains elaborating the AAC(3)-I enzyme. Data previously reported by Mori et al. (5) suggest that the acute toxicity of sporaricin A is very similar to that of 2-deoxyfortimicin A. Thus, 2-deoxygenation in the fortimicins seems to effect an increase of about 50% in antibacterial potency and an increase of about 100% in toxicity. Epimerization at C-1 seems to cause little change in the biological properties of the molecule; in this respect structural analogy between the fortimicins and the gentamicins is lost, as 3-*epi*-gentamicins have been reported by McCombie (4) to have greatly reduced activity compared with the parents.

1. **Barton, D. H. R., and S. W. McCombie.** 1975. A new method for the deoxygenation of secondary alcohols. J. Chem. Soc. Perkin Trans. 1 **1975**:1574–1585.

2. **Daum, S. J., R. A. Dobson, W. A. Gross, and D. Rosi.** 1976. New aminoglycoside antibiotics obtained from idotrophs of *Micromonospora purpurea*—characterization and biological evaluation. Program Abstr. Intersci. Conf. Antimicrob. Agents Chemother. 16th, Chicago, Ill., abstr. no. 43.

3. **Deushi, T., M. Nakayama, I. Watanabe, T. Mori, H. Naganawa, and H. Umezawa.** 1979. A new broad-spectrum aminoglycoside antibiotic complex, sporaricin III. The structures of sporaricins A and B. J. Antibiot. **32:**187–192.

4. **McCombie, S. W.** 1978. Chemical modification of aminoglycoside antibiotics at positions associated with bacterial inactivation. Abstr. IX International Symposium on Carbohydrate Chemistry, London, paper no. 839.

5. **Mori, T. et al.** 1978. A new aminoglycoside antibiotic, sporaricin. 210th Meeting of the Japanese Antiobiotics Research Association, Tokyo.

6. **Sato, S., T. Iida, R. Okachi, K. Shirahata, and T. Nara.** 1977. Enzymatic acetylation of fortimicin A and seldomycin factor 5 by aminoglycoside-3-acetyltransferase I. [AAC(3)-I] of *E. coli* KY8348. J. Antibiot. **30:**1025–1027.

Acute and Subacute Toxicity Studies with Fortimicin A Sulfate (ABBOTT-44747), a New Aminoglycoside Antibiotic

EUGENE T. KIMURA,* SAIT TEKELI, JAMES P. LEWKOWSKI, KENNETH R. MAJORS, AND JAMES W. KESTERSON

Division of Drug Safety Evaluation, Abbott Laboratories, North Chicago, Illinois 60064, U.S.A.

Fortimicin A sulfate (test drug no. ABBOTT-44747) is a pseudo-disaccharide antibiotic with bactericidal activity against a broad spectrum of gram-negative and some gram-positive pathogenic bacteria. Its isolation, chemical identity, and antimicrobial activities have been described (1–4). Whereas most aminoglycoside antibiotics have three rings in their structures, fortimicin A has only two, consisting of the amino sugar 6'-*epi*-purpurosamine B and a unique aminocyclitol (Fig. 1). This report describes the acute intravenous (i.v.) and intramuscular (i.m.) toxicity in mice, rats, and guinea pigs; acute i.m. symptomatology in cats; acute muscle and vein irritation in rabbits; and 1-month i.m. toxicity in rats and dogs.

Acute toxicity studies. Table 1 presents the acute LD_{50} of fortimicin A sulfate, expressed as the base. Decreased activity, dyspnea, ataxia, jerks, and clonic convulsions occurred in animals dosed i.v.; deaths occurred within minutes after injection. Decreased activity, dyspnea, and ataxia occurred in animals dosed i.m.; all deaths occurred within 1 h after injection.

All three cats injected i.m. in both hind legs with either 141, 282, or 563 mg base of fortimicin A per kg showed transient discomfort during injection. The lowest-dosage animal remained asymptomatic during the remaining 24-h observation period. Although the mid-dose cat showed an unsteady gait and the high-dose cat showed generalized flaccidity, neither lost its righting reflex.

Acute tissue irritation studies. No gross or microscopic changes were induced in either the

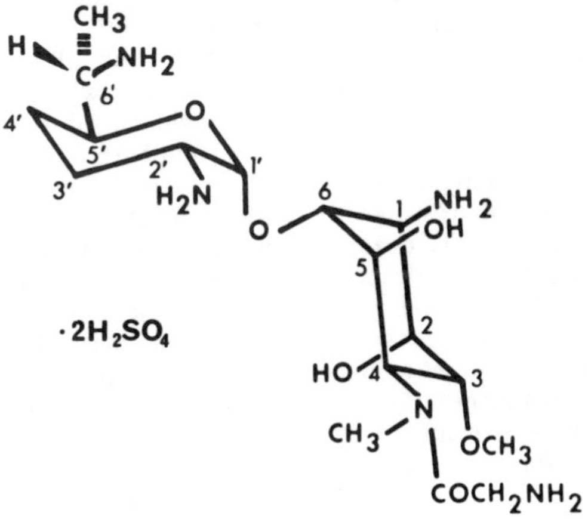

FIG. 1. *Structure of fortimicin A.*

TABLE 1. *Acute i.v. and i.m. LD$_{50}$ values for fortimicin A sulfate in mice, rats, and guinea pigs*

Test species (strains)	Fortimicin A lot no.	LD$_{50}$ (mg base/kg)			
		i.v.		i.m.	
		Males	Females	Males	Females
Mouse[a]	75-094-AL	94 (83–101)[b]	100 (93–105)	546 (481–713)	436 (396–467)
Rat[c]	75-094-AL	86 (79–92)	90 (86–94)		
Rat[d]	66-937-AL			1,042 (962–1,129)	1,009 (956–1,064)
Guinea pig[e]	75-094-AL			663 (569–707)	611 (539–666)

[a] Ten of each sex in four or five dosage groups. Strain ICR, ARS Sprague-Dawley, Madison, Wis.
[b] Numbers in parentheses are 95% confidence limits.
[c] Ten of each sex in four or five dosage groups. Strain Sprague-Dawley, Blue Spruce Farms, Altamont, N.Y.
[d] Ten of each sex in four or five dosage groups. Strain Long-Evans, Blue Spruce Farms, Altamont, N.Y.
[e] Six of each sex in four or six dosage groups. Scientific Small Animals, Arlington Heights, Ill.

ear veins or the sacrospinalis muscles of rabbits injected with fortimicin A. One, 2.5, and 5% solutions in saline were injected into the marginal ear veins at 2 ml/kg per 10 min, equivalent to 20, 50, and 100 mg base/kg. One and 0.5 ml of either 10, 18.5, or 25% aqueous solutions of fortimicin A were injected into the left and right sacrospinalis muscles, respectively.

One-month i.m. toxicity studies. Two i.m. toxicity studies, each 1 month in duration, were carried out in both dogs and rats. In the first of these studies, the toxicological profile of fortimicin A was studied in dogs at 30, 45, and 60 mg base/kg per day and in rats at 50, 75, and 100 mg base/kg per day. In the second study, fortimicin A (dogs: 7.5, 15, and 30 mg base/kg per day; rats: 12, 25, and 50 mg base/kg per day) was compared with gentamicin (dogs: 4.1, 8.2, and 16.4 mg base/kg per day; rats: 7, 14, and 28 mg base/kg per day). Lameness and edema at the injection sites (hind legs) in dogs were dose related for both fortimicin A and gentamicin. In rats, vocalization or withdrawal, or both, of the injected legs were seen in about half of the animals of each group in the first study, whereas a dose-related increase in the incidence of irritability during injection was seen in both fortimicin A- and gentamicin-treated rats in the second study. Microscopically, dose-related fasciitis and myositis with degeneration and necrosis in both dogs and rats ranged from mild to marked. In both dogs and rats, the clinical signs at the injection sites were more severe in the gentamicin-treated animals (30 mg base of fortimicin A per kg per day was comparable to 4.1 mg base of gentamicin per kg per day in dogs; 50 mg base of fortimicin A per kg per day was comparable to 7 mg base of gentamicin per kg per day in rats).

Fortimicin A at 7.5 mg base/kg per day did not produce any significant light-microscope renal lesions in dogs with the exception of minimal renal tubular hyaline droplet degeneration. Various degrees of dose-related renal lesions (tubular cell necrosis, hyaline droplet degeneration, and peritubular inflammation) were seen in the dogs given 15 through 60 mg base of fortimicin A per kg per day and in all gentamicin-treated dogs. In rats, fortimicin A from 25 through 100 mg base/kg per day induced dose-related renal tubular necrosis with peritubular inflammation and tubular cell degeneration, but not at 12 mg base/kg per day. The renal lesions in the male dogs treated with gentamicin at 16.4 mg base/kg per day correlated with the statistically significant increase in relative kidney weights, as did the renal lesions in the rats treated with gentamicin at 14 and 28 mg base/kg per day. In both dogs and rats, the degree of renal lesions was more severe in the gentamicin-treated animals (4.1 and 7 mg base of gentamicin per kg per day in dogs and rats, respectively, were comparable to 30 and 50 mg base of fortimicin A kg per day in dogs and rats, respectively). Urinary casts occurred in all gentamicin-treated rats (7, 14, and 28 mg base/kg per day) but only in the rats given fortimicin at 50 mg base/kg per day.

No relevant changes were observed in the hematology, blood chemistry, or urinalysis values of fortimicin A-treated dogs or rats. However, statistically significant treatment-related increases in blood urea nitrogen and creatinine values, decreases in serum sodium and potassium, and low urinary specific gravity were seen in some mid- and high-dose gentamicin-treated dogs. The mean hematocrit and hemoglobin values in the high-dose gentamicin-treated rats were significantly lower than those of other groups. Dose-related increases in the serum and kidney tissue levels of both fortimicin A and gentamicin were seen in dogs. In rats, there were dose-related increases in the kidney tissue concentrations of fortimicin A but not of gentamicin.

1. Egan, R. S., R. S. Stanaszek, M. Cirovic, S. L. Mueller, J. Tadanier, J. R. Martin, P. Collum, A. W. Goldstein, R. L. De Vault, A. C. Sinclair, E. E. Fager, and L. A. Mitscher. 1977. Fortimicins A and B, new aminoglycoside antibiotics. III. Structural identification. J. Antibiot. 30:552–563.

2. Girolami, R. L., and J. M. Stamm. 1977. Fortimicins A and B, new aminoglycoside antibiotics. IV. In vitro study of fortimicin A compared with other aminoglycosides. J. Antibiot. 30:564–570.

3. Nara, T., M. Yamamoto, I. Kawamoto, K. Takayama, R. Okachi, S. Takasawa, T. Sato, and S. Sato. 1977. Fortimicins A and B, new aminoglycoside antibiotics. I. Producing organism, fermentation and biological properties of fortimicins. J. Antibiot. 30:533–540.

4. Okachi, R., S. Takasawa, T. Sato, S. Sato, M. Yamamoto, I. Kawamoto, and T. Nara. 1977. Fortimicins A and B, new aminoglycoside antibiotics. II. Isolation, physico-chemical and chromatographic properties. J. Antibiot. 30:541–551.

Experimental Studies on the Ototoxicity and Nephrotoxicity of Fortimicin A

ATSUSHI SAITO, YASUSHI UEDA,* AND MASATOYO AKIYOSHI

Department of Internal Medicine, The Jikei University School of Medicine, Tokyo, Japan,* and Department of Pathology, Tsurumi University School of Dental Medicine, Yokohama, Japan

Fortimicin A (test drug number, KW-1070) is a new aminoglycoside which was developed at Tokyo Research Laboratory of Kyowa Hakko Kogyo Co., Ltd., and has a broad antibacterial spectrum against gram-positive and -negative bacteria (2). Furthermore, this substance is stable to all aminoglycoside-inactivating enzymes except acetyltransferase (3)-I and exhibits excellent antibacterial activity against gram-negative bacilli resistant to gentamicin. It is known that fortimicin A does not interact with amikacin in enzymatic inactivation (2, 3). In this study, the effect of fortimicin A on the auditory system and the kidneys was evaluated in animal experiments.

Ototoxicity. Eighty female Hartley guinea pigs weighing about 350 g and 58 newborn guinea pigs were used. In the short-term test, fortimicin A was given intramuscularly to 20 animals at doses of 200 and 400 mg/kg for 28 days each. As a control drug, ribostamycin was administered to 10 animals at 400 mg/kg for 30 days. The differential frequency pinna reflex (1) in frequency range (0.5 to 20 kHz) was measured before, during, and after administration, and the inner ears were examined histopathologically after treatment. In the long-term test, fortimicin A was given intramuscularly to 20 animals at 10 and 100 mg/kg for 90 days each. In these animals, a consecutive pinna reflex test was performed. In the transplacental ototoxicity test, the transplacental ototoxic effect of fortimicin A was investigated by short-term administration of the drug at doses of 100 and 200 mg/kg in the

early period of gestation, and the pinna reflex was measured on 58 newborn litters for 2 weeks after birth. In the tests using combined administration with furosemide, the effect of intravenous injection of furosemide (100 mg/kg) on the inner ears in the animals treated with fortimicin A (200 mg/kg, intramuscularly) 2 h previously was examined by the pinna reflex test and supravital reduction of nitroblue tetrazolium of the hair cells.

Results. In the short-term test, no animal showed loss of the pinna reflex; histopathologically, absence of outer hair cells was found at the basal end of the first turn of the unilateral cochlea in only 1 of 10 animals receiving 200 mg of fortimicin A per kg. However, all of these animals showed scattered loss of hair cells in the vestibular organs. The pinna reflex and changes in the inner ears were not significantly enhanced in the group treated with 400 mg of fortimicin A per kg. At this dose there was no distinct difference in ototoxicity between fortimicin A and ribostamycin (1), an aminoglycoside with the lowest audiotoxicity (Table 1). In the long-term test, neither an increase in threshold nor loss of the pinna reflex was seen in any of the animals given fortimicin A. None of 58 newborn guinea pigs whose mothers received fortimicin A indicated any transplacental ototoxic effect on the pinna reflex. A single intravenous injection of furosemide induced a continuous loss of the pinna reflex in higher frequencies in animals treated previously with fortimicin A, beginning 1 day after furosemide administration. These

TABLE 1. *Ototoxic effect of short-term (30 days) intramuscular administration of fortimicin A on pinna reflex and inner ear in 28 guinea pigs, 10 animals per group*

Antibiotic	Dose (mg/kg)	Loss of pinna reflex[a]	Cochlear damage as loss of:			Vestibular damage[c]
			Outer hair cells	Inner hair cells	Spiral ganglion cells	
Fortimicin A	200	0	1[b]	0	0	10
Fortimicin A	400	0	1[b]	0	0	10
Ribostamycin	400	3	1[a]	0	0	10

[a] Loss of outer hair cells at basal end of bilateral cochleas.
[b] Loss of outer hair cells at basal end of unilateral cochlea.
[c] Slight damage.

TABLE 2. *Histological score on renal lesions in rats treated with fortimicin A, amikacin, and gentamicin[a]*

Antibiotic	Dose (mg/kg)	During administration			After administration, 28th day[c]
		7th day[b]	14th day[b]	21st day[c]	
Control		0	0	0	0
Fortimicin A	80	1.0 ± 0.00	1.4 ± 0.25	1.9 ± 0.18	1.0 ± 0.26
Amikacin	80	1.4 ± 0.25	1.4 ± 0.25	2.1 ± 0.23	1.1 ± 0.18
Gentamicin	24	1.6 ± 0.25[d]	1.8 ± 0.20	2.4 ± 0.22	1.5 ± 0.17
Fortimicin A	160	1.2 ± 0.20	1.8 ± 0.20	2.7 ± 0.15	2.2 ± 0.33
Amikacin	160	1.6 ± 0.24	2.8 ± 0.37[d]	5.3 ± 0.33[e]	4.0 ± 0.45[f]
Gentamicin	48	1.8 ± 0.20	4.6 ± 0.75[f]	5.0 ± 0.37[e]	2.5 ± 0.27
Fortimicin A	320	1.6 ± 0.25	3.8 ± 0.58	3.9 ± 0.28	2.3 ± 0.45
Amikacin	320	1.8 ± 0.20	6.0 ± 0.00[f]	6.5 ± 0.19[e]	5.6 ± 0.56[e]
Gentamicin	96	3.0 ± 0.00[e]	6.0 ± 0.00[f]	6.4 ± 0.24[e]	3.8 ± 0.37[d]

[a] Histological score was determined as grade of I (degenerative findings) + grade of II (alterative findings), mean ± SE. Grade 0: I, almost normal; II, no alterative findings. Grade 1: I, patchy swelling and desquamation of tubular epithelial cells; II, small clusters of round cells surrounding altered tubules. Grade 2: I, grade 1 with patchy necrosis of tubular epithelial cells and rare mitosis; II, wider distribution of round cell infiltrations surrounding altered tubules. Grade 3: I, widespread necrosis of tubular epithelial cells and presence of regenerative cells; II, grade 2 with focal distribution of dilatated tubules. Grade 4: I, extensive necrosis of tubules and regenerative changes; II, diffuse distribution of dilatated tubules and presence of interstitial fibrosis.
[b] Five animals in study group.
[c] Ten animals per study group (eight received amikacin at 320 mg/kg; five received gentamicin at 320 mg/kg).
[d] $P = 0.05$.
[e] $P = 0.001$.
[f] $P = 0.01$.

results indicate that fortimicin A has mild toxicity in the vestibular organ and, like ribostamycin, belongs to the aminoglycoside group with the lowest audiotoxicity. The enhanced impairment of the pinna reflex in animals given fortimicin A and then furosemide may be attributed to an increase in permeability of outer hair cells by furosemide-induced inhibition of membrane adenosine triphosphatase. The latter change may allow penetration of fortimicin A with potential ototoxicity in extracellular cortilymph into the outer hair cells, resulting in impairment of energy metabolism and pinna reflex.

Nephrotoxicity. Male Wistar rats weighing about 150 g were used in this experiment. In single-dose tests, fortimicin A and amikacin were given intramuscularly at doses of 80, 160, and 320 mg/kg for 21 days (4) each. Gentamicin was given at 24, 48, and 96 mg/kg in the same way. In these animals, the following determinations were made: measurement of body weight and intake of food and water; autopsy; biochemical analysis of serum and urine; measurement of drug concentration in the serum and kidney; and histopathological examination of the kidneys. In the recovery test, the serum and urine were continuously examined biochemically for 28 days after administration of the three drugs for 21 days. The kidneys were investigated histopathologically after the end of the experiments. In combined-administration tests, furosemide (30 mg/kg) was given in combination with fortimicin A and amikacin at 160 and 320 mg/kg for 14 days each. As a control, each antibiotic was given at the same dose for 14 days. In these animals, the same examinations as in the single-dose test were carried out.

Results. In the single-dose test, dose dependency of renal damage was noted in animals treated with fortimicin A, amikacin, and gentamicin at different doses. Fortimicin A was found to be the lowest of the three drugs in nephrotoxicity in the following cases: fortimicin A and amikacin at 160 mg/kg each and gentamicin at 48 mg/kg, and the former two at 320 mg/kg each and the latter at 96 mg/kg (Table 2). After cessation of drug administration, fortimicin A showed a tendency to disappear more rapidly from the kidneys than amikacin. The examination made in this study showed that renal damage was milder in animals treated with fortimicin A than in those receiving the other drugs. Combined administration with furosemide enhanced renal damage by fortimicin A and, especially, amikacin. The recovery test indicated that renal damage persisted longer in animals receiving amikacin than in those treated with fortimicin A. These results indicate that fortimicin A is one of the drugs lowest in oto- and nephrotoxicity among the current aminoglycosides.

1. **Akiyoshi, M.** 1977. Evaluation of ototoxicity and safety of aminoglycoside antibiotics in the guinea pig. Adv. Clin. Pharmacol. **13**:374–386.
2. **Girolami, R. L., and J. M. Stamm.** 1977. Fortimicins A and B, new aminoglycoside antibiotics. IV. In vitro study of fortimicin A compared with other aminoglycosides. J. Antibiot. **30**:564–570.
3. **Nara, T., M. Yamamato, I. Kawamoto, K. Takayama, R. Okachi, S. Takasawa, T. Sato, and S. Sato.** 1977. Fortimicins A and B, new aminoglycoside antibiotics. I. Producing organism, fermentation and biological properties of fortimicins. J. Antibiot. **30**:533–540.
4. **Ueda, Y., A. Saito, and G. Uchiura.** 1975. Nephrotoxicity of antibiotics. Pharm. Monthly (Tokyo) **17**:1867–1871.

Evaluation of New 1-N-Substituted Aminoglycosides Against Strains with Known Resistance Mechanisms

ROBERTA S. HARE,* THOMAS W. SCHAFER, PETER J. CHIU, FRANK J. SABATELLI, EUGENE L. MOSS, JR., AND GEORGE H. MILLER

Schering-Plough Corporation, Bloomfield, New Jersey 07003, U.S.A.

New synthetic capabilities have recently been described for the preparation of aminoglycosides with either novel substituents on the 1-amino group (5) or epimerization at the 5 position (2) of the 2-deoxystreptamine ring. Preliminary in vitro tests indicated that several derivatives of sisomicin and gentamicin B prepared by these methods maintained potency with increased activity against strains containing aminoglycoside-modifying enzymes. (A. Afonso and F. Hon, A. K. Mallams et al., D. F. Rane and P. J. L. Daniels, and T. Nagabhushan et al., this volume). This paper presents a more extensive analysis of their in vitro and in vivo activities and of their acute toxicities and nephrotoxicities. The methods for all tests have been described by Waitz et al. (6).

The in vitro activities of the aminoglycosides are summarized in Table 1. The compounds were tested not only against normal or susceptible strains but also against a large group of resistant organisms that have been classified according to their aminoglycoside resistance patterns (4). All of the compounds maintained potency similar to or better than that of gentamicin and amikacin against the normal strains with the exception of the L-seryl derivative, which was significantly less active against *Providencia*, *Proteus*, and *Pseudomonas*.

Aminoglycosides were tested against three main classes of acetylating strains. Against all types of 3- and 2'-N-acetylating strains, aminoglycosides with 1-N-S-3-amino-2-hydroxypropionyl (HAPA) and 1-N-2-aminoethoxycarbonyl (AEC) substitutents had activity, whereas the L-seryl derivative (Sch 23002) was only active against one type of 3-N-acetylator. Varying degrees of activity against 6'-acetylating strains were observed. Sch 23002 was not active against either type. Compounds with a 1-N-AEC substituent were generally less active than those with a 1-N-HAPA side chain against this class of acetylators. Combinations of 1-N-HAPA and 5-epimerization led to compounds with the best activity against 6'-acetylators (Sch 27082 and Sch 27598).

All the tested aminoglycosides were active against 2''-adenylylating strains, including those *Serratia* in which this activity was combined with low levels of 6'-acetylating activity. None

TABLE 1. *Comparative in vitro activities of selected aminoglycosides*[a]

Organism	Geometric mean MIC (µg/ml)[b]									
	Genta-micin	Sch 23002	Sch 26128	Sch 26361	Sch 27083	Sch 27082	Ami-kacin	Sch 21420	Sch 24628	Sch 27598
Normal (90)[c]	0.6	6.2	0.7	0.7	0.9	0.5	1.0	1.1	1.3	0.8
AAC(3)-I (17)	114	5.5	1.5	1.1	0.9	0.7	2.6	2.5	4.0	1.8
AAC(3)-Ia (10)	139	17	3.6	2.5	1.5	0.8	2.0	3.3	7.3	2.2
AAC(3)-II (8)	139	10	0.7	0.5	0.6	0.6	1.5	0.8	1.5	0.9
AAC(2′) (21)	39	96	3.4	1.3	2.4	0.6	2.7	2.5	3.4	1.2
AAC(6′)-I (4)	1.7	76	14	2.5	13	1.1	23	8.0	27	2.8
AAC(6′)-II (10)	125	60	42	12	5.4	1.1	4.3	5.3	25	3.0
ANT(2″) (30)	59	2.7	0.8	0.7	0.7	0.5	1.1	1.1	1.4	0.9
ANT(2″) and AAC(6′) (10)	61	8.0	2.7	1.7	1.8	1.7	4.3	3.1	5.0	1.7
APH(2″) and AAC(6′) (2)	90	—[d]	0.5	0.5	0.2	0.3	5.6	5.6	45	2
ANT(4′) (2)	0.8	—	0.8	1.0	1.4	2.0	32	28	32	32
APH(3′)-IV (1)	0.5	—	0.5	0.5	0.7	1.4	8	25	16	32
Permeability (10)	83	95	70	64	70	28	60	68	102	39

[a] Sch 23002, L-serylsisomicin; Sch 26128, AEC-sisomicin; Sch 26361, AEC-5-episisomicin; Sch 27083, HAPA-sisomicin; Sch 27082, HAPA-5-episisomicin; Sch 24628, AEC-gentamicin B; Sch 27598, HAPA-5-epigentamicin B; Sch 21420, HAPA-gentamicin B.

[b] Measured at 24 h after culture in Mueller-Hinton agar.

[c] Numbers in parentheses indicate minimum number of strains tested.

[d] —, Not tested.

of the compounds which have a 4′-hydroxyl group were active against the 4′-adenylylating strains.

As expected from their activity against the aminoglycoside-2″-*O*-nucleotidyltransferase [ANT(2″)] strains, all of the compounds except Sch 24628 were active against the *Staphylococcus* with 2″-phosphorylating activity. All compounds having a 3′-OH group had poor activity against the *Staphylococcus* with 3′-IV phosphorylating activity. None of the tested compounds were active against the high-level-permeability strains. The combination of a 1-*N*-HAPA side chain and 5-epimerization led to the compounds with the broadest spectrum and the greatest potency.

Mouse protection tests with a variety of resistant strains confirmed the spectrum and potency of HAPA-5-episisomicin (Sch 27082) and HAPA-5-epigentamicin B (Sch 27598). Comparative 50% protective dose values (PD$_{50}$) with gentamicin, tobramycin, sisomicin, netilmicin, and amikacin showed Sch 27082 and Sch 27598 to be active in vivo against strains containing the following resistance patterns: ANT(2″), four strains; aminoglycoside-6′-*N*-acetyltransferase [(AAC(6′)]-I, two strains; AAC(3)-I, one strain; AAC(2′), one strain; and AAC(6′)-II, one strain. PD$_{50}$ values obtained with Sch 27082 were either lower than those of all other tested compounds or equal to that of the most active compound, confirming the high potency of this derivative. Similarly, PD$_{50}$ values of Sch 27598 were either lower than or equal to those observed with Sch

21420 and amikacin, confirming that this compound would seem to be the most potent gentamicin B derivative prepared to date.

Preliminary values for acute toxicities were determined, using groups of three to five mice. The intravenous LD$_{50}$ values for the sisomicin derivatives were as follows: Sch 23002, 125 mg/kg; Sch 26128, 65 mg/kg; Sch 26361, 45 mg/kg; Sch 27083, 90 mg/kg; and Sch 27082, 35 mg/kg. As expected, the values for the gentamicin B derivatives were higher, with Sch 24628 being 210 mg/kg and Sch 27598 being 325 mg/kg.

The effect on renal function of these compounds is shown in Fig. 1, which is a plot of glomerular filtration rate (GFR) remaining after 7 days of dosing versus the total daily dose. The dose at which GFR was reduced to 0.5 ml/min per 100 g (~50% reduction) was chosen as an estimate of nephrotoxicity. The 1-*N*-HAPA and 1-*N*-AEC derivatives of sisomicin seemed to have a nephrotoxic potential similar to that observed with gentamicin. This was not unexpected, since 1-*N*-HAPA-gentamicin B (Sch 21420) has been reported to have a nephrotoxicity similar to that of gentamicin B (3). In contrast, the 1-*N*-seryl derivative of sisomicin seemed to have a nephrotoxic potential in rats similar to that of amikacin. Thus, it seemed to be behaving more like 1-*N*-alkyl derivatives of sisomicin (e.g., netilmicin), which are approximately four times less nephrotoxic than the parent compound (1).

Since 5-episisomicin (Sch 22591) has been reported to be similar in nephrotoxic potential to

spectrum of activity against resistant strains, they also enhance nephrotoxicity.

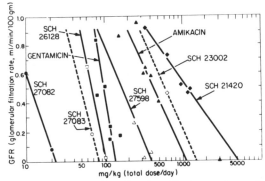

FIG. 1. *Effect of aminoglycosides on rat renal function. Rats weighing 200 g were dosed intramuscularly twice daily for 7 days, at which time the state of renal function was determined by measuring ^{14}C-inulin clearance (GFR).*

sisomicin (6), it was surprising to find that the 1-N-HAPA derivatives of 5-episisomicin and 5-epigentamicin B were about five times more nephrotoxic than their parent compounds. It would seem that although these two modifications lead to outstanding potency and a broad

1. **Chiu, P. J. S., G. H. Miller, A. D. Brown, J. F. Long, and J. A. Waitz.** 1977. Renal pharmacology of netilmicin. Antimicrob. Agents Chemother. **11:**821–825.
2. **Daniels, P. J. L., and D. F. Rane.** 1979. Synthetic and mutasynthetic antibiotics related to sisomicin, p. 314–317. *In* D. Schlessinger (ed.), Microbiology—1979. American Society for Microbiology, Washington, D.C.
3. **Miller, G. H., P. J. S. Chiu, and J. A. Waitz.** 1978. Biological activity of *Sch 21420*, the 1-N-S-α-hydroxy-β-amino-propionyl derivative of gentamicin B. J. Antibiot. **31:**688–696.
4. **Miller, G. H., F. J. Sabatelli, R. S. Hare, and J. A. Waitz.** Survey of aminoglycoside resistance patterns. Dev. Ind. Microbiol., in press.
5. **Nagabhushan, T. L., A. B. Cooper, W. N. Turner, J. Tsai, S. McCombie, A. K. Mallams, D. Rane, J. J. Wright, P. Reichert, D. L. Boxler, and J. Weinstein.** 1978. Interaction of vicinal and nonvicinal amino-hydroxy group pairs in aminoglycoside-aminocyclitol antibiotics with transition metal cations. Selective N protection. J. Am. Chem. Soc. **100:**5253–5254.
6. **Waitz, J. A., G. H. Miller, E. Moss, Jr., and P. J. Chiu.** 1978. Chemotherapeutic evaluation of 5-episisomicin (Sch 22591), a new semisynthetic aminoglycoside. Antimicrob. Agents Chemother. **13:**41–48.

Synthesis of 1-*N*-Peptidyl Derivatives of Sisomicin

ADRIAN AFONSO* AND FRANK HON

Schering-Plough Corporation, Bloomfield, New Jersey 07003, U.S.A.

Several 1-*N*-α-aminoacyl, 1-*N*-dipeptidyl, and 1-*N*-tripeptidyl derivatives (I) of the aminoglycoside antibiotic sisomicin (II) (3) were prepared in order to evaluate the effects produced by such modifications on the antibacterial spectrum of II (Fig. 1). The general method used in the synthesis of these compounds is described below.

II was converted to 6'-*N*-*tert*-butyloxycarbonyl sisomicin (III) by reaction with *t*-butyloxycarbonyl azide. Alternatively, II was converted to the fully protected 3,2',6'-tris(trichloroethoxycarbonyl)-sisomicin (IV), using a procedure described previously (2). Acylation of the 1-amino group was effected by reacting either III or IV with the 2,4,5-trichlorophenyl ester of the appropriate *N*-butyloxycarbonyl amino acid or peptide. The latter compounds were prepared by conventional peptide chemistry techniques (1). The products resulting from the condensation of III with the active esters were deprotected with trifluoroacetic acid (V) to afford I. When IV was used in the condensation with the

active esters, the products were treated with zinc-acetic acid in order to remove the trichloroethoxycarbonyl protective groups followed by debocylation with V to afford I. The aminoacyl units used in this series of compounds were derived from glycine, L-α,γ-diaminobutyric acid,

FIG. 1. *Structure of 1-N-peptidyl derivatives of sisomicin.*

L-leucine, L-alanine, L-methionine, L-serine, L-valine, L-tyrosine, and L-threonine.

Among the 1-N-α-aminoacyl derivatives, Ia, the L-valyl, L-alanyl, and L-tyrosyl analog, showed weak antibacterial activity; the L-leucyl, L-methionyl, L-threonyl, and glycyl analogs possessed moderate activity, and the L-seryl analog (Ia, R = $-CH_2OH$) showed high activity. Seven dipeptidyl derivatives (Ib) containing glycine, L-α,γ-diaminobutyric acid, L-leucine, and L-serine were prepared; weak activity was observed for compounds Ib when a L-α,γ-diaminobutyric acid or L-leucine unit acylated the 1-amino group, and moderate activity was observed when these units were L-serine or glycine. The 1-N-diglycyl derivative (Ib, R = R″ = H) showed high activity, whereas the 1-N-triglycyl derivative (Ic, R = H) had reduced activity. From this series, 1-N-L-serylsisomicin (Ia, R = $-CH_2OH$) and 1-N-diglycylsisomicin (Ib, R = R″ = H) showed an improved antibacterial spectrum in vitro and unusually low LD_{50} values relative to the parent antibiotic. More detailed biology of Ia (R = $-CH_2OH$) is included in the preceding paper (R. S. Hare et al.).

1. **Bodansky, M., and M. Ondetti.** 1966. Peptide synthesis. John Wiley & Sons, New York.
2. **Nagabhushan, T. L., A. B. Cooper, W. N. Turner, J. Tsai, S. McCombie, A. K. Mallams, D. Rane, J. J. Wright, P. Reichert, D. L. Boxler, and J. Weinstein.** 1978. Interaction of vicinal and nonvicinal amino-hydroxy group pairs in aminoglycoside-aminocyclitol antibiotics with transition metal cations. J. Am. Chem. Soc. **100**:5253–5254.
3. **Reimann, H., et al.** 1974. The structure of sisomicin, a novel unsaturated aminocyclitol antibiotic from *Micromonospora inyoensis.* J. Org. Chem. **39**:1451–1457.

Synthesis of Novel 1-N-Aminoalkyloxycarbonyl and 1-N-Aminoalkylcarboxamido Derivatives of Sisomicin, Gentamicin B, Gentamicin C1a, and Kanamycin A

ALAN K. MALLAMS,* PAUL REICHERT, AND JAMES B. MORTON

Research Division, Schering-Plough Corporation, Bloomfield, New Jersey 07003, U.S.A.

The discovery of amikacin (1) and netilmicin (3) gave a considerable impetus to the search for other novel 1-N-substituted aminoglycosides, and we describe here the synthesis, conformations, and antibacterial properties of a series of 1-N-aminoalkyloxycarbonyl and 1-N-aminoalkylcarboxamido derivatives of 5-episisomicin, sisomicin, gentamicin B, gentamicin C1a, and kanamycin A (Fig. 1).

Synthesis. Suitable 3,(2′),6′-N-protected aminoglycosides were prepared by the type 1 transition metal complexing method (2), and these were reacted with the succinimide-active ester of the desired side chain, prepared by standard methods, to give after deprotection a variety of 1-N-alkyloxycarbonyl derivatives (Table 1).

In some instances it was necessary to protect the 3″-amino group as well, and this was accomplished as follows. 3,6′-Di-N-benzyloxycarbonylgentamicin B was treated with N-(2,2,2-trichloroethoxycarbonyloxy)succinimide to give 3,6′-di-N-benzyloxycarbonyl-1-N-(2,2,2-trichloroethoxycarbonyl)gentamicin B. The latter was reacted with benzylchloroformate and treated with zinc in acetic acid to give 3,6′,3″-tri-N-benzyloxycarbonylgentamicin B. The latter was reacted with 2-azidoethylisocyanate, and the product was subjected to hydrogenation to give 1-N-

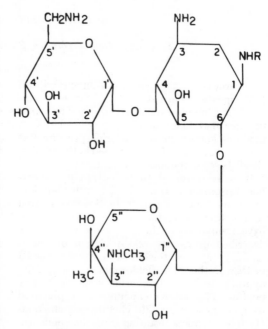

R = $COOCH_2CH_2NH_2$

R = $CONHCH_2CH_2NH_2$

FIG. 1. *Structure of 1-N-substituted aminoglycoside derivatives.*

TABLE 1. MICs (24 h) in Mueller-Hinton broth[a]

Substrate: 1-NHR	MIC (µg/ml)[b]																LD₅₀ (mg/kg) i.v. in mice
	Staphylococcus aureus Wood, susceptible	Escherichia coli ATCC 10536, susceptible	Proteus mirabilis Harding, susceptible	P. rettgeri Membel, susceptible	Pseudomonas aeruginosa Stone 20, susceptible	E. coli JR 66, ANT(2″)	Klebsiella pneumoniae Georgetown 3694, ANT(2″)	E. coli JR 88, AAC(3)-I	P. aeruginosa Maryland 8327, AAC(3)-Ia	P. aeruginosa Travers, AAC(3)-II	Proteus rettgeri 012360S, AAC(2′)	E. coli W677/R5, AAC(6′)-I	P. aeruginosa Shreveport, AAC(6′)-II	Serratia Dalton, APH(3′)-I	K. pneumoniae Adler 17, APH(3′)-II	P. aeruginosa Shriners 10099, permeability	LD_{50} (mg/kg) i.v. in mice
5-Episisomicin																	
H	<0.06	0.25	2	1	<0.06	2	0.25	0.25	0.25	8	0.5	4	32	<0.06	0.125	>16	45
COOCH₂CH₂NH₂	0.06	0.06	0.5	0.25	0.03	0.25	0.06	0.25	0.25	0.06	0.5	2	>16	0.06	1	>16	45
Sisomicin																	
H	<0.06	0.25	0.5	4	0.25	32	8	8	128	128	32	4	128	<0.06	0.125	>16	50
COOCH₂CH₂NH₂	<0.015	0.06	0.25	1	0.03	0.125	0.03	0.125	4	1	1	1	>16	0.125	0.5	>16	65
COOCH₂CH₂NHCH₂CH₃	0.25	0.25	1	2	0.25	0.5	0.5	0.25			16				2	>16	60
CSOCH₂CH₂NH₂	8	0.5	8	16	0.5	2	2	8				8	>32	2	8	>32	140
COOCH₃	0.5	0.5	1	1	0.5	1	0.5	1	>32	>32	>32	>32	>32	>32	4	>32	130
COOCH₂CH₃	4	0.5	4	16	0.5	2	2	2	8	8	8	16	>32	4	8	>32	130
CONH₂	0.3	0.3	17.5	7.5	0.3	3	7.5	17.5	>32	>32	>32	>32	>32	32	3	>25	
CONHCH₃	0.3	0.75	>25	>25	0.3	7.5	0.3	>25				>25	>25	3	0.75	>25	
Gentamicin B																	
H	0.25	0.5	2	2	2	>16	>16	2	>16	>16	2	>16	>16	>16	>16	>16	228
COOCH₂CH₂NH₂	0.5	0.5	1	2	0.25	1	0.5	2	16	4	2	>16	>16	8	8	>16	210
COOCH₂CH₂CH₂NH₂	<0.015	0.25	4	1	0.25	0.25	2	1	1	0.5	1	>16	8	4	4	>16	210
COOCH₂CH₂CH₂NH₂	0.5	1	8	2	0.25	1	1	2	16	4	16	>16	>16	4	4	>16	240
COOCH₂CH(NH₂)CH₂CH₃	0.5	0.25	1	1	0.25	0.5	0.25	0.5	8	2	8	>16	>16	>16	4	>16	160
COOCH₂CH(NH₂)CH₂CH(CH₃)₂	1	0.5	2	2	0.06	1	1	0.5	>16	8	4	>16	>16	1	4	>16	165
CONHCH₂CH₂NH₂	0.03	0.5	1	1	0.25	2	1	17.5	4	1		>25	16	>25	>16	>25	195
CONH₂	1	7.5	>25	17.5	3	>25	>25	16		>25			>25		>25	>16	70
Gentamicin	3	0.25	1	8	0.5	32	16	0.125	>128	128	64	1	128	0.125	0.25		65
Gentamicin C1a																	
COOCH₂CH₂NH₂	<0.015	0.03	0.125	0.5	0.03	0.125	0.03	>25	0.25	0.125	2	0.5	4	0.25	0.25	>16	65
CSNHCH₂CH₃	0.75	3	>25	>25	3	17.5	25		>25	>25		>25	>25	>25	>25	>25	
Kanamycin A																	
COOCH₂CH₂NH₂	0.03	0.5	1	0.5	0.06	4	1	1	1	0.25	2	>16	>16	1	>16	>16	175
Amikacin	0.5	1	16	8	0.25	8	1	1	4	0.25	4	64	2	0.25	1	>16	400

[a] MICs are noncomparative in most instances.

[b] ANT(2″), aminoglycoside-2″-O-nucleotidyltransferase; AAC(3), aminoglycoside-3-N-acetyltransferase; AAC(2′), aminoglycoside-2′-N-acetyltransferase; AAC(6′), aminoglycoside-6′-N-acetyltransferase; APH(3′), aminoglycoside-3′-O-phosphotransferase; i.v., intravenous.

(2-aminoethylcarboxamido)gentamicin B (Table 1). The other 1-N-carboxamido derivatives were prepared in a similar manner.

Conformations. A detailed study of the ^{13}C nuclear magnetic resonance parameters of these 1-N-substituted aminoglycosides revealed interesting conformational differences about the O-C_6 glycosidic bond between 1-N-acyl-substituted aminoglycosides (acyl, aminohydroxybutyryl [HABA], aminohydroxypropionyl [HAPA], alkyloxycarbonyl, and alkylcarboxamido) and the parent unsubstituted aminoglycosides. Introduction of the 1-N-acyl-type substituent resulted in a clockwise rotation of the 6-O-glycoside about the O-C_6 glycosidic bond. Thus gentamicin B exhibited $\Delta\delta c_{\text{deoxystreptamine} \to \text{trisaccharide}}$ for C_6 of 9.0, whereas 1-N-(2-aminoethoxycarbonyl)gentamicin B exhibited $\Delta\delta c_{\text{1-}N\text{-(2-aminoethoxycarbonyl)de-}}$
$_{\text{oxystreptamine} \to \text{1-}N\text{-(2-amino-ethoxycarbonyl)gentamicin B}}$ for C_6 of 5.6. The strong shielding component evident at C_6 in these 1-N-substituted derivatives indicated clockwise rotation of the 6-O-glycoside about the O-C_6 glycosidic bond. Reduced dipolar repulsion between the C_6 glycosidic oxygen and the 1-NH-acyl group was most likely responsible for the observed conformational change. No change was observed in the solution conformation about the O-C_4 glycosidic bonds relative to the unsubstituted aminoglycosides.

Antibacterial activity and toxicity. In general, the 1-N-(2-aminoethoxycarbonyl), 1-N-(3-aminopropyloxycarbonyl), and 1-N-(2-aminoethylcarboxamido) derivatives were the most potent in the series. In all cases, the above derivatives were as potent as the parent aminoglycosides against all gentamicin-susceptible organisms (Table 1). These derivatives were also as potent as the corresponding 1-N-HAPA de-

rivatives against gentamicin-susceptible organisms. Against resistant strains, the above derivatives were highly potent against all of the resistance mechanisms with the exception of *Pseudomonas* strains carrying the aminoglycoside 6'-N-acyltransferase [AAC(6')]-II inactivating enzyme and permeability-resistant strains. In general, the above derivatives were one to two tubes less potent against resistant organisms and three to five tubes less potent against AAC(6')-II-producing *Pseudomonas* than the corresponding 1-N-HAPA derivatives. Removal of the terminal amino group in the side chain resulted in compounds having reduced potency. Similarly, extension of the alkyl side chain also resulted in compounds with lower potency. The thio analogs were also less potent.

The 1-N-substituted derivatives in general showed similar acute toxicities to the parent aminoglycosides, as shown by the LD_{50} values determined by intravenous administration of the drugs to mice (Table 1).

Thanks are due to G. H. Miller, T. W. Schafer, and E. L. Moss, Jr., for permission to quote their biological data.

1. Kawaguchi, H., T. Naito, S. Nakagawa, and K. Fujisawa. 1972. BB-K8, a new semisynthetic aminoglycoside antibiotic. J. Antibiot. **25**:695–708.
2. Nagabhushan, T. L., A. B. Cooper, W. N. Turner, H. Tsai, S. McCombie, A. K. Mallams, D. Rane, J. J. Wright, P. Reichert, D. L. Boxler, and J. Weinstein. 1978. Interaction of vicinal and nonvicinal aminohydroxy group pairs in aminoglycoside-aminocyclitol antibiotics with transition metal cations. Selective N protection. J. Am. Chem. Soc. **100**:5253–5254.
3. Wright, J. J. 1976. Synthesis of 1-N-ethylsisomicin: a broad-spectrum semisynthetic aminoglycoside antibiotic. Chem. Commun., p. 206–208.

Synthesis and In Vitro Microbiological Properties of the 1-N-(3-Amino-2-Hydroxypropionyl) Derivatives of Sisomicin and 5-Episisomicin

DINANATH F. RANE* AND PETER J. L. DANIELS

Schering-Plough Corporation, Bloomfield, New Jersey 07003, U.S.A.

Sisomicin, a new *Micromonospora*-derived aminoglycoside antibiotic discovered in our laboratories, has recently been introduced into clinical practice in a number of countries. Like all naturally occurring aminoglycoside antibiotics, sisomicin experiences bacterial resistance to some extent. The majority of this resistance is due to inactivation of the antibiotic by aminoglycoside-modifying enzymes specified by R-fac-

tor genes. A minor resistance problem arises from bacterial impermeability, which is probably chromosomally specified, and occurs predominantly in species of *Pseudomonas aeruginosa*.

We have carried out a number of semisynthetic and microbiological modifications of sisomicin in search of broader-spectrum compounds which would be unable to serve as substrates for one or more aminoglycoside-inactivating enzymes. The best known of these is netilmicin (8), which is active against bacterial strains possessing aminoglycoside-2″-O-nucleotidyltransferase [ANT(2″)] enzymes as well as some strains harboring aminoglycoside-3-N-acetyltransferase [AAC(3)] enzymes (3). A broader-spectrum compound, pentisomicin (5-episisomicin; see Fig. 1), resulted from inversion of the 5-hydroxyl group of the antibiotic, which can be done microbiologically by the process of mutasynthesis (1) or more efficiently by chemical semisynthesis (D. F. Rane and P. J. L. Daniels, unpublished data). 5-Episisomicin adopts a solution conformation different from that of sisomicin and netilmicin, demonstrated by carbon magnetic resonance studies, and this most likely explains its inability to serve as a substrate for several aminoglycoside-modifying enzymes and hence its broader spectrum.

Acylation at nitrogen 1 of the aminocyclitol unit of aminoglycosides has proved to be a reliable means of preparing broader-spectrum semisynthetic antibacterials. This was first demonstrated by the synthesis of amikacin (2) and has been confirmed by the preparation of many similar derivatives of other aminoglycoside antibiotics. Along these lines we recently reported the synthesis of 1-N-(S-3-amino-2-hydroxypropionyl)gentamicin B (Sch 21420) (5), a broad-spectrum aminoglycoside with reduced toxicity compared with amikacin (4). We now report the synthesis and antimicrobial properties of the analogous derivatives of sisomicin and 5-episisomicin.

The method of synthesis of these compounds was based on the selective N-protection method of Nagabhushan et al. (6), using divalent transition metal complexes. Thus, reaction of sisomicin with cobaltous acetate in dimethyl sulfoxide resulted in a type I complex (6) between $N(3″)-O(4″)$ and $N(1)-O(2″)$ (see Fig. 1 for numbering). Selective acylation of the uncomplexed amines with an active ester of p-methoxybenzylcarbonate, followed by removal of the cobaltous ions with hydrogen sulfide, gave

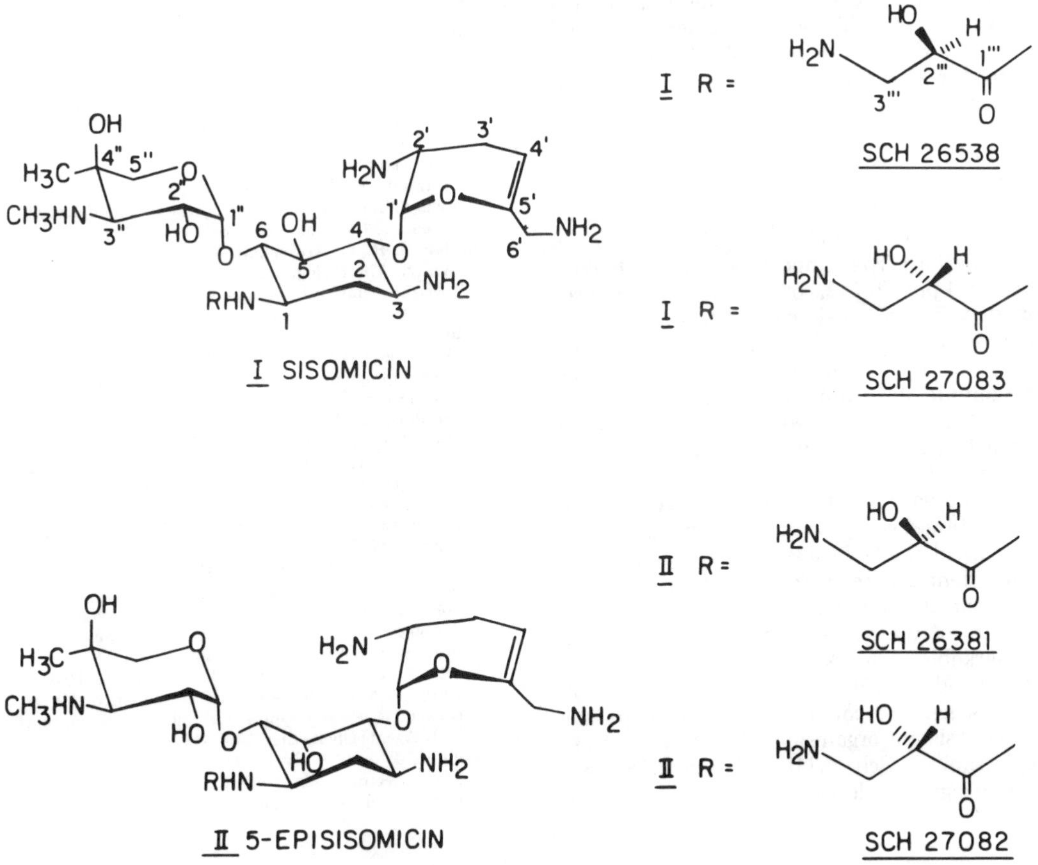

FIG. 1. Novel aminoglycosides.

TABLE 1. *In vitro antibacterial activities of 1-N-hydroxyaminopropionyl derivatives of sisomicin and 5-episisomicin*

Organism	Resistance mechanism	MIC (µg/ml, 24 h)			
		Sch 26538	Sch 27083	Sch 26381	Sch 27082
Staphylococcus aureus	Susceptible	<0.015	0.03	<0.015	<0.03
Escherichia coli 10536	Susceptible	0.125	0.125	0.06	<0.03
Proteus mirabilis	Susceptible	1.0	1.0	0.125	0.5
Proteus rettgeri	Susceptible	0.5	0.5	0.125	0.5
Pseudomonas aeruginosa Stone 20	Susceptible	0.03	0.25	0.03	<0.03
Escherichia coli JR66	ANT(2")	0.25	1.0	0.06	0.5
Klebsiella pneumoniae 3694	ANT(2")	0.25	0.125	0.06	0.5
Escherichia coli JR88	AAC(3)-I	0.25	0.5	0.125	0.25
Pseudomonas aeruginosa 8327	AAC(3)-Ia	0.125	0.25	0.06	0.25
P. aeruginosa Travers 1	AAC(3)-II	0.125	0.125	0.06	0.5
Providencia 164	AAC(2')	0.5	4.0	0.25	0.5
Serratia 0323605	AAC(6')-I	4.0	16.0	0.5	1.0
Pseudomonas aeruginosa 3796	AAC(6')-II	0.25	16.0	0.06	0.5
P. aeruginosa 1136	Permeability	>16.0	>16.0	16.0	16.0

$3,2',6'$-tri-N-p-methoxybenzyloxycarbonylsisomicin in very high yield. Selective acylation at N-1 with active esters of R and S-3-amino-2-hydroxypropionic acid, followed by removal of the N-protecting groups by brief treatment with trifluoroacetic acid, gave the desired products shown in Fig. 1. These were assigned the code numbers Sch 26538 and Sch 27083. Identical procedures starting with 5-episisomicin gave the corresponding derivatives, Sch 26381 and Sch 27082, also shown in Fig. 1.

The structures of these derivatives were confirmed by comparison of their carbon magnetic resonance spectra with those of reference compounds at acidic and basic pH. In particular, protonation of the compounds caused a shielding of only 4 ppm in C-2, compared with an approximately 7 ppm shielding in the unsubstituted parent antibiotic, indicating acylation at nitrogen 1 or 3 of the deoxystreptamine ring. The magnitude of the protonation-induced shielding of C-4 and the reduced shielding of C-6 confirmed N-1 as the site of substitution of the compounds in Fig. 1.

Preliminary in vitro antimicrobial properties of the target compounds are shown in Table 1. In general, the 1-N-substituted compounds were equivalent in potency to their parent antibiotics (comparative data not shown); the antibacterial spectra of the new derivatives, however, were remarkable. The sisomicin derivatives, Sch 26538 and Sch 27083, were relatively weak only against AAC(6')-containing strains and permeability-resistant organisms. The derivatives of 5-episisomicin, Sch 26381 and Sch 27082, were active against all bacterial strains possessing

aminoglycoside-modifying enzymes and, moreover, retained the very high potency of 5-episisomicin. These compounds are the most potent, broadest spectrum aminoglycoside antibiotics made to date. Further properties of these compounds are described by R. S. Hare et al. (this volume).

1. **Daniels, P. J. L., and D. F. Rane.** 1979. Synthetic and mutasynthetic antibiotics related to sisomicin, p. 314–317. *In* D. Schlessinger (ed.), Microbiology—1979. American Society for Microbiology, Washington, D.C.
2. **Kawaguchi, H., T. Naito, S. Nakagawa, and K. Fujisawa.** 1972. BB-K8, a new semisynthetic aminoglycoside antibiotic. J. Antibiot. **25**:695–708.
3. **Miller, G. H., G. Arcieri, M. J. Weinstein, and J. A. Waitz.** 1976. Biological activity of netilmicin, a broad-spectrum semisynthetic aminoglycoside antibiotic. Antimicrob. Agents Chemother. **10**:827–836.
4. **Miller, G. H., P. J. S. Chiu, and J. A. Waitz.** 1978. Biological activity of Sch 21420, the 1-N-S-α-hydroxy-β-aminopropionyl derivative of gentamicin B. J. Antibiot. **31**:688–696.
5. **Nagabhushan, T. L., A. B. Cooper, H. Tsai, P. J. L. Daniels, and G. H. Miller.** 1978. The synthesis and biological properties of 1-N-(S-4-amino-2-hydroxybutyryl)-gentamicin B and 1-N-(S-3-amino-2-hydroxypropionyl)-gentamicin B. J. Antibiot. **31**:681–687.
6. **Nagabhushan, T. L., A. B. Cooper, W. N. Turner, H. Tsai, S. McCombie, A. K. Mallams, D. Rane, J. J. Wright, P. Reichert, D. L. Boxler, and J. Weinstein.** 1978. Interaction of vicinal and nonvicinal aminohydroxy group pairs in aminoglycoside-aminocyclitol antibiotics with transition metal cations. Selective N protection. J. Am. Chem. Soc. **100**:5253–5254.
7. **Waitz, J. A., G. H. Miller, E. Moss, Jr., and P. J. S. Chiu.** 1978. Chemotherapeutic evaluation of 5-episisomicin, a new semisynthetic aminoglycoside. Antimicrob. Agents Chemother. **13**:41–48.
8. **Wright, J. J.** 1976. Synthesis of 1-N-ethylsisomicin: a broad-spectrum semisynthetic aminoglycoside antibiotic. J. Chem. Soc. Commun., p. 206–208.

Syntheses and Biological Properties of 5-*epi*-Gentamicin B, 1-*N*-(*S*-3-Amino-2-Hydroxypropionyl)-5-*epi*-Gentamicin B, and Their Kanamycin A Analogs

TATTANAHALLI L. NAGABHUSHAN, ALAN B. COOPER,* AND GEORGE H. MILLER

Schering-Plough Corporation, Bloomfield, New Jersey 07003, U.S.A.

We have recently published the biological properties of a semisynthetic broad-spectrum aminoglycoside-aminocyclitol antibiotic, 1-*N*-(*S*-3-amino-2-hydroxypropionyl)-gentamicin B (Sch 21420) (1, 2). Our objective in the present work was to enhance its potency by further chemical modification.

It was shown by D. F. Rane and P. J. Daniels (U.S. patent 4,000,261, December 1976) that epimerization at C-5 of sisomicin enhanced the potency as well as the spectrum of antibacterial activity. We have made a similar change at the 5 position of Sch 21420 and examined its effect on the biological activity. These results are compared with those obtained in the kanamycin A series.

The synthesis of 1-*N*-(*S*-3-amino-2-hydroxypropionyl)-5-*epi*-gentamicin B (Sch 27598) followed the sequence gentamicin B → 5-*epi*-gentamicin B → Sch 27598. The transformation of gentamicin B to its 5-*epi* derivative was carried out by a modification of the method of Rane and Daniels. Treatment of gentamicin B with methoxycarbonyl chloride under buffered conditions followed by sodium methoxide produced the tri-*N*-methoxycarbonyl-3″,4″-*N*,*O*-carbonyl derivative. Protection of all but the 5-hydroxyl group of this compound was carried out with acetic anhydride in pyridine at room tempera-

ture. The 5-hydroxyl group was next mesylated, and the mesylate was displaced with acetate ion. Base hydrolysis of the product gave 5-*epi*-gentamicin B in a overall yield of 50%. It is interesting to note that *O*-benzoyl protecting groups prevented mesylation at the 5 position. This is not surprising, since in the preferred conformation the benzoate carbonyl group at the 2′ position should be nearly *syn*-periplanar with the C-2′—H bond. This places the phenyl ring in the proximity of the already hindered 5-hydroxyl group, causing further steric shielding. 5-*epi*-Kanamycin A was synthesized in a similar manner; however, in this case it was not necessary to form the 3″,4″-oxazolidinone.

The proton-decoupled-^{13}C magnetic resonance spectrum of 5-*epi*-gentamicin B clearly indicated a change in the conformational preference about the glycosidic linkages relative to gentamicin B. This is evident from the 4.4-, 6.9-, and 6.4-ppm shielding of C-1′ (100 → 95.7), C-4 (87.7 → 80.8), and C-5 (74.9 → 68.5), respectively. The shielding effects on C-4 (or C-6) and C-5 upon inversion of configuration at C-5 of deoxystreptamine are considerably smaller, viz., 2 and 2.6 ppm, respectively. Despite the conformational change similar to the one observed in the sisomicin series, the antibacterial spectrum or potency of 5-*epi*-gentamicin B did not change

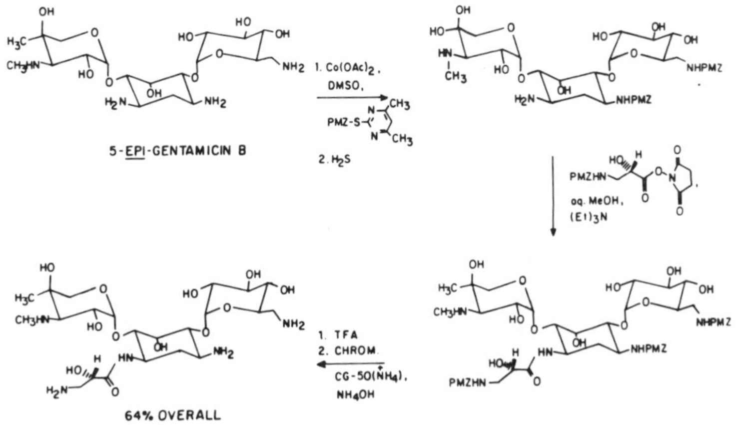

FIG. 1. *Synthesis of 1-N-(S-3-amino-2-hydroxypropionyl)-5-epi-gentamicin B. Abbreviations: Ac, acetyl; DMSO, dimethyl sulfoxide; aq. MeOH, aqueous methyl hydroxide; Et, ethyl.*

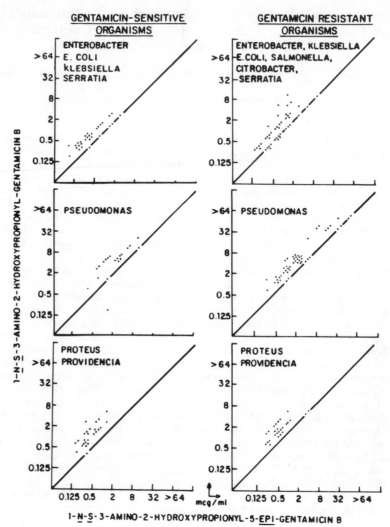

FIG. 2. *Comparison of the potencies of 1-N-(S-3-amino-2-hydroxypropionyl)-gentamicin B and its 5-epimer.*

significantly from that of its equatorial analog. A similar effect was observed with kanamycin A.

Using the transition metal complexing technique developed by Nagabhushan and co-workers (3) (type I, see Fig. 1), the 3,6'-di-N-p-methoxybenzyloxycarbonyl-5-epi-gentamicin B was synthesized in high yield. Reaction of this compound with the N-hydroxysuccinimid ester of S-3-p-methoxybenzyloxycarbonylamino-2-hydroxypropionic acid yielded, after de-N-protection with trifluoroacetic acid and chromatographic purification, Sch 27598 in an overall yield of 64% from 5-epi-gentamicin B. Sch 27598 maintained the broad spectrum of activity of Sch 21420 but was clearly two to four times more potent (Fig. 2). It is apparent, therefore, that in addition to a change in the rotameric

population about the glycosidic linkages effected through inversion of configuration at C-5, other structural features are needed to obtain potency enhancement. In this connection, it is interesting to note that 1-N-S-(3-amino-2-hydroxypropionyl)-5-epi-kanamycin A (Sch 28576) synthesized in a similar manner from 5-epi-kanamycin A by way of a type II complex was only similar to or slightly less potent than amikacin.

1. **Miller, G. H., P. J. S. Chiu, J. A. Waitz,** 1978. Biological activity of Sch 21420, the 1-N-S-α-hydroxy-β-aminopropionyl derivative of gentamicin B. J. Antibiot. **31**:688–696.

2. **Nagabhushan, T. L., A. B. Cooper, H. Tsai, P. J. L. Daniels, and G. H. Miller.** 1978. The synthesis and biological properties of 1-N-(S-4-amino-2-hydroxybutyryl)-gentamicin B and 1-N-(S-3-amino-2-hydroxypropionyl)-gentamicin B. J. Antibiot. **31**:681–687.

3. **Nagabhushan, T. L., A. B. Cooper, W. N. Turner, H. Tsai, S. McCombie, A. K. Mallams, D. Rane, J. J. Wright, P. Reichert, D. L. Boxler, and J. Weinstein.** 1978. Interaction of vicinal and non-vicinal amino-hydroxy group pairs in aminoglycoside-aminocyclitol antibiotics with transition metal cations. Selective N-protection. J. Am. Chem. Soc. **100**:5253–5254.

BB-K311: a Derivative of Amikacin Resistant to Inactivation by All Known Aminoglycoside-Modifying Enzymes

P. A. KRESEL,* T. A. PURSIANO, K. E. PRICE, M. MISIEK, AND F. LEITNER

Departments of Microbiological Research and Research Administration, Bristol Laboratories, Syracuse, New York 13201, U.S.A.

The ability to elaborate drug-modifying enzymes is a prevalent mode of bacterial resistance to aminoglycoside antibiotics. Six types of aminoglycoside-modifying enzymes confer resist-

TABLE 1. *Relative susceptibilities of amikacin, 4'-deoxyamikacin, 6'-N-methylamikacin, and 4'-deoxy-6'-N-methylamikacin to modification by 4'-O-nucleotidyltransferase and 6'-N-acetyltransferase*

Substrate	Relative uptake of label by:						
	4'-O-Nucleotidyltransferase from:			6'-N-Acetyltransferase from:			
	Staphylococcus aureus A22050	S. aureus A21978	Staphylococcus epidermidis A22152	Enterobacter cloacae A21136	Serratia marcescens A21974	S. marcescens A22302	S. aureus A22153
Kanamycin A	100	100	100	100	100	100	100
Amikacin	87	109	67	147	161	56	114
4'-Deoxyamikacin (BB-K160)	3	4	8	382	190	94	65
6'-N-methylamikacin (BB-K28)	86	86	59	1	2	1	13
4'-Deoxy-6'-N-methylamikacin (BB-K311)	<1	<1	4	3	3	2	1

TABLE 2. *Antibacterial spectra of amikacin, 4'-deoxyamikacin (BB-K160), 6'-N-methylamikacin (BB-K28), and 4'-deoxy-6'-N-methylamikacin (BB-K311)*

Strain	Resistance mechanism[a]	MIC (µg/ml)[b]			
		Amikacin	BB-K160	BB-K28	BB-K311
S. aureus (3 strains)		1.3	4	1.6	5
Enterobacteriaceae (12 strains)		1.6	4.8	2.9	4.6
Pseudomonas aeruginosa (3 strains)		4	16	16	20
Escherichia coli A20895	AAC(3)-I[c]	2.8	8	4	8
S. marcescens A22478	AAC(3)-II	4	—	4	8
E. coli A22045	AAC(3)-III	1.4	8	1	8
Proteus rettgeri A21207	AAC(2')	2	4	4	4
S. marcescens A21226	AAC(6')	8	>16	1	4
S. marcescens A21974	AAC(6')	22.6	>16	2.8	8
S. aureus A22231	ANT(4')-I	4	4	32	4
S. aureus A22058	ANT(4')-II	22.6	2	125	2
E. coli A20732	ANT(2")	1	1.4	4	2.5
E. coli A20665	APH(3')-I	2	8	4	4
E. cloacae A21006	APH(3')-II	4	8	8	8
E. coli A22356	APH(3')-III	2	4	4	8

[a] AAC(3), 3-N-acetyltransferase; AAC(2'), 2'-N-acetyltransferase; AAC(6'), 6'-N-acetyltransferase; ANT(4'), 4'-O-nucleotidyltransferase; ANT(2"), 2"-O-nucleotidyltransferase; APH(3'), 3'-O-phosphotransferase.

[b] Geometric mean where applicable. Assays were performed in Mueller-Hinton medium.

[c] Roman numerals refer to isozymes.

TABLE 3. *Relative susceptibilities of 4'-deoxy-6'-N-methylamikacin (BB-K 311) and various aminoglycosidic drugs to alteration by aminoglycoside-modifying enzymes*

Relative uptake of label by[a]:

Substrate	Acetyltransferase from:							Nucleotidyltransferase from:		Phosphotransferase from:				
	P. aeruginosa GN 315 [AAC(6')]	S. marcescens A22668 [AAC(6')]	E. coli W677/R-5 [AAC(6')]	Providencia stuartii 164 [AAC(2')]	P. aeruginosa 209 [AAC(3)-I]	Klebsiella pneumoniae A22479 [AAC(3)-II]	E. coli LA290/R176 [AAC(3)-III]	E. coli JR66/W677 [ANT(2")]	S. aureus Ap01 [ANT(4')]	S. aureus Palm [APH(2")]	E. coli ML1630 [APH(3')-I]	P. aeruginosa A22428 [APH(3')-II]	P. aeruginosa 21-75 [APH(3')-III]	S. aureus EK 142 [APH(3')-IV]
Paromomycin	6	<1	10	38	<1	165	<1	15	77	7	100	100	100	100
Tobramycin	100	100	100	100	7	100	100	100	100	38	<1	<1	7	<1
Gentamicin	33	83	36	51	100	89	69	42	12	100	8	4	20	2
Amikacin	63	48	251	2	<1	1	<1	3	77	6	11	2	14	24
BB-K311	9	1	11	<1	<1	3	<1	2	4	4	7	<1	7	<1
Kanamycin A	31	84	180	8	<1	172	36	41	80	33	40	72	32	43

[a] See footnote *a* of Table 2 for abbreviations.

ance to kanamycin A, but only two of these—4'-O-nucleotidyltransferase and 6'-N-acetyltransferase—protect the organism against amikacin, the 1-N-(S)-2-hydroxy-4-aminobutyryl derivative of kanamycin A. Additional alterations of the molecule were undertaken in an attempt to further reduce its vulnerability to modifying enzymes.

Modification by 4'-O-nucleotidyltransferase, an enzyme found to date only in staphylococci, was circumvented by preparing an amikacin derivative that lacks the 4'-hydroxyl group: BB-K160. Radioenzymatic assays (1) indicated that 4'-deoxyamikacin was unaffected by 4'-O-nucleotidyltransferase (Table 1). Although organisms elaborating 4'-O-nucleotidyltransferase were susceptible to BB-K160, the intrinsic activity of the compound was only about one-third that of amikacin (Table 2).

Another chemically prepared derivative, 6'-N-methylamikacin (BB-K28), was unaffected by 6'-N-acetyltransferase obtained from several sources (Table 1) and active against organisms producing this enzyme. However, its intrinsic

activity was only about one-half that of the parent compound (Table 2).

Finally, a dual modification was undertaken, yielding 4'-deoxy-6'-N-methylamikacin, BB-K311. This compound was refractory to the two enzymes that affect amikacin (Table 1). The radioenzymatic studies were extended to other modifying enzymes and to additional substrates. The results of those studies appear in Table 3. Tobramycin was affected by six groups of enzymes, gentamicin was affected by five, and amikacin was affected by two; BB-K311, on the other hand, was inert to all seven groups of enzymes. This amikacin derivative was active against the strains producing these enzymes, but its intrinsic activity was less than that of amikacin (Table 2).

BB-K28, BB-K160, and BB-K311 were obtained from H. Kawaguchi of the Bristol-Banyu Research Institute, Tokyo, Japan.

1. Benveniste, R., and J. Davies. 1971. R-factor mediated gentamicin resistance. A new enzyme which modifies aminoglycoside antibiotics. FEBS Lett. 14:293.

In Vitro Comparison of Rosaramicin and Erythromycin Against Urinary Bacterial Isolates

PAULINE K. W. YU* AND JOHN A. WASHINGTON II

Mayo Clinic and Mayo Foundation, Rochester, Minnesota 55901, U.S.A.

In 1972, Wagman et al. (4) reported the isolation of rosaramicin, a macrolide antibiotic, from the fermentation broth of *Micromonospora rosaria*. Waitz and co-workers (5) demonstrated that rosaramicin was active in vitro against gram-positive cocci and was more active than erythromycin against gram-negative bacilli. This study compares the in vitro activities of rosaramicin and erythromycin under different pH conditions against urinary isolates.

MICs of rosaramicin sulfate (batch 9825-148 I; Schering Corp., Bloomfield, N.J.) and erythromycin gluceptate (lot S1-72-8C; Eli Lilly & Co., Indianapolis, Ind.) were determined by the ICS agar dilution technique on Mueller-Hinton agar (lot BODFXR; BBL Microbiology Systems, Cockeysville, Md.) at pH values of 6.0, 7.4, and 8.0 with an inoculum of 10⁴ colony-forming units.

A total of 45 group D streptococci, 50 *Escherichia coli* strains, 51 *Klebsiella* strains, 84 *Enterobacter* strains, 29 *Serratia marcescens* strains, 81 *Proteeae*, and 26 *Pseudomonas aeruginosa* strains were tested.

At pH 6.0, rosaramicin or erythromycin had little or no activity against gram-negative bacilli except *E. coli* strains, 58% of which were inhibited by 32 μg of rosaramicin per ml. The cumulative percentages of inhibition of the gram-negative bacilli by increasing concentrations of the two antimicrobials at pH 7.4 and pH 8.0 are shown in Tables 1 and 2. Activities of both rosaramicin and erythromycin were enhanced at least two- to fourfold at the higher pH, with rosaramicin being at least two to four times more active than erythromycin. At pH 8.0, 8 μg of rosaramicin or erythromycin per ml inhibited 100% or 70% of 50 strains of *E. coli*, respectively. The MICs of rosaramicin and erythromycin were higher for *Klebsiella*, *Enterobacter*, and *S. marcescens*. At pH 8.0, 16 μg of rosaramicin per ml inhibited 98% of *Klebsiella* strains, 67% of *Enterobacter* strains, and 80% of *S. marcescens* strains; the corresponding figures for erythromycin were 43, 20, and 0%, respectively.

Elevation of pH from 7.4 to 8.0 did not im-

TABLE 1. *Activities of rosaramicin and erythromycin in Mueller-Hinton agar, pH 7.4*

Strains (no.)	Cumulative % inhibition									
	Rosaramicin concn (µg/ml)					Erythromycin concn (µg/ml)				
	4	8	16	32	64	4	8	16	32	64
E. coli (50)	8	76	100				2	36	92	100
Klebsiella (51)			18	92	100			2	24	77
Enterobacter (84)		1	17	77	95				13	43
S. marcescens (29)			3	90	100					7
Proteeae (81)				19	65					0
P. aeruginosa (26)				8	31					0

TABLE 2. *Activities of rosaramicin and erythromycin in Mueller-Hinton agar, pH 8.0*

Strains (no.)	Cumulative % inhibition									
	Rosaramicin concn (µg/ml)					Erythromycin concn (µg/ml)				
	4	8	16	32	64	4	8	16	32	64
E. coli (50)	80	100				4	70	100		
Klebsiella (51)		49	98	100			6	43	88	98
Enterobacter (84)		12	67	99	100			20	55	98
S. marcescens (29)		3	80	100					14	72
Proteeae (81)		10	73	100						5
P. aeruginosa (26)		8	65	92						39

prove the activity of erythromycin against the *Proteeae* at the concentrations tested, but MICs of rosaramicin were greatly decreased, so that 73% were inhibited by 32 µg/ml.

Even though the activities of rosaramicin and erythromycin were enhanced against *P. aeruginosa* by alkalinization of the medium, only 65% of the strains were inhibited by 32 µg of rosaramicin per ml, and all strains required ≥64 µg of erythromycin per ml for inhibition.

Both antimicrobials showed the greatest activities at pH 7.4 and pH 8.0 against group D streptococci, with rosaramicin being the more active agent. At pH 8.0, 0.5 µg of rosaramicin per ml inhibited twice as many strains (22 of 45, or 71%) as did erythromycin.

Our data indicate that rosaramicin is more active than erythromycin against common urinary isolates. Its activity, like that of other macrolides, is enhanced by alkalinization of medium. Against enteric bacteria, our results are consistent with those reported by Eickhoff and Ehret (2), although 43% of *P. aeruginosa* strains that they tested were inhibited by 31 µg of erythromycin per ml and none of our strains had MICs of <64 µg/ml. The lower range of MICs reported by Crowe and Sanders (1) could be related to differences in geographic location, variations in methodology, and slight changes in pH.

There is considerable disagreement regarding the relative susceptibility of group D streptococci to rosaramicin and erythromycin. Rosaramicin had activity similar to or greater than

that of erythromycin in studies by Wagman et al. (4) and Waitz et al. (5), using Mueller-Hinton broth or yeast-beef broth. With Mueller-Hinton agar supplemented with 5% sheep blood and the ICS method, Shadomy et al. (3) found that rosaramicin inhibited more than twice as many strains of enterococci as did erythromycin at 0.39 µg/ml. Crowe and Sanders (1) found that erythromycin was at least twice as active as rosaramicin in brain heart infusion broth. Eickhoff and Ehret showed that erythromycin was more active than rosaramicin at pH 8.0 in Mueller-Hinton broth (2). Our data indicated that at pH 7.4 and pH 8.0, 0.5 µg of rosaramicin per ml was at least twice as active as erythromycin against group D streptococci.

In conclusion, rosaramicin was 2 to 4 times more active than erythromycin at pH 7.4 and pH 8.0, inhibiting nearly all *Enterobacteriaceae* tested, except for the *Proteeae*, at concentrations of ≤32 µg/ml at pH 8.0. At this pH, 32 µg of rosaramicin per ml inhibited approximately two-thirds of strains of *P. aeruginosa*, whereas 0.5 µg/ml inhibited nearly three-quarters of strains of group D streptococci. The activities of both compounds were highly pH dependent.

1. **Crowe, C. C., and W. E. Sanders, Jr.** 1974. Rosamicin: evaluation in vitro and comparison with erythromycin and lincomycin. Antimicrob. Agents Chemother. 5:272–275.
2. **Eickhoff, T. C., and J. M. Ehret.** 1979. In vitro comparison of rosamicin and erythromycin against urinary

tract pathogens. Antimicrob. Agents Chemother. **16:** 69–73.

3. **Shadomy, S., M. Tipple, and L. Paxton.** 1976. Josamycin and rosamicin: in vitro comparisons with erythromycin and clindamycin. Antimicrob. Agents Chemother. **10:**773–775.

4. **Wagman, G. H., J. A. Waitz, J. Marguez, A. Mur-**

awski, E. M. Oden, R. T. Testa, and M. J. Weinstein.** 1972. A new micromonospora-produced macrolide antibiotic, rosamicin. J. Antibiot. **25:**641–646.

5. **Waitz, J. A., C. G. Drube, E. L. Moss, Jr., and M. J. Weinstein.** 1972. Biological studies with rosamicin, a new micromonospora-produced macrolide antibiotic. J. Antibiot. **25:**647–652.

Comparative Study of the Effects of Rosaramicin, Rifampin, and Placebo on Meningococcal Carriers

STUART M. POLLY,* CHRISTINE C. SANDERS, AND W. EUGENE SANDERS, JR.

Infectious Disease Division, Department of Medical Microbiology, School of Medicine, Creighton University, Omaha, Nebraska 68178, U.S.A.

Sulfadiazine was relied upon for postexposure chemoprophylaxis of meningococcal infection until the emergence of resistant strains. Rifampin and minocycline are currently recommended in postexposure situations, but neither drug is ideal. Consequently, a search for an effective alternative continues.

Rosaramicin is a macrolide antibiotic similar to erythromycin. Its in vitro activity against *Neisseria meningitidis* is good. In a study with 25 strains, Sanders and Sanders (1) showed rosaramicin to be as active as penicillin G and more active than rifampin, minocycline, erythromycin, or chloramphenicol. MICs were 0.25 μg/ml or less. Human tolerance studies revealed no significant adverse reactions, but gastrointestinal side effects were frequent. The present study was designed to compare the effectiveness of rosaramicin with rifampin in eradication of the meningococcal carrier state.

A total of 514 college students underwent nasopharyngeal culture, and 56 were positive for *N. meningitidis*, a carrier rate of 10.9%. Forty-five subjects were selected for the study, but one dropped out for personal reasons. Criteria for acceptance into the study included a normal physical examination and laboratory screen (SMAC-20, blood urea nitrogen, complete blood count, and urinalysis) and a history of no antibiotic use for 2 weeks. Subjects with an allergy to macrolides or rifampin, gastrointestinal intolerance to erythromycin, or pregnancy were not considered. A negative nasopharyngeal culture immediately before therapy, the intercurrent use of antibiotics, or incomplete follow-up would have excluded a subject from further evaluation, but these did not occur.

Pretreatment cultures were obtained 2 and 1 week before and on day 1 of therapy. Subsequent cultures were obtained on days 2 to 4, 7 to 11, and 14 to 18. Nasopharyngeal swabs were streaked onto modified Thayer-Martin agar and were incubated at 37°C in 10% CO_2 in air for 48 h. Colonies resembling *N. meningitidis* were selected and Gram stained, and their identity was confirmed by sugar fermentations. A "positive" culture was one in which at least one colony was isolated from a specimen. Colony counts were semiquantitated. Isolates from subjects that transiently lost the microorganism were serogrouped to differentiate persistent carriers from those that had acquired another strain. Susceptibility of the isolates to rosaramicin, rifampin, and minocycline was determined by the agar dilution technique with an inoculum of 10^4 colony-forming units per cm^2 on Mueller-Hinton agar at pH 7.4.

Tolerance to the medications was evaluated by pre- and poststudy laboratory testing. Subjective evaluation was based on daily interviews. When a subject had specific complaints, these were evaluated carefully, and an attempt was made to classify them as "doubtfully," "possibly," or "probably" drug related.

Subjects were assigned to either the placebo, rifampin, or rosaramicin group in a randomized, double-blind manner. Sixteen sequentially numbered capsules were taken over a 4-day period. The rosaramicin group received 500 mg twice daily, and the rifampin group received 600 mg/day as a single a.m. dose. The placebo capsules contained lactose.

Table 1 shows the effect of treatment in reduction of the meningococcal carrier rate. In the placebo group, two subjects (13%) lost the microorganism. During drug administration, all 15 subjects in the rifampin group stopped carrying the meningococcus. However, one subject relapsed immediately. A second subject reacquired *N. meningitidis* on day 7 and a third reacquired

TABLE 1. *Efficacy of treatment in reduction of meningococcal carrier rate*

Drug[a]	No. of subjects treated	Carrier rate (% with positive cultures)	
		Day 1	Day 18
Placebo	15	100	87
Rifampin	15	100	7
Rosaramicin	14	100	79

[a] Administered days 1 to 4.

TABLE 2. *Effect of rosaramicin dose on meningococcal recovery and side effects*

Drug dose (mg/kg/day)	Meningococcal count	Subjects studied	Reported side effects
<14	No change	5	2
	Suppression[a]	0	0
	Eradication[b]	1	0
>14	No change	1	0
	Suppression	5	4
	Eradication	2	2

[a] Suppression = <10 colonies per culture recovered during treatment (day 2 to 4).
[b] Eradication = Absence of carrier state at day 18.

the organism on day 18. In each case, this represented acquisition of a different serogroup. Thus, rifampin resulted in an 80% loss of the carrier state and a 93% change from the initial microorganism.

Of 14 subjects in the rosaramicin group, 7 (50%) lost the microorganism during drug administration. In four cases, meningococci returned and were of the same serogroup. Three subjects (21%) lost carriage completely. Careful examination of the data suggested that rosaramicin had some effect, and that this was dose related. "Suppression" of growth was defined as 10 or less colony-forming units per specimen and was seen in eight subjects during rosaramicin administration. When dose-weight ratios were determined, two distinct groups appeared (Table 2). Six subjects received less than 14 mg/kg per

day. Within this group, five showed no change in the colony count, and one lost the carrier state. Eight subjects received more than 14 mg/kg per day. One subject showed no change in colony count, five showed suppression, and two had eradication of the microorganism. Also, 75% of the reported side effects occurred in the latter group.

All meningococci were susceptible to rosaramicin, rifampin, and minocycline. The MICs of posttreatment isolates were unchanged from pretreatment values. This was true whether the microorganism was unaffected by treatment, relapsed, or was a new acquisition.

Twelve subjects complained of side effects during drug administration. Two subjects from the placebo (lactose) group complained of nausea and loose stools. Two subjects from the rifampin group reported vague uneasiness which was not considered drug related. Of 14 subjects from the rosaramicin group, 8 (57%) complained of adverse effects. These were nausea (5/8), abdominal cramps (4/8), and loose stools (4/8).

Although rosaramicin has shown excellent in vitro activity against *N. meningitidis,* it was not effective in eradicating the carrier state. However, it suppressed recovery of the microorganism during therapy, and this appeared to be dose related. Side effects were common but not severe.

After the completion of this study, a new tablet preparation was developed that reportedly produces higher serum levels than the capsules and has a half-life of 4 h. Side effects are decreased when the drug is taken with food and absorption is not affected. Based upon our findings, future studies should be designed with this new formulation, with four-times-a-day dosing, to determine whether rosaramicin can be effective in postexposure prophylaxis.

1. **Sanders, C. C., and W. E. Sanders, Jr.** 1977. In vitro activity of rosamicin against *Neisseria* and *Haemophilus,* including penicillinase-producing strains. Antimicrob. Agents Chemother. **12:**293–294.

Susceptibilities of *Ureaplasma urealyticum* and *Mycoplasma hominis* to Rosaramicin

R. B. KUNDSIN* AND S. A. POULIN

Department of Microbiology and Molecular Genetics, Harvard Medical School, and Department of Medicine, Peter Bent Brigham Hospital, Boston, Massachusetts 02115, U.S.A.*

In a laboratory that processes 5,000 cultures per year for *Mycoplasma hominis* and *Urea-* *plasma urealyticum*, resistance to four tetracyclines (demeclocycline, doxycycline, minocy-

TABLE 1. *Susceptibilities of U. urealyticum and M. hominis to four tetracyclines[a]*

Results	U. urealyticum (523 strains)	M. hominis (158 strains)
Susceptible to all	448 (86)[b]	106 (67)
Resistant to all	53 (10)	17 (11)
Partially susceptible[c]	22 (4)	35 (22)

[a] The broth-disk method was used with doxycycline (1 μg/ml), minocycline (1 μg/ml), demeclocycline (1 μg/ml), and tetracycline (6 μg/ml).

[b] Data in parentheses are percentage of strains susceptible.

[c] Resistant to at least one tetracycline.

TABLE 2. *MIC of rosaramicin for U. urealyticum and M. hominis patient isolates*

Strains	No. tested	Initial MIC (μg/ml)	Final MIC (μg/ml)
U. urealyticum	38	0.03–0.125 (0.06)[a]	0.125–0.5 (0.25)
M. hominis	4	0.06–0.125 (0.125)	0.125–0.5 (0.5)

[a] Data in parentheses are median MICs.

cline, and tetracycline) has been encountered. Source of isolates for testing was the urine sediment of patients coming to the laboratory for problems of reproductive failure or genitourinary tract infections. As shown in Table 1, 10% (53/523) of *U. urealyticum* strains were found resistant to all four tetracyclines at the levels tested. Of *M. hominis* strains, 11% (17/158) were found resistant to all four tetracyclines. Because of this resistance, an antibiotic is urgently needed which would be useful for treating patients with these strains.

A broth susceptibility test with urine sediment as the inoculum has been developed in our laboratory (1). Mycoplasmas and ureaplasmas are known to alter membrane constituents by acquisition of components from the media in which they are grown. Therefore, laboratory-cloned and -grown isolates do not reflect the characteristics of the microorganisms in their natural environment. For this reason, use of urine sediments as the inoculum furnishes the best approximation of antibiotic susceptibilities in situ. Urine titers for both microorganisms ranged from 10^1 to 10^5/ml.

Two types of tests were done: broth disk tests with two levels of rosaramicin (1.5 and 3 μg/ml) and tests for initial and final MICs with gradations of rosaramicin.

All 127 strains of *U. urealyticum* tested at the 3-μg/ml level were susceptible to rosaramicin. This included 105 tetracycline-susceptible strains and 22 tetracycline-resistant strains.

All 144 strains of *U. urealyticum* tested were susceptible to 1.5 μg of rosaramicin per ml; 119 of these were tetracycline susceptible, and 25 were tetracycline resistant.

M. hominis strains tested against rosaramicin showed a similar susceptibility. All 29 strains tested were susceptible to 3 μg/ml. The five strains resistant to all tetracyclines tested were also susceptible.

Thirty-eight strains of *M. hominis* were susceptible to 1.5 μg of rosaramicin per ml. Six strains resistant to all tetracyclines tested were susceptible to rosaramicin.

Table 2 indicates the initial and final MICs of rosaramicin for *U. urealyticum* and *M. hominis*. For *U. urealyticum*, initial MICs ranged from 0.03 to 0.125 μg/ml, a median of 0.06 μg/ml. Final MICs at 6 days ranged from 0.125 to 0.5 μg/ml, a median of 0.25 μg/ml.

These findings are noteworthy because tetracycline-susceptible *U. urealyticum* and *M. hominis* patient isolates as well as isolates resistant to all tetracyclines tested were all susceptible to rosaramicin. MICs were low, with a median final MIC of 0.25 μg/ml for *U. urealyticum* and 0.5 μg/ml for *M. hominis*.

If in vivo results can be correlated with in vitro results, a new effective antibiotic will be available for patient use to combat infections with these newly recognized agents of genitourinary tract infections.

1. **Spaepen, M. S., R. B. Kundsin, and H. W. Horne.** 1976. Tetracycline-resistant T-mycoplasmas (*Ureaplasma urealyticum*) from patients with a history of reproductive failure. Antimicrob. Agents Chemother. **9:** 1012–1018.

Activity of the New Compound Tetroxoprim Against Gram-Positive and Gram-Negative Microorganisms

KLAUS HÖXER

Department of Microbiology, Heumann Pharma, D-8500 Nürnberg, Federal Republic of Germany

A connection between chemical structure and pharmacological effect is already known for the group of antibacterial 2,4-diaminobenzylpyrimidines. The 2,4-diaminopyrimidine residue is essential for the antibacterial effect. For chemical variations, only the benzyl residue is available.

With tetroxoprim (TXP) (chemical structure in Fig. 1) it has been possible to synthesize a further compound from the group of the 2,4-diaminobenzylpyrimidines with good antibacterial activity without harmful side effects.

The MIC of TXP was established from 15 clinically important bacterial species by means of the tube dilution method in microtiter plates with Iso-sensitive broth. Altogether, 404 strains were tested. Shortly before starting the experiment, bacteria were isolated from different clinical sources. The results have been summarized in Table 1.

Proteus rettgeri and *Proteus inconstans* proved to be less susceptible to TXP. *Pseudomonas aeruginosa* proved to be resistant. The other bacterial species were susceptible to TXP.

For the bacterial strains listed in Table 1, the MIC for trimethoprim (TMP) has been measured. If the antibacterial activity of TXP is compared with TMP, then it can be established that the antibacterial activity of the two substances in vitro is qualitatively but not quantitatively the same. TXP is approximately two to eight times less active than TMP.

The effect of the inoculum size on the MIC for seven different bacterial strains, namely *Staphylococcus aureus* SG 511, *Streptococcus pyogenes* ATCC 8668, *Sarcina lutea* ATCC 15957, *Escherichia coli* ATCC 9637, *Klebsiella pneumoniae* ATCC 10031, *Proteus mirabilis* Hbg, and *Proteus vulgaris*, was examined in a further experiment.

With an inoculum which results in 10^4 and 10^5 germs per ml, the MIC differs in four cases by one dilution step. However, if an inoculum is used which results in 10^6 germs per ml, then the MIC shifts by four and more dilution steps. The same effect can also be observed with TMP.

The affinity of TXP to the plasma proteins is slight. It is between 10 and 14%. The range for TMP is approximately 31%. An experiment was made to test whether the addition of 8% human albumin to the culture medium would have an effect on the antibacterial activity. In this experiment the growth of *E. coli* ATCC 9637 was continuously controlled by photometry. The ad-

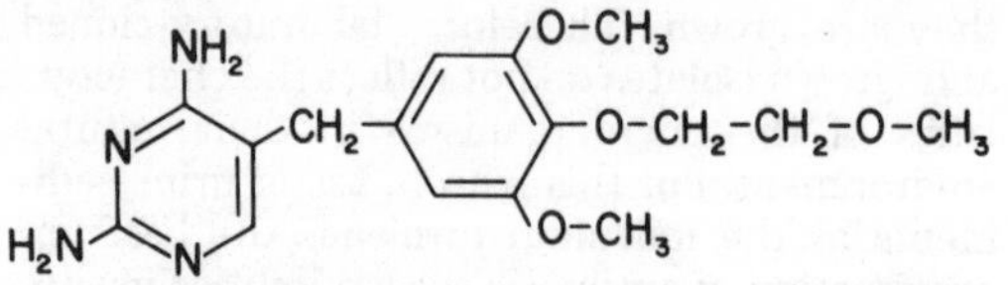

Fig. 1. *Chemical structure of 2,4-diamino-5-[3,5-dimethoxy-4-(2-methoxyethoxy)benzyl]pyrimidin (TXP).*

TABLE 1. *Cumulative percentage of strains out of some species inhibited by TXP*

Species	No.	% of strains with MIC (µg/ml) of:									
		0.5	1	2	4	8	16	32	64	128	>128
E. coli	40		2.5	7.5	50	70	87.5	90	90	92.5	100
Citrobacter	21			19	62	86	96	96	96	96	100
Klebsiella	40			2.5	15	47.5	75	80	85	90	100
Enterobacter	40		5	5	22.5	47.5	87.5	92.5	92.5	95	100
S. marcescens	21				9.5	19	48	67	77	77	100
Shigella	21				5	24	58	67	82	91	100
Salmonella	21			5	72	91	96	100			
P. mirabilis	21					9.5	19	53	77	96	100
P. vulgaris	20					5	40	65	85	95	100
P. morganii	40					10	30	70	82.5	85	100
P. rettgeri	18				5.5	11	28	45	50	67	100
P. inconstans	21					5	10	24	29	43	100
P. aeruginosa	20									10	100
S. faecalis	40	35	55	82.5	95	97.5	100				
S. aureus	20		10	90	100						

dition of 8% human albumin had no influence on the antibacterial activity of TXP, whereas for TMP a significant reduction of the activity could be confirmed.

The results show that in TXP a potent antibacterial substance similar to TMP has been found.

Comparative Evaluation of the New Compound Tetroxoprim with Co-Trimoxazole and Trimethoprim Alone for Treatment of Prostatitis

GERD RIEDASCH,* KLAUS MOHRING, AND H. FERBER

Urological Department, University of Heidelberg, Heidelberg, and Clinical Research Department, Heumann Pharmaceutical Co., Nuerenberg, Federal Republic of Germany*

The antimicrobial treatment of a chronic bacterial disease such as pyelonephritis and bronchitis still poses unanswered questions concerning proper isolation and identification of the causative organism, the definition of the drug of choice on the basis of pharmacokinetic considerations, and last but not least the proper dose regimen and adequate length of treatment.

One of the parenchymal diseases that urologists find themselves confronted with is chronic bacterial prostatitis. The pathomorphological findings in chronic prostatitis are basically similar to those of other chronic diseases. The inflammation occurs both inside the excretory ducts or acini of the prostate and closely around the excretory ducts. The identification of the causative organism demands stringent criteria for the localization of the infection within the prostate. We achieved this by ruling out patients suffering from concomitant infection of the bladder, urethra, or epididymis and by use of the antibody-coating test in semen as described by Riedasch et al. (4). Only those isolated organisms showing antibody coating with immunoglobulin G were accepted as causing chronic prostatitis. Antibody coating of at least 30% of the bacteria was considered a positive antibody-coating test.

The pathomorphological findings mentioned before and basic pharmacokinetic considerations are the primary factors for proper drug selection. In addition to being active against the isolated organism in vitro, the antimicrobial drug of choice should yield effective interstitial levels, particularly at the excretory site of the prostate. Commonly recommended drugs, according to Stamey et al. (5), yield "tissue levels" only on the interstitial side of the inflamed gland. Only lipophilic drugs, basic in character and/or having a favorable pK_a, can diffuse from the interstitial side to the excretory side of the prostatic acini and thus reach effective levels at both loci of infection.

Mohring et al. (3) showed that sulfa drugs such as sulfadiazine and sulfamethoxazole can achieve only minor concentrations in prostatic fluid, whereas the partition coefficient of trimethoprim is much more favorable, yielding levels at least as high as corresponding plasma levels. The new dihydrofolate antagonist tetroxoprim, which has similar structure and pharmacokinetic behavior, is available both as a monosubstance and in combination with sulfadiazine.

A prospective, randomized study was performed with four groups of patients to evaluate the effects of the monosubstances trimethoprim and tetroxoprim and the combination of trimethoprim with sulfamethoxazole versus tetroxoprim with sulfadiazine in the treatment of chronic bacterial prostatitis. Treatment groups established for the study were comparable as far as age, body weight, and causative organisms were concerned. The treatment was usually carried out for 21 days since this length of time was expected to be adequate for treatment of a chronic disease. After a 7-day treatment-free interval, all bacterial studies, including the antibody-coating test, were repeated for proof of cure (Table 1).

The organisms most often found were enterococci, followed by *Escherichia coli*, *Proteus*, staphylococci, and *Pseudomonas* in one case. *Mycoplasma* was found in two instances, whereas *Chlamydia* could be excluded in all treated patients.

The results and side effects of treatment are shown in Table 2. Treatment with the monosubstances tetroxoprim or trimethoprim led to an average cure rate of approximately 60%. Treatment with 300 mg of tetroxoprim in two divided daily doses or with trimethoprim at 200 mg per day over 3 weeks caused no side effects.

The combination of tetroxoprim and sulfadiazine led to the symptoms of urticaria in one case and a typical Steven-Johnson syndrome in

TABLE 1. *Causative organisms in four treatment groups of patients with prostatitis*[a]

Organism	No. of isolates				
	TXP	TMP	TXP/ SDZ	TMP/ SMZ	Total
Enterococci	4	8	7	6	25
Escherichia coli	2	4	5	1	12
Proteus spp.	2	2	—	1	5
Staphylococcus albus.	—	—	1	1	2
Pseudomonas	—	—	1	1	2
Mycoplasma	2	—	1	2	5
Chlamydia	—	—	—	—	—

[a] The disk concentrations were as follows: 10 μg of tetroxoprim (TXP) or trimethoprim (TMP) when used alone and 5 μg of TXP or TMP combined with 45 μg of sulfadiazine (SDZ) or sulfamethoxazole (SMZ) in the combinations.

TABLE 2. *Results and side effects causing discontinuation of treatment in four groups of patients with prostatitis*[a]

Effect	No. of patients			
	TXP	TMP	TXP/SDZ	TMP/SMZ
Cured	4	7	8	6
Not cured	3	2	4	3
Side effects	0	0	4[b]	1[c]

[a] Patients were treated with tetroxoprim (TXP) or trimethoprim (TMP) alone or with these drugs in combination with sulfadiazine (SDZ) or sulfamethoxazole (SMZ).

[b] Steven-Johnson syndrome in 1, exanthema in 1, and nausea in 2.

[c] Itching in one.

another case. Two other patients of this group discontinued treatment because of nausea. Co-trimoxazole treatment with 160 mg of trimethoprim plus 800 mg of sulfamethoxazole (twice daily) showed side effects in only one patient in whom itching led to discontinuation of treatment.

Pharmacokinetic data collected by Dabhoiwala et al. (2) demonstrate that the dihydrofolate antagonists trimethoprim and tetroxoprim yield effective concentrations on both sides of the prostatic acini. If a conventional treatment is carried out with penicillins, cephalosporins, or even aminoglycosides, the bacterial infection will persist on the excretory side of the prostate. The different pharmacokinetic behavior of the folic acid antagonists trimethoprim and tetroxoprim seems to be the key for the reported treatment results.

Whether or not the combination of tetroxoprim with sulfadiazine or trimethoprim with sulfamethoxazole has an additional curative effect in treatments of chronic prostatitis, as reported by Chesley and Dow (1), could not be substantiated by our study.

In summary, the treatment of bacterial prostatitis has to be based on proper identification and isolation of the causative organism. The antibody-coating test has been shown to be practical for this purpose. Trimethoprim and tetroxoprim yield adequate interstitial as well as intra-acinal concentrations to counteract bacterial infection. Whether the addition of sulfa drugs is justified from a microbiological standpoint only or causes synergistic effects clinically has to be proven, preferably under controlled conditions.

1. Chesley, A. E., and D. Dow. 1973. Use of trimethoprim-sulfamethoxazole in chronic prostatitis. Urology 2:280.
2. Dabhoiwala, N. F., A. Bye, and M. Claridge. 1976. A study of concentrations of trimethoprim-sulfamethoxazole in the human prostate gland. Br. J. Urol. 48:77.
3. Mohring, K., N. Christiansen, J. F. Pedersen, and P. O. Madsen. 1971. The concentration of various antibiotics, sulfonamides and trimethoprim in prostatic fluid in dogs. Abstract, American Urological Association Meeting.
4. Riedasch, G., E. Ritz, K. Mohring, and U. Ickinger. 1977. Antibody-coated bacteria in the ejaculate—a possible test for prostatitis. J. Urol. 118:787.
5. Stamey, Th.A., E. M. Meares, D. G. Winningham. 1970. Chronic bacterial prostatitis and the diffusion of drugs into prostatic fluid. J. Urol. 103:187.

Tetroxoprim in the Treatment and Prophylaxis of Recurrent, Nonobstructive Urinary Tract Infection

H. PICHLER,* W. GRANINGER, S. BREYER, K. H. SPITZY, E. NEUMANN, E. BALZAR, R. PÜSPÖK, H. KÖCK, AND N. NÜRNBERGER

School of Medicine, University of Vienna, Vienna, Austria

Recurrent, nonobstructive urinary tract infections (UTI) in children and females are more than 80% reinfections. In asymptomatic episodes of UTI where congenital malformations or acquired abnormalities of the urinary tract have been excluded by careful radiological and urological examinations, it is nowadays well established that treatment of frequent reinfections is not imperative. However, there are some cases in which antibacterial prophylaxis after curative treatment is necessary: (i) frequent symptomatic reinfections, (ii) recurring UTI in children and pregnant women, and (iii) frequent reinfections associated with vesicoureteral reflux or neurogenic bladder dysfunction.

Trimethoprim-sulfamethoxazole (TMP-SMX) and nitrofurantoin are the two most useful drugs for the low-dosage prophylactic treatment. TMP-SMX, even when given in a prophylactic dosage of 40 mg of TMP and 200 mg of SMX daily, greatly reduced the coliforms of the fecal flora and prevented vaginal colonization (3). But TMP-SMX induced a marked increase in sulfonamide-resistant coliform strains in the feces which was not observed when TMP was given alone (2). TMP alone has shown equal efficacy in the curative treatment (1, 2) and was superior to nitrofurantoin in the prophylactic treatment (2). Additionally, side effects occurred with TMP alone at a considerably lower rate than with TMP-SMX. Because TMP as a monosubstance is not available in Austria, we were interested in investigating the therapuetic efficacy of tetroxoprim, a derivative of TMP with less antibacterial activity, in patients with recurrent UTI.

Sixteen girls ranging in age from 3 to 13 years and five females ranging in age from 20 to 39 years with recurrent, nonobstructive UTI with at least four documented reinfections during the preceding year received tetroxoprim. UTI was defined as bacteriuria of greater than 10^5 organisms per ml of urine with or without symptoms referable to the urinary tract. In asymptomatic patients two separate urine specimens with significant bacteriuria were required before the diagnosis of UTI was established. In all patients complete urological examination including intravenous pyelogram, voiding cystourethrogram, cystoscopy, and cysto-manometry were carried out. Tetroxoprim was administered, when the causative bacteria were susceptible to it, in a curative dosage of 200 mg twice daily to adults and 3 mg/kg twice daily to children for 10 days. Otherwise, an appropriate chemotherapeutic substance according to susceptibility testing was given for 10 days. After the end of treatment all patients received tetroxoprim in a prophylactic dosage of 100 mg once daily at night to adults and 1.5 mg/kg once daily to children over a period of 3 months. The urine was examined bacteriologically at the end of therapy, monthly during the period of prophylaxis, and 2 and 6 weeks after the end of prophylaxis. Erythrocyte and leukocyte counts, platelet counts, reticulocytes, serum creatinine, blood urea nitrogen, transaminases, and alkaline phosphatase were assessed monthly during the prophylaxis. Serum folate was estimated by a radioimmunoassay method at the beginning and at the end of tetroxoprim medication.

Six of the 16 children treated with tetroxoprim had undergone previous operations in the urinary tract, 3 for meatotomy, two for bilateral ureteral reimplantation for reflux, and one for nephrectomy as well as unilateral ureteral reimplantation for reflux. At the time of tetroxoprim administration, three children had renal scars and three had bilateral reflux. One child had renal scars and reflux and another child had malformation of the kidneys. The causative bacteria were *Escherichia coli* 15 times and *Staphylococcus epidermidis* once. Tetroxoprim was given in a curative dosage to 14 children and eradicated the infection in all of them. In two children with symptomatic UTI the susceptibility testing showed resistance, but the drug was not discontinued because of good clinical and bacteriological results. There was only one breakthrough infection caused by a resistant *E. coli* strain among the 16 patients receiving tetroxoprim prophylaxis, which occurred at the end of the third month. Four of 16 patients had reinfections within a period of 6 weeks, all of them caused by tetroxoprim-susceptible *E. coli* strains. This finding is in good agreement with those of others (3). Regarding side effects, there was only one patient with nausea, which subsided during the continuation of the drug.

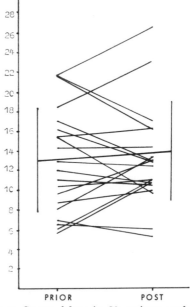

FIG. 1. *Serum folate in 20 patients undergoing tetroxoprim treatment. Numbers on the ordinate represent nanomoles of folic acid per liter.*

The findings and results of tetroxoprim administration in five females were as follows. There were two patients with renal scars and unilateral reflux as well. One patient had neurogenic bladder dysfunction caused by multiple sclerosis, but had no retention of urine at the time of examination. The causative organisms were enterococci three times and *E. coli* twice; both were successfully eradicated by tetroxoprim treatment. During prophylaxis there was one breakthrough infection at the end of the second month with a resistant hemolytic *Streptococcus*. No reinfection occurred within the follow-up of 6 weeks. Only one patient had a transitory episode of nausea, which did not require discontinuation of tetroxoprim administration.

There was no change of the erythrocyte and leukocyte counts, platelet count, and reticulocytes in any of the patients. The concentration of serum folate, which was assessed in 20 of 21 patients, showed no decrease either in children or in adults at the 3-month control (Fig. 1). The

above-mentioned parameters of kidney and liver function showed no change during the administration of tetroxoprim. There were no allergic side effects observed. Gastronintestinal side effects occurred in the two previously described patients as nausea which required no discontinuation of the drug. According to our results tetroxoprim showed a good efficacy in the curative and prophylactic treatment of UTI and had a remarkably low incidence of side effects.

1. **Brumfitt, W., and R. Pursell.** 1973. Trimethoprim-sulfamethoxazole in the treatment of bacteriuria in women. J. Infect. Dis. **128**:657–663.
2. **Kasanen, A., M. Anttila, R. Elfving, P. Kahela, H. Saarimaa, H. Sundquist, R. Tikkanen, and P. Toivanen.** 1978. Trimethoprim. Pharmacology, antimicrobial activity and clinical use in urinary tract infections. Ann. Clin. Res. **10**(Suppl. 22):1–39.
3. **Stamey, T. A., M. Condy, and G. Mihara.** 1977. Prophylactic efficacy of nitrofurantoin macrocrystals and trimethroprim-sulfamethoxazole in urinary infections. Biologic effects on the vaginal and rectal flora. N. Engl. J. Med. **296**:780–783.

Experimental Model of *Escherichia coli* Renal Infections in Rats

V. PRÁT, M. HATALA, AND H. FERBER*

Institute of Clinical and Experimental Medicine, Prague 4, Czechoslovakia, and Department of Clinical Research, Ludwig Heumann & Co. GmbH, Nürnberg, Federal Republic of Germany

In the treatment of urinary tract infections, antibacterial substances play an important part. The questions that have to be answered with respect to such substances can frequently be dealt with better in animal experiments than would be possible clinically. Animal experiments represent the most reliable basis for assessing in vivo effectiveness.

In recent years, we have established the usefulness of two model infections in rats for dealing with therapeutic problems: a pyelonephritis model and an infection model for the lower urinary tract with prolonged bacteriuria. We have employed the pyelonephritis model for a comparative investigation of the new inhibitor of dehydrofolate reductase, tetroxoprim (TXP), and the well-known trimethoprim (TMP), employed alone and also in a combination of TXP with sulfadiazine (SDZ).

TXP is a new dehydrofolate reductase inhibitor (1) which, in combination with SDZ in the form of a tablet (Sterinor/Tibirox) containing 100 mg of TXP and 250 mg of SDZ, has proved successful in the clinical sector as described by

Ferber et al., Korn et al., Pines et al., Reeves et al., and Reutter et al. (J. Antimicrob. Chemother., in press). The object of this investigation was to determine whether there is any difference in the antibacterial effect of TXP alone, TMP alone, and the combination TXP/SDZ.

The experimental induction of pyelonephritis in the rat is simple to effect. After performing medial laparotomy, three injections of 0.02 ml of a concentrated suspension of bacteria were made into each kidney, approximately 2 mm beneath the surface of the organ. The bacterial inoculum was a fresh suspension of *Escherichia coli* haemolyticus strain, serotype O4-H6 containing 1.5 × 10^9 living bacteria per ml. The experimental animals were female albino Wistar rats weighing between 175 and 195 g. The bacterial suspension was injected into both kidneys in all the animals. An autopsy of control animals performed in the first 10 days after infection revealed purulent foci on the surface of the kidneys. Histologically, these changes in the cortex extended, stripewise, into the medulla.

The animals were divided into four groups, a

control group of 18 animals which were given only a solution of 10 ml of methylcellulose per kg and three experimental groups of 40 animals each. The latter three groups were given 16 mg of TXP/kg per dose, 8 mg of TMP/kg per dose, or a combination of 16 mg of TXP plus 40 mg of SDZ/kg per dose. Each group of animals was divided into two equal parts in which therapy was instituted 24 or 48 h after injections of the bacterial suspension. The substances under study were suspended in a methylcellulose solution (10 ml/kg) and administered every 12 h via a stomach tube. For all animals, the duration of the therapy was 10 days. At 24 to 48 h after completion of the therapy phase, the animals were killed and autopsied. At autopsy, urine was collected by puncturing the filled bladder, and both kidneys were removed. The kidneys were then homogenized. The number of organisms was determined within the urine and in the kidney homogenates by means of quantitative bacteriological techniques. The results obtained with the individual experimental groups were analyzed and compared, one with the other.

Figure 1 clearly shows that in the animals treated 24 h after inoculation with bacteria no significant difference in the reduction of the number of organisms could be observed within the treated groups; in comparison with the un-treated group, however, the reduction in the number of pathogens was highly significant ($P = 0.001$). Therapy with TMP, TXP, or TXP/SDZ did not, however, eliminate the renal infection completely. As compared with the controls, however, the infection was kept within bounds (number of organisms, 10^4 to 10^5 pathogens/g of tissue).

In the control group the number of organisms found in the urine collected by puncturing the bladder was smaller than that found in the renal tissue.

After therapy with TMP and TXP, the degree of bacteriuria was significantly lower ($P = 0.05$) than in the control group. No significant difference could be demonstrated between the TMP and the TXP groups. Therapy with the combination of TXP/SDZ, however, resulted in a highly significant ($P = 0.01$) reduction in the number of pathogens. In this group, 12 of 20 animals were free from organisms.

Similar results were also obtained in the animals in whom treatment had been instituted 48 h after inoculation with bacteria (Fig. 1). The degree of infection was lower in the treated animals than in the untreated controls. It was, however, higher than in the animals in whom treatment had been initiated 24 h after inoculation. No significant differences were observed

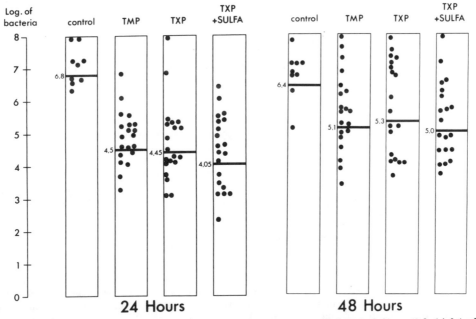

FIG. 1. *Log of bacterial count in renal tissue when therapy was started 24 h (left) or 48 h (right) after infection. The decrease of bacteria in the treatment groups in comparison with the control group was highly significant (P = 0.001) in the group that started treatment at 24 h and was significant (P = 0.01) in the group that started treatment at 48 h (Wilcoxon-Rang test). TMP, trimethoprim; TXP, tetroxoprim; SULFA, sulfadiazine.*

among the treated groups. The urinary findings were also similar to those seen in the animals first treated 24 h after induction of infection. Here, too, the lowest mean number of organisms was seen in the group treated with the combination of TXP and SDZ. In the majority of these animals, the urine was free from pathogens.

The model of inoculation pyelonephritis described above, which was the basis for this investigation, has been employed to study the action of antibacterial substances on numerous occasions. This study has demonstrated that the effects of TXP, TMP, and a combination of TXP and SDZ do not differ significantly within the groups with respect to the reduction of organisms in the renal tissue. This result was to be expected, since studies on the distribution of TXP and SDZ in the tissue revealed that, after oral administration, TXP is distributed within the renal tissue to a degree that is higher than its concentration in plasma by a factor of 11, and thus manifests a behavior similar to that of TMP (3) in contrast to SDZ (2). A striking fact is the difference in the distribution of TXP within the compartments of the kidney. The medulla manifests a 5- to 10-fold higher affinity for TXP than the renal cortex (H. Vergin, personal communication).

The urinary findings revealed a greater efficacy of the combination as compared with TXP or TMP alone. Since, in the majority of acute urinary tract infections, there is no involvement of the renal parenchyma, combination of a sulfonamide with a dehydrofolate reductase inhibitor should not be dispensed with. The situation appears somewhat different in the case of an infection with involvement of the renal parenchyma. Here, in particular in the case of prophylactic therapy of chronic pyelonephritis in children, we have been able to demonstrate that the combination is not associated with any decisive advantage as compared with single-drug treatment with TXP or TMP.

1. **Liebenow, W., and J. Prikryl.** 1976. 2,4 Diamino-5-(3′,5′-dimethoxy-4-methoxyalkoxybenzyl-pyrimidine. German patent PS 23 13 361.
2. **Rieder, J.** 1963. Physikalisch-chemische und biologische Untersuchungen an Sulfonamiden. Arzneim.-Forsch. **13**:89–95.
3. **Schwartz, B. D., and J. Rieder.** Pharmacokinetics of sulfamethoxazole + trimethoprim in man and their distribution in the rat. Chemotherapy (Basel) **15**:337–335.

Clinical Study of Tetroxoprim in Recurrent, Nonobstructive Urinary Tract Infections in Children

M. KIENITZ

Children's Department, Municipal Hospital, Offenbach/Main, Federal Republic of Germany

The discussion as to the effectiveness of prophylaxis of long-term reinfections by administering substances with an antibacterial action, in children with chronic pyelonephritis, has certainly not yet come to an end. In our experience, for those patients with frequently recurring, nonobstructive urinary tract infections, prophylactic measures, frequently extending over a period of years, represent the most reliable means of preventing reinfection or recurrences in the majority of cases. For such prophylactic measures, we have, to date, employed co-trimoxazole, nitrofurantoin, and nalidixic acid. Each of these substances has well-known side effects which not infrequently lead the parents of the patient to discontinue medication and thus, with a high degree of probability, to provoke a new attack of pyelonephritis. In the search for a suitable alternative, my attention was drawn to tetroxoprim.

On the basis of a knowledge of the properties of tetroxoprim, and dispensing with the simultaneous administration of sulfonamides, my objective was to establish the curative and prophylactic efficacy of tetroxoprim administered alone. I hoped that tetroxoprim would prove to be well tolerated—and thus lead to improved patient compliance—while manifesting equally good, or at worst only slightly poorer, efficacy with respect to the number of relapses within a given period of time.

Twenty girls aged 2 to 16 years with chronic, nonobstructive pyelonephritis, who had been known to the examiner for at least 1 year, but on average somewhat more than 3 years, were admitted to this study with the consent of their parents (group A). Both these girls and also the 20 2- to 10-year-old female patients of group B (reinfection prophylaxis with nitrofurantoin or co-trimoxazole) had been subjected to a careful nephrological examination in our department beforehand. On this occasion, all the parameters important for an assessment of pyelonephritis, including radiological examinations and isotope procedures, had been carried out. Characteristic for these girls is the lack of obstructive changes and the fact that the disease manifests at least four to five acute phases per year.

All the patients were examined and treated exclusively within the framework of the special consultation facility for children with renal disease, on an outpatient basis. Before treatment with tetroxoprim was initiated, a thorough examination which included the establishment of all the important parameters (hematology, serum alkaline, phosphatase, total bilirubin, serum transaminase, etc.) was performed. To improve reliability, we always repeated these examinations on the occasion of the subsequent, predetermined follow-up dates. All the patients were under my exclusive personal supervision, and I was personally responsible for checking their condition.

At the beginning of the study, 15 patients of group A presented with an acute attack of their chronic pyelonephritis, which was confirmed bacteriologically and, in some cases, also clinically. The distribution of the pathogens demonstrated was as follows: Escherichia coli strains susceptible to tetroxoprim and trimethoprim in 12, an E. coli strain not susceptible to either drug in 1, and B. proteus strains susceptible to both drugs in 2. These 15 girls received tetroxoprim at a dose of 3 mg/kg of body weight per day for a period of 10 days. When multiple bacteriological examinations of the urine revealed that the urine was sterile, we reduced the dose of tetroxoprim to 1.5 mg/kg per day and continued with this dose until the end of the study. The remaining five patients who, at the start of the study, had no significant concentrations of organisms in the urine, were treated primarily with a dose of 1.5 mg of tetroxoprim/kg per day. In addition to the total of seven follow-up dates, the examiner was available to the parents, to provide information and answer questions by telephone, throughout the entire study.

Throughout the course of the 3 months, it was not possible to examine the 20 girls comprising group B with identical thoroughness. These participants were patients we are continually following up in a normal rhythm in the outpatient department and who complied with all the requirements of the study. As a rule, the hematological and serological parameters were established on two occasions during the 3 months; the bacteriological examination of the urine, however, was performed at least three times within the period of this study. None of the girls in

group B was in an acute phase of the chronic pyelonephritis when the study was initiated, so that the dose of nitrofurantoin or co-trimoxazole was continued unchanged.

As was expected, the acute flare-up of the chronic pyelonephritis was eliminated with the indicated dose of tetroxoprim in all 15 children in group A. The subsequent long-term prophylactic administration of tetroxoprim was well tolerated, without exception. Three girls, to whom we had previously administered nitrofurantoin, had, according to their parents, a markedly improved appetite and put on up to 1 kg of weight within the course of the study. All the hematological and serological parameters investigated remained unchanged. With the exception of two girls who had moved to Italy, we believe we are justified in continuing the administration of tetroxoprim, retaining the follow-up examinations.

The decisive question as to the number of acute attacks during therapy can be answered by Table 1. In view of the small number of patients, however, any assessment should not be a final one. Accordingly, I should merely like to establish that, within the framework of this short-term study, tetroxoprim was inferior to neither nitrofurantoin nor co-trimoxazole. When we examined each individual case, we established that, in at least two of the girls manifesting a relapse under tetroxoprim, their mothers had simply stopped the administration of the drug on their own responsibility when the symptoms had improved. Following this, as was to be expected, clinical bacteriological signs of a relapse were established a few days later. Also, in the case of the 20 girls comprising group B, close questioning of the parents revealed faulty compliance on the part of four patients, so that here, too, the acute attacks cannot be said to have occurred despite the drug. Reinfection by enterococci in the children treated with co-trimoxa-

TABLE 1. *Treatment of chronic, nonobstructive pyelonephritis in two groups of 20 female patients with tetroxoprim, nitrofurantoin, or co-trimoxazole*

Group	Age (yr)	Treatment	No. of patients	Relapses No.	Relapses Organism
A	2–16	Tetroxoprim	20	3	Escherichia coli
				1	Enterococci
B	2–10	Nitrofuran-toin	10	2	E. coli
				1	Proteus mirabilis
				1	Staphylococcus
		Co-tri-moxazole	10	1	E. coli
				1	Klebsiella
				4	Enterococci

zole occurred in all four cases under thorough-going therapy. It might be a coincidence that in group A only one child was seen with a relapse due to enterococci.

The value of an open pilot study limited to 3 months should not be overestimated. The small number of our patients, alone, permits no absolutely binding statement. The thoroughgoing adherence to the planned seven follow-up dates involving a complete examination of the girls does, however, permit the conclusion that tetroxoprim was well tolerated by all the patients and, taking into account the laboratory results, gave rise to no side effects. An improvement in appetite and a desirable increase in weight, as also in two cases the elimination of enuresis, were noted by the parents with satisfaction.

The decisive question as to the number of acute attacks under tetroxoprim in comparison with nitrofurantoin and co-trimoxazole can be answered with appropriate caution. Taking into account the cases of noncompliance, equally good results were obtained with all three substances. With the consent of the parents we shall continue to administer tetroxoprim and, if possible, shall increase the number of patients in order, after a minimum period of 12 months, to be able to assess the long-term tolerance and efficacy of this new substance. Tetroxoprim, which has proved to be well tolerated and, according to the results of this present study, was hardly less effective than comparable preparations, would certainly seem suitable for administration to the doubtless particularly problematic group of patients with chronic, nonobstructive, but frequently recurring, pyelonephritis, that is, for patients who at intervals of 6 weeks to a maximum of 12 weeks enter the hospital with an acute attack. Investigations in larger groups of patients and over a longer period of time are, therefore, both justified and necessary, in order to correct or confirm our preliminary evaluation.

Pharmacokinetic Studies in Dogs with Antibacterial 2,4-Diaminobenzylpyrimidines, Tetroxoprim, Ethanesulfonate Derivatives of Trimethoprim, and Related Compounds

DIANE PRESLAR, MICHAEL E. GRACE, AND CARL W. SIGEL*

Department of Medicinal Biochemistry, Wellcome Research Laboratories, Research Triangle Park, North Carolina 27709, U.S.A.

The pharmacokinetics of several antibacterial benzylpyrimidines related to trimethoprim [TMP, 2,4-diamino-5-(3,4,5-trimethoxybenzyl)-pyrimidine] have been studied in dogs. The compounds were of interest for human or veterinary medicine either because of their spectrum of antibacterial activity or their physicochemical properties, which were expected to alter their disposition relative to TMP. The TMP analogs studied differed structurally from TMP at the C-4 of the 5-benzyl group: BW19U has a 4-allyloxy group; BW245U, a 4-(γ-chloropropyloxy) group; and BW32U, a 4-(2-methoxyethoxy) group (for compounds BW19U and BW245U, see B. Roth and J. Strelitz, U.S. Patent 3,819,629, 1974).

The pharmacokinetics of TMP and sulfamethoxypyridazine (SMP) after administration as their bis-ethanesulfonic acid derivatives were studied also. Although the bis-ethanesulfonate derivatives of TMP and SMP are present in a commercial preparation (Amphoprim, pH 7, Virbac Laboratories), the disposition of these compounds has not been reported. The rationale for preparation of these derivatives was based (presumably) upon the work of Ikeda et al., who reported that the water-soluble methanesulfonic acid derivatives of sulfonamides were rapidly hydrolyzed in vivo, and therefore should act as "pro-drugs" after intravenous (i.v.) administration (2).

The pharmacokinetic profile of TMP administered to dogs was described in detail previously by Kaplan et al. (3). Blood level data (i.v. administration) for two dogs was fitted to a biexponential equation; the slow disposition rate constants (β-phase) corresponded to half-lives ($t_{1/2}$) of 2.5 and 3.7 h. The mean absolute bioavailability was 103%, which was indicative that the drug was absorbed completely.

In the current work, the pharmacokinetic profile of TMP in the dog was compared directly with those for the related benzylpyrimidines. Serial blood and cumulative urine samples were obtained during the first 24 h after each dose. The concentrations of SMP, TMP, and the related benzylpyrimidines were measured by making appropriate modifications to the sensitive and specific quantitative thin-layer chromatography methods developed by this laboratory for TMP (1) and sulfonamides (4).

In the first study, three male beagle dogs received a single oral dose (5 mg/kg) of TMP in a gelatin capsule on one day and 2 weeks later received (i.v.) the same quantity in a propylene glycol solution. The average β-phase $t_{1/2}$ was 4.2 h (Fig. 1), and the absolute bioavailability was 107%, which compared well with the data of Kaplan. An average of 7.6% of the dose was recovered as TMP in the 24-h cumulative urine.

In a second study, two groups of three male beagle dogs received a single oral dose (5 mg/kg) of BW19U or BW245U on one day and the same quantity i.v. 2 weeks later. The mean serum half-lives (i.v. dose) were 1.43 h for BW19U and 0.91 h for BW245U. Peak serum concentrations occurred within 1 h and were ~0.5 µg/ml (Fig. 1); the absolute bioavailabilities were 95% for BW19U and 68% for BW245U. Both compounds were extensively metabolized; on the average, <2% of the dose was found as intact drug in the 24-h cumulative urine sample.

The third TMP analog studied was BW32U,

which was introduced recently for human medicine as an antibacterial agent (tetroxoprim, Ludwig Heumann & Co.). Three dogs received TMP (5 mg/kg) orally on day 1, BW32U (5 mg/kg) orally on day 7, and BW32U (5 mg/kg) as an i.v. dose on day 15. Peak serum concentrations of BW32U and TMP were reached within 1 h (oral dose) and were 1 to 2 µg/ml (Fig. 1). BW32U was eliminated from serum more rapidly than TMP, with an average $t_{1/2}$ of 0.98 h for BW32U and 2.01 h for TMP. The absolute bioavailability for BW32U was 61%, which was suggestive of either incomplete absorption or extensive first-pass metabolism. An average of 10.6 ± 1.23% of the BW32U dose was recovered as intact drug in the 24-h cumulative urine.

Thus, these studies in dogs indicated that TMP and the three related compounds were rapidly absorbed and extensively metabolized with <10% of the dose excreted in the urine as intact drug in 24 h. TMP had a longer plasma $t_{1/2}$ than any of the analogs and the greatest absolute bioavailability.

In studies with the bis-ethanesulfonate derivatives of TMP and SMP, two dogs received (i.v.) the equivalent of 5 mg of TMP per kg and 25 mg of SMP per kg (as Amphoprim, which by quantitative thin-layer chromatography analysis was found to have <2% of the label strengths of either SMP or TMP). Significant concentrations of SMP were found in plasma from 0.12 to 31 h (Table 1), which implied that there was a facile conversion in vivo of the SMP ethanesulfonic acid derivative to SMP; however, only trace quantities of TMP (<0.1 µg/ml) were found in plasma samples for the 30 min after administration (Table 1). Following these observations in

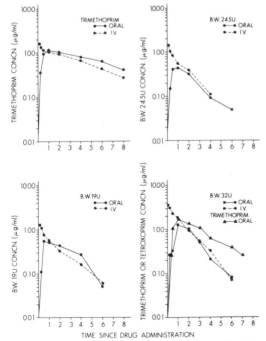

FIG. 1. Pharmacokinetic profiles for trimethoprim, BW245U, BW19U, and BW32U after administration of oral and intravenous doses (5 mg/kg) to dogs. Time since drug administration is given in hours.

TABLE 1. Plasma concentrations of trimethoprim (TMP) and sulfamethoxypyridazine (SMP) after intravenous administration of their bis-ethanesulfonate derivatives

Time (h)	SMP (µg/ml)		TMP (µg/ml)	
	Dog GXD 8	Dog EFB 8	Dog GXD 8	Dog EFB 8
0.0	<0.20	<0.20	<0.02	<0.02
0.12	62.1	82.3	0.065	0.049
0.25	58.7	56.4	0.042	0.034
0.50	45.4	48.7	0.031	0.025
1.0	47.2	44.9	<0.02	<0.02
2.0	41.9	39.1	<0.02	<0.02
3.0	40.8	42.3	<0.02	<0.02
4.0	41.4	39.1	<0.02	<0.02
6.0	32.1	30.8	ND[a]	ND
7.0	26.9	22.4	ND	ND
24.0	14.4	7.4	ND	ND
31.0	7.1	4.8	ND	ND

[a] ND, Not determined.

vivo, the stability of the bis-ethanesulfonate derivative of SMP in fresh dog plasma was studied in vitro. When the parenteral formulation was added to dog plasma and extracted within 2 min, approximately 34% of the SMP-related material was already free SMP. Additional SMP was generated by incubation (37°C) in dog plasma; ~84% of the SMP-related material was converted to SMP in 2 h. These studies indicated that the SMP bis-ethanesulfonate was rapidly converted to an active form of the drug in dog plasma, but the TMP derivative was more stable and was probably eliminated rapidly by excretion. It is unlikely that therapeutically effective TMP concentrations are reached by administration of TMP in this form to dogs, and therefore any antibacterial activity for the combined eth-

anesulfonates is apparently due to the sulfonamide component.

1. **DeAngelis, R. L., and C. W. Sigel.** 1979. Diaminopyrimidine folate antagonists, p. 251-273. In J. C. Touchstone and J. A. Sherma (ed.), Densitometry in thin layer chromatography. John Wiley & Sons, Inc., New York.
2. **Ikeda, K., Y. Kurono, and T. Tukamoto.** 1972. Methanesulfonic acid derivative of sulfonamides. I. Hydrolysis rate in vitro and pharmacokinetics in vivo. Chem. Pharm. Bull. **20**:863-870.
3. **Kaplan, S. A., R. E. Weinfeld, S. Cotler, C. W. Abruzzo, and K. Alexander.** 1970. Pharmacokinetic profile of trimethoprim in dog and man. J. Pharm. Sci. **59**:358-363.
4. **Sigel, C. W., and J. L. Woolley.** 1979. Sulfonamides, p. 677-694. In J. C. Touchstone and J. A. Sherma (ed.), Densitometry in thin layer chromatography. John Wiley & Sons, Inc., New York.

Rifaprim (Rifampin plus Trimethoprim): a Comparative Trial with Cephradine in Patients with Recurrent Urinary Infection

WILLIAM BRUMFITT,* JOHN COOPER, AND JEREMY HAMILTON-MILLER

Renal Polyclinic and Department of Medical Microbiology, Royal Free Hospital, London, England

The failure rate in patients with recurrent urinary infections remains high, despite recent advances in antibacterial agents. We have now tested a novel combination, Rifaprim (rifampin plus trimethoprim), in comparison with cephradine, in a highly selected group of "difficult" patients (J. Cooper, W. Brumfitt, and J. Hamilton-Miller, J. Antimicrob. Chemother., in press), namely, those with recurrent infections who have recently failed treatment.

Rifampin is an antibiotic of extremely wide antimicrobial activity, but its use at present is confined almost exclusively to the treatment of tuberculosis. We have proposed that, in combination with trimethoprim (as Rifaprim), rifampin could be a useful drug for treating other infections also. Our in vitro experiments (3) suggested that trimethoprim would prevent the rapid emergence of rifampin-resistant strains, which up to now has proved a major obstacle. We (1) have been able to refute the fear (4) that extra-tuberculosis use of rifampin might encourage the emergence of rifampin-resistant strains of Mycobacterium tuberculosis. We nevertheless advocate restricting the use of Rifaprim, especially for the first few years of its use in practice, for certain specific indications, such as severe and chronic urinary infections.

Eighty episodes of urinary infection were treated in 50 patients. All the outpatients had a

history of recurrent urinary infection, often for many years, and all had recently failed treatment, usually with co-trimoxazole or ampicillin. The patients thus make up a group who have a predictably high failure rate (2). Table 1 shows the comparability of the treatment groups, which were similar except for the incidence of radiological abnormalities.

Outpatients were seen at the Urinary Infection Clinic. At the first attendance a full clinical examination was made, the history was taken, and a wide range of radiological, biochemical, and hematological tests were carried out. One or two midstream specimens of urine (MSU) were taken under the supervision of an experienced nurse.

Quantitative counts of cells (made with a counting chamber) and bacteria (surface viable counting on CLED agar) were made on each MSU. Organisms isolated in significant numbers ($\geq 10^5$ bacteria/ml) were identified, their susceptibility patterns were determined, and, if *Escherichia coli*, they were serotyped.

Patients with a significant bacteriuria were allocated at random to either Rifaprim (one tablet [300 mg of rifampin and 80 mg of trimethoprim] in the morning, two tablets at night) or cephradine (1 g [two 500-mg capsules] in the morning, 1 g at night). Each course was for 7 days. The reason for choosing this dosage schedule was to have the highest concentration of the antibiotics in the urinary system overnight (2).

Patients were recalled to the Clinic 6 to 7 days after the end of treatment and again 4 weeks later. They were examined and questioned as to symptoms and side effects, and an MSU was taken.

Reinfection (presence in the MSU of a new species or serotype in significant numbers) was distinguished from relapse (reappearance of the original infecting organism in significant numbers) by careful speciation and serotyping. Relapse was recorded as a failure of antibiotic treatment. By contrast, reinfection was regarded as a cure since the original infecting organisms had been eradicated.

After 2 weeks, cure rates were 83% in the Rifaprim group and 70% in the cephradine group. This difference is not significant. After 6 weeks seven patients given Rifaprim had relapsed, as had two given cephradine. Cure rates at this stage were 65% and 63%, respectively.

E. coli (55%), *Proteus mirabilis* (15%), fecal streptococci (10%), and *Staphylococcus epidermidis/Micrococcus* spp. (7.5%) were the most common species of infecting organism isolated. The incidence of *E. coli* was considerably lower than that we have found in simple infections (85%) and in unselected patients with recurrent

urinary infections (76%; Cooper et al., in press), and the proportion of gram-positive strains was higher, 20% against 10% in other trials reported by us.

Susceptibility patterns are shown in Table 2. In only a single case did resistance to rifampin emerge during therapy: this was in a strain of *Citrobacter freundii* isolated from a patient with Down's syndrome, with scarred kidneys and calculi.

Only one patient in each group had to discontinue treatment as a result of side effects. The most common single side effect after Rifaprim was nausea, reported in five patients. For cephradine, vaginal irritation was complained of by four patients. This incidence of vaginal irritation was very much lower than that we experienced in two earlier trials using cephradine every 6 h (Brumfitt, Franklin, Hamilton-Miller, and Anderson, Scand. J. Infect Dis., in press; Cooper et al., in press).

Eight patients had more than one course of Rifaprim, at intervals varying from 6 to 26 weeks apart. No adverse effects were observed in this group.

In many of the patients in whom bacteriuria persisted in spite of treatment, the failure could be explained. Thus, of the seven 2-week failures given Rifaprim, three had a radiological abnormality and one had prostatitis. Of the 11 in this category who had been given cephradine, five had a radiological abnormality and three were over 70 years of age.

This very difficult group of patients responded well to treatment with either cephradine or Rifaprim. The cure rate at 2 weeks was higher after Rifaprim than after cephradine, although not significantly so. We are considerably encouraged by the fact that it is possible to eradicate bacteriuria in this type of patient; once this goal has been achieved, we continue the clinical man-

TABLE 1. *Comparability of patients treated with Rifaprim and cephradine*[a]

Drug	No. of patients (M/F)	Age (yr)	X-ray abnormalities (%)	Symptomatic/asymptomatic
Rifaprim	42 (6/36)	46.6 ± 20.9	32.5	30/12
Cephradine	38 (3/35)	41.4 ± 20.8	20	20/18

[a] All patients had recently failed conventional treatment (usually ampicillin or co-trimoxazole).

TABLE 2. *Susceptibility patterns of infecting bacteria*[a]

Bacterial species	Treatment group	Percent resistant to antibiotic							
		Tmp	Su	Ceph	Nitro	Amp	Tet	Rif	Mec
Escherichia coli	Rif	4	39	0	0	13	26	0	0
	Ceph	4	45	0	4	23	36	0	0
	Total	4.5	42	0	2	18	31	0	0
Others	Rif	25	55	40	30	20	55	0	40
	Ceph	19	31	19	38	38	81	19	38
	Total	22	44	31	33	28	61	8	39
All species		12	43	13.5	16	22	35	4	17

[a] The number of species susceptible to both rifampin and trimethoprim was 68 of 81 (85%). Among the *E. coli* strains, 49% were fully susceptible, 20% were mono-resistant, 18% were di-resistant, 11% were tri-resistant, and 2% were tetra-resistant. Tmp, Trimethoprim; Su, sulfadiazine; Ceph, cephradine; Nitro, nitrofurantoin; Amp, ampicillin; Tet, tetracycline; Rif, rifampin; Mec, mecillinam.

agement of the patient by starting long-term prophylaxis with a suitable agent. Of special importance is that the patient is treated with oral drugs at home, thus avoiding the need both for expensive hospitalization and for the use of parenteral therapy.

1. **Acocella, G., J. M. T. Hamilton-Miller, and W. Brumfitt.** 1977. Can rifampicin use be safely extended? Evidence for nonemergence of resistant strains of *Mycobacterium tuberculosis*. Lancet **1**:740–742.
2. **Brumfitt, W., and D. S. Reeves.** 1969. Recent developments in the treatment of urinary tract infection. J. Infect. Dis. **120**:61–81.
3. **Kerry, D. W., J. M. T. Hamilton-Miller, and W. Brumfitt.** 1975. Trimethoprim and rifampicin: *in vitro* activities separately and in combination. J. Antimicrob. Chemother. **1**:417–427.
4. **Morrison-Smith, J.** 1975. Rifampicin in clinical use. J. Antimicrob. Chemother. **1**:353–354.

Interactions Between Rifampin and Trimethoprim: an In Vitro Study

SALVADOR ALVAREZ, ALFRED DeMARIA, JR.,* JEROME O. KLEIN, AND WILLIAM R. McCABE

The Maxwell Finland Laboratory for Infectious Diseases, Boston City Hospital, Boston, Massachusetts 02118, U.S.A.

Rifampin is active against virtually all pathogenic bacteria, but the development of resistant strains has limited its use. Recent reports (1–5) indicate that the combination of rifampin and trimethoprim (TMP) has a synergistic action against some bacteria and that the combination can prevent the emergence of resistance since both drugs owe their antibacterial activity to their effect on different metabolic steps in nucleic acid biosynthesis.

MICs for 440 organisms isolated from clinical specimens at Boston City Hospital were determined for rifampin, TMP, and their combination in 7:1, 7:2, and 1:1 ratios (rifampin/TMP). Synergism and antagonism were defined as an increase or decrease of fourfold or more of the MIC of the most active drug in the combination. Rifampin and TMP alone and in the various ratios were incorporated into solid media to determine the MIC. Inoculum size was approximately 2×10^4 to 3×10^4 organisms. For none of the 203 *Enterobacteriaceae* was the rifampin MIC <6.25 µg/ml. All *Pseudomonas aeruginosa* were uniformly resistant to TMP and most of *Proteus mirabilis*, *Serratia marcescens*, and *Providencia stuartii* were resistant to the drug in concentrations similar to those achievable in serum. However, most gram-negative bacilli with the exception of *Pseudomonas* were susceptible to concentrations that can be obtained in the urine. MICs for the gram-negative bacilli with the combination of antibiotics at 7:1, 7:2, and 1:1 ratios were similar to those of the most active drug in the combination.

All gram-positive cocci except enterococci were susceptible to 1.5 µg of rifampin per ml. MICs for both *Streptococcus pneumoniae* and *Staphylococcus aureus* were well below the serum concentration achievable with this drug. The MICs for the gram-positive organisms with the combinations were very similar to those for the most active drug in the combination.

All strains of *Haemophilus influenzae*, *Neisseria gonorrhoeae*, and *N. meningitidis* tested were susceptible to rifampin, including β-lactamase-producing strains. With the combinations, *H. influenzae* and *N. gonorrhoeae* had a fourfold decrease in median MIC as compared with the median MIC of rifampin.

Synergy was present in 25% of 40 strains of *Escherichia coli*, 15% of 40 strains of *Klebsiella pneumoniae*, 30% of 27 strains of *Enterobacter* sp., and 30% of 30 strains of *N. gonorrhoeae* with the 1:1 combination when TMP was the most active drug and in 21% of 19 strains of enterococci, 33% of 21 strains of group B streptococci, 20% of 30 strains of *N. gonorrhoeae*, 39% of 17 strains of group A streptococci, and 43% of 21 strains of *S. aureus* when rifampin was the most active drug in the combination at the 1:1 ratio. With the 7:2 ratio, with TMP as the most active drug in the combination, synergism was present in 23% of 30 strains of *N. gonorrhoeae* and antagonism was present in 15% of 40 strains of *Klebsiella* sp., 30% of 27 strains of *Enterobacter* sp., 42% of 19 strains of enterococci, and 20% of 30 strains of *N. gonorrhoeae*. At the 7:1 ratio, 19% of 21 strains of group B streptococci showed synergism but 19% of 21 strains of *S. aureus* manifested antagonism when rifampin was the most active drug in the combination and 52% of 19 strains of enterococci plus 20% of 30 strains of *N. gonorrhoeae* demonstrated antagonism with this combination when TMP was the most active drug. The other strains were indifferent to the antibiotic combination.

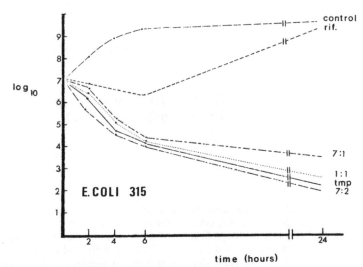

FIG. 1. *"Killing curve" demonstrating the effect of rifampin (rif.), trimethoprim (tmp), and combinations of the two in 7:1, 7:2, and 1:1 ratios (rif/tmp) on a strain of E. coli, using concentrations of the drugs of 4× the MIC. Numbers of organisms are represented as the log₁₀ concentration.*

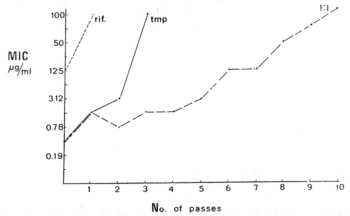

FIG. 2. *Emergence of resistance to rifampin (rif.), trimethoprim (tmp), and a 1:1 combination in E. coli 367. The organisms were exposed to subinhibitory concentrations of the drugs, and each "pass" represents transfer of organisms to new broth dilutions of the drugs.*

Killing curves for selected organisms were done using 4× the MIC with rifampin alone, TMP alone, and combinations at the same ratios as above and failed to show any significant synergistic action against *H. influenzae, S. aureus, E. coli,* and *Enterobacter* sp. strains (see Fig. 1).

To induce the development of resistance, *N: meningitidis, S. pneumoniae* (penicillin G resistant), *S. aureus,* and *E. coli* strains were exposed to subinhibitory concentrations of rifampin alone, TMP alone, and a combination in a 1:1 ratio. The combination of rifampin and TMP did not prevent the appearance of resistance in these strains but did delay its occurrence in some strains of *E. coli* (see Fig. 2).

The combination of rifampin and TMP showed both synergistic and antagonistic activity in a low percentage of strains tested and failed to prevent the development of resistance to rifampin in the organisms tested.

1. **Arioli, V. M. Berti, G. Carniti, and L. G. Silvestri.** 1977. Interactions between rifampicin and trimethoprim in vitro and in experimental infections. J. Antimicrob. Chemother. **3:**87–94.
2. **Brumfitt, W., and J. M. T. Hamilton-Miller.** 1978. The possible clinical value of rifampicin and trimethoprim in combination. Infection **6**(Suppl. 1):53–56.
3. **Gruneberg, R. N., A. M. Emerson.** 1977. The interactions between rifampicin and trimethoprim: an *in vitro* study. J. Antimicrob. Chemother. **3:**453–457.

4. **Farrell, W., M. Wilks, and F. A. Drasar.** 1977. The action of trimethoprim and rifampicin in combination against Gram-negative rods resistant to gentamicin. J. Antimicrob. Chemother. **3**:459–462.

5. **Kerry, D. W., J. M. T. Hamilton-Miller, and W. Brumfitt.** 1975. Trimethoprim and rifampicin: *in vitro* activities separately and in combination. J. Antimicrob. Chemother. **1**:417–427.

Effect of Bicyclomycin (CGP 3543/E) on Enterobacterial Flora in Humans and Experimental Animals

W. SACKMANN,* RAWEWAN JARUMILINTA, K. VOSBECK, AND F. KRADOLFER

Research Department, Pharmaceuticals Division, Ciba-Geigy Ltd., Basel, Switzerland

The antibiotic bicyclomycin, first described in 1971 (1), is a product of *Streptomyces sapporonensis* ATCC 21532 and displays a distinctive antibacterial spectrum. Its activity in vitro and in vivo is directed preferentially at clinically important members of the *Enterobacteriaceae* family. Laboratory studies on its activity in vitro against fresh enterobacterial isolates from patients with acute diarrhea of nonparasitic origin (R. Jarumilinta, F. Kradolfer, K. Vosbeck, and V. Viranuvatti, this volume) and on its chemotherapeutic effects in animals are reported.

Susceptibility of enterobacterial strains (Table 1). The MICs of bicyclomycin and of some other selected antibiotics were determined in an agar dilution test. Enterotoxin production was assessed in the rabbit jejunal loop model. Two series of strains were studied: one from Thailand (A; Jarumilinta et al., this volume) and the other from Ethiopia (B; by courtesy of T. Wadström, Uppsala, Sweden).

Of a total of 192 different strains of *Escherichia coli* originating from 119 patients, 172 (89.6%) were inhibited by bicyclomycin at a concentration of 64 µg/ml or lower. The distribution pattern of susceptible, less susceptible, and resistant strains was comparable in the two series and in enterotoxigenic as well as in nontoxigenic cultures. Susceptibility testing with ampicillin, tetracycline, chloramphenicol, and neomycin revealed a considerable percentage (28 to 47%) of strains resistant to one or more of these drugs (MIC > 64 µg/ml). No correlation pointing to cross-resistance between bicyclomycin and other antibiotics was noted.

The isolates belonging to taxonomic groups other than *E. coli* were also predominantly (83%) susceptible to bicyclomycin, with the exception of *Proteus* spp. (Table 1). Six laboratory strains of *Vibrio cholerae*, 20 of *Yersinia enterocolitica* (by courtesy of S. Toma, Toronto, Canada), 6 of *Aeromonas* spp., and 4 of *Campylobacter* spp. (by courtesy of J. P. Butzler, Brussels, Belgium) were also found to be predominantly (86%) susceptible to bicyclomycin.

Anti-enterobacterial activity in animals. In albino rats treated orally with bicyclomycin a numerical reduction of susceptible bacteria was clearly demonstrated in their feces. Whereas the numbers of nonsusceptible fecal bacteria such as gram-positive cocci, lactobacilli, and anaerobic organisms did not change, the *Enterobacteriaceae* strains, as cultured on violet red bile agar, significantly diminished to about one-thirtieth during treatment with 3 mg/kg, given four times within 40 h. Differential counts showed that lactose-fermenting enterobacterial species were greatly reduced.

TABLE 1. *Number of clinical isolates susceptible to bicyclomycin*

Organism[a]	Geographical area	
	A	B
Escherichia coli		
Total	135/145[b]	37/47
Ent+	24/26	12/15
Klebsiella pneumoniae		
Total	33/36	2/3
Ent+	3/3	0/0
Enterobacter		
Total	37/49	2/3
Ent+	0/0	1/1
Citrobacter		
Total	11/14	2/3
Ent+	1/2	0/0
Salmonella		
Total	2/3	
Ent+	0/0	
Shigella		
Total	19/19	
Ent+	2/2	
Proteus		
Total	0/24	
Ent+	0/3	

[a] Ent+, Enterotoxigenic.
[b] Number of strains susceptible (MIC ≤ 64 µg/ml)/total.

TABLE 2. *Test organisms implanted into rat jejunum*

Chemothera-peutic agent	Minimal effective dose (mg/kg)[a]				MIC (μg/ml) for strains suscepti-ble in vivo
	E. coli strain			S. ty-phimu-rium 1189B	
	1249B	1312B	3B		
Bicyclomycin	3	1	1	10	32–64
Ampicillin	>10	2	0.3	>10	1–4
Neomycin	10	2	3	10	2–8
Metronidazole	5	20	10	>30	32–128
Furazolidone	>100	10	50	100	0.25–2.0

[a] Oral doses (repeated four times) giving >90% reduction in average bacterial count, equivalent to $P < 0.05$ in Wilcoxon's rank order test with individual counts (five animals per group).

In an attempt to induce in the small intestine of rats a pathological colonization akin to human disease, the animals were artificially infected: the test organisms, marked by rifampin resistance, were implanted into the jejunum by surgical introduction and fixation of a silk thread carrying the organisms. As these bacteria multiplied on the thread, they were excreted in the feces over a period of weeks. Rats infected by this method were treated orally four times during the 40 h after implantation. Six hours after the last treatment they were sacrificed. Average counts of viable bacteria on the threads taken from treated animals were significantly lower than those from control animals (<10%). There was a clear dose-response relationship. The minimal effective doses of bicyclomycin and of some other drugs commonly used as intestinal chemotherapeutics were determined for three strains of E. coli and one strain of Salmonella typhimurium. In this respect, bicyclomycin compared well with neomycin and ampicillin, and it was superior to metronidazole and furazolidone (Table 2).

Bicyclomycin exerts its anti-enterobacterial activity, as illustrated in the rat intestine, when administered orally; when used parenterally, it displays in addition the properties of a systemic antibiotic. The protective doses (ED_{50}) for mice infected with E. coli, Klebsiella pneumoniae, Shigella flexneri, or Salmonella typhimurium ranged from 10 to 50 mg/kg subcutaneously.

The results of chemotherapeutic animal experiments with bicyclomycin, together with the susceptibility pattern found in enterobacterial isolates from patients with acute diarrhea of various nonparasitic origins, indicate that further clinical trials with this drug are warranted.

1. Miyoshi, T., N. Miyari, H. Aoki, M. Kohsaka, H. Sakai, and H. Imanaka. 1972. Bicyclomycin, a new antibiotic. I. Taxonomy, isolation and characterization. J. Antibiot. 25:569–575.

Effect of Bicyclomycin (CGP 3543/E) in Acute Diarrhea of Various Nonparasitic Origins

RAWEWAN JARUMILINTA,* F. KRADOLFER, K. VOSBECK, AND V. VIRANUVATTI

Research Department, Pharmaceuticals Division, Ciba-Geigy Ltd., Basel, Switzerland, and Department of Gastroenterology, Medical School, Siriraj Hospital, Bangkok, Thailand*

Interest in intestinal chemotherapy has been greatly stimulated by the recent discovery that enterotoxigenic enteric bacilli are a major cause of diarrhea in some areas. The new antibiotic bicyclomycin, which is unique in being specifically active against important genera of Enterobacteriaceae (1; W. Sackmann, R. Jarumlina, K. Vosbeck, and F. Kradolfer, this volume), appears particularly well suited for the treatment of diarrheal disease. It is of very low toxicity when given parenterally to animals and is only slightly absorbed from the gastrointestinal tract in humans and in animals. There is no intrinsic cross-resistance with other antibiotics. These properties prompted us to study its efficacy in patients.

Bicyclomycin has been tested clinically, at Siriraj University Hospital, Bangkok, Thailand, in 82 hospitalized patients suffering from acute diarrhea of less than 2 days' duration (54 women and 26 men aged 16 to 83 years and 2 children both aged 13). The diarrhea was nonparasitic (i.e., no trophozoites of Entamoeba histolytica or Giardia lamblia in the stools) in all cases and was nondysenteric (i.e., no blood or mucus) in 67 and dysenteric in 15. Patients who had received antibacterial drugs during the week before admission to the hospital, those with severe dehydration or other concomitant disease, and pregnant women were not included in the trial.

As a rule, all the patients received intravenous replacement therapy. Bicyclomycin was given in doses of 500 mg orally every 6 h for 36 h in nondysenteric patients and for 5 days in dysenteric patients.

Tolerability. Bicyclomycin was very well tolerated without side effects by all patients. Organ functions (liver, kidney, and hemopoietic system) were not influenced.

Duration of diarrhea, symptomatological response. In the 67 nondysenteric patients, diarrhea was initially severe (more than eight evacuations/24 h) in 61 and moderate (four to eight evacuations/24 h) in 6. It was associated with fever in 13 patients, abdominal pain in 56, and vomiting in 57. The duration of diarrhea before treatment ranged from 3 to 46 h (median, 12 h) but was <24 h in most cases (81%). After the start of treatment, diarrhea ceased within 24 h in 69% of the patients and within 36 h in 93%. The duration of diarrhea after treatment (i.e., the time between the start of treatment and the last loose stools) ranged from <1 to 57 h (median, 17 h). Statistically, there was no correlation between the duration after and that before treatment. In 29 patients with enterotoxigenic bacilli and 7 with *Shigella* or *Salmonella*, the duration of diarrhea after treatment ranged from <1 to 54 h (median, 14 h) and from 5 to 28 h (median, 20 h), respectively. Fever and vomiting ceased in all patients and abdominal pain ceased in 82% during the first day.

In the 15 patients with dysenteric diarrhea,

TABLE 1. *Enteric bacilli isolated before treatment from patients with acute nonparasitic, nondysenteric diarrhea*

Bacterial species	No. of patients[a]	Avg no. of strains/patient	
		Examined[b]	Isolated
Escherichia coli	58 (17)[c]	2.1	3.5
Klebsiella pneumoniae	31 (4)	1.9	2.8
Proteus spp.	14 (7)	1.4	2.1
Enterobacter spp.	13 (2)	1.7	2.6
Shigella spp.	6	1.2	2.5
Salmonella spp.	1	1.0	3.0
Citrobacter freundii	7 (2)	1.7	2.4
Providencia spp.	2 (0)	1.0	2.0
Aeromonas hydrophila	1 (1)	1.0	2.0

[a] Number of patients, from a total of 60, in whom the species was present.

[b] Differentiated by antibiograms and enterotoxigenicity.

[c] The numbers in parentheses show the number of patients with enterotoxigenic bacteria.

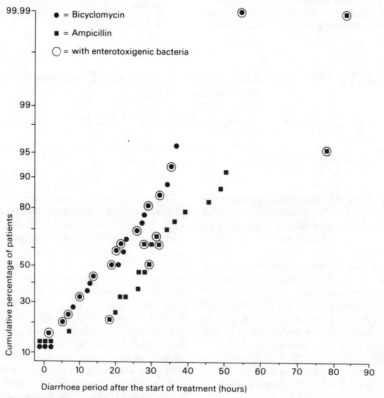

FIG. 1. *Distribution of diarrhea periods after treatment in 26 patients treated with bicyclomycin and 24 patients treated with ampicillin.*

diarrhea was initially severe in all cases; 10 had fever. After the start of treatment, diarrhea lasted 16 to 126 h (median, 66 h). Fever disappeared mostly within 1 day.

Bacteriological diagnosis and follow-up. Stool cultures for enteric bacilli were made on selective media before and after treatment. The isolated bacilli were identified, and their antibiotic susceptibility and enterotoxigenicity were tested. The latter tests were performed within 2 months after isolation by the rabbit jejunal loop method on the isolates of 60 of the 67 nondysenteric patients.

In these 60 nondysenteric patients, enterotoxigenic bacilli were found in 29 (48%), and *Shigella* or *Salmonella* was found in 7 (12%) (*Shigella flexneri* in 5, *S. boydii* in 1, *Salmonella* group E in 1). In the rest (40%), no bacteria of probable etiological significance were found. The toxigenic organisms present were *Escherichia coli* in 14 patients, non-*E. coli* in 12, and both *E. coli* and non-*E. coli* in 3 (Table 1). After treatment, stool examinations could be made in 44 cases. In all but 2 of the patients with toxigenic bacilli before treatment (23 of the 44), none was present 2 or 3 days after the start of treatment. In all those with *Shigella* or *Salmonella* initially, the organisms were eliminated after treatment. The predominant enterobacterial flora isolated before and after treatment were similar, as also were the numbers of strains susceptible to bicyclomycin (MIC ≤ 64 μg/ml) isolated before and 5 to 7 days after treatment (85% and 84%, respectively).

In the 15 dysenteric patients, *S. flexneri* was initially found in 10 cases, and both *S. flexneri* and *Salmonella* group E were found in 1. Stool culture could be made after treatment in all but 1 patient. The organisms were no longer present on the fifth day of treatment in 9 cases. In these patients neither *Shigella* nor *Salmonella* was found during follow-up (14 days). In one case *Shigella* was still present on the fifth day of treatment.

Comparative trial with bicyclomycin and ampicillin. In the early phase of the trial, 26 cases of acute nondysenteric diarrhea were treated with bicyclomycin and 24 were treated with ampicillin under the same conditions, including dosage. The treatments were allocated at random. The distributions of sex, age, fever, and pretreatment duration of diarrhea were comparable. After the start of treatment, diarrhea persisted for <1 to 54 h (median, 20 to 21 h) in the bicyclomycin group and for <1 to 82 h (median, 29 to 31 h) in the ampicillin group (Fig. 1). The difference was statistically significant ($P < 0.05$; Kruskal Wallis rank test). This was true for all patients (irrespective of bacteriological diagnosis) and also for patients with enterotoxigenic bacilli only.

In view of these satisfactory therapeutic results, further study of the effects of bicyclomycin in intestinal infection is warranted.

1. Nishida, M., M. Yasuhiro, and T. Matsubara. 1972. Bicyclomycin, a new antibiotic. III. In vitro and in vivo antimicrobial activity. J. Antibiot. **25**:582–593.

Sorbistin A₁: a New Non-Nephrotoxic Aminoglycoside

G. VIOTTE,* J. P. MORIN, J. P. BENDIRDJIAN, M. GODIN, AND J. P. FILLASTRE

Groupe de Physiopathologie Tissulaire, Université de Rouen, Service de Néphrologie, Hôpital de Bois Guillaume, 76230 Bois Guillaume, France

Sorbistin A₁ (Sor A₁) is a new aminoglycoside antibiotic produced by *Pseudomonas sorbicinii* sp. nov. The presence of a linear aglycone chain (1,4-diamino-1,4-dideoxy-D-sorbitol) renders this molecule rather unique among the aminoglycoside antibiotics. This molecule exhibits a wide antibacterial spectrum, is active against most of the aminoglycoside-resistant bacterial strains, and is not sensitive to the known aminoglycoside-inactivating enzymes (4).

All aminoglycosides are known to induce, in various animal species and in humans, renal tubular lesions which are predominant in the proximal part of the nephron. We have shown important modifications of the behavior of isolated kidney lysosomes and mitochondria (2, 3). This work reports the action of Sor A₁ on the renal structure and function as compared to the action of gentamicin.

Methods. Sor A₁ (50 to 100 and 250 mg/kg) and gentamicin (50 mg/kg) prepared in 9% NaCl were injected intraperitoneally daily for 8 days to Fischer 344 female rats weighing 170 to 190 g. Rats were killed 14 h after the last injection by a blow to the head. Blood samples were taken for blood urea nitrogen and creatinine assays. The cortex of one kidney was rapidly dissected and frozen for biochemical analyses: alanine-aminopeptidase, N-acetyl-β-D-glucosaminidase, acid α-D-galactosidase, and sphingomyelinase (sphingo) assays.

Histological examinations were performed on the contralateral kidney on 3-μm-thick slices after fixation with the Dubosc Brasyl, paraffin embedding, and staining by the periodic acid-Schiff stain, trichrome, and eosin-hematein. Ultrastructural studies were performed after fixation with glutaraldehyde and osmium tetroxide.

Lysosomal-enriched fractions were prepared by centrifuging kidney cortex homogenates on a linear sucrose concentration gradient. The lysosomal membrane integrity was estimated by the measure of the structural latency (free/total activity ratio) of N-acetyl-β-D-glucosaminidase. The mitochondrial fraction was prepared by differential centrifugation. The O_2 consumption by mitochondria was measured by oxypolarography. The in vitro studies were performed on the kidneys from female Wistar rats weighing 200 to 250 g.

Results. For all treatments with Sor A_1 (50 and 100 mg/kg) and gentamicin (50 mg/kg), blood urea nitrogen and blood creatinine were elevated. However, blood creatinine was affected more by gentamicin treatment than by both 50- and 100-mg/kg Sor A_1 treatments.

Histological studies showed that after 8 days' treatment of Fisher 344 rats with Sor A_1 at 50 and 100 mg/kg, no tubular alteration could be seen in the inner cortex. All tubes were well juxtaposed, the interstitium was normal, and no lesions could be seen in the tubular epithelium. In the outer cortex, glomeruli were unaffected, and the only alteration seen from cell to cell was a slight decrease of the size of the brush border microvilli. These lesions were discrete and much less severe than those induced by gentamicin treatment at 50 mg/kg for 8 days.

Ultrastructural studies of kidney cortices after 50- and 100-mg/kg Sor A_1 treatments revealed only the presence of a slight extracellular edema at the basal pole of the proximal tubule

cells; however, cell ultrastructure appeared similar to control samples. On the other hand, the administration of 250 mg of Sor A_1 per kg for 8 days induced focal necrosis of proximal tubule cells, an increase in the size of mitochondria, the presence of numerous cytosomes containing cytoplasmic residues, the appearance of large masses of smooth membranes and dense bodies, and a diminution of brush border and basolateral membrane microvilli. However, we did not observe the presence of myeloïd bodies induced by gentamicin treatment.

Biochemical study. In vitro studies. No modification of lysosomal structural latency was observed when adding Sor A_1 lysosomal suspension in concentrations ranging from 5 to 100 μg ml^{-1}, whereas gentamicin at a concentration of 5 μg ml^{-1} induced a decreased structural latency as measured by the free/total activity ratio of either N-acetyl-β-D-glucosaminidase cathepsin B. The respiratory control of isolated mitochondria remained unaffected by the presence of Sor A_1 in concentrations ranging from 100 to 800 μg ml^{-1}, whereas gentamicin induced an activation of state 4 and an inhibition of state 3 described by Chance and Williams (2a). Maximal effect was reached at gentamicin concentrations of 50 μg ml^{-1} and 100 μg ml^{-1} with regard to lysosomal structural latency and mitochondrial respiration, respectively.

In vivo studies. Treatment of rats by Sor A_1 50 and 100 mg/kg for 8 days did not affect the activities of alanine-aminopeptidase and N-acetyl-β-D-glucosaminidase; acid α-D-galactosidase was affected only after 100-mg Sor A_1 treatment while sphingomyelinase was decreased by both treatments (Table 1). Gentamicin treatment induced a decrease in the activity of alanine-aminopeptidase, acid α-D-galactosidase, and sphingomyelinase; however, sphingomyelinase is affected to a larger extent after gentamicin than after Sor A_1 therapies.

Sor A_1 treatments did not induce any modification of the lysosomal structural latency except

TABLE 1. *Effect of Sor A_1 and gentamicin administration on Fischer 344 rats during 8 days on four renal cortex hydrolases*[a]

Treatment	Alanine-aminopeptidase	N-acetyl-β-D-glucosaminidase	α-Galactosidase (mU/g of protein)	Sphingomyelinase (mU/g of protein)
Control ($n = 11$)	112 ± 3.6	60 ± 4.5	$1,995 \pm 77$	701 ± 78
Gentamicin				
50 mg/kg/day ($n = 4$)	93 ± 6.7	41.5 ± 1.7	$1,261 \pm 75$	396 ± 79
Sorbistin				
50 mg/kg/day ($n = 4$)	113.5 ± 3.12	65.25 ± 4.98	$2,207.5 \pm 196.9$	641.5 ± 50.8
100 mg/kg/day ($n = 4$)	109.7 ± 8.02	79.75 ± 5.36	$1,284.5 \pm 273$	451.7 ± 56.7

[a] Results expressed as units per gram of protein (mean ± standard error of the mean).

TABLE 2. *Effect of intraperitoneal Sor A$_1$ and gentamicin administration for 8 days on blood urea nitrogen, serum creatinine, lysosomal latency, and sensitivity to the thermal shock of Fischer 344 rats*

Treatment	BUN[a] (mmol/liter)	Creatinine (μmol/liter)	Lysosomal latency[b]	
			Without incubation	60-min incubation at 37°C
Control (n = 4)	6.65 ± 0.25	48.0 ± 2.00	0	23.3 ± 2.6
Gentamicin				
50 mg/kg/day (n = 4)	8.56 ± 1.08	87.5 ± 7.5	26.16 ± 3.61	53.85 ± 0.92
Sorbistin				
50 mg/kg/day (n = 4)	11.06 ± 1.6	60.0 ± 4.08	4.1 ± 2.9	26.3 ± 0.45
100 mg/kg/day (n = 4)	9.16 ± 2.05	56.6 ± 0.00	4.0 ± 1.0	26.6 ± 8.5
250 mg/kg/day (n = 1)			42.9	55.3

[a] BUN, Blood urea nitrogen.

[b] Results are expressed as the percentage of the issued lysosomal suspension from control rats without incubation.

for the 250-mg/kg treatment, whereas gentamicin at 50 mg/kg induced a decreased structural latency (Table 2).

Discussion. Sorbistin A$_1$ treatments of Fischer 344 rats at 50 and 100 mg/kg for 8 days induced less elevation of blood creatinine than gentamicin treatment at 50 mg/kg. We did not observe any histological alterations after Sor A$_1$ at 50 and 100 mg/kg, whereas tubular lesions were prominent after gentamicin at 50 mg/kg. A five times higher dosage of Sor A$_1$ than of gentamicin has to be given to observe proximal tubule cell necrosis. However, this high dose of Sor A$_1$ does not induce the accumulation of myeloïd bodies within the lysosomes of these cells, as can be seen after gentamicin therapy, which suggests that the mechanisms involved in the toxicity of both drugs are different. This is further supported by the biochemical study; except for acid α-D-galactosidase, the enzymatic activities were much less affected after Sor A$_1$ than after gentamicin treatments.

We pointed out earlier (2) in accordance with other authors (1) that a structure-activity relationship might exist for the nephrotoxicity of aminoglycosides. Sor A$_1$ is actually the aminoglycoside which has the smallest number of amino groups, three, whereas gentamicin has five. Our present in vitro and in vivo results confirm the hypothesis of a relation between the number of amino groups and the severity of ultrastructural and functional alteration of the kidney proximal tubule cells.

We want to thank D. Falize and D. Doublet for excellent technical assistance. We are greatly indebted to Bristol Myers Laboratories for financial support and for providing us Sorbistin A$_1$. This work was also supported in part by the French Institut National de la Santé et de la Recherche Médicale (grant 76-1176-5) and Fondation de la Recherche Médicale Française.

1. **Appel, G. B., and H. C. Neu.** 1977 Nephrotoxicity of antimicrobial agents. N. Engl. J. Med. **296:**723–726.
2. **Bendirdjian, J. P., B. Foucher, and J. P. Fillastre.** 1978. Influence des aminoglycosides sur le métabolisme respiratoire des mitochondries isolées de foie et de rein de rat, p. 315–332. In J. P. Fillastre (ed.), Nephrotoxicity: interactions of drugs with membrane systems mitochondria-lysosomes. Masson Publishing U.S.A., Inc., New York.
2a. **Chance, B., and G. R. Williams.** 1956. The respiratory chain and oxidative phosphorylation. Adv. Enzymol. **17:**65–134.
3. **Morin, J. P., J. Fresel, J. P. Fillastre, and R. Vaillant.** 1978. Aminoglycoside actions on rat kidney lysosomes "in vivo" and "in vitro," p. 253–263. In J. P. Fillastre (ed.), Nephrotoxicity: interactions of drugs with membrane systems mitochondria-lysosomes. Masson Publishing U.S.A., Inc., New York.
4. **Tsukiura, H., M. Hanada, K. Saito, K. Fujisawa, T. Miyaki, H. Koshiyama, and H. Kawaguchi.** 1976. Sorbistin, a new aminoglycoside antibiotic complex of bacterial origin. J. Antibiot. **29:**1137–1146.

Rosoxacin, a New Synthetic Agent for the Treatment of Systemic Gram-Negative Infections

JOHN R. O'CONNOR,* RICHARD A. DOBSON, PAUL E. CAME, AND ROLAND B. WAGNER

Department of Microbiology, Sterling-Winthrop Research Institute, Rensselaer, New York 12144

Despite continued advances in the development of new chemotherapeutic agents, systemic infections produced by certain strains of *Pseudomonas, Serratia,* and *Providencia* continue to cause serious clinical problems in the immunosuppressed, the elderly, and in burn patients. The addition of a new member to an antibiotic series may encompass additional strains within an already susceptible bacterial species. Meanwhile, however, bacteria with multiple resistance to potent and once effective antibiotics are being confronted with increasing frequency. A new drug with a structure that is unrelated to the frequently used antibiotics could be especially useful for antibiotic-resistant organisms as well as for those that have not yet developed resistance patterns.

Rosoxacin, 1-ethyl-1,4-dihydro-4-oxo-7-(4-pyridyl)-3 quinoline carboxylic acid, is a new structure with potential utility as a systemic antibacterial agent. Its spectrum includes a broad range of aminoglycoside-susceptible and -resistant gram-negative organisms including *Serratia, Providencia,* and many problem-causing strains of *Pseudomonas.*

The antibacterial spectrum of rosoxacin is well defined by the MICs of the drug against known reference strains of 18 gram-negative and 7 gram-positive organisms. The *Enterobacteriaceae* are uniformly susceptible to rosoxacin: MICs range from 0.1 µg/ml for the most susceptible *Escherichia coli* to 1.6 µg/ml for *Serratia, Providencia,* and *Klebsiella.* The single strain of *Pseudomonas* tested was susceptible to 4.0 µg of the drug per ml. The MICs for two *Salmonella* and the two *Shigella* species, at 0.8 and 0.4 µg/ml, respectively, are comparable to those for the other enteric organisms.

Neisseria gonorrhoeae, Neisseria meningitidis, and *Haemophilus influenzae* are particularly susceptible to the action of rosoxacin (MIC, 0.02 µg/ml). *Bacteroides fragilis,* with a rosoxacin MIC of 15.6 µg/ml, is the least susceptible of the gram-negatives and, in fact, of the other anaerobic organisms tested.

Among the gram-positive cocci tested, *Staphylococcus aureus,* represented by strain ATCC 6538 (FDA 209), was susceptible to 0.8 µg/ml. *Streptococcus pyogenes* and *Streptococcus pneumoniae* were resistant to rosoxacin at 25 µg/ml or more. *Streptococcus faecalis* was moderately susceptible at 4.0 µg/ml. *Clostridium perfringens* was susceptible to <0.1 µg/ml. This susceptibility was not typical for other anaerobic organisms. The MIC for *Propionibacterium acnes* was 2.0 µg/ml.

Gram-negative study. The MICs for 338 clinically isolated gram-negative organisms were determined by tube dilution or agar inclusion tests (Table 1). The seven strains of *H. influenzae* that have been tested in vitro against rosoxacin indicate that this species is most highly susceptible to its antibacterial action. Four of the seven strains tested were inhibited by 0.015 µg of the drug per ml. The agar inclusion method was reserved for 29 strains of *N. gonorrhoeae,* another species found to be highly susceptible to rosoxacin. Even the least susceptible strain of this species was inhibited by 0.06 µg/ml. Among the species of *Enterobacteriaceae* tested, a small percentage of the strains of *E. coli,* indole-positive *Proteus,* and *Serratia* were not susceptible to 7.8 µg or more of the drug per ml. Although the sample size is small, the strains of *Proteus mirabilis* were uniquely uniform in their response to rosoxacin. The MICs for these *Proteus* strains range from 0.5 to 1.95 µg/ml. MICs for indole-positive *Proteus* range from highly susceptible at 0.5 µg/ml to resistant at 31.3 µg/ml. Of 123 strains of *Pseudomonas* tested, 82.9% were susceptible to 7.8 µg/ml or less. A total of 7.5% of the *Pseudomonas* strains and 11% of the indole-positive *Proteus,* with MICs of 31.3 µg/ml or greater, were the most resistant of the entire series tested in these experiments.

In another in vitro experiment, 114 consecutive cultures of gram-negative rods were collected in the laboratory of a 450-bed hospital, identified to species, and tested by tube dilution for susceptibility to rosoxacin, gentamicin, and amikacin. *Pseudomonas* cultures were not included in this particular study. The organisms were identified as 41 strains of *E. coli,* 26 strains of *Klebsiella pneumoniae,* 1 *Klebsiella oxytoca,* 9 *Serratia marcescens,* 21 *P. mirabilis,* 6 *Proteus vulgaris,* 3 *Proteus morganii,* 2 *Citrobacter freundii,* 1 *Citrobacter diversus,* 3 *Providencia stuartii,* and 1 *Providencia alcalifaciens.* The cumulative percentage of organisms inhibited at

TABLE 1. *Clinical isolates susceptible to indicated concentration of rosoxacin*

Organism (no. of strains)	Cumulative % of strains with MICs (µg/ml) at or below:													
	≤0.008	0.015	0.03	0.06	0.125	0.25	0.5	1.0	1.95	3.9	7.8	15.6	31.3	≥62.5
H. influenzae (7)	28.6	57.1	85.7	100										
N. gonorrhoeae (29)[a]		13.8	58.6	100										
Escherichia (54)						37	85.2	94.4	94.4	94.4	96.3	100		
Klebsiella (54)					1.9	1.9	20.4	79.6	96.3	100				
Enterobacter (4)							50	100						
Proteus, indole negative (26)							11.5	92.3	100					
Proteus, indole positive (9)							66.7	66.7	77.8	77.8	88.9	88.9	100	
Providencia (4)							50	100						
Serratia (24)						8.3	20.8	58.3	66.7	66.7	91.7	100		
Citrobacter (4)						50	75	100						
Pseudomonas (123)							0.8	1.6	8.9	30.9	82.9	93.5	95.1	100

[a] Agar dilution.

TABLE 2. *Chemotherapeutic effect of rosoxacin against systemic bacterial infections in mice*

Infection	Length of medication (days)	Inoculum size	Lethal dose control	Rosoxacin ED$_{50}$ (mg/kg per day)[a]	
				Oral	Subcutaneous
H. influenzae	Single dose	1.9×10^7	LD$_{90}$	1.0	
E. coli (Vogel)	Single dose	1.0×10^7	LD$_{95}$	7.5	3.1
K. pneumoniae	1	1.2×10^7	LD$_{100}$	9.4	1.5
E. aerogenes	1[b]	6.2×10^2	LD$_{90}$	6.7	8.25
S. typhosa (Hopkins)	1	1.6×10^5	LD$_{90}$	12.5	6.5
S. flexneri (1070)	1	1.7×10^6	LD$_{100}$	4.9	3.1
S. marcescens (1)	1	4.0×10^5	LD$_{90}$	7.6	4.4
P. rettgeri (3141)	1	9.3×10^6	LD$_{100}$	16	9.7
P. mirabilis (MGH-1)	1	1.5×10^4	LD$_{100}$	4.7	4.25
P. aeruginosa (12-4-4)	1	1.2×10^6	LD$_{100}$	22.4	25.0
P. aeruginosa (MGH-2)	1	1.5×10^6	LD$_{100}$	10.6	15.3
S. aureus (Smith)	3	1.0×10^4	LD$_{100}$	25.0	35.0
S. pyogenes (C-203)	3	1.4×10^2	LD$_{85}$	>200	>200
S. pneumoniae (type II)	3	1.6×10^2	LD$_{100}$	>200	>200

[a] ED$_{50}$ calculated by Reed and Muench method (Am. J. Hyg. **27**:493–497, 1938).

[b] Three doses.

each dilution concentration were statistically analyzed, and log MICs were plotted. The MIC$_{50}$ (95% confidence limits) was determined to be 0.36 µg/ml for rosoxacin, 1.1 µg/ml for gentamicin, and 3.5 µg/ml for amikacin.

Systemic infections in mice produced by the intraperitoneal inoculation of a series of gram-negative and three gram-positive species were treated orally or subcutaneously with rosoxacin (Table 2). Differences in therapeutic effect produced by different routes of administration of the drug are minor, if in fact they exist. The ED$_{50}$'s range from 1 mg/kg for *H. influenzae,* the most susceptible species tested in vitro, to >200 mg/kg for the streptococcal infections, which were also found to be the most resistant in vitro. The two pseudomonal infections, with

oral ED$_{50}$'s of 22.4 and 10.6 mg/kg, were the most difficult of the gram-negative infections to control.

Rosoxacin concentrations in the sera of mice, rats, dogs, and monkeys after oral administration of various dose levels of the drug were determined at several time intervals. Peak levels generally occurred at 1 h after medication, and the half-life was found to be 4 to 6 h. After a single dose of 25 mg/kg, the peak serum level for mice was 7.3 µg/ml; for rats it was 15.7 µg/ml, for dogs, 7.9 µg/ml, and for monkeys, 21.2 µg/ml. Monkeys always responded with higher levels than the other species. It was impossible to obtain an accurate determination in dogs after doses of 25 or 50 mg/kg because of an emetic response. The time of this response after medication varied from 10 min to 4.5 h and was not affected by the physical state of the drug. No emetic response was seen in monkeys that received rosoxacin in doses up to 400 mg/kg.

In single-dose human tolerance studies rosoxacin was administered to five normal male volunteers per dose. After doses of 50, 100, 150, or 200 mg, average peak plasma levels of 1.36, 2.39, 3.88, and 6.20 µg/ml, respectively, were produced and each peak was reached at 1 h after oral medication. A dose of 250 mg (3.29 mg/kg, average) produced a peak level of 6.40 µg/ml at 2 h after medication. Doses of 500 (6.25 mg/kg), 1,000 (13 mg/kg), or 1,500 (20.5 mg/kg) mg produced average peak plasma levels of 10.4, 16.2, and 26.0 µg/ml at 4 h after oral medication. Emesis was not seen at any dose in these human trials and, therefore, did not interfere with the development of plasma levels.

Conclusion. Rosoxacin has been shown to be an effective antibacterial agent, both in vitro and in vivo, against most gram-negative pathogens and staphylococci. In these studies, 83% of 123 strains of *Pseudomonas* were inhibited in vitro by 7.8 µg of rosoxacin per ml. It would not be unreasonable to expect a therapeutic response in humans against these strains with multiple daily doses of 200 or 250 mg since a single 200-mg capsule has been found to provide a peak plasma level of 6.2 µg/ml.

Multiple-dose tolerance studies in humans have been completed and clinical studies are in progress. Results of these studies are now being evaluated and will be reported elsewhere.

Novel Class of Chloramphenicol Analogs with Activity Against Chloramphenicol-Resistant and Chloramphenicol-Susceptible Organisms

TATTANAHALLI L. NAGABHUSHAN,* DURAISAMY KANDASAMY, HSINGAN TSAI, WILLIAM N. TURNER, AND GEORGE H. MILLER

Schering-Plough Corporation, Bloomfield, New Jersey 07003, U.S.A.

Chloramphenicol is a drug of choice in the treatment of infections caused by *Salmonella typhi*. The world-wide emergence of bacterial resistance to this drug, especially in *Salmonella* species, prompted us to re-examine the structure-activity relationships of the amphenicols.

The clinically important resistance to chloramphenicol in bacteria is usually due to the presence of specific inactivating enzymes, chloramphenicol acetyltransferases, which catalyze an acetyl–coenzyme A-dependent acetylation of the 1 or 3 hydroxyl group, or both (3). It is presumed that acetylation of the 1,3-propanediol moiety proceeds through initial acetylation of the primary hydroxyl group. This is followed by intramolecular migration of the acetyl group to the secondary one and reacetylation of the primary hydroxyl group. If this were indeed the case, then prevention of the enzymatic O-acetylation at the 3-position by replacement of that hydroxyl group by a suitable non-acylatable function should theoretically block both modes of inactivation. However, modifications of chloramphenicol at the 3-position in the past have led to no therapeutically useful derivatives, and it is generally accepted that the 1,3-propanediol moiety is absolutely necessary for amphenicol-type activity (2). For example, replacement of the primary hydroxyl group of chloramphenicol by a hydrogen, chlorine, or bromine atom results in complete or significant loss of potency.

We speculate the existence of specific dipolar attractive interactions in chloramphenicol to rationalize the conformational properties. The three important conformers of chloramphenicol are shown in Fig. 1. In solution, like in the crystalline state, the amide carbonyl group is expected to be near *syn*-periplanar with the C-2—H bond. This situation must be maintained in all three rotameric forms. The requirement of a strongly electron-withdrawing substituent in the *para*-position of the phenyl ring for high antibacterial activity and inspection of the solid-state conformation using molecular models suggested to us that strong dipolar attractive forces may be operative between the carbonyl oxygen and the nitroaromatic ring. This indeed may be the dominant factor deciding the stability of rotamer I. In the solid state, chloramphenicol displays conformation I, and the two hydroxyl groups are in a *syn*-periplanar orientation to allow hydrogen bonding between them. This may merely be a consequence of crystal forces. Indeed, studies in solution have shown that the preferred conformer of chloramphenicol is I and that no intramolecular hydrogen bonding is detectable (1). Furthermore, theoretical calculations suggest net polar stabilizing effects in con-

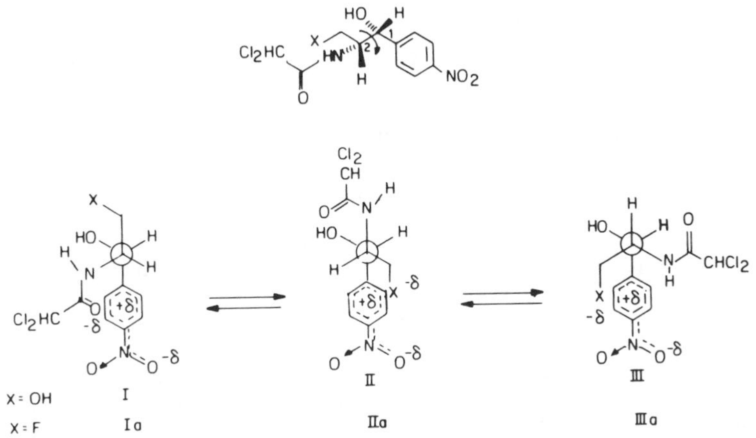

FIG. 1. *Conformers of chloramphenicol and 3-fluoro-3-deoxychloramphenicol (Sch 24893).*

formation I (1). Dipolar attraction between the carbonyl oxygen and the nitroaromatic system cannot occur in rotamer III unless the carbonyl group is forced out of its preferred orientation. Attraction between the 3-oxygen atom and the nitrophenyl ring is, however, conceivable, but a relatively low barrier to rotation about the C-2—C-3 bond and strong solvation effects could shift the equilibrium towards I. The stereochemistry in rotamer II is unfavorable for establishing attractive forces between the carbonyl group and the nitroaromatic ring. The situation with the 3-oxygen atom in this conformation is similar to the one in rotamer III. In the absence of extraneous steric effects, it is not surprising, therefore, that conformer I should be preferred to II and III in solution.

In the absence of an absolute knowledge of the biologically active form, it was necessary that any 3-substituted derivative of chloramphenicol retain the stabilizing dipolar attractions discussed above to attain an equilibrium population of conformers similar to chloramphenicol. The size and nature of the 3-substituent, low barrier to rotation about the C-2—C-3 bond, and the length of the C-3-substituent bond were, therefore, highly critical. Since the van der Waals radii of the fluorine and oxygen atoms are the same (0.14 nm) and the average C—O and C—F bond lengths are close (0.141, 0.138 nm), we replaced the 3-hydroxyl group of chloramphenicol with a fluorine atom, although it had been described in the literature that the 3-chloro- and the 3-bromo-3-deoxy-chloramphenicols were inactive. Optical rotatory and nuclear magnetic resonance measurements of 3-fluoro-3-deoxy-chloramphenicol (Sch 24893) and chlor-

amphenicol in protic and dipolar aprotic solvents clearly indicated close similarities in conformational properties. Single crystal X-ray structure analysis (Nagabhushan and McPhail, manuscript in preparation) showed that Sch 24893 crystallized in two conformations (Ia and IIa) in the asymmetric crystal unit. The preferred conformation of the amide carbonyl was maintained in both conformations. In rotamer I, the carbonyl and the nitrophenyl rings were the same as in chloramphenicol. The proximity of the fluorine atom and the aromatic ring in conformer IIa suggested strong dipolar attraction. To examine if electrostatic repulsive effects would have opposite effects, the solid-state conformation of the desnitro analog of Sch 24893 was studied. The compound crystallized in the rotameric form similar to IIa, and indeed the fluorine atom was deflected away from the aromatic ring.

Sch 24893 is highly active against both chloramphenicol-susceptible and chloramphenicol acetyltransferase-producing resistant organisms. Similar analogs of thiamphenicol (Sch 25298) and fluorthiamphenicol (Sch 25393) are also highly active against these strains. It is interesting to note that the latter two compounds are more potent than thiamphenicol.

1. **Bustard, T. M., R. S. Egan, and T. J. Perun.** 1967. Conformational studies on chloramphenicol and related molecules. Tetrahedron Lett. **29:**1961–1967.
2. **Hahn, F. E.** 1967. Chloramphenicol, p. 321. *In* D. Gottlieb and P. D. Shaw (ed.), Antibiotics, vol. I. Springer-Verlag, New York.
3. **Shaw, W. V.** 1967. The enzyme acetylation of chloramphenicol by extracts of R factor resistant Escherichia coli. J. Biol. Chem. **242:**687–693.

Novel Fluorine-Containing Analogs of Chloramphenicol and Thiamphenicol: Antibacterial and Biological Properties

THOMAS W. SCHAFER,* EUGENE L. MOSS, JR.,
TATTANHALLI L. NAGABHUSHAN, AND GEORGE H. MILLER

Schering-Plough Corporation, Bloomfield, New Jersey 07003, U.S.A.

The chemical structures of a novel chloramphenicol (Cm) analog (Sch 24893) and two novel thiamphenicol (Tm) derivatives (Sch 25298 and Sch 25393) have been described elsewhere (T. L. Nagabhushan, D. Kandasamy, H. Tsai, W. N. Turner, and G. H. Miller, this volume). This paper gives the results of in vitro and in vivo activity determinations as well as some preliminary serum levels and acute toxicities.

The MICs of these compounds against Cm-susceptible and Cm-resistant isolates are shown in Table 1. In general, strains of *Streptococcus*, *Staphylococcus*, and *Shigella* were the most susceptible to the new analogs and to Cm. MICs for most gram-negative organisms were only slightly higher, whereas for *Serratia* and *Pseudomonas* isolates MICs were much higher. Against gram-negative Cm-susceptible strains, the most potent compound, Sch 25298, was equipotent to Cm and 32 to 128 times more potent than Tm. Against these isolates, Sch 25393 and Sch 24893 were twofold less potent than Sch 25298. MICs obtained with a small number of Cm-susceptible staphylococci suggested that Sch 24893 is two- to eightfold more potent than the other compounds tested.

All isolates resistant to Cm were also resistant to Tm, but most were susceptible to the fluorine analogs. MICs obtained with 103 strains (*Enterobacter*, *Escherichia coli*, *Klebsiella*, *Providencia*, *Proteus*, *Serratia*, *Salmonella*, and *Staphylococcus*) exhibited this pattern. Cm and Tm MICs ranged from 64 to 1,024 μg/ml, with mean MICs of 256 and 512 μg/ml, respectively. Those for the new analogs ranged from 1 to 64 μg/ml, with median values of 8 and 16 μg/ml (Table 1).

Several of the Cm-resistant isolates used in the in vitro assay (Table 1) are known to produce Cm-acetyltransferase which is the most commonly encountered Cm resistance mechanism. This enzyme is responsible for the acetylation of the primary hydroxyl group of the Cm propanediol moiety. Such enzymatic acetylation of the Schering antibiotics is prevented because a fluorine atom has been substituted for this hydroxyl in each analog.

Strains of *Pseudomonas* and a few strains of *Acinetobacter*, *Citrobacter*, and *Serratia* had high MICs to one or more of the new analogs as well as to Cm and Tm. These strains are probably resistant to Cm by some means other than Cm-acetyltransferase, presumably via a permeability resistance mechanism.

These data indicate that Sch 25298 was the most potent compound against Cm-susceptible and -resistant isolates, followed by Sch 25393 and Sch 24893, respectively.

In contrast, mouse protection tests suggested that Sch 25393 was the most potent antibiotic in vivo. In these studies, mice were treated with a single subcutaneous or oral dose of drug 1 h before intraperitoneal infection, and observed for 5 to 7 days for survival. The dose of antibiotic which protected 50% of the mice (PD$_{50}$) was determined by probit analysis. All antibiotics were evaluated concurrently against each strain. These included a Cm-susceptible *Enterobacter* and *Shigella* and 10 Cm-resistant isolates, including one strain each of *Enterobacter*, *Providencia*, and *Serratia*, two *Klebsiella*, two *Salmonella*, and three *Staphylococcus*. In general, the PD$_{50}$'s for Cm against resistant strains were approximately 200 mg/kg, whereas the three analogs demonstrated much lower PD$_{50}$'s (5 to 50 mg/kg). Similar results were obtained by either subcutaneous or oral administration of drug, suggesting good adsorption in mice of the three analogs.

Acute toxicity studies in mice revealed that Tm was least toxic by all routes tested. For example, the LD$_{50}$'s (milligrams per kilogram) for intravenous administration were: Cm, 90; Tm, 370; Sch 24893, 75; Sch 25298, 100; and Sch 25393, 135. By other routes one of the Tm analogs, Sch 25298, had toxicity similar to that of Tm, whereas the other Tm analog, Sch 25393, was more toxic than either Cm or its analog, Sch 24893.

These results could not be attributed solely to differences in serum binding, since Cm and the three analogs were moderately bound (32 to 70% as determined by equilibrium dialysis), whereas the binding affinity for Tm was 16%. These data, taken together, imply that the analogs might have a different pharmacokinetic profile than the parent compounds.

This possibility was further substantiated by pilot serum level studies in mice, rats, and dogs. Peak serum levels of the analogs, after oral administration, were very similar to those seen

TABLE 1. *Median in vitro susceptibilities*

Strain/no. tested	Susceptibility[a]	Median MIC (µg/ml)				
		Cm	Tm	Sch 24893	Sch 25298	Sch 25393
Enterobacter						
4	S	4	64	8	4	4
14	R	512	1,024	16	8	8
Citrobacter						
3	S	4	32	8	4	8
3	R	512	1,024	128	128	128
E. coli						
9	S	4	64	8	4	8
20	R	256	1,024	8	8	8
Klebsiella						
9	S	4	64	16	8	8
20	R	512	1,024	16	8	4
Providencia						
4	S	16	128	8	16	8
12	R	128	1,024	16	16	8
Pseudomonas						
13	R	128	128	256	>128	256
Serratia						
6	S	16	512	16	16	64
18	R	512	1,024	32	32	64
Salmonella						
15	S	4	32	16	4	8
7	R	256	1,024	8	8	8
Shigella						
9	S	1	2	4	1	2
Proteus						
23	R	256	512	16	8	8
Acinetobacter						
4	R	64	512	4	64	128
Staphylococcus aureus						
9	S	4	8	1	2	8
7	R	64	512	1	2	8
Streptococcus pneumoniae						
3	R	8	64	1	2	4

[a] S, Susceptible; R, resistant.
[b] Agar dilution, 24 h. Mueller-Hinton agar.

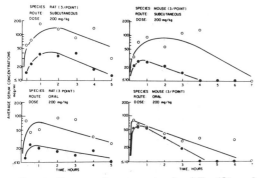

FIG. 1. *Comparative serum levels of Tm (●) and Sch 25393 (○).*

after parenteral dosing. However, peak serum levels were different for each of the five antibiotics and were species dependent. For example, Fig. 1 demonstrates that the Tm analog Sch 25393 produced peak serum levels in rats and mice three to four times higher than did Tm and that, in mice, the serum levels of Sch 25393 were significantly prolonged, as compared with Tm. Moreover, peak serum levels of Sch 25393 were as much as 100 times higher than that observed for Cm in rats and mice. These data seem consistent with the structure of Sch 25393, since three known metabolic sites of Cm have been altered (i.e., the primary hydroxyl group, the nitro group, and the dichloracetamide group). Serum levels with Sch 24893 and Sch 25298 were either similar to or lower than those seen with Sch 25393, depending on the species and presumably on the importance of metabolism in that species. The apparent contradiction that Sch 25298 was the most potent of the analogs in vitro but that Sch 25393 offered the best protection in vivo may be partially explained by the high serum levels Sch 25393 attained in mice.

These novel synthetic analogs possess microbiological advantages over their parent compounds which may make them clinically useful. However, rare but frequently fatal aplastic anemia is associated with Cm and possibly Tm. Because these derivatives possess several distinct structural differences, their propensity for causing aplastic anemia cannot be assumed. Cm and Tm have also been associated with reversible bone marrow depression. Since metabolism of the new analogs appears different from Cm, they could also differ with regard to this less serious type of toxicity. Evaluation of these derivatives for these serious side effects awaits development of appropriate animal models.

Fluorinated Chloramphenicol Analogs Active Against Bacteria Resistant to Chloramphenicol

HAROLD C. NEU,* KWUNG P. FU, AND KET KUNG

Departments of Medicine and Pharmacology, College of Physicians and Surgeons, Columbia University, New York, New York 10032, U.S.A.

In recent years the appearance of increasing numbers of bacteria resistant to chloramphenicol had decreased the utility of this agent. Chemical preparation of structural variants of chloramphenicol in which the hydroxyl group at position 3 is replaced with a fluorine atom has provided agents which might show activity against bacteria which were resistant to chloramphenicol on the basis of a chloramphenicol transacetylase enzyme.

This study is an evaluation of the fluorine analogs of chloramphenicol and thiamphenicol. The activities of SCH 24893, SCH 25298, and SCH 25393 were compared with the in vitro activities of chloramphenicol and thiamphenicol against 399 bacterial isolates. MICs were determined by agar dilution with Mueller-Hinton agar and an inoculum on 10^5 colony-forming units. Anaerobic isolates were incubated in GasPak (BBL Microbiology Systems) jars for 48 h. *Haemophilus* and *Neisseria* were tested by tube dilution, using Levinthal broth. Synergy studies were performed using antibiotic combinations similar to those that could be achieved in humans after intravenous administration.

The antibacterial activities of SCH 24893, SCH 25298, and SCH 25393 as compared with those of chloramphenicol and thiamphenicol are shown in Table 1. Overall, at a concentration of 12.5 µg/ml, chloramphenicol inhibited 70% of the isolates; thiamphenicol, 24%; SCH 24893, 74%; SCH 25298, 91%; and SCH 25393, 89%. Against *Escherichia coli*, SCH 24893, SCH 25298, and SCH 25393 had similar activities, inhibiting 94% of the isolates tested, including thiamphenicol- and chloramphenicol-resistant *E. coli* isolates. SCH 25298 and SCH 25393 inhibited all the *Shigella* isolates tested at a concentration of 6.3 µg/ml. Five *Shigella* isolates with chloramphenicol MICs >200 µg/ml were inhibited. Chloramphenicol was the most active agent at a low concentration (≤3.1 µg/ml) against *Klebsiella*. However, at a concentration of 12.5 µg/ml, the three analogs were equal in activity, inhibiting more than 75% of the isolates and some of the chloramphenicol-resistant isolates. Chloramphenicol, SCH 24893, SCH 25298, and SCH 25393 were similar in activity against *Enterobacter*, *Citrobacter*, and *Proteus mirabilis* and more active than thiamphenicol. However, SCH 25298 and SCH 25393 were the most active against indole-positive *Proteus*. They inhibited more than 90% of isolates tested and were active against both chloramphenicol-susceptible and -resistant isolates. All of the *Serratia* and most of the *Pseudomonas* isolates tested were resistant to all five antibiotics. SCH 25393 was the most active agent tested against *Salmonella*. At a concentration of 6.3 µg/ml, SCH 25393 inhibited all of the isolates tested, whereas chloramphenicol inhibited 69%, SCH 25298 inhibited 94%, and thiamphenicol and SCH 24893 did not inhibit any. Most *Providencia* isolates were resistant to chloramphenicol, thiamphenicol, and SCH 24893. However, 82 and 68% of *Providencia* isolates were inhibited by SCH 25393 and SCH 25298, respectively. At a concentration of 12.5 µg/ml, SCH 24893 inhibited 92% of *Acinetobacter* tested. Forty percent were inhibited by SCH 25298 and SCH 25393; only 15% were inhibited by chloramphenicol, and none were inhibited by thiamphenicol. SCH 24893 inhibited all of the *Staphylococcus aureus* isolates at a concentration of 3.1 µg/ml. SCH 24893 was threefold more active than chloramphenicol and SCH 25393. Among 51

TABLE 1. *Comparative in vitro activities of chloramphenicol, thiamphenicol, and fluorinated analogs*

Organism (no. tested)	Chloramphenicol		Thiamphenicol		SCH 24893		SCH 25298		SCH 25393	
	3.1 µg/ml	12.5 µg/ml	3.1 µg/ml	12.5 µg/ml	3.1 µg/ml	12.5 µg/ml	3.1 µg/ml	12.5 µg/ml	3.1 µg/ml	12.5 µg/ml
E. coli (51)	8	74	2	2	0	55	0	75	3	66
Shigella (32)	47	88	75	78	19	100	88	100	31	100
Klebsiella (35)	49	61	0	6	3	71	6	77	23	83
Enterobacter (10)	20	80	0	0	10	70	0	70	10	80
Serratia (16)	0	0	0	0	0	0	0	0	0	0
Salmonella (32)	6	78	0	0	0	41	38	100	10	100
Citrobacter (16)	6	75	0	6	6	44	0	81	0	75
P. mirabilis (13)	0	38	0	0	0	46	8	100	0	100
Proteus, indole positive (32)	0	59	0	22	0	66	56	96	52	92
Providencia (28)	0	4	0	28	0	0	7	82	7	68
P. aeruginosa (10)	0	20	0	0	0	30	0	0	0	10
Acinetobacter (13)	8	23	0	0	23	92	8	31	15	31
S. aureus (15)	33	80	7	50	100	100	80	100	60	100
Enterococcus (15)	0	80	0	0	20	80	0	100	100	100
H. influenzae (15)	100	100	0	0	100	100	91	100	100	100
Neisseria (15)	38	92	0	0	100	100	54	92	100	100
Bacteroides (51)	3	87	0	71	100	100	3	100	93	100

TABLE 2. *Activities of fluorinated chloramphenicol and thiamphenicol against chloramphenicol-resistant bacteria[a]*

Organism	MIC (µg/ml)		
	SCH 24893	SCH 25298	SCH 24393
S. aureus	3.1	3.1	6.3
E. coli	6.3	3.1	3.1
K. pneumoniae	6.3	3.1	6.3
E. cloacae	12.5	12.5	12.5
C. freundii	25	12.5	12.5
S. marcescens	>200	>200	>200
S. typhimurium	6.3	3.1	3.1
S. sonnei	6.3	3.1	6.3
P. rettgeri	12.5	12.5	12.5
P. stuartii	6.3	6.3	3.1
A. anitratus	6.3	100	100
P. aeruginosa	200	100	200

[a] MICs of chloramphenicol and thiamphenicol, >200 µg/ml.

Bacteroides tested, SCH 24893 was the most active agent, inhibiting all the isolates tested at a concentration of 3.1 µg/ml. At the same concentration SCH 25298 inhibited 94% of the isolates, but only 3% were inhibited by chloramphenicol, thiamphenicol, and SCH 25393. SCH 24893 and SCH 25298 were equal in activity against *Haemophilus*, inhibiting all the isolates tested at a concentration of 0.8 µg/ml, twofold more active than chloramphenicol and eightfold more active than SCH 25393. All 16 *Neisseria* isolates tested were inhibited by SCH 24893 and

SCH 25298 at a concentration of 3.1 µg/ml. At the same concentration SCH 25393 inhibited only 22% and chloramphenicol inhibited 85%.

The activities of the analogs against isolates resistant to chloramphenicol and thiamphenicol are given in Table 2. MICs for all isolates were 12.5 µg/ml or less, with the exception of those for *P. aeruginosa* and *S. marcescens*.

Combination of the chloramphenicol analogs with gentamicin did not result in any increase in the MIC of either agent when treated against 11 isolates which included *Salmonella*, *E. coli*, *Klebsiella*, *Enterobacter*, *Shigella*, and *S. aureus*. In fact, there was a reduction in the MICs of the chloramphenicol analog against all but one organism so tested. This was seen with organisms susceptible or resistant to either the gentamicin or the chloramphenicol analogs.

The excellent activities of these three new agents against many chloramphenicol-resistant isolates suggest that these new agents are resistant to inactivation by chloramphenicol acetyltransferase. Like chloramphenicol, all three new agents were inactive against *Pseudomonas*, in which resistance is due to a failure of entry of the compound.

These agents may prove useful in treating infections due to chloramphenicol-resistant bacteria in selected settings. They may prove to be useful particularly in veterinary medicine where chloramphenicol-resistant enteric organisms are a particular problem.

Pharmacokinetic Evaluation of Ceforanide in Laboratory Animals and Humans

ROBERT D. SMYTH,* FRANCIS H. LEE, MORRIS PFEFFER, DONALD R. VAN HARKEN, AND
GIRARD H. HOTTENDORF

Bristol Laboratories, Syracuse, New York 13201, U.S.A.

Ceforanide [7-(2 aminomethylphenylacetamido)-3-(1-carboxymethyl-tetrazol-5-ylthiomethyl)-3-cephem-4 carboxylic acid, lysine salt] is a new parenteral cephalosporin with broadspectrum activity (1). Clinical pharmacokinetic and efficacy studies (2) have indicated that the usual adult dose is 0.5 to 1.0 g administered twice daily. The proposed dosage interval is based on the intrinsic antimicrobial activity and extended half-life of ceforanide as compared to other cephalosporins. The present studies are a comparison of the pharmacokinetics of ceforanide and cefazolin in laboratory animals and humans.

Single-dose plasma and renal pharmacokinetics (Table 1) indicated that the elimination of ceforanide was slower than that of cefazolin in laboratory animals and humans. The half-lives ($t_{1/2}$) of ceforanide and cefazolin were 1.1 and 0.5 h in rats, 5 and 0.3 h in rabbits, 1 and 0.8 h in dogs, and 3 and 2.0 h in humans, respectively. Higher ceforanide peak plasma concentrations (C_{max}) and areas under the plasma concentration time curve (AUC) were attributed to the slower plasma (Cl_p) and renal (Cl_r) clearances of ceforanide.

Ceforanide and cefazolin were not metabolized prior to elimination in urine. No antibiotically active metabolites were found on bioautographic analysis of urine. Rats, dogs, and humans excreted 80 to 90% of the cephalosporin dose as intact drug in urine within 24 h. Rabbits excreted 50% of the ceforanide dose and 90% of the cefazolin dose in urine in the same period. The lower value for ceforanide was due to the extended $t_{1/2}$ in rabbits. Tubular secretion accounted for 50% of ceforanide renal excretion in dogs, rabbits, and humans, and for 87% in rats. Cefazolin was excreted primarily by tubular secretion (82 to 97%) in all species except dogs (64%).

In vitro plasma protein binding of the two cephalosporins, as determined by centrifugal ultrafiltration, was 95% in rat and rabbit plasma over a range of 25 to 100 µg/ml. Cefazolin was more highly bound to dog (51% versus 31%) and human (91% versus 82%) plasma proteins than was ceforanide. The similarity in volume of distribution (V_d) was also indicative of similar tissue distribution of these cephalosporins.

The multiple-dose pharmacokinetics of ceforanide were studied after intravenous (i.v.) administration of 1 and 2 g as 30-min constant rate infusions and intramuscular (i.m.) administration of 500 and 1,000 mg in normal human subjects. The C_{max} values after i.v. administration were 136 and 222 µg/ml at termination of infusion; 12-h trough concentrations were 5.9 and 9.0 µg/ml, respectively. The MICs of ceforanide were in the range of 1 to 4 µg/ml for common pathogens. The C_{max} values after i.m. administration of 500 and 1,000 mg were 38 and 74 µg/ml at 1.0 to 1.3 h after dosing; 12-h trough concentrations were 3.9 and 6.7 µg/ml, respectively. Comparison of plasma AUC after i.v. and i.m. administration indicated that the i.m. dose was 100% bioavailable and the absorption rate constant (k_a) was 1.2 h⁻¹. There was no change in plasma pharmacokinetics and no tendency toward drug accumulation after the administration of these doses twice daily for 9.5 days. The major route of drug elimination was urinary excretion; 85% of the dose was excreted unchanged in the urine within 12 h. The mean terminal plasma $t_{1/2}$ was 3 h by both routes, the steady-state volume of distribution (Vd_{ss}) was 12 liters, Cl_p was 46 ml/min per 1.73 m², and Cl_r was 35 ml/min per 1.73 m².

The pharmacokinetics and safety of ceforanide and cefazolin were compared in normal subjects after 30-min i.v. infusions of 2-, 3-, and 4-g single doses and doses of 4 g twice daily for 10 days. No significant differences were observed in plasma-renal pharmacokinetic parameters between single and multiple doses of ceforanide (Table 2). The $t_{1/2}$ (2.8 h), Cl_p (48 ml/min per 1.73 m²), Cl_r from 0 to 12 h (47 ml/min per 1.73 m²; tubular secretion, 44%; glomerular filtration, 56%) did not change with increased dose or on multiple dosing. No significant change was observed in $t_{1/2}$ (1.9 h), AUC, or Cl_r (60 ml/min per 1.73 m²) with a 4-g single dose as compared to twice daily administration of cefazolin. A small increase in cefazolin clearance (Cl_r) from 0 to 2 h was observed during the intervals when plasma concentrations were greater than 100 µg/ml, as the single dose increased from 2 to 4 g. Analysis of individual (0 to 2 h) clearance of cefazolin indicated that mean Cl_r increased from 61 ml/min per 1.73 m² at a plasma concentration

TABLE 1. *Single-dose pharmacokinetics of ceforanide and cefazolin in laboratory animals and humans*[a]

Species	Antibiotic	Dose (mg/ kg)	Route[b]	k_a (h^{-1})	C_{max} (μg/ml)	T_{max} (h)	$t_{1/2}$ (h)	AUC ($\mu g \cdot h$/ ml)	CL_p (ml/ min per kg)	Cl_r (ml/ min per kg)	V_d (liters/ kg)
Rat	Ceforanide	100	s.c.	1.5	169	0.5	1.1	416	5.4	4.4	0.5
	Cefazolin	100	s.c.	2.0	235	0.3	0.5	269	9.7	5.6	0.4
Rabbit	Ceforanide	30	i.v.	—	369	—	5.0	1,440	0.4	0.2	0.2
	Cefazolin	20	i.v.	—	230	—	0.3	59	5.3	4.7	0.1
Dog	Ceforanide	25	i.v.	—	46.5^d	—	1.0	72	6.5	5.0	0.5
	Cefazolin	25	i.v.	—	31.2^d	—	0.8	41	10.4	5.9	0.7
Human	Ceforanide	30^c	i.v.	—	246^d	—	2.6	707	0.7	0.7	0.2
	Cefazolin	30^c	i.v.	—	256^d	—	2.0	559	0.9	0.9	0.2

[a] The parameters measured were absorption rate constant (k_a), peak plasma concentration (C_{max}), time of peak plasma concentration (T_{max}), half-life ($t_{1/2}$), area under the plasma concentration time curve (AUC), plasma clearance (CL_p), renal clearance (Cl_r), and volume of distribution (V_d).

[b] Routes: s.c., subcutaneous; i.v., intravenous. Doses in rabbits were administered as an i.v. bolus, and those in dogs and humans were administered as i.v. infusions.

[c] A 2-g i.v. dose.

[d] C_{max} at the end of the 30-min i.v. infusion.

TABLE 2. *Pharmacokinetic parameters for ceforanide and cefazolin after single intravenous doses*[a]

Compound	Dose (g)	C_{max} (μg/ ml)	$t_{1/2}$ (h)	AUC ($\mu g \cdot h$/ ml)	Clearance (ml/min per 1.73 m^2)	
					Cl_p	Cl_r
Ceforanide	2	246	2.6	707	45	45
	2	247	2.8	724	48	41
	3	336	2.6	980	56	44
	4	396	2.7	1,238	56	47
Cefazolin	2	256	2	559	62	54
	2	241	2	509	78	52
	3	309	2	679	80	75
	4	423	1.9	878	79	66

[a] The parameters measured were peak plasma concentration at the end of the 30-min intravenous infusion (C_{max}), half-life ($t_{1/2}$), area under the plasma concentration time curve (AUC), plasma clearance (Cl_p), and mean 0- to 12-h renal clearance based on individual urine collections at 0 to 2, 2 to 4, 4 to 6, 6 to 8, 8 to 10, and 10 to 12 h (Cl_r).

of 50 μg/ml to 92 ml/min per 1.73 m^2 at 200 μg/ ml. Ceforanide Cl_r only increased from 45 to 50 ml/min per 1.73 m^2 as the plasma concentration increased from 50 to 200 μg/ml. This was a result of a decrease in the percentage of plasma protein binding and increased Cl_r due to increased glomerular filtration at high plasma concentrations. This increase in Cl_r resulted in a lack of linear proportionality of AUC with dose over a range of 2 to 4 g for both cephalosporins, although this effect was much less marked with ceforanide. Moderate, transient elevations in serum transaminases and one incidence of allergic rash were observed with each cephalosporin. There was no evidence of any change in renal function based on clearances of drug, *p*-aminohippurate, and creatinine or other standard clinical parameters.

The pharmacokinetic and presently available clinical efficacy studies have indicated that the antimicrobial and pharmacokinetic properties of ceforanide could provide the potential for safe and effective therapy at a 0.5- to 1.0-g i.v. or i.m. dose administered on a twice daily schedule.

1. Leitner, F., M. Misiek, T. A. Pursiano, R. E. Buck, D. E. Chisholm, R. G. DeRegis, Y. H. Tsai, and K. E. Price. 1976. Laboratory evaluation of BL-S786, a cephalosporin with broad-spectrum antibacterial activity. Antimicrob. Agents Chemother. **10**:426–435.
2. Lutz, F., and W. Mogabgab. 1978. A long acting cephalosporin in various infections. *In* Program Abstr. Intersci. Conf. Antimicrob. Agents Chemother. 18th, Atlanta, Ga., abstr. no. 163.

Comparison of Ceforanide and Cefazolin Treatment of Bacterial Pneumonia

DANIEL RAWSON, DONNA S. JONES, DORIS CRAIN, AND CARL A. PERLINO*

Emory University Department of Medicine, Division of Infectious Disease, Atlanta, Georgia 30303, U.S.A.

Cephalosporin antibiotics are commonly used as empiric therapy for presumed bacterial infection before the results of cultures are available. Ceforanide, a newly developed cephalosporin, has an in vitro antibacterial spectrum similar to cefazolin, but has the apparent advantage of a comparatively longer half-life (3 h), enabling an every-12-h dosage schedule (1).

In the present study the efficacy and safety of ceforanide were compared with those of cefazolin in the treatment of hospitalized patients with bacterial pneumonia. Patients with a chest X-ray compatible with pneumonia were considered for admission to the study. A pretreatment Gram stain of expectorated sputum demonstrating polymorphonuclear leukocytes and gram-positive cocci or small pleomorphic gram-negative bacilli was also necessary. Gram stains suggesting the presence of Enterobacteriaceae, Pseudomonas, or an anaerobic (mixed) flora were excluded from the study because of the known limited spectrum of antibacterial activity of the cephalosporins against these organisms.

Definitive diagnosis of the bacterial cause of the pneumonia was made using standard aerobic culture of blood, sputum, and pleural fluid. The quellung stain of sputum smears and the detection of pneumococcal polysaccharide in the sputum by counterimmunoelectrophoresis using pneumococcal antisera were also done (2).

Patients were randomized to receive either cefazolin or ceforanide. Twenty-four patients received cefazolin, 0.5 to 1.0 g parenterally every 8 h. The ages of these patients ranged from 22 to 80 years (median, 54). There were 13 men and 11 women in this group. Twenty-seven patients received ceforanide (Bristol Laboratories), 0.5 to 1.0 g parenterally every 12 h. Ages of these patients ranged from 23 to 104 (median, 49). Fifteen men and 12 women comprised this group. The character of symptoms, age distribution, race, sex, associated illnesses, and bacterial etiology of the pneumonia were comparable between the two treatment groups.

Upon admission to the study, additional tests including SMA-12, blood urea nitrogen, creatinine, serum electrolytes, CBC with differential and platelet counts, a Coombs test, and urinalysis were performed. These studies, along with a chest X-ray, were repeated at the end of ther-

apy. The patients were judged to have a satisfactory response to therapy if fever returned to normal within 72 to 96 h of beginning therapy and if cough and sputum production decreased. Unsatisfactory responses included persistence or worsening of symptoms, a worsening of pulmonary infiltrates on chest X-ray, or adverse reactions to the antibiotic. The antibiotic susceptibility to ceforanide and cefazolin of the isolated pathogens was determined using the agar dilution method of Steers et al. (3).

Results. The bacterial etiology of the pneumonia was determined for 19 of the 24 patients in the cefazolin treatment group (79%) and for 20 of the 27 patients in the ceforanide group (74%). In the cefazolin group, 12 cases were caused by *Streptococcus pneumoniae*; 6 of these patients were bacteremic. Four infections were due to *Haemophilus influenzae*. More than one pathogen was isolated from two patients: *S. pneumoniae* and *H. influenzae*; *Staphylococcus aureus* and *S. pneumoniae*. In the ceforanide treatment group there were 15 cases due to *S. pneumoniae*, one case due to *H. influenzae*, and four cases due to more than one organism: *S. pneumoniae* and *H. influenzae* in each case. Seven patients had no pathogens documented in this group. Five of the patients in the ceforanide treatment group had pneumococcal bacteremia.

The MIC of cefazolin and ceforanide necessary to inhibit the growth of pneumococcal isolates was 0.3 to 0.13 µg/ml for cefazolin and 0.13 to 0.5 µg/ml for ceforanide (Table 1). The level of cefazolin inhibiting the growth of *H. influenzae* was 2.0 to 16.0 µg/ml. Similar values were obtained for ceforanide. Thus, although pneumococci appear slightly less susceptible to ceforanide, the susceptibility of *H. influenzae* to each of the drugs was equivalent. These levels of antibiotic are easily achieved in serum with the doses of antibiotic used in this study.

A satisfactory response was observed in 23 of 24 patients receiving cefazolin and in 26 of the 27 ceforanide-treated patients (Table 2). One patient treated with cefazolin, a 68-year-old woman with pneumococcal pneumonia, died within 48 h after therapy was started. One ceforanide-treated patient with pneumococcal pneumonia, and bacteremia diagnosed initially by cultures obtained by transtracheal aspiration,

TABLE 1. *Pneumococcal antibiotic susceptibility*

Drug	No. of organisms inhibited at MIC (μg/ml):				
	0.03	0.06	0.13	0.25	0.5
Ceforanide	0	0	29	2	1
Cefazolin	2	25	5	0	0

TABLE 2. *Results of therapy*

Determination	No. of patients	
	Cefazolin group	Ceforanide group
Total number of patients	24	27
Satisfactory response	23	26
Death	1	0
Treatment failure	0	1
Side effects		
Phlebitis	0	1
Hemolysis	1	0
Rise in SGOT[a]	1	3
Rise in alk. phos.[b]	7	1
Rise in both	3	0

[a] SGOT, Serum glutamic oxalacetic transaminase; rise $\geq$10 units.

[b] Alk. phos., Alkaline phosphatase; rise $\geq$10 units.

remained febrile for 7 days of therapy and experienced no improvement of cough. Gram stain of the sputum still showed leukocytes and gram-positive diplococci. Pneumococcal polysaccharide was not detected in the sputum at this time, however. Therapy was changed to penicillin and resulted in rapid improvement.

Eleven of the 24 patients treated with cefazolin had significant elevations of serum glutamic oxalacetic transaminase or alkaline phosphatase during therapy, whereas only 4 of the ceforanide-treated patients had similar changes. By Fischer's exact test this difference is statistically significant ($P < 0.02$). No correlation was found between these abnormalities and infection with *S. pneumoniae*. A history of alcohol abuse also did not correlate with these changes. Three of the 11 patients with liver enzyme abnormalities in the cefazolin treatment group received other medications including cimetidine, diphenylhydantoin sodium (Dilantin), digoxin, and a thiazide diuretic. Three of the four patients in the ceforanide group were receiving other drugs including isoniazid and ethambutol (two patients). This incidence of abnormal liver function tests associated with cefazolin therapy is higher than that reported previously and is unexplained.

Other side effects related to drug therapy were uncommon. One cefazolin-treated patient experienced a significant drop in his hematocrit early in therapy, associated with evidence of hemolysis. A Coombs test was negative. One ceforanide-treated patient experienced phlebitis.

Discussion. From the experience of this study we are able to conclude that parenteral ceforanide is an effective alternative to cefazolin in the treatment of bacterial pneumonia due to *S. pneumoniae* or *H. influenzae* and offers the advantage of an every-12-h dosage schedule. The drug is well tolerated by patients, with few side effects. Our study also found a higher incidence of liver enzyme abnormalities with cefazolin than has previously been reported, which did not appear to be related to underlying illnesses or the type of bacterial infection. These abnormal values were transient and did not require the cessation of the drug in any patient.

1. Leitner, F., M. Misiek, T. A. Pursiano, R. E. Buck, D. R. Chisholm, R. G. DeRegis, Y. H. Tsai, and K. E. Price. 1976. Laboratory evaluation of BL-S786, a cephalosporin with broad-spectrum antibacterial activity. Antimicrob. Agents Chemother. 10:426–435.
2. Perlino, C., and J. A. Shulman. 1976. Detection of pneumococcal polysaccharide in the sputum of patients with pneumococcal pneumonia by counterimmunoelectrophoresis. J. Lab. Clin. Med. 87:496–502.
3. Steers, E. E., E. L. Foltz, B. S. Graves, and J. Riden. 1959. An inocula replicating apparatus for routine testing of bacterial susceptibility to antibiotics. Antibiot. Chemother. 9:307–311.

AT-2266, a New Oral Antipseudomonal Agent

M. SHIMIZU, Y. TAKASE, S. NAKAMURA, H. KATAE, S. INOUE, A. MINAMI, K. NAKATA, AND Y. SAKAGUCHI

Department of Chemotherapy, Research Laboratories, Dainippon Pharmaceutical Co., Ltd., Enoki 33-94, Suita, Osaka 564, Japan

AT-2266, 1-ethyl-6-fluoro-1,4-dihydro-4-oxo-7-(1-piperazinyl)-1,8-naphthyridine-3-carboxylic acid (J. Matsumoto et al., this volume), is a new antipseudomonal agent structurally related to pipemidic acid (5). It has a broad and potent antibacterial activity and is almost as effective as gentamicin in experimental infections in mice. This compound is well absorbed by the oral route, is metabolized slightly, and is distributed to most tissues at concentrations higher than the plasma levels (S. Nakamura et al., this volume). These properties suggest that AT-2266 might be useful for the treatment of infections in various tissues, being different from the related compounds such as nalidixic acid (2), oxolinic acid (1), and piromidic acid (3), whose application is generally restricted to urinary, biliary, and intestinal tract infections. The present report summarizes the results of studies on antibacterial properties of AT-2266.

Table 1 shows the antibacterial spectrum of AT-2266 compared with that of commercially available antibacterial agents. The MIC was determined by the twofold agar dilution method (5). The MICs of AT-2266 were between 0.1 and 0.78 µg/ml against some gram-positive bacteria such as staphylococci and Bacillus subtilis and against most gram-negative bacteria such as Escherichia coli, Shigella sonnei, Salmonella enteritidis, Klebsiella pneumoniae, Proteus vulgaris, Vibrio parahaemolyticus, Serratia marcescens, Enterobacter cloacae, Citrobacter freundii, Haemophilus influenzae, Pseudomo-

nas aeruginosa, etc. AT-2266 inhibited the other gram-positive pathogens, e.g., streptococci, Corynebacterium pyogenes, Listeria monocytogenes, etc., and glucose-nonfermentative organisms, e.g., Pseudomonas putida, Acinetobacter calcoaceticus, Moraxella bovis, Alcaligenes faecalis, and Flavobacterium sp. at concentrations between 1.56 and 12.5 µg/ml. None of the tested organisms was highly resistant to AT-2266. Therefore, the antibacterial spectrum of AT-2266 was considered to be broader than that of pipemidic acid, nalidixic acid, oxolinic acid, cephalexin, ampicillin, and carbenicillin and comparable to that of gentamicin. The activity of AT-2266 was less potent against gram-positive bacteria but generally more potent against gram-negative bacteria than that of gentamicin.

Similar results were obtained with recent clinical isolates of staphylococci, streptococci, E. coli, indole-positive and -negative Proteus species, K. pneumoniae, Enterobacter sp., S. marcescens, and P. aeruginosa.

AT-2266 was not cross-resistant with antibiotics such as tetracycline, streptomycin, chloramphenicol, ampicillin, and cephalexin. Cross-resistance between AT-2266 and nalidixic acid was incomplete; most strains highly resistant to nal-

TABLE 1. Comparison of antibacterial spectra of AT-2266 and commercially available antibacterial agents

Organism	MIC (µg/ml)[a]							
	AT-2266	PPA	NA	OA	CEX	ABPC	CBPC	GM
Staphylococcus aureus 209P, JC-1	0.78	12.5	100	1.56	1.56	0.05	0.39	0.1
S. epidermidis no. 8	0.39	25	50	3.13	3.13	6.25	6.25	0.05
Streptococcus pyogenes A65	12.5	200	400	100	0.78	0.05	0.2	3.13
S. pneumoniae I Neufeld	6.25	200	>400	100	3.13	0.05	0.39	6.25
S. faecalis 2473	12.5	>200	>200	100	200	1.56	50	50
Bacillus subtilis PCI 219	0.2	6.25	6.25	0.2	1.56	0.39	0.39	<0.05
Corynebacterium pyogenes C-21	1.56	25	400	6.25	1.56	1.56	3.13	3.13
Erysipelothrix rhusiopathiae Agata	3.13	100	400	25	1.56	0.05	0.39	12.5
Listeria monocytogenes LI-2402	3.13	200	>400	25	25	0.39	6.25	0.1
Escherichia coli NIHJ, JC-2	0.2	1.56	12.5	0.39	6.25	6.25	12.5	6.25
Shigella sonnei EW33	0.1	1.56	3.13	0.2	6.25	0.2	0.78	0.78
Salmonella enteritidis no. 1891	0.1	1.56	3.13	0.2	3.13	0.2	0.78	0.78
Klebsiella pneumoniae no. 13	0.2	6.25	12.5	0.78	6.25	100	>200	1.56
Proteus vulgaris OX19	0.2	6.25	6.25	0.39	100	200	6.25	0.78
Vibrio parahaemolyticus S-1	0.1	3.13	1.56	0.1	25	200	>200	0.78
Serratia marcescens IFO 3736	0.39	3.13	6.25	0.78	>200	25	6.25	1.56
Enterobacter cloacae 2540	0.2	1.56	6.25	0.39	>200	>200	6.25	3.13
Citrobacter freundii 3433	0.2	1.56	6.25	0.39	6.25	3.13	6.25	1.56
Pseudomonas aeruginosa Tsuchijima	0.39	12.5	100	6.25	>200	>200	12.5	0.78
P. putida 3682a	6.25	50	>100	50	>200	>200	100	50
Brucella abortus Kusayanagi	6.25	200	>400	100	50	0.2	3.13	<0.05
Yersinia enterocolitica MY-79	0.2	1.56	1.56	0.39	50	200	100	0.78
Pasteurella multocida M-17	0.1	1.56	1.56	0.39	3.13	0.2	0.39	0.39
Neisseria meningitidis P-6002	0.2	3.13	6.25	0.2	25	0.78	50	0.78
Haemophilus influenzae 6568	0.1	3.13	6.25	0.39	50	>100	>100	0.78
Acinetobacter calcoaceticus 3125b	1.56	50	25	1.56	>200	25	25	0.78
Moraxella bovis 444	3.13	25	>100	100	>200	>200	>200	0.78
Alcaligenes faecalis 767	3.13	50	25	6.25	>200	>200	>200	50
Flavobacterium sp. 43	12.5	200	100	12.5	>200	>200	>200	>200

[a] PPA, Pipemidic acid; NA, nalidixic acid; OA, oxolinic acid; CEX, cephalexin; ABPC, ampicillin; CBPC, carbenicillin; GM, gentamicin.

Table 2. *Comparative activities of AT-2266 and commercially available antibacterial agents against systemic and urinary bladder-kidney infections in mice*

Infecting organism	ED50: mg/kg per dose (MIC: μg/ml)							
	AT-2266[a]	PPA[a]	NA[a]	OA[a]	CEX[a]	ABPC[a]	CBPC[b]	GM[b]
Systemic infection								
S. aureus no. 50774	10.0	238	>800	53.2	12.1	2.2	—[c]	—
	(0.78)	(25)	(50)	(1.56)	(1.56)	(0.1)		
E. coli P-5101	1.8	21.2	33.7	19.7	213	120	—	—
	(0.1)	(3.13)	(3.13)	(0.2)	(12.5)	(6.25)		
K. pneumoniae no. 13	3.5	28.6	49.8	47.1	8.2	383	—	—
	(0.2)	(6.25)	(12.5)	(0.78)	(6.25)	(100)		
P. morganii Kono	2.5	67.3	87.3	20.3	>800	>1,600	—	—
	(0.2)	(3.13)	(6.25)	(0.2)	(>200)	(100)		
S. typhimurium S-9	2.5	11.7	24.8	8.1	53.8	5.2	—	—
	(0.1)	(3.13)	(3.13)	(0.2)	(6.25)	(0.39)		
S. marcescens S-9	2.0	8.0	—	—	—	—	>1,600	1.1
	(0.39)	(1.56)					(>400)	(1.56)
P. aeruginosa no. 12	9.0	99.5	—	—	—	—	122	6.3
	(0.78)	(25)					(100)	(1.56)
P. aeruginosa Ky-22	17.7	218	—	—	—	—	>1,600	>100
	(1.56)	(25)					(>400)	(50)
Urinary bladder-kidney infection								
E. coli P-5101	1.5	4.8	6.6	9.1	44.2	36.3	—	—
K. pneumoniae no. 13	3.1	11.9	40.8	57.8	35.4	>800	—	—
S. marcescens S-9	5.0	18.6	—	—	—	—	>800	7.3
P. aeruginosa no. 12	2.4	30.6	—	—	—	—	130	1.7

[a] Oral route (PPA, pipemidic acid; NA, nalidixic acid; OA, oxolinic acid; CEX, cephalexin; ABPC, ampicillin).
[b] Subcutaneous route (CBPC, carbenicillin; GM, gentamicin).
[c] —, Not tested.

idixic acid (MIC: >100 μg/ml) were inhibited by AT-2266 at 0.78 to 3.13 μg/ml.

The MICs of AT-2266 were not changed significantly by the addition of horse serum into nutrient broth to 40% or of sodium cholate into nutrient agar up to 5%. However, the values rose slightly when nutrient broth was made acid or larger inocula were employed.

AT-2266 was found to be bactericidal around its MIC when colony-forming ability of *Staphylococcus aureus*, *E. coli*, and *P. aeruginosa* was checked after exposure to the compound for various periods.

Spontaneous mutants resistant to AT-2266 were not detected in all tested pathogens such as *S. aureus*, *E. coli*, *Shigella flexneri*, *Salmonella typhi*, *K. pneumoniae*, *Proteus morganii*, and *P. aeruginosa*, when over 10^8 colony-forming units were plated with heart infusion agar containing 10 μg of the agent per ml. This was in contrast with the results of nalidixic acid, rifampin, and streptomycin, with which highly resistant spontaneous mutants (MIC: >100 μg/ml) were observed in some of the pathogens.

Table 2 shows comparative activities of AT-2266 and commercially available antibacterial agents against systemic and urinary bladder-kidney infections in mice. The experimental conditions were generally the same as those described by Shimizu et al. (4). AT-2266, pipemidic acid,

nalidixic acid, oxolinic acid, cephalexin, and ampicillin were administered by the oral route, and carbenicillin and gentamicin were given by the subcutaneous route. AT-2266 showed 50% effective doses (ED50) ranging from 1.8 to 17.7 mg/kg per dose against systemic infections with *S. aureus*, *E. coli*, *K. pneumoniae*, *P. morganii*, *Salmonella typhimurium*, *S. marcescens*, and *P. aeruginosa*. The ED50 values of AT-2266 were always lower than those of orally administered reference drugs, with one exception: AT-2266 was, dose for dose, superior to carbenicillin and almost comparable to gentamicin against the *P. aeruginosa* no. 12 infection. It was noted that AT-2266 was also effective on the infection due to the *P. aeruginosa* strain that was simultaneously resistant to both carbenicillin and gentamicin. The ED50 values of AT-2266 in urinary bladder-kidney infections were similarly lower than those of the oral reference drugs and carbenicillin, and the same as those of gentamicin.

These therapeutic accomplishments of AT-2266 indicate that this compound is worth further study as a possible potent oral antipseudomonal agent.

1. **Kaminsky, D., and R. I. Meltzer.** 1968. Quinolone antibacterial agents. Oxolinic acid and related compounds. J. Med. Chem. **11:**160–163.
2. **Lesher, G. Y., E. J. Froelich, M. D. Gruett, J. H.**

Bailey, and R. P. Brundage. 1962. 1,8-Naphthyridine derivatives. A new class of chemotherapeutic agents. J. Med. Pharm. Chem. **5**:1063–1065.

3. **Shimizu, M., S. Nakamura, and Y. Takase.** 1971. Piromidic acid, a new antibacterial agent: antibacterial properties, p. 117–122. Antimicrob. Agents Chemother. 1970.

4. **Shimizu, M., Y. Takase, S. Nakamura, H. Katae, A.**

Minami, K. Nakata, and N. Kurobe. 1976. Pipemidic acid: its activity against various experimental infections. Antimicrob. Agents Chemother. **9**:569–574.

5. **Shimizu, M., Y. Takase, S. Nakamura, H. Katae, A. Minami, K. Nakata, S. Inoue, M. Ishiyama, and Y. Kubo.** 1975. Pipemidic acid, a new antibacterial agent active against *Pseudomonas aeruginosa*: in vitro properties. Antimicrob. Agents Chemother. **8**:132–138.

Structure-Activity Relationships of 4-Oxo-1,8-Naphthyridine-3-Carboxylic Acids Including AT-2266, a New Oral Antipseudomonal Agent

JUN-ICHI MATSUMOTO,* TERUYUKI MIYAMOTO, AKIRA MINAMIDA, YOSHIRO NISHIMURA, HIROSHI EGAWA, AND HARUKI NISHIMURA

Research Laboratories, Dainippon Pharmaceutical Co., Ltd., Suita, Osaka, Japan

During recent years compounds with a pyridone-carboxylic acid moiety have increasingly attracted the attention of medicinal chemists. Since the development of piromidic acid (Ia) and pipemidic acid (Ib) from our laboratories, we have continuously studied the pyridone-carboxylic acid derivatives including 1,7-disubstituted 1,4-dihydro-4-oxo-quinoline- and -1,8-naphthyridine-3-carboxylic acids (II and III: R₃ = H) to find some structure-activity relationships associated with changes in the nucleus (S. Minami et al., British patent 1426070, 1976). A comparative biological study on the representatives of II and III (R₃ = H) revealed that the 1,8-naphthyridines (III: R₃ = H), in most cases, were superior to the corresponding quinoline derivatives (II) in oral effects on experimental systemic infections caused by gram-negative bacteria in mice, whereas, in in vitro activity, III (R₃ = H) was slightly inferior to II. This finding stimulated an effort to investigate the naphthyridine derivatives (III) having a further substituent at position 6 in hopes of obtaining an improved antibacterial agent. The present work is concerned with a synthesis and structure-activity relationship of the 6-substituted 1,8-naphthyridines (III) with variations of the groups R₁, R₂, and R₃.

Although a number of the 1,8-naphthyridine derivatives without a substituent at position 6 have been prepared and claimed to have antibacterial activity, little appears to be known about the 6-substituted analog (III) (1). An attractive intermediate for the synthesis of III would be a 6-diazonium salt (VI) of the naphthyridine, which might be converted into the 6-cyano (VII) and 6-chloro (VIII) analogs by means of Sandmeyer reaction as shown in general formulas in Fig. 1. The diazonium salt (VI) was readily accessible by diazotization of the corresponding 6-amino derivative (V) through the 6-nitro compound (IV) prepared by nitration of the ethyl ester of III (R₃ = H). In fact, replacement of the diazo group by cyano and chloro groups was accomplished in good yields by treatment of the diazonium sulfate (VI: X = ½ SO₄) with potassium cyanide in the presence of cuprous cyanide and by decomposition of the diazonium chloride (VI: X = Cl) in a hydrochloric acid solution, respectively. The reaction was successfully extended to the synthesis of 6-fluoro derivatives (IX), involving the thermal decomposition (Schiemann reaction) of the diazonium tetrafluoroborate (VI: X = BF₄). Another route to the 6-fluoro compounds (IX) involved the thermal cyclization (Gould-Jacobs reaction) of diethyl N-(2-substituted 3-fluoro-6-pyridyl)-aminomethylenemalonates which were derived from 2,6-dichloro-3-nitropyridine in several steps including Schiemann reaction. When the 7-substituents (R) on the 1,8-naphthyridines (VII, VIII, and IX) thus prepared were groups such as chloro, methoxy, and ethylsulfonyl, they were replaced by various secondary amino functions such as pyrrolidinyl, piperazinyl, and morpholino groups.

The 6-substituted 1,8-naphthyridines (III) (not all compounds prepared) and their antibacterial activities are listed in Table 1; the data for pipemidic acid (Ib) are included for comparison. The activity was given as geometrical mean values of the MICs (micrograms per milliliter) taken for 6 gram-positive organisms (4 strains of *Staphylococcus aureus*, 1 of *Streptococcus epidermidis*, and 1 of *Corynebacterium pyogenes*) and 21 gram-negative organisms (6 strains of

Table 1. *Antibacterial activity of the 1,8-naphthyridines*

$$R_3 \diagdown \diagup \diagdown \diagup \diagdown COOH$$
$$R_2 \diagup N \diagup N$$
$$R_1$$

III

Com-pound	R_1	R_2	R_3	Mp (°C)	Formula[a]	MIC (µg/ml)[b] Gram-positive	MIC (µg/ml)[b] Gram-negative
IIIa	C_2H_5	HN N-	H	273–274	$C_{15}H_{18}N_4O_3$	39.7	9.02
IIIb	C_2H_5	HN N-	NH_2	254–256	$C_{15}H_{19}N_5O_3$	178	9.60
IIIc	C_2H_5	HN N-	NO_2	234–236	$C_{15}H_{17}N_5O_5$	41.0	8.14
IIId	C_2H_5	HN N- (HCl)	CN	265–273	$C_{16}H_{17}N_5O_3 \cdot HCl$	19.8	3.29
IIIe	C_2H_5	HN N- (HCl)	Cl	290–300	$C_{15}H_{17}ClN_4O_3 \cdot HCl$	4.42	1.38
IIIf	C_2H_5	HN N-	F	225–227	$C_{15}H_{17}FN_4O_3$	0.88	0.26
IIIg	C_2H_5	HN N-	F	238–240	$C_{16}H_{19}FN_4O_3$	3.51	0.69
IIIh	C_2H_5	HO-pyrrolidinyl N-	F	291–293	$C_{15}H_{16}FN_3O_4$	0.50	0.73
IIIi	C_2H_5	$(CH_3)_2N-$	F	273–276	$C_{13}H_{14}FN_3O_3$	0.78	1.51
IIIj	C_2H_5	N-	F	299–300	$C_{15}H_{16}FN_3O_3$	0.35	1.78
IIIk	C_2H_5	O N-	F	261–263	$C_{15}H_{16}FN_3O_4$	1.24	3.29
IIIl	C_2H_5	N-	F	211–213	$C_{16}H_{18}FN_3O_3$	0.98	8.69
IIIm	C_2H_5	CH_3N N-	F	227–230	$C_{16}H_{19}FN_4O_3$	1.24	0.64
IIIn	C_2H_5	C_2H_5N N-	F	193–194	$C_{17}H_{21}FN_4O_3$	1.23	0.95
IIIo	C_2H_5	$n\text{-}C_3H_7N$ N-	F	208–209	$C_{18}H_{23}FN_4O_3$	2.48	3.34
IIIp	C_2H_5	$n\text{-}C_4H_9N$ N-	F	184–185	$C_{19}H_{25}FN_4O_3$	2.78	5.30
IIIq	C_2H_5	$C_6H_5CH_2N$ N-	F	220–222	$C_{22}H_{23}FN_4O_3$	1.10	8.14
IIIr	$CH=CH_2$	HN N-	F	256–260 (dec.)	$C_{15}H_{15}FN_4O_3$	1.97	0.13
IIIs	$CH=CH_2$	CH_3N N-	F	205–207	$C_{16}H_{17}FN_4O_3$	1.97	0.42
Ib	Pipemidic acid					22.3	0.58

a All compounds were analyzed for C, H, N and, where present, Cl and F; analytical results were within ± 0.3% of the theoretical values.

b The activities are presented as geometrical mean values of the MIC taken for the strains given in the text by the twofold agar dilution method.

Escherichia coli, 2 of *Salmonella* spp., 2 of *Shigella flexneri*, 1 of *Klebsiella pneumoniae*, 2 of *Enterobacter* spp., 4 of *Pseudomonas aeruginosa*, 1 of *Serratia marcescens* and 3 of *Proteus* spp.).

Introduction of the 6-substituent (R_3) into 1-ethyl-1,4-dihydro-4-oxo-7-(1-piperazinyl)-1,8-naphthyridine-3-carboxylic acid (IIIa) influenced markedly the antibacterial activity. One may compare the activities of the amino (IIIb), nitro (IIIc), cyano (IIId), chloro (IIIe), and fluoro (IIIf) derivatives, which increase in that order, with those of the parent compound (IIIa). The

fluoro compound (IIIf) is about 45 and 35 times greater in activity against gram-positive and gram-negative organisms, respectively, than IIIa. The same situation prevailed in a series of 1-ethyl-1,4-dihydro-7-(4-methyl-1-piperazinyl)-4-oxo-1,8-naphthyridine-3-carboxylic acids with amino, nitro, cyano, chloro, and fluoro groups at position 6.

In variations of the 7-substituent (R_2), keeping the 6-substituent (R_3) constant as the most active fluoro group, piperazinyl (IIIf), hexahydro-1H-1,4-diazepinyl (IIIg), and 3-hydroxypyrrolidinyl (IIIh) groups, which have hydrophilic

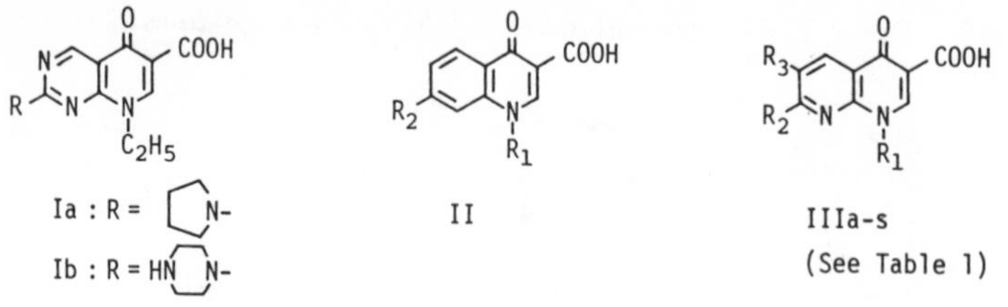

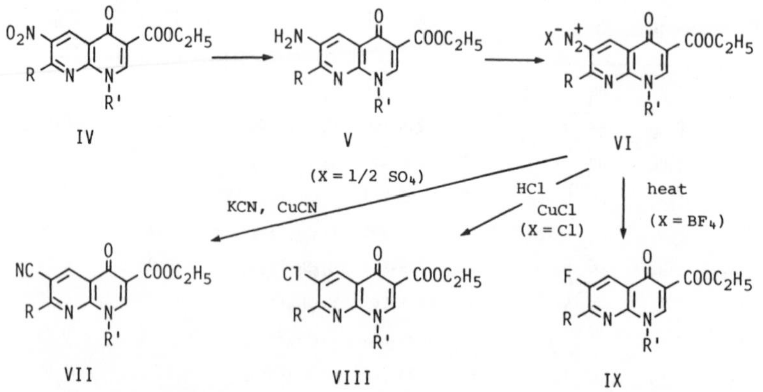

FIG. 1. *General synthetic routes to the 6-substituted 1,8-naphthyridine derivatives.*

character, lead to the compounds with a high activity against gram-negative organisms. However, when R_2 is a dimethylamino (IIIi), pyrrolidinyl (IIIj), morpholino (IIIk), or piperidino (IIIl) group, the gram-negative activity of the compounds considerably decreases in that order; in this case the gram-positive activity is less affected than the gram-negative activity. Further introduction of an alkyl chain into the nitrogen atom of the piperazinyl ring in compound IIIf causes a decrease in the gram-negative activity with increase in the number of carbon atoms (e.g., IIIm-IIIq). It seems that, in general, increasing the lipophilicity of R_2 decreases the gram-negative activity more strongly than it does the gram-positive activity.

Regarding the 1-substituent (R_1), replacement of the ethyl group in compound IIIf by a vinyl group results in a slight increase in the gram-

negative activity, whereas it reduces considerably the gram-positive activity (compare IIIf and IIIm with IIIr and IIIs, respectively).

On the basis of the broad and potent in vitro antibacterial activity, along with preliminary biological results showing an excellent oral effect on experimental infections and weak acute toxicity, compound IIIf, named AT-2266 [1-ethyl-6-fluoro-1,4-dihydro-4-oxo-7-(1-piperazinyl)-1,8-naphthyridine-3-carboxylic acid], was selected as a promising candidate for further research. Details of biological properties of AT-2266 will be presented in this volume (M. Shimizu et al. and S. Nakamura et al.).

1. **Albrecht, R.** 1977. Development of antibacterial agents of the nalidixic acid type, p. 51–69. *In* E. Jucker (ed.), Progress in drug research, vol. 21. Birkhauser Verlag, Basel.

Pharmacological Properties of AT-2266

S. NAKAMURA,* Y. TAKASE, N. KUROBE, S. KASHIMOTO, AND M. SHIMIZU

Department of Chemotherapy, Research Laboratories, Dainippon Pharmaceutical Company, Ltd., Enoki 33–94, Suita, Osaka 564, Japan

AT-2266 (J. Matsumoto et al., this volume) is a new antipseudomonal agent structurally related to pipemidic acid (2). It has a broad and

potent antibacterial activity in vitro and shows excellent therapeutic effects by the oral route, comparable to subcutaneously injected gentamicin in experimental infections in mice (M. Shimizu et al., this volume). These therapeutic effects seem to be related to its pharmacological properties. This report describes bioassay data on the absorption, distribution, and excretion of AT-2266 and the results of preliminary tests on its toxicity.

The experimental methods used were essentially the same as those described by Shimizu et al. (1). Figure 1 shows the plasma levels of AT-2266 in mice, rats, and dogs given a single oral dose of 50 mg/kg. In mice and rats given AT-2266 dissolved in water with hydrochloric acid, the peaks of average plasma levels, which were 2.4 µg/ml in both animals, were seen 15 or 30 min after administration. The half-life of AT-2266 in plasma was 2.2 h in both animals. In dogs given AT-2266 packed in a capsule, the average plasma level rose to a maximum of 11.4 µg/ml 4 and 5 h after administration, with a half-life of 6.6 h. Compared with mice and rats, dogs showed relatively high plasma levels and relatively long half-lives in plasma. A dose response was observed in the plasma levels of rats given AT-2266 at doses of 25, 50, and 100 mg/kg; the average plasma level at 50 mg/kg was about twofold higher than that at 25 mg/kg, and that at 100 mg/kg was about fourfold higher. In dogs serially receiving 25-mg/kg doses every 12 h, the curve of average plasma levels after the third dose was about 1.4 times higher than that after the first dose and about equal to that after the

TABLE 1. *Organ and tissue levels of AT-2266 in rats given a single dose of 50 mg/kg orally*

Body part	Concn (µg/ml or g)[a] at time after administration (h):					
	0.5	1	2	4	6	8
Plasma	2.4	2.1	0.99	0.70	0.40	0.22
Brain	0.11	0.16	0.094	ND[b]	ND	ND
Heart	6.7	4.9	2.3	1.4	0.86	0.38
Lung	4.6	4.6	2.4	1.5	0.91	0.36
Liver	21.3	19.1	8.8	4.0	2.6	1.2
Kidney	33.9	22.1	11.6	6.0	3.5	1.7
Spleen	5.1	5.9	2.8	2.0	1.1	0.54
Muscle	4.2	5.4	3.4	2.4	1.4	0.74

[a] Average of three rats.
[b] ND, Not detected.

fifth dose, as expected from a pharmacokinetic analysis.

The protein binding of AT-2266 was measured by ultrafiltration, and the rate of unbound AT-2266 was found to be about 60% in rat, dog, and human plasma or serum, almost independent of the drug concentrations used. The protein binding of AT-2266 was reversible and rapidly broken down by dilution.

Table 1 shows the concentrations of AT-2266 in the organs and tissues of rats given a single oral dose of 50 mg/kg. The peak concentrations, which were 2.4, 0.16, 6.7, 4.6, 21.3, 33.9, 5.9, and 5.4 µg/ml or g in plasma, brain, heart, lung, liver, kidney, spleen, and muscle, respectively, were observed 30 min or 1 h after administration. Except in brain, the concentrations were about 2 to 14 times higher than the peak plasma level. The half-lives of AT-2266 in these organs and tissues ranged between 2.0 and 2.8 h, not significantly different from that in plasma (2.2 h).

Biliary excretion of AT-2266 was tested in rats receiving a single oral dose of 50 mg/kg. An average bile level reached a peak of 27 µg/ml 6 to 8 h after administration, and about 2.5% of the dose was recovered over 24 h on the average.

Urinary excretion of AT-2266 was so abundant that about 57, 41, and 65% of the dose was recovered over 24 h from urine of mice, rats, and dogs given a single oral dose of 50 mg/kg. The peak urine levels of AT-2266 were about 1,000 µg/ml in these three animal species. In the case of rats, fecal excretion was examined at the same time and found to be about 53% of the dose. Thus, the total recovery from urine and feces of rats came to about 93%, indicating that most of AT-2266 administered was in a bacteriologically active form.

To determine the active principle in vivo, deproteinized plasma and urine of rats and dogs receiving AT-2266 were spotted on a silica gel plate (Merck, no. 5714) and developed in a sol-

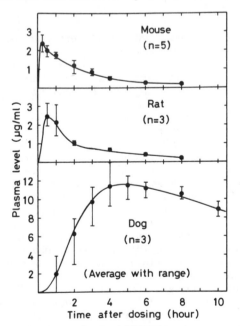

FIG. 1. *Plasma levels of AT-2266 in mice, rats, and dogs given a single oral dose of 50 mg/kg.*

vent mixture of dioxane and 28% ammonia water (3:2). After development, bacteriologically active spots were detected by bioautography (1). Only one active spot with an R_f value corresponding to authentic AT-2266 was seen in rat plasma, dog plasma, and rat urine. In dog urine, however, two active spots, one large and one small, were detected: the substance of the large active spot with an R_f value corresponding to AT-2266 was purified and identified as AT-2266 by mass spectrometry, whereas the substance of the small active spot with a slightly higher R_f value has not been identified yet.

The LD_{50}'s of AT-2266 after a single administration to mice were about 330 mg/kg intravenously, about 1,100 mg/kg subcutaneously, and more than 5,000 mg/kg orally, irrespective of sex. No significant abnormalities possibly due to AT-2266 were observed in mice given AT-2266 orally once a day for 16 days at doses of 500, 1,000, and 2,000 mg/kg per day, except for the dilatation of cecum which is often seen in rodents given antibacterial agents of various kinds.

The results obtained may be summarized as follows: AT-2266 is well absorbed by the oral route, distributed to most tissues at high concentrations, stable to metabolic inactivation, excreted into urine in quantity, and weak in oral toxicity. Given these results together with antibacterial properties, one can imagine that AT-2266 might be orally applicable to infections of various sites of the body. This possibility is worth examining.

1. **Shimizu, M., S. Nakamura, Y. Takase, and N. Kurobe.** 1975. Pipemidic acid: absorption, distribution, and excretion. Antimicrob. Agents Chemother. **7**:441–446.
2. **Shimizu, M., Y. Takase, S. Nakamura, H. Katae, A. Minami, K. Nakata, S. Inoue, M. Ishiyama, and Y. Kubo.** 1975. Pipemidic acid, a new antibacterial agent active against *Pseudomonas aeruginosa*: in vitro properties. Antimicrob. Agents Chemother. **8**:132–138.

DJ-6783, a New Synthetic Antimicrobial Agent: Comparison with Miloxacin, Pipemidic Acid, and Nalidixic Acid

YASUAKI OSADA,* TSUTOMU UNE, HIDEMASA OGAWA, AND KENICHI SATOH

Research Institute, Daiichi Seiyaku Company, Ltd., Tokyo, and Department of Microbiology, School of Medicine, Gunma University, Gunma, Japan*

DJ-6783 (DJ), 5-ethyl-5,8-dihydro-8-oxo-furo[3,2-b][1,8]naphthyridine-7-carboxylic acid (Fig. 1), is a new synthetic antimicrobial agent. It is chemically analogous to miloxacin (MIL), pipemidic acid (PPA), and nalidixic acid (NA), which, as a partial structure, contain 4-pyridone-3-carboxylic acid. This paper is a primary presentation of the in vitro and in vivo antimicrobial activities of DJ compared with those of MIL, PPA, and NA.

In vitro antimicrobial activity. The in vitro antimicrobial activity is represented as the MIC. MICs were measured according to the agar (heart infusion agar) dilution method. The antimicrobial spectrum was tested using a total of 56 laboratory strains of bacteria (44 gram negatives and 12 gram positives). DJ had a broad spectrum of antimicrobial activity and was more active against these strains than MIL, PPA, and NA, the MICs of DJ for *Enterobacteriaceae*, *Pseudomonas*, *Bordetella*, *Haemophilus*, *Neisseria*, and *Staphylococcus* being 0.05 to 0.39, 0.78 to 3.13, 0.10 to 1.56, ≤0.025, 0.025 to 0.10, and 0.78 μg/ml, respectively. It was characteris-

tic that DJ was highly active against gram negatives, i.e., *Escherichia coli, Proteus* spp., *Enterobacter cloacae, Serratia marcescens, Pseudomonas aeruginosa, Pseudomonas cepacia, Pseudomonas maltophilia, Bordetella pertussis,* and *Haemophilus influenzae.*

The antimicrobial potency of DJ against clinical isolates of gram-negative and gram-positive organisms was compared with those of the other three drugs on the basis of cumulative percentages of strains inhibited by various concentrations of the drugs. The concentrations of these drugs inhibiting growth of 50 and 75% of the strains used and median MICs are presented in Table 1. Overall, DJ was the highest in antimicrobial potency against the clinical isolates used, followed by MIL, PPA, and NA in that order. DJ was significantly more active than the other three drugs against *Proteus, P. aeruginosa, S. marcescens,* and staphylococci. Large differences in MIC distributions for *Staphylococcus epidermidis* were demonstrated between DJ and MIL, which was nearest to DJ in potency among the control drugs; the median MICs of DJ and

MIL were 0.78 and 12.5 $\mu g/ml$, respectively. The strains of clinical isolates of *E. coli*, *Proteus* spp., *S. marcescens*, and *Klebsiella pneumoniae* resistant to NA were also highly susceptible to DJ; namely, no cross-resistance between DJ and NA has been found so far.

The bactericidal activity of DJ was compared with that of PPA. The cells of *E. coli* NIHJ used as a representative organism were completely killed within 4 h by DJ at a concentration twofold the MIC, whereas they were not killed completely by PPA. MBCs of DJ against 10 strains each of *E. coli*, *K. pneumoniae*, *Proteus mirabilis*, *Proteus vulgaris*, *E. cloacae*, *S. marcescens*, *P. aeruginosa*, and *S. aureus* were almost identical to the MICs; the mean ratio of MBC to MIC against these organisms was 1.1 ± 0.2.

In vivo antimicrobial activity. The protective effect of a single dose of DJ on sepsis-type infection in mice with *E. coli*, *Citrobacter freundii*, *K. pneumoniae*, *E. cloacae*, *P. vulgaris*, *P. mirabilis*, *S. marcescens*, *P. aeruginosa*, *S. aureus*, and *Streptococcus pyogenes* was compared with that of MIL, PPA, and other antibiotics such as amoxicillin, carbenicillin, cefazolin, and gentamicin. Among the drugs used, DJ was the most effective on the infections with the gram negatives, except for gentamicin. The effectiveness was significantly elevated when double

doses (1 and 4 h after infection) were applied. Although not comparable to the effectiveness of the β-lactam antibiotics on infections with gram positives, DJ was more active than MIL, PPA, and NA.

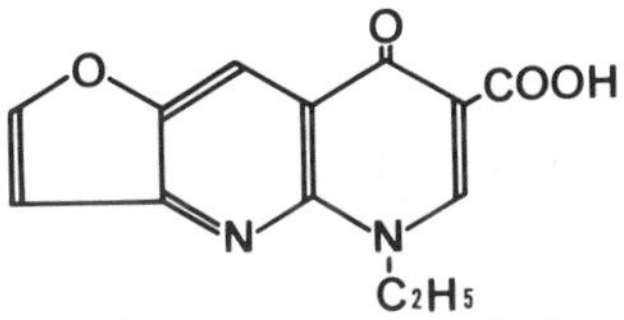

The curative effect of DJ on experimental urinary and respiratory tract infections in mice and rats was compared with that of PPA, NA, and other antibiotics. Urinary tract infection was made by intracystic inoculation with *E. coli* O6, E77156, in rats and with *S. marcescens* 339 in mice. In both infections, the organisms gradually multiplied in the kidneys by day 7 to 10 and provoked acute-phase ascending pyelonephritis in both animals. DJ, PPA, or NA was used in treating these infections once or twice a day for 4 to 5 consecutive days, and the effect of these drugs was primarily estimated as the clearance rate of bacilli from the kidneys, $<10^2$ colony-forming units being considered as complete recovery. On *E. coli* infection in rats, DJ completely cleared the organisms from the kidneys at a dose of 40 mg/kg twice daily for 4 consecutive days, whereas PPA and NA did not; the ED_{50}'s of DJ, PPA, and NA were 12.6, 46.8, and 100 mg/kg, respectively. On urinary tract infection with *S. marcescens* in mice, DJ was also more effective than PPA; the ED_{50}'s were 101 and >200 mg/kg, respectively. The active concentration of DJ was retained in the kidneys of the affected mice for a surprisingly longer time than that of PPA. In addition to the higher activity of DJ than of PPA against the organisms, this fact should contribute to its higher effectiveness. DJ was also more effective than carbenicillin on respiratory tract infections in rats with *K. pneumoniae* SK, although it was less so than gentamicin.

FIG. 1. *Chemical structure of DJ-6783.*

TABLE 1. *Antimicrobial potency against clinical isolates[a]*

Organism	No. of strains	ID_{50} ($\mu g/ml$)				ID_{75} ($\mu g/ml$)				Median MIC ($\mu g/ml$)			
		DJ	MIL	PPA	NA	DJ	MIL	PPA	NA	DJ	MIL	PPA	NA
E. coli	100	0.11	0.27	1.13	3.09	0.17	0.37	1.49	4.85	0.19	0.39	1.56	3.13
K. pneumoniae	100	0.28	0.59	1.39	5.20	0.37	0.70	2.26	8.44	0.39	0.78	1.56	6.25
E. cloacae	100	0.06	0.13	0.65	3.00	0.09	0.19	1.39	5.50	0.10	0.19	0.78	3.13
C. freundii	26	0.19	0.30	1.10	3.72	0.56	0.65	3.72	11.9				
S. marcescens	100	0.46	1.56	4.23	9.70	3.87	9.70	58.9	>100	0.19	0.78		
P. mirabilis	98	0.13	0.61	1.97	4.85	0.17	1.21	2.79	6.40	0.19	0.78	3.13	6.25
P. vulgaris	52	0.04	0.18	1.21	2.60	0.06	0.30	1.49	3.72	0.05	0.19	1.56	3.13
P. morganii	59	0.06	0.14	0.75	1.49	0.09	0.18	1.30	2.79	0.10	0.19	0.78	1.56
P. rettgeri	31	0.12	0.15	2.11	3.94	0.19	0.30	5.20	6.18	0.10	0.10	1.56	6.25
P. aeruginosa	100	1.97	5.97	7.88	44.6	2.79	11.1	11.9	58.8	3.13	6.25	12.5	50
S. aureus	58	0.49	3.72	23.9	22.3	0.65	5.97	44.6	31.5	0.78	3.13		25
S. epidermidis	89	0.49	7.35	12.5	33.8	0.67	9.70	22.3	77.5	0.78	12.5	25	

[a] The test was conducted with the agar dilution method, at an inoculum size of 10^6 colony-forming units/ml. The antimicrobial potency is represented as the concentration of each antibiotic inhibiting growth of 50 and 75% of the strains (ID_{50} and ID_{75}) and the median MICs.

These data suggest that DJ is a broad-spectrum antimicrobial agent significantly more active than MIL, PPA, and NA against *Pseudomonas, Proteus, Enterobacter, Klebsiella, Serratia, Citrobacter, Haemophilus,* and *Staphylococcus.* Of special interest is the potent activity of this agent against *Pseudomonas* other than *P. aeruginosa,* such as *P. cepacia, P. putida,* and *P. maltophilia,* which have been studied as the nosocomial pathogens resistant to many chemotherapeutics and disinfectants. The laboratory studies of protection and remedy for infections in animals in part validated the high effectiveness of DJ.

DJ-6783, a New Synthetic Antimicrobial Agent: Absorption and Excretion in Animals and Humans

M. SANO,* N. TAKASUGI, K. ABE, M. TSUMURA, H. NOMURA,
H. OGAWA, AND Y. OSADA

Research Institute, Daiichi Seiyaku Co., Ltd., Edogawa-ku, Tokyo, 132 Japan

DJ-6783-Na, sodium 5-ethyl-5,8-dihydro-8-oxofuro[3,2-*b*][1,8]naphthyridine-7-carboxylate hydrate, was a new synthetic ketocarboxylic acid-type compound developed by our institute, which had a broad antibiotic spectrum against gram-positive and gram-negative bacteria. This paper describes the metabolic fate of DJ-6783 in animals and humans to clarify the disposition of the drug and to estimate the therapeutic potency for humans.

Animal studies: blood levels. After oral administration of [^{14}C]DJ-6783-Na, the maximum serum levels of radioactivity in rats, dogs, and monkeys were 10.9 (whole blood), 33.2, and 51.9 μg-equivalents of free drug per ml, at 4, 3, and 4 h, respectively (Fig. 1). The radioactivity levels decreased slowly, with half-lives of approximately 2.8, 6.5, and 7.0 h in rats, dogs, and monkeys, respectively. Among the animals used here, the serum levels of radioactivity and intact drug in monkeys were higher than those in others.

Protein binding. Sera obtained from 0.5 to 24 h after oral administration of the drug in rats, dogs, and monkeys were subjected to ultrafiltration and to gel filtration by Sephadex G-25. Percentages bound by ultrafiltration and gel filtration were 93.8 and 89.7 in rats, 87.6 and 70.8 in dogs, and 95.8 and 89.5 in monkeys, respectively. According to the data obtained from both methods, most of the drug was firmly associated with serum protein.

Distribution. The distribution was quantitatively examined at several times after administration in rats and also studied by autoradiography in rats and immature dogs. The levels of radioactivity were high in the blood, liver, kidneys, lungs, and heart and slightly high in the adrenals, thyroid, pituitary gland, prostate gland, and testes. The disappearance curves of radioactivity in tissues were similar to that of whole blood, and most tissue levels reached maximums at 2 to 8 h after dosing. The tissue distribution of radioactivity by autoradiograph suggested that most activity was observed in the gastric intestine, liver, and kidneys. Specific observations were presence of radioactivity on the epiphyseal cartilage, especially in immature dogs.

Urinary, fecal, and biliary excretions. Excretions of radioactivity into urine and feces in rats, dogs, and monkeys were 34 and 60%, 29 and 58%, and 58 and 2% of the dose, respectively. Species differences in main excretion route were observed. About 38% of the dose was excreted into the bile within 24 h in bile duct-cannulated rats.

Metabolism. Many radioactive metabolites were observed in urine in all animals, but the biologically active metabolite isolated so far has proved to be unchanged drug. *N*-Hydroxyethyl metabolite was detected as the main metabolite in dogs. Urinary metabolites contained glucuronides of the drug and other polar metabolites.

Human studies. The studies in humans were carried out by use of liquid chromatographic determination and bioassay.

Blood levels. Three doses of DJ-6783-Na (250, 500, and 1,000 mg-equivalents of free acid per man) were examined in healthy male volunteers, and good dose responses of the drug in serum levels were observed. The absorption of the drug in fasted men was compared with that in nonfasted men, and the maximum concentrations appeared 2 h faster in fasted than in nonfasted individuals (Fig. 2). Repeating administrations were carried out at a dose of 500 mg equivalents of free acid per man twice daily for

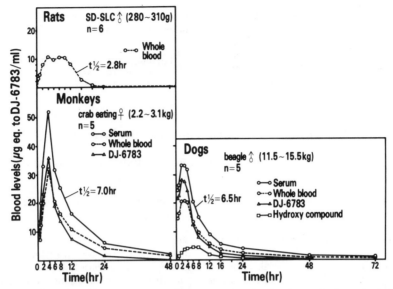

FIG. 1. *Blood levels of radioactivity and DJ-6783 in several animals after a single oral administration of 23.1 mg of [^{14}C]DJ-6783-Na (99.0%, 0.68 mCi/mmol) per kg (20 mg equivalent of free drug per kg). Monkeys and dogs were fasted for 16 h before dosing, but rats were nonfasted.*

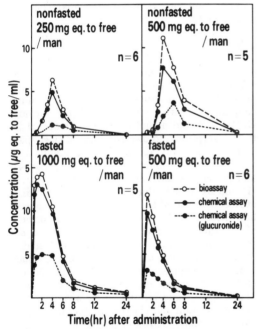

FIG. 2. *Serum concentrations of DJ-6783 and its glucuronide after a single oral administration of DJ-6783-Na in humans.*

3 days. No specially noticeable accumulation of the drug was observed during the trial. Pharmacokinetic studies were performed, using repeating-trial data. In the first medication, K_a,

K_d, V_d, $t_{1/2}$, T_{max} and C_{max} were 1.140, 0.468, 0.409, 1.937, 3.065, and 10.952, respectively; in the second medication they were 0.937, 0.329, 0.588, 2.298, 2.498, and 7.911, respectively. Slower absorption and excretion were recognized in the second medication (at night).

Protein binding. Protein binding examinations in vitro were performed with human serum albumin solution and human serum in several concentrations of DJ-6783-Na. Percentages of drug bound were 83 with human serum albumin and 93 with human serum.

Excretion. Seventy to eighty percent of the dose was totally excreted into urine in the form of intact free acid and ester-type glucuronide within 48 h. Urinary levels of the intact drug reached to 33 μg-equivalents of free drug per ml in the urine excreted from 2 to 4 h after oral administration of DJ-6783-Na at 500 mg-equivalents of free drug per man.

Metabolism. The main metabolite in human urine and serum was glucuronide of the drug. Other metabolites have not been detected so far.

Ratio of values by chemical assay versus bioassay. Apparent discrepancies were found between the values by bioassay and by chemical assay in serum and urine. The reason for these seems to be hydrolysis of a part of the glucuronide in the sample during the incubation in bioassay.

Conclusion. The above results suggested that DJ-6783-Na was well absorbed from the intestine and excreted almost completely within

48 h in humans and animals. But species differences in drug behaviors in blood levels, excretion routes, and metabolism were observed among rats, dogs, monkeys, and humans. Especially, a higher concentration of DJ-6783 in serum was shown to be characteristic behavior when compared with those of similar compounds which have appeared in some publications (1).

1. **Edelson, J., C. Davison, and D. P. Benziger.** 1977. Quinolone and "azaquinolone" antimicrobial agents. Drug Metab. Rev. **6**:105–148.

A6888, a New Macrolide Antibiotic Complex Related to the Cirramycins

STEPHEN M. NASH,* LAVERNE D. BOECK, PAUL W. ENSMINGER, MARVIN M. HOEHN, AND KAY F. KOCH

The Lilly Research Laboratories, Eli Lilly and Company, Indianapolis, Indiana 46206, U.S.A.

The A6888 complex of macrolide antibiotics was active against gram-positive aerobic and anaerobic bacteria. This paper describes the fermentation, isolation, structural properties, and biological evaluation of the four major factors. Factors A and F have been identified as cirramycins B and A_1, and factors C and X have been shown to be new macrolides.

Fermentation. *Streptomyces flocculus* NRRL 11459 was grown in a fermentation medium that contained 1.5% glucose, 1.5% soybean meal, 0.1% acid-hydrolyzed casein, 0.3% blackstrap molasses, and 0.25% $CaCO_3$. Fermenters were incubated for 4 to 5 days at 25°C. The fermentation was characterized by a highly unusual antibiotic production profile. Antibiotic production began at approximately 30 h, midway in the trophophase, and peaked within an extremely short time, sometimes less than 2 h. Maximum antibiotic, in terms of activity and number of components, appeared in the broth before biomass proliferation ceased. Factors A and F were isolated, primarily, from 35- to 40-h broth filtrates. The isolation of A6888C was facilitated by allowing the fermentation to continue until approximately 90 h, when the quantities of factors A and F were greatly reduced. Disappearance of some factors appeared to result from degradation or bioconversion, or both, by the cell mass of *S. flocculus.*

Broth potency was monitored by a photometric method, using liquid cultures of *Staphylococcus aureus* NRRL B-314 as the test organism.

Isolation. The fermentation broth (pH ~ 6.5) was adjusted to pH 3.0 to 3.5 and filtered with filter aid (Johns-Manville, Hyflo Super Cel). The filtrate was extracted with ethyl acetate to remove, at low pH, the inactive acidic and neutral extractables. The extracted filtrate was adjusted to pH 7.0 and extracted with ethyl acetate to obtain the complex of macrolides. Factors were partially fractionated by countercurrent distribution with five transfers, using benzene and Sorenson citrate buffer at pH 5.8. The factor-enriched preparations were subjected to high-performance liquid chromatography, using Quantum LP-1 silica gel (dry packed). Gradient elution with chloroform to 9:1 chloroform-methanol (each solvent containing 0.01% ethanolamine) gave rise to purified preparations of A6888 factors. Thin-layer chromatography of the A6888 factors established the following R_f values on Merck silica gel 60 F254 plates in 3:1 chloroform-methanol: A6888A, 0.86; A6888C, 0.58; A6888X, 0.53; A6888F, 0.24.

Physicochemical characteristics. Factor A of A6888 was isolated as a white crystalline compound with the empirical formula $C_{37}H_{59}O_{12}N$ and a molecular weight of 709 by field desorption and electron impact mass spectrometry. A6888A appeared to be identical to the macrolide antibiotics cirramycin B, B-58941, and possibly acumycin as described by Suzuki (1) and by Von Keller-Schierlein (3). Factor F of A6888 appeared to be identical to the macrolide cirramycin A_1, having an empirical formula of $C_{31}H_{51}O_{10}N$ (molecular weight, 597) as described by Tsukiura et al. (2). Factors C and X of A6888 were shown to be 16-membered macrolides of empirical formulas $C_{37}H_{61}O_{12}N$ and $C_{37}H_{63}O_{12}N$, respectively. Molecular weights of 711 (factor C) and 713 (factor X) were found by field desorption and electron impact mass spectrometry. Both factors displayed a UV λ_{max} of 240 nm (ϵ 14,500), which is characteristic of this series of macrolides. The nuclear magnetic resonance (NMR) spectral data were consistent with a 16-membered aglycone, the sugar mycaminose, and a sugar identified as the reduction product of cinerulose. ^{1}H-NMR, ^{13}C-NMR, circular dichroism, and mass spectral data were used to establish that A6888C differs from

A6888A at the terminal sugar (cinerulose). ^{13}C-NMR for A6888A showed a chemical shift at 211.0 ppm for the carbonyl function in the terminal sugar. Chemical shifts of 67.3 and 67.2 ppm were found for factors C and X, respectively. The mass spectra gave an $m/e = 115$ (factors C and X) and an $m/e = 113$ (factor A) which were assigned to the terminal sugar fragments. Circular dichroism displayed ellipticities at 240 and 297 nm for factor A and at 240 nm for factors C and X. These data established the 4″-dihydrocinerulose sugar in A6888 factors C and X. A6888X was shown to differ from A6888C in the aglycone portion of the molecule. ^{1}H-NMR, ^{13}C-NMR, and mass spectral data established that the aldehyde moiety present in factor C was not present in factor X, but had been replaced by an alcohol moiety. The ^{1}H-NMR displayed a chemical shift at δ 9.70 for the aldehyde in A6888C which was not present in the spectrum of A6888X. The mass spectra contained the following mass ions: $m/e = 407$ (factors A and C, aldehyde moiety) and $m/e = 409$ (factor X,

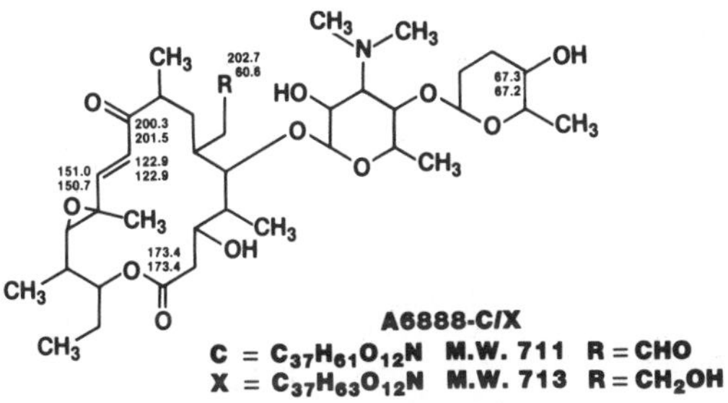

TABLE 1. *Biological evaluation*

Disc-Plate Zone Sizes (mm) of A6888 Factors

Bacteria		Erythromycin 100 μg Discs	A6888-C 100 μg Discs	A6888-X 300 μg Discs
S. aureus	3055	30.8	21.6	27.8
	3074*	11.6	18.8	24.2
	3130**	15.2	23	28.6
S. pyogenes C203		27	21	24.2
Group D. Strep.		22.2	18.4	22.5
S. pneumoniae I		31	24	36
E. coli EC-14		13.2	0	14
P. rettgeri PR-2		0	0	8.6
K. pneumoniae KL-14		12.3	0	11.3
Sh. flexneri SH-4		14.4	13.2	12.5
S. typhosa SA-12		13.3	0	8.8

* Penicillin-Resistant
** Methicillin-Resistant

A-6888 Therapy in Experimental Mouse Infections

Mouse Infection	PD$_{50}$ Values—mg/kg x 2 (S.C.)		
	Erythromycin	A6888C	A6888X
S. aureus 3055	2.9	5.0	>70
S. pyogenes C203	2.6	4.7	>70

alcohol moiety). Figure 1 compares the structures of A6888 factors C and X with key ^{13}C-NMR chemical shifts.

Biological evaluation. A6888 factors C and X inhibited a variey of gram-positive bacteria, including *Staphylococcus aureus*, *Streptococcus pyogenes*, *Streptococcus pneumoniae*, and group D *Streptococcus*. Both factors also inhibited anaerobic organisms. In vivo activity of factors C and X is shown in Table 1.

A6888-C/X

C = C$_{37}$H$_{61}$O$_{12}$N M.W. 711 R = CHO
X = C$_{37}$H$_{63}$O$_{12}$N M.W. 713 R = CH$_2$OH

FIG. 1. *Comparison of ^{1}H- and ^{13}C-NMR and mass spectral data indicated that the structures of factors C and X differ in the aldehyde moiety of factor C being replaced by an alcohol in factor X.*

1. **Suzuki, T.** 1970. The structure of an antibiotic, B-58941. Bull. Chem. Soc. Jpn. **43**:292.
2. **Tsukiura, H., M. Konishi, M. Saka, T. Naito, and H. Kawaguchi.** 1969. Studies on cirramycin A$_1$. III. Structure of cirramycin A$_1$. J. Antibiot. **22**:89–99.
3. **Von Keller-Schierlein, W.** 1973. Chemie der Makrolid-Antibiotica. Fortschr. Chem. Org. Naturst. **30**:314–445.

Bu-2313, a New Antibiotic Complex Active Against Anaerobes: Structure Determination of Bu-2313A and Bu-2313B

MITSUAKI TSUNAKAWA, SOICHIRO TODA, TAKA-AKI OKITA, MINORU HANADA, SUSUMU NAKAGAWA,* HIROSHI TSUKIURA, TAKAYUKI NAITO, AND HIROSHI KAWAGUCHI

Bristol-Banyu Research Institute, Ltd., Meguro, Tokyo, Japan

Bu-2313 is a new anti-anaerobic antibiotic complex produced by an unidentified actinomycete, strain E864-61. The production, isolation, and various properties of Bu-2313 have been reported by H. Tsukiura, K. Tomita, M. Hanada, S. Kobaru, M. Tsunakawa, K. Fujisawa, and H. Kawaguchi (this volume). Two components of the antibiotic complex, Bu-2313A (I; C$_{27}$H$_{35}$NO$_9$) and Bu-2313B (II; C$_{26}$H$_{33}$NO$_9$), are acidic substances obtained as pale yellow crystals, giving a positive reaction with ferric chloride.

The UV spectrum of I in acidic solution exhibited absorbance maxima at 242, 358, and 375 nm ($E_{1\,cm}^{1\%}$ values of 170, 645, and 555) and that of II exhibited absorbance maxima at 237, 353, and 370 nm ($E_{1\,cm}^{1\%}$ values of 170, 668, and 580). In alkaline solution, absorbance maxima occurred at 262, 286, and 337 nm ($E_{1\,cm}^{1\%}$ values of 375, 393, and 430) in I and at 253, 286, and 331 nm ($E_{1\,cm}^{1\%}$ values of 345, 411, and 467) in II. These UV absorptions with pH-dependent shifts observed for I and II are similar to those reported for tirandamycin (3) and streptolydigin (1), suggesting that Bu-2313A and Bu-2313B are $\alpha,\beta,\gamma,\delta$-dienoyltetramic acid antibiotics.

The nuclear magnetic resonance (NMR) spectrum of I showed three $>$CH—CH$_3$, two $\geqslant$C—CH$_3$, one N—CH$_3$, and one COOCH$_3$ signals, whereas II exhibited three $>$CH—CH$_3$, two $\geqslant$C—CH$_3$, and one COOCH$_3$ (appeared as a 5H singlet combined with another 2H signal) signals, but no N—CH$_3$ signal. The NMR spectrum of II showed an amide NH at δ 6.98 which disappeared by D$_2$O addition. This NH signal was not present in the spectrum of I. In other respects, the NMR spectra of I and II were alike. This, coupled with the molecular formulas, indicated that I was an N-methyl derivative of II. The presence of a methyl ester group was confirmed by hydrolysis of II with 1 N NaOH-CH$_3$OH (1:1) at room temperature to afford the acid (III) whose NMR spectrum showed no O-methyl signal at around δ 3.76.

In support of the presence of the $\alpha,\beta,\gamma,\delta$-dienoyl chromophore, the NMR spectrum of II showed two deshielded sharp doublets ($J = 15.6$ Hz) at δ 6.96 (2-H) and δ 7.41 (3-H) owing to vicinal *trans* protons on the α,β-unsaturated carbonyl with no proton in the γ position. The γ-methyl (4-CH$_3$) signal was found at δ 1.87, and the olefinic δ-proton (5-H) appeared at δ 5.96 as

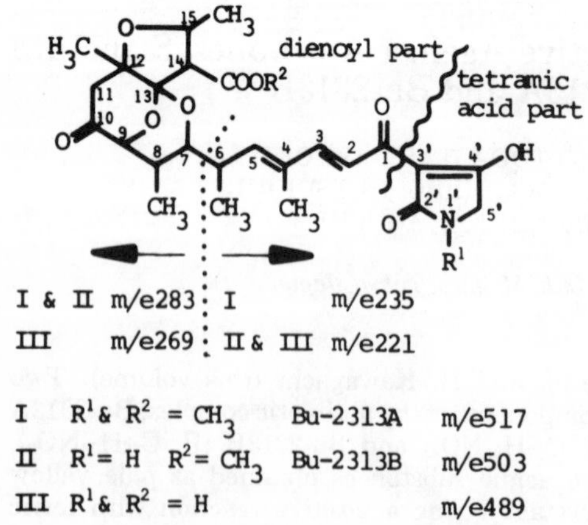

FIG. 1. *Structures of compounds I, II, and III.*

TABLE 1. *Spin decoupling experiment on IV*

Proton (δ in ppm)		Multiplicity change	Splitting decoupled (Hz)
Irradiated	Observed		
6-H (2.76)	6-CH$_3$ (1.03)	d → s	7.0
	5-H (5.89)	d → s	10.0
	7-H (3.36)	dd → d	2.0
8-H (2.07)	7-H (3.36)	dd → d	11.0
	8-CH$_3$ (0.87)	d → s	7.0
	9-H (4.01)	d → s	5.0
15-CH$_3$ (1.31)	15-H (4.49)	dq → d	6.0
15-H (4.49)	15-CH$_3$ (1.31)	d → s	6.0
	14-H (2.92)	d → s	7.5
14-H (2.92)	15-H (4.49)	dq → q	7.5

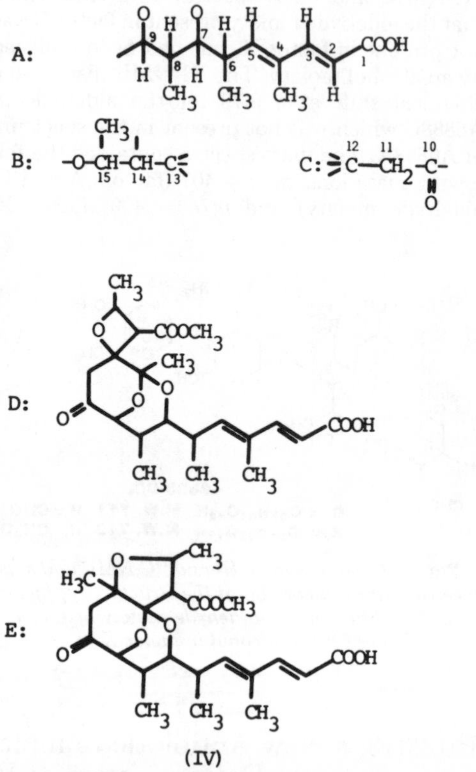

FIG. 2. *Structural units A through C and two possible structures, D and E, for IV.*

a doublet ($J = 10$ Hz) broadened by coupling with the γ-methyl protons. The above-mentioned signals were also observed in the spectrum of I.

A two-proton methylene singlet (5'-H) was observed in the NMR spectra of both I and II. This methylene signal and the amide proton mentioned above were assigned to those of the tetramic acid moiety in comparison with the NMR spectrum of tirandamycin (2). In the mass spectra of I, II, and III, the common fragmentations which occurred between C-6 and C-7 were in good agreement with the respective structures (Fig. 1).

Periodate oxidation of II afforded the dienoic acid (IV) which retained three $>$CH—CH$_3$ (δ 0.87, 1.03, and 1.31), two $\geqq$C—CH$_3$ (δ 1.42 and 1.79), one COOCH$_3$ (δ 3.76), and three olefinic protons, at δ 5.72 and 7.25 (AB quartet, J = 15.5 Hz) and at 5.89 (broad doublet, J = 10 Hz). The UV absorbance resulting from a γ,δ-disubstituted *trans,trans-α,β,γ,δ*-dienoic acid occurs at 257 nm (ϵ 26,000), which is consistent with those of tirandamycic acid (2) and streptolic acid (4). The carboxylic acid (IV) was hydrolyzed with aqueous NaOH-methanol to give the dibasic acid (V), whose infrared and NMR spectra showed a lack of carbonyl at 1,740 cm^{-1} and O-methyl signal at 3.76 owing to the COOCH$_3$ group.

The preceding spectral data and the NMR spin-decoupling results (Table 1) showed that IV had the partial structures A and B. A further three-carbon unit, C, in the structure of IV was deduced from the NMR data of the NaBH$_4$ reduction product, VI, and its acetyl derivative, VII. The doublet at δ 4.01 owing to the 9-methine changed to a multiplet in VI (δ 3.90) and VII (δ 4.00). One new proton multiplet appeared in the spectrum of VI at around δ 4.2 and shifted to δ 5.25 in the O-acetate (VII). In addition, two

doublets at δ 2.56 and δ 2.95, with a large J value (17.5 Hz) owing to the isolated, geminal methylene protons (11-CH$_2$) of IV, collapsed to multiplets and shifted to around δ 1.8 in VI and δ 2.2 in VII. Assembling of the structural units A, B, and C together with a tertiary carbon-linked methyl and a methoxycarbonyl gives the compound IV the two possible structures, D and E (Fig. 2).

X-ray diffraction analysis of the *p*-bromophenacyl ester of IV (VIII), performed by K. Sasaki (Nagoya University, Nagoya, Japan; personal communication), revealed the structure of the dienoyl part. Hence, the structure E was assigned to IV, which in turn established the gross structure of Bu-2313A and Bu-2313B.

1. Eble, T. E., C. M. Large, W. H. DeVries, G. F. Crum, and J. W. Shell. 1956. Streptolydigin. A new antimicrobial antibiotic. II. Isolation and characterization. Antibiot. Annu. **1955/1956**:893–896.
2. MacKellar, F. A., M. F. Grostic, E. C. Olson, R. J. Wnuk, A. R. Branfman, and K. L. Rinehart, Jr. 1971. Tirandamycin. I. Structure assignment. J. Am. Chem. Soc. **93**:4943–4945.
3. Meyer, C. E. 1971. Tirandamycin, a new antibiotic. Isolation and characterization. J. Antibiot. **24**:558–560.
4. Rinehart, K. L., Jr., J. R. Beck, W. W. Epstein, and L. D. Spicer. 1963. Streptolydigin. I. Streptolic acid. J. Am. Chem. Soc. **85**:4035–4037.

Bu-2313, a New Antibiotic Complex Active Against Anaerobes: Production, Isolation, and Properties of Bu-2313A and Bu-2313B

HIROSHI TSUKIURA,* KOJI TOMITA, MINORU HANADA,
SEIKICHI KOBARU, MITSUAKI TSUNAKAWA, KEI-ICHI FUJISAWA,
AND HIROSHI KAWAGUCHI

Bristol-Banyu Research Institute, Ltd., Meguro, Tokyo, Japan

In the antibiotic screening program using *Bacteroides fragilis* of the assay test species, an oligosporic actinomycete strain, E864-61, was found to produce a new antibiotic complex, Bu-2313. It was extracted from the fermentation broth and separated into two components, A and B. Both components showed antibiotic activities against various anaerobic and some aerobic bacteria. As reported by M. Tsunakawa, S. Toda, T. Okita, M. Hanada, S. Nakagawa, H. Tsukiura, T. Naito, and H. Kawaguchi (this volume), Bu-2313A and Bu-2313B belong to the dienoyl tetramic acid group of antibiotics, which includes streptolydigin (1), tirandamycin (3), and nocamycin (2).

The producing strain, E864-61, formed single

spores and spore chains bearing 2 to 8 spores. The color of the aerial mycelium was dull bluish green or light grayish green. Two types of pigment, violet and dark green, were produced in agar media. The spores had a smooth surface. It grew at 20 to 50°C. The cell wall of strain E864-61 contained *meso*-diaminopimelic acid. The characteristics of strain E864-61 are very similar to those of the genus *Microtetraspora*.

Strain E864-61 was fermented in shake flasks and stir jars. Vegetative medium contained 3% glucose, 3% soybean meal, 1% corn steep liquor, and 0.5% CaCO$_3$. Fermentation medium for shake flasks was composed of 3% sucrose, 3% linseed meal, 0.3% (NH$_4$)$_2$SO$_4$, 0.003% ZnSO$_4$·7H$_2$O, and 0.5% CaCO$_3$, whereas that for jar fermentors contained 3% glucose, 3% soybean meal, 1% corn steep liquor, and 0.5% CaCO₃. Antibiotic production reached the maximum on day 6 by shaking culture and after 72 h in jar fermentors. The antibiotic activity in the fermentation broth was determined by a paper disk-agar plate method, using *B. fragilis* A20928 as the test strain, which was grown on a GAM (Gifu anaerobe medium) agar plate under anaerobic conditions in a GasPak jar (BBL).

The harvested broth was filtered. The filtrate was adsorbed on a column of porous adsorption resin (DIAION HP-20) at pH 8, and the activity was eluted with 95% methanol. The activity in the mycelium was extracted by methanol. The

methanol extract and active fractions from the HP-20 process were combined, concentrated, and extracted with ethyl acetate. The extract was concentrated to an oily solid which was purified by carbon chromatography. The active eluates were evaporated to leave a brown solid which was crystallized from methanol to give a crystalline mixture of components A and B. The mixture was separated by HP-20 chromatography developed with 90% methanol. The first active fractions, containing component B, were evaporated, and the residue was crystallized from methanol to give pale yellow needles. The second active fractions contained components A and B, which were separated from each other by

TABLE 1. *Physicochemical properties of Bu-2313A and Bu-2313B*[a]

Bu-2313 component	Melting point (°C)	Optical rotation ($[\alpha]_D^{26}$)	pKa' (50% EtOH)	Mol wt (mass spectroscopy, m/e)	Formula	UV l_{max} in nm ($E_{1\,cm}^{1\%}$) in: 0.01 N HCl– 95% EtOH	UV l_{max} in nm ($E_{1\,cm}^{1\%}$) in: 0.01 N NaOH– 95% EtOH
A	116 ~ 118	−58 (c 0.5, MeOH)	5.2	517	$C_{27}H_{35}NO_9$	242 (170) 358 (645) 375 (555, sh)	262 (375) 286 (393) 337 (430)
B	160 ~ 162	−69.9 (c 0.3, MeOH)	4.9	503	$C_{26}H_{33}NO_9$	237 (170) 353 (668) 370 (580, sh)	253 (345) 286 (411) 331 (467)

[a] Abbreviations: EtOH, ethyl hydroxide; MeOH, methyl hydroxide.

TABLE 2. *Antibacterial spectra of Bu-2313 A and Bu-2313 B*

Test species	Strain	Test medium[a]	MIC (μg/ml)[b] Bu-2313A	MIC (μg/ml)[b] Bu-2313B
Aerobic bacteria				
Staphylococcus aureus	209P	A	25	25
Staphylococcus aureus	Smith	A	12.5	12.5
Sarcina lutea	PCI 1001	A	25	12.5
Streptococcus pyogenes	A9604	B	0.8	0.4
Bacillus subtilis	PCI 219	A	1.6	1.6
Bacillus cereus	ATCC 10702 A	A	0.8	0.8
Escherichia coli	Juhl	A	>100	>100
Klebsiella pneumoniae	A9678	A	>100	>100
Proteus morganii	A9553	A	>100	>100
Neisseria meningitidis	A20049	B	1.6	0.8
Haemophilus influenzae	A9832	B	0.8	0.4
Anaerobic bacteria				
Bacteroides fragilis	A20926	C	0.2	0.1
Bacteroides fragilis	A20928-1	C	0.1	0.1
Sphaerophorus necrophorus	A15202	C	0.2	0.1
Fusobacterium varium	ATCC 8501	C	0.1	0.1
Acidoaminococcus fermentans	ATCC 25085	C	0.2	0.1
Veillonella parvula	ATCC 17745	C	0.2	0.1
Clostridium perfringens	A9635	C	0.4	0.2
Clostridium perfringens	A21284	C	0.4	0.2
Propionibacterium acnes	A21933	C	0.2	0.2
Peptococcus prevotii	ATCC 9321	C	0.2	0.1
Peptostreptococcus anaerobius	B43	C	0.4	0.4

[a] A, Nutrient agar (Eiken); B, Gonococcus medium (Eiken); C, GAM medium (Nissui) in a GasPak jar.
[b] Twofold agar dilution method.

silica gel chromatography developed with chloroform. The fractions containing component A were concentrated and crystallized from methanol to give pale yellow needles.

Bu-2313A and Bu-2313B were acidic substances. They were readily soluble in most organic solvents, such as lower alcohols, ethyl acetate, chloroform, and benzene; slightly soluble in hexane and alkaline water; and practically insoluble in water. Both components reacted positively with ferric chloride but gave negative reactions in ninhydrin, anthrone, Sakaguchi, and Tollen tests. The physicochemical properties of Bu-2313A and Bu-2313B are summarized in Table 1.

The in vitro antibacterial activities of Bu-2313A and Bu-2313B were determined by the serial twofold agar dilution method. Bu-2313A and Bu-2313B inhibited the growth of aerobic organisms, such as streptococci, *Neisseria* species, and *Haemophilus influenzae*, but only weakly inhibited strains of staphylococci and *Enterobacteriaceae*. However, Bu-2313A and Bu-2313B showed strong inhibitory activities against a wide range of anaerobic bacteria, including gram-positive and gram-negative rods and cocci (Table 2). The intrinsic activity of Bu-2313B was approximately two times stronger than that of Bu-2313A.

The in vivo activities of Bu-2313A and Bu-2313B were evaluated in experimental infections in mice produced by two anaerobic bacteria, *B. fragilis* and *Clostridium perfringens*, and by one aerobic pathogen, *Streptococcus pyogenes*. Bu-2313A and Bu-2313B were nearly equally active against systemic infections caused by *C. perfringens* and *S. pyogenes* when the animals were treated subcutaneously, the 50% protective doses being 6.3 mg/kg for *C. perfringens* and 7.6 ~ 9.0 mg/kg for *S. pyogenes*. When the treatment was made by the oral route, Bu-2313B showed greater efficacy than did Bu-2313A. Against a localized infection of *B. fragilis*, Bu-2313B was effective by subcutaneous and oral administrations, the 50% protective doses being 60 and 200 mg/kg, respectively. The acute subcutaneous LD$_{50}$'s determined in mice were 90 mg/kg for Bu-2313A and 320 mg/kg for Bu-2313B.

1. Eble, T. E., C. M. Large, W. H. DeVries, G. F. Crum, and J. W. Shell. 1956. Streptolydigin. A new antimicrobial antibiotic. II. Isolation and characterization. Antibiot. Annu. 1955/1956:893–896.
2. Gauze, G. F., M. A. Sveshnikova, R. S. Ukholina, G. N. Komarova, and V. S. Bazhanov. 1977. Production of nocamycin, a new antibiotic by *Nocardiopsis syringae* sp. nov. Antibiotiki (Moscow) 22:483–486.
3. Meyers, C. E. 1971. Tirandamycin, a new antibiotic. Isolation and characterization. J. Antibiot. 24:558–560.

Structure of U-54,702 Using Computer-Assisted Structure Elucidation

L. A. DOLAK* AND M. E. MUNK

The Upjohn Company, Research Laboratories, Kalamazoo, Michigan 49001, and
Arizona State University, Tempe, Arizona 85281, U.S.A.

Structure elucidation is one of the primary functions of organic chemistry. When products of natural origin are considered, the chemist is faced with the possibility of having one of numerous known structural families or with proposing entirely novel structural classes. The array of spectroscopic and chemical methodology which provides the clues whereby the structure problem is solved has grown considerably in the past 20 years and promises to continue to do so. In the case of antibiotics it is now a relatively simple matter to determine if a given antibiotic is a known compound or if it belongs to a known family. Whenever this is not true, the structure chemist must present sound reasons for proposing new structural classes. The classical method to accomplish this consists of "doodling" until

one generates a structure which fits all the data available. This is generally, but not always, the correct structure. Computer programs are now available which draw all possible structures for a given molecular formula. Because of the large number of isomers possible for even small molecules, this is an exercise in futility unless the program draws only those structures consistent with data normally available to the chemist (1, 5).

Such a program has been developed at Arizona State University which allows interaction between the machine and the chemist. The program consists of a molecular assembler and a Draw program. The structure of U-54,702 has been limited to two possibilities using CASE (computer-assisted structure elucidation). We believe this to be the first example of a structure solution for an unknown compound by a computer program. We have used CASE on several other new antibiotics with some success.

The molecular formula ($C_7H_9ClN_2O$) of U-54,702 (2) was derived from high-resolution mass spectroscopy of its mono- and di-trimethylsilyl (TMS) derivatives prepared for gas chromatography-mass spectrometry. Since trimethylsilylylimidazole produced only the mono-TMS derivative, which could then be acylated with a variety of reagents, the molecule must contain one hydroxyl and one NH moiety. The C-13 spectrum showed seven lines which could be generally assigned using correlation tables. ^{13}C magnetic resonance [CMR], D_2O, ext TMS, pH 2: 44.0 δ, t; 54.6, t; 61.1, d; 104.7, s; 124.1, d; 154.7, d; 169.8, s. The proton magnetic resonance spectrum indicated that the molecule consisted of two isolated fragments: a vinyl group (CH=CH) and a 3-carbon fragment, CH_2—CHX—CH_2, where X had to be a hetero atom. (Proton magnetic resonance, D_2O, ext TMS, pH 2: 7.5 δ, 1H, $J = 5.5$ cps; 6.5, 1H, $J = 5.5$; 5.0, 1H; 4.0, 2H; 2.5, 2H. Couplings for CH_1H_2—CH_3X—CH_4H_5: $J_{12} = -12$, $J_{13} = 6$, $J_{45} = -14$, $J_{13} = 6$, $J_{23} = 4$, $J_{34} = 6$, $J_{35} = 7$.) Since the UV spectrum (maxima at 250 and 212 nm) disappeared on reduction to dihydro U-54,702, the vinyl group had to be conjugated to a second double bond. The second double bond was resistant to catalytic reduction. The UV spectrum did not change with pH so an enol or nitrogen attached to a vinyl group seemed unlikely. The chemical shifts of the new triplets observed in the C-13 spectrum of dihydro U-54,702 were consistent with this reasoning. (CMR, D_2O, ext TMS, 33.6 δ, t; 35.8 δ, t; 47.8 δ, t; 53.5 δ, t; 58.8 δ, d; 103.7 δ, s; 170.3 δ, s.)

The above data must be reduced to statements which the program can accept. The actual input statements for the molecular assembler can be varied, with resultant families of structures generated. These were examined for numerous attempts, and certain structural features were routinely rejected because of expected lack of stability. The input for one run which was useful is reproduced below with an explanation of the notations used. The prompt from the program is underlined.

(1) Molecular Formula: C7H9N2OX
    USER MESSAGE THE FORMULA CORRESPONDS TO 4 UNSATURATION(S)
(2) Fragment: CH2⟨OØØ⟩—CH⟨CØØ⟩—CH2⟨OØØ⟩
    This states that neither methylene group can be attached to oxygen and that the methine cannot be attached to carbon.
(3) Fragment: C⟨HØØ⟩—CH=CH⟨=11⟩—C⟨HØØ⟩
    Neither end of the vinyl group may be attached

to a hetero atom. The carbons so attached may not bear protons. The vinyl group must be conjugated.

(4) Constraint: Atom OH1 1 1; Atom NH1 1 1; Atom CH3 Ø Ø
    This requires the presence of exactly one hydroxyl and one NH group and forbids the presence of a methyl group.
(5) Constraint:
    HYBRID C   SP1 Ø Ø; HYBRID CH1 SP2 2 2
    HYBRID CHØ SP2 1 2; HYBRID CHØ SP3 Ø 1
    These statements forbid formation of a triple bond, require the presence of exactly two vinylic protons, and allow the singlets in the CMR spectrum to be due to either two SP2 carbons or one SP2 and one SP3 hybridized carbon.
(6) Constraint: CSIZE 3 4 Ø Ø
    This forbids the formation of 3- or 4-membered rings.
(7) Constraint: SPRUNE: 7 7
    This requires that all the carbons be in different environments since seven lines were observed in the CMR spectrum.
(8) Command: Start
(9) **USER MESSAGE** ASSEMBLY COMPLETE, 23 STRUCTURES ASSEMBLED

The structures are now saved on a temporary file and displayed on a CRT terminal or printed out using the Draw program. Of these 23 structures, 9 violated Bredt's Rule. Certain strained molecules are eliminated by the program (e.g., cyclobutadienes), but bridgehead double bonds have not been. Another 10 structures contained Cl—C≡N or HO—C≡N groups and were not considered further. The prohibition of small rings was considered in a separate run in which their presence was required. The appearance of unlikely functional groups such as N-chloramines can be eliminated by the use of an additional constraint called Substructure.

The structures considered further are shown in Fig. 1. No decision can be made regarding these two structures, which differ only in the placement of the hydroxyl and chlorine functions. Theoretical calculations indicated that

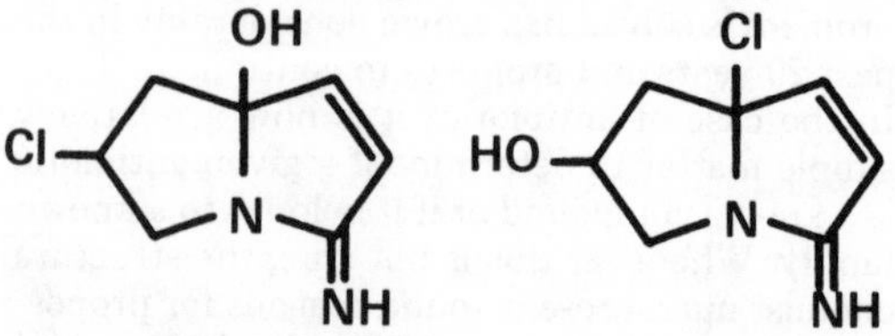

FIG. 1. *(Left)* Structure 1. U-54,702. *(Right)* Structure 2. Alternate structure.

structures 1 and 2 could give the observed UV spectrum (4). U-54,702 gave a positive nitroprusside but a negative Sakaguchi test, as expected for a cyclic amidine. We favored 2 over 1 since 1 resembles a hemiaminal, which would be unstable in acid. However, the structure of U-54,702 has been shown to be 1 by X-ray crystallography (3).

1. Djerassi, C., D. H. Smith, and T. H. Varkony. 1979. A novel role of computers in the natural products field. Naturwissenschaften **66**:9–21.

2. DeBoer, C., L. A. Dolak, and D. H. Peterson. 1978. U.S. Patent 4,113,855.

3. Horiuchi, Y., S. Kondo, T. Ikeda, D. Ikeda, K. Miura, M. Hamada, T. Takeuchi, and H. Umezawa. 1979. New antibiotics, clazamycins A and B. J. Antibiot. **32:** 762–764.

4. Kornilov, M. Yu, and V. P. Makovetskii. 1975. Electronic structure and spectra of 1,3-diaminoisoindoline, 1-imino-3-aminoisoindole, their derivatives and analogs. Ukr. Khim. Zh. (Russ. Ed.) **41**:933–939.

5. Smith, D. H., (ed.). 1977. Computer-assisted structure elucidation. ACS Symposium Series no. 54. American Chemical Society, Washington, D.C.

CP-47,433 and CP-47,434, New Polycyclic Ether Antibiotics Produced by a New Species of *Actinomadura*

J. TONE, R. SHIBAKAWA, H. MAEDA, K. INOUE, Y. YAMAUCHI, K. TSUKUDA, M. YAMADA, W. P. CULLEN, L. R. CHAPPEL, C. E. MOPPETT, J. R. OSCARSON, C. J. LAPLANTE, L. H. HUANG, AND W. D. CELMER*

Pfizer Central Research, Nagoya, Japan, and Groton, Connecticut 06340, U.S.A.

During the course of our antibiotic screening program, we isolated from a soil sample collected in Okayama, Japan, a strain of *Actinomadura* which produced CP-47,433 and CP-47,434, new members of the acidic polycyclic ether group of antibiotics, as major (95 to 96%) and minor components (4 to 5%), respectively (U.S. Patent 4,148,882, April 1979). The producing culture was taxonomically studied in accordance with the procedure described by Lechevalier and Lechevalier (3). The cultural characteristics were observed after 2 weeks of incubation at 28°C on the designated media. Regarding its morphological properties, hyphae were narrow, branched, 0.4 to 0.6 μm in diameter; hyphal swellings produced on tyrosine agar, terminal or intercalary; spores produced in short chains on the aerial mycelium, 4 to 15 spores per spore chain. The spore chains were straight, flexuous, hooked, or once or twice coiled. The spores were oval to elliptical and measured 1.2 to 2 by 0.8 to 1 μm. The culture is classified as *Actinomadura macra* Huang sp. nov. based on cell wall analysis indicating cell wall type III, sugar pattern B, and the morphological features showing short spore chains, and it has been deposited at the American Type Culture Collection under the accession number ATCC 31286. To our knowledge, this culture is the second case in which polyether antibiotics were isolated from a genus other than *Streptomyces*. The first case, CP-44,161, from the genus *Dactylosporangium*, was reported by us last year (U.S. Patent 4,081,532, March 1978; J. Tone, R. Shibakawa, H. Maeda, K. Inoue, S.

Nishiyama, M. Ishiguro, W. P. Cullen, J. B. Routien, L. R. Chappel, C. E. Moppett, M. T. Jefferson, and W. D. Celmer, Program Abstr. Intersci. Conf. Antimicrob. Agents Chemother. 18th, Atlanta, Ga., Abstr. no. 171, 1978).

Cells from a slant of the CP-47,433- and CP-47,434-producing culture grown on ATCC 172 medium were transferred to a 300-ml Erlenmeyer flask containing 50 ml of the inoculum medium which consisted of (in grams per liter): glucose, 10; starch, 20; yeast extract, 5; casein digest, 5; meat meal, 5; K_2HPO_4, 0.5; $CoCl_2 \cdot 6H_2O$, 0.002; $CaCO_3$, 4; at pH 7.1 to 7.2. The inoculum was shaken on a rotary shaker for 72 to 96 h at 28°C, and 5 to 10% of the grown inoculum was transferred to a 4-liter jar fermentor containing 2 liters of fermentation medium which consisted of (in grams per liter): glucose, 20; soy flour, 30; $Fe_2(SO_4)_3$, 0.3; $MnCl_2 \cdot 6H_2O$, 0.3; $CoCl_2 \cdot 6H_2O$, 0.002; at pH 6.9 to 7.1. It was stirred at 1,700 rpm, 30°C, with 1 vol/vol per min of air. Antibiotic titers of about 100 μg/ml were obtained in the final fermentor stage in approximately 72 to 120 h. The whole (unfiltered) broth was extracted with methylisobutyl ketone. The solvent extract was processed by a series of batch and chromatographic fractionations to afford a mixture of crystalline sodium salts of CP-47,433 and CP-47,434 (15:1, respectively). The individual components were isolated as crystalline-free acid and/or sodium salts (cf. physicochemical properties, Table 1). The crystalline silver salt of CP-47,433 proved suitable for X-ray structural analysis (performed by J.

TABLE 1. *Physicochemical properties of CP-47,433 and CP-47,434*

	CP-47,433 Free Acid	CP-47,433 Sodium Salt	CP-47,434 Sodium Salt
Molecular Weight	871.2	893.1	879.1
Elemental Analysis			
(C)	64.92	62.75	62.31
(H)	9.73	9.21	9.12
(O)	25.35	–	–
Molecular Formula	$C_?H_{??}O_{??}$	$C_?H_?O_{??}Na$	$C_?N_?O_{??}Na$
Specific Rotation $[\alpha]_D^{?}$	+16° (c = 1.0, methanol)	-0.2° (c = 1.0, methanol)	-1.3° (c = 1.0, methanol)
Melting Point	89-99 °C	226-232 °C	230-238 °C
UV Absorption	–	–	–
Solubility	Soluble in $CHCl_3$, Acetone, EtOAc and MeOH. Insoluble in H_2O.	same	same
IR (μ)	2.87, 3.42, 5.77, 6.85, 7.30, 8.05, 8.60, 9.20, 10.15, 10.53 and 11.45	3.40, 6.40, 6.85, 7.12, 7.25, 8.02, 8.38, 8.60, 9.40, 10.05, 10.49, 11.45, 12.65 and 13.25	3.40, 6.40, 6.85, 7.14, 7.27, 7.75, 8.05, 8.40, 8.62, 9.10, 9.40, 10.07, 10.50, 11.49, 12.65, and 13.25

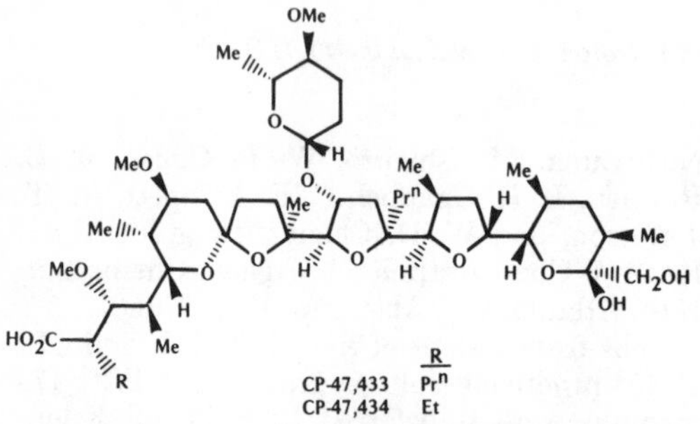

FIG. 1. *Structures of CP-47,433 and CP-47,434.*

Bordner), and the structure of CP-47,434 was elucidated by ^{13}C-nuclear magnetic resonance spectral analyses (performed by E. R. Whipple) (Fig. 1).

Various biological activities of the new ionophores have been investigated (U. S. Patent 4,148,882, April 1979). MICs of CP-47,433, CP-47,434, and their 15:1 mixtures were determined against a number of aerobic microorganisms in accordance with the standard broth dilution method. They showed relatively fair to good in vitro activity against most of the gram-positive organisms tested; little activity was observed against the gram-negative organisms. Good MIC values were determined for many gram-positive and gram-negative anaerobic microorganisms. CP-47,433, CP-47,434, and their 15:1 mixture exhibited activity against coccidial infections in poultry when we utilized published procedures (1, 4); when incorporated into the diet of chickens at levels of 10 to 20 ppm, these compounds were comparable to monensin at 100 ppm in controlling infections due to *Eimeria tenella, E. acervulina, E. maxima, E. brunetti,* and *E. necatrix.* CP-47,433, a 15:1 mixture of CP-47,433

and CP-47,434, and monensin exhibited comparable activities in Kellogg's (2) in vitro rumen propionic acid test system.

In conclusion, CP-47,433 and CP-47,434 are new polycyclic ether antibiotics from *A. macra* which are produced as a 15:1 mixture of major and minor components, respectively. These antibiotics were isolated as individual entities in crystalline form, and their chemical structures were determined by X-ray and ^{13}C-nuclear magnetic resonance spectral methods and shown to be monovalent monoglycoside polyethers (type 1b) according to Westley's classification scheme (5). Although the structures of the two new ionophores are quite similar, their biological activities are measurably different; i.e., CP-47,433 exhibits greater in vivo anticoccidial activity whereas CP-47,434 shows much more in vitro antibacterial potency, especially against strains of staphylococci.

We are very grateful to J. Bordner, North Carolina State University, and many of our colleagues in Nagoya, Japan, Groton, Connecticut, and Sandwich, England, for their cooperation.

1. **Johnson, J., and W. H. Reid.** 1970. Anticoccidial drugs. Lesion scoring techniques in battery and floor pen experiments in chicks. Exp. Parasitol. **28**:30–36.
2. **Kellogg, D. W.** 1969. Analysis of rumen fluid volatile fatty acids by chromatography with Porapak QS. J. Dairy Sci. **52**:1690–1692.
3. **Lechevalier, H. A., and M. P. Lechevalier.** 1970. A critical evaluation of the genera of aerobic actinomycetes, p. 393–405. *In* H. Prauser (ed.), The actinomycetales. Gustav Fischer, Jena.
4. **Lynch, J. E.** 1961. A new method for the primary evaluation of anticoccidial activity. Am. J. Vet. Res. **22**:324–326.
5. **Westley, J. W.** 1977. Polyether antibiotics: versatile carboxylic acid ionophores produced by *Streptomyces,* p. 177–223. *In* D. Perlman (ed.), Advances in applied microbiology, vol. 22. Academic Press Inc., New York.

Ethyl Monate A: a Semisynthetic Antibiotic Derived from Pseudomonic Acid A

MICHAEL J. BASKER, KEITH R. COMBER, J. PETER CLAYTON, PETER C. T. HANNAN, LINDA W. MIZEN, NORMAN H. ROGERS,[1]* BRIAN SLOCOMBE, AND ROBERT SUTHERLAND

Beecham Pharmaceuticals Research Division, Brockham Park, Betchworth, Surrey, England

Pseudomonic acid A, the major active fermentation metabolite produced by submerged cultures of *Pseudomonas fluorescens* NCIB 10586, was first described by Fuller et al. (6). The structure was elucidated by Chain and Mellows (2, 3), and the absolute configuration was clarified by Alexander et al. (1). (The structure of pseudomonic acid A is shown in Fig. 1.) The compound is active mainly against gram-positive bacteria, but also has antimycoplasmal activity as described by Sutherland et al. (7). It is highly bound to serum protein and is rapidly metabolized in vivo to an inactive compound. After oral administration of sodium pseudomonate A to humans, the blood levels attained were of insufficient duration for further progression of this antibiotic.

Considerable chemical modification of pseudomonic acid has been carried out with the aim of producing a derivative with (i) lower binding to serum protein, (ii) improved pharmacokinetic properties, and (iii) an extended spectrum of antimicrobial activity. One of the most important chemical changes to be made to this molecule has been the hydrolysis of the nonanoic acid side chain to give the nucleus, monic acid A, which was prepared in good yield in a four-step, one-pot process by Clayton et al. (4). It is interesting to note that monic acid A has neither antibacterial nor antimycoplasmal activity. In contrast, the ethyl ester of monic acid A, which represents one of many derivatives prepared, has an in vitro spectrum of activity comparable with that of the parent compound and shows improved in vivo biological properties.

Ethyl monate A and sodium pseudomonate A are active primarily against gram-positive bacteria, but also have activity against *Haemophilus influenzae* and *Neisseria gonorrhoeae*. The *Enterobacteriaceae*, *Pseudomonas aeruginosa*, and enterococci are resistant. As a rule, ethyl monate A showed activity similar to, or only slightly less than, that of sodium pseudomonate A against most of the bacteria tested, but was from 5- to 20-fold less active against streptococci. Both compounds were active against mycoplasmal pathogens of humans and animals, with

ethyl monate A generally being the more active (Table 1). The high serum binding (95%) of sodium pseudomonate A was apparent in MIC tests in the presence of 50% human serum, where its activity against staphylococci and streptococci was considerably reduced. In contrast, ethyl monate A is only 30% bound to human

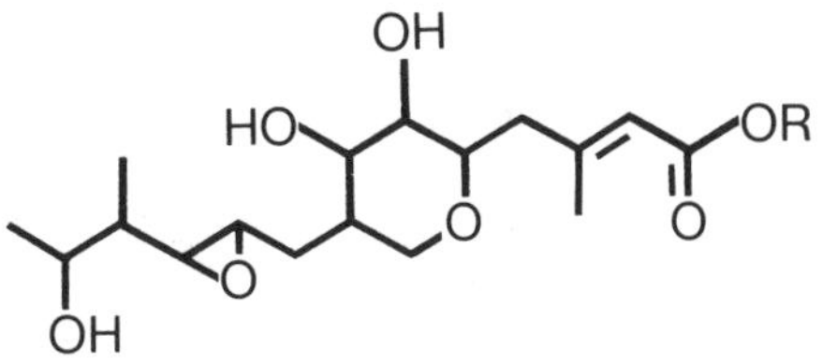

R=(CH$_2$)$_8$ CO$_2$ H - Pseudomonic Acid A
=H   - Monic Acid A
=C$_2$H$_5$ - Ethyl Monate A

FIG. 1. *Structures.*

TABLE 1. *Antibacterial and antimycoplasmal activity of ethyl monate A and sodium pseudomonate A*

Organism	Typical MIC[a] (µg/ml)	
	Ethyl monate A	Sodium pseudo-monate A
Escherichia coli	100	50
Pseudomonas aeruginosa	>100	>100
Haemophilus influenzae	0.12	0.12
Neisseria gonorrhoeae	0.05	0.01
Bacillus subtilis	0.12	0.12
Staphylococcus aureus	0.25	0.12
Streptococcus faecalis	>100	50
Streptococcus pyogenes	2.5	0.12
Streptococcus pneumoniae	1.0	0.25
Mycoplasma pneumoniae (I)[b]	1.25	2.5
Mycoplasma suipneumoniae (I)	0.156	1.25
Mycoplasma hyorhinis (II)	0.156	0.156
Mycoplasma bovis (II)	<0.02	0.039
Mycoplasma dispar (I)	≤0.02	0.625

[a] MICs for bacteria were determined by serial dilutions in nutrient agar with 5% chocolated horse blood. Inoculum was 0.001 ml of overnight broth culture. MICs were determined after incubation at 37°C for 18 h.

[b] MICs for mycoplasma were (I) determined by serial dilution in Friis' broth (5) in microtiter plates using a modification of the metabolite inhibition test (8) or (II) determined in Friis' broth solidified with 1.3% agar. The inoculum was 10^3 to 10^5 colony-forming units, and MICs were recorded after 7 days of incubation at 37°C.

[1] Present address: Beecham Pharmaceuticals Research Division, Walton Oaks, Tadworth, Surrey, England.

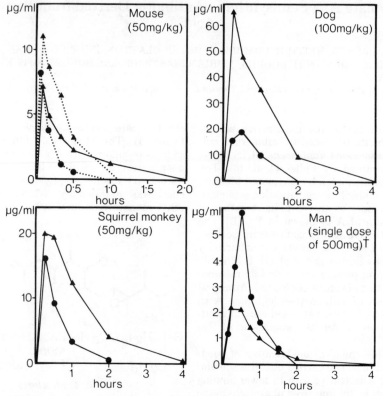

FIG. 2. *Blood levels of ethyl monate A and sodium pseudomonate A in the mouse, dog, and squirrel monkey, and serum levels in humans. Symbols:* ▲, *ethyl monate A;* ●, *sodium pseudomonate A;* †, *study supervised by D. Staniforth;* ——, *oral;* ·····, *subcutaneous.*

serum, and consequently its activity against both streptococci and staphylococci was relatively unaffected in the presence of serum.

Generally, ethyl monate A gives rise to higher and more prolonged blood levels in animals (e.g., mouse, dog, and squirrel monkey) than the parent compound (Fig. 2). In the mouse, due to rapid metabolic deactivation, no levels of pseudomonic acid A were detected after oral administration. In the dog and squirrel monkey, both compounds were rapidly absorbed after oral administration, with ethyl monate A giving rise to higher and more prolonged levels than those for sodium pseudomonate A.

In mouse protection tests, ethyl monate A given orally was effective against intraperitoneal staphylococcal and *Streptococcus pyogenes* infections, with 50% protective dose values of 10 and 35 mg/kg, respectively. In contrast, sodium pseudomonate was not active against these infections when given orally, but was effective after subcutaneous administration against the staphylococcal infection only, with a 50% protective dose value of 160 mg/kg. However, neither

ethyl monate A nor sodium pseudomonate A was effective against an intraperitoneal infection with the highly mice-virulent pneumococcus tested. Ethyl monate A was also very effective against a *Staphylococcus aureus* 1555 thigh lesion infection in mice when administered orally.

In contrast to the blood level profiles in experimental animals, human serum levels of ethyl monate A were disappointingly and unpredictably lower than those of sodium pseudomonate A after 500-mg single oral doses of each compound to volunteers. The serum levels of these antibiotics in humans are too low and of insufficient duration to preclude their progression for the treatment of human infections. However, their use in treating mycoplasmal and bacterial infections in animals is currently being investigated.

1. **Alexander, R. G., J. P. Clayton, K. Luk, N. H. Rogers, and T. J. King.** 1978. The absolute configuration of pseudomonic acid A. J. Chem Soc. Perkin Trans. I, p. 561.
2. **Chain, E. B., and G. Mellows.** 1974. Structure of pseudomonic acid, an antibiotic from *Pseudomonas fluores-*

cens. Chem. Commun., p. 847.

3. **Chain, E. B., and G. Mellows.** 1977. The structure of pseudomonic acid A, a novel antibiotic produced by *Pseudomonas fluorescens.* J. Chem Soc. Perkin Trans. I, p. 294.

4. **Clayton, J. P., K. Luk, and N. H. Rogers.** 1979. The conversion of pseudomonic acid A into monic acid A and its esters. J. Chem. Soc. Perkin Trans. I, p. 308.

5. **Friis, N. F.** 1975. Nord. Vet. Med. **27**:337.

6. **Fuller, A. T., G. Mellows, M. Woolford, G. T. Banks, K. D. Barrow, and E. B. Chain.** 1971. Pseudomonic

acid: an antibiotic produced by *Pseudomonas fluorescens.* Nature (London) **234**:416.

7. **Sutherland, R., K. R. Comber, L. W. Mizen, B. Slocombe, and J. P. Clayton.** 1976. Pseudomonic acid, an antibiotic produced by *Pseudomonas fluorescens. In* Program Abstr. Intersci. Conf. Antimicrob. Agents Chemother. 16th, Chicago, Ill., abstr. no. 52.

8. **Taylor-Robinson, D.** 1967. Mycoplasmas of various hosts and their sensitivities. Postgrad Med. J. Suppl. **43**:100.

A38533, a New Antipseudomonal Antibiotic: Fermentation, Isolation, and Structure Studies

RONALD D. JOHNSON,* LAVERNE D. BOECK, HAROLD R. PAPISKA, Y.-H. BERNICE CHAO, AND R. NAGARAJAN

The Lilly Research Laboratories, Eli Lilly and Company, Indianapolis, Indiana 46206, U.S.A.

The A38533 complex was discovered in the course of screening for inhibitors of gram-negative bacteria with emphasis on *Pseudomonas aeruginosa.* Taxonomic studies on the producing organism, NRRL 11298, identified it as a *Streptomyces* species. The complex, consisting of four factors (A$_1$, A$_2$, B, and C), was shown to be related to the R.P. 6798 complex (British Patent 846,801, August 1960) and the FR3383 complex (K. Umehara et al., 1977, 207th Meeting

of the Jpn. Antibiot. Res. Assoc.). The A38533 factors differed in chromatographic and/or physicochemical characteristics from these complexes. Interest in the antipseudomonal activity led to further investigation of the structure and biological properties of these antibiotics.

This paper describes the fermentation, isolation, and physical properties of the four factors and some structural data on the two major factors, A$_1$ and B.

TABLE 1. *Physicochemical characteristics of A38533 factors*

A 38533 Factors

Physical Data	A$_1$	A$_2$	B	C
Melting point, °C	189-193	206-209	187-190	197-200
High resolution FDMS Data	840.2738		863.2900	
Plasma desorption MS	841 (M + 1)	823 (M + 1)	864 (M + 1)	846 (M + 1)
Molecular formula	$C_{37}H_{44}N_8O_{13}S$	$C_{38}H_{46}N_8O_{13}$	$C_{39}H_{45}N_9O_{12}S$	$C_{40}H_{47}N_9O_{12}$
Titration pKa (66% DMF)	6.0; 7.8; 10.8; 12.8; > 12.8	6.1; 7.8; 10.8; >12.0; > 13.0	6.1; 7.8; 10.8; 12.7	6.2; 7.8; 10.8; 12.7
UV Spectrum λmax (ϵ) acid and neutral	256 (21,500) 222 (28,500)	258 (20,500) 222 (26,500)	290 (6,150) 258 (22,600) 222 (48,000)	290 (6,000) 259 (21,100) 222 (46,100)
basic	290 (7,500) 260(S) (22,400) 242(S) (35,500)	290 (6,400) 260(S) (21,600) 242 (32,000)	290 (8,600) 260(S) (23,000) 243 (25,000) 222(S) (53,800)	290 (8,500) 260(S) (21,600) 243 (25,400) 222(S) (51,700)
Optical rotation [α]$_D^{25}$; DMSO	+ 59.7°	+ 46.3°	+ 57.1°	+ 40.2°
^{13}C-nmr (DMSO-d$_6$)	37-38 carbons 3-phenolic grps 1 alcohol uracil	—	39-40 carbons 2-phenolic grps. uracil	40-41 carbons 2-phenolic groups uracil

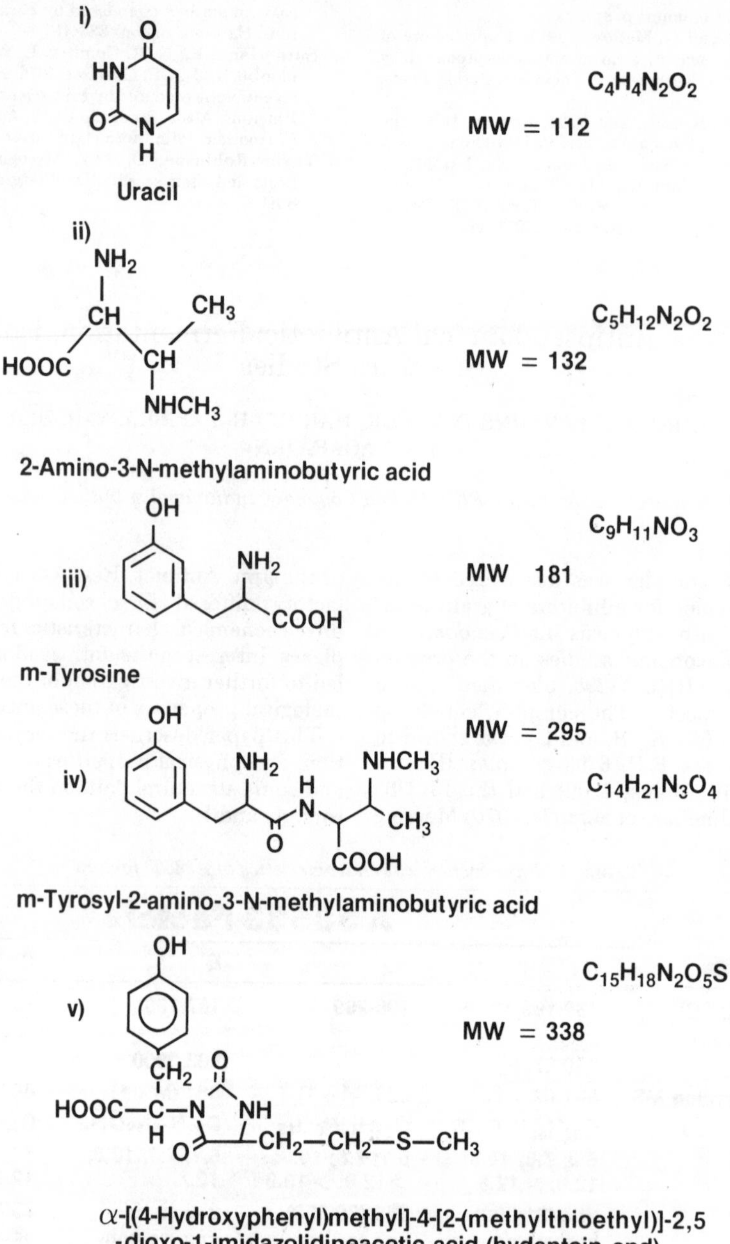

i)

$C_4H_4N_2O_2$

MW = 112

Uracil

ii)

$C_5H_{12}N_2O_2$

MW = 132

2-Amino-3-N-methylaminobutyric acid

iii)

$C_9H_{11}NO_3$

MW   181

m-Tyrosine

iv)

MW = 295

$C_{14}H_{21}N_3O_4$

m-Tyrosyl-2-amino-3-N-methylaminobutyric acid

v)

$C_{15}H_{18}N_2O_5S$

MW = 338

HOOC—C—N   NH

CH₂—CH₂—S—CH₃

α-[(4-Hydroxyphenyl)methyl]-4-[2-(methylthioethyl)]-2,5
-dioxo-1-imidazolidineacetic acid (hydantoin cpd)

FIG. 1. *Structural components of A38533 factors A_1 and B.*

Fermentation. Stock cultures of NRRL 11298 were maintained either in the vapor phase of liquid nitrogen or as lyophilized pellets. Cultures for the first-stage seed flasks were grown in wide-mouth 250-ml Erlenmeyer flasks containing 50 ml of a medium composed of 3.0% Trypticase soy broth (BBL Microbiology Systems), 1.5% glycerol, and 0.2% calcium carbonate. The flasks were incubated for 48 h at 30°C on a shaker rotating in a 5-cm-diameter circle at 250 rpm. A second seed stage, employing 400 ml of the same medium in a wide-mouth 2-liter Erlenmeyer flask, was incubated for 24 h. Fermentors were inoculated with a 1% (vol/vol) seed volume. The fermentor medium was composed of 2.5% glucose, 2.0% soybean meal, 0.1% casein, 0.3% molasses, 0.02% $MgSO_4 \cdot 7H_2O$, 0.02% KCl, 0.004% $FeSO_4 \cdot 7H_2O$, and 0.25%

CaCO$_3$ in deionized water. The incubation temperature was maintained at 34°C, whereas dissolved oxygen was maintained between 50 and 70% of air saturation at atmospheric pressure. Peak antibiotic levels were produced after 40 to 50 h.

Isolation. The filtered broth was chromatographed over XAD-4 (Rohm and Haas), and the activities were eluted with 50 and 90% methanol in water. The 50% methanol preparation (A$_1$ enriched) and the 90% methanol preparation (B enriched) were chromatographed separately over Florisil (Merck) using 10 and 15% water in acetonitrile. Resulting active preparations were passed over a sodium acetate-buffered silica gel 950 (Grace-Davison) column and eluted with 10 and 12.5% water in acetonitrile. Active preparations were separated into their component factors by reverse-phase preparative high performance liquid chromatography using 1% ammonium carbonate-buffered acetonitrile-water mixtures (pH 8.5). The resulting purified factor preparations were desalted over XAD-4. The minor factors, A$_2$ and C, were further purified by a second preparative high performance liquid chromatography step followed by a second XAD-4 desalting step.

Physiochemical properties. The A38533 factors were shown to be water-soluble, noncrystalline white compounds that were stable for 16 days at room temperature between pH 3 and 10. Under strongly acidic conditions, the compounds were inactivated by hydrolysis with loss of a uracil group. All factors showed positive Pauly and Molisch tests. Factors B and C showed a positive Erlich test.

The factors were shown to be paired in their structural relationship, with A$_1$ similar to A$_2$ and B similar to C. Table 1 shows selected physiochemical data for each of the factors.

Nuclear magnetic resonance (NMR) data for the A38533 factors were complicated by peak doubling probably due to conformational change in a tertiary amide. Acid solution or sodium bicarbonate solution forced the equilibrium to one side (~80%) and simplified the spectra somewhat. From the ^{1}H-NMR and ^{13}C-NMR spectra of A$_1$, it was shown that A$_1$ has one carboxyl, three phenols (or enols), one alcohol, one —N—CH$_3$, and two C—CH$_3$ groups.

Structural studies. Factors A$_1$ and B were subjected to 6 N HCl hydrolysis at 110°C for 21 h. The resulting reaction mixture was neutralized with ammonium hydroxide. The precipitate was removed by filtration, and the filtrate was subjected to Bio-Rex 70 (Bio-Rad) chromatography followed by cellulose (Avicel Ph101; FMC Corp.) chromatography. The resulting components (Fig. 1) were identified by combinations of mass spectrometry, ^{1}H-NMR, ^{13}C-NMR, UV, infrared, titration, and amino acid analysis data.

Discussion. The structural studies conducted on A$_1$ and B have indicated a novel class of peptide antibiotics. The structural components found in factor A$_1$ included uracil, 2-amino-3-N-methylaminobutyric acid, m-tyrosine, and the hydantoin compound. These components accounted for nearly 90% of the molecular weight of factor A$_1$.

The same components were found in factor B with the exception of the hydantoin compound. However, amino acid analysis showed the presence of methionine and ^{13}C-NMR data suggested the presence of a modified tyrosine moiety of unknown structure. These components accounted for 85% of the molecular weight of factor B.

The novel structural type and antipseudomonal activity led to biological studies, which will be discussed in subsequent papers.

A38533, a New Antipseudomonal Antibiotic: Resistance Development and Mechanism of Action

JOE N. HOBBS, JR., AND NORRIS E. ALLEN*

The Lilly Research Laboratories, Eli Lilly and Company, Indianapolis, Indiana 46206, U.S.A.

A38533 is a new narrow-spectrum antibiotic discovered at the Lilly Research Laboratories in the course of screening for inhibitors of gram-negative bacteria. Although good activity against *Pseudomonas* was observed, development of high-level resistance to this antibiotic was also noticed. These observations led to further studies on the mechanisms of action and resistance.

Development of resistance. When *Pseudomonas aeruginosa* was plated on Mueller-Hinton agar supplemented with A38533 (0.05 to 5.0 mg/ml), resistant colonies appeared at a frequency of approximately 2×10^{-6}. This one-step resistance to high concentrations was similar to that seen with streptomycin except that the frequency of streptomycin resistance was much lower (4×10^{-9}).

Resistance to A38533 appeared to be constitutive rather than inducible since inhibition of peptidoglycan synthesis (see following section) did not require preexposure to antibiotic. Moreover, resistance was not lost when resistant strains were subcultured in the absence of A38533.

A38533-resistant strains showed cross-resistance to chemically related antibiotics. Several mutants selected on A38533 factor A_1 were cross-resistant to factors A_2, B, and C, which are produced in the same fermentation. The mutants were also resistant to the chemically similar RP6798 (Rhone-Poulenc) and FR3383 (Fujisawa). There was no cross-resistance to streptomycin, tobramycin, carbenicillin, polymyxin B, or fosfomycin.

Mechanism of action. A38533 had a negligible effect on [^{14}C]leucine and [^{14}C]uracil incorporation by intact *P. aeruginosa* X577 (A38533 susceptible) (Table 1). Incorporation of exogenous [^{14}C]thymidine in the presence of deoxyadenosine could not be measured in this strain.

TABLE 1. *Effects of A38533 on protein, RNA, and peptidoglycan synthesis in P. aeruginosa*

Precursor	Additions (μg/ml)	X577[a]		X577R[b]	
		dpm/A_{600}[c]	% Inhibited	dpm/A_{600}	% Inhibited
[^{14}C]leucine[d]	None	14,001		ND[e]	ND
	A38533 (50)	11,912	15		
[^{14}C]uracil[f]	None	8,869		ND	ND
	A38533 (50)	9,228	<1		
[^{14}C]alanine[g]	None	5,023		4,549	
	A38533:				
	(100)	1,631	68	5,640	<1
	(10)	1,764	65	4,210	8
	(1)	3,754	25	5,688	<1
	(0.1)	5,031	<1	5,022	<1

[a] A38533-susceptible *P. aeruginosa*.
[b] A38533-resistant *P. aeruginosa*.
[c] A_{600}, Absorbance at 600 nm.
[d] Hot trichloroacetic acid-insoluble incorporation of [^{14}C]-leucine (0.2 μCi/ml; 5.3 μCi/μmol) during 15-min incubation was measured with cells that had reached an optical density at 600 nm of 0.55 in Davis minimal broth supplemented with 50 μg of methionine per ml.
[e] ND, Not determined.
[f] Trichloroacetic acid-insoluble incorporation of [^{14}C]uracil (0.2 μCi/ml; 4.4 μCi/μmol) was measured by the same procedure used for leucine incorporation.
[g] Trichloroacetic acid-insoluble incorporation of [^{14}C]alanine (1.0 μCi/ml; 18.5 μCi/μmol) during a 15-min incubation was measured with cells grown to an optical density at 600 nm of 0.5, washed, and resuspended in cell wall synthetic broth (1) containing 100 μg of chloramphenicol per ml.

TABLE 2. *Effect of A38533 on peptidoglycan synthesis by permeabilized P. aeruginosa (A38533-susceptible and -resistant strains)*[a]

Strain	Antibiotic	μg/ml	dpm	% Inhibition
X48 (A38533 susceptible)	None		3,966	0
	A38533	100	79	98
	A38533	10	69	98
	A38533	1	24	95
	A38533	0.1	1,327	66
X48R (A38533 resistant)	None		8,339	0
	A38533	100	<1	100
	A38533	10	<1	100
	A38533	1	218	97
	A38533	0.1	1,782	79

[a] Trichloroacetic acid-insoluble incorporation of UDP-*N*-acetyl [^{14}C]glucosamine during a 180-min incubation was measured using ether-treated cells prepared by the methods of Vosburg and Hoffmann-Berling (2). Reactions contained, in a total volume of 75 μl: 15 μmol of Tris-hydrochloride (pH 7.5), 3 μmol of $MgCl_2$, 0.06 μmol of adenosine 5'-triphosphate, 5 nmol of UDP-*N*-acetylmuramyl pentapeptide, 0.43 nmol of UDP-*N*-acetyl [^{14}C]glucosamine (46.7 μCi/μmol), and 0.8 to 1.2 mg of ether-treated cell protein.

Trichloroacetic acid-insoluble incorporation of [^{14}C]alanine in the presence of 100 μg of chloramphenicol per ml was inhibited by A38533 at concentrations as low as 1.0 μg/ml. By contrast, [^{14}C]alanine incorporation by *P. aeruginosa* X577R (A38533 resistant) was unaffected by 100 μg of A38533 per ml, suggesting that this antibiotic was a selective inhibitor of peptidoglycan synthesis.

Incorporation of radiolabeled nucleotide precursors (uridine 5'-diphosphate [UDP]-*N*-acetyl [^{14}C]glucosamine and UDP-*N*-acetylmuramyl-[^{14}C]diaminopimelic acid-pentapeptide) into peptidoglycan was measured using permeabilized (ether-treated) *P. aeruginosa* (A38533 susceptible). A38533 inhibited incorporation of both precursors into peptidoglycan as indicated by the lack of radioactivity remaining at the origin after chromatography in isobutyric acid–1 N NH_4OH (5:3). In addition, there was no increase in radioactivity appearing in material assumed to represent the lipid-bound intermediate. Comparison with vancomycin, which causes accumulation of the lipid-bound intermediate, indicated that A38533 does not interfere with the vancomycin-susceptible step.

The effect of A38533 on peptidoglycan synthesis in A38533-susceptible and A38533-resistant *P. aeruginosa* was determined by measuring UDP-*N*-acetyl [^{14}C]glucosamine incorporation by permeabilized cells (Table 2). Unlike intact cells, peptidoglycan synthesis in permeabilized cells was susceptible to A38533 regardless of whether susceptible or resistant strains were used. In addition, A38533 was a potent inhibitor of UDP-N-acetyl [^{14}C]glucosamine incorporation by a cell-free particulate enzyme preparation from *Bacillus megaterium*.

Discussion. Based on measurements of [^{14}C]alanine incorporation by intact cells and [^{14}C]nucleotide precursor incorporation by permeabilized cells, A38533 appears to selectively inhibit peptidoglycan synthesis in *Pseudomonas*. The specific step sensitive to A38533 is not known. Although A38533 must inhibit a step occurring subsequent to precursor formation, it does not affect the vancomycin-susceptible transfer reaction.

The fact that peptidoglycan synthesis in a cell-free *B. megaterium* system was susceptible to A38533 suggests that the narrow spectrum of antimicrobial activity for this drug may be due to an exclusion mechanism. Impermeability to A38533 is the most likely explanation for the nonsusceptibility of strains other than *Pseudomonas*.

High-level resistance to A38533 develops in one step at a relatively high frequency. Peptidoglycan synthesis in resistant mutants is not inhibited by A38533 when measurements are made on intact cells. However, peptidoglycan synthesis in permeabilized cells is inhibited by A38533, regardless of whether susceptible or resistant strains are used. Thus, resistance to this antibiotic does not seem to result from an alteration affecting a target enzyme. Rather, resistance to A38533 is more likely due to a change that prevents penetration of the antibiotic to the target site.

1. **Lugtenberg, E. J. J., and P. G. De Haan.** 1971. A simple method for following the fate of alanine-containing components in murein synthesis in *Escherichia coli*. Antonie von Leeuwenhoek J. Microbiol. Serol. **37**:537–552.

2. **Vosburg, H. P., and H. Hoffmann-Berling.** 1971. DNA synthesis in nucleotide-permeable *Escherichia coli*. I. Preparation and properties of ether-treated cells. J. Mol. Biol. **58**:739–753.

Structure of Povidone-Iodine

HANS UWE SCHENCK,* PETR SIMAK, WOLFGANG SCHWARZ, AND DIETER HORN

BASF Aktiengesellschaft, D-6700 Ludwigshafen, Federal Republic of Germany

Povidone-iodine has for years been used in the form of various formulations as a multivalent, local, broad-spectrum antiseptic having bactericidal, fungicidal, sporicidal, protocidal, and virucidal properties.

It has now been shown by spectroscopic investigations of commercial povidone-iodine (USP XIX) in comparison with corresponding complexes of low-molecular-weight substances that povidone-iodine in the solid state is an adduct of polyvinylpyrrolidone (PVP) with HI$_3$ (H. U. Schenck, P. Simak, and E. Haedicke, Makromol. Chem., in press). In this adduct, a proton is bonded between the carbonyl groups of two pyrrolidone rings. The I$_3^-$ anion is substantially ionically coordinated with the resulting complex ion (Fig. 1).

The good solubility of the product in water results from the substantial number of pyrrolidone rings which are free, i.e., which are not involved in complexing. If the proportion of HI$_3$ in the adduct is increased to the point that the predominant proportion of the pyrrolidone rings participates in adduct formation, the complex loses its good solubility characteristics.

Hence, in commercial povidone-iodine, about one-third of the total amount of iodine is already present as iodide (I^{-1}), namely in combination with molecular iodine, i.e., as the I$_3^-$ ion. The amount of iodine of oxidation level −1 can be measured as the difference between the total amount of iodine, determined by the method of USP XIX, and the amount of available iodine, i.e., iodine which can be titrated with thiosulfate.

A product completely identical in its spectroscopic properties to commercial povidone-iodine can therefore also be obtained, inter alia, from the corresponding amounts of PVP, iodine, and hydrogen iodide.

We have been unable to find any indication that solid commercial povidone-iodine contains any substantial amounts of iodine in oxidation levels −1 and +1, e.g., I$^-$ and IO$^-$, alongside one another.

The quality of a povidone-iodine complex is critically affected by whether a sufficient amount of iodide ions is present. These ions repress the amount of free iodine, i.e., of iodine not present as I$_3^-$, to a minimum and hence eliminate the danger of possible irritant effects.

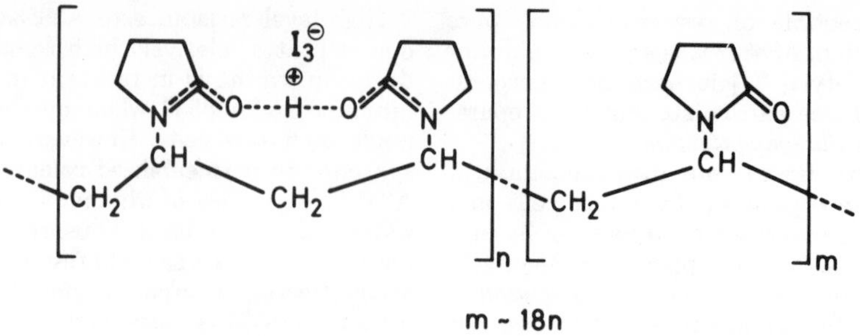

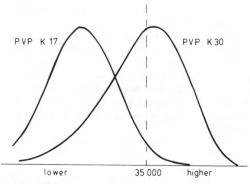

m ~ 18n

FIG. 1. *Structure of povidone-iodine.*

As regards aqueous solutions of povidone-iodine, equilibrium dialysis experiments (cellulose hydrate membranes) using aqueous povidone-iodine solutions (1.0%) showed an equilibrium constant at 25°C and pH 5.0 of 813 liters/mol (povidone-iodine based on PVP with K value of 30) and of 958 liters/mol (povidone-iodine based on PVP with K value of 17) for the following equilibrium: $I_3^\theta + PVP \rightleftharpoons I_3^\theta \cdot PVP$. This means that 99% of the iodine is in the complexed state.

Furthermore, we investigated the kinetics of the release of available iodine from povidone-iodine by a stopped-flow method in aqueous solution.

For this purpose we studied the kinetics of the iodine amylose reaction as a biological model by spectrophotometric methods. The selection of this model reaction is based on the concept that, for the formation of the iodine-amylose compound, as in the case of the antiseptic action of the iodine, the available iodine must at first be freed from the iodine-PVP complex at a sufficiently high velocity.

At a pH of from 3 to 7 we observed the changes in transmission at 600 nm and calculated the extinction-time relationship from these data. The time at which the extinction reaches half the amount of the total change is within the range of milliseconds (20 ms at pH 5, 300 ms at pH 7; concentrations: I_2, $2.5 \cdot 10^{-5}$ mol/liter; PVP, 50 mg/liter).

These results show that povidone-iodine acts as a stable depot for iodine from which iodine is released very quickly if it is consumed by reduction as is the case when it acts as a disinfectant.

We found no basic difference between povidone-iodine based on PVP with a K value of 30 and PVP with a K value of 17 as regards stability of the aqueous solutions and the kinetics of iodine release.

Figure 2 shows the molecular weight distribution of PVP ($K = 17$) and PVP ($K = 30$).

Only recently has it proved possible to prepare an iodine complex of excellent stability from a

FIG. 2. *Molecular weight distribution of povidone-iodine.*

PVP having a K value of 17 and a mean molecular weight of about 10,000 (with about 98% of the constituent molecules having a molecular weight of less than 40,000).

From the point of view of the excretion of molecules which, after resorption, pass into the blood circulation, an important question is therefore which macromolecules are still small enough to pass through the kidneys. The upper limit has been stated to be a molecular weight of 40,000 (3), this figure being based on various investigations (1, 2).

The recent development, discussed above, using PVP with a K value of 17 may open up new and improved therapeutic possibilities for the treatment of large wounds and for use of the product in those body cavities where questions of resorption and excretion are relevant.

1. **Ashwood-Smith, M. J.** 1971. Polyvinylpyrrolidone solutions used in plasma expanders: potential carcinogens? Lancet, June 19, p. 1304.
2. **Dupon, A., and J. M. Lachapelle.** 1968. The fate of foreign macromolecules. Br. J. Dermatol. **80**:543–544.
3. **Rice, J. M.** 1973. Toxicity and carcinogeniety of polyvinylpyrrolidone (PVP) for experimental animals and its toxicity to man. OTC Volume 020149. Food and Drug Administration, Washington, D.C.

A40104, a New Group of Pleuromutilin-Related Antibiotics: Isolation, Characterization, and Structures of A40104A and A40104B

KARL H. MICHEL,* DOUGLAS E. DORMAN, AND JOHN L. OCCOLOWITZ

The Lilly Research Laboratories, Eli Lilly and Company, Indianapolis, Indiana 46206, U.S.A.

A strain of *Cliptopilus pseudo-pinsitus*, NRRL 11179, a basidiomycete, produces a complex of antibiotics: A40104C (pleuromutilin, *A* in structure I [Fig. 1]), A40104D (14-acetylmutilin, *B* in structure I), and two new antibiotics, designated A40104A (*C* in structure I) and A40104B (structure II [Fig. 2]). A40104A and A40104C (3) are major components of the complex, whereas A40104B and A40104D are minor factors. All four factors were found to be structurally related, and they were separated from the filtered fermentation broth by extraction procedures.

The filtered broth (3,640 liters) of a fermentation medium (4,560 liters) was extracted at broth pH (6.5) with toluene. The extract (2,500 liters) was concentrated to a volume of 23 liters whereby 1.94 kg of A40104C crystallized. The mother liquor contained more A40104C in addition to small quantities of A40104B and A40104D. The aqueous solution remaining after the toluene extraction was further extracted with chloroform. The chloroform was concentrated to a volume of 10 liters and chilled to 4°C. Approximately 590 g of A40104A crystallized within 72 h.

A40104A is a white compound, mp 117–120°C, $[\alpha]_D^{25}$ −14° (*c* 1.0, ethyl alcohol). The empirical formula, $C_{27}H_{42}O_9$ (molecular weight, 510), was established by elemental analysis and was confirmed by mass spectrometry. Potentiometric titration showed no titratable group, and the compound showed no significant absorbance in the UV spectrum.

The structure of A40104A was elucidated by a combination of chemical degradation and spectroscopic methods. Base hydrolysis in methanol-water at room temperature produced mutilin (*D* in structure I), and acidic hydrolysis in methanol-water at room temperature gave pleuromutilin and a pentose, which subsequently was identified as D-xylose. Treatment of A40104A with acetic anhydride in pyridine yielded a tetraacetyl derivative, $C_{35}H_{50}O_{13}$ (molecular weight, 678). The deuteroacetyl derivative (molecular weight, 690) was also prepared under similar reaction conditions.

The electron impact mass spectrum of A40104A is like that of A40104C. The highest mass peak in both spectra occurs at m/z 378, which corresponds to the molecular ion of A40104C. The field desorption spectrum of A40104A, however, shows three main peaks, m/z 510, 303, and 133, confirming a molecular weight of 510, as calculated from elemental analysis data. The difference in composition of A40104A and A40104C, which is $C_5H_9O_4$, together with the fact that A40104A has four acetylable groups, suggested that A40104A was pleuromutilin (A40104C) with a pentose moiety attached. This hypothesis was strengthened by the observation of an intense m/z 73 peak in the mass spectrum of A40104A not present in the spectrum of A40104C. Fragment m/z 73 is the base peak in the spectrum of, e.g., DL-xylose (1).

Proton and ^{13}C nuclear magnetic resonance spectroscopy confirmed the presence of a pentose. Chemical shifts corresponded more closely to a pentopyranose than to a pentofuranose with β-D or β-L glycosidic bond (4). Comparison of the $C_5H_9O_4$ fragment in the ^{13}C spectrum to spectra of known α-D pentopyranose sugars resulted in data corresponding closely to xylose (2). The pentose was subsequently identified as D-xylose.

There are two likely points of attachment of a pentose moiety to the pleuromutilin molecule. The presence of a peak at m/z 317 having the composition $C_{13}H_{17}O_9$ in the mass spectrum of the tetraacetyl A40104A supports the attachment of the acetylated pentose to the glycolic acid unit. In the absence of skeletal rearrangements, it would not be possible to have an ion having 9 oxygen atoms associated with 13 carbon atoms if the acetylated pentose was attached to the eight-membered ring.

Carbon nuclear magnetic resonance measurements showed that the resonance assigned to the hydroxymethyl of the glycolic acid fragment of pleuromutilin is deshielded by ca. 5 ppm in A40104A. This is consistent with the usual β-effect associated with etherification of alcohols (5) and supports the conclusion based on mass spectrometry that the $C_5H_9O_4$ moiety is attached to the glycolic acid hydroxyl group.

A40104B (see structure II), the new minor antibiotic factor, was isolated in small quantities by liquid chromatography from mother liquors of the A40104C crystallization. The electron impact spectra gave a molecular ion of m/z 394. The empirical formula $C_{22}H_{34}O_6$ was established

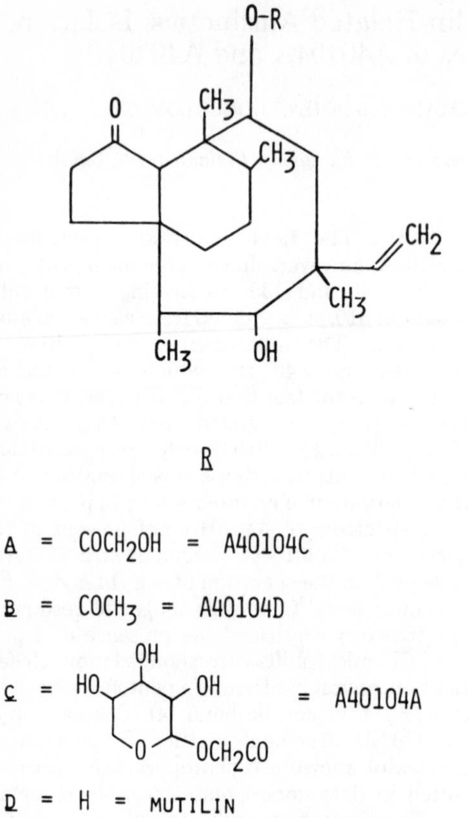

A = COCH$_2$OH = A40104C

B = COCH$_3$ = A40104D

C = [structure] = A40104A

D = H = MUTILIN

FIG. 1. *Structure I.*

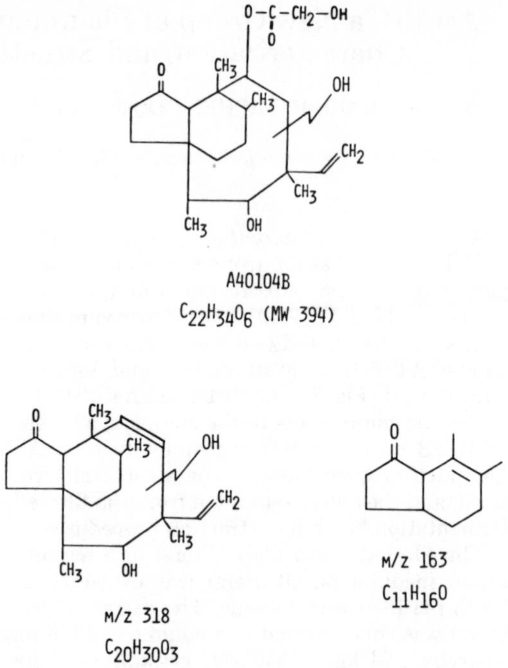

A40104B

C$_{22}$H$_{34}$O$_6$ (MW 394)

M/z 318

C$_{20}$H$_{30}$O$_3$

M/z 163

C$_{11}$H$_{16}$O

FIG. 2. *Structure II.*

by peak matching. The acetyl derivative, C$_{28}$H$_{40}$O$_9$, was prepared with acetic anhydride in pyridine. Mass spectrometry confirmed the presence of three acetyl groups. A fragment m/z 318 (C$_{20}$H$_{30}$O$_3$) is the analog of m/z 302 in the pleuromutilin spectrum and indicates that this extra oxygen atom is part of the nucleus rather than located on the side chain. Fragment m/z 163 is common to both A40104B and pleuromutilin. This new antibiotic is unique because it is the first member of this class of compounds known to have an additional hydroxyl group in the

tricyclic diterpene ring system. A40104A, A40104B, and A40104C are inhibitory to gram-positive and gram-negative bacteria, whereas A40104D has shown no such activity.

1. **Biemann, K.** 1962. Mass spectrometry, p. 350. McGraw-Hill Book Co., New York.
2. **Dorman, D. E., and J. D. Roberts.** 1970. Nuclear magnetic resonance spectroscopy. Carbon-13 spectra of some pentose and hexose aldopyranoses. J. Am. Chem. Soc. **92:**1355–1361.
3. **Kavanaugh, F., et al.** 1951. Antibiotic substances from basidiomycetes. VIII. *Pleurotus mutilis* (Fr) Sacc. and *Pleurotus passeckerianus* Pilat. Proc. Natl. Acad. Sci. U.S.A. **37:**570–574.
4. **Ritchie, R. G. S., et al.** 1975. Carbon-13 chemical shifts of furanosides and cyclopentanols. Configurational and conformational influences. Can. J. Chem. **53:**1424.
5. **Stothers, J. B.** 1972. Carbon-13 NMR spectroscopy, p. 143–144. Academic Press Inc., New York.

B. In Vitro Studies

Synergism of Mezlocillin or Cefotaxime with Sisomicin in Strains of Indole-Positive *Proteus* spp.

C. TAUCHNITZ* AND R. EZOLD

Evangelisch-Lutherisches Diakonissenhaus and Institut für Medizinische Mikrobiologie der Karl-Marx-Universität, Leipzig, German Democratic Republic

Mezlocillin is one of the acylureido penicillins which was discussed in detail during an international symposium held in 1978 in Stuttgart (5). It is in clinical use now as Baypen. HR-756 received the generic name cefotaxime in the meantime and can be regarded as a very potent cephalosporin. The antibacterial activity against enterobacteria exceeds that of other compounds, such as cefuroxime or cefoxitin, 100 to 1,000 times (1). The substance is twice as active as carbenicillin against *Pseudomonas aeruginosa*, and *Bacteroides fragilis* belongs to the spectrum also (3).

The introduction of new antibacterial drugs for clinical use should raise the question of combination effects, if they are used simultaneously with other drugs, especially one of the aminoglycosides. Extensive studies which we have done during more than 10 years (6, 7) showed that the newer β-lactam antibiotics and the newer aminoglycosides very often act synergistically against the majority of susceptible strains, very similar to the long-known synergism of penicillin and streptomycin. The latter, for instance, is very important for the successful therapy of streptococcal endocarditis.

It is most regrettable that one cannot give general rules, and new drugs therefore must be tested for combination effects with aminoglycosides against a sufficient number of strains of all clinically important species of bacteria. The main questions are: Against how many strains of a species does a given combination act synergistically? How many strains do show indifference? Are there examples of antagonism? How large is the degree of synergism regarding bacteriostatic and bactericidal activities?

Of 30 strains of indole-positive *Proteus* spp. which had been isolated recently from clinical specimens, especially from urine samples, 17 were identified as *Proteus rettgeri*. They all were resistant to carbenicillin in disk diffusion tests. Eight strains belonged to *P. morganii*, one of them being resistant to carbenicillin, and five were *P. vulgaris*. Thus, 12 of the strains showed

susceptibility and 18 showed resistance to carbenicillin.

Combination tests of mezlocillin and cefotaxime were done as tube dilution tests in geometric steps. In parallel, second series of the same concentrations contained a subinhibitory concentration of sisomicin, 1 µg/ml. MICs and MBCs of sisomicin had been determined before. They ranged from 2 to >8 µg/ml (see Table 1). Technical details of our mode in combination tests are described elsewhere (6). The inoculum dose was about 10^5 germs. The tubes with the inoculated nutrient broth were stored for 18 h at 37°C. Subcultures were done from all clear tubes on solid media (Gassner substrate) for determination of MBCs.

The results with mezlocillin are summarized in Table 1. The 12 strains which had proved to be susceptible to carbenicillin were susceptible to mezlocillin too. MICs were between 1 and 32 µg/ml and MBCs were between 1 and 64 µg/ml. The subinhibitory concentration of sisomicin used in these experiments, 1 µg/ml, reduced MICs of mezlocillin to 0.12 to 2 µg/ml and MBCs to 0.12 to 8 µg/ml. This correlates with a diminution of 3.8 geometric steps for the MBC and 3.7 steps for the MIC (arithmetic mean). The geometric mean of the MBC fell from 5.65 to 0.36 and that for the MIC fell from 3.17 to 0.29 µg/ml.

All strains of *P. rettgeri* in our study proved to be resistant to 64 µg of mezlocillin per ml, as well as one strain of *P. morganii*. No synergistic effect of 1 µg of sisomicin per ml was seen, and only minimal effects in two strains (MBC) and four strains (MIC) were seen using 4 µg/ml (Table 1). The values for these strains remained above the 32-µg/ml level, which is regarded as the breakpoint of susceptibility.

On the other hand, cefotaxime alone showed MICs between 0.015 and 8 µg/ml for all the strains, independently of their resistance or susceptibility to mezlocillin or carbenicillin. MBCs were between 0.03 and 32 µg/ml. The addition of sisomicin, 1 µg/ml, reduced MICs and MBCs

TABLE 1. *Mezlocillin and sisomicin singly and in combination: MBCs and MICs of 30 strains of indole-positive Proteus spp.*

Antibiotic[a]	MBC or MIC (µg/ml):											Geometric mean
	0.12	0.25	0.5	1	2	4	8	16	32	64	>64	
Car[s] strains (12)												
Mezlocillin												
MBC				1[b]	5		2	2	1	1		5.7
MIC				2	5		3		2			3.2
Mezlocillin + sisomicin (1 µg/ml)												
MBC	5	2	2	1	1	1						0.4
MIC	6	1	2	1	2							0.3
Car[r] strains (18)												
Mezlocillin												
MBC											18	
MIC											18	
Mezlocillin + sisomicin (4 µg/ml)												
MBC										2	16	
MIC										4	14	

	Geometric step:										Arithmetic mean
	+1	±0	−1	−2	−3	−4	−5	−6	−7	−8	
Mezlocillin + sisomicin (1 µg/ml) (12)			1[b]	2	2	4	1		2		3.8
				3	2	5	1		1		3.7

	MBC or MIC (µg/ml):						
	0.25	0.5	1	2	4	8	>8
Sisomicin (30)							
MBC				2[b]	3	6	19
MIC				5	1	5	19

[a] Car[s], Carbenicillin-susceptible strains; Car[r], carbenicillin-resistant strains. Number in parentheses is number of strains tested.

[b] Number of strains.

considerably, ranging now between 0.0075 and 8 µg/ml (MIC) and 0.015 and 8 µg/ml (MBC). The amount of reduction on the average was 4.7 geometric steps for the MBC and 3.3 for the MIC regarding the carbenicillin-susceptible strains and 2.3 steps for the MBC and 1.4 steps for the MIC regarding the resistant ones. Looking at all the 30 strains tested, cefotaxime reduced the MBC for 3.3 and the MIC for 2.3 steps (arithmetic mean). The geometric mean of MBCs fell from 2.0 to 0.08 µg/ml and that of the MICs fell from 0.5 to 0.05 µg/ml in the carbenicillin-susceptible strains and from 5.6 to 1.2 (MBC) and 2.2 to 0.8 µg (MIC) in the resistant strains. For details, see Table 2. Five strains demonstrated indifference in the MBC and three strains demonstrated it in the MIC. Antagonism was not seen at all.

From these results we concluded that the combination of mezlocillin and sisomicin may be useful in the therapy of serious infections induced by strains of indole-positive *Proteus* spp., which are susceptible to mezlocillin. The reduc-

tion of MICs will help to avoid maximal dosages of both antibiotics. Reduction of the MBC may be important for a better bactericidal effect in vivo and for eradicating bacterial persisters which otherwise can lead to antibiotic failure, not only in the therapy of bacterial endocarditis but also in other life-threatening or chronic infections.

The high rate of resistance of *P. rettgeri* to mezlocillin is somewhat surprising and contrasts to the results of Knothe (2). According to Potel (4), however, *P. rettgeri* seems to be the least susceptible species compared with *P. morganii* and *P. vulgaris*. Cefotaxime proved to be superior to mezlocillin because all the strains tested were susceptible. The median reductions of MBCs and MICs are impressive also and should be used in clinical chemotherapy. We believe that reduction of MBCs may be more important from a clinical point of view, especially for eradicating persisters. It is noteworthy that the absolute values of MBC and MIC were higher in the strains resistant to carbenicillin, and the

TABLE 2. *Cefotaxime singly and in combination with sisomicin: MBCs and MICs of 30 strains of indole-positive Proteus spp.[a]*

Antibiotic	MBC or MIC (µg/ml):													Geometric mean
	0.0075	0.015	0.03	0.06	0.12	0.25	0.5	1	2	4	8	16	32	
Car[s] strains (12)[a]														
Cefotaxime														
MBC			1[b]	1			2	1	1	1	2	1	2	2.0
MIC		1	1		2	1	2	2		1	2			0.5
Cefotaxime + sisomicin (1 µg/ml)														
MBC		3	4	1		1	2			1				0.08
MIC	3	3	2		1	1	1			1				0.05
Car[r] strains (18)														
Cefotaxime														
MBC							2	1	3	2	3	3	4	5.6
MIC							3	3	4	4	4			2.2
Cefotaxime + sisomicin (1 µg/ml)														
MBC					2	2	2	2	5	4	1			1.2
MIC					3	3	2	3	6		1			0.8

Antibiotic	Geometric step:													Arithmetic mean
	+1	±0	−1	−2	−3	−4	−5	−6	−7	−8	−9	−10	−11	
Car[s] strains (12)[a]														
Cefotaxime + sisomicin (1 µg/ml)														
MBC		2[b]	1	1		3	1		1	1		1	1	4.7
MIC		1	2	3		2	1	2	1					3.3
Car[r] strains (18)														
Cefotaxime + sisomicin (1 µg/ml)														
MBC		3	4	2	4	3	2							2.3
MIC		2	7	6	2		1							1.4
All strains (30)														
Cefotaxime + sisomicin (1 µg/ml)														
MBC		5	5	3	4	6	3		1	1		1	1	3.3
MIC		3	9	9	2	2	2	2	1					2.3

[a] Car[s], Carbenicillin-susceptible strains; Car[r], carbenicillin-resistant strains. Number in parentheses is number of strains tested.
[b] Number of strains.

reduction rates were less. The observation of single strains with indifference to the cefotaxime-sisomicin combination does not justify the abandonment of combined chemotherapy using cefotaxime and an aminoglycoside such as sisomicin, if the clinical situation requires such a combination. Not one example of antagonism could be found.

1. **Hamilton-Miller, J. M. T., W. Brumfitt, and A. V. Reynolds.** 1978. Cefotaxime (HR 756), a new cephalosporin with exceptional broad-spectrum activity in vitro. J. Antimicrob. Chemother. 4:437–444.
2. **Knothe, H.** 1978. Die antibakterielle Aktivität von Mezlocillin and Azlocillin unter besonderer Berücksichtigung von β-Laktamase-bildenden Enterobakterien, p. 11–17. *In* Internationales Symposium Acylureido-Penicilline, Stuttgart, 1978. Verlag für angewandte Wissenschaften, Munich.
3. **Neu, H. C., N. Aswapokee, P. Aswapokee, and K. P. Fu.** 1979. HR756, a new cephalosporin active against gram-positive and gram-negative aerobic and anaerobic bacteria. Antimicrob. Agents Chemother. 15:273–281.
4. **Potel, J.** 1978. Resistenzsituation im Bereich der Medizinischen Hochschule Hannover, p. 101–103. *In* Internationales Symposium Acylureido-Penicilline, Stuttgart, 1978. Verlag für angewandte Wissenschaften, Munich.
5. **Spitzy, K. H., H. Weuta, and E. Wiechert (ed.).** 1978. Internationales Symposium Acylureido-Penicilline, Stuttgart, 1978. Verlag für angewandte Wissenschaften, Munich.
6. **Tauchnitz, C.** 1974. Untersuchungen über synergistische Antibiotikakombinationen. Promotion-B-Schrift, Leipzig.
7. **Tauchnitz, C.** 1976. Rationelle antimikrobielle Chemotherapie. J. A. Barth, Leipzig.

In Vitro Synergism with the Use of Three Antibiotics Simultaneously Against *Pseudomonas maltophilia*

V. L. YU,* T. P. FELEGIE, AND R. B. YEE

Department of Medicine, Division of Infectious Diseases, University of Pittsburgh School of Medicine, Pittsburgh, Pennsylvania 15261, U.S.A.

We devised an abbreviated three-dimensional checkerboard titration method to test combinations of three antimicrobials for determination of synergy against multi-drug-resistant bacteria. *Pseudomonas maltophilia* was used as the test organism because of its resistance to most of the commercially available antimicrobials, including those active against *Pseudomonas aeruginosa*.

Our abbreviated method uses 192 dilutions (thus only two microtiter plates are required) and yields individual MIC values for three drugs (X, Y, Z), synergy determination for each of the two-drug combinations (i.e., drugs X + Y, Y + Z, X + Z), and finally synergy determination for all three drugs (X + Y + Z). Fourteen clinical isolates of *P. maltophilia* were studied using various three-drug combinations. Synergy was defined as a fractional inhibitory concentration (FIC) index ≤0.5 according to the formula:

$$FIC\ index = FIC_X + FIC_Y + FIC_Z$$

$$= \frac{MIC_X}{MIC_{XYZ}} + \frac{MIC_Y}{MIC_{XYZ}} + \frac{MIC_Z}{MIC_{XYZ}}$$

We found the triplet combinations of gentamicin-carbenicillin-rifampin (mean FIC index, 0.32) and trimethoprim/sulfamethoxazole-car-benicillin-rifampin (mean FIC index, 0.16) were consistently synergistic against all *P. maltophilia* isolates studied.

Figure 1 is a schematic representation of our three-dimensional checkerboard. Each plane represents a fixed concentration of drug Z added to a standard checkerboard titration for drugs X + Y. Three-dimensional isobolograms with concave surfaces are formed if the antibiotic combination is synergistic. Figure 2 depicts an actual isobologram for one isolate of *P. maltophilia* using carbenicillin, gentamicin, and rifampin.

With the appearance of multi-drug-resistant bacteria, this in vitro method may have clinical relevance. Correlation with in vivo models and actual clinical cases need to be made.

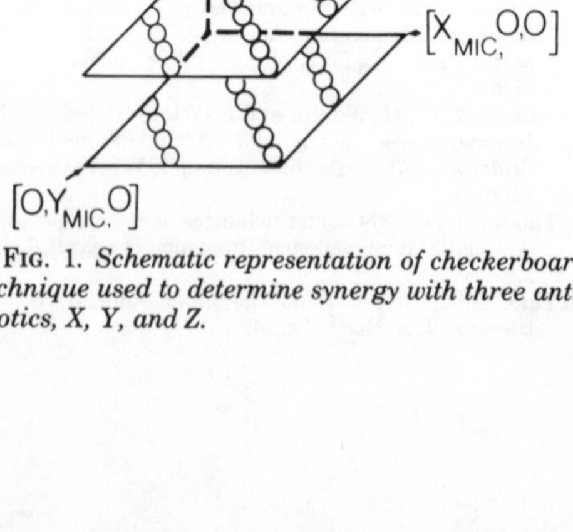

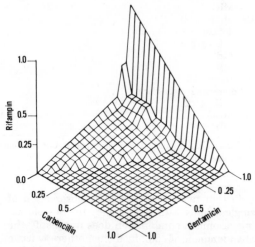

FIG. 2. *Computer-generated isobologram for one isolate of P. maltophilia. Note that rifampin and carbenicillin interact together in an "additive" fashion as demonstrated by the additive line in the rifampin-carbenicillin plane. The double combinations of gentamicin + rifampin and gentamicin + carbenicillin interact in a synergistic fashion, which is visually expressed as a concave isobologram in the gentamicin-rifampin and gentamicin-carbenicillin plane. However, when all three antibiotics are combined in vitro, the isobologram "sinks" further toward the origin (i.e., lowering the FIC index and depicting marked synergistic interaction).*

FIG. 1. *Schematic representation of checkerboard technique used to determine synergy with three antibiotics, X, Y, and Z.*

Synergy Between Some Newer Aminoglycoside and Beta-Lactam Antibiotics

HAROLD GAYA,* THEODORE SACKS, ANN GOOD, CHRISTOPHER UPTON, AND CAROLINE GLICKSMAN

Bacteriology Department, Wright-Fleming Institute, St. Mary's Hospital Medical School, London W2 1PG, England

Patients with severe sepsis in hospital, particularly those whose natural defenses against infection are impaired, may die before the results of laboratory tests become available. As the commonest causes of such infections are *Escherichia coli, Pseudomonas aeruginosa, Klebsiella*, and *Staphylococcus aureus*, and as mixed infections are not uncommon, therapy with a broad-spectrum combination of antibiotics is frequently commenced as soon as appropriate specimens have been taken for culture.

Combinations of an aminoglycoside with one or two β-lactam antibiotics have been most widely used as initial empirical therapy because of the breadth of cover such combinations offer against both gram-positive and gram-negative bacteria and because of the possibilities of synergism between the compounds. When culture and susceptibility results become known, treatment is often continued with one antibiotic alone, usually an aminoglycoside in the United Kingdom but more usually a cephalosporin, particularly cephalothin, in other parts of the world.

The present study was undertaken to determine the activities of a number of aminoglycoside and β-lactam antibiotics, alone and in combination, against a selection of clinical isolates of gram-negative bacilli in an attempt to identify useful agents and their combinations for the treatment of severe gram-negative sepsis.

Clinical isolates of *P. aeruginosa, E. coli, Klebsiella* spp., and *Proteus mirabilis* were tested with the following antibiotics: gentamicin, amikacin, Schering compounds 21420 and 22591, BBK-28, carbenicillin, cefuroxime, cefamandole, cefotaxime, and Glaxo compound 826/359. MICs for the individual compounds and fractional inhibitory concentration (FIC) indices (measures of synergy; sums of the fractions of the inhibitory concentrations) for each aminoglycoside–β-lactam pair were determined using the classical checkerboard method.

The results are summarized in Tables 1 and 2. Median MICs (MIC$_{50}$) are used to summarize the activities of the individual compounds against the four bacterial genera; geometric mean FIC indices are used to summarize the degree of synergy between compounds in a combination for each genus. FIC indices < 1 denote

TABLE 1. *Median MICs of the various antibiotics against four bacterial genera*

Antibiotic	Median MIC (μg/ml)			
	E. coli	Klebsiella	P. mirabilis	P. aeruginosa
Gentamicin	0.5	0.5	1.0	1.0
Amikacin	2.0	1.0	2.0	2.0
SCH-21420	2.0	1.0	4.0	2.0
SCH-22591	1.0	0.5	2.0	0.5
BBK-28	2.0	2.0	8.0	4.0
Carbenicillin	4.0		1.0	32.0
Cefuroxime	4.0	4.0	2.0	
Cefamandole	1.0	2.0	2.0	
Cefotaxime	0.06	0.06	<0.06	16.0
Glaxo-826/359	1.0	1.0	0.125	8.0

TABLE 2. *Geometric mean FIC indices for the various combinations against four bacterial genera*

Combination	Geometric mean FIC index			
	E. coli	Klebsiella	P. mirabilis	P. aeruginosa
Gentamicin +				
Carbenicillin	1.46		0.66	0.94
Cefuroxime	0.69	0.91	0.47	
Cefamandole	1.18	0.73	0.36	
Cefotaxime	0.65	0.77	0.71	0.76
826/359	0.64	0.82	0.60	0.68
Amikacin +				
Carbenicillin	0.62		0.38	0.73
Cefuroxime	0.65	0.61	0.30	
Cefamandole	0.46	0.52	0.33	
Cefotaxime	0.82	0.67	0.73	0.68
826/359	0.86	0.87	0.68	0.77
SCH-21420 +				
Carbenicillin	0.85		0.93	0.66
Cefuroxime	0.80	0.77	0.58	
Cefamandole	0.71	0.73	0.61	
Cefotaxime	0.97	0.88	0.78	0.77
SCH-22591 +				
Carbenicillin	0.72		0.94	0.79
Cefuroxime	0.90	0.91	0.64	
Cefamandole	0.95	0.86	0.59	
Cefotaxime	0.86	0.91	0.74	0.83
BBK-28 +				
Carbenicillin	0.78		0.81	0.84
Cefuroxime	0.86	0.91	0.66	
Cefamandole	0.84	0.87	0.67	
Cefotaxime	0.86	0.84	0.78	0.72
826/359	0.85	0.82	0.67	0.71

synergy, whereas those > 1 denote antagonism.

Synergy could be demonstrated with many of the combinations, but it must be remembered that there is considerable variation between species and within species for any particular combination. It would seem reasonable, nevertheless, that one should use data on synergy only as a guide to the probability of a particular combination being synergistic against a particular microorganism and as a pointer to which combinations to test in clinical situations where combination chemotherapy is indicated.

Synergy data cannot be used without taking into account the MICs of the agents in the combination against the infecting microorganism, as highly active compounds in additive combination (ΣFIC = 1) can have a better real activity, at least in vitro, than synergistic combinations of less active compounds.

In vivo, the levels of each antibiotic which can be achieved in blood and at the site of infection are obviously of paramount importance, and serum antibacterial activity (measured by back titration) against the offending pathogen gives a good indication of the interaction of all these factors. However, knowing the serum levels (L) of the antibacterial agents (A and B) that one can expect and their MICs and FIC index (ΣFIC) against the infecting organism, the expected degree of serum antibacterial activity (maximum inhibitory dilution [MID]) can easily be predicted from the equation: MID = $[(L_A/\mathrm{MIC}_A) + (L_B/\mathrm{MIC}_B)]/\Sigma$FIC.

Thus, where pharmacokinetic data are available and serum levels can be predicted, it is possible to identify those antibiotic combinations which will produce adequate serum antibacterial activity well in excess of the eightfold dilution known to be associated with good clinical response.

Comparative Activity of Dibekacin or Gentamicin in Combination with Sulbenicillin, Carbenicillin, or Ticarcillin Against *Pseudomonas aeruginosa* and *Escherichia coli* In Vitro

YOSHIO KOBAYASHI,* SUSUMU TOMIOKA, AND KEISUKE TOYAMA

Department of Internal Medicine, School of Medicine, Keio University, Tokyo, Japan

We have already shown that dibekacin has a more pronounced effect than gentamicin against *Pseudomonas aeruginosa* when used in combination with antipseudomonal penicillins (Y. Kobayashi and S. Tomioka, Program Abstr. Intersci. Conf. Antimicrob. Agents Chemother., 18th, Atlanta, Ga., abstr. no. 113). In this paper, comparative activities of gentamicin or dibekacin in combination with sulbenicillin, carbenicillin, or ticarcillin against *P. aeruginosa* and *Escherichia coli* were studied by the twofold agar dilution method, with the use of the checkerboard technique described elsewhere (1). The inoculum was a 100-fold dilution of a heart infusion broth overnight culture. All strains of *P. aeruginosa* and *E. coli* used for this study were isolated from sera of patients admitted to Keio University Hospital.

Synergistic effects were observed against 9 of 25 strains of *P. aeruginosa* between gentamicin and sulbenicillin and against 13 strains between dibekacin and sulbenicillin (Table 1). This suggests that dibekacin has better activity than gentamicin against *P. aeruginosa* when used in combination with sulbenicillin.

A further study was done to detect whether dibekacin would show a better effect than gentamicin against *E. coli* when used in combination with antipseudomonal penicillins. No synergistic effects of sulbenicillin and gentamicin or dibekacin were detected against any of the 25 strains of *E. coli* (Table 2). Synergistic effects

TABLE 1. *Effects of combination of sulbenicillin and gentamicin or dibekacin on P. aeruginosa*

Effect	Sulbenicillin plus:	
	Gentamicin	Dibekacin
Indifferent		
Additive	1[a]	
Superadditive	15	12
Synergistic	9	13

[a] Number of strains affected.

TABLE 2. *Effects of combination of sulbenicillin and gentamicin or dibekacin on E. coli*

Effect	Sulbenicillin plus:	
	Gentamicin	Dibekacin
Indifferent	4[a]	
Additive	5	7
Superadditive	16	18
Synergistic		

[a] Numbers of strains affected.

between carbenicillin and gentamicin or dibekacin were observed in only four or five strains of *E. coli*, respectively. Combined effects of gentamicin or dibekacin and sulbenicillin or carbenicillin were superadditive against most strains of *E. coli*. Combined effects of gentamicin or dibekacin and ticarcillin were superadditive against 16 strains of *E. coli*. Synergistic effects of gentamicin or dibekacin and ticarcillin were detected against only 2 or 1 *E. coli* strain, respectively.

In conclusion, we have detected a better effect of dibekacin than gentamicin when the drug is used in combination with sulbenicillin against *P. aeruginosa*, but not when it is used against *E. coli*. Moreover, synergistic effects of these antibiotics were observed in only a few strains of *E. coli*.

1. **Kobayashi, Y.** 1976. Effect of combined use of antibiotics against Pseudomonas aeruginosa in vitro. Keio J. Med. **25**:151–161.

In Vitro Antibacterial Activity of Dibekacin

JEAN R. DUVAL,* CLAUDE J. SOUSSY, AND LIONEL P. DEFORGES

Centre Hospitalier Universitaire Henri Mondor, Creteil, France

Dibekacin is derived semisynthetically from kanamycin B (dideoxy-3′,4′-kanamycin B). Presented here are the results of a study on the antibacterial activity of this new aminoglycoside.

Comparison of bacteriostatic activities of dibekacin and other aminoglycosides of the deoxystreptamine group on reference strains. With 18 gram-negative bacillus reference strains susceptible to all deoxystreptamine aminoglycosides, the MICs if dibekacin, determined by using the dilution method in an agar medium, ranged from 0.25 to 1 μg/ml, the majority lying between 0.32 and 0.63 μg/ml. The relative activity of dibekacin thus appears to be quite close to those of gentamicin (MIC, 0.16 to 0.78 μg/ml), sisomicin and netilmicin (0.19 to 1.25 μg/ml), and tobramycin (0.16 to 1.56 μg/ml). Amikacin, kanamycin, and particularly lividomycin had higher MICs. The MICs for the six staphylococcal susceptible strains studied ranged between 0.12 and 0.25 μg/ml. The relative activities of the different drugs are equivalent, thus, only for the gram-negative bacilli.

With the deoxystreptamine-inactivating gram-negative bacillus reference strains, the data show that dibekacin is inactivated by 2″-nucleotidyl transferase (2″-ANT) and all acetyltransferases (AAC) with the exception of 3.I-AAC. It escapes the action of 3′-phosphotransferases (3′-APH), as it lacks the required action site. Dibekacin is therefore inactivated by the same group of enzymes that inactivate tobramycin. With resistant *Staphylococcus aureus* reference strains, the 3′-APH does not break down dibekacin. In contrast, the strains that produce the polyfunctional inactivating enzyme recently described (1), breaking down the de-

oxystreptamine molecules by phosphorylation at the 2″ position and acetylation at position 6′, are resistant to dibekacin, albeit at various levels. The 4′-ANT-producing strains showed variable behavior, with elevated to normal MICs; dibekacin does not possess a 4′-hydroxyl radical, but it has been demonstrated elsewhere, following these present observations, that this enzyme is indeed capable of inactivating dibekacin by adenylation of another hydroxyl radical in the 2″ (2) or 4″ (3) position. With resistant *S. aureus* strains, we see once again that dibekacin and tobramycin are sensitive to the same enzymes.

Activity of dibekacin on clinical isolates and comparison with activities of other aminoglycosides. A total of 588 clinical isolates were studied by dibekacin MIC measurement. We found for most of the species of gram-negative bacilli that two distinct populations existed: one population of dibekacin-susceptible strains with MICs comparable to those of the susceptible reference strains (0.5 or 1 μg/ml) and a second population of resistant strains whose frequency varied with the species considered (*Escherichia coli*, 1 of 67; *Klebsiella pneumoniae*, 2 of 50; *K. oxytoca*, 2 of 26; *Enterobacter* spp., 17 of 50; *Serratia*, 17 of 26; *Proteus mirabilis*, 2 of 52; *P. morganii*, 1 of 23; *Citrobacter*, 11 of 25; and *Pseudomonas aeruginosa*, 5 of 59). In a few of the species, represented by a small number of samples, no resistance was seen; *P. vulgaris*, *Salmonella*, *Shigella*, *Levinea*, and *Aeromonas hydrophila*. The *Providencia* organisms studied appeared to make up an apparently homogeneous population in a zone of intermediate concentrations (2 to 32 μg/ml). Finally, in two groups of organisms, *P. rettgeri* and *Acinetobacter*, we noted that the strains were

TABLE 1. Study of 1,000 clinical isolates using the disk method[a]

Antibiotic	No. of strains susceptible															
	E. coli (284)[b]	K. pneumoniae (100)	K. oxytoca (31)	Enterobacter (125)	Serratia (35)	P. mirabilis (106)	Proteus, indole positive (50)	Providencia (10)	Citrobacter (30)	Salmonella (6)	Shigella (4)	Levinea (2)	Yersinia (1)	Aeromonas (5)	Pseudomonas (159)	Acinetobacter (52)
Amikacin	284	100	31	125	26	106	50	10	30	6	4	2	1	5	154	48
Tobramycin	279	90	28	79	14	100	45	4	15	6	4	2	1	5	129	43
Dibekacin	279	90	28	79	14	99	45	4	15	6	4	2	1	5	129	43
Gentamicin	277	80	27	68	10	99	45	4	13	6	4	2	1	5	111	25
Lividomycin	236	74	21	99	17	87	42	3	23	6	4	2	1	5	22	25
Kanamycin	234	73	21	63	9	93	39	4	13	6	4	2	1	5	13	21

[a] Diameter of inhibition, ≥20 mm.
[b] Number in parentheses is total number of strains studied.

TABLE 2. Frequency of resistance phenotypes encountered among clinical isolates of gram-negative bacilli

Phenotypes[a]	Probable enzymatic mechanism	No. of isolates showing phenotype												
		E. coli	K. pneumoniae	K. oxytoca	Enterobacter	Serratia	P. mirabilis	P. vulgaris	P. morganii	P. rettgeri	Providencia	Citrobacter	P. aeruginosa	Acinetobacter
K	APH 3'-II	1											8	
KL	APH 3'-I	44	9	6	8	1	6	1	3	1	1		91	1
G	AAC 3-I	2	2		3					1			1	1
KGTD	ANT 2" or AAC 3-II	1	1		36	8	3		1			10		
KATD	AAC 6'													4
LGTD	AAC 2'										1			
KGD							1							
KLG			8	1	8	4						2	17	21
KLGTD		4	9	3	10	4	3		2		5	5	24	5
KLAGTD					9								5	

[a] K, L, G, T, A, D = Resistant to Kanamycin, Lividomycin, gentamicin, tobramycin, amikacin, and dibekacin, respectively.

spread over a wide range of MICs. Of the *S. aureus* isolates, 51 of the 60 samples studied (85%) had MICs comparable to those of the susceptible reference strains (i.e., 0.12, 0.25, and 0.50 µg/ml). Nine of the strains (15%) were resistant and two of these showed very marked resistance. With the exception of one group A strain, the dibekacin MICs are high for the streptococci (≥8 µg/ml); most of the strains have MICs of 16 or 32 µg/ml. Thus, dibekacin, like other aminoglycosides, has little activity against streptococci.

A total of 1,146 clinical isolates (1,000 aerobic gram-negative bacilli and 146 *S. aureus*) were tested with six aminoglycosides by the agar diffusion method. For gram-negative bacilli (Table 1), we note that 84.3% of the strains were susceptible to dibekacin, which is exactly equal to that observed with tobramycin. Furthermore, this is consistent with the results obtained from the study of the reference strains, i.e., common sensitivity of both drugs to the same inactivating enzymes. Amikacin was active more often (98.2% of the strains were susceptible), but the three other drugs were active in a lower proportion of instances: gentamicin (77.7% of susceptible strains), lividomycin (67.7%), and kanamycin (60.1%). Those species showing the highest percentage of dibekacin resistance were *Enterobacter, Serratia, Providencia, Citrobacter*, and, to a lesser extent, *Pseudomonas* and *Acinetobacter*; in other studies, these species have been shown to exhibit multiresistance. For each bacterial species, a comparison of the six preparations always shows amikacin to be the antibiotic that encounters the least number of resistant strains. Dibekacin and tobramycin followed second in their activity, except with *Enterobacter, Serratia*, and *Citrobacter*, where lividomycin appeared to show an advantage. Table 2 illustrates the frequency of resistance phenotypes encountered per species studied.

Among the 146 strains of *S. aureus*, 115 (79%) were found to be susceptible to all the deoxystreptamines. The 31 strains found to be resistance carriers may be categorized as follows: 12 strains (8%) resistant to kanamycin, lividomycin, and weakly resistant to amikacin were dibekacin

susceptible; 16 strains (11%) resistant to kanamycin, gentamicin, tobramycin, and amikacin (low grade) were also dibekacin resistant; 3 strains (2%) resistant to kanamycin, tobramycin, amikacin (low grade), and lividomycin (low grade) varied in their behavior with regard to dibekacin. One of these appeared to be dibekacin resistant, but for the remaining two strains we were unable to detect potential resistance. In all, 13% of the *S. aureus* strains were potentially resistant to dibekacin. This was consistent with our findings for the limited number of strains studied by MIC determination.

Complementary studies. The bactericidal activity of dibekacin was assessed by organism survival counts in liquid media with three susceptible strains provided by the Pasteur Institut: *S. aureus* 7625, *E. coli* 7624, and *P. aeruginosa* 76110. The MBC was defined as 0.01% surviving organisms after 24 h of incubation with the drug. MBCs were equal to the MICs for *E. coli* and *P. aeruginosa* and were twice the MIC for *S. aureus*.

Serum does not appear to influence dibekacin activity significantly. Thus, the MIC for the *E. coli* strain does not vary in the presence of 25 or 50% serum. Under the same conditions, the MICs for the *S. aureus* and *P. aeruginosa* strains are doubled. This result is consistent with the level of protein-bound dibekacin, which was found to be near zero.

For the 18 strains tested, we observed dibekacin activity to be greater in alkaline than in acid medium. As the pH was decreased from 8.4 to 6.4, there was a four- or eightfold increase in the MIC.

1. Le Goffic, F., N. Moreau, and M. Masson. 1977. Are some aminoglycoside antibiotics inactivating enzymes polyfunctional? Ann. Microbiol. (Inst. Pasteur) **128B:** 465–469.
2. Le Goffic, F., N. Moreau, C. J. Soussy, and J. Duval. 1977. How can DKB and tobramycin be inactivated on two different sites by the same enzyme? Ann. Microbiol. (Inst. Pasteur) **128B:**459–463.
3. Santanam, P., and F. H. Kayser. 1978. Purification and characterization of an aminoglycoside inactivating enzyme from Staphylococcus epidermidis FK 109 that nucleotidylates the 4'- and the 4″-hydroxyl groups of the aminoglycoside antibiotics. J. Antibiot. **31:**343–351.

Antagonism of Carbenicillin by Cephalosporins in Gram-Negative Bacilli

WILLIAM C. GRAHAM AND ANTONE A. MEDEIROS*

The Miriam Hospital and Brown University, Providence, Rhode Island 02906, U.S.A.*

By chance, we observed that cefoxitin disks blunted the zone of inhibition around carbenicillin disks on routine Kirby-Bauer test plates of clinical isolates of *Enterobacter cloacae*. In a previous report, the action of carbenicillin had been antagonized by ampicillin in a single isolate of *E. cloacae* (4), and in another, cephaloridine and 6-aminopenicillanic acid antagonized carbenicillin in five isolates of *Proteus* and in one each of *Escherichia coli* and *Pseudomonas aeruginosa* (1). We examined the effect of several newer cephalosporins on the action of carbenicillin in a representative sample of recent clinical isolates of gram-negative bacilli.

The gram-negative bacilli were isolated from clinical specimens by the Microbiology Laboratory of the Miriam Hospital and identified by the API method. A 3-h broth growth was streaked onto Mueller-Hinton agar, and antibiotic disks were placed next to each other at distances corresponding to the sum of their inhibition zone radii ± 5 mm. We interpreted blunting of the carbenicillin zone as "antagonism," extension as "synergy," and neither effect as "indifference." As another test of antagonism, cephalosporin disks were applied to agar containing the test organism and a concentration of carbenicillin sufficient to inhibit its growth. Growth around the disks indicated antagonism. "Two-way" serial dilution antibiotic susceptibility determinations were done using 10^5 organisms per ml in 100 μl of Mueller-Hinton broth. The results after 18 to 20 h of growth at 37°C were plotted as isobolograms. β-Lactamase activity was measured iodometrically as described previously (3).

Sixty-five consecutive clinical isolates of gram-negative bacilli susceptible to carbenicillin were tested using the disk approximation method with cefoxitin versus carbenicillin. Antagonism occurred with all isolates of *E. cloacae* (5 isolates), *Enterobacter aerogenes* (2), *Serratia marcescens* (2), *Morganella morganii* (5), and *Citrobacter freundii* (3) and in none of *E. coli* (23), *Serratia liquefaciens* (1), *Proteus mirabilis* (9), *P. aeruginosa* (12), *Acinetobacter calcoaceticus* (2), and *Providencia stuartii* (1). Other cephalosporins antagonized carbenicillin in some but not all isolates (Table 1). The patterns of interaction between the cephalosporins and carbenicillin appeared to be species specific. In representative isolates, cefoxitin antagonized the actions of ticarcillin and piperacillin as well.

The isobologram plot of the effects of cefoxitin plus carbenicillin on *E. cloacae* 760D (Fig. 1) demonstrates antagonism of carbenicillin, with its peak MIC being 62.5 μg/ml in the presence of 7.8 μg of cefoxitin per ml, a 16-fold increase over the MIC of carbenicillin alone. Antagonism of carbenicillin occurred at concentrations of cefoxitin as low as 1 μg/ml. At high concentrations of cefoxitin, antagonism occurred, but to a lesser degree. With other organisms, high con-

centrations of cephalosporins resulted usually in an indifferent effect (antagonism, I pattern), whereas continued antagonism (antagonism, A pattern) or synergy (antagonism, S pattern) occurred less commonly.

Growth patterns around cephalosporin disks placed on agar containing test organisms plus an inhibitory concentration of carbenicillin reflected the isobologram curves. When high concentrations of cephalosporins caused synergy or indifference in the isobolograms, a clear zone appeared between the ring of bacterial growth and the disk. Peripheral colonies often appeared larger and more mucoid; Gram stains of direct smears of these organisms showed very long filaments. Subcultures of these colonies reverted to normal bacterial morphology and colony appearance.

Under phase-contrast microscopy, we examined the morphology of *E. cloacae* 760D grown in broth containing different concentrations of both carbenicillin and cefoxitin. At a carbenicillin concentration of 3.9 μg/ml cell lysis occurred, whereas subinhibitory concentrations (1 to 2 μg/ml) produced long filaments. Concentrations of cefoxitin as high as 125 μg/ml had little effect on cell shape. However, when low concentrations of cefoxitin (1 to 125 μg/ml) were added to concentrations of carbenicillin as high as 31.3 μg/ml, long filaments were formed.

Cell lysis has been shown to result from inhibition of penicillin-binding protein (PBP) 1A/B, whereas filament formation results from inhibition of PBP 3 (5). The data above suggest that cefoxitin, which has high affinity for PBP 1A (2), may block the effect of carbenicillin on PBP 1A, thus preventing cell lysis. However, another possibility is that the concentration of carbenicillin in the medium was lowered by a cefoxitin-induced β-lactamase. To test this we added 10 μg of cefoxitin per ml to a log-phase culture of *E. cloacae* 760D. β-Lactamase activity of sonic extracts of these cells was at least eightfold greater than that of cells grown in the absence of cefoxitin. However, the induced β-lactamase was a cephalosporinase which hydrolyzed cefamandole, cephalothin, and cephaloridine but not carbenicillin.

In summary, cefoxitin antagonized carbenicillin in 26.2% of carbenicillin-susceptible gram-negative bacilli isolated from clinical specimens over a 1-week period. The antagonism occurred only with isolates of *E. cloacae*, *E. aerogenes*, *S. marcescens*, *M. morganii*, and *C. freundii*. Other cephalosporins caused antagonism in some, but not all, of these isolates. Maximal antagonism of carbenicillin occurred at low concentrations of cephalosporins, whereas higher concentrations resulted in further antagonism,

TABLE 1. *Results of disk approximation studies of antagonism in 17 clinical isolates*[a]

Organism/strain no.	Effect of: FOX on: CARB	MAN CARB	KEF CARB	LOR CARB	FOX MAN	FOX PIP	FOX TICAR
E. cloacae							
329C	A	I	S	A	A		
760D	A	I	S	A	A	A	A
1051	A	I	S	A	A		
1123	A	I	S	A	A		
1571	A	I	S	a	A		
E. aerogenes							
1056	A	I	S	s	A		
1058	A	I	S	S	A	a	A
S. marcescens							
432C	A	a	a	A			
614B	A	A	a	a		A	A
M. morganii							
130D	A	I	A	A	A		
155B	A	I	A	A	A		
288B	A	I	A	A	A		
343	A	I	A	A	A		
597C	A	I	A	A	A	A	A
C. freundii							
103B	A	I	S	A	A		
123B	A	I	S	A	A		
323D	A	I	S	A	A	A	A

[a] Abbreviations: CARB, Carbenicillin; PIP, piperacillin; TICAR, ticarcillin; FOX, cefoxitin; MAN, cefamandole; KEF, cephalothin; LOR, cephaloridine; A, antagonism; S, synergy; I, indifference; a, slight antagonism; s, slight synergy.

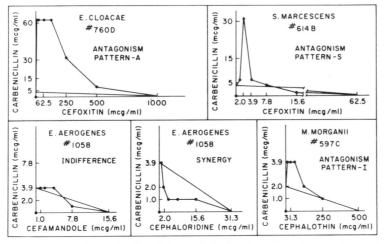

FIG. 1. *Isobologram plots of "two-way" serial antibiotic dilution susceptibilities demonstrating the five representative patterns of interaction between carbenicillin and cephalosporins.*

indifference, or synergy depending on the species tested and the antibiotic used. Preliminary studies of morphology and β-lactamase induction with *E. cloacae* suggest that the antagonism resulted from inhibition of cell lysis, possibly due to a blocking of the effect of carbenicillin by cefoxitin on PBP 1A.

1. Acar, J. F., L. D. Sabath, and P. A. Ruch. 1975. Antagonism of the antibacterial action of some penicillins by other penicillins and cephalosporins. J. Clin. Invest. 55:446–453.

2. Birnbaum, J., E. O. Stapley, A. K. Miller, H. Wallick, D. Henlin, and M. B. Woodruff. 1978. Cefoxitin, a semi-synthetic cephamycin: a microbiologic overview. J. Antimicrob. Chemother. 4(Suppl. B):15–32.

3. Perret, C. J. 1954. Iodometric assay of penicillinase. Nature (London) 174:1012–1013.

4. Seligman, S. J. 1968. Antagonism between penicillin combinations. Clin. Res. 16:355.

5. Spratt, B. G. 1977. Properties of the penicillin-binding proteins of *E. coli* K12. Eur. J. Biochem. 72:341–352.

Thienamycin: In Vitro Studies

ANTONIO RODRÍGUEZ,* TRÁNSITO OLAY, AND MARIA VICTORIA DE VICENTE

Instituto de Farmacología Española, Madrid, Spain

Thienamycin is the first member of a new family of β-lactam antibiotics produced by *Streptomyces cattleya*. With a carbapenem nucleus, its chemical structure is different from the natural and semisynthetic penicillins and cephalosporins. The 6-α-hydroxyethyl side chain confers high resistance to β-lactamases (1). Thienamycin exhibits a broad spectrum of antibacterial activity, including activity against bacteria resistant to β-lactam antibiotics (2–4).

We studied the in vitro activity of thienamycin against facultative aerobic and anaerobic bacteria, both gram positive and gram negative, isolated in Madrid hospitals. The in vitro activity of thienamycin was compared with that of the other antibiotics against certain species of both groups of bacteria.

Aerobic bacteria. The susceptibility of aerobic bacteria to thienamycin was determined by the dilution agar method, following the criteria of Ericsson and Sherris (International Collaborative Study). The inoculum was applied with a Steers replicator. A total of 779 aerobic gram-positive and gram-negative strains were tested. All isolates were susceptible to 10 μg or less per ml, with the exception of one strain of methicillin-resistant *Staphylococcus* and one of *Pseudomonas aeruginosa* (Fig. 1).

Staphylococcus spp., *Streptococcus pneumoniae,* and *Neisseria meningitidis* were very susceptible to thienamycin, with 100% of strains susceptible to 0.078 μg/ml. A notable difference of susceptibility was seen between *S. pneumoniae* and *Streptococcus faecalis*, as well as between methicillin-susceptible and methicillin-resistant *Staphylococcus*.

The median thienamycin MICs against all strains of 17 bacterial groups tested were between 0.009 and 5.0 μg/ml. These results confirm the very wide spectrum of thienamycin, includ-

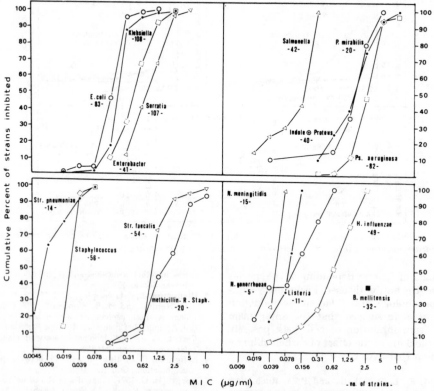

FIG. 1. *Susceptibility of aerobic bacteria to thienamycin.*

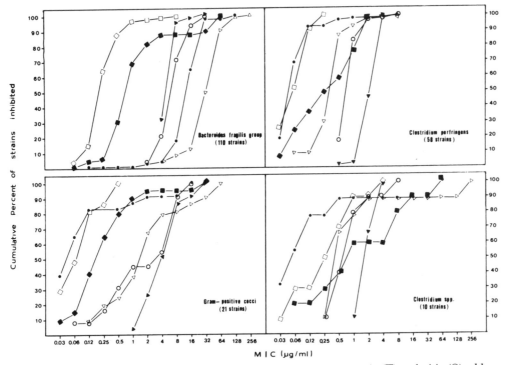

FIG. 2. *Susceptibility of anaerobic bacteria to thienamycin (□), clindamycin (■), cefoxitin (○), chloramphenicol (▲), penicillin G (●), and carbenicillin (△).*

ing *Pseudomonas, Serratia,* indole-positive *Proteus,* and *Brucella melitensis,* all of which are resistant to most β-lactam antibiotics.

We compared the thienamycin activity against four bacterial species with several other antibiotics. Thienamycin was found to be more active than ampicillin, carbenicillin, cephalothin, fosfomycin, and gentamicin against *Staphylococcus, Serratia,* and *Pseudomonas* and equally active as ampicillin and fosfomycin against *Haemophilus.*

Anaerobic bacteria. The susceptibility of anaerobic bacteria to thienamycin was determined by the dilution agar method according to the procedures described in the *Wadsworth Anaerobic Bacteriology Manual.* A total of 209 anaerobic bacterial strains were tested.

Thienamycin was very active against all anaerobic bacteria tested. All strains were inhibited at concentrations less than or equal to 1 µg/ml, with the exception of three strains of *B. fragilis* and one strain of *Clostridium* sp., which were susceptible to 8 µg or less per ml.

We compared the thienamycin in vitro activity with penicillin G, carbenicillin, cefoxitin, chloramphenicol, and clindamycin against all anaerobic bacteria tested (Fig. 2).

Thienamycin was more active than carbenicillin, chloramphenicol, cefoxitin, and clinda-

mycin against all isolates tested. Thienamycin was equally as active as penicillin against *Clostridium perfringens* and gram-positive cocci and less active than penicillin against other clostridia.

The results obtained in this study show that this antibiotic is very active against the following aerobic and anaerobic bacteria: *Staphylococcus* spp., *S. faecalis, S. pneumoniae, Escherichia coli, Klebsiella* spp., *Enterobacter* spp., *Serratia marcescens, Proteus* spp., *Salmonella* spp., *P. aeruginosa, Haemophilus influenzae, Listeria monocytogenes, Neisseria gonorrhoeae, N. meningitidis, B. melitensis, Bacteroides fragilis, Clostridium* spp., gram-positive anaerobic cocci, and nonsporeforming gram-positive anaerobic bacilli.

Thienamycin is more active than ampicillin, carbenicillin, chloramphenicol, gentamicin, and fosfomycin against aerobic bacteria, with the exception of *Haemophilus* which is equally susceptible to ampicillin and fosfomycin. Against anaerobes, thienamycin is more active than carbenicillin, chloramphenicol, cefoxitin, and clindamycin.

1. Kahan, J. S., F. M. Kahan, R. Goegelman, S. A. Currie, M. Jackson, E. O. Stapley, T. W. Miller, A. K. Miller, D. Hendlin, S. Mochales, S. Hernández, H. B. Woodruff, and J. Birnbaum. 1979. Thiena-

mycin, a new β-lactam antibiotic. I. Discovery, taxonomy, isolation and physical properties. J. Antibiot. **32:** 1–12.

2. **Kropp, H., J. S. Kahan, F. M. Kahan, J. Sundelof, G. Darland, and J. Birnbaum.** 1976. Thienamycin. A new β-lactam antibiotic. II. *In vitro* and *in vivo* evaluation. Progr. Abstr. Intersci. Conf. Antimicrob. Agents Chemother. 16th, Chicago, Ill., Abstr. no. 228.

3. **Tally, F. P., N. V. Jacobus, and S. L. Gorbach.** 1978. In vitro activity of thienamycin. Antimicrob. Agents Chemother. 14:436–438.

4. **Weaver, S. S., G. P. Bodey, and B. M. LeBlanc.** 1979. Thienamycin: new beta-lactam antibiotic with potent broad-spectrum activity. Antimicrob. Agents Chemother. **15:**518–521.

Antibacterial Activity of Thienamycin Compared with β-Lactamase-Stable Compounds Against Multiresistant Bacteria

MARIO F. ROMAGNOLI,* KWUNG P. FU, AND HAROLD C. NEU

Division of Infectious Diseases, Departments of Medicine* and Pharmacology, College of Physicians and Surgeons, Columbia University, New York, New York 10032, U.S.A.

Thienamycin was described in 1976 (J. S. Kahan, F. M. Kahan, R. Goegelman, S. A. Currie, M. Jackson, E. O. Stapley, T. W. Miller, A. K. Miller, D. Hendlin, S. Mochales, S. Hernandez, and H. B. Woodruff, Program Abstr. Intersci. Conf. Antimicrob. Agents Chemother. 16th, Chicago, Ill., abstr. no. 227, 1976) as a new β-lactam antibiotic with a markedly extended spectrum of in vitro activity. It has been evaluated by several groups who have found that it has activity against anaerobes comparable to that of metronidazole (1) and that it inhibits *Pseudomonas aeruginosa* at lower concentrations than do the anti-*Pseudomonas* penicillins (2). None of the studies has compared its activity with other β-lactamase-stable cephalosporins or cefamycins against multiresistant bacterial isolates. This study was an attempt to evaluate the in vitro activity of thienamycin compared with cefoxitin, cefamandole, and cefotaxime.

Thienamycin and cefoxitin were supplied by Merck, Sharpe and Dohme Research Laboratories. Cephalothin and cefamandole were gifts from Eli Lilly and Co., and cefotaxime was supplied by Hoechst-Roussel Inc. Carbenicillin and ticarcillin were from Beecham Laboratories. Antibiotics were prepared fresh daily. Susceptibility tests were performed in Mueller-Hinton broth with a final inoculum of 10^5 colony-forming units. Anaerobic tests were performed in GasPak jars (BBL Microbiology Systems). Bactericidal concentrations were determined by plating clear tubes to agar. Organisms tested had been saved because of their resistance to multiple antibiotics.

Thienamycin was tested against 32 multiresistant bacteria which were ampicillin, carbenicillin, and cephalothin resistant (Table 1). Thienamycin inhibited *Proteus mirabilis* at 12.5 μg/ml which were resistant to cefoxitin and cef-

amandole, but cefotaxime inhibited both organisms at 0.1 μg/ml. Indole-positive *Proteus* resistant to cefoxitin and cefamandole were inhibited at 25 μg/ml by thienamycin, but were inhibited by 3.1 μg/ml by cefotaxime. *Enterobacter cloacae* resistant to cefamandole were inhibited by 25 μg/ml of thienamycin, including one isolate resistant to cefotaxime. Thienamycin inhibited *Klebsiella pneumoniae* resistant to cefamandole at 3.1 μg/ml, but it was less active on a microgram-per-milliliter basis than was cefotaxime. Against resistant *Providencia stuartii*, thienamycin had activity similar to cefoxitin and cefamandole. Thienamycin was less active than cefotaxime against *P. aeruginosa* at low concentrations, but it inhibited a strain resistant to cefotaxime and inhibited carbenicillin-resistant isolates.

Thienamycin had excellent activity against penicillin-resistant staphylococci. It inhibited 67% of *Staphylococcus aureus* at 0.2 μg/ml and 100% at 0.4 μg/ml. Likewise, 83% of *Staphylococcus epidermidis* were inhibited at 0.1 μg/ml, and 100% were inhibited at 0.4 μg/ml. This included *S. epidermidis* resistance to methicillin.

TABLE 1. *Comparative activity of thienamycin and other β-lactamase-resistant agents*

Organism (no.)	Concn at which 90% of isolates were inhibited (μg/ml)			
	Thienamycin	Cefotaxime	Cefoxitin	Cefamandole
P. mirabilis (2)	12.5	0.1	>50	>50
Proteus, indole-positive (3)	25	3.1	50	>400
E. cloacae (5)	12.5	>50	>400	>400
K. pneumoniae (5)	3.1	0.2	25	400
P. stuartii (4)	12.5	0.8	6.3	12.5
P. aeruginosa (13)	25	>400	>400	>400

TABLE 2. *Comparative activity of thienamycin against B. fragilis*

Agent	% Inhibited at MIC (µg/ml) of:		
	6.3	12.5	25
Thienamycin	43	86	100
Cefotaxime	83	83	83
Cefoxitin	43	57	86
Ticarcillin	14	43	57

Thienamycin also inhibited enterococci at a concentration of 1.6 µg/ml.

The MBCs were, in a number of cases, many-fold greater than the MICs for several of the multiply resistant, β-lactamase-producing bacteria.

Thienamycin was more active than either cefoxitin or ticarcillin in inhibiting *Bacteroides fragilis* subsp. *fragilis*; 86% of the isolates were inhibited at 12.5 µg/ml and 100% were inhibited at 25 µg/ml, whereas 86% of isolates were in-

hibited by cefoxitin and 57% inhibited by ticarcillin (Table 2).

This study demonstrates that thienamycin is a highly active agent which will inhibit bacteria resistant to cefamandole and cefoxitin. However, it is not more active than cefotaxime, and we found rather large differences between MICs and MBCs. Hopefully further studies of the stable derivatives of thienamycin will clarify the position of thienamycin in relation to other new cephalosporins. The anti-staphylococcal activity of thienamycin combined with its excellent activity against *Pseudomonas* and *B. fragilis* makes it comparable to these other agents.

1. **Talley, F. P., N. V. Jacobus, and S. L. Gorbach.** 1978. In vitro activity of thienamycin. Antimicrob. Agents Chemother. **14:**436–438.
2. **Weaver, S. S., G. P. Body, and B. M. LaBlanc.** 1979. Thienamycin: a new beta-lactam antibiotic with potent broad-spectrum activity. Antimicrob. Agents Chemother. **15:**518–521.

Antimicrobial Susceptibility Testing of Pneumococci by Disk Diffusion

M. R. JACOBS[1]* AND H. J. KOORNHOF

Department of Microbiology, School of Pathology of the South African Institute for Medical Research and the University of the Witwatersrand, Johannesburg, South Africa

Resistance to antimicrobial agents developed rapidly after their introduction and soon became a major problem in infections caused by staphylococci and enteric gram-negative bacilli. Recently, antimicrobial resistance has become clinically important in infections caused by *Haemophilus influenzae, Neisseria gonorrhoeae, Streptococcus pneumoniae,* and viridans group streptococci. Much resistance has been to the β-lactam antibiotics, the mechanism of resistance being due to either β-lactamase production or membrane permeability barriers to the drugs. *Streptococcus pyogenes* and *Neisseria meningitidis* have not yet shown any tendency to become resistant to the penicillins, but the potential for this development probably exists.

Monitoring the antimicrobial susceptibility of bacteria continues to be important in determining changes that may occur. Changes in resistance do not have to be large to be clinically significant, and several minor increases in resistance can result in eventual complete resistance. For many of the organisms mentioned above, determination of antimicrobial susceptibility is

still not routinely advocated, and techniques for screening such organisms have only recently been approved by the National Committee for Clinical Laboratory Standards (6).

With many of the above factors concerning resistance to antimicrobial agents applying to resistant strains of *S. pneumoniae* isolated in South Africa since 1977 (1, 3), a simple, reliable technique was required to enable pneumococci to be screened for antimicrobial susceptibility, based on the Kirby-Bauer method of disk diffusion. For this purpose, recommended Kirby-Bauer MIC breakpoints (6) for erythromycin, clindamycin, tetracycline, and chloramphenicol were used to assess the use of disks containing these agents. For penicillin G, MIC breakpoints were chosen at 0.1 and 1 µg/ml to reflect any increase in the susceptibility of pneumococci to penicillin from their exquisite susceptibility of ≤0.02 µg of penicillin G per ml. Pneumococci of intermediate penicillin resistance by these criteria (MICs of 0.1 to 1 µg/ml) have not responded clinically to penicillin G therapy when causing meningitis, and resistant strains with MICs of penicillin G of 2 to 10 µg/ml have caused many serious infections in South Africa (5).

Initial results in our laboratories showed that

[1] Present address: Institute of Pathology, Case Western Reserve University, Adelbert Road, Cleveland, OH 44106, U.S.A.

TABLE 1. *Disk diffusion zone diameters obtained with penicillin G, methicillin, oxacillin, erythromycin, clindamycin, tetracycline, chloramphenicol, and rifampin, with recommended zone diameter cut-offs*

Antibiotic	MIC breakpoints			Disk content (µg)	Zone diam (mm)					
					Mean ± 2 SD			Recommended cut-off zones		
	S[a]	I	R		S	I	R	S	I	R
Penicillin G	<0.1	0.1–1	>1	6	43 ± 9	31 ± 7	19 ± 8	>35	22–35	<22
				0.6	8 ± 7	22 ± 6	31 ± 6	>25	15–25	<15
				0.15	27 ± 4	13 ± 9	≤6 ± 0	>22	7–20	≤6
				0.018	20 ± 4	7 ± 5	≤6 ± 0	>15	6–12	≤6
Methicillin[b]	<0.1	0.1–1	>1	5	34 ± 7	19 ± 8	7 ± 4	>25	16–25	<16
Oxacillin[b]	<0.1	0.1–1	>1	1	28 ± 7	11 ± 8	≤6 ± 0	>21	7–20	≤6
Erythromycin	≤2	4	≥8	15	34 ± 10		7 ± 5	>20		<20
Clindamycin	≤1		≥2	2	29 ± 9		8 ± 8	>20		<20
Tetracycline	≤4	8	≥12	30	27 ± 8		10 ± 8	>19		<19
Chloramphenicol	≤12	16	≥25	30	28 ± 8		13 ± 4	>19		<19
Rifampin	≤1	2–8	≥16	5	30 ± 6		7 ± 4	>20		<20

[a] S, Susceptible; I, intermediate resistant; R, resistant.

[b] Methicillin and oxacillin disks are used to reflect susceptibility to penicillin G, and MIC breakpoints are those of penicillin G and not those of methicillin or oxacillin.

reliable results could be obtained on 5% horse blood agar plates (Columbia base) for erythromycin, clindamycin, tetracycline, chloramphenicol, and rifampin using Kirby-Bauer disks, but that detection of penicillin susceptibility with 6-µg penicillin G disks was not entirely reliable (3). Methicillin disks reflected penicillin G susceptibility more accurately than did 6-µg penicillin G disks (3), confirming the similar report by Dixon et al. (2), using oxacillin disks.

Further investigations of disk susceptibility testing on Mueller-Hinton agar with 5% horse blood was undertaken on 168 strains of pneumococci using a modified Kirby-Bauer technique (plates were 3.5 mm and not 4 mm deep). Disk diffusion breakpoints between susceptible and resistant strains were found to be (4): erythromycin (15-µg disks), 20 mm; clindamycin (2-µg disks), 20 mm; tetracycline (30-µg disks), 19 mm; chloramphenicol (30-µg disks), 19 mm; and rifampin (5-µg disks), 20 mm (Table 1). Resistance to these agents was usually marked, and clear separation of strains occurred with both MIC and disk diffusion methods, with good correlation between the methods. Very few intermediate resistant strains were found to these agents.

The investigation of the optimal method of testing susceptibility to penicillin G by disk diffusion was then undertaken on 159 strains. On determination of their MICs of penicillin G, 44 were susceptible (MICs <0.1 µg/ml), 29 intermediate (MICs 0.1 to 1 µg/ml), and 86 resistant (MICs 1 to 10 µg/ml) (Fig. 1). Disk diffusion testing was performed on Mueller-Hinton agar

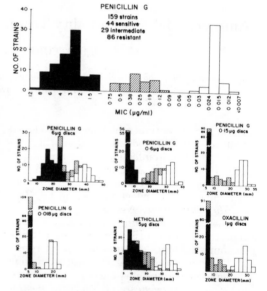

FIG. 1. *Histograms of frequency distribution of MICs of penicillin G and zone diameters obtained with various penicillin G, methicillin, and oxacillin disks. Division of strains into sensitive (susceptible), intermediate, and resistant groups is based on MICs of penicillin G throughout. Symbols:* □, *susceptible;* ▨, *intermediate resistant;* ■, *resistant to the antimicrobial agent based on MICs.*

containing 5% lysed horse blood, and various disks were used, including penicillin G (0.018, 0.15, 0.6, 1.2, 2.4, and 6 µg), methicillin (2, 5, and 10 µg), cloxacillin (5 µg), oxacillin (1 µg), nafcillin

(1 μg), and ampicillin (2 and 10 μg). Optimal separation of strains occurred with 0.15-μg penicillin G, 1-μg oxacillin, and 5-μg methicillin disks (Table 1 and Fig. 1). Disks containing 0.6 μg of penicillin G gave reasonable separation of strains, while those containing 6 μg produced considerable overlap of intermediate strains into both the susceptible and resistant ranges. The 0.018-μg penicillin G disks separated susceptible from both intermediate and resistant groups and may be useful if used for this purpose (Fig. 1). Similar results were obtained on strains tested on Mueller-Hinton agar with 5% whole sheep and horse blood, and on Columbia agar with 5% horse blood.

These investigations have shown that the widely used Kirby-Bauer disk diffusion technique can be easily modified to screen pneumococci for antimicrobial resistance. For penicillin G susceptibility screening, oxacillin or methicillin disks appear to be the most reliable and are readily available as they contain the recommended amounts of these agents used for testing of staphylococci by the Kirby-Bauer method. Confirmation of resistance must be obtained by MIC determination, and the testing of susceptibility of pneumococci to antimicrobial agents should be routinely performed on all clinically significant isolates.

1. Appelbaum, P. C., A. Bhamjee, J. N. Scragg, A. F. Hallet, A. A. Bowen, and R. C. Cooper. 1977. Streptococcus pneumoniae resistant to penicillin and chloramphenicol. Lancet ii:995–997.
2. Dixon, J. M. S., A. E. Lipinski, and M. E. P. Graham. 1977. Detection and prevalence of pneumococci with increased resistance to penicillin. Can. Med. Assoc. J. 117:1159–1161.
3. Jacobs, M. R., H. J. Koornhof, R. M. Robins-Browne, C. M. Stevenson, Z. A. Vermaak, I. Freiman, G. B. Miller, M. A. Witcomb, M. Isaacson, J. I. Ward, and R. Austrian. 1978. Emergence of multiply resistant pneumococci. N. Engl. J. Med. 299:735–740.
4. Jacobs, M. R., Y. Mithal, R. M. Robins-Browne, M. N. Gaspar, and H. J. Koornhof. 1979. Antimicrobial susceptibility testing of pneumococci: determination of Kirby-Bauer breakpoints for penicillin G, erythromycin, clindamycin, tetracycline, chloramphenicol and rifampin. Antimicrob. Agents Chemother. 16:190–197.
5. Koornhof, H. J., M. R. Jacobs, J. I. Ward, P. C. Appelbaum, and A. F. Hallett. 1979. Therapy and control of antibiotic-resistant pneumococcal disease, p. 286–289. In D. Schlessinger (ed.), Microbiology—1979. American Society for Microbiology, Washington, D.C.
6. National Committee for Clinical Laboratory Standards. 1979. Performance standards for antimicrobial disc susceptibility tests. NCCLS publication no. ASM 2. National Committee for Clinical Laboratory Standards, Villanova, Pa.

Comparison of Antimicrobial Susceptibility Between Isolates from Doctorless Areas and from Hospitals

WOO-HYUN CHANG,* KWANG-HO RHEE, HEE-SUP SHIN, IK-SANG KIM, AND JUNG-KYU LIM

College of Medicine, Seoul National University, Seoul, Korea

Besides the benefits of antimicrobial agents in the control of various infectious diseases, widespread and prolonged use of a particular antimicrobial agent brought about the increase of drug-resistant strains in a community and profound changes in the pattern of infectious diseases. Bacteria may become resistant to antimicrobial agents by transduction, transformation, mutation, and conjugation, but selection out also accounts for an increase in number of resistant strains in a community (2). In Korea, there are some remote villages where no clinics and drug stores are available, and the residents in those areas are assumed to have fewer contacts with antimicrobial agents. We studied the differences in susceptibilities to 14 antimicrobial agents between the isolates from doctorless areas, (L), and Seoul National University Hospital (SNUH), (H). The isolates and their number were Staphylococcus aureus (L;55, H;68), Streptococcus pneumoniae (L;28, H;30), Enterococcus spp. (L;28, H;30), Haemophilus influenzae (L;31, H;23), Escherichia coli (L;40, H;40), Enterobacter aerogenes (L;25, H;21), and Klebsiella pneumoniae (L;58, H;67). MICs of penicillin, ampicillin, carbenicillin, cephalexin, tetracycline, oxytetracycline, doxycycline, minocycline, gentamicin, kanamycin, streptomycin, erythromycin, troleandomycin, and co-trimoxazole were determined by the agar dilution method (1).

Comparison of MIC. With E. coli, E. aerogenes, and K. pneumoniae, the mean MIC of penicillin, tetracycline, oxytetracycline, doxycycline, kanamycin, streptomycin, and co-trimoxazole to the isolates from SNUH were significantly higher than the mean MIC to the isolates from doctorless areas. However, with S.

aureus, S. pneumoniae, Enterococcus spp., and *H. influenzae,* significant differences in the mean MIC were found only in streptomycin (*S. aureus*), carbenicillin (*S. pneumoniae*), or kanamycin (*S. aureus* and *S. pneumoniae*). The mean MIC of tetracycline to *S. aureus* isolated from doctorless areas was higher than *S. aureus* isolated at SNUH.

In general, differences in susceptibility to these antimicrobial agents between the isolates from doctorless areas and SNUH were greater and broader in gram-negative enteric bacteria. There were no species showing differences in susceptibility to recently introduced gentamicin. In this connection, it was very interesting that *E. coli* and *E. aerogenes* from SNUH were more resistant to newly introduced minocycline than the isolates from doctorless areas. This appears to be due to cross-resistance of bacteria to chemically related antimicrobial agents (Table 2).

Multiple drug resistance patterns. Since 1960 the proportion of multiply drug-resistant gram-negative enteric bacteria isolated from the environment has sharply increased, and in most, resistance is mediated by R factors (3). In this study, multiple drug resistance patterns and their incidence were studied in ampicillin, tetracycline, cephalexin, gentamicin, streptomycin, kanamycin, and co-trimoxazole among *E. coli, E. aerogenes,* and *K. pneumoniae* (Table 1). Significant differences appeared in the incidence of multiply drug-resistant strains and multiple

drug resistance patterns between the isolates from SNUH and doctorless areas in all three bacteria. The incidence of multiply drug-resistant strains and the diversity of their patterns were highest with *E. coli* isolated from SNUH, and there were no multiply drug-resistant strains in *K. pneumoniae* isolated from doctorless areas. The number of drug-resistance determinants was also different in the isolates from doctorless areas and those from SNUH. Most of the multiply drug-resistant strains of *E. coli, E. aerogenes,* and *K. pneumoniae* isolated from SNUH were resistant to more than three kinds of antimicrobial agents, most frequently to ampicillin, tetracycline, and streptomycin, while multiply drug-resistant strains from doctorless areas were resistant to two kinds of antimicrobial agents.

With drug-resistant *E. coli* strains, resistance to tetracycline, which was used most widely from 1951 in Korea, was the most frequent factor in multiple drug resistance, followed by resistance to ampicillin and streptomycin. This suggests strongly that emergence of a drug-resistant population in a community is directly dependent on the selective pressure exerted by the antimicrobial agent used.

Cross-resistance. Cross-resistance of bacteria was studied among tetracycline, oxytetracycline, doxycycline, and minocycline by analyzing the correlation coefficients of susceptibility. Results are shown in Table 2. With these bacteria, there was high correlation of susceptibility to

TABLE 1. *Comparison of multiple resistance pattern*

Combination of antibiotics[a]	Resistance incidence (%)					
	E. coli		*E. aerogenes*		*K. pneumoniae*	
	SNUH	Local	SNUH	Local	SNUH	Local
Am + Tc + Gm + Sm + Km	2.5		23.8		7.5	
Am + Tc + Sm + Km	20		14.3		9.0	
Am + Tc + Sm + Ct	2.5					
Am + Tc + Sm + Cx	2.5					
Am + Tc + Sm	25				3.0	
Tc + Sm + Cx	2.5					
Tc + Sm + Km	2.5					
Am + Tc	5					
Tc + Sm	7.5	7.5		4	1.5	
Am + Sm		2.5			1.5	
Am + Cx		2.5			1.5	
Gm + Sm	2.5					
Km + Sm			4.8			
Am + Ct		2.5				
Total incidence of resistant strains (%)	72.5	15	42.8	4	23.9	0

[a]Am, Ampicillin; Tc, tetracycline; Gm, gentamicin; Sm, streptomycin; Km, kanamycin; Cx, cephalexin; Ct, co-trimoxazole.

TABLE 2. *Correlation coefficients of susceptibility among tetracycline derivatives*

Organism	Combination of antibiotics[a]					
	Tc/Oc	Tc/Dc	Tc/Mc	Oc/Dc	Oc/Mc	Dc/Mc
S. aureus	0.93	0.86	0.76	0.70	0.75	0.95
S. pneumoniae	0.91	0.92	0.95	0.86	0.88	0.91
Enterococcus	0.98	0.97	0.88	0.96	0.87	0.86
H. influenzae	0.85	0.96	0.85	0.76	0.72	0.80
E. coli	0.97	0.97	0.91	0.95	0.88	0.90
E. aerogenes	0.97	0.88	0.82	0.91	0.76	0.80
K. pneumoniae	0.94	0.89	0.57	0.87	0.57	0.65

[a] Tc, Tetracycline; Oc, oxytetracycline; Dc, doxycycline; Mc, minocycline.

tetracycline derivatives. One exception was the correlation of susceptibility to minocycline with that of three other tetracyclines in *K. pneumoniae*. This relatively low correlation in susceptibility appeared to be due to intrinsic resistance of *K. pneumoniae* to minocycline, because the mean MIC of minocycline to *K. pneumoniae* isolated from doctorless areas was higher than the mean MICs of three other tetracyclines, and there was no significant difference in susceptibility to minocycline between *K. pneumoniae* isolated from doctorless areas and those from SNUH.

1. **Ericsson, H. M., and J. C. Sherris.** 1971. Antibiotic sensitivity testing. Acta Pathol. Microbiol. Scand. Sect. B **217**(Suppl.):1–90.
2. **Goodman, L. S., and A. Gilman.** 1970. Chemotherapy of microbial diseases. *In* The pharmacological basis of therapeutics, 4th ed. The MacMillan Co., New York.
3. **Wilson, G. S., and A. A. Miles.** 1975. Topley and Wilson's principles of bacteriology, virology and immunity, 6th ed., p. 206–209. Edward Arnold Ltd., London.

Development of Resistance to Trimethoprim, Trimethoprim-Sulfamethoxazole, Sulfamethoxazole, Ampicillin, and Nitrofurantoin in Urinary Tract Pathogens: a 20-Month Epidemiological Study in Stockholm and Turku

PAAVO TOIVANEN* AND KATHRINE DORNBUSCH

Department of Medical Microbiology, Turku University, Turku, Finland, and Department of Bacteriology, National Bacteriological Laboratory, Stockholm, Sweden

The combination trimethoprim-sulfamethoxazole (TMP-SMZ) has been successfully used in the control of urinary tract infections. In recent years, certain advantages of TMP therapy have also become apparent (1, 2). However, concern has arisen that TMP alone may cause increased TMP resistance. In Finland, plain TMP has been used in the long-term control of recurrent urinary tract infections since 1973, whereas in Sweden only the combination TMP-SMZ has been available. This forms the basis of the present study in which resistance of urinary tract pathogens against TMP, TMP-SMZ, SMZ, ampicillin, and nitrofurantoin was investigated in hospitalized patients in Stockholm, Sweden, and in Turku, Finland. The design of the study included routine use of TMP-SMZ in Stockholm and that of TMP in Turku whenever medically indicated during a 20-month follow-up.

Urinary pathogens ($>10^5$/ml) were collected during 1-month periods in Stockholm and during 2-month periods in Turku as follows: period I, February–March 1977; period II, September–October 1977; period III, February–March 1978; and period IV, September–October 1978. The strains were tested for susceptibility to antibacterial drugs by a standardized agar dilution method. Five of the six hospitals in Stockholm were for geriatrics and one for lung diseases. In Turku, one of the participating hospitals was for oncology, one for geriatrics, and one for psychiatry. Only hospitalized patients were included in the study. Altogether 230 patients (mean age, 79 years) participated in Stockholm and 332 patients (mean age, 73 years) in Turku.

Among the 287 strains isolated in Stockholm, 41.1% were *Escherichia coli*, 26.5% *Proteus mirabilis*, and 4.3% *Pseudomonas aeruginosa*. In

TABLE 1. *Percentage of TMP-resistant strains (MIC ≥ 8 µg/ml) among urinary pathogens in Turku during the four collection periods*

Organism	% Resistant (period)					No. studied (period)				
	I	II	III	IV	Total	I	II	III	IV	Total
E. coli	7	13	9	27	15	30	38	22	41	131
Klebsiella	30	37	60	42	46	10	8	20	12	50
P. mirabilis	86	82	56	74	72	7	11	16	19	53
Streptococcus faecalis	47	0	27	30	32	15	4	11	10	40
Others	40	60	75	74	66	10	38	24	27	99
Achromobacter			100		100			3		3
Citrobacter	33	90	25	100	70	3	10	4	3	20
Enterobacter	33	56	0	33	44	3	9	1	3	16
P. morganii		67		0	50		3		1	4
P. rettgeri		0			0		1			1
P. vulgaris		100	0	0	33		1	1	1	3
Providencia stuartii		100	100	100	100		1	6	6	13
Serratia		0		100	50		1		1	2
Staphylococcus aureus	0	33	100		40	1	3	1		5
Staphylococcus epidermidis	67	50	87	75	71	3	8	8	12	31
Streptococcus viridans		0			0		1			1
Total	30.6	40.4	47.3	48.6	42.6	72	99	93	109	373

Turku, out of 454 strains isolated 28.8% were *E. coli*, 11.7% *P. mirabilis*, and 17.8% *P. aeruginosa*. All strains of *P. aeruginosa* in both centers were TMP resistant.

With *Pseudomonas* excluded, the majority (269/275) of the bacteria collected in Stockholm were susceptible to TMP (MIC ≤4 µg/ml). Six strains (2.2%) of the Stockholm material were TMP resistant (MIC ≥8 µg/ml), comprising one strain each of *P. mirabilis, Enterobacter cloacae, Klebsiella pneumoniae, Staphylococcus epidermidis, E. coli,* and *Streptococcus faecalis.* No difference in the occurrence of TMP-resistant strains was observed during the four periods of the Stockholm study.

In Turku, 159 (42.6%) of the 373 strains (with *Pseudomonas* excluded) were TMP resistant (MIC ≥8 µg/ml; Table 1). The majority of resistant strains comprised *P. mirabilis* (38 strains), *Klebsiella* spp. (23), *S. epidermidis* (22), and *E. coli* (20). The frequency of TMP resistance increased from 30.6% in period I to 48.6% in period IV, showing a linear trend. During the later periods (II to IV) of the study, the frequency of *P. mirabilis, Providencia,* and *S. epidermidis* was higher than initially, indicating a shift to the occurrence of more resistant strains (Table 1). Such a shift was not observed in Stockholm.

In the Stockholm material, resistance to TMP-SMZ was about the same as to TMP alone and significantly lower than in Turku (Fig. 1). In contrast, the frequency of strains resistant to SMZ, nitrofurantoin, or ampicillin was roughly on the same level in both centers. No significant changes were observed during the Stockholm

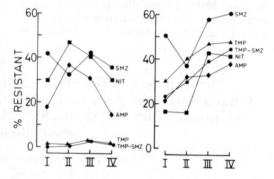

FIG. 1. *Percentage of resistant strains among urinary pathogens in Stockholm (left) and Turku (right) during the four collection periods. Resistance is defined with the following MICs: trimethoprim (TMP) ≥8 µg/ml, trimethoprim-sulfamethoxazole (TMP-SMZ) ≥64 µg/ml, sulfamethoxazole (SMZ) ≥512 µg/ ml, ampicillin (AMP) ≥32 µg/ml, and nitrofurantoin (NIT) ≥64 µg/ml.*

study in the resistance to any of the five drugs tested. In Turku, the increase in the resistance did not involve only TMP but also all the other drugs tested: the resistance to SMZ increased from 50.8% to 60.6%, to TMP-SMZ from 23.7% to 45.0%, to ampicillin from 22.0% to 38.5%, and to nitrofurantoin from 16.9% to 42.2% (Fig. 1). In these calculations all strains of *Pseudomonas* were excluded.

The increase in resistance to TMP or TMP-SMZ observed in Turku could be due to the heavy use of plain TMP; 22% of all prescribed antibacterial treatments in the participating wards in Turku were TMP. Further, use of plain

TMP is generally heavy in the Turku area, per inhabitant 67% more than in the whole country on average (H. Sundquist, personal communication). On this basis, the increase in TMP resistance could represent the natural time-dependent increase in resistance. However, in light of the overall increase in bacterial resistance, including ampicillin and nitrofurantoin, this alternative becomes unlikely.

A probable explanation for the overall increase in bacterial resistance in Turku appears to be the generally heavy use of antibacterial drugs in the participating Turku hospitals. During the study, on average 0.90 antibacterial treatment per patient was used in the participating wards in Stockholm, whereas 1.19 per patient was used in Turku. The difference between Stockholm and Turku is also apparent from the corresponding data regarding the participating hospitals in total. During a 3-month period at a final stage of the study, 0.52 antibacterial treatment per patient was used on average in Stockholm and 0.98 per patient in Turku. Other factors contributing to the overall increase in resistance include a change in the use of nitrofurantoin during the study; 0.07 to 0.10 nitrofurantoin treatment per patient was used in the participating Turku wards during periods I–II and 0.20 to 0.28 per patient during periods III–IV. It should also be noted that in a Turku hospital, with the shortest time of hospitalization (mean 2.9 months per patient), no increase in TMP resistance occurred (18.7% for period I and 17.6% for period IV). In this hospital, none of the 38 isolated *E. coli* strains was TMP resistant.

In conclusion, a high frequency of strains resistant to TMP or TMP-SMZ was demonstrated in Turku (where plain TMP has been used since 1973) but not in Stockholm. During a 20-month follow-up, an overall increase in bacterial resistance, including ampicillin and nitrofurantoin, was observed in Turku but not in Stockholm. This increase is related rather to the heavy use of antibacterial drugs in general than to the use of plain TMP.

1. **Brumfitt, W., and R. Pursell.** 1972. Double-blind trial to compare ampicillin, cephalexin, co-trimoxazole and trimethoprim in treatment of urinary infection. Br. Med. J. i:673–676.
2. **Kasanen, A., M. Anttila, R. Elfving, P. Kahela, H. Saarimaa, H. Sundquist, R. Tikkanen, and P. Toivanen.** 1978. Trimethoprim; pharmacology, antibacterial activity and clinical use in urinary tract infections. Ann. Clin. Res. 10(Suppl. 22):1–39.

Activity of Sulfamethoxazole/Trimethoprim Against Aerobic and Anaerobic Bacteria

J. WÜST* AND F. H. KAYSER

Institute of Medical Microbiology, University of Zurich, CH-8028 Zurich, Switzerland

Sulfamethoxazole/trimethoprim (SMZ/TMP) is one of the most used drugs in hospitals as well as in medical practice in Switzerland. The drug is applied not only in urinary tract infections but also in many other bacterial diseases. Because of this frequent use of SMZ/TMP in our country, a continuous survey of resistance against the agent is necessary. Such a survey became feasible with the introduction of an electronic data-processing system in 1974. The data were obtained with the standardized single disk method recommended by the U.S. Food and Drug Administration. An inhibition zone of 16 mm around the 25-µg disk was used as breakpoint between resistant and susceptible organisms (2).

Table 1 shows the susceptibility to SMZ/TMP in all gram-positive and gram-negative strains (including OF bacteria) isolated since 1974. Only a very slight decrease in susceptibility over these years could be observed, despite the presence of SMZ/TMP plasmids in part of the resistant gram-negative bacteria (3). Presently, SMZ/TMP is a broad-spectrum antimicrobial,

TABLE 1. *Susceptibility to sulfamethoxazole/trimethoprim (June 1974–June 1979)*

Yr	Outpatients[a]		Hospitalized patients	
	No. of strains	% of susceptible strains	No. of strains	% of susceptible strains
1974	1,893	87	12,135	76
1975	3,322	85	19,125	74
1976	3,471	87	18,651	77
1977	4,938	82	20,643	69
1978	4,243	85	20,500	72
1979	1,990	85	9,780	70

[a] Relation to prior hospitalization not determined.

TABLE 2. *Susceptibility of anaerobic bacteria*

Organism	% of susceptible strains[a]					
	131 VPI strains	218 Zurich strains				
	SXT[b]	SXT	Clindamycin	Cefoxitin	Metronidazole	Chloramphenicol
B. fragilis group	100	99	93	94	100	100
Bacteroides spp.	77	100	100	100	100	100
Fusobacterium spp.	92	100	100	100	100	100
Anaerobic cocci	78	50	100	95	100	100
Clostridium perfringens	100	83	100	100	100	100
Clostridium spp.	62	92	93	64	100	100

[a] MICs: SXT, ≤ 16 μg/ml; clindamycin, ≤ 4 μg/ml; cefoxitin, ≤ 16 μg/ml; metronidazole, ≤ 8 μg/ml; chloramphenicol, ≤ 16 μg/ml.

[b] SXT, Sulfamethoxazole/trimethoprim (19:1).

to which a high percentage of susceptible strains is observed; e.g., *Enterobacteriaceae* isolated from hospitalized patients show the following susceptibilities: SMZ/TMP, 75%; ampicillin, 54%; meclocillin, 73%; cefalotin, 69%; cefamandol, 86%; cefoxitin, 91%; cefuroxim, 87%; chloramphenicol, 77%; tetracycline, 60%; gentamicin, 97%; amikacin, 100%.

Despite its widespread use in Europe, relatively little is known about the effect of SMZ/TMP on anaerobic bacteria. There are only few reports on in vitro susceptibility. Rosenblatt and Stewart (5) found little activity of SMZ/TMP against anaerobes. In contrast to this, other workers, among them Phillips and Warren (4), reported good susceptibility of the *Bacteroides fragilis* group to SMZ alone and to SMZ/TMP, whereas most strains were resistant to TMP alone.

Two further MIC studies were performed to determine the susceptibility of a variety of anaerobic bacteria to SMZ/TMP. In a first study done at the Anaerobe Laboratory of the Virginia Polytechnic Institute (6), 58% of 144 anaerobic strains were susceptible to SMZ alone, only 12% were susceptible to TMP alone, and 85% were susceptible to the combination of SMZ and TMP at a ratio of 19:1. All 45 strains of the *B. fragilis* group were susceptible to the combination. Synergy of the combination was often observed by a checkerboard MIC determination of 123 strains, usually most markedly when the ratio of the two components was near 1:1. However, there was also synergism at the ratio of SMZ to TMP of 16:1 in 54% of the strains.

Because the selective pressure of SMZ/TMP in Europe is much higher than in the United States, 218 anaerobes isolated from clinical material in Zurich were studied. Table 2 shows the susceptibility of these strains to SMZ/TMP and some other antimicrobial agents used in treatment of anaerobic infections. No important difference in susceptibility to SMZ/TMP could be found between strains isolated in the United States and in Switzerland.

The main factor that led to the conclusion by Rosenblatt and Stewart that the majority of anaerobes are resistant to SMZ/TMP appears to have been the higher inoculum that they used and other differences in methods as discussed in detail by Phillips and Warren (4). The inoculum used in the present study corresponds to the one recommended in the ICS study by Ericsson and Sherris (1) and also used by Phillips and Warren.

The in vitro results of the activity of SMZ/TMP against anaerobic bacteria are promising. SMZ/TMP might represent an alternative for therapy of anaerobic infections, especially in mixed infections of obligate anaerobes with facultatively anaerobic bacteria susceptible to it. The value of SMZ/TMP for treatment of anaerobic infections needs further evaluation by animal studies and carefully controlled clinical trials.

1. **Ericsson, H. M., and J. C. Sherris.** 1971. Antibiotic sensitivity testing: report of an international collaborative study. Acta Pathol. Microbiol. Scand. **217**(Suppl.): 1–90.

2. **Kayser, F. H., and I. Müller.** 1978. Resistance of bacteria to sulfamethoxazole/trimethoprim, p. 657–658. *In* Current chemotherapy, Proceedings of the 10th International Congress of Chemotherapy. American Society for Microbiology, Washington, D.C.

3. **Kayser, F. H., and J. Wüst.** 1973. Determination of bacterial resistance to trimethoprim/sulfamethoxazole using the single disk diffusion method. Chemotherapy (Basel) **18**:162–168.

4. **Phillips, I., and C. Warren.** 1976. Activity of sulfamethoxazole and trimethoprim against *Bacteroides fragilis*. Antimicrob. Agents Chemother. **9**:736–740.

5. **Rosenblatt, J. E., and P. R. Stewart.** 1974. Lack of activity of sulfamethoxazole and trimethoprim against anaerobic bacteria. Antimicrob. Agents Chemother. **6**: 93–97.

6. **Wüst, J., and T. D. Wilkins.** 1978. Susceptibility of anaerobic bacteria to sulfamethoxazole/trimethoprim and routine susceptibility testing. Antimicrob. Agents Chemother. **14**:384–390.

Epidemiology of Methicillin-Resistant *Staphylococcus aureus* Infections

JOHN M. BOYCE,[1]* MARTHA LANDRY, THOMAS R. DEETZ, AND HERBERT L. DuPONT

University of Texas Medical School, Houston, Texas 77030, U.S.A.

In June 1978, a burned patient at Hermann Hospital, Houston, Tex., developed bacteremia caused by *Staphylococcus aureus* resistant to methicillin and gentamicin (MRSA). Similar strains soon infected other patients in the surgical intensive care unit (SICU) and intermediate care unit (SIMU). This report describes the epidemiology of the MRSA outbreak that followed.

Patients were considered infected when MRSA was isolated from normally sterile body fluids, purulent wound drainage, or sputum of patients with increased sputum production and chest X-ray findings of pneumonia. Antimicrobial susceptibility tests of MRSA were performed using standard agar diffusion and agar dilution techniques. Phage lysis and phage inhibition typing were performed by the Center for Disease Control, Atlanta, Ga.

From June through December 1978, MRSA was isolated from 61 patients (Fig. 1). Fifty-seven (93%) of the patients were on surgical services; 38 (62%) of cases were in the SICU or SIMU when MRSA were first isolated; only 15% of cases had never been in SICU or SIMU before becoming colonized. Twenty-two patients had burns, 19 had multiple trauma, 4 had head injuries, and 16 had other surgical or medical problems. In the outbreak period, 39% of all burned patients, 6% of multiple trauma patients, and 4% of head injury patients admitted to the hospital acquired MRSA ($P < 0.001$). At the time the outbreak began, burned patient census, emergency surgery admissions, and SICU and SIMU occupancy rates were higher than at any previous time in 1978.

MRSA isolates from all 61 patients were susceptible to cephalothin and resistant to methicillin, penicillin, ampicillin, erythromycin, and tetracycline by agar diffusion techniques. Fifty-seven patients had MRSA resistant to gentamicin, and in 41 patients MRSA was also resistant to chloramphenicol and clindamycin. Twenty-three strains were tested for methicillin susceptibility by agar dilution techniques and all were resistant (MIC >12.5 µg/ml). Thirty-eight of 41 strains tested by phage lysis techniques were untypable. Thirty-two of 38 strains without lytic phage reaction showed phage inhibition reactions to 47/53/54/85 or closely related patterns.

The mean interval between admission and the first MRSA isolate was 27.2 ± 5.6 days in burned patients and 34.4 ± 8.2 days in patients without burns ($P > 0.05$). The median duration of MRSA colonization was 32 days (range 1–127) for burned patients and 10 days (range 1–134) in patients without burns ($P > 0.05$). MRSA was commonly recovered from wounds (42 patients), sputum (31 patients), blood (22 patients), and central venous catheter tips (16 patients). Overt infections due to MRSA occurred in 64% of burned patients and 51% of patients without burns. MRSA bacteremia was documented in 45% of burned patients and 31% of patients without burns. In 6 of 61 patients, MRSA infection was a primary or contributing cause of death.

Fifteen patients with MRSA infections were compared with 15 age- and sex-matched control patients with methicillin-susceptible *S. aureus* (MSSA) infections. In addition, burned patients were matched by percent total body surface area burned, and patients without burns were matched by admitting diagnosis and extent of surgery prior to becoming colonized with *S. aureus*. The mean time between admission and first *S. aureus* isolate, the number of antibiotics received, and the duration of antibiotic therapy before becoming colonized were significantly greater for MRSA cases than for MSSA controls (Table 1).

Comparison of patients with MRSA and randomly selected SICU controls did not implicate exposure to a common source but did reveal associations between acquiring MRSA and ex-

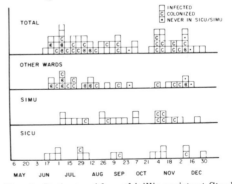

FIG. 1. *Patients with methicillin-resistant Staphylococcus aureus, by date of onset and location, Hermann Hospital, 1978.*

[1] Present address: Division of Infectious Diseases, University of Mississippi Medical Center, Jackson, MS 39216, U.S.A.

TABLE 1. *Matched-pair analysis of patients with MRSA and patients with methicillin-susceptible Staphylococcus aureus (MSSA) infections (N = 15)*

Determination	MRSA	MSSA	P value
Admission to first isolate interval (days)	40.3 ± 8.7^a	15.0 ± 4.8	0.02
No. of antibiotics received[b]	5.1 ± 0.6	1.4 ± 0.5	0.01
Duration of antibiotic therapy (days)[b]	21.8 ± 5.0	9.4 ± 2.9	0.01
Bacteremic (%)	60	80	
Duration of colonization (days)	47.3 ± 15.3	53.6 ± 30.8	
Duration of hospitalization (days)	101.7 ± 20.6	96.3 ± 34.8	
Mortality rate (%)	33.3	13	
Cost of hospitalization	$\$64,370 \pm 11,191$	$\$24,380 \pm 3,178$	0.02

[a] Mean ± standard error.
[b] Interval between admission and first *S. aureus* isolate.

posure to five different hospital personnel ($P < 0.05$). Nasal swab cultures performed on 220 hospital personnel revealed that 14 (6%) harbored MRSA. Three personnel carried MRSA for at least 3 months despite attempts to eradicate carriage with topical bacitracin therapy. None of 37 hospital personnel examined carried MRSA on their hands. All 59 cultures of respiratory therapy equipment and solutions and air sample cultures were negative for MRSA. Culture surveys of SICU and SIMU patients failed to uncover MRSA carriers not already identified by cultures obtained for clinical reasons.

Control measures included strict isolation of patients with MRSA, transfer of critically ill MRSA patients to the SIMU, use of cohort nursing, treatment of MRSA-positive personnel with topical bacitracin, and curtailment of admissions to SIMU in December 1978. These measures reduced the incidence of new cases (5 cases in January and February 1979) but did not end the outbreak.

S. aureus isolates from this outbreak resembled MRSA reported previously, i.e., resistant to methicillin, penicillin, erythromycin, tetracycline, and gentamicin (1). Although standard phage-typing studies were inconclusive, the evidence suggested that this outbreak involved a limited number of strains. The heterogeneity of antibiograms seen in this outbreak has been observed in other hospitals (1, 2).

MRSA infections frequently affect patients with burns or preceding surgery (1, 2). The frequent use of antimicrobials in such patients promotes colonization of patients with multiply resistant organisms including MRSA (1). About 50% of patients who acquire MRSA become clinically infected, 13 to 36% develop bacteremia, and in 10% of patients from this outbreak, MRSA infection was a primary or contributing cause of death (1, 2). Results of our matched-pair analysis, and clinical and experimental data reported by others, suggest that MRSA and methicillin-susceptible *S. aureus* are of comparable virulence (1). Unlike strains susceptible to methicillin, MRSA colonize a small proportion (2–8%) of hospital personnel (1, 2).

1. Crossley, K., D. Loesch, B. Landesman, et al. 1979. An outbreak of infections caused by strains of *Staphylococcus aureus* resistant to methicillin and aminoglycosides. I. Clinical studies. J. Infect. Dis. **139**:273–279.
2. Klimek, J. J., F. J. Marsik, R. C. Bartlett, et al. 1976. Clinical, epidemiologic and bacteriologic observations of an outbreak of methicillin-resistant *Staphylococcus aureus* at a large community hospital. Am. J. Med. **61**:340–345.

Novel Aspects of an Aminoglycoside-Resistant Mutant of *Staphylococcus aureus* with Deficient Oxidative Metabolism and Decreased Gentamicin Uptake

STEPHEN G. WILSON* AND CHRISTINE C. SANDERS

Department of Medical Microbiology, Creighton University School of Medicine, Omaha, Nebraska 68178, U.S.A.

In a previous study (1), a mutant (M) of *Staphylococcus aureus* 29/52/80 (wild type [WT]) was selected with gentamicin (GM) at concentrations eightfold above the MIC for WT (0.2 µg/ml). M was eightfold more resistant than WT to kanamycin, tobramycin, GM, amikacin, and sisomicin. The present study attempts to relate the GM resistance of M to a deficiency in oxidative metabolism.

The susceptibility of M and WT to GM was determined in Mueller-Hinton broth by a standard serial twofold tube dilution method. The uptake of [³H]GM was determined in Mueller-Hinton broth by a centrifugation method. Logarithmic-phase cells were incubated with [³H]-GM. Portions of 25 ml were removed at various time intervals and added to centrifuge tubes containing 10 ml of cold 0.1 M Mg^{2+} solution. The tubes were centrifuged at 25,000 × g. The pellet was resuspended in 15 ml of the Mg^{2+} solution, recentrifuged, resuspended in 1.0 ml of water, and counted in 15 ml of scintillation cocktail. The effect of hemin on the growth of M and

WT in basal medium was determined spectrophotometrically at 450 nm. The basal medium consisted of Casamino Acids, vitamins, and salts. Cell viability in kill curves with GM and in [³H]GM uptake studies was quantified by agar dilution plate counts. Anaerobic growth in Mueller-Hinton broth was studied in an anaerobic chamber with an atmosphere of 10% CO_2, 10% H_2, and 80% N_2. O_2 uptake by M and WT was determined by Warburg respirometry with 10^9 colony-forming units of the organism per ml in basal medium with 0.005 M glucose.

To assess the relationship between GM resistance of M and deficiencies in oxidative metabolism, agents which block oxidative metabolism were tested for their effects on the susceptibility of WT and M to GM. KCN, an electron trans-

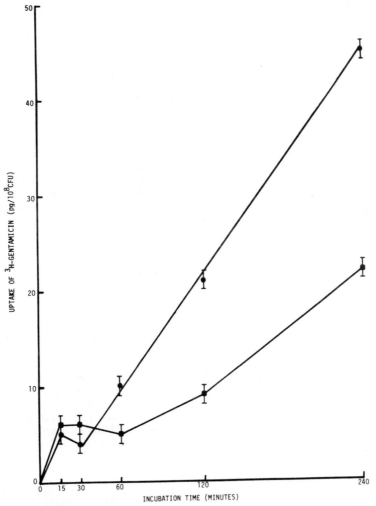

FIG. 1. *Uptake of [³H]GM (0.05 µg/ml) by Staphylococcus aureus 29/52/80 WT (●) and M (■) in Mueller-Hinton broth. Each point represents the mean ± two standard deviations.*

port inhibitor, and dinitrophenol, an oxidative phosphorylation uncoupler, increased the MIC and MBC of GM for WT approximately fourfold but decreased the MIC for M without effect on the MBC. Thiamine, an inhibitor of heme synthesis, increased the MIC for both M and WT four- to eightfold but had little effect on the MBCs. These results suggested that the GM resistance of M was due to defective oxidative metabolism. M should thus be less able to oxidize its sulfhydryl groups and should be more susceptible than WT to $HgCl_2$. Accordingly, the susceptibilities of WT and M to $HgCl_2$ were inversely related to their GM susceptibilities.

To determine whether the defective oxidative metabolism of M resulted in decreased uptake of GM, the kinetics of [^{3}H]GM uptake by M and WT were compared. Uptake of [^{3}H]GM by both M and WT followed triphasic kinetics (Fig. 1). Phase 1 was a 15-min period of rapid uptake. Phase 2 was a 15-min period of no uptake. This was followed by phase 3, a period of sustained, rapid uptake. Although uptake by WT and M was similar in phases 1 and 2, the rate of uptake by WT in the third phase was significantly greater than uptake by M. This suggested that phase 3 was the most dependent upon a functional oxidative metabolism and that the GM resistance of M was reflected by a reduced ability to take up GM. To further substantiate this, the effects of increasing concentrations of GM on the accumulation of [^{3}H]GM by M and WT over a 60-min period were compared (Table 1). The greatest difference in the amount of [^{3}H]GM accumulated by M and WT (10-fold) occurred at a concentration of 2.0 μg of GM per ml, the MBC for WT and the point of greatest difference in susceptibility between the two organisms. Thiamine significantly decreased the amount of [^{3}H]GM accumulated by WT at this concentration while hemin increased the amount of [^{3}H]GM accumulated by M to equal that of WT (Table 1). At concentrations above and below 2.0 μg of GM per ml, thiamine had little effect on the uptake of [^{3}H]GM by WT.

The oxidative metabolism of WT and M was studied further by evaluating their growth and susceptibility to GM under aerobic and anaerobic conditions. The growth of M and WT in Mueller-Hinton broth aerobically and anaerobically was similar. The growth of M was unaffected by a concentration of GM eightfold above the MIC for WT in both atmospheres. WT was killed by this concentration of GM under aerobic conditions but was unaffected by GM under anaerobic conditions that block oxidative metabolism by WT. The growth of M in basal medium without glucose aerobically was much slower than that of WT, suggesting that M was unable to oxidize amino acids, the only carbon source in the medium. By 24 h, WT had grown from an optical density of 0 to 0.34, whereas M had only reached an optical density of 0.14 by 48 h. Hemin (0.001 mM) increased the growth of M significantly to an optical density of 0.43 by 48 h. In basal medium with glucose, the growth of M was not affected by hemin but the resistance of M to GM was greatly decreased. Without hemin, M grew to 10^6 colony-forming units per ml by 24 h in concentrations of GM eightfold above the MIC for WT. In hemin, M was completely killed by this concentration of GM by 24 h.

To determine whether hemin enhanced the oxidative metabolism of M, the rates of O_2 uptake by M in basal medium with and without hemin were compared with the rate of O_2 uptake by WT. The rate of O_2 uptake by M was 1.26 μl/min, or 53% of the rate of WT (2.36 μl/min). The addition of hemin plus acetate increased the rate of O_2 uptake by M to 1.87 μl/min, or 79% of the rate of WT. Acetate alone had no effect upon the rates of O_2 uptake.

The results of this study suggested the following: (i) M is deficient in oxidative metabolism; (ii) this deficiency is due to either a deficiency in heme synthesis or an inability to incorporate heme into the cytochromes; and (iii) the level of GM susceptibility is directly related to both the rate of GM uptake and the rate of oxidative metabolism.

TABLE 1. Effects of GM concentration, hemin, and thiamine on the uptake of [^{3}H]GM by WT and M

Organism	GM concn in medium (μg/ml)	[^{3}H]GM accumulated (ng/10^8 CFU/60 min ± 2 standard deviations)[a]
WT	0.2	0.079 ± 0.005
	2.0	2.400 ± 0.080
	20.0	11.450 ± 0.020
M	0.2	0.049 ± 0.010
	2.0	0.210 ± 0.130
	20.0	8.220 ± 0.420
WT with 2.0 mg of thiamine per ml	2.0	1.260 ± 0.120
M with 0.01 mM hemin	2.0	2.630 ± 0.410

[a] CFU, Colony-forming units.

1. Wilson, S. G., and C. C. Sanders. 1976. Selection and characterization of strains of Staphylococcus aureus displaying unusual resistance to aminoglycosides. Antimicrob. Agents Chemother. 10:519–525.

Susceptibility of *Nocardia asteroides* to 25 Antimicrobial Agents

M. C. SAENZ-GONZALEZ, A. C. GOMEZ-GARCIA, J. IGLESIAS, AND F. MARTIN-LUENGO*

Department of Microbiology, Faculty of Medicine, University of Salamanca, Salamanca, Spain

The first human infection by *Nocardia* was reported by Eppinger in 1890 (4). Since then, the cases of human nocardiosis published in the world literature have been quite numerous. The clinical cases caused by several species of the genus *Nocardia* have been various, ranging from benign infections limited to cutaneous levels to disseminated processes.

It is difficult to establish the real frequency of these processes because they are not usually reported to the sanitary authorities. However, several publications which estimate the severity and incidence of nocardiosis exist (5, 6).

Three species within the genus *Nocardia* are currently regarded as responsible for pathological cases in the human species: *N. asteroides, N. brasiliensis*, and *N. caviae*.

A total of 40 strains of *N. asteroides* of human and soil origin were used during this study.

Each one of the strains was smeared in brain heart infusion agar, and incubation was carried out at 35°C for 5 days.

Flasks (85 by 30 mm) containing 20 ml of Middlebrook 7H9 broth were inoculated with each one of the strains grown in brain heart infusion agar. Incubation took place in an incubator with constant stirring (150 oscillations per min) at 35°C during 5 days.

After the incubation stage, the bacterial growth of each of the strains was made equal in turbidity to a no. 1 MacFarland standard by the addition of sterile distilled water with subsequent dilution to 1/100. A small portion of each dilution was deposited in the wells of the Steers replicator used for the inoculation.

Middlebrook 7H10 agar was used as the culture medium for the study of the susceptibility of *N. asteroides* to the 25 antimicrobial agents tested (see Tables 1 and 2). The antimicrobial agents were added, starting from filtered dilutions, to the aforementioned medium so as to obtain concentrations from 0.3 to 200 µg/ml. Plates of the Middlebrook 7H10 agar without antibiotics were used as controls.

After inoculation, the plates were kept at room temperature for approximately 30 min so that the inoculum drops would not touch each other.

Incubation took place for 4 days at 35°C, after which the reading was taken.

The MIC was regarded as the lowest concentration of each antibiotic which caused inhibition of bacterial development.

The MICs of the various drugs are recorded in Tables 1 and 2.

Within the beta-lactam group, the most active were amoxicillin, cephaloridin, and cefoxitin, the latter showing the highest overall activity, inhibiting 90% of the strains at 12.5 µg/ml. In the beta-lactam group, the rest of the antibiotics studied (flucoxacillin, cephalexin, cefazolin, and cephapirin) were less active; of these, flucoxacillin and cephalexin were the least active.

Within the aminoglycosides, the three most active drugs were amikacin, tobramicin, and dibekacin. The first inhibited 75% of the strains studied at 3.1 µg/ml; the least effective aminoglycoside was streptomycin.

Concerning the activity of the remaining antibiotics against *Nocardia asteroides*, their low level of activity should be noted. Thus, clindamycin and lincomycin at concentrations of 25 µg/ml inhibited only 35 and 25% of the strains studied, respectively.

Although some authors (1, 2) have observed

TABLE 1. *In vitro susceptibility of 40 strains of N. asteroides to miscellaneous agents*

Drug	Cumulative % of strains inhibited at concn (µg/ml):									
	0.3	0.75	1.5	3.1	6.2	12.5	25	50	100	200
Clindamycin	0	0	7.5	15	22.5	25	35	42.5	50	60
Erythromycin	0	0	0	0	25	32.5	40	47.5	55	62.5
Spiramicin	0	0	0	0	0	7.5	15	20	30	40
Ethambutol	0	0	12.5	27.5	35	40	45	50	55	67.5
Isoniazid	0	0	0	0	0	0	0	12.5	20	30
Josamycin	0	0	0	0	0	15	15	20	25	40
Lincomycin	0	0	0	15	20	25	25	30	35	35
Rifampicin	0	0	12.5	27.5	35	40	45	50	55	67.5
Vancomycin	0	12.5	25	25	32.5	45	45	57.5	75	87.5

TABLE 2. *In vitro susceptibility of 40 strains of N. asteroides to β-lactams and aminoglycosides*

Drug	Cumulative % of strains inhibited at concn (µg/ml):									
	0.3	0.75	1.5	3.1	6.2	12.5	25	50	100	200
Amoxicillin	0	12.5	25	55	67.5	80	87.5	100	100	100
Ampicillin	0	0	20	55	67.5	80	80	100	100	100
Cephalexin	0	0	12.5	12.5	12.5	25	25	57.5	62.5	87.5
Cephaloridin	0	12.5	43	57.5	62.5	75	75	75	82.5	100
Cephapirin	0	0	0	0	12.5	37.5	57.5	70	87.5	87.5
Cefazolin	0	0	20	20	20	25	45	62.5	62.5	75
Cefoxitin	0	0	8	28	60	90	92	92	100	100
Flucoxacillin	0	0	0	7.5	12.5	12.5	20	32.5	62.5	75
Amikacin	45	50	62.5	75	82.5	87.5	95	100	100	100
Streptomycin	0	0	12.5	22.5	25	32.5	37.5	45	75	80
Dibekacin	30	40	50	60	70	75	82.5	87.5	95	100
Gentamicin	10	15	17.5	22.5	32.5	45	50	70	82.5	87.5
Kanamycin	25	30	37.5	45	50	55	62.5	67.5	75	80
Ribostamicin	25	32.5	40	45	55	60	65	70	75	85
Sisomicin	0	12.5	17.5	37.5	50	62.5	87.5	100	100	100
Tobramycin	40	50	50	70	75	77.5	80	80	87.5	92.5

a diversity of results in the susceptibility tests for the genus *Nocardia*, such tests are necessary to ascertain which drugs have the highest activity against such microorganisms.

On the other hand, improved standardization of the susceptibility tests would yield more consistent and reliable results. In the past, the use of certain methods was a contributing factor in the contradictory results obtained.

This study has basically employed the Wallace technique (7), although some changes regarding the inoculum, incubation time, culture medium, etc., were introduced.

Even though the in vitro activity of a drug against a certain microorganism does not necessarily mean that the drug might be used therapeutically, it can be an initial indication to be considered together with the pharmacokinetic properties of the drug. Therefore, it would be desirable to develop in vivo studies with laboratory animals to know which of the most active antibiotics might be of therapeutic use in humans.

Likewise, the development of studies of the activity of nocardiae with combinations of different drugs would certainly be useful in the treatment of nocardiosis. The administration of several antimicrobials is recommended (3).

1. Bach, M. C., O. Gold, and M. Finland. 1973. Activity of mynocycline against *Nocardia asteroides*: comparison with tetracycline in agar-dilution and standard disc-diffusion tests and with sulfadiazine in an experimental infection of mice. J. Lab. Clin. Med. 81:787–793.
2. Bach, M. C., L. D. Sabath, and M. Finland. 1973. Susceptibility of *Nocardia asteroides* to 45 antimicrobial agents in vitro. Antimicrob. Agents Chemother. 3: 1–8.
3. Emmons, C. W., H. B. Chapman, J. P. Utz, and K. J. Kwon-Chung. 1977. Medical mycology, p. 107. Lea and Febiger, Philadelphia.
4. Eppinger, H. 1890. Ueber eine neue Pathogene Cladothrix und eine durch die hervorgerufene Pseudotuberculosis (Cladothrichia). Beitr. Pathol. Anat. Allg. Pathol. 9:287–328.
5. Palmer, D. L., R. L. Harvey, and J. K. Wheller. 1974. Diagnostic and therapeutic considerations in *Nocardia asteroides* infection. Medicine (Baltimore) 53:391–401.
6. Presant, C. A., P. H. Wiernik, and A. A. Serpick. 1973. Factors affecting survival in nocardiosis. Am. Rev. Respir. Dis. 108:1444–1448.
7. Wallace, R. J., E. J. Septimus, D. M. Mushen, and R. R. Martin. 1977. Disk diffusion susceptibility testing of *Nocardia* species. J. Infect. Dis. 135:568–575.

In Vitro Susceptibilities of Bacteria from Human Periodontal Pockets to 13 Antimicrobial Agents

CLAY B. WALKER,* THEODORE A. NIEBLOOM, JEFFREY M. GORDON, AND SIGMUND S. SOCRANSKY

Department of Microbiology, Forsyth Dental Center, Boston, Massachusetts 02115, U.S.A.

Periodontal diseases are a group of inflammatory diseases having different clinical manifestations and different microbiotas that affect supporting tissues of the teeth. Antimicrobial therapy can be effective in the treatment of periodontal disease either alone (1, 2; A. Haffajee, C. Walker, J. M. Goodson, and S. S. Socransky, J. Dent. Res. **57A**:266, abstr. no. 767, 1978) or in conjunction with mechanical or surgical debridement (1; R. Genco, S. Singh, G. Krygier, and M. Levine, J. Dent. Res. **57A**:266, abstr. no. 768, 1978; H. Reynolds, P. Mashimo, J. Slots, N. Sedransk, and R. Genco, J. Dent. Res. **57A**:267, abstr. no. 769, 1978). Unfortunately, there have been few controlled studies to determine which antibiotics are most effective. The selection of the most appropriate antibiotic can be improved if data are available concerning the susceptibility patterns of the organisms most likely to be present. Investigators have determined the in vitro effects of antimicrobial agents on some of the bacteria encountered (3; S. Osterberg and B. L. Williams, J. Dent. Res. **57A**:318, abstr. no. 976, 1978; G. Sundquist, Ph.D. thesis, University of Umeå, Umeå, Sweden, 1976). However, interpretation of these results is difficult because of differences in methodology, the limited number of antibiotics tested, or the limited number of bacteria tested. In the study reported here, the susceptibilities to 13 antimicrobial agents were determined by standardized methods for approximately 150 strains representing 25 to 30 species or groups of bacteria commonly isolated from periodontal pockets. MICs were determined by an agar dilution technique, using a blood-free agar medium specifically developed for susceptibility testing of periodontal bacteria (4). Cultivation, preparation, and standardization of inocula, incubation, and other manipulations were performed as previously described by us (4).

Results of this study are summarized in Table 1. The data are presented as the percentages of each bacterial species or group that would be expected to be susceptible to antibiotic levels that are normally achieved in the blood after recommended dosage.

With the exceptions of vancomycin, kanamycin, and neomycin, most bacteria were relatively susceptible to the majority of the antibiotics.

Eikenella corrodens, which is often found in certain forms of periodontal disease, demonstrated the most widely resistant profile of any particular group. Individual strains were relatively resistant to penicillin, cephalothin, clindamycin, erythromycin, metronidazole, and tetracycline. Many of these resistant strains were isolated from patients who had been treated with tetracycline. However, a few strains resistant to penicillin, cephalothin, and erythromycin were recovered from patients with no history of antimicrobial therapy within the preceding year. Resistance to clindamycin and metronidazole is found in most *E. corrodens* strains and appears to be characteristic of the species.

Actinobacillus actinomycetemcomitans is often recovered from periodontal pockets of young adults with juvenile periodontitis. Many of these strains were resistant to erythromycin, and approximately one-half were resistant to tetracycline, clindamycin, and metronidazole. The majority of tetracycline-resistant strains were isolated from young patients who either had been treated with the antibiotic for periodontitis or had been on long-term tetracycline for the treatment of acne.

Bacteroides asaccharolyticus and the subspecies of *B. melaningoenicus* have been implicated in different forms of periodontal disease. Unlike clinical isolates from other regions of the body, oral strains were relatively susceptible to both the β-lactam antibiotics and to the tetracyclines. It may be that as more strains are examined, resistance may be noted; or it may be that oral strains differ from nonoral strains.

Tetracycline, penicillin, and, to a lesser extent, erythromycin are the antibiotics most commonly used in periodontal practice. In this study, penicillin and tetracycline were about equally effective in vitro, based on comparing MICs to concentrations which can be achieved in blood. The bacteria in the periodontal pocket are bathed in gingival crevice fluid, which is derived from serum and interstitial fluid. It has been assumed that antibiotic concentrations would be approximately the same in gingival fluid as in blood. We have found, however, that tetracycline concentrations are typically 2 to 10 times higher in the gingival fluid (J. M. Gordon, C. B. Walker, J. M. Goodson, and S. S. Socransky, manuscript submitted for publication). This would mean that tetracycline concentrations may range from 4 to 20 µg/ml in the periodontal pocket. Penicillin appears to be approximately the same in the gingival fluid as in the blood. This difference may very well account for the higher efficacy of tetracycline noted in periodontal practice. At present there is not an assay available that is sensitive enough to quantitate the amount of erythromycin that is present in gingival crevice fluid. However, clindamycin has been measured in gingival fluid and has been found to be approximately the same as in blood. It is assumed that erythromycin concentrations in gingival fluid would probably be about the same as blood concentrations as well. Since in vitro data indicate that erythromycin, at concentrations readily achievable in the blood, is not extremely effective against a number of periodontal organisms, it is not likely that this drug would be particularly effective in vivo.

Both ampicillin and carbenicillin appear to be effective based on in vitro data. Clindamycin may be of use in patients that do not respond to

TABLE 1. *Susceptibilities of periodontal bacteria to 13 antibiotics*

Bacteria	No. of strains	% Susceptible to antibiotic at achievable blood levels (μg/ml)[a]												
		Penicillin (≤2)	Ampicillin (≤4)	Carbenicillin (≤64)	Cephalothin (≤8)	Tetracycline (≤2)	Minocycline (≤2)	Clindamycin (≤4)	Erythromycin (≤2)	Metronidazole (≤8)	Chloramphenicol (≤8)	Vancomycin (≤8)	Kanamycin (≤64)	Neomycin (≤64)
Actinomyces species	11	100	91	100	100	64	91	100	100	0	91	75	50	0
Actinobacillus actinomycetemcomitans	8	88	100	100	100	50	100	50	13	50	100	0	100	100
Bacteroides asaccharolyticus	15	100	100	93	100	100	100	100	100	100	100	0	0	0
Bacteroides melaninogenicus	24	96	100	100	100	100	100	100	67	100	92	0	0	0
Bacteroides gracilis[b]	6	33	100	100	0	0	0	100	67	100	100	0	100	100
Campylobacter concisus[c]	6	100	100	100	75	100	0	100	50	50	100	—[d]	—	—
Capnocytophaga species	14	100	100	100	50	100	100	100	100	79	100	0	0	0
Elkenella corrodens	17	53	94	100	24	59	71	6	17	6	88	0	0	0
Eubacterium species	6	100	100	100	100	100	100	100	100	67	100	0	0	0
Fusobacterium nucleatum	22	91	27	100	100	91	100	100	0	100	100	0	—	0
Selenomonas sputigena	2	100	100	100	100	100	100	100	0	100	100	100	100	100
Streptococcus species	19	100	100	100	100	21	58	100	100	0	84	100	50	0
Peptostreptococcus species	10	100	100	100	100	75	75	100	50	100	100	100	100	100
Wolinella recta[e]	8	100	100	100	100	100	100	100	100	100	100	0	100	100

[a] This arbitrary designation is based on the assumption that strains are susceptible when the MIC is equivalent to or less than blood levels readily achieved with conventional dosage.
[b] Proposed name for "corroding" Bacteroides (A. Tanner, personal communication).
[c] Proposed name for oral Campylobacter (A. Tanner, personal communication).
[d] —, Not tested.
[e] Proposed name for anaerobic Vibrio (A. Tanner, personal communication).

either tetracycline or penicillin therapy. Metronidazole does not appear to be particularly useful due to the number of facultative and capnophilic species present in the periodontal pocket that are relatively resistant to this drug. However, it may be of use when more is known about which species are directly implicated in periodontal diseases.

This investigation was supported by a grant from the Upjohn Co., Kalamazoo, Mich., and by periodontal disease clinical research grant DE-04881 from the National Institute of Dental Research, U.S. Public Health Service.

1. Listgarten, M. A., J. Lindhe, and L. Hellden. 1978. Effect of tetracycline and/or scaling on human periodontal disease. Clinical microbiological and histological observation. J. Clin. Periodontol. 5:246–271.

2. Listgarten, M. A., J. Lindhe, and L. Hellden. 1979. The effect of systemic antimicrobial therapy on plaque and gingivitis in dogs. J. Periodontol. Res. 14:65–75.

3. Newman, M. G., C. Hulem, J. Colgate, and C. Anselmo. 1979. Antibacterial susceptibility of plaque bacteria. J. Dent. Res. 58:1722–1732.

4. Walker, C. B., T. A. Niebloom, and S. S. Socransky. 1979. Agar medium for use in susceptibility testing of bacteria from human periodontal pockets. Antimicrob. Agents Chemother. 16:452–457.

C. Laboratory Methodology

Assay of Gentamicin by Enzyme Immunoassay

DENIS PHANEUF,* ELLIOT L. FRANCKE, AND HAROLD C. NEU

Division of Infectious Diseases, Departments of Medicine and Pharmacology, College of Physicians and Surgeons, Columbia University, New York, New York 10032, U.S.A.

Aminoglycoside antibiotics are widely used to treat serious infections caused by aerobic gram-negative bacteria. However, the toxic-therapeutic ratio for these agents is fairly narrow, and it has proved necessary to monitor serum levels in order to avoid undue toxicity and to achieve adequate therapeutic concentrations (1). Bioassays of serum levels of aminoglycosides are reliable if run in volume by skilled technicians, but the delay in obtaining results precludes their usefulness in making rapid changes in dosage programs. Adenylating enzyme assays with [^{14}C]ATP have been limited mainly to research laboratories. Radioimmunoassay (RIA) is the most common assay currently used, but it also requires expensive equipment and generates radioactive waste.

Homogeneous enzyme immunoassay (EIA) was introduced in 1972 (2) and has been used to monitor serum levels of cardiac, asthma, and epileptic agents. Since the EIA has proved useful to monitor these agents and provides rapid information, we compared the EIA and RIA methods to determine serum gentamicin levels.

The EIA method employs a bacterial glucose-6-phosphate dehydrogenase to which gentamicin has been linked. The assay follows the conversion of NAD to NADH when enzyme acts on substrate. Antigentamicin antibody is prepared, and the assay detects free gentamicin, which competes for antibodies with gentamicin bound to the glucose-6-phosphate dehydrogenase. The reaction is run with 50-μl samples and a thermally regulated spectrophotometer set at 340 nm. Standard curves are prepared with gentamicin in concentrations of 1 to 16 μg/ml. Use of logit function graph paper permits conversion of data to a straight line from which concentrations of serum samples can be calculated.

The results of samples tested 20 times on the same day and on separate days are given in Table 1. The standard deviation of 20 assays of the same sample was 0.16 μg/ml, and the coefficient of variation was only 4.1%. Assay of the same samples over 25 successive days showed that the EIA method had a coefficient of varia-

tion of only 3.6%, compared with a variation within the same day of 5.7% for the RIA.

Assays were run on serum samples to which other antibiotics had been added and on samples of serum which contained other agents but no aminoglycoside. None of the penicillins or cephalosporins, nor chloramphenicol, nor trimethoprim-sulfamethoxazole interfered with the EIA assay. The results of initial assays for gentamicin by the EIA and RIA were similar when assayed immediately and when the assays were performed 72 h later (Table 2). Other aminoglycosides, such as kanamycin, neomycin, amikacin, and tobramycin, showed no cross-reaction with gentamicin by EIA. Netilmicin and sisomicin

TABLE 1. *Precision of EIA gentamicin assay system*

Assay	No. of assays	Concn of standard (μg/ml)	Assayed concn (μg/ml)		Coefficient of variation (%)
			Mean	SD	
EIA					
Within a day[a]	20	4	3.88	0.16	4.1
Day to day[b]	25	6	5.89	0.21	3.6
RIA					
Within a day[a]	20	6	7.72	0.44	5.7

[a] All assays done the same day.
[b] Assays done on 25 consecutive days.

TABLE 2. *Comparison of EIA and RIA results in the presence of other antimicrobials and cross-reactions with other aminoglycosides*

Condition	Compound concn (μg/ml)	Gentamicin concn (μg/ml)	
		EIA	RIA
Gentamicin mixed with other agents	4	3.73	3.88
Mixed, assay at 72 h	4	3.69	3.88
Other aminoglycosides			
Amikacin	10–16	<1	<1
Tobramycin	1–16	<1	<1
Neomycin	20	<1	<1
Netilmicin	12	3.3	3.5
Sisomicin	4	4.9	4.8

showed cross-reactions in both EIA and RIA, as would be expected since both are essentially derivatives of gentamicin C_{1A}.

Sera, 111 samples, from 51 patients receiving gentamicin were analyzed by EIA and RIA. The concentrations ranged from <1 to 16 µg/ml, with the majority between 2 and 8 µg/ml. The coefficient of correlation of the methods was 0.97 for samples of ≥ 1 µg/ml by both methods. The level found for 17 sera was <1 µg/ml by both methods. Reassay of those samples with readings below 0.5 µg/ml gave similar results for both methods.

The EIA could be set up in 25 min, with tests run in 2 min. The RIA required a setup time of 95 min and 5 min for each sample. The EIA standard curve was reproducible in a 12-h period as long as the spectrophotometer was left on. As a result we were able to provide results to the physician within 30 min of obtaining a sample. The EIA was simpler, and its precision and specificity were similar to those of the RIA. For laboratories using this equipment to assay theophylline and anticonvulsants, the EIA offers an alternative method to provide rapid aminoglycoside serum level results to the physician.

1. **Appel, G. B., and H. C. Neu.** 1978. Gentamicin in 1978. Ann. Intern. Med. **89**:528–538.
2. **Rubenstein, K., R. Schneider, and E. Ullman.** 1972. Homogenous enzyme immunoassay, a new immunochemical technique. Biochem. Biophys. Res. Commun. **47**:846–851.

Enzyme Immunoassay for Gentamicin and Comparison with Other Methods

PETER J. WILLS AND RICHARD WISE*

Department of Medical Microbiology, Dudley Road Hospital, Birmingham, England

We here describe an enzyme immunoassay for gentamicin and its use in a clinical laboratory. Performance of the method was compared with that of the bioassay, acetyltransferase assay, radioimmunoassay (RIA), quenching fluoroimmunoassay (quenching FIA), and polarization fluoroimmunoassay (polarization FIA). Sera from patients receiving gentamicin therapy, and also gentamicin-free sera to which a known concentration of gentamicin was added, were assayed by these methods.

The enzyme immunoassay was as described by Wills and Wise (4). It uses a conjugate of gentamicin with glucose 6-phosphate dehydrogenase. This enzyme-gentamicin conjugate is inhibited by antiserum specific for gentamicin, which binds it via the gentamicin ligands. Gentamicin from a test or standard will also bind antibody and thus leaves less available for binding and inhibiting the enzyme. Therefore, the enzyme activity is directly related to gentamicin concentration in the sample. The method is similar in principle to the E.M.I.T. kits (Syva Corp., Palo Alto, Calif.), but it is designed for manual operation rather than for use with a reaction rate analyzer. The assay procedure is as follows:

(i) Pipette 20-µl sample and 100 µl of substrate-antibody reagent into plastic tubes.

(ii) Warm tubes to 37°C.

(iii) Pipette 100 µl of enzyme-gentamicin conjugate at timed intervals, and then mix.

(iv) After 10 min, add 2.5 ml of borate to stop the reaction. Blank tubes contain a similar mixture but with the enzyme reagent omitted.

(v) Measure absorbance at 340 nm.

(vi) Subtract corresponding blanks from test values.

(vii) Use the net absorbance to construct a calibration curve, and calculate the unknown gentamicin concentrations.

The bioassay was an agar well diffusion technique using *Klebsiella edwardsii* var. *atlantae* as indicator, which is resistant to most antibiotics except the aminoglycosides, colistin, and certain cephalosporins.

The quenching FIA (2) and the polarization FIA (3) were performed using a filter fluorimeter with an excitation wavelength of 439 nm and an emission wavelength of 535 nm. The polarization FIA was a modification of the published method using a larger sample volume of 10 µl, which simplified the assay by eliminating the sample dilution stage. Albumin had to be added to one reagent to give a final concentration of 5 mg/liter in the assay mixture, in order to overcome serum effects. Polarization measurements were made by placing polarizing filters in the excitation and emission light beams in such a way that it was possible to rotate one filter by 90° every time a measurement was made. The signal was measured on each sample with the filters parallel and with the filters perpendicular. The difference between these readings divided by their

TABLE 1. *Correlation coefficients between assay methods*

Method	Bioassay	Acetylase	RIA	Quenching FIA	Polarization FIA
Enzyme immunoassay	0.91	0.94	0.99	0.94	0.98
Polarization FIA	0.89	0.90	0.98	0.93	
Quenching FIA	0.84	0.91	0.95		
RIA	0.92	0.93			
Acetylase	0.94				

sum is the polarization, which depends on gentamicin concentration.

The acetyltransferase technique was that of Broughall and Reeves (1), and the radioimmunoassay was a diagnostic kit supplied by New England Nuclear Corp., using standards prepared in our laboratory.

The results show that there is good correlation between the immunoassays and reasonable correlation of these assays with the bioassay and acetyltransferase methods (Table 1). In order to test the assays further, gentamicin-free sera were taken, mixed with gentamicin at 100 mg/liter, to give a final concentration of 5 mg/liter, and assayed by the different methods. The mean percentage of error and its standard deviation were calculated, and the 95% confidence limits were deduced. For the enzyme immunoassay, this was 21% for a series of 41 different sera. Similar experiments gave the following 95% confidence limits with the other assays: RIA, 23%; quenching FIA, 29%; polarization FIA, 16%; bioassay, 17%; and acetyltransferase, 28%.

The enzyme immunoassay required that the incubation time with enzyme was the same in all the tubes of a particular batch, so the additions of enzyme and borate were timed with a stopwatch. Reading of the results was on a simple spectrophotometer capable of measurements at 340 nm. In order to make allowance for the variable absorbance of different sera at this wavelength, it was necessary to prepare serum blanks. These had the same reagents as the tests, but with enzyme reagent omitted. The difference between tests and their corresponding blank was a measure of enzyme activity, which depended on gentamicin concentration.

All these assays, except the bioassay, require a small sample volume, are very specific, and show no interference by antibiotics other than aminoglycosides. The quenching FIA overestimated the result of a grossly hemolyzed specimen by 50%, but normally encountered levels of hemolysis did not affect the assay.

The enzyme immunoassay therefore compares well with other techniques for gentamicin assay, particularly the radioimmunoassay and polarization fluoroimmunoassay. It is sufficiently rapid, accurate, and specific for clinical use.

1. **Broughall, J. M., and D. S. Reeves.** 1975. The acetyltransferase enzyme method for the assay of serum gentamicin concentrations and a comparison with other methods. J. Clin. Pathol. 28:140–145.
2. **Shaw, E. J., R. A. A. Watson, J. Landon, and D. S. Smith.** 1977. Estimation of serum gentamicin by quenching fluoroimmunoassay. J. Clin. Pathol. 30:526–531.
3. **Watson, R. A. A., J. Landon, E. J. Shaw, and D. S. Smith.** 1976. Polarisation fluoroimmunoassay of gentamicin. Clin. Chim. Acta 73:51–55.
4. **Wills, P. J., and R. Wise.** 1979. A rapid, simple enzyme immunoassay for gentamicin. Antimicrob. Agents Chemother. 16:40–42.

Substrate-Labeled Fluorometric Immunoassay for Serum Gentamicin Determination

JOHN E. van HAMONT,* RENATE F. KLEIN, AND LAWRENCE B. SENTERFIT

New York Hospital-Cornell Medical Center, New York, New York 10021, U.S.A.

Aminoglycosides such as gentamicin are invaluable as broad-spectrum antibiotics in the treatment of severe gram-negative infections. Therapeutic levels for gentamicin lie between 4 and 12 µg/ml. Treatment, however, is complicated by the fact that levels above the therapeutic range can cause ototoxicity and nephrotox-

icity. Patients, therefore, must be carefully monitored to insure that safe, effective therapy is achieved. When such a monitoring system is lacking, there is an unfortunate tendency to undertreat the patient in order to avoid the risk of creating a toxic condition. The resulting subtherapeutic serum levels are of no help to the patient and may lead to the development of resistant strains. It is, thus, important that there be a variety of procedures suited to the various testing facilities present in hospitals in order to insure the availability of an accurate gentamicin monitoring system. The procedure which has been investigated is a substrate-labeled fluorescent immunoassay (SLFIA) developed by the Ames Division of Miles Laboratories.

The Ames SLFIA employs β-galactosyl-umbelliferone-sisomicin (G-U-S), a conjugate consisting of galactose, umbelliferone (a fluorescent dye), and sisomicin (a compound immunochemically similar to gentamicin). Under initial test conditions, this conjugate is not fluorescent. Addition of β-galactosidase to the test system cleaves the galactose from the fluorescent dye, yielding an actively fluorescing umbelliferone-sisomicin product.

Antibody directed against gentamicin/sisomicin blocks the cleaving of the galactose from the conjugate by β-galactosidase. Consequently, the more antibody there is available to bind with the conjugate, the lower the resulting level of fluorescence upon the addition of the β-galactosidase.

Thus, using the principles of competitive inhibition, one can construct a test system in which the concentration of gentamicin in a sample is directly proportional with the final amount of fluorescence:

$$
\left.
\begin{array}{l}
\text{G-U-S + Ab + Gentamicin} \\
\updownarrow \\
\text{G-U-S-Ab + Gentamicin-Ab}
\end{array}
\right\}
\xrightarrow{\text{Beta-Galactosidase}}
$$

$$\xrightarrow{\text{Beta-Galactosidase}}$$

Fluorescence in proportion to the drug level

When performing the Ames SLFIA, the antibody and enzyme are combined in one reagent. To assay for gentamicin, the following steps are performed: (i) 3 ml of antibody/enzyme are placed into a disposable cuvette; (ii) 100 μl of diluted serum or gentamicin standard is added to the cuvette; (iii) 100 μl of G-U-S conjugate is added and the contents of the cuvette are mixed; (iv) after a fixed time interval of 20 min at room temperature, the fluorescent intensity is measured. A standard curve of fluorescent intensity versus standard concentration is constructed and the serum gentamicin levels are determined by comparing their fluorescent intensities with those of the standard curve.

The Ames SLFIA was studied in terms of its accuracy, reproducibility, and clinical correlation with a routine radioimmunoassay procedure. Accuracy and reproducibility were determined by assaying three gravimetrically calibrated controls, in replicates of 10, daily for 3 days. In order to monitor the consistency of the assay system, the three controls were included with the clinical specimens assayed in the second phase of the study. The results produced by the fluorometric procedure demonstrated a precision and accuracy similar to that obtainable by radioimmunoassay. Overall precision and composite variabilities for the two assay systems are presented in Tables 1 and 2.

A close correlation was demonstrated between the performance of the fluorescent and radio assays in the determination of serum gentamicin levels of 88 clinical specimens.

Conclusion. Though the procedures are equally rapid, providing results within 45 min, the fluorescent assay has the advantage of not containing isotopes, thus eliminating the complications of a shortened shelf life and of disposal.

TABLE 1. *Composite variabilities of two assay systems*

Method	Specimen concn (μg/ml)	Mean[a]	Overall SD[b]	90% Tolerance interval[c] Low	90% Tolerance interval[c] High
Ames gentamicin	2	2.05	0.08	1.91	2.18
	6	6.51	0.24	6.10	6.91
	10	11.10	0.39	10.45	11.74
RIA[d]	2	1.92	0.08	1.78	2.05
	6	5.81	0.12	5.60	6.02
	10	10.41	0.35	9.82	10.99

[a] The mean was determined from a total of 106 assays performed over 22 runs.
[b] SD, Standard deviation.
[c] For a future observation.
[d] RIA, Radioimmunoassay.

TABLE 2. *Overall precision of two assay systems*

Method	Specimen concn (μg/ml)	Mean[a]	Overall SD[b]	Overall coefficient of variation	95% Upper confidence[c]
Ames gentamicin	2	2.05	0.08	4.1	4.6
	6	6.51	0.24	3.7	4.4
	10	11.10	0.39	3.5	4.0
RIA[d]	2	1.92	0.08	4.2	4.8
	6	5.81	0.12	2.1	2.5
	10	10.41	0.35	3.4	3.9

[a] The mean was determined from a total of 106 assays performed over 22 runs.
[b] SD, Standard deviation.
[c] Bound for coefficient of variation.
[d] RIA, Radioimmunoassay.

New Method for Activation of Aminoglycoside Antibiotics for Coupling to Proteins: Application to Homogeneous Enzyme Immunoassay of Tobramycin

D. K. LEUNG, Y. TSAY, P. SHERIDAN, A. JAKLITSCH, P. SINGH,* AND D. S. KABAKOFF

Syva Company,[1] Palo Alto, California 94304, U.S.A.

Monitoring plasma concentrations of aminoglycoside antibiotics is frequently practiced as an aid to therapy with these antimicrobial agents. The EMIT homogeneous enzyme immunoassay has been widely applied for measurement of drugs in body fluids (4). Extension of the technique to monitoring antibiotic plasma levels will increase its utility in routine therapeutic drug monitoring. The EMIT method utilizes drug-specific antibodies and a drug-enzyme conjugate as the key reagents. The drug-enzyme conjugate is commonly prepared by reacting an activated carboxylic acid derivative of a suitably functionalized drug with amino groups of the enzyme. This method cannot be readily applied to aminoglycosides since activation of their appropriate acid derivatives would result in polymerization. During the course of development of an EMIT assay for gentamicin (5), we solved this problem by application of a three-stage heterobifunctional coupling method. We have now extended this coupling method for the development of an EMIT tobramycin assay.

Chemical modification of tobramycin. Of the five amino groups in tobramycin (Fig. 1) the C_6'-NH_2 group is most readily acylated. We have taken advantage of this reactivity to introduce a sulfhydryl group at this position. Tobramycin was carefully reacted with N-acetyl-homocysteinethiolactone under argon at pH 10.2 and 4°C. The product, adduct **2**, characterized as **3** by derivatization with ω-bromoacetophenone, could be directly coupled with suitably modified proteins.

Modification of glucose 6-phosphate dehydrogenase and its coupling to sulfhydryl-tobramycin. Electrophilic bromoacetyl groups were introduced into the enzyme, glucose 6-phosphate dehydrogenase, by labeling with bromoacetylglycine-N-hydroxysuccinimide ester. The bromoacetylglycyl-glucose 6-phosphate dehydrogenase was then reacted at 0°C under inert atmosphere with the nucleophilic sulfhydryl tobramycin derivative **2** at pH 8.5 to give the drug-enzyme conjugate (see Fig. 2). This drug-enzyme conjugate had ~25% of the activity of the native enzyme. The residual activity of the conjugate

could be substantially reduced by antitobramycin antibodies.

Tobramycin antibodies. Previous workers prepared a tobramycin immunogen by coupling the drug to bovine serum albumin using 1-ethyl-3(3-dimethylaminopropyl)carbodiimide (EDCI) (1). Such a method should lead to random coupling of tobramycin, resulting in a heterogeneous mixture of immunogens. We found that such a mixture elicited low-titer antitobramycin antibodies. Superior titer antibodies were obtained from a specifically labeled tobramycin BSA immunogen prepared as outlined in Fig. 2.

Homogeneous enzyme immunoassay for tobramycin. The drug-enzyme conjugate and antibodies prepared as described above were used to develop a homogeneous enzyme immunoassay for tobramycin (3). Reagent concentrations were optimized to yield an assay in the

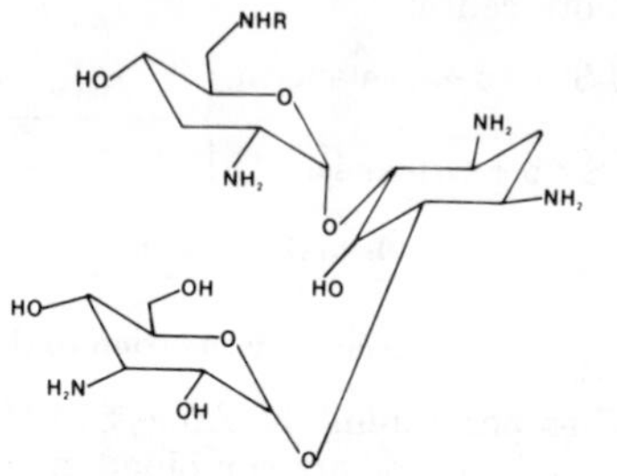

1 R = H
2 R = CO(CH₂)₂CH(NHCOCH₃)SH
3 R = CO(CH₂)₂CH(NHCOCH₃)SCH₂COC₆H₅

FIG. 1. *Chemical structure of tobramicin.*

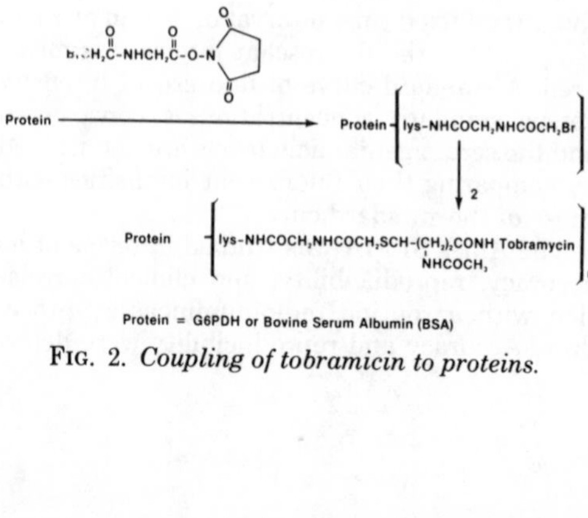

Protein = G6PDH or Bovine Serum Albumin (BSA)

FIG. 2. *Coupling of tobramicin to proteins.*

[1] Contribution no. 83.

range of 1 to 16 μg of tobramycin per ml. This assay utilizes the usual convenient protocol of the EMIT assays (4) and provides sample quantitation in less than 1 min.

To perform an assay, 50 μl of serum is prediluted sixfold. A sample of the diluted serum is combined with antibody, substrates (nicotinamide adenine dinucleotide, glucose 6-phosphate), and enzyme-drug conjugate. The reaction mixture is aspirated into the flowcell of a standard laboratory spectrophotometer, and the enzyme activity is measured kinetically at 340 nm. The drug is quantitated from a calibration curve of enzyme activity versus drug concentration.

The within-day and day-to-day precision of the tobramycin assay are less than 10% and recovery of the drug added to negative serum is 97 to 98%. Cross-reactivity of other antibiotics was studied to determine assay specificity. When evaluated at concentrations of the cross-reactant sufficient to give the same rate as 4 μg of tobramycin per ml, the ratios of concentrations of tobramycin to the related aminoglycosides were: amikacin, 2.0%; kanamycin, 77%; gentamicin, <0.1%. No other antibiotics showed interference in the assay at 1,000-μg/ml levels. The cross-reactivity of kanamycin is not unexpected because of its structural similarity to tobramycin. This cross-reactivity is not clinically significant because the two aminoglycosides are usually not co-administered. Patient sample quantitation was assessed by comparison of the EMIT assay with three alternative methods for the assay of tobramycin (2). Excellent correlation data were obtained: EMIT = 0.95(RIA) −0.03, r = 0.97, n = 34; EMIT = 1.02 (radioenzymatic), r = 0.97, n = 62; EMIT = 0.99 (bioassay) −0.02, r = 0.92, n = 29. The relatively larger scatter in the comparison with bioassay is probably due to inherent problems in the latter methods.

1. Broughton, A., J. E. Strong, L. K. Pickering, and G. P. Brody. 1976. Radioimmunoassay of iodinated tobramycin. Antimicrob. Agents Chemother. 10:652–656.
2. Kahlmeter, G. 1979. Gentamicin and tobramycin clinical pharmacokinetics and nephrotoxicity. Aspects on assay techniques. Scand. J. Infect. Dis. Suppl. 18:7–40.
3. Leung, D., Y. Tsay, P. Singh, A. Jaklitsch, and D. S. Kabakoff, 1979. Homogeneous enzyme immunoassay for tobramycin in serum. Clin. Chem. 25:1094.
4. Rubenstein, K. E. 1978. Homogeneous enzyme immunoassay today. Scand. J. Immunol. 8 (Suppl. 7):57–72.
5. Singh, P., D. K. Leung, and E. F. Ullman. 1978. Homogeneous enzyme immunoassay for gentamicin. Xth Int. Congr. Clin. Chem., Mexico City, Abstr. 51, 69.

Substrate-Labeled Fluorescent Immunoassays for Measuring Levels of the Aminoglycoside Antibiotics, Gentamicin, Sisomicin, Netilmicin, Tobramycin, Kanamycin, and Amikacin

JOHN F. BURD,* STEPHAN G. THOMPSON, AND CAROL A. MILLER

Ames Company, Miles Laboratories, Inc., Elkhart, Indiana 46514, U.S.A.

The measurement of serum levels of aminoglycoside antibiotics during therapy is extremely important, since these drugs have a narrow therapeutic concentration range and toxic side effects are associated with their use. Consequently, after therapy has begun, serum concentrations should be measured to facilitate appropriate adjustments to dosage schedule. We have developed a series of rapid and simple substrate-labeled fluorescent immunoassays (SLFIA) to quantitatively measure the levels of aminoglycoside antibiotics and other drugs in human serum (1–7). These assays are also useful for the measurement of aminoglycoside levels in fermentation broths.

The SLFIA uses the principles of competitive protein binding to quantitatively measure drug levels in human serum. To establish the assay for a drug, we synthesize a conjugate which has the drug covalently attached to a derivative of the fluorogenic enzyme substrate, umbelliferyl-β-D-galactoside. This fluorogenic drug reagent (FDR) is nonfluorescent under the conditions of the assay; however, hydrolysis catalyzed by β-galactosidase yields a fluorescent product. When antibody (Ab) to the drug reacts with the FDR, the complex is virtually inactive as a substrate for the β-galactosidase. Competitive binding reactions are set up with a constant amount of FDR and a limiting amount of antibody to the drug:

$$\text{FDR} + \text{Ab} + \text{Drug} \left.\begin{array}{c} \\ \updownarrow \\ (\text{Ab/FDR}) + (\text{Ab/Drug}) \end{array}\right\} \xrightarrow{\beta\text{-galactosidase}}$$

Fluorescence produced in proportion to the drug level

The drug in the serum sample competes with

the FDR for antibody binding sites. The unbound FDR is hydrolyzed with β-galactosidase to produce the fluorescent product. The fluorescence intensity is related to the drug level by means of a standard curve.

The structure of the fluorogenic enzyme substrate used as the label in the SLFIA is shown in Fig. 1. Antiserum specific for the individual drugs is produced in animals (rabbits or goats) by immunization with an immunogen composed of a protein, e.g., bovine serum albumin, to which the drug has been covalently attached.

The antibody and enzyme are combined in one reagent. To assay for a drug, the following steps are performed: (i) 3 ml of antibody/enzyme reagent is placed into a disposable cuvette; (ii) 100 μl of diluted serum or drug standard is added to the cuvette; (iii) 100 μl of fluorogenic drug reagent is added, and the contents of the cuvette are mixed; (iv) after a fixed time interval (10 to 30 min) at room temperature, the fluorescence intensity is measured in a fluorometer.

Unknown serum drug levels are determined from a standard curve such as that shown in Fig. 2. The assay of as many as 20 unknown specimens can easily be performed in less than 1 h.

To validate the SLFIA for a drug, we perform studies to assure recovery, parallelism, sensitivity, stability, precision, accuracy, and cross-reactivity of metabolites and other drugs in the assay. We also compare the values obtained in the SLFIA to those determined with accepted reference methods. The precision of the assay is typically 5 to 7% (Fig. 2).

The amikacin SLFIA was compared to a radioimmunoassay (RIA) for amikacin with 93 clinical serum samples. A correlation coefficient of 0.987 was observed with a standard error of estimate of 1.55 μg/ml. The regression line was SLFIA = 0.95 RIA + 0.15.

Because certain of the aminoglycoside antibiotics are structurally similar, it is possible to design SLFIA systems which allow a given set of antiserum and FDR to measure more than one drug. This is accomplished by simply employing the appropriate drug standards in the assay. The antiserum and FDRs employed in the various aminoglycoside drug assays are presented in Table 1. The specificity of the SLFIA resides in both the antiserum and the FDR.

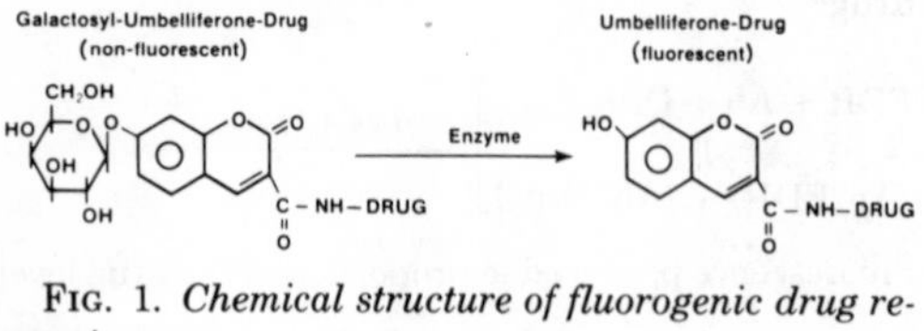

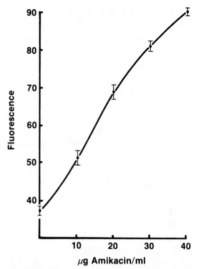

FIG. 2. *Standard curve for amikacin SLFIA. Error bars indicate one standard deviation of the mean for 10 assays (n = 5 per assay).*

TABLE 1. *Substrate-labeled fluorescent immunoassays (SLFIA) for aminoglycoside antibiotics*

Assay	Drug in fluorogenic drug reagent	Drug for antiserum
Gentamicin	Sisomicin	Gentamicin
Sisomicin	Sisomicin	Gentamicin
Netilmicin	Sisomicin	Gentamicin
Tobramycin	Tobramycin	Kanamycin
Kanamycin	Tobramycin	Kanamycin
Amikacin	Amikacin	Amikacin

Conclusion. The SLFIA offers several advantages over other techniques currently employed for drug level measurement. The SLFIA is rapidly and easily performed, uses very stable reagents and inexpensive instrumentation, has high sensitivity and specificity, and does not require stringent temperature control. Furthermore, the same simple assay format can be used to measure a variety of drugs and other biologically important molecules.

1. **Burd, J. F.** 1979. Substrate-labeled fluorescent immunoassays (SLFIA) for measuring therapeutic drug levels in human serum. Clin. Chem. **25**:1077.
2. **Burd, J. F., R. J. Carrico, H. M. Kramer, and C. E. Denning.** 1978. Homogeneous substrate-labeled fluorescent immunoassay for determining tobramycin concentrations in human serum, p. 387–403. *In* Enzyme-labeled immunoassay of hormones and drugs. Walter de Gruyter and Co., New York.
3. **Burd, J. F., R. C. Wong, J. E. Feeney, R. J. Carrico, and R. C. Boguslaski.** 1977. Homogeneous reactant-

Galactosyl-Umbelliferone-Drug
(non-fluorescent)

Umbelliferone-Drug
(fluorescent)

Enzyme

FIG. 1. *Chemical structure of fluorogenic drug reagent.*

labeled fluorescent immunoassay for therapeutic drugs exemplified by gentamicin determination in human serum. Clin. Chem. **23**:1402–1408.

4. **Krausz, L. M., J. B. Hitz, and J. F. Burd.** 1979. A homogeneous substrate-labeled fluorescent immunoassay (SLFIA) for the determination of phenobarbital levels in human serum. Fed. Proc. **38**:661.

5. **Li, T. M., and J. F. Burd.** 1979. Determination of theophylline concentrations in human serum using the sub-

strate-labeled fluorescent immunoassay (SLFIA). Abstr. XIth Int. Congr. Biochem. 522.

6. **Wong, R. C., and J. F. Burd.** 1979. Phenytoin determination by the substrate-labeled fluorescent immunoassay (SLFIA). Clin. Biochem. **12**:p4.

7. **Wong, R. C., J. F. Burd, R. J. Carrico, R. T. Buckler, J. Thoma, and R. C. Boguslaski.** 1979. Substrate-labeled fluorescent immunoassay for phenytoin in human serum. Clin. Chem. **25**:686–691.

In Vitro and In Vivo Interaction Between Carbenicillin and Aminoglycosides

JOHN A. PIEPER, RONALD A. VIDAL, AND JEROME J. SCHENTAG*

Department of Pharmaceutics, School of Pharmacy, State University of New York at Buffalo, and Clinical Pharmacokinetics Laboratory, Millard Fillmore Hospital, Buffalo, New York 14209, U.S.A.*

The combined use of carbenicillin and aminoglycosides for life-threatening gram-negative infections, especially those caused by *Pseudomonas aeruginosa*, has been advocated on the basis of clinical and experimental evidence. However, McLaughlin and Reeves (3) demonstrated that gentamicin is inactivated by carbenicillin in vitro, and suggested an in vivo antagonism. Various penicillins can inactivate gentamicin in vitro, with the rate influenced by temperature, concentration, and medium composition (4).

In patients with renal dysfunction, a reduction in gentamicin half-life has been reported when concomitantly administered with therapeutic doses of carbenicillin (1, 2), suggesting that in vivo inactivation also occurs. However, because these studies have not employed sampling and assay techniques which reliably differentiate inactivation occurring prior to assay from actual in vivo inactivation, this study was performed to develop methods which would distinguish in vitro from in vivo interactions, and to determine the effects of carbenicillin on aminoglycosides in an animal model of renal failure.

We studied seven bilaterally nephrectomized mongrel dogs. Three dogs received an i.v. bolus (75 mg/kg) and infusion (4.5 mg per kg/h) of carbenicillin followed in 2 h by an i.v. bolus composed of a gentamicin (2 mg/kg), tobramycin (2 mg/kg), and amikacin (6 mg/kg) mixture. These doses were chosen to achieve therapeutic serum concentrations of gentamicin (10 µg/ml), tobramycin (10 µg/ml), amikacin (30 µg/ml), and carbenicillin (400 µg/ml). An additional three dogs received an i.v. bolus of tobramycin followed in 10 h by a bolus and infusion of carbenicillin. The seventh dog received a single i.v.

bolus dose of gentamicin, tobramycin and amikacin, and served as a control.

At blood sampling times, one-third of the sample was collected into a Vacutainer containing penicillinase (5,000 units/ml of sample), and one-third was collected into a test tube containing cellulose phosphate powder (100 mg/ml of sample) (5). The third aliquot was collected and refrigerated. Cellulose phosphate powder had previously been shown to selectively bind aminoglycosides without binding or inactivating carbenicillin.

These samples were assayed immediately (10 min), again after being refrigerated for 24 h and again after 7 days. A microbioassay, using *Bacillus subtilis*, was performed to quantitate carbenicillin concentrations, and radioimmunoassay (RIA) was used to assay aminoglycosides.

Figure 1 depicts mean serum aminoglycoside concentrations in the first three dogs after immediate, 24-h and 7-day RIA. When compared to immediate RIA, concentrations of gentamicin and tobramycin were reduced in vitro by 40% when assayed after refrigeration for 24 h and by 85% when assayed after 7 days. Tobramycin concentrations determined by immediate microbioassay were approximately 65% of those determined by immediate RIA. This reduction in tobramycin concentrations was similar to that observed in samples stored for 24 h before assay. Because inactivation occurs during microbioassay incubation (in spite of sample pretreatment with 5,000 units of penicillinase per ml), either immediate RIA or larger penicillinase concentrations must be employed to accurately determine concentrations in the presence of carbenicillin.

In contrast to gentamicin and tobramycin, no

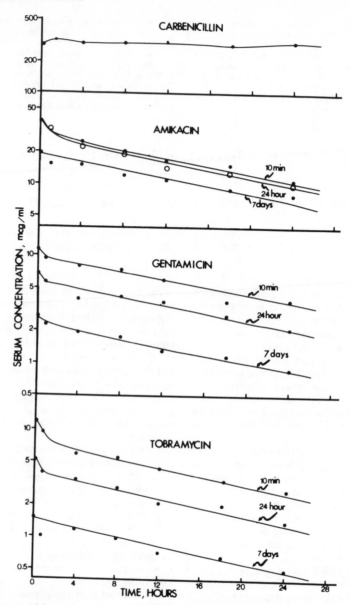

FIG. 1. *Mean gentamicin, tobramycin, and amikacin concentrations in dogs 1, 2, and 3 in the presence of carbenicillin after immediate (10 min), 24-h and 7-day RIA.*

significant change in amikacin concentrations was observed when samples were assayed at 24 h, and only a 30% decrease occurred when samples were assayed after 7 days of refrigeration. Amikacin appears to be the most resistant aminoglycoside to the inactivating effects of carbenicillin, both in vitro and in the anephric dog, and may be a compound of choice in those patients with *renal failure* who require the combination of an aminoglycoside and carbenicillin.

Table 1 shows the effect of carbenicillin on the in vivo half-lives of gentamicin, tobramycin, and amikacin. The three aminoglycosides were administered simultaneously to dogs 1, 2, and 3 so that relative in vivo properties of these drugs could be assessed under identical physiological conditions. Immediate RIA demonstrated that the in vivo serum half-lives of gentamicin and tobramycin, in the presence of carbenicillin, were significantly less than control in dogs 1, 2,

TABLE 1. *In vivo half-life values in dogs 1 to 7 (in hours)*

Aminoglyco-side	Control (dog 7)	During carbenicillin (dogs 1, 2, 3)	Before carbenicillin (dogs 4, 5, 6)	After carbenicillin (dogs 4, 5, 6)	% Decrease on carbenicillin
Gentamicin	30.4	18.2 ± 2.6^a			40.1
Tobramycin	29.2	17.5 ± 2.3^a	27.8 ± 1.2	16.9 ± 1.8^b	39.3
Amikacin	33.8	28.6 ± 2.6			15.4

[a] Statistical significance, $P < 0.05$, control versus "during carbenicillin."
[b] Statistical significance, $P < 0.01$, before versus "after carbenicillin."

and 3 ($P < 0.05$). Mean tobramycin half-life in dogs 4, 5, and 6 was similarly reduced by approximately 40% and again was significantly less ($P < 0.01$) after carbenicillin administration as compared to before treatment.

Based on these in vivo findings, tobramycin and gentamicin doses should be increased by 40% in the uremic patient given carbenicillin in similar doses, *if* blood levels must be maintained in a predetermined range. However, we caution that aminoglycoside dosage increases based on microbioassay or delayed RIA results may not reflect actual in vivo concentrations, and such increases may elevate *actual* in vivo levels into the toxic range.

The significance of these findings for patients with normal renal function deserves further in-vestigation, using our more precise methodology.

1. **Davis, M., J. R. Morgan, and C. Anand.** 1975. Inter-actions of carbenicillin and ticarcillin with gentamicin. Antimicrob. Agents Chemother. **7**:431–434.
2. **Ervin, F. R., W. E. Bullock, and C. E. Nuttall.** 1976. Inactivation of gentamicin by penicillins in patients with renal failure. Antimicrob. Agents Chemother. **9**:1004–1011.
3. **McLaughlin, J. E., and D. S. Reeves.** 1971. Clinical and laboratory evidence for inactivation of gentamicin by carbenicillin. Lancet **1**:261–264.
4. **Riff, L. J., and G. G. Jackson.** 1972. Laboratory and clinical conditions for gentamicin inactivation by car-benicillin. Arch. Intern. Med. **130**:887–891.
5. **Stevens, P., and L. S. Young.** 1977. Simple method for elimination of aminoglycosides from serum to permit bioassay of other antimicrobial agents. Antimicrob. Agents Chemother. **12**:286–287.

Evaluation of a Radioimmunoassay for Measurements of Serum Vancomycin Concentration

JOHN ROTSCHAFER, KAREN MEAD, M. MYRA CHERN, AND KENT CROSSLEY*

Department of Internal Medicine and Section of Clinical Pharmacy, St. Paul-Ramsey Medical Center, St. Paul, Minnesota 55101; and Department of Medicine and Division of Health Computer Sciences, University of Minnesota Medical School, and College of Pharmacy, University of Minnesota, Minneapolis, Minnesota 55455, U.S.A.*

Vancomycin, a bactericidal antistaphylococ-cal antibiotic introduced in the mid-1950s, has been associated with both ototoxicity and neph-rotoxicity (1, 3). Ototoxicity has been reported in patients with vancomycin serum concentra-tions in excess of 80 μg/ml but is uncommon when serum concentrations are 30 μg/ml or less (1, 2). Serum concentrations of vancomycin have been reported to vary widely even in patients with normal renal function after administration of the 500-mg dose recommended by the manu-facturer (D. E. Zaske, K. B. Crossley, R. J. Sawchuk, D. L. Uden, and K. E. Mead, Program Abstr. Intersci. Conf. Antimicrob. Agents Chem-other. 17th, New York, N.Y., abstr. no. 157, 1977). The apparent patient-to-patient variation in antibiotic serum concentration after a given dosage and concern about potential ototoxicity make it appropriate to monitor serum concen-trations of vancomycin in patients being treated with this antibiotic.

Disk diffusion microbiological assay (MA) techniques have been widely used for the meas-urement of serum vancomycin concentrations. A recently developed radioimmunoassay (RIA) (Monitor Science Corp., Newport Beach, Calif.) for the measurement of serum vancomycin con-centrations was made available to us for evalu-ation. This study reports a comparison between the traditional MA and this RIA.

The RIA was used to measure concentrations of vancomycin in 137 specimens of serum from patients being treated with this antibiotic. Eighty-four of the sera were also analyzed by using a modification of the MA technique described by Sabath et al. (4). Duplicate determinations were done with each specimen by both RIA and MA. The individual values and the averaged values for both methods were used in the statistical analyses.

The correlation coefficients between all possible combinations of individual and averaged values for RIA and MA results for the 84 sera were ≥0.99 ($P \ll 0.01$). Values of the regression coefficients of RIA results on MA results ranged from 0.98 ± 0.01 to 1.03 ± 0.01. The correlation between the averaged RIA and the averaged MA results for the 84 samples is shown in Fig. 1. The deviation of the MA results from the RIA results (expressed as a percentage of the RIA results) was examined to establish an estimate of the range of deviation. The distribution of the percent deviation of MA results from RIA results for the 84 samples is shown in Fig. 2. The 95% confidence range of the percent deviation (estimated by the 2.5th percentile and the 97.5th percentile) is −14.92 + 5%. Therefore, 95% of the time, the concentration of vancomycin determined by MA will be within −15% and +5% of the corresponding RIA result.

The two possible sources of variability for the MA (use of locally prepared solutions and the need to generate a separate standard curve for each batch of samples) were also studied. RIA was used to measure the concentrations of vancomycin in the standard solutions used in the MA. The correlation coefficient between the average of the two RIA determinations for each of the standard solutions and the assumed concentration of the standard is 0.99 ($P < 0.01$).

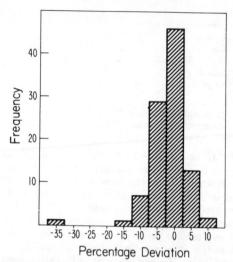

FIG. 2. *Frequency distribution of the percent deviation of MA results from RIA results (expressed as a percentage of the RIA results).*

However, the measured concentration of vancomycin in the standard solutions (as determined by RIA) was somewhat higher than the expected concentration (mean difference, 1.68 ± 0.73 μg/ml). Additional analyses indicated that there is no difference in percent deviation when MA results obtained from different batches of samples assayed using the same lot of standard solutions were compared with RIA results.

These studies indicate that the RIA for vancomycin yields results essentially identical to those obtained by MA. We have also demonstrated that laboratory preparation of standard solutions of vancomycin and the use of MA in batches with different standard curves does not alter the reliability and repeatability of results obtained with the MA technique.

There are inherent disadvantages to the MA for vancomycin. Presence of antimicrobial agents other than vancomycin in the serum specimen requires chemical inactivation of the other antibiotics. Some antimicrobial agents cannot be inactivated, and the MA for vancomycin cannot be used if one of these drugs is present in the serum. The MA is also considerably slower than the RIA. Moreover, unknown antimicrobial agents in the serum of patients receiving vancomycin may yield false-positive results with the MA, but this would not be expected to occur with the RIA.

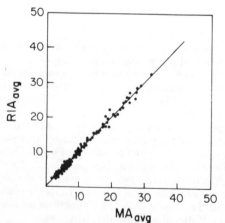

FIG. 1. *Correlation between values of RIA$_{avg}$(Y) and MA$_{avg}$(X) for 84 specimens of serum (r = 1.00; Y = 0.08 + 1.01X).*

1. **Geraci, J. E.** 1977. Vancomycin. Mayo Clin. Proc. **52:** 631–634.
2. **Geraci, J. E., F. R. Heilman, D. R. Nichols,** and **W. E. Wellman.** 1958. Antibiotic therapy of bacterial endo-

carditis. VII. Vancomycin for acute microbial endocarditis. Proc. Staff Meet. Mayo Clin. **33**:172–181.

3. **Louria, D. B., T. Kaminski, and J. Buchman.** 1961. Vancomycin in severe staphylococcal infections. Arch. Intern. Med. **107**:225–240.

4. **Sabath, L. D., J. I. Casey, P. A. Ruch, L. L. Stumpf, and M. Finland.** 1971. Rapid microassay of gentamicin, kanamycin, neomycin, streptomycin, and vancomycin in serum or plasma. J. Lab. Clin. Med. **78**:457–463.

Rapid Assay of Gentamicin in Serum by the Enzyme Multiplied Immunoassay Technique

CHARLES V. SANDERS,* LUCILLE M. SHAIK, ROBERT L. MARIER, AND H. PETER LEHMANN

Department of Medicine, Division of Infectious Diseases, and Department of Pathology, Louisiana State University Medical Center, New Orleans, Louisiana 70112, U.S.A.

Gentamicin, like all other aminoglycosides, is potentially ototoxic and nephrotoxic and has a low therapeutic index; toxic effects are more common if the serum concentration exceeds 10 μg/ml, whereas therapeutic effects are decreased if the serum concentration is less than 2 μg/ml (2, 5). These toxicities may be decreased or prevented by serial monitoring of the serum level of gentamicin and adjusting the dosage accordingly (4).

Recently, a homogeneous enzyme immunoassay (EMIT; Syva Co., Palo Alto, Calif.) for gentamicin has been described (3). In this assay the patient's sample (50 μl) is mixed with enzyme (glucose-6-phosphate dehydrogenase-labeled gentamicin [ELG]), antibody to gentamicin, enzyme substrate (glucose-6-phosphate), and the coenzyme NAD. If gentamicin is present it will compete with ELG for antibody binding sites; if not, the ELG will bind to antibody, leaving no free ELG in the mixture. Only free ELG can act on glucose-6-phosphate and convert NAD to NADH (conversion measured by a spectrophotometer). Enzyme activity is directly proportional to the concentration of free gentamicin in the sample.

We evaluated the precision and accuracy of the EMIT assay for gentamicin and compared it with the radioimmunoassay (RIA) and microbiological assay (MBA) methods to measure gentamicin in duplicate serum samples obtained from 100 patients receiving gentamicin.

In the EMIT assay for gentamicin, each volume measurement of the pipetter was automatically diluted with 250 μl of buffer with a Syva pipetter-diluter (model 2500). Fifty microliters of one of the gentamicin calibrators (0, 1.0, 2.0, 4.0, 8.0, and 16.0 μg/ml), gentamicin control (6.0 μg/ml), or serum sample was transferred to a 2-ml disposable plastic beaker. Fifty microliters of this diluted sample was transferred to a second beaker, followed by 50 μl of reagent A (containing antibodies specific for gentamicin, enzyme substrate glucose-6-phosphate, and the coenzyme NAD) and 50 μl of reagent B (containing gentamicin coupled to glucose-6-phosphate dehydrogenase). The contents of the second beaker were immediately aspirated into the flow cell of a Gilford Stasar III spectrophotometer (Gilford Instrument Laboratories, Inc., Oberlin, Ohio), and the Syva CP-1000 EMIT Timer-Printer was automatically activated. Duplicate determinations were performed for each sample and all calibrators. The increase in absorbance (ΔA) over a 30-s period was used to calculate the results. The difference ($\Delta A - \Delta A_0$) between the average EMIT calibrator zero reading (ΔA_0) and the average reading (ΔA) of the gentamicin calibrators was determined, and a standard curve was plotted on graph paper supplied by Syva. The results ($\Delta A - \overline{\Delta A_0}$) of unknown samples were converted to concentrations (micrograms per milliliter) by extrapolation from the standard curve.

RIA of gentamicin was accomplished by using the [^{125}I]gentamicin RIA kit (Diagnostic Products Corp., Los Angeles, Calif.). The MBA for gentamicin was that described by Alcid and Seligman (1), except that Mueller-Hinton agar was substituted for Trypticase soy agar.

Results of the within-day reproducibility of the EMIT assay (obtained with serum samples spiked with 2.0, 4.0, and 12.0 μg of gentamicin per ml) and the day-to-day reproducibility (determined with a control serum spiked with 6.0 μg of gentamicin per ml) are shown in Table 1.

The accuracy of the EMIT assay for gentamicin was determined by analyzing 10 drug-spiked serum samples prepared by Syva which contained known amounts of gentamicin. Correlation analysis comparing known concentrations with experimental concentrations gave: slope = 1.02; intercept = 0.10, r = 0.996, SE of the estimate = 0.38.

TABLE 1. *Precision data for EMIT gentamicin assay*

Replications	Gentamicin (μg ml)	n	Mean	SD	CV (%)[a]
Within day	2.0	10	2.6	0.16	6.5
	4.0	10	4.3	0.16	3.8
	12.0	10	12.5	0.23	1.8
Day to day	6.0	10	5.7	0.21	3.6

[a] Coefficient of variation = (SD/mean) $\times$ 100.

The specificity of the EMIT assay was determined by adding measured amounts of tobramycin, amikacin, sisomicin, kanamycin, and streptomycin to sera and analyzing for gentamicin. Sisomicin, a 4,5-dehydrogentamicin C_{1A}, reacted very much like gentamicin except that at the highest concentration tested (12.0 μg/ml) it was less than 50% reactive. When gentamicin was added to serum samples containing carbenicillin, ticarcillin, and cephalothin and the EMIT assay for gentamicin was repeated, there was no significant interference from any of these drugs.

Finally, we compared the EMIT assay, RIA, and MBA for measuring gentamicin (Table 2). The EMIT assay compared more favorably with the RIA ($r = 0.97$) than with the MBA ($r = 0.83$).

The EMIT assay for gentamicin requires only 50 μl of serum and has the following advantages over currently available assays. First, it is rapid. The standard curve, which requires approximately 30 min to generate, is stable up to 8 h, and only 5 min is required for each assay. Second, as with the RIA and radioenzymatic assay, the EMIT assay has excellent specificity, preci-

TABLE 2. *Comparison of EMIT, RIA, and MBA for gentamicin in serum samples from patients receiving gentamicin*

Methods	n	Slope	Intercept	r	SE of estimate
EMIT vs RIA	100	1.078	−0.28	0.969	0.39
EMIT vs MBA	100	0.902	+0.05	0.832	0.97

sion, and accuracy. However, unlike the RIA and radioenzymatic assay, the EMIT assay does not require the use of radioisotopes (and the associated potential health hazards) or expensive radioisotope counters. Third, the EMIT assay, unlike the RIA, does not require an incubation period or separation of free and bound labeled material.

In summary, the EMIT assay for gentamicin is a simple, convenient, rapid, sensitive, specific, safe, and inexpensive method for the analysis of gentamicin in serum.

1. **Alcid, D. V., and S. J. Seligman.** 1973. Simplified assay for gentamicin in the presence of other antibiotics. Antimicrob. Agents Chemother. 3:559–561.
2. **Dahlgren, J. G., E. T. Anderson, and W. L. Hewitt.** 1975. Gentamicin blood levels: a guide to nephrotoxicity. Antimicrob. Agents Chemother. 8:58–62.
3. **Kabakoff, D. S., D. K. Leung, and P. Singh.** 1978. An EMIT® assay for gentamicin. Clin. Chem. (Winston-Salem, N.C.) 24:1055.
4. **Maitra, S. K., T. T. Yoshikawa, L. B. Guze, and M. C. Schotz.** 1979. Determination of aminoglycoside antibiotics in biological fluids: a review. Clin. Chem. (Winston-Salem, N.C.) 25:1361–1367.
5. **Riff, L. J., and G. G. Jackson.** 1971. Pharmacology of gentamicin in man. J. Infect. Dis. 124(Suppl.):S98–S105.

Antimicrobial Susceptibility Test: a Comparison of the Results of Four Methods

JOHN E. DEGENER,* IWAN P. THONUS, AND MARC F. MICHEL

Department of Clinical Microbiology and Antimicrobial Therapy, Erasmus University, Rotterdam, The Netherlands

Two semiautomatic systems for testing the antimicrobial susceptibility of bacteria, the Autobac-I (Pfizer) and the MS-2 (Abbott), were tested together with the agar diffusion method and the agar dilution method (ADM). In all four methods the same two sets of 55 *Escherichia coli* strains and 33 *Staphylococcus aureus* strains were used. Test results of Autobac-I and MS-2 were interpreted according to susceptibility criteria set by the manufacturers. The agar

diffusion test was interpreted according to the criteria recommended by the Food and Drug Administration (FDA) and the National Committee for Clinical Laboratory Standards (NCCLS) (1). The ADM was interpreted with criteria set by FDA/NCCLS and by criteria recommended by a Dutch Working Group for the Standardization of Susceptibility Tests (WRG) (Table 1).

The different criteria set by FDS/NCCLS and

TABLE 1. *MIC interpretive criteria, zone diameter interpretive standards, and disk loads*

Antibiotic	MIC (µg/ml) Susceptible				MIC (µg/ml) Resistant				Zone diam (mm) FDA/NCCLS Diffusion test		Disk load (µg)		
	FDA/NCCLS	WRG	MS-2	Auto-bac-I	FDA/NCCLS	WRG	MS-2	Auto-bac-I	S	R	Diffusion test	MS-2	Auto-bac-I
Ampicillin (Beecham)	≤8	≤1	≤10	≤16	≥32	>8	≥20	>16	≥14	≤11	10	2.5	7.5
Carbenicillin (Beecham)	≤16	≤16	≤34	≤16	≥32	>128	≥44	>16	≥23	≤17	100	16	24
Cephalothin (Lilly)	≤10	≤1	≤18	≤16	≥32	>8	≥24	>16	≥18	≤14	30	10	20
Gentamicin (Schering)	≤6	≤1	≤4.8	≤4	≥6	>4	≥11	>4	≥13	≤12	10	4	6
Kanamycin (Brocades)	≤6	≤4	≤10		≥25	>16	≥22		≥18	≤13	30	8	
Tobramycin (Lilly)	≤6	≤1	≤4.8		≥6	>4	≥11		≥14	≤13	10	4	
Tetracycline (Pfizer)	≤4	≤1	≤6.2	≤4	≥12	>4	≥11.4	>4	≥19	≤14	30	5	0.4
Clindamycin (Upjohn)	≤1	≤1	≤1.6		≥2	>4	≥1.8		≥17	≤14	2	1	
Erythromycin (Upjohn)	≤2	≤1	≤3.8	≤4	≥8	>2	≥5.5	>4	≥18	≤13	15	3	0.4
Methicillin (Beecham)	≤3	≤4	≤6	≤2	>3	>4	≥12	>2	≥14	≤9	5	5	7
Penicillin G (Specia)	≤0.1	≤0.15	≤1.5	≤16	>0.1	>0.15	>1.5	>16	≥29	≤20	6	1.5	24
Co-trimoxazole = sulfamethoxazole-trimethoprim 19:1 (Roche)	≤35	≤20	≤40	?	≥200	>20	≥43	?	≥16	≤10	25	25	24

WRG gave rise to a substantial shift in the distribution of susceptible (S), intermediate (I), and resistant (R) strains in the *E. coli* set. For instance: cephalothin gives 83% S, 13% I, and 4% R strains under FDA/NCCLS criteria, whereas these figures are 0% S, 84% I, and 16% R under the WRG criteria. In the *S. aureus* set no major shift was seen in susceptibility interpretation when comparing FDA/NCCLS and WRG criteria for any antimicrobial agent.

The percentage of agreement with ADM was expressed as satisfactory (≥95%), moderate (86 to 94%), or insufficient (≤85%). The agreement scores for the diffusion test, Autobac-I, and MS-2 compared with the ADM are shown in Table 2.

According to FDA/NCCLS criteria, the diffusion test gave a satisfactory overall agreement score with all antibiotics for both sets of strains, but there were moderate scores for *E. coli* strains with cephalothin and kanamycin and for *S. aureus* strains with methicillin and penicillin G. According to WRG criteria, the diffusion test gave an insufficient overall agreement score; only carbenicillin and co-trimoxazole scored satisfactorily with *E. coli*. The *S. aureus* set, however, did score satisfactorily for all antibiotics.

Autobac-I scored insufficiently with the *E. coli* set according to FDA/NCCLS criteria, except for gentamicin and co-trimoxazole, which scored moderately. When WRG criteria were used, we found a shift to more insufficient results with the *E. coli* set from 73% agreement according to FDA/NCCLS criteria to 55% according to

TABLE 2. *Overall agreement with the E. coli set for eight antibiotics and with the S. aureus set for six antibiotics with the diffusion method, Autobac-I, and MS-2 compared with the ADM, according to FDA/NCCLS and WRG criteria*

Method	% Agreement E. coli set		% Agreement S. aureus set	
	FDA/NCCLS	WRG	FDA/NCCLS	WRG
Diffusion test	96	70	99	99
Autobac-I	73	55	90	91
MS-2	95	70	92	92

WRG criteria. With the *S. aureus* set Autobac-I gave moderate results.

According to FDA/NCCLS criteria, MS-2 scored satisfactorily with the *E. coli* set except with kanamycin and cephalothin, which scored moderately. The overall agreement score according to WRG criteria was insufficient, in particular with cephalothin and tetracycline. The *S. aureus* set gave a satisfactory score with both FDA/NCCLS and WRG criteria.

Because the agar diffusion test is related via regression analysis to the ADM, it was expected that the results for both sets of strains according to FDA/NCCLS criteria would be satisfactory. Moderate results were found for cephalothin and kanamycin with the *E. coli* strains. These deviating results may be explained as follows. The MIC criteria (FDA/NCCLS) for these antibiotics, to discriminate the susceptible from the in-

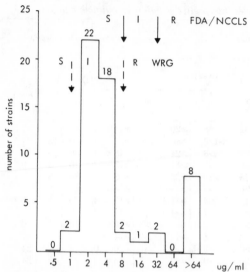

FIG. 1. *MIC distribution of E. coli strains for ampicillin using FDA/NCCLS and WRG interpretive criteria.*

termediately susceptible strains, fall within the continuous MIC distribution of the strains, thus making it very difficult to assign borderline cases to the exact category. For any method it will be difficult to produce correctly such an artificial separation. The insufficient scores found for the *E. coli* set, when shifting from FDA/NCCLS to WRG criteria, can be understood by studying the place of the MIC breakpoints within the MIC distribution curves. In Fig. 1 this is shown for ampicillin. The criteria shift (8 µg/ml for FDA/NCCLS to 1 µg/ml for WRG) causes an interpretive shift for 40 strains, which is in good agreement with the occurrence of 41 minor discrepancies.

Autobac-I was developed with the criteria set in the International Cooperative Study (2). These criteria differ from those of the FDA/NCCLS and WRG, and it was therefore expected that there would be discrepancies. However, in our hands the Autobac-I system showed a substantial number of unexplainable discrepancies for ampicillin, carbenicillin, and methicillin.

The criteria used for the development of MS-2 are similar to FDA/NCCLS criteria, and therefore a good performance under FDA/NCCLS criteria was expected and found. The same kind of discrepancies for the *E. coli* set as seen with the diffusion test were met with MS-2. With the *S. aureus* strains problems were met with erythromycin, methicillin, and tetracycline.

Conclusion. Setting of interpretive criteria for the susceptibility of bacteria may differ from country to country and is more or less arbitrary. As can be seen from our data, the difference between FDA/NCCLS and WRG criteria is larger for some antibiotics. It appears from this study that setting different criteria gives rise to serious discrepancies in interpretation. Diffusion tests can readily be adjusted to different criteria by doing regression analysis. Adaption of the Autobac-I and MS-2 to different criteria cannot be accomplished in such a simple manner. The user should take into account substantial discrepancies in interpretation when his criteria differ from the apparatus' interpretive criteria.

1. **Barry, A. L.** 1976. The antimicrobic susceptibility test. Lea & Febiger, Philadelphia.
2. **Ericsson, H. M., and J. C. Sherris.** 1971. Antibiotic sensitivity testing: report of an International Collaborative Study. Acta Pathol. Microbiol. Scand. Suppl. **217:**1–19.

Clinical Laboratory Feasibility Study of Antibiotic Susceptibility Determined by the Auto Microbic System

HENRY D. ISENBERG* AND J. SAMPSON-SCHERER

Long Island Jewish-Hillside Medical Center, New Hyde Park, New York 11042, U.S.A.

The versatility of the Auto Microbic System (AMS; Vitek Systems, Inc.; 1, 4) in the automation of diagnostic procedures for the clinical microbiology laboratory has been demonstrated by its application to the analysis of urine specimens (2, 3), susceptibility testing of bacteria isolated from urine specimens (H. D. Isenberg and J. Scherer, Program Abstr. Intersci. Conf.

Antimicrob. Agents Chemother. 17th, New York, N.Y., abstr. no. 383, 1977; H. D. Isenberg, T. L. Gavan, and W. Taylor, 17th ICAAC, abstr. no. 386, 1977), and the biochemical species identification of *Enterobacteriaceae* (M. C. Meyer, J. J. Underwood, R. Wilkinson, and L. V. Woods, Abstr. Annu. Meet. Am. Soc. Microbiol. 1979, C142, p. 333; H. D. Isenberg, J. Scherer, and S.

Freedman, Abstr. Annu. Meet. Am. Soc. Microbiol. 1979, C143, p. 334). The 30-compartment card, used for the biochemical reaction profile, provided sufficient separate wells for the design of several, distinct means of using the AMS to assess the antibiotic susceptibility of bacteria isolated in the clinical laboratory in terms of general susceptibility as well as the MICs for such organisms.

The feasibility of this approach was applied to gram-negative bacteria, examined simultaneously with manual agar diffusion and microtiter dilution modalities. Standardized suspensions of bacteria in 0.5% NaCl were tested in three separate systems: a general susceptibility card which contained amikacin, ampicillin, cefamandole, carbenicillin, cephalothin, chloramphenicol, gentamicin, kanamycin, tetracycline, tobramycin, cefoxitin, trimethoprim-sulfamethoxazole, and nitrofurantoin in low and high concentrations as well as two compartments of a modified Eugon broth (BBL Microbiology Systems, Cockeysville, Md.) without any agent; a general MIC card containing selected concentrations of ampicillin, cefamandole, gentamicin, tobramycin, cephalothin, chloramphenicol, tetracycline, and cefoxitin, as well as modified Eugon broth without antibiotics; and a card with selected concentrations of amikacin, chloramphenicol, gentamicin, kanamycin, carbenicillin, colistin, and tobramycin, in addition to control components. Several colonies were transferred to modified Eugon broth, incubated for 1 h at 35°C, diluted with 0.5% NaCl, introduced into the various cards by vacuum, and placed into the computerized incubator-reader, which reported the results in 4 h on a print-out form. The control studies involved the transfer of several colonies to brain heart infusion broth (BBL), preincubation at 35°C for 2 to 4 h, incubation of the appropriate media for 18 h, and recording of results.

We examined 206 bacteria, isolated from clinical specimens. These were: *Escherichia coli*, 33; *Pseudomonas aeruginosa*, 25; enterococci, 21; *Streptococcus bovis*, 2; *Citrobacter freundii*, 9; *Enterobacter* sp., 26; *Klebsiella* sp., 29; *Proteus mirabilis*, 16; other *Proteus* and *Providencia* sp., 11; *Salmonella* and *Shigella* sp., 17; *Serratia* sp., 9; miscellaneous gram-negative rods including *Arizona* sp., *C. diversus*, *Edwardsiella tarda*, and *Yersinia enterocolitica*, 8.

Computer print-out of the general susceptibility card reported the range of susceptibility in micrograms per milliliter and the appropriate interpretation, i.e., susceptible, intermediate (equivocal), or resistant. The two MIC cards reported the MIC if values fell within the range

of concentrations incorporated. MICs higher than the greatest or less than the smallest concentrations were designated as such.

Comparison of AMS findings with manual techniques was governed by the following criteria. The AMS results were considered correct when manual results equaled automated findings, the manual results were equal or less than the lowest concentration tested in the AMS, or the manual results were equal or greater than the highest AMS concentration. Variations of one dilution between the methods were considered acceptable. Disagreement was considered very major if the standard finding indicated resistance and the AMS reported susceptibility, major if the manual determination indicated susceptibility and the AMS resistance, and minor if the manual methods designated the organism's response as intermediate and the AMS as either susceptible or resistant, as well as the converse of these results. Finally, differences of two dilutions or greater that did not alter the category of bacteria response were included in the minor discrepancy category.

Tables 1 and 2 summarize the comparison. The discrepancies observed fall into several categories which can be corrected by adjustments of the computer-controlled functions or of the concentrations of antibiotics or medium components in the card itself. The results indicate that *P. aeruginosa* and the group D streptococci required 1- to 2-h-longer incubation or a denser inoculum for drugs such as amikacin, cephalothin, chloramphenicol, kanamycin, tetracycline, and tobramycin. For other bacteria, discrepancies can be resolved by lowering or increasing the threshold level in the computer. This ad-

TABLE 1. *Percent agreement of manual MIC versus AMS general susceptibility card*

Test substance	Gram-negative rods other than *Pseudomonas*	*P. aeruginosa*	Group D streptococci
Amikacin	97 (93)[a]	96 (96)	95 (85)
Ampicillin	96.5 (84)	100 (96)	94 (94)
Carbenicillin	90 (70)	66 (40)	51 (51)
Cefamandole	97 (86)	100 (76)	100 (85)
Cefoxitin	95 (80)	92 (92)	100 (95)
Cephalothin	97.5 (84)	96 (64)	90 (75)
Chloramphenicol	87.5 (85)	96 (92)	90 (50)
Gentamicin	100 (99)	92 (88)	75 (70)
Kanamycin	97 (97)	70 (52)	65 (50)
Nitrofurantoin	68.5 (68.5)	100 (100)	85 (85)
Tetracycline	92 (83)	100 (96)	95 (55)
Tobramycin	100 (84)	96 (52)	80 (70)
Trimethoprim-sulfamethoxazole	91 (91)	92 (92)	60 (60)

[a] Number in parentheses is percent agreement including minor discrepancies.

TABLE 2. *Percent agreement of manual MIC versus MIC cards I and II*

Test substance	Gram-negative rods other than Pseudomonas	P. aeruginosa	Group D streptococci
Ampicillin	93 (74)[a]	100 (100)	95 (85)
Cefamandole	96 (86)	100 (96)	96 (92)
Cefoxitin	94 (83)	96 (92)	100 (100)
Cephalothin	98 (91)	100 (100)	100 (76)
Chloramphenicol	96 (91)	100 (92)	100 (95)
Gentamicin	100 (96)	92 (88)	65 (65)
Tetracycline	95 (80)	92 (92)	75 (50)
Tobramycin	99 (76)	100 (100)	65 (55)
Amikacin	99 (86)	100 (72)	100 (70)
Carbenicillin	94 (84)	100 (88)	100 (90)
Colistin	97 (93)	92 (92)	100 (100)
Kanamycin	98 (84)	60 (50)	95 (85)
Chloramphenicol	98 (92)	100 (76)	100 (95)
Gentamicin	100 (90)	96 (92)	70 (50)
Tobramycin	99 (83)	100 (96)	100 (80)

[a] Number in parentheses is percent agreement including minor discrepancies.

justment would resolve observed differences, mostly minor, with ampicillin, carbenicillin, cefoxitin, chloramphenicol, nitrofurantoin, kanamycin, and tobramycin. With kanamycin and tobramycin drug levels at the lower concentration can also be adjusted.

Although only 206 bacteria were tested in the study, the responses between the various AMS cards and the two manual methods were of the same order if not slightly better than the comparison between the manual diffusion and dilution modalities. Therefore, one can conclude that the AMS is a useful instrument for the assessment of bacterial susceptibility to antibiotics and chemotherapeutic agents and that the instrument has the versatility to perform a two-concentration screen helpful in categorizing the bacterial response and a determination of the MICs. The two MIC cards need not be used together, but should be used in keeping with the organisms isolated, the clinical situation of the patient, and his therapeutic regimen. AMS has minimal demands on personnel time and completes the antibiotic profile in 4 h. This investigation indicates convincingly that the instrument can perform antibiotic susceptibilities accurately.

1. **Aldridge, C., P. W. Jones, S. Gibson, J. Lanham, M. Meyer, R. Vannest, and R. Charles.** 1977. Automated microbiological detection/identification system. J. Clin. Microbiol. **6:**406–413.
2. **Isenberg, H. D., T. L. Gavan, A. Sonnenwirth, W. I. Taylor, and J. A. Washington II.** 1979. Clinical laboratory evaluation of automated microbial detection/identification system in analysis of clinical urine specimens. J. Clin. Microbiol. **10:**226–230.
3. **Smith, P. B., T. L. Gavan, H. D. Isenberg, A. Sonnenwirth, W. I. Taylor, J. A. Washington II, and A. Balows.** 1978. Multi-laboratory evaluation of an automated microbial detection/identification system. J. Clin. Microbiol. **8:**657–666.
4. **Sonnenwirth, A. C.** 1977. Preprototype of an automated microbial detection and identification system: a developmental investigation. J. Clin. Microbiol. **6:**400–405.

Susceptibility Testing with the Plate Dilution Method, Diffusion Methods, and Autobac

V. FRØLUND THOMSEN,[1]* IDA MORTENSEN, VIGGO PERRIARD, OLE B. JEPSEN, SEVERIN O. LARSEN, AND JØRGEN BANG

Statens Seruminstitut and Copenhagen County Hospital, Copenhagen, Denmark

Testing of bacterial susceptibility to antibiotics may in many ways be regarded as the basic procedure in a clinical microbiological laboratory. An extensive literature deals with the problems of the technical performance of susceptibility testing; all these studies aim to establish a fast, simple, and cheap method with the highest possible specificity, reproducibility, and clinical relevance.

In this report results obtained by five different performances are evaluated comparatively. A

[1] Present address: Clinical Microbiology Department, Lundtofrej 5, DK 2800, Lyngby, Denmark.

plate dilution method (2) was selected as the reference method. Results were obtained simultaneously by two diffusion methods, the predffusion method of Thomsen (3) and the Biodisc method of Ericsson (1), and by an automated method, Autobac 1 (Pfizer), performed in two different laboratories (Statens Seruminstitut and Lyngby, Copenhagen, Denmark) (4).

The susceptibilities of 451 strains belonging to more than 10 bacterial species isolated from daily clinical routine were grouped as susceptible or resistant according to selected "breakpoints" (Table 1).

TABLE 1. *Selected breakpoints between susceptibility and resistance*

Method	MIC (µg/ml)								
	Penicillin	Strepto-mycin	Genta-micin	Tetracy-cline	Ampicil-lin	Cephalo-thin	Nalidixic acid	Carbeni-cillin	Clinda-mycin
Plate dilution	16	8	2	4	16	16	32	16	4
Autobac	16	8	2	4	16	16	32	16	4
Prediffusion	16	8	2	4	16	16	32	16	4
Biodisc	16	8	8	4	16	16	32	16	8

TABLE 2. *Susceptibility testing with Autobac performed simultaneously in two different laboratories*

Antibiotic	Overall agreement (%)[a]
Penicillin	95.6
Ampicillin	93.8
Carbenicillin	89.6
Cephalothin	91.3
Streptomycin	90.9
Gentamicin	87.1
Tetracycline	89.4
Clindamycin	93.6
Nalidixic acid	90.9

[a] Percentage of tested strains showing identical results in the two laboratories.

The reproducibility of Autobac 1 was illustrated by testing the same strains in two different laboratories (Table 2). The highest consistency was obtained with penicillin, and the lowest was obtained with gentamicin. Overall it was expected that about 10% of the results could differ by repeated determinations.

In reproducing results obtained by the plate dilution method, it was found that a diffusion method using 20 h of prediffusion showed the highest consistency. Six percent of the results were in disagreement (Table 3). Nine percent of the results obtained by the Biodisc method deviated from results obtained by the plate dilution

method. In both Autobac determinations the disagreements rose to 15%, or nearly double that of either of the diffusion methods.

Evaluation of in vitro methods for testing bacterial susceptibility to antibiotics may in principle be based upon a direct comparison with the clinical result of the actual treatment. As such an evaluation is difficult to conduct, a plate dilution method is often used as a standard reference method. The prerequisite is that there be a close parallelism between the concentration of antibiotic inhibiting bacterial growth in the substrate and the infected organism.

For practical purposes the agar diffusion method for semiquantitative determination of bacterial susceptibility is the most widespread. It is known that a correlation to results obtained by a plate dilution method varies with the different diffusion methods. The correlation depends on multiple factors, partly on factors connected with diffusion (diffusion factors in the substrate, preincubation, prediffusion, amount of antibiotic in diffusion center, size of diffusion center) and partly on the size of the inoculum and the bacterial growth rate. Most of these factors are more or less eliminated in Autobac 1, especially is the result corrected for the actual bacterial growth rate, because the inhibition is related to the degree of growth in the antibiotic-free control chamber. Autobac 1 correlates less with the plate dilution method than with what

TABLE 3. *Disagreement between the plate dilution method (ICSO) and the prediffusion method, the Biodisc method, and Autobac*

Method	Disagreement (%)[a]									
	Antibiotic									
	Penicil-lin	Strepto-mycin	Genta-micin	Tetra-cycline	Ampi-cillin	Cepha-lothin	Nali-dixic acid	Carben-icillin	Clinda-mycin	Avg
Prediffusion	3	6	8	4	4	5	8	8	8	6
Biodisc	3	13	10	14	6	6	9	14	9	9
Autobac										
Statens Serum-institut	10	11	20	20	10	11	20	20	11	15
Lyngby	9	12	23	21	8	15	21	17	11	15

[a] Percentage of strains giving different susceptibility-resistance results from those obtained with the plate dilution method.

is obtained by the diffusion methods. It seems, too, that disagreements are different for gram-positive cocci and gram-negative rods.

It is not possible from these experiments to explain these differences, but they may be related to differences in the growth rate. Further experiments seem necessary to solve the technical problems before automated methods are able to give results which correlate to the plate dilution method to the same extent as do the traditional diffusion methods.

1. **Ericsson, H.** 1960. Rational use of antibiotics in hospitals. Scand. J. Clin. Lab. Invest. **12**(Suppl. 50).
2. **Reyn, A., M. W. Bentzon, and H. Ericsson.** 1963. Comparative investigations of the sensitivity of *N. gonorrhoeae* to penicillin. Acta Pathol. Microbiol. Scand. **57**:235–255.
3. **Thomsen, V. F.** 1967. Resistensbestemmelse. Busck, Copenhagen.
4. **Thornsberry, C., T. L. Gavan, J. C. Sherris, A. Balows, J. M. Matsen, L. D. Sabath, F. Schoenknecht, L. D. Thrupp, and J. A. Washington II.** 1975. Laboratory evaluation of a rapid, automated susceptibility testing system: report of a collaborative study. Antimicrob. Agents Chemother. **7**:466–480.

Agar Dilution Procedure for Antimicrobial Susceptibility Testing of Anaerobic Bacteria Isolated from Clinical Specimens

CHARLES W. HANSON[1]* AND WILLIAM J. MARTIN

Departments of Pathology and Microbiology and Immunology, UCLA School of Medicine, Clinical Microbiology Laboratory, Los Angeles, California 90024, U.S.A.

A 2-year evaluation of the antimicrobial susceptibility patterns of 2,126 anaerobic bacteria isolated from properly obtained clinical specimens was carried out in a test system which, except for minor modifications, was similar to a recommended reference standard agar dilution procedure (6). The test was found to be easy to perform on a weekly basis and to yield reliable and reproducible results. In addition, the accumulated data can be used as guidelines to help assess trends in susceptibility patterns and thereby facilitate the management of anaerobic infections. Control organisms included two *Bacteroides fragilis* isolates and one anaerobic *Lactobacillus* species that were determined to have MICs in the middle dilution range of one or more of the antibiotics tested. The antibiotics and serial twofold dilutions used in this investigation were: carbenicillin, 128 to 8.0 μg/ml; chloramphenicol, 16.0 to 0.5 μg/ml; clindamycin, 4.0 to 0.015 μg/ml; penicillin, 8.0 to 0.031 μg/ml; and tetracycline, 16.0 to 0.5 μg/ml.

Pure cultures of anaerobic isolates were inoculated on blood agar plates and incubated aerobically and anaerobically (GasPak jars [BBL Microbiology Systems]) at 35°C for 72 h. These cultures served, respectively, as aerobic contamination and anaerobic viability controls. In addition, the anaerobic plate provided a fresh inoculum for the remainder of the procedure. Viable anaerobic bacteria were then incubated anaerobically in Schaedler broth for 24 h, adjusted

[1] Present address: Abbott Laboratories, Department 481, North Chicago, IL 60064.

to the turbidity of a no. 1 McFarland standard in fresh Schaedler broth, and dispensed into wells of a Steers replicator (5).

Frozen stock solutions (2,560 μg/ml) of each antibiotic were thawed and diluted, using standard procedures (2).

Wilkins-Chalgren (WC) agar medium (8), prepared in advance, was melted in a microwave oven (3) and cooled to 50°C. An 18-ml amount of cooled agar was added to respective tubes containing 2 ml of the appropriately diluted antibiotic, mixed, and poured into round petri dishes (100 by 15 mm). The plates were inoculated with a Steers replicator and incubated at 35°C in GasPak jars for 48 h. Duplicate blood agar and WC agar plates without antibiotics were inoculated at the beginning and end of each run. One of each type of medium was incubated aerobically and anaerobically to serve as respective contamination and growth controls. MICs were determined relative to the WC agar control (6).

Other than incubation in GasPak jars, all procedures were carried out in air at the bench.

At least one of the three control strains used in every test over the 2-year period consistently showed >95% agreement to within one dilution of the organism's known MIC of one or more of the antibiotics tested. In addition, repeat testing (a minimum of three and usually four times) was done on selected isolates. These results showed 100% reproducibility to within one dilution of the original MIC and 98% absolute agreement in all of the repeat tests.

It was found that substantial numbers of *Bac-*

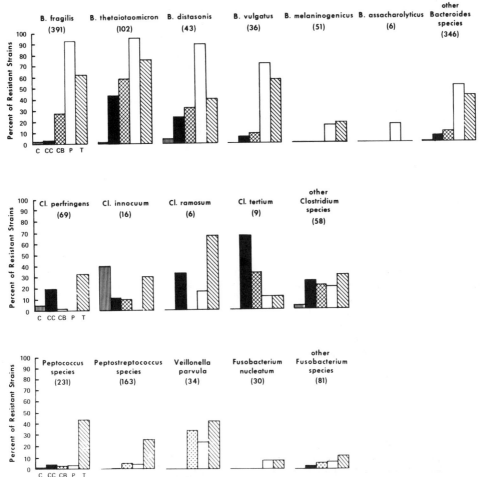

FIG. 1. *Percentage of strains from selected groups of anaerobic bacteria resistant to readily achievable levels of the antibiotics tested. Endpoints for the antibiotics were: chloramphenicol (C), >8 µg/ml; clindamycin (CC), >2 µg/ml; carbenicillin (CB), >64 µg/ml; penicillin (P), >2 µg/ml; tetracycline (T), >8 µg/ml. Numbers in parentheses after the name of the organism refer to the number of strains tested.*

teroides melaninogenicus and *Fusobacterium* species would not grow on WC agar medium (Table 1) and smaller percentages yielded poor growth on this medium relative to the growth obtained on blood agar plates. In addition, poor growth or no growth on WC agar medium was observed with members of a number of other groups of anaerobic isolates listed in Table 1. The occurrence of poor growth was considered to be less serious than no growth because the MICs obtained from antibiotic-containing WC agar plates were always determined by comparison to growth obtained on antibiotic-free WC agar control plates. However, the failure to obtain growth from some of the *Bacteroides* species on WC medium was of concern since these organisms generally show a higher degree of resistance than other groups of anaerobic bac-

teria which failed to grow or grew poorly on that medium. If such an isolate is implicated in a pathogenic process and susceptibility testing is necessary, then an agar dilution method using blood agar medium is recommended.

A significant number of *Propionibacterium* species were found to grow aerobically on WC medium (Table 1, last column), whereas parallel cultures of the same organism on blood agar failed to show aerobic growth. This phenomenon was also observed with a few strains of *Peptococcus* and *Peptostreptococcus* species. On the other hand, pinpoint aerobic growth was a common occurrence with "anaerobic" *Lactobacillus* species when subcultured subsequent to primary isolation.

Evaluation of susceptibility patterns for various members of the penicillin-resistant *Bacte-*

TABLE 1. *Comparison of anaerobic bacterial isolates on blood agar (BA) and Wilkins-Chalgren (WC) medium in situations where growth characteristics on the two media differed*

Organism	Total no. evaluated	% Negative on WC relative to 4+ growth on BA	% Showing 2+ growth on WC relative to 4+ growth on BA	% of anaerobes showing aerobic growth on WC medium and negative for aerobic growth on BA
Bacteroides sp.	187	25.7	1.6	
Fusobacterium nucleatum	23	21.7		
Fusobacterium sp.	43	48.8	2.3	
Bacteroides melaninogenicus	19	47.4	5.3	
Peptococcus sp.	130	17.7	6.2	3.1
Peptostreptococcus sp.	89	33.7	4.5	5.6
Propionibacterium acnes	64			51.6
Propionibacterium sp.	31			22.6
Eubacterium sp.	53	18.9	1.9	
Bifidobacterium sp.	16	12.5		
Lactobacillus sp.	13	53.9	15.4	92.3[a]

[a] Most *Lactobacillus* sp. encountered were found to yield pinpoint colonies on the aerobically incubated control BA and WC agar plates.

roides group showed *B. thetaiotaomicron* and *B. distasonis* to be markedly more resistant to clindamycin (Fig. 1) than was expected in light of the results of earlier investigations (1, 4, 7). These data suggest an emerging resistance pattern to clindamycin by *B. thetaiotaomicron* and *B. distasonis*. Future surveillance studies will be necessary to follow this trend since these organisms are not uncommon isolates from serious clinical situations.

A wide divergence was noted in the susceptibility patterns among members of various *Clostridium* species tested (Fig. 1). The respective endpoints for each of the *Clostridium* species were so variable that we feel general statements about the overall susceptibilities of this group of organisms would be unwise. A more cautious approach would be to test each isolate on an individual basis when the organism is suspected to be involved in a pathogenic process.

1. **Blazevic, D. J.** 1976. Antibiotic susceptibility of the subspecies of *Bacteroides fragilis*. Antimicrob. Agents Chemother. 9:481–484.

2. **Ericsson, H. M., and J. C. Sherris.** 1971. Antibiotic sensitivity testing. Report of an international collaborative study. Acta Pathol. Microbiol. Scand. Sect. B, Suppl. no. 217.

3. **Hanson, C. W., and W. J. Martin.** 1978. Microwave oven for melting laboratory media. J. Clin. Microbiol. 7:401–402.

4. **Jones, R. N., and P. C. Fuchs.** 1976. Identification and antimicrobial susceptibility of 250 *Bacteroides fragilis* subspecies tested by broth microdilution methods. Antimicrob. Agents Chemother. 9:719–721.

5. **Steers, E., E. L. Folty, B. S. Graves, and J. Riden.** 1959. An inocula replicating apparatus for routine testing of bacterial susceptibility to antibiotics. Antibiot. Chemother. (Basel) 9:307–311.

6. **Sutter, V. L., A. L. Barry, T. D. Wilkins, and R. J. Zabransky.** 1979. Collaborative evaluation of a proposed reference dilution method of susceptibility testing of anaerobic bacteria. Antimicrob. Agents Chemother. 16:495–502.

7. **Sutter, V. L., and S. M. Finegold.** 1976. Susceptibility of anaerobic bacteria to 23 antimicrobial agents. Antimicrob. Agents Chemother. 10:736–752.

8. **Wilkins, T. D., and S. Chalgren.** 1976. Medium for use in antibiotic susceptibility testing of anaerobic bacteria to 23 antimicrobial agents. Antimicrob. Agents Chemother. 10:736–752.

Comparison of Serodiagnosis by Hemagglutination Inhibition, Indirect Hemagglutination, and Enzyme Immunoassay in Human Respiratory Coronavirus Infections

GREGORY W. HAMMOND,* HAROLD S. KAYE, AND GARY R. NOBLE

Center for Disease Control, Public Health Service, U.S. Department of Health, Education, and Welfare, Atlanta, Georgia 30333, U.S.A.

An enzyme immunoassay (EIA) was established with ratio comparisons of optical density (OD) between acute- and convalescent-phase sera for the diagnosis of infection by human coronavirus strains OC43 and 229E.

Sera of children and adults previously shown to have a significant rise in antibody titer to OC43 (4) (47 patients) and 229E (3) (25 patients) were tested by hemagglutination inhibition (HI) (2), indirect hemagglutination (IHA) (5), and EIA. Control sera for the EIA tests included 34 patients with serologically documented non-coronaviral respiratory infections and, in addition, sera of children from the same environment as the coronavirus infected patients, including sera positive patients who had seroconverted to the alternate coronavirus strain. All sera were inactivated at 56°C for 30 min.

OC43 purified by the protamine sulfate method from infected suckling mouse brain had a titer of 1,280 hemagglutinating units per 0.1 ml. Five hemagglutinating units per 50 µl were used in the EIA. Standard procedures were used for HI. Five of six serum pairs positive by HI but negative by EIA were treated with phospholipase C and 1,10-phenanthroline (1) and were retested by HI.

229E harvested from RU-1 cells (diploid human lung fibroblasts) had a titer of $10^{4.2}$ log/0.1 ml. A 1:5 dilution of this clarified virus stock was used in the EIA and IHA tests, and uninfected RU-1 cells were used as an EIA control.

Virus and antigen control for the EIA were incubated in Cooke micro-ELISA (enzyme-linked immunosorbent assay) plates overnight at 4°C; the plates were then washed three times with phosphate-buffered saline, pH 7.2. Each acute and convalescent serum was tested in duplicate. Sera diluted 1:101 were incubated at room temperature for 1 h and washed three times with phosphate-buffered saline containing Tween 20. Horseradish peroxidase to goat anti-human immunoglobulin G (Cappel) was diluted in phosphate-buffered saline, Tween 20, and bovine serum albumin 1:2,000 and 1:1,000 for OC43 and 229E antibody testing, respectively. After incubation with conjugate for 1 h, the plates were washed three times, and substrate (1% o-phenylenediamine and 0.003% H_2O_2) was added for 30 min at 25°C. The reaction was stopped with H_2SO_4, and the OD was read at 490 nm with a Gilford Stasar III spectrophotometer. The mean OD of duplicate readings was used to calculate EIA seroconversions, where a ratio of the (mean convalescent-phase serum OD/mean acute-phase serum OD) of ≥ 1.5 was considered indicative of recent infection. A comparison of EIA OD ratio versus EIA endpoint titers was determined with twofold dilutions of serum from 75 patients, 43 of whom had seroconverted by the HI test to OC43. The EIA endpoint titer was the highest serum dilution with an OD ≥ 0.25.

The EIA ratio method showed 97% (37 of 38) sensitivity and 97% (36 of 37) specificity versus the EIA endpoint method for OC43. The 38 serum pairs which demonstrated $\geq$4-fold rise in antibody titer by the EIA endpoint titer method represented 88% (38 of 43) sensitivity when compared with the HI test for OC43. However, of the sera from the five patients who failed to show significant antibody rises by EIA, four were shown to have nonspecific serum inhibitors which were removed by phospholipase C, suggesting false-positive HI results for OC43.

Comparisons of mean EIA ratios with fold

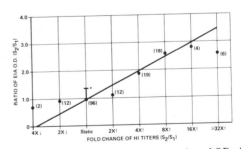

FIG. 1. *Comparison of the mean ratios of OD obtained by EIA measurement of OC43 antibodies in convalescent- to acute-phase sera with fold changes in titers of acute- to convalescent-phase serum by HI for OC43. Symbols: ●, mean ratio of OD measured by EIA for OC43 antibody in convalescent- to acute-phase sera; *, an EIA OD S_2/S_1 ratio of 1.36 was the upper 95% confidence limit for 96 patients with no titer change between acute- and convalescent-phase serum by the HI test for OC43.*

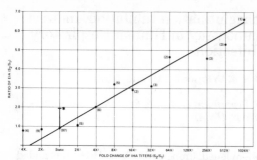

FIG. 2. *Comparison of the mean ratios of OD obtained by EIA measurement of 229E antibodies in convalescent- to acute-phase sera with fold changes in titers of acute- to convalescent-phase serum by IHA for 229E. Symbols:* ●, *mean ratio of OD measured by EIA for 229E antibody in convalescent- to acute-phase sera;* *, *mean EIA OD S_2/S_1 ratio of 1.91 was the upper 95% confidence limit for 97 patients with no titer change for 229E between acute- and convalescent-phase sera by the IHA test.*

changes in titer for the HI and IHA tests are shown in Figs. 1 and 2, respectively. EIA ratios showed a 87% (41 of 47) sensitivity and 99% (120 of 121) specificity with the HI test in the diagnosis of OC43 infections and 96% (24 of 25) sensitivity and 95% (108 of 114) specificity for 229E infections diagnosed by the IHA test.

Conclusions. EIA OD ratios of convalescent- to acute-phase sera correlate with EIA endpoint titers, as shown for OC43 infections. EIA results for the serodiagnosis of coronavirus OC43 and 229E infections correlate well with the HI and IHA tests. Only two patients showed evidence of infection with both OC43 and 229E, suggesting no significant cross-reacting antibodies between these two human coronaviruses (6). The use of single serum dilutions in EIA allows economy of reagents, avoids errors with serial dilutions, and provides objective results. Favorable results with the serodiagnosis of coronavirus infections suggest that EIA could be used to rapidly screen for antibody rises to other virus infections, using OD ratios obtained with single serum dilutions of acute- and convalescent-phase sera. Four of five patients who showed rises in antibody titer to OC43 by HI, but not by EIA, may reflect false-positive HI results due to the presence of nonspecific serum inhibitors.

1. **Hovi, T.** 1978. Nonspecific inhibitors of coronavirus OC43 hemagglutination in human sera. Med. Microbiol. Immunol. **166**:173–176.
2. **Kaye, H. S., and W. R. Dowdle.** 1969. Some characteristics of hemagglutination of certain strains of "IBV-like" virus. J. Infect. Dis. **119**:282–290.
3. **Kaye, H. S., and W. R. Dowdle.** 1975. Seroepidemiologic survey of coronavirus (strain 229E) infections in a population of children. Am. J. Epidemiol. **101**:238–244.
4. **Kaye, H. S., H. B. Marsh, and W. R. Dowdle.** 1970. Seroepidemiologic survey of coronavirus (strain OC43) related infections in a children's population. Am. J. Epidemiol. **94**:43–49.
5. **Kaye, H. S., S. B. Ong, and W. R. Dowdle.** 1972. Detection of coronavirus 229E antibody by indirect hemagglutination. Appl. Microbiol. **24**:703–707.
6. **Pederson, N. C., J. Ward, and W. L. Mangeling.** 1978. Antigenic relationship of feline infectious peritonitis virus to coronavirus of other species. Arch. Virol. **58**: 45–53.

Improved Fluorescent Antibody-to-Membrane Antigen Test Using Frozen, Infected Tissue Culture Cells

MARK FISHAUT,[1]* RICHARD YANAGIHARA, NEVA BLACK, AND KENNETH McINTOSH

Department of Pediatrics, University of Colorado Medical Center, Denver, Colorado, 80262 U.S.A.

Many viruses introduce antigens into and through the plasma membrane of infected cells (1). This phenomenon has been exploited through the use of infected tissue culture cells as targets for immunofluorescence assay of antibodies directed against varicella-zoster virus (VZV; 7) and respiratory syncytial virus (RSV; 5) and for the rapid subtyping of strains of influenza A viruses (2). As noted by other investigators (9), problems associated with the use of live infected cells in fluorescence tests include limited availability of tissue culture and virus culture facilities in many institutions, lot variability, and the possible risk of infection to personnel performing serological tests. Glutaraldehyde fixation of infected tissue culture cells has been used to overcome these limitations for the VZV fluorescent antibody-to-membrane antigen (FAMA) test (9). Cryopreservation with glycerol or with dimethyl sulfoxide has been successfully applied to erythrocytes for use in both transfusion (4) and hemolysis-in-gel antibody titration tests (6) and for lymphocyte preservation (3).

[1] Present address: Clinical Infectious Diseases–Virology, Children's Hospital of Buffalo, Buffalo, NY 14222.

We herein describe our experience with preservation of viral antigens on the surface of infected cells by freezing them in the presence of 20% glycerol and the general application of the technique to FAMA assays for antibodies directed against several viruses.

Tissue culture targets were infected for specified times chosen for maximum antigenic expression with the several viruses, as summarized in Table 1. Infected cells were then harvested by (i) washing the monolayer with phosphate-buffered saline, (ii) exposure to trypsin-EDTA to disperse the cells, (iii) exposure to UV light to inactivate viruses, (iv) washing in Hanks balanced salt solution with 10% fetal calf serum, (v) resuspension in Hanks balanced salt solution with 2% fetal calf serum (4 parts) and glycerol (1 part), and (vi) storage at −90°C without graded freezing.

For performance of a FAMA test, cells were quick-thawed at 37°C, washed in Hanks balanced salt solution with 2% fetal calf serum, sedimented, and resuspended in the same medium. The FAMA test was performed in micro-

titer plates, using 10 to 25 μl of reconstituted cell suspension first with an equal volume of test sample dilution and then with class-specific anti-human fluorescein isothiocyanate-conjugated rabbit immunoglobulin G (IgG). Specimens tested included serum, nasal secretions, and breast milk. Uninfected frozen cells and fresh living infected and uninfected cells were used as controls and for comparisons. For some specimens, comparisons were also made with titers obtained using a fixed-cell slide method (8) and by hemagglutination inhibition.

Results are summarized in Table 2. Overall sensitivity (ratio of frozen cell positives to total positives by standard methods) and specificity (ratio of frozen cell negatives to total negatives by standard methods) in comparison with the other tests were excellent. Nonspecific fluorescence was less with frozen than with live infected tissue culture cells. There was never greater than a twofold difference in end points of positive titers for any virus tested. Stability of the frozen cells' surface antigens was tested by titrating several sera (VZV-IgG; influenza A-IgM) and breast milk samples (RSV-IgA) with targets of various ages. Titers remained constant over extended periods of time; VZV-infected cells were usable for at least 6 months, those infected with RSV were usable for more than 3 months, and those infected with influenza A were usable for at least 1 month.

In summary, the results of these studies with glycerol cryopreservation of a variety of cells infected with several common viruses applied to an assortment of antibody-containing fluids were equivalent to those obtained with the currently used fresh cell methods. Cryopreservation makes the FAMA test safe, easy to perform, and inexpensive, permitting its possible use in routine serology laboratories.

TABLE 1. *Infection of cells for cryopreservation*

Virus	Strain/type/subtype	Input (TCID$_{50}$ × 10^{-6})	Target[a]	Time to harvest (h)
VZV	Ellen	0.5	HEL	96
RSV	Long	1.0	HEp-2	24
Parainfluenza	1	1.5	HEp-2	48
	2	0.1	HEp-2	48
	3	1.0	HEp-2	24
Influenza	A/Texas/1/77	320	2°MK	72
	A/USSR/90/77	320	2°MK	48

[a] HEL, Human embryonic lung; 2°MK, secondary rhesus monkey kidney.

TABLE 2. *Comparison of frozen cell FAMA with other tests*

Virus	Strain/type/sub-type	Specimen	No.	Antibody class	Comparison test(s)[a]	Sensitiv-ity[b]	Specific-ity[c]
VZV	Ellen	Serum	80	IgG	LFAMA	100	100
RSV	Long	Serum	25	IgA	LFAMA	96	100
		Nasal wash	25	IgA	LFAMA	92	96
		Breast milk	200	IgA, IgG, IgM	LFAMA	100	100
Parainfluenza	1	Nasal wash	9	IgA	LFAMA; SFA	89	100
	2	Nasal wash	10	IgA	LFAMA; SFA	90	100
	3	Serum	10	IgA, IgG, IgM	LFAMA; SFA	100	100
Influenza	A/Texas/1/77	Serum	10	IgM, IgG	LFAMA; HI	90	100
	A/USSR/90/77	Serum	15	IgM, IgG	LFAMA; HI	94	94
		Nasal wash	5	IgA, IgG, IgM	LFAMA	100	100

[a] LFAMA, Fluorescent antibody-to-membrane antigen assay, using fresh, live cells; SFA, fixed-cell slide fluorescent-antibody assay; HI, hemagglutination inhibition.
[b] Sensitivity = ratio of positives using frozen cells to total true positives by comparison tests.
[c] Specificity = ratio of negatives using frozen cells to total true negatives by comparison tests.

1. **Blough, H. A., and J. M. Tiffany.** 1975. Theoretical aspects of structure and assembly of virus envelopes. Curr. Top. Microbiol. Immunol. **70**:1–30.

2. **Fishaut, M., K. McIntosh, and G. Meiklejohn.** 1979. Rapid subtyping of influenza A isolates by membrane fluorescence. J. Clin. Microbiol. **9**:269–272.

3. **Ford, C. H. J., C. E. Newman, and A. B. Carter.** 1979. The effect of cryopreservation of lymphocytes on E rosetting ability: a study in lung cancer patients and controls. J. Immunol. Methods **26**: 113–124.

4. **Meryman, H. T., and M. Hornblower.** 1972. A method of freezing and washing red blood cells using a high glycerol concentration. Transfusion **12**:145–156.

5. **Scott, R., M. D. Landazuri, P. S. Gardner, and J. H. T. Owen.** 1976. Detection of antibody to respiratory syncytial virus by membrane fluorescence. Clin. Exp. Immunol. **26**:78–85.

6. **Wesslen, L.** 1978. Hemolysis-in-gel (HIG) test for antibodies to influenza A, measles, and mumps using liquid nitrogen freezed erythrocytes coupled with the respective viral antigen. J. Immunol. Methods **24**:1–8.

7. **Williams, V., A. Gershon, and P. Brunell.** 1974. Serologic response to varicella-zoster membrane antigens measured by indirect immunofluorescence. J. Infect. Dis. **130**:669–672.

8. **Yanagihara, R., I. Orr, and K. McIntosh.** 1979. Secretory antibody response in infants and children to parainfluenza virus types 1 and 2. Pediatr. Res. **13**:471.

9. **Zaia, J. A., and M. N. Oxman.** 1977. Antibody to varicella-zoster virus-induced membrane antigen: immunofluorescence assay using monodisperse glutaraldehyde-fixed target cells. J. Infect. Dis. **136**:519–530.

Detection of Herpes Simplex Virus Type 1-Infected Cells by Bacterial Adherence

JOHN F. MODLIN[1]* AND ALICE S. HUANG

Childrens Hospital Medical Center and Harvard Medical School, Boston, Massachusetts 02115, U.S.A.

Many strains of *Staphylococcus aureus* possess a cell wall protein, protein A, which avidly binds to the Fc portion of immunoglobulin G of most mammals (1, 4). Protein A has been widely used as a tool in immunology research but has only recently come to the attention of the clinical virologist. Recently, Huang and Okorie showed that vesicular stomatitis virus-infected cells could be detected by the surface analysis by bacterial adherence (SABA) technique (2). They also have shown that the SABA technique detects virus-specific cell membrane antigens, but not viral antigens within the cell (3). In this paper we describe a simple modification of the SABA technique.

HSV-1-infected and uninfected control 350-Q (human fetal foreskin fibroblast) cells were gently dispersed with trypsin and EDTA, fixed in glutaraldehyde, and allowed to dry on a glass slide. Duplicate infected and control cells were each incubated with rabbit anti-herpes simplex virus type 1 (HSV-1) serum and normal rabbit serum, each diluted 1:20. A suspension of *S. aureus* was added, and the cells were Gram stained and examined by light microscopy.

Bacteria-adhering cells (SABA positive) were easily distinguished from cells which failed to bind bacteria (SABA negative) (Fig. 1). Uninfected cells incubated with HSV-1 antiserum and control serum and HSV-1-infected cells incubated with specific antiserum were SABA pos-

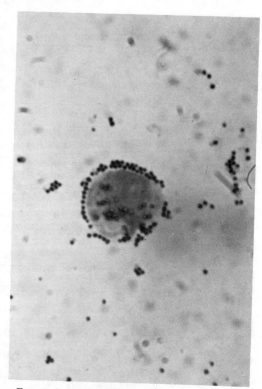

FIG. 1. *S. aureus bound by SABA to 350-Q cell infected with HSV-1 for 24 h.*

itive. Both the number of bacteria per positive cell and the proportion of infected cells that were SABA positive increased with duration of

[1] Present address: Virus Laboratory, Beth Israel Hospital, Boston, MA 02115.

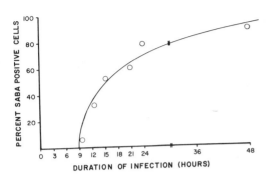

FIG. 2. *Percentage of SABA-positive cells as a function of time after infection of 350-Q cell monolayer by HSV-1 at multiplicity of infection of 5:1.*

cell infection (Fig. 2). HSV-2-infected cells were SABA positive when HSV-1 antiserum was used as the ligand, but cells infected with varicella-zoster virus and cytomegalovirus were SABA negative.

This modification of the SABA technique is simple and can be performed easily in less than 4 h. It is an early and specific indicator of HSV-1 infection of tissue culture cells. The technique is potentially applicable to rapid identification of cell infection by any virus which produces cell membrane viral antigen.

1. **Goding, J. E.** 1978. Use of staphylococcal protein A as an immunological reagent. J. Immunol. Methods **20**:241–253.
2. **Huang, A. S., and T. Okorie.** 1978. Rapid diagnosis using surface analysis by bacterial adherence. Lancet **ii**:1146.
3. **Huang, A. S., and T. Okorie.** 1979. Surface analysis by bacterial adherence to virus infected cells. J. Infect. Dis. **140**:147–151.
4. **Kronvall, G., U. S. Seal, J. Finstad, and D. C. Williams.** 1970. Phylogenetic insight into evolution of mammalian Fc fragment of G globulin using Staphylococcal protein A. J. Immunol. **104**:140–147.

Effect of Calcium Alginate Wool and Other Swab Materials upon the Isolation of Herpes Simplex Virus Type 2 from Genital Ulcers

LAWRENCE R. CRANE,* PAUL A. GUTTERMAN, THOMAS CHAPEL, AND A. MARTIN LERNER

Departments of Medicine and Dermatology, Wayne State University School of Medicine, Detroit, Michigan 48201, U.S.A.

Genital herpes is the most common cause of penile or vulvar ulcerations which are seen in sexually transmissible disease clinics in the United States. The best method for diagnosis is to swab the base of an ulcer and insert the swab with agitation into a sterile screw-capped vial containing a transport medium and antibiotics. Most clinics must send these specimens to another virus laboratory for processing. In transit, titers of herpes simplex virus type 2 (HSV-2) may decrease markedly, and to alleviate this, Earle-lactalbumin hydrolysate-yeast extract, Leibovitz-Emory (agarose-charcoal), Amies, or Stuart transport medium and rabbit kidney (RK-13) or Vero renal tissue cultures are recommended (2, 4, 6). No one has questioned the effect of swab materials upon the isolation of HSV-2. We were stimulated to do this by the report that an animal herpesvirus, infectious bovine rhinotracheitis virus, is inactivated by calcium alginate wool in Eagle medium (1).

When cotton, rayon, Dacron, or polyester swab material was shredded and incubated at 4°C in Eagle medium with HSV-2, infectious virus persisted comparably over 72 h. A similar infectious virus decay occurred in control Eagle medium without swab material. In contrast, $10^{3.5}$ PFU of HSV-2 in 0.1 ml was completely noninfectious after a 48 h of incubation in shredded calcium alginate wool (Fig. 1). Likewise, specimens from fresh genital ulcers harboring HSV-2 yielded virus in Vero renal cell cultures significantly less frequently when calcium alginate rather than Dacron swabs were used. This reduced virus isolation rate for calcium alginate swabs was the case whether the transport medium for the swabs was Eagle medium or agarose-charcoal medium (Table 1). Calcium alginate swabs should not be used to determine either the natural history or the effects of antiviral therapy in genital herpes (5). Whether this admonition applies to other human and animal herpesviruses in addition to infectious bovine rhinotracheitis requires study.

A series of experiments was done to examine the interactions of calcium alginate, HSV-2, and Vero renal tissue cultures. Calcium alginate appeared to bind firmly to the HSV-2 virion, and the union was noninfectious. Shaking in 10% fetal calf serum or sonication did not separate virus from alginate. The calcium alginate polysaccharide did not, however, bind to Vero renal

TABLE 1. *Recovery of HSV-2 from duplicate calcium alginate and Dacron swabs in Eagle or agarose-charcoal medium*

Time in transport before inoculation to Vero renal tissue cultures (h)	No. of virus-positive cultures[a] in:			
	Eagle medium		Agarose-charcoal medium	
	Dacron swab	Calcium alginate Swab	Dacron swab	Calcium alginate swab
None	10/10	9/10	Not done	Not done
24	10/10	8/10	10/10	9/10
48	9/10	4/10[b]	10/10	4/10[b]
72	8/10	0/10[b]	9/10	2/10[b]

[a] Forty patients with genital ulcers presenting to the Wayne State University Infectious Diseases Clinic or the Detroit Social Hygiene Clinic (Detroit, Mich.) paticipated in this study.

[b] Difference is significant ($P > 0.05$) by chi-square test with Yates' correction.

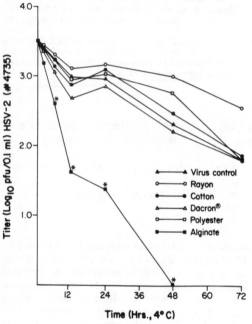

FIG. 1. *Incubation of swab materials with HSV-2 (strain 4735), 4°C. Swab materials (rayon, cotton, Dacron, polyester, and calcium alginate) were shredded with fine scissors, and 0.1 g of each was mixed in 4 ml of Eagle medium. Then 0.1 ml of HSV-2 (4735) containing 8.4 × 10^4.5 to 1.97 × 10^6 PFU/ml was added to each suspension (4°C). Suspensions were agitated with a magnetic stirrer, and at several times 0.3-ml samples were taken and centrifuged (1,000 × g, 15 min, 4°C) and residual virus was quantitated in Vero renal tissue culture microtiter plates. Each point is the mean of eight experiments. Significant differ-*

tissue cultures. Preincubation of Vero renal cells with calcium alginate inhibited absorption of HSV-2, but the effect was easily reversible by washing.

Alginic acid is a hydrophilic colloidal carbohydrate extracted from various species of brown seaweed. The structure of the polymer is related to cellulose and is composed of L-guluronic and D-manuronic residues (S. W. Metz, Inolex Corp., Glenwood, Ill.; personal communication). Rayon, Dacron, and polyester are esters prepared from cotton by reactions utilizing the hydroxyl groups of cellulose. Free hydroxyl groups of alginic acid may react with the HSV-2 capsid, inactivating the virus (3).

1. **Hanson, B. R., and I. A. Schipper.** 1976. Effects of swab materials on infectious bovine rhinotracheitis virus. Am. J. Vet. Res. **37**:707–708.

2. **Nahmias, A., C. Wickliffe, J. Pipkin, A. Leibovitz, and R. Hutton.** 1971. Transport media for herpes simplex virus types 1 and 2. Appl. Microbiol. **22**:451–454.

3. **Pigman, W.** 1957. The carbohydrates; chemistry, biochemistry, physiology. Academic Press Inc., New York.

4. **Rodin, P., M. J. Hare, C. F. Barwell, and M. J. Withers.** 1971. Transport of herpes simplex virus in Stuart's medium. Br. J. Vener. Dis. **47**:198–199.

5. **Spruance, S. L., J. C. Overall, E. R. Kern, G. G. Krueger, V. Pliam, and W. Miller.** 1977. The natural history of recurrent herpes simplex labialis. Implications for antiviral therapy. N. Engl. J. Med. **297**:69–75.

6. **Taka, A., N. Sekine, M. Toba, and K. Yoshino.** 1977. An analysis of factors influencing the isolation rate of herpes simplex virus. Microbiol. Immunol. **21**:219–229.

ences (*, P < 0.01, Wilcoxan signed-ranks test) from all other points occurred only with calcium alginate after incubations of 6 to 48 h.

Teichoic Acid Antibody Levels in Two High-Risk Populations for Invasive *Staphylococcus aureus* Infections

LEON SMITH, JR., JOHN BOGDEN, BARRY WIENER, CAROL PALMIERI, LEON SMITH, SR., ANTHONY MINNEFOR, AND JAMES OLESKE*

St. Michael's Medical Center, College of Medicine and Dentistry of New Jersey, Newark, New Jersey 07102, and Jersey City Medical Center, Jersey City, New Jersey 07304, U.S.A.*

Staphylococcus aureus (SA) is a common pathogen in both noninvasive and life-threatening infections. It is at times difficult to determine when blood cultures signify transient bacteremia in superficial infection or significant deep-tissue infection. White and Crouder (5) demonstrated that normal individuals have low levels of teichoic acid antibody (TAA) undetectable by gel diffusion techniques. In response to deep-tissue SA infection, in particular, endocarditis, a secondary immunoglobulin G response with TAA titers greater than 1:2 dilution in a gel diffusion assay are often seen.

The major antigenic determinant of TAA has been shown to be *N*-acetylglucosamine in a β-glycoside linkage as side chains connected by phosphate diester to ribitol. Polymers of this make up teichoic acid, the major cell wall component of SA (2).

The measurement of TAA has been useful in the rapid diagnosis of patients with SA endocarditis as well as in follow-up studies to measure therapeutic effectiveness (4). This investigation was undertaken to study the sensitivity and specificity of this assay when applied to two populations at high risk of developing deep-tissue infections with SA. Ninety-one parenteral drug addicts (DA) and 38 patients on chronic hemodialysis (HD) simultaneously had blood taken for TAA while they were free of clinically apparent SA infection. Nasopharyngeal cultures for SA were taken as well as plasma for zinc levels. In addition, seven DA and eight HD patients had TAA levels performed during the initial phase of deep-tissue SA infection.

As a control, data from 109 non-DA, non-HD patients who had TAA performed were used for comparison. Of this group, 6 had SA endocarditis, 12 had SA osteomyelitis, 34 had other SA infections including abscess, cellulitis, and pneumonia, and 41 had no evidence of SA infection (Table 1).

TAA levels were performed in 1% agarose gel by standard Ouchterlony techniques. The Wood strain of *Staphylococcus* supplied by Arthur White (5) was used to prepare the teichoic acid antigen. Commercial gamma globulin was used as a positive antibody control. In our laboratory the TAA assays are initially determined with undiluted sera and, when positive, repeated in twofold dilutions. In our control group, when a specimen was positive at a $\geq$1:2 dilution, this was associated with deep-tissue SA infection, in particular, endocarditis and less often with osteomyelitis. Control patients with positive TAA in only undiluted sera usually had more superficial SA infections or pneumonia. A negative TAA level almost always suggested the absence of SA infection in our control group. Plasma zinc was determined by atomic absorption spectrophotometry (N = 65 − 125 mg/ml). Nasopharyngeal cultures for SA were done by routine bacteriological techniques.

The data showing the correlation of SA nasal carrier rate (SNCR) with TAA levels in DA and HD patients is shown in Table 2. Among the 91 DAs, there was a direct correlation between SNCR and TAA levels. TAA levels of $\geq$1:2 dilutions, undiluted, or negative were associated with SNCRs of 40, 10, and 3%, respectively. Over 10% of these DAs had $\geq$1:2 dilution TAA levels and thus represented false positives. There was a 9% SNCR in this DA population. HD patients, on the other hand, had an SNCR of 16%, but there was no correlation of SNCR and TAA levels. All seven DA patients had TAA levels of $\geq$1:2 when they developed deep-tissue SA infections. In the nine HD patients who had TAA levels done during SA endocarditis and osteomyelitis, 50% had false-negative TAA responses. In our non-DA, non-HD control population, there were no false-negative TAA responses in the 14 patients with endocarditis, although 6 had only undiluted TAA. The sensitivity of TAA was 60% for SA osteomyelitis in this control population, when undiluted titers of TAA were considered as a positive test. Of the 33 patients in the control group with SA abscess, cellulitis, or pneumonia, only 6 (18%) developed TAA, and then only in undiluted serum titers.

The zinc levels in 91 DAs were normal compared with controls. The 35 HD patients, however, showed abnormally high levels of plasma zinc which increased after dialysis. These data have been reported elsewhere (1). Zinc is an essential trace metal which has been shown to

TABLE 1. *TAA levels correlated with diagnosis in control (C), DA, and HD populations*

TAA levels	SA endocarditis			SA osteomylitis			Other SA infections[a]			No SA infections		
	C	DA	HD	C	DA	HD	C	DA	HD	C	DA	HD
Positive (1:2 dilution)	10	4	1	2	2	1	0	0	0	0	10	0
Positive (undiluted)	6	1	1	6	0	1	6	0	0	2[b]	20	0
Negative	0	0	2	4	0	2	27[c]	0	9	39	61	34[d]

[a] Diagnosis: Abscess/cellulitis/pneumonia with *S. aureus*.

[b] Diagnosis: One case with γ-hemolytic streptococcal endocarditis; one case with SA epidermitis or osteomylitis.

[c] Includes 14 patients with recent influenza A infection associated with pneumonia, 4 with SA bacteremia and with pure cultures of SA in sputum.

[d] No cases of any form of endocarditis or osteomylitis.

TABLE 2. *Correlation of TAA levels with S. aureus nasopharyngeal carrier (NPC) state of DA and HD patients*

TAA levels	No. of patients		TAA (%)		No. with NPC (*S. aureus*)		NPC/TAA (%)	
	DA	HD	DA	HD	DA	HD	DA	HD
Positive (1:2 dilution)	10	0	11	0	4	0	40	0
Positive (undiluted)	20	4	22	10	2	2	10	33
Negative	61	34	67	90	2	4	3.3	66

have direct effects on primary immune functions (3). It is possible that part of the known immunodeficiency of uremic patients on HD may be related to this disturbance in zinc hemostasis and that this may also partially explain their inability to form TAA in response to deep-tissue SA infections.

This study demonstrates that TAA studies in these two high-risk populations for deep-tissue SA infection must be interpreted cautiously since in DA there is at least a 10% false-positive rate (at TAA dilution ≥1:2), whereas 50% of HD patients may have false-negative tests.

1. Bogden, J. D., J. M. Oleske, B. Weiner, and L. G. Smith. 1979. Elevated plasma zinc concentrations in renal dialysis patients. Abstr. 63rd Annu. FASEB, Dallas, Tex.

2. Martin, R. R., H. Daughorthy, and A. White. 1966. Staphylococcal antibodies and hypersensitivity to teichoic acids in man, p. 91–96. Antimicrob. Agents Chemother. 1965.

3. Oleske, J. M., M. L. Westphal, S. Shore, D. Gorden, J. D. Bogden, and A. Nahmias. 1979. Correction with zinc therapy of depressed cellular immunity in Aerodermatitis enteropathica. **133**:195–918.

4. Tuazon, C. U., and J. N. Shagren. 1976. Teichoic acid antibodies in the diagnosis of serious infections with *Staphylococcus aureus*. Ann. Intern. Med. **84**:543–546.

5. White, A., and J. G. Crouder. 1972. Teichoic acid antibody in staphylococcal endocarditis. Ann. Intern. Med. **77**:87–90.

Direct Gas-Liquid Chromatography of Clinical Material as an Aid in the Diagnosis of Anaerobic Lung Infections

JOHN GRAY,* WARREN H. PERKS, AND JANET BIRCH

Public Health Laboratory and North Staffordshire Medical Centre, Stoke-on-Trent, England

Anaerobic bacteria have been implicated in many types of lung infection, especially when associated with putrid sputum and necrosis of lung parenchyma (3). However, not all patients with anaerobic pneumonitis show these characteristic features (2), and the clinical presentation may be similar to that of pneumococcal pneumonia. The diagnosis is especially difficult in this group of patients because invasive techniques are needed to obtain valid specimens for culture. Expectorated sputum is coated with saliva containing indigenous anaerobic organisms and does not represent the true flora of the infected lung. Transtracheal aspiration (TTA) is a way of obtaining uncontaminated specimens for anaerobic culture (4). Those who use the technique regularly find that complications are rare. However, many physicians are reluctant to use the technique. Some advocate lung aspiration, but this too can cause complications. We hoped to find an alternative noninvasive technique.

Gas-liquid chromatography (GLC) of clinical specimens, especially pus, is an established technique for the diagnosis of anaerobic infections (5). The short-chain fatty acids produced by anaerobic organisms serve as markers of infection. GLC of sputum has been used in two patients with anaerobic lung infections (1). In these patients the volatile fatty acids (VFA) produced corresponded to those produced by cultures of the infecting organisms.

We used GLC to examine sputum samples from patients with varied lung infections. We considered the following questions: (i) Do patients with anaerobic lung infections have VFA in the sputum? (ii) Is the VFA pattern the same as in the infected tissue? (iii) Is GLC of sputum a valid technique or does the saliva contain VFA from its anaerobic flora which would invalidate it? (iv) Would GLC of sputum enable selection of those patients for whom a TTA would be appropriate or would it remove the necessity for TTA?

Five patients with anaerobic lung infections were examined. Specimens of sputum and lung or pleural aspirates were transported rapidly to the laboratory and plated on routine media for aerobic and anaerobic culture. These specimens were prepared for GLC by acidified ether extraction and examined on a Pye-Unicam GCD with flame ionization detectors and an internal standard of 10 mmol of caproic acid per liter.

Patient A was a 69-year-old male who pre-

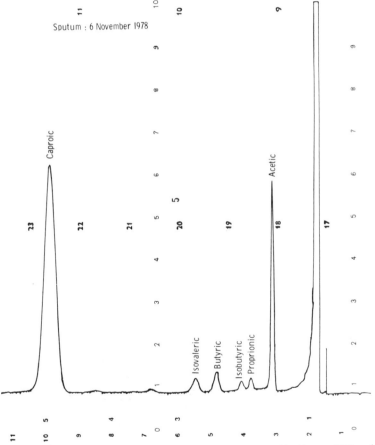

FIG. 1. *Patient A. Chromatographic pattern of sputum. Caproic acid, 10 mmol/liter, is the internal standard.*

sented with severe pneumonia and multiple lung abscesses. The sputum contained VFA including isobutyric, butyric, and isovaleric acids (Fig. 1). Pus aspirated from one of the lung abscesses also contained these fatty acids (Fig. 2). Both samples yielded a mixed growth including *Citrobacter koseri*, *Bacteroides fragilis*, *B. melaninogenicus*, and anaerobic cocci.

Patient B was a 25-year-old male who had been treated for aspiration pneumonia. Multiple sputum samples yielded VFA including isobutyric, butyric, and isovaleric acids. Cultures grew *B. fragilis* and *B. melaninogenicus*. While awaiting pneumonectomy and despite treatment with penicillin and metronidazole, the patient developed a brain abscess. *B. fragilis*, *Streptococcus salivarius*, and *S. dysgalactiae* were isolated from the brain abscess, and *B. fragilis*, *B. melaninogenicus*, and microaerophilic streptococci were isolated from the lung tissue.

In both these patients the VFA in the sputum gave a good indication of the infecting organisms.

Patient C was an 11-year-old girl who developed a solitary lung abscess after polyneuritis associated with infectious mononucleosis. TTA yielded no growth and no VFA. The abscess was aspirated and contained large amounts of butyric and isovaleric acids and a smaller amount of isobutyric acid. *Fusobacterium nucleatum* and microaerophilic streptococci grew from the pus. TTA was unhelpful because the abscess did not communicate with the bronchus.

Patient D was a 57-year-old man with an empyema and carcinoma of the bronchus. The empyema fluid contained VFA, mainly butyric acid, and grew *B. fragilis* and anaerobic cocci. Sputum did not yield VFA because the bronchus was occluded by carcinoma and the infected material was not expectorated. TTA is unlikely to have been helpful in this patient. After drainage and treatment with benzyl penicillin and metronidazole, the fluid became sterile and VFA could not be detected.

Patient E was a 66-year-old female with an empyema for which no underlying cause was

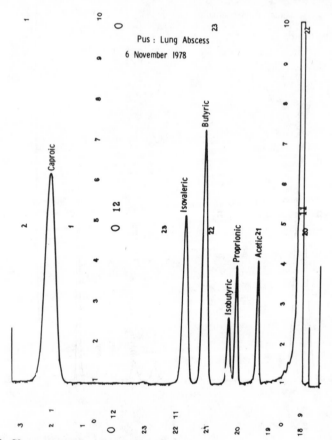

FIG. 2. *Patient A. Chromatographic pattern of pus aspirated from lung abscess. Caproic acid, 10 mmol/ liter, is the internal standard.*

found. Aspirated pus yielded VFA, mainly iso-butyric, butyric, and isovaleric acids, and *B. fragilis*, *B. melaninogenicus*, and microaero-philic streptococci were grown. VFA were not found in the sputum. The patient died of a pulmonary embolus. At postmortem the lung tissue was found to be unaffected. Again, TTA is unlikely to have been helpful.

Ten patients had TTA, sputum, and saliva cultured. GLC was performed on the sputum. GLC was also performed on the five patients whose TTA and salivary specimens were of sufficient volume. None of these patients had anaerobic infections and none had VFA in the sputum or saliva. Fifty patients with chronic bronchitis were examined. None had VFA in the sputum and none had evidence of anaerobic lung infection. This suggests that sputum does not normally contain VFA and that saliva does not contaminate expectorated sputum with VFA.

The number of patients studied is small but we feel that the presence of VFA in sputum is a good indication of anaerobic infection. The investigation is rapid, results being available in 30 min. The results can be helpful as a guide to the choice of initial antibiotic therapy. If desired, TTA can be undertaken but in some cases, especially empyema, aspiration and GLC analysis of the pus is of more value.

1. **Abeysundere, R. L., M. E. Hodson, M. Szawatkowski, and P. Noone.** 1978. Pleuropulmonary lung infection by anaerobic bacteria. Br. J. Dis. Chest **72**:187–195.
2. **Bartlett, J. G.** 1979. Anaerobic bacterial pneumonitis. Am. Rev. Respir. Dis. **119**:19–23.
3. **Bartlett, J. G., and S. M. Finegold.** 1972. Anaerobic pleuropulmonary infections. Medicine (Baltimore) **51**: 413–450.
4. **Bartlett, J. G., J. E. Rosenblatt, and S. M. Finegold.** 1973. Percutaneous transtracheal aspiration in the diagnosis of anaerobic pulmonary infection. Ann. Intern. Med. **79**:535–540.
5. **Gorbach, S. L., J. W. Mayhew, J. G. Bartlett, H. Thadepalli, and A. B. Onderdonk.** 1976. Rapid diagnosis of anaerobic infections by direct gas liquid chromatography of clinical specimens. J. Clin. Invest. **57**: 478–484.

Microtiter Enzyme-Linked Immunosorbent Assay for Measurement of Cholera Antitoxin in Humans

CHARLES R. YOUNG, ROY ROBINS-BROWNE,* MYRON M. LEVINE, MARGARET B. RENNELS, AND JOHN P. CRAIG

The Center for Vaccine Development, Division of Infectious Diseases, University of Maryland School of Medicine, Baltimore, Maryland 21201, and the Department of Microbiology and Immunology, Downstate Medical Center, State University of New York, New York, New York 11203 U.S.A.*

A serological diagnosis of infection with *Vibrio cholerae* can be made by assaying antibodies against the somatic O antigens or the heat-labile enterotoxin. Current techniques for estimating cholera antitoxin measure antibodies which either bind the toxin or neutralize its biological activity. Toxin-neutralizing antibodies can be demonstrated by the rabbit skin permeability factor (PF), Y-1 adrenal cell (AC), and rabbit ileal loop tests, and toxin-binding antibodies can be shown by using passive hemagglutination or radioimmunoassay.

Each method suffers from one or more of the following disadvantages: is not readily adaptable to large numbers of specimens, is expensive, requires tissue culture or radioisotope counting facilities, does not measure specific immunoglobulin class, requires relatively large volumes of serum. Microtiter enzyme-linked immunosorbent assay (ELISA), currently used for measuring antibodies to a wide range of antigens, provides a method that could overcome all these disadvantages.

We have recently developed a microtiter ELISA for cholera antitoxin which makes use of commercially available reagents, requires as little as 5 μl of serum, permits estimation of antibody titer in serum at a single dilution (1:200) and, if desired, can be read without using a colorimeter.

The sensitivity and specificity of the assay and its correlation with established techniques have been determined. For these investigations, sera were obtained from informed community volunteers admitted to the 22-bed isolation ward of the Center for Vaccine Development during studies to evaluate cholera vaccines and to investigate the mechanisms of cholera immunity. Sera from 92 volunteers were collected before and 10, 21, and 28 days after the volunteers ingested 10^3 to 10^6 *V. cholerae* of Ogawa or Inaba serotype and classical or El Tor biotype. Pre-

and postchallenge sera were also obtained from a negative control population comprising 30 volunteers who ingested nontoxigenic *Escherichia coli* or *E. coli* that produced heat-stable (ST) but not heat-labile enterotoxin.

Sera were examined for cholera toxin-neutralizing antibodies by the PF and AC techniques and for immunoglobulin G (IgG)-binding antibodies by ELISA as previously described (C. R. Young, M. M. Levine, J. P. Craig, and R. Robins-Browne, Infect. Immun., in press). Induced cholera infections were classified clinically and bacteriologically as follows: class 0 denoted no diarrhea with repeated negative stool and rectal swab cultures; class 1 signified no diarrhea but at least one stool or rectal swab yielding *V. cholerae*; class 2 indicated the development of diarrhea with a positive stool culture; and class 3 signified diarrhea in excess of 5 liters.

In 162 serum samples from 49 volunteers who ingested classical *V. cholerae*, levels of cholera antitoxin measured by ELISA and expressed as net optical density (OD) correlated closely with toxin-neutralizing antibodies determined by PF assay ($r = 0.86$, $P < 0.001$) (Fig. 1). Correlation

between ELISA values and antitoxin units was also demonstrated with 165 sera from 43 volunteers before and after ingestion of *V. cholerae* El Tor ($r = 0.83$, $P < 0.001$). At net OD values greater than 0.9, however, this relationship was no longer demonstrable ($r = 0.24$, $P > 0.1$). Reexamination of the high-titer sera (net OD > 0.9) diluted 1:800, however, showed that linearity to the relationship between OD and PF antitoxin units was restored ($r = 0.64$, $P < 0.001$).

From these data, it was apparent that although IgG ELISA for cholera antitoxin does not measure neutralizing antibodies directly, it provides a valuable in vitro correlate of in vivo toxin-neutralizing capacity.

In the AC and PF assays, the demonstration of a significant rise in antitoxin titer in pre- and postchallenge sera corresponded with the class of illness. Of 54 volunteers who developed overt illness (class 2 or 3) after ingesting *V. cholerae*, 46 (85%) showed a rise in antitoxin titer by the AC technique (fourfold or greater), and 42 (77%) showed a rise by the PF method (twofold or greater comprising a net rise of at least 2 antitoxin units/ml). Of 12 individuals with subclini-

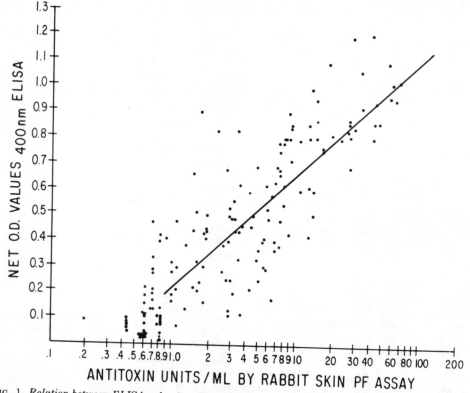

Fig. 1. *Relation between ELISA value (net OD) and antitoxin units measured by the PF assay in 162 sera from 49 volunteers before and after ingestion of V. cholerae. The regression equation is $Y = 0.44 \log_{10} X + 0.23$, $r = 0.86$.*

TABLE 1. *Correlation between severity of induced cholera and serological response to infection measured by the AC and PF techniques and by ELISA*

Class of illness	No. of volunteers	No. (%) showing significant rise in antitoxin titer[a] by:		
		AC	PF	ELISA
0	26	4 (15)	4 (15)	3 (12)
1	12	6 (50)	5 (42)	8 (67)
2	44	38 (86)	33 (75)	40 (91)
3	10	8 (80)	9 (90)	10 (100)
Total	92	56 (61)	51 (55)	61 (66)

[a] See text for definitions.

cal (class 1) infection, six and five, respectively, were positive by these assays. In contrast, only 4 of 26 (15%) individuals who ingested *V. cholerae* and who failed to develop clinical or subclinical cholera (class 0) exhibited a rise by either assay. Overall, results of the AC and PF assays concurred in 79 of 92 sets of sera, whereas in 9 only the AC assay and in 4 only the PF assay showed a rise. Both assays were negative in all 30 volunteers who ingested *E. coli* and who comprised the negative control population.

Matched sera from 47 individuals in whom antitoxin rises were detected by both AC and PF assays were designated a positive reference sample for comparison with ELISA. All 47 paired sera also showed rises by ELISA, with values (net OD) from 0.26 to 1.15 (mean ± SD = 0.72 ± 0.22) higher in postchallenge than in prechallenge specimens. In contrast, paired sera from the 30 persons who ingested *E. coli*, all of which were negative in both the AC and PF assays, showed a rise of between −0.09 and 0.12 (mean ± SD = 0.03 ± 0.06). Based on these observations, a rise in net OD of 0.20 or greater between matched pre- and postchallenge sera was taken to denote a significant rise in antitoxin titer. This value, which exceeded the mean of the negative control population by 3 SD, was approximately midway between the lowest rise in net OD in the positive control population

(0.26) and the highest in the negative control population (0.12).

By this criterion, 61 of 92 (66%) volunteers who ingested *V. cholerae*, including 50 of 54 (93%) who developed overt clinical illness, showed a rise in circulating antitoxin titer by ELISA. Rises in IgG-binding antibody titers measured by ELISA corresponded closely with rises in neutralizing antibody titers. For all classes of illness except class 0, however, ELISA demonstrated significant rises in antitoxin more frequently than either neutralization assay (Table 1). The superiority of ELISA in detecting antibody rises was consistent in sera from all volunteers regardless of their history of prior exposure to cholera toxin or toxoids or of the challenge strain biotype. Increased sensitivity of ELISA was achieved without any loss of specificity. Thus ELISA was positive no more frequently than either neutralization assay in people with class 0 cholera (no diarrhea, negative cultures) or in volunteers who ingested nontoxigenic or ST-producing *E. coli*.

Assays that measure binding or neutralizing antibodies to cholera toxin also detect antibodies to *E. coli* LT, which is immunologically related to cholera toxin. It would be anticipated, therefore, that persons infected with LT-producing *E. coli* might demonstrate antitoxin rises by ELISA.

In summary, microtiter ELISA provides a practicable method for screening single serum samples for the presence of cholera antitoxin and for demonstrating antitoxin rises in paired sera. The technique is relatively easy to perform, requires only minute quantities of serum, and is readily adapted to use in field studies. Its ability to deal with large numbers of specimens, moreover, makes it particularly well suited to seroepidemiological surveys.

This work was supported by research contracts N01 AI42553 with the National Institute of Allergy and Infectious Diseases and DAMD 17-78-C-8011 with the U.S. Army Research and Development Command and by a grant from the World Health Organization. R.R.-B. is an Overseas Traveling Fellow of the South African Medical Research Council.

Radioimmunoassay for Detection of Antigenemia in Granulocytopenic Rabbits with *Pseudomonas aeruginosa* Sepsis

RICHARD KOHLER,* L. JOSEPH WHEAT, AND ARTHUR WHITE

Indiana University Medical Center, Indianapolis, Indiana 46202, U.S.A.

Pseudomonas aeruginosa infections appear to require early institution of specific antibiotic combinations for maximal cure rates. Such antibiotic combinations are not optimal for certain other common pathogens. Additionally, some *P. aeruginosa* infections are difficult to diagnose with confidence, especially *P. aeruginosa* nosocomial pneumonias. For these reasons we believe that a rapid, sensitive assay which detects circulating *P. aeruginosa* antigens would be a useful adjunct in the management of *P. aeruginosa* infections. As a preliminary step in the development of such an assay, we studied the ability of a solid-phase radioimmunoassay to detect circulating *P. aeruginosa* antigens in granulocytopenic rabbits with *P. aeruginosa* septicemia.

The radioimmunoassay used in these experiments has been previously described (1). In brief, in vitro antigen-solvent mixtures or test sera were incubated in antibody-coated tubes and then aspirated. Antigens adherent to the tubes were then detected with radioiodinated antibodies. Antibodies were obtained as the immunoglobulin G fraction of serum from rabbits immunized with whole serotype 6 *P. aeruginosa* organisms. Rabbits were made granulocytopenic with nitrogen mustard, and *P. aeruginosa* sepsis was induced by providing the rabbits with drinking water and daily eye drops containing serotype 6 *P. aeruginosa* (3). Blood samples from most rabbits were cultured quantitatively. Control samples consisted of serum from normal rabbits. Culture-negative specimens from granulocytopenic rabbits were used as an additional control.

When serotype 6 *P. aeruginosa* lipopolysaccharide was added to normal human serum, the antigen detection sensitivity was 10 μg/ml; in buffered saline, the sensitivity was 0.05 μg/ml. Thus, serum components diminished the assay's sensitivity 200-fold. Attempts were therefore made to diminish these inhibitory effects of serum. Deproteinization of serum or plasma with chloroform (2), addition of heparin to a final concentration of 1,000 U/ml, or heating at 56°C for 30 min all partially diminished the inhibitory effects of serum (Fig. 1). With no treatment, antigen was detected in serum at 10 μg/ml. Treatment with chloroform or heparin improved the sensitivity to 1.25 μg/ml; heating improved the sensitivity to 0.625 μg/ml.

Residual chloroform in the deproteinized serum or plasma sometimes caused partial dissolution of the polystyrene assay tubes, resulting in nonspecific binding of the iodinated antibodies to the tubes. With heparin treatment, sensitivity enhancement was noted at a final heparin concentration of 10 U/ml but not a 1 U/ml. Marked additional enhancement occurred at 100 U/ml, and some further enhancement occurred at 1,000 U/ml. Above 1,000 U/ml, sensitivity

declined due to dilutional effects. Attempts to prolong heating at 56°C for longer periods or to heat at higher temperatures resulted in coagu-

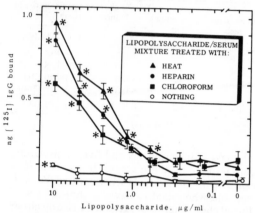

FIG. 1. *Effect of treating serum-lipopolysaccharide mixtures with heat, heparin, chloroform, or nothing on the ability of solid-phase radioimmunoassay to detect P. aeruginosa lipopolysaccharide. The units of the y-axis represent the amount of radioiodinated immunoglobulin G bound to the tubes after the final step of the assay. Each point represents the mean of four tubes; each vertical bar represents ±1 SD. Asterisks denote points which differed from the zero-antigen control as analyzed by t-testing at the P < 0.05 level of sensitivity.*

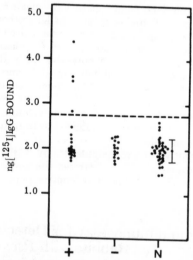

FIG. 2. *Detection of P. aeruginosa antigens by radioimmunoassay in the serum or plasma of granulocytopenic rabbits. Symbols: +, 20 culture-positive (P. aeruginosa) granulocytopenic rabbits; −, 15 culture-negative granulocytopenic rabbits; N, 38 normal control rabbits; dotted line, 3 SD above the normal control group mean, used to divide positive from negative results; vertical bar, ±1 SD.*

lation of some specimens. Because of its simplicity and relative effectiveness, therefore, all test sera were treated by heating at 56°C for 30 min.

Serum or plasma specimens from 20 bacteremic, granulocytopenic rabbits, from 15 nonbacteremic, granulocytopenic rabbits, and from 38 normal control rabbits were tested in the radioimmunoassay. Serum or plasma from 20% of the bacteremic rabbits were positive for *P. aeruginosa* antigens; no specimens from the other two groups were positive (Fig. 2). Of five rabbits with 10^3 or more colony-forming units per ml of blood, four were positive in the assay. Colony counts ranged from 2 to 300 per ml in 12 rabbits; none were positive in the assay. In the remaining three rabbits, only qualitative cultures were performed.

We conclude from these studies that the inhibitory activity of serum for detecting *P. aeruginosa* antigens by solid-phase radioimmunoassay can be diminished, but not completely eliminated, by treatment of the serum with chloroform deproteinization, addition of heparin, or heating. Of these, heating is most desirable because of its simplicity and relative effectiveness. Circulating antigens are present in the blood of rabbits with overwhelming *P. aeruginosa* bacteremia and can be detected by radioimmunoassay. We doubt that the assay in its present form is sensitive enough to be used as a reliable indicator of systemic *P. aeruginosa* infections. Ongoing work in our and other laboratories to eliminate entirely the inhibitory effects of serum and to further enhance the assay's sensitivity will, we hope, result in an assay that is sensitive enough to be of clinical value.

1. **Kohler, R. B., L. J. Wheat, and A. White.** 1979. Rapid diagnosis of *Pseudomonas aeruginosa* urinary tract infections by radioimmunoassay. J. Clin. Microbiol. **9:** 253–258.
2. **Levin, J., P. A. Tomasulo, and R. S. Oser.** 1970. Detection of endotoxin in human blood and demonstration of an inhibitor. J. Lab. Clin. Med. **75:**903–911.
3. **Ziegler, E. J., H. Douglas, and A. I. Braude.** 1974. Experimental bacteremia due to Pseudomonas in agranulocytic animals. J. Infect. Dis. **130**(Suppl.):S145–S148.

D. Mechanism of Action and Toxicity

Rate of Bacterial Killing by Ribostamycin and Other Aminoglycosides

A. FERRARA AND G. GIALDRONI GRASSI*

Chair of Chemotherapy, University of Pavia, Pavia, Italy

The need to know more about the characteristics of the activity of antibiotics has been largely recognized. The significance of MIC and MBC values has been critically reexamined, and it is agreed that they often offer only a partial view of drug activity. In order to obtain more information, it seems that determination of the rate of killing of bacteria exposed to antibiotics as well as study of the activity of so-called subinhibitory concentrations can be helpful (2).

In previous experiments by Gialdroni Grassi et al. (1), the rate of killing of different grampositive and gram-negative bacteria by aminoglycosides was studied. Sisomicin and gentamicin killed *Escherichia coli* and *Pseudomonas aeruginosa* most rapidly, and ribostamycin was generally the most active on *Staphylococcus aureus*. In the present study, we further investigated the activity of ribostamycin, determining the killing curves against *S. aureus* under different conditions and the ratio of MIC and MBC for ribostamycin and other aminoglycosides.

Killing of *S. aureus*. Experiments were performed on 20 strains of *S. aureus*. The time-kill curve method was used to study the dynamics of killing by ribostamycin and gentamicin at concentrations equal to 1 × MIC, 2 × MIC, and 5 × MIC as well as at sub-MIC and sub-MBC concentrations. *S. aureus* was grown overnight in Trypticase soy broth (BBL Microbiology Systems, Cockeysville, Md.) and then diluted to give between 10^5 and 10^6 organism per ml in the cultures with antibiotic; the cultures were then incubated at 37°C. At 0.5, 1, 2, 4, 6, and 8 h of incubation, viable organisms were enumerated by making serial 10-fold dilutions and plating on Trypticase soy agar (BBL). The effects of adding antibiotic to cultures in the stationary or logarithmic phase of growth, of different pH, and adding 50% horse serum were determined.

Susceptibility tests. The MIC and MBC values of 12 clinical isolates of *S. aureus* were determined by serial broth dilution in Trypticase soy broth (BBL). An inoculum of approximately 10^4 colony-forming units from an overnight culture was added. After incubation for 18 to 24 h, 0.01 ml from all the clear tubes was transferred on Trypticase soy agar (BBL) by means of a microtiter apparatus dispensing 0.01 ml. The agar plates were incubated at 37°C for 24 h. The MBC was defined as the minimal concentration of antibiotic in the tube from which no colonies grew in subculture.

Results. Ribostamycin added in both stationary and logarithmic phases rapidly killed 20 strains of *S. aureus* at concentrations equal to 1 × MIC, 2 × MIC, and 5 × MIC. The addition of 50% horse serum to the cultures increased the rate of killing (Fig. 1). A reduction in viable cells usually exceeding 99.9% was achieved in 2 to 4 h and, after addition of horse serum, in 1 to 2 h. Gentamicin showed less rapid action; in addition, horse serum did not substantially affect its activity.

Alkalinization of the medium (from pH 7.2 to 8.3) increased the activity of both antibiotics, apparently more markedly for ribostamycin. In fact, complete eradication with 1 × MIC of gentamicin was reached in 8 h at pH 7.2 and in 6 h at pH 8.3; with 2 × MIC of ribostamycin, complete eradication was reached in 6 h at pH 7.2 and in 2 h at pH 8.3. No difference in the rate of killing susceptible and resistant strains was observed.

In most instances, the MIC and MBC values for microorganisms susceptible to aminoglycosides are equal. Sometimes, however, a twofold and, rarely, a greater increase in MBC is observed. For 12 strains of *S. aureus* recently isolated in hospital, determination of MIC and MBC values of gentamicin, tobramycin, amikacin, and ribostamycin showed that the differences between MIC and MBC values for the same strain varied according to the aminoglycoside.

Table 1 shows the ratio between MBC and MIC values of the *S. aureus* strains examined. Eleven of 12 strains had MIC = MBC for ribostamycin, and one strain had an MBC twofold higher than the MIC; for the other aminoglycosides, a wider discrepancy in values was observed. In a few cases the MBC was 8- to 16-fold higher than the MIC. To test whether the subinhibitory or sub-bactericidal concentrations of

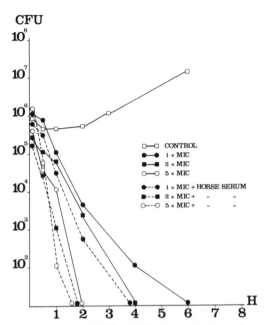

CFU

- □—□ CONTROL
- ●—● 1 × MIC
- ■—■ 2 × MIC
- ○—○ 5 × MIC
- ●--● 1 × MIC + HORSE SERUM
- ■--■ 2 × MIC + "   "
- ○--○ 5 × MIC + "   "

FIG. 1. *Rate of killing of S. aureus (mean values of 20 strains) determined by ribostamycin in the presence or absence of 50% horse serum. CFU, Colony-forming units.*

TABLE 1. *Difference between MIC and MBC of gentamicin, tobramycin, amikacin, and ribostamycin for 12 strains of S. aureus*

Antibiotic	No. of strains with MBC/MIC ratio of:				
	1	2	4	8	16
Gentamicin	4 (2)[a]	5 (2)		3	
Tobramycin	1	5 (3)	4 (1)	1	1
Amikacin	2 (1)	3 (3)	7		
Ribostamycin	11 (3)	1 (1)			

[a] Numbers in parentheses indicate the number of beta-lactamase-producing strains.

ribostamycin could affect the growth of *S. aureus*, the killing rate against a strain with MIC = 12.5 µg/ml and MBC = 25 µg/ml was determined in the presence of 10 and 5 µg/ml. After the first 6 h, in which a 2- to 3-log decrease in viable organisms was obtained, regrowth occurred.

Conclusion. Study of antibacterial activity by means of different tests, in addition to determining MIC and MBC, can provide more information on the effectiveness of an antibiotic. In our experiments, the rate of killing of ribostamycin against 20 strains of *S. aureus* was more rapid than that of gentamicin, and, as was previously demonstrated, than that of other aminoglycosides.

We found that for some strains the MBC of aminoglycosides was 4- to 16-fold higher than the MIC. Even in our limited experience, it seems that this phenomenon occurs less frequently with ribostamycin than with other aminoglycosides. Similar findings were interpreted by Watanakunakorn (3) as examples of a phenomenon of tolerance to aminoglycosides, similar to that observed for penicillins. Finally, it has been demonstrated that subinhibitory concentrations can also have a profound effect on the growth curve. In conclusion, it seems advisable to consider that many components determine the final antibacterial activity of an antibiotic. It is not clear whether the behavior observed in vitro may be important in clinical practice. It seems likely, however, that in some infections the difference in activity shown by the wide range of concentrations obtainable in biological fluid and tissues as a function of time can play a role in determining the clinical outcome.

1. **Gialdroni Grassi, G., A. Ferrara, and P. Sala.** 1979. Velocità di battericidia di alcuni aminoglicosidici. Chemiot. Antimicrob. **2**:30–36.
2. **Lorian, V.** 1978. Effects of subinhibitory concentrations of antibiotics on bacteria, p. 72–78. *In* Current chemotherapy, Proceedings of the 10th International Congress of Chemotherapy. American Society for Microbiology, Washington, D.C.
3. **Watanakunakorn, C.** 1978. Antibiotic-tolerant *Staphylococcus aureus*. J. Antimicrob. Chemother. **4**:561–568.

Effect of Silver Sulfadiazine on Human Spermatozoa

P. S. LIN* AND T. W. CHANG

Tufts-New England Medical Center, Boston, Massachusetts 02111, U.S.A.

Silver sulfadiazine (Ag-SD), an antibacterial agent, has been used successfully to prevent and treat burn sepsis (4–6). In addition, it has been demonstrated to possess antifungal (7), antitreponemal (2), and antiherpesviral (1, 3) activities. Many of these organisms are involved in sexually transmitted diseases, and the possibility arises that the drug may be used topically for prevention of these diseases. The present study describes the damaging effects of Ag-SD on human spermatozoa.

Methods. Stock solutions of Ag-SD (10,000 μg/ml in 0.3% xantham gum) were supplied by Marian Laboratories, Inc., Kansas City, Mo. Dilution was made in medium 199. For controls, xantham gum was added to medium 199 at a

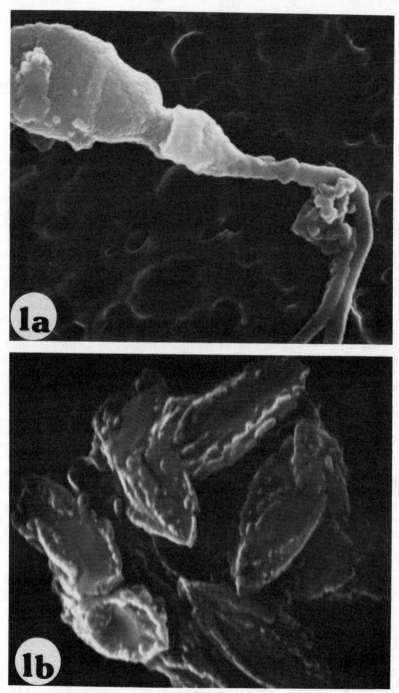

FIG. 1. *(a) Scanning electron micrograph of a sperm with swelling at the junction between the tail and the head (×8,400). (b) Tailless sperm with formation of bloblike structures on the surface (×6,000).*

TABLE 1. *Morphological changes in the tail of human sperm after exposure to Ag-SD*

Changes observed	% Showing change at Ag-SD concn (µg/ml) of:					
	0	5	10	25	50	100
Tailless	6	8	10	8	18	22
Swelling and/or shortening of tail ...	8	8	24	36	57	64
Normal appearance ..	86	84	66	56	25	14

concentration equivalent to that found in the Ag-SD suspension.

Fresh human semen from healthy donors was collected into sterile tubes. The specimens were allowed to stand at room temperature for 30 min for autoliquefication to take place. Fifteen milliliters of medium 199 containing no antibiotics was added to each specimen. After mixing gently, the specimens were again allowed to stand at room temperature for an additional 5 min before centrifugation at 1,000 rpm for 10 min. The sediment was resuspended in medium 199 to make the sperm count about 10^6/ml.

Small drops of sperm suspension were placed on microscopic slides and were used to determine the sperm motility. After drying, the slides were fixed in absolute methanol and stained with Giemsa for morphological observation. For scanning electron microscopic (SEM) study, the sperm suspensions were fixed in 2% glutaraldehyde at a 1:10 ratio. After washing twice, small drops were placed on a membrane filter. Dehydration was carried out in ethanol. After washing, the specimens were dried by Anderson's critical method with CO_2 as the transition fluid, coated with gold-palladium (60:40), and viewed with a JSM-U3 microscope.

Results. (i) Effect of Ag-SD on sperm motility. Although no quantitative data were recorded, it was noted that the number of motile spermatozoa became increasingly reduced as the time of exposure to Ag-SD increased. It was also noted that the loss of motility was dependent on the Ag-SD concentration.

(ii) Morphological changes in sperm after exposure to Ag-SD. Giemsa-stained slides showed that the earliest changes occurred in the tail portion of the sperm. The changes included local and diffuse swelling, formation of bloblike structures, and shortening of the tail length. Most of the swelling was seen at the junction between the tail and the head. Table 1 summarizes the morphological changes in spermatozoa after exposure to Ag-SD.

SEM observation confirmed the interpreta-

tion made from Giemsa-stained preparations. Figure 1a shows the changes seen at the junction between the head and the tail; Fig. 1b shows the changes seen on the surface of the tailless heads. Besides local swelling, there were many bloblike structures of various sizes scattered over the entire surface of the plasma membranes.

Discussion. We found in our laboratory that after exposure of cultured mammalian cells (e. g., human amnion and WI-38 cells) to 20 µg or more of Ag-SD per ml, morphological changes were regularly observed. These included granularity, loss of cell processes, and sometimes rounding of the cell body. The morphological changes in human spermatozoa after exposure to Ag-Sd appeared within 20 to 30 min, whereas those observed in tissue cultures began after 20 h of exposure. Under the light microscope, changes consisted of swelling and bubble formation involving various lengths of the tail portion of the sperm. As the swelling or bubbles enlarged, the involved portion vanished, resulting in loss of tails, either partially or completely. SEM observation confirmed these findings. In addition, there were diffuse bloblike structures of various sizes covering the surface of the plasma membrane, indicating a membrane-damaging effect of Ag-SD. As the tail portion of the sperm was damaged or vanished as a consequence, sperm motility was lost.

Whether similar changes may occur in animals remains to be studied. In humans, topical application of the drug is not accompanied by any appreciable amount of absorption. Its effect on sperm motility, therefore, is unlikely to occur. However, if the drug is to be used intravaginally for prevention of sexually transmitted disease, the damaging effects of Ag-SD on spermatozoa are probably unavoidable.

1. **Chang, T.-W., and L. Weinstein.** 1975. In vitro antiherpesviral activity of silver sulfadiazine. J. Infect. Dis. **132**:79–81.

2. **Chang, T.-W., and L. Weinstein.** 1975. Inactivation of *Treponema pallidum* by silver sulfadiazine. Antimicrob. Agents Chemother. **7**:538–539.

3. **Chang, T.-W., and L. Weinstein.** 1975. Prevention of herpes keratoconjunctivitis in rabbits by silver sulfadiazine. Antimicrob. Agents Chemother. **8**:677–678.

4. **Baxter, C. R.** 1971. Topical use of 0.1% silver sulfadiazine, p. 217–225. *In* H. H. Stone (ed.), Contemporary burn management. Little Brown and Co., Boston.

5. **Fox, L. L., Jr.** 1968. Silver sulfadiazine—new topical therapy for pseudomonas in burns. Arch. Surg. **96**:184–188.

6. **Limber, R. B., J. A. Moncrief, W. E. Switzer, S. E. Order, and W. Mills, Jr.** 1965. The successful control of burn sepsis. J. Trauma **5**:601–616.

7. **Wlodkowski, T. J., and H. D. Rosenbranz.** 1973. Antifugal activity of silver sulfadiazine. Lancet ii:738–740.

Sulfonamide Crystalluria: Isolation and Identification of Sulfamethoxazole and Four Metabolites in Urinary Calculi

JOSEPH L. WOOLLEY, JR., ARIS RAGOUZEOUS, DAVID A. BRENT, AND CARL W. SIGEL*

Departments of Organic Chemistry and Medicinal Biochemistry,* Wellcome Research Laboratories, Research Triangle Park, North Carolina 27709, U.S.A.

The antibacterial sulfonamides have been prescribed for over 40 years. During the first decade of use, renal injury due to sulfonamide crystalluria was widely reported (1). It is generally believed that the urinary calculi result from the poor aqueous solubility of the sulfonamides or their N^4-acetyl metabolites, or both (3). Over the years, crystalluria has been circumvented by using triple-sulfa combinations, alkalinizing the urine by administering sodium bicarbonate, introducing sulfonamides with greater solubility, or combining the sulfonamide with a potentiator so that the quantity of sulfonamide administered can be decreased.

In 1977, Siegel reported that he observed crystalluria in a patient treated with trimethoprim (TMP)-sulfamethoxazole (SMX) for chronic prostatitis (5). Infrared spectral analysis of the calculi provided evidence that the material was sulfonamide related, and it was described as a "pure metabolite of the combination of sulfamethoxazole and trimethoprim."

Subsequently, our laboratory obtained (L. Herring & Co., Orlando, Fla.) seven samples of urinary calculi for analysis. The samples were from patients who had been treated with either SMX or TMP-SMX. Infrared spectral analysis of the crystals by L. Herring & Co. indicated that these calculi were similar to the one studied by Siegel. Of the seven samples, five were easily dissolved in an acetone-methanol (1:1) solution and two were partially soluble (Table 1). The solutions were analyzed qualitatively by thin-layer chromatography (TLC), using solvent systems that separate TMP, SMX, and their respective metabolites (4). The soluble calculi showed at least five spots with similar R_f values. To isolate and identify the compounds in the calculi, the largest sample (78-11971) was ground to a fine powder, sonicated for 5 min in methanol-acetone (1:9) solution, and filtered. The funnel was washed with methanol-acetone (1:1). All of the sample was dissolved by this treatment. The combined filtrate was evaporated, and the residue was streaked onto 0.5-mm Silica Gel G plates, which were developed in a methanol-chloroform (15:85, vol/vol) solvent system. Five bands were visible by fluorescence quench (254-nm ultraviolet [UV] light). Bands A ($R_f = 0.51$),

B ($R_f = 0.41$), and C ($R_f = 0.31$) were resolved, and the silica gel was scraped from the plate and eluted with ethyl acetate. The eluate was washed (1 M phosphate buffer, pH $\cong$ 5.5) and evaporated, and the residues were analyzed by mass spectrometry (Varian MAT CH 5 DF double-focusing mass spectrometer) and nuclear magnetic resonance (NMR) spectrometry (Varian XL-100 spectrometer in d_6-dimethyl sulfoxide). Bands D ($R_f = 0.17$) and E ($R_f = 0.14$) were isolated as a mixture, and the residue was resolved by chromatography on Silica Gel G plates with an ethyl acetate-methanol-water (95:5:1, vol/vol) solvent system.

Band A and the major compound, band B, cochromatographed with and had NMR and mass spectra data identical to those of SMX (I) and N^4-acetyl SMX (II), respectively (Fig. 1).

Band C did not react with fluorescamine or with potassium ferricyanide-ferric chloride, which indicates a substituted N^4-amino group with no aromatic hydroxyl groups. Hydrolysis of C (6 N hydrochloric acid, 10 min, 100°C) yielded a compound which cochromatographed with I in three TLC systems. Field desorption mass spectral data provided evidence for a molecular weight for C of 311 (addition of $C_2H_2O_2$ to II). The UV spectrum of C had a λ_{max} at 263 nm, as did that of II (λ_{max} SMX = 270 nm). The NMR spectrum did not show the characteristic 3H acetate methyl signal at $\delta = 2.0$, but rather a 2H singlet at $\delta = 4.0$, suggesting a $OCH_2C{=}O$ group. N^4-glycolyl-N^1-(5-methyl-3-isoxazolyl)-sulfanilamide was proposed as the structure for C, and it was shown to be identical to synthetic III by TLC cochromatography and NMR and mass spectral comparisons. The method of Fries et al. for the synthesis of N^4-glycolylsulfanilamide (2) was used to prepare III.

Band D had a λ_{max} at 270 nm and reacted with fluorescamine, which suggested a free amino group. Since the NMR spectrum, which did not show a signal for the isoxazole-5-methyl group, was directly comparable to that previously reported (7) for N^1-(5-hydroxymethyl-3-isoxazolyl)sulfanilamide (IV), D was assigned that structure.

Band E did not react with fluorescamine, and the UV spectrum had a λ_{max} at 263 nm, suggest-

BAND A:

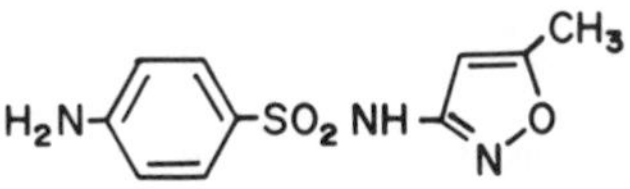

sulfamethoxazole (I)

BAND B:

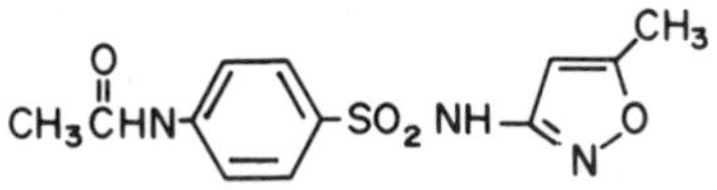

N⁴-acetylsulfamethoxazole (II)

BAND C:

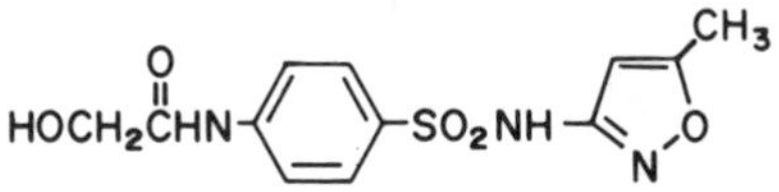

N⁴-glycolylsulfamethoxazole (III)

BAND D:

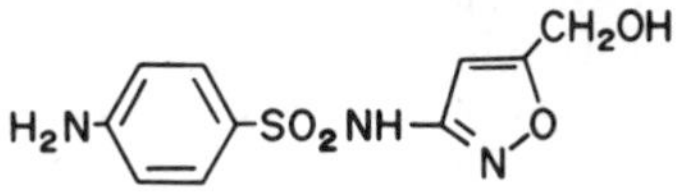

N'-(5-hydroxymethyl-3-isoxazolyl) sulfanilamide (IV)

BAND E:

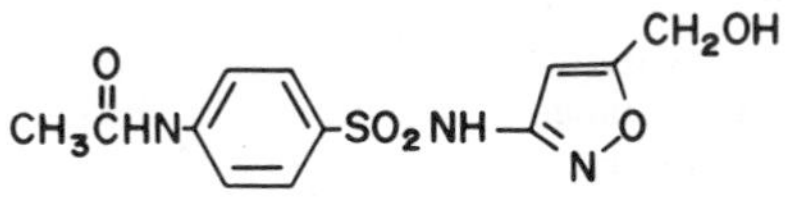

N⁴-acetyl-N'-(5-hydroxymethyl-3-isoxazolyl)-
sulfanilamide (V)

FIG. 1. *Structures of sulfamethoxazole and metabolites isolated from urinary calculi.*

TABLE 1. *Quantitative analysis of urinary calculi*[a]

| Sample | % Wt as: | |
	Sulfamethoxazole (I)	N⁴-acetylsulfamethoxazole (II)
78-06101	5.0	59
78-09642	1.1	98
78-11971	0.37	75
78-14391	0.23	67
78-17086	0.13	78

[a] The quantities of I and II in calculi were measured by application of the specific quantitative TLC procedure of Sigel et al. (6). Quantities of the metabolites III through V were not measured, but qualitatively (TLC, fluorescence quench) appeared to be at or below the concentration of I in the samples.

ing an N⁴-substituent. Hydrolysis (6 N HCl, 10 min, 100°C) afforded a compound that cochromatographed by TLC with IV, which suggested that E was an N⁴-substituted analog of IV. The NMR spectrum showed a 3H singlet at δ = 2.07 consistent with an N⁴-acetyl group. On this basis,

E was assigned the structure N⁴-acetyl-N¹-(5-hydroxymethyl-3-isoxazolyl)sulfanilamide (V).

Thus, the current work has led to identification of two new metabolites of SMX, III and V. The glycolamide metabolite III is novel for SMX; however, Fries et al. reported identification of a glycolamide metabolite of sulfanilamide for both rabbits and humans (2). Ueda et al. (7) studied the pattern of SMX urinary metabolites in humans and did not report finding V; however, Rieder in 1973 postulated that V was formed by humans (4).

Finally, even though SMX is considered to be one of the more soluble sulfonamides, the present study indicates that crystalluria still occurs and that it is mainly a result of crystallization of the N⁴-acetyl metabolite. In these urinary calculi, there was no evidence for the presence of TMP or its known metabolites.

1. **Dorfman, L. E., and J. P. Smith.** 1970. Sulfonamide crystalluria: a forgotten disease. J. Urol. **104**:482–483.

2. **Fries, W., M. Kiese, and W. Lenk.** 1971. Additional route in the metabolism of sulfanilamide. Xenobiotica 1:241–55.
3. **Krüger-Thiemer, E., and P. Bünger.** 1965. Evaluation of the risk of crystalluria with sulfa drugs. Proc. Eur. Soc. Study Drug Toxic. 6:185–207.
4. **Rieder, J.** 1973. Metabolism and techniques for assay of trimethoprim and sulfamethoxazole. J. Infect. Dis. 128: S567–573.

5. **Siegel, W.** 1977. Unusual complication of therapy with sulfamethoxazole-trimethoprim. J. Urol. 117:397.
6. **Sigel, C. W., and J. L. Woolley.** 1979. Sulfonamides, p. 677–694. In J. C. Touchstone and J. A. Sherma (ed.), Densitometry in thin layer chromatography. John Wiley and Sons, Inc., New York.
7. **Ueda, M., I. Takegoshi, and T. Koizumi.** 1971. Studies on metabolism of drugs X. New metabolite of sulfisomezole in man. Chem. Pharm. Bull. 19:2041–2045.

Comparison of the Effects of Two Groups of Polyene Antibiotics on Human Erythrocytes

G. MEDOFF,* J. BRAJTBURG, G. S. KOBAYASHI, S. ELBERG, AND C. FINEGOLD

Washington University School of Medicine, St. Louis, Missouri 63110, U.S.A.

All of the macrolide polyene antibiotics (polyenes) bind to cholesterol in the membrane of erythrocytes (RBC), altering membrane permeability and inducing hemolysis. Despite the similarities in their effects, there are important differences among the polyenes when the permeabilizing and hemolytic effects are studied in detail. We have recently proposed classifying the polyenes into two groups, based on these differences (2). The small polyenes (group I, those which have fewer than seven double bonds in the macrolide ring) induce no K^+ leakage without hemolysis. In contrast, the large polyenes (group II, heptaenes and the tetraene nystatin, which is considered a "degenerate heptaene") induce K^+ leakage at low concentrations and hemolysis at high.

The distinction between the two classes of polyenes is important because it implies different mechanisms of action. Furthermore, the permeabilizing effects of the large polyenes may be responsible for (i) the synergistic relationships these drugs have with other antibiotics and antitumor agents and (ii) the immunoadjuvant properties that are characteristic of this class of polyenes. For these reasons, we studied in detail the dose-response relationships between the permeabilizing and hemolytic effects of the large polyenes and then compared these results with those obtained with the small polyenes.

Amphotericin B (AmB) was purchased from Calbiochem, San Diego, Calif. The sources of other polyene antibiotics are reported elsewhere (2).

Human RBC drawn from one donor were separated from citrate-anticoagulated venous blood and added to NaCl containing 10 mM tris(hydroxymethyl)aminomethane buffer (pH 7.4) supplemented with the antibiotic to be assayed, incubated for 1 h at 37°C, centrifuged, and rinsed. Cell pellets were lysed in water. The Na^+ and K^+ remaining in cells were measured by a flame photometer, and hemoglobin was determined by absorbance at 550 nm. All data were expressed as percentage of control values found in untreated cells.

For all large-polyene antibiotics (group II), a decrease in cellular K^+ occurred at much lower concentrations than hemolysis and was accompanied by an increase in Na^+. Table 1 shows the specific concentration of each polyene which produced the maximal increase in Na^+. At this concentration, the cellular K^+ content decreased to 80 to 90% of initial values and the Na^+ content increased to about 400% of initial values. Further increases in polyene concentrations resulted in a decrease in Na^+ concentration and then hemolysis.

The results obtained with the large polyenes were in marked contrast to those obtained with filipin, etruscomycin, and chainin (polyenes in group I), which did not induce any change in cellular cation content before hemolysis.

The increase in cellular Na^+ seen with the large polyenes, but not with the small, may therefore be used as a criterion for classifying a polyene of unknown structure into either group I or group II. This notion has been tested in our laboratory and found to be reliable.

In the above experiments, it was observed that the Na^+ content in cells, when incubated with antibiotic concentrations higher than those shown in Table 1, decreased before the beginning of hemolysis. To better define these changes, we examined the effects of polyenes under conditions in which hemolysis did not occur. Sucrose, which has been shown to protect RBC against the hemolytic action of polyenes (1), was added to the incubation mixture. Figure 1 presents the AmB effect on RBC dispersed in buffer containing sucrose. Under these conditions, hemolysis occurred only after prolonged

TABLE 1. *Concentrations of large-polyene antibiotics (group II), and their semisynthetic derivative, inducing maximal increases in Na$^+$ content of RBC^a*

Polyene	Concn (µg/ml)
Candicidin	0.2
Amphotericin B	4.0
Nystatin	20.0
Candicidin methyl ester	2.5
N-acetyl amphotericin B	15.0
N-acetyl nystatin	300.0

^{a} RBC (5 × 10^7 cells/ml) were incubated with the antibiotics in buffer containing 0.155 M NaCl and rinsed with 0.2 M sucrose solution.

incubation (3 h) with AmB at 100 µg/ml, and within the shown concentration the RBC did not lyse. Up to an AmB concentration of 7.5 µg/ml, the K$^+$ content in rinsed cells decreased and the Na$^+$ content increased. At higher AmB concentrations, cellular Na$^+$ decreased; at 40 µg of AmB per ml, Na$^+$ fell to its initial value.

The simplest explanation for these observations is that Na$^+$ entered cells incubated with high and low concentrations of AmB equally well, but cells incubated with lower concentrations retained Na$^+$ when rinsed (stage I), whereas cells incubated with higher concentrations did not (stage II). Thus, at stage I the permeabilizing effect was reversed after the antibiotic was removed from the cell environment, but at stage II the effect was irreversible. Sucrose blocked hemolysis (stage III), but did not influence permeability changes to cations. Similar effects of sucrose on antibiotic action were seen when cells were treated with other large polyenes such as candicidin and nystatin.

We compared the protective action of three carbohydrates of different molecular size against polyene-induced hemolysis. In order to produce hemolysis even in the presence of carbohydrate, we used higher antibiotic concentrations and lower cell concentrations than in the experiments shown in Fig. 1. The effectiveness of carbohydrates in inhibiting hemolysis increased as the size of the carbohydrate molecules increased (melezitose > sucrose > mannitol).

Under carefully controlled conditions, the carbohydrates could partially decrease the hemolysis caused by filipin, etruscomycin, and chainin, and the potency of this protection increased in the same order as the blocking of AmB-induced hemolysis. However, the extent to which carbohydrates could block hemolysis caused by the small polyenes was markedly less than the extent to which they could block hemolysis induced by large polyenes. When hemolysis by the group I polyenes was inhibited by carbohydrates, leakage of Na$^+$ and K$^+$ was inhibited to

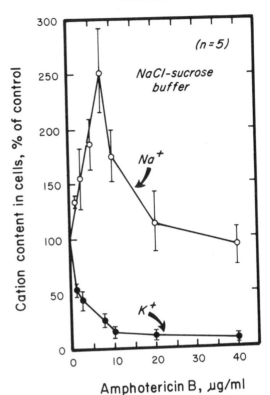

FIG. 1. *Effect of amphotericin B on RBC (11 × 10^8 cells/ml) dispersed in buffer containing 0.116 M NaCl and 0.062 M sucrose. After incubation with AmB, cells were rinsed with 0.25 M sucrose, and Na$^+$ (○) and K$^+$ (●) remaining in cells were measured.*

the same extent. Therefore, the permeabilizing effect did not occur with this group of polyenes, and hemolysis was the only discernible effect.

Delineation of the three stages of large-polyene action may be important in understanding differences in the biological effects of polyenes shown by us and others. First, the reversible permeabilizing (stage I) action of large polyenes has been exploited to introduce drugs and macromolecules into animal cells. Similar effects cannot be produced by small polyenes. Second, the large polyenes have immunoadjuvant properties, and the small do not. This implies that these properties are related to the permeabilizing effects of large polyenes.

1. **Cass, A., and M. Dalmark.** 1973. Equilibrium dialysis of ions in nystatin-treated red cells. Nature (London) New Biol. **244:**41–49.
2. **Kotler-Brajtburg, J., G. Medoff, G. S. Kobayashi, S. Boggs, D. Schlessinger, R. C. Pandey, and K. L. Rinehart, Jr.** 1979. Classification of polyene antibiotics according to chemical structure and biological effects. Antimicrob. Agents Chemother. **15:**716–722.

Mechanism of Action of Microcins

A. AGUILAR, A. F. DURO, A. CANDELA, M. RODRIGUEZ, D. FERNANDEZ-JORGE, C. ASENSIO,
AND F. BAQUERO*

*Instituto de Enzimologia, Facultad de Medicina, Universidad Autónoma, and Servicio de Microbiologia,
Centro Ramon y Cajal,* Madrid, Spain

Microcins constitute a new group of antimicrobial agents produced and excreted into culture medium by *Enterobacteriaceae.* They are low-molecular-weight compounds (in general less than 500), thermoresistant, soluble in methanol-water (5:1), and generally insensitive to proteases (pronase and subtilisin). Some microcins seem to have an amino acid derivative or oligopeptide structure, but the group in general appears as chemically diversified (1). There is good evidence that certain plasmids (M plasmids) code for synthesis of microcins. The plasmid coding for microcin 15 has a molecular weight of 3.4×10^6 and about 20 copies per cell (J. C. Perez Diaz, D. Bouanchaud, and F. Baquero, personal communication), and the plasmid coding for microcin 17 has a molecular weight of 26×10^6 and only one to two copies per cell (3). As for chemical structure, until now the better-known microcin was microcin 15, whose antibiotic action can be reversed by L-methionine. Methionine itself appears as a biosynthetic precursor of microcin 15, as has been shown by isotopic labeling. Microcin 15 is, on the other hand, different from other already known (mostly artificial) methionine analogs.

The mechanism of action of microcin 15 is related to the inhibition of the enzyme homoserine *O*-transsuccinilase (HTS), the first specific enzyme in the bacterial biosynthesis of methionine. Microcin 15 acts as a false end product, replacing methionine at the allosteric site of this enzyme and thus blocking methionine synthesis. A synergistic effect on the inhibition of HTS by microcin 15 can be shown by the use of *S*-adenosylmethionine (Fig. 1). This effect corresponds to the physiological cooperation of methionine and *S*-adenosylmethionine in the normal feedback inhibition of HTS. Available data indicate that microcin 15 works with the same efficacy as methionine in inhibiting HTS. Other effects of microcin 15 include the inhibition of the methionyl-transfer RNA-synthetase, but kinetic studies indicated that this probably is not the in vivo mechanism of action. We isolated mutants resistant to microcin 15, and its corresponding HTS enzymes were insensitive to inhibition by both methionine and microcin 15. Very strong inhibition of HTS by microcin 15 was observed

if the assay was performed at 42°C. Similarly, microcin 15-producing strains exerted a more powerful antibiotic effect on susceptible strains if they were incubated at 42°C. Unexpectedly, it was found that the amino acid D-serine also stimulated the in vivo inhibition of microcin 15 in susceptible strains, but the mechanism of this action is still under investigation.

Microcin 140 interfered with the energy-transducing process of the bacterial cell by rapidly depleting the adenosine triphosphate pool of susceptible *Escherichia coli* strains. This effect seemed to be caused by stimulation of adenosine triphosphatase (ATPase) since it was not observed either in a mutant strain (*E. coli* N144) that lacked this enzyme activity or in the presence of the ATPase inhibitor dicyclohexylcarbodiimide.

Under these conditions, microcin 140 did not affect the incorporation of labeled glucose into macromolecules. Microcin 140 also produced a strong inhibition of proline and phenylalanine transport, which is known to be coupled to the proton gradient across the bacterial membrane. Therefore, stimulation of the bacterial ATPase can be a consequence of collapsing the proton gradient maintained by this enzyme through a

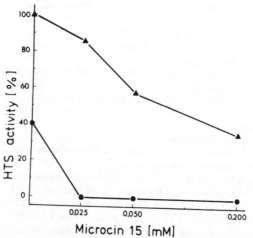

FIG. 1. *Inhibition of the HTS activity of E. coli 405 by microcin 15 (▲) and by association of microcin 15 with S-adenosylmethionine, 0.1 mM (●).*

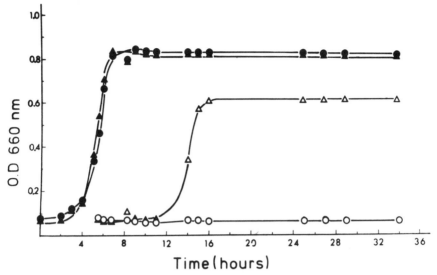

FIG. 2. *Inhibition of the growth of E. coli 405 (microcin-susceptible strain, ○) by E. coli Mcc 15+ (microcinogenic strain, ●). Isolated cultures of both strains (△, ▲) served as controls.*

proton-pumping activity. These results point to a similar mechanism of action for both microcin 140 and colicin K, despite their great difference in molecular size (4).

Microcin 509$_a$ apparently has a peptidic structure, but its antibiotic action could be antagonized by a wide variety of compounds. Pantothenic acid seemed to be the most powerful inhibitor of microcin 509$_a$. Methionine also exerted some antagonistic activity on microcin 509$_a$, but the mechanism of action of this microcin was not related to that of microcin 15, because microcin 509$_a$ did not inactivate HTS at all. Microcin 509$_n$ (produced by the same wild strain as microcin 509$_a$) could induce protoplasts in susceptible *E. coli* strains. Since it interfered with the incorporation of labeled 2,6-diaminopimelic acid into the bacterial cell, this is probably the mechanism of action of microcin 509$_n$ in cell wall synthesis.

There are some data suggesting that microcins could act as ecological effectors in complex microbial ecosystems like intestinal flora (2). To determine whether microcin-producing microorganisms can inhibit the growth of susceptible strains under conditions which simulate natural growth and a natural environment, we used a mixed-culture apparatus (Ecologen model E40), mounted on a shaker, using multiple growth chambers which can be connected by membrane filters or isolated by stainless-steel pieces. In the first case, cells are permitted to grow in pure

culture while microcin diffuses freely from the chamber of the producing strain to the vessel of the susceptible one. Figure 2 shows a typical assay of activity, in minimal medium Davis at 37°C, of *E. coli* 15 (microcin 15 producer) and *E. coli* 405 (susceptible strain) after a 42°C pulse. If the susceptible strain was inoculated after some delay, complete inhibition of growth of the latter was observed. No inhibition was seen with microcin-resistant mutants.

These results show the diversified mechanisms of action of microcins and point again to their potential as interbacterial ecological modulators.

1. **Asensio, C., J. C. Perez-Diaz, M. C. Martinez, and F. Baquero.** 1976. A new family of low molecular weight antibiotics from Enterobacteria. Biochem. Biophys. Res. Commun. **69**:7–14.
2. **Baquero, F., and C. Asensio.** 1979. Microcins as ecological effectors in human intestinal flora: preliminary findings, p. 90–94. *In* D. van der Waaij and J. Verhoef (ed.), New criteria for antimicrobial therapy: maintenance of digestive tract colonization resistance. Excerpta Medica, Amsterdam and Oxford.
3. **Baquero, F., D. Bouanchaud, M. C. Martinez-Perez, and C. Fernandez.** 1978. Microcin plasmids: a group of extrachromosomal elements coding for low molecular weight antibiotics in *Escherichia coli.* J. Bacteriol. **135**:342–347.
4. **Duro, A. F., R. Serrano, and C. Asensio.** 1979. Effect of the antibiotic microcin 140 on the ATP level and amino acid transport of *Escherichia coli.* Biochem. Biophys. Res. Commun. **88**:297–304.

Effect of Clindamycin on Protein Synthesis in *Bacteroides fragilis*

MURIEL LEDERMAN* AND TRACY D. WILKINS

Anaerobe Laboratory, Virginia Polytechnic Institute and State University, Blacksburg, Virginia 24061, U.S.A.

Although clindamycin is extensively used for treating infections caused by anaerobic bacteria, little is known about its mechanism of action. The related antibiotic lincomycin has been shown in other bacteria to inhibit protein synthesis (2), bind to the 50S ribosomal subunit (1), and, in in vitro systems, inhibit peptide bond formation (4). Neither drug has been studied in anaerobic bacteria with respect to effects on protein synthesis.

We have investigated the effect of clindamycin on in vivo protein synthesis in susceptible and resistant strains of *Bacteroides fragilis*. The MICs of clindamycin and lincomycin for the susceptible strain VPI 2553 (ATCC 25285) were 0.2 μg/ml and 1.6 to 3.2 μg/ml, respectively. The MIC of both drugs for the resistant strain VPI 12256 (ATCC 29763) was >500 μg/ml. All experiments were carried out in a modification of the minimal medium of Varel and Bryant (6) which omitted sodium bicarbonate and included 0.1 M potassium phosphate buffer, pH 7.0.

To study incorporation of radioactive amino acid into trichloroacetic acid-insoluble product, cells from an overnight chopped-meat culture were pelleted at 12,000 × g for 10 min and suspended in the equivalent volume of modified minimal medium. For each experimental culture, the suspended material was further diluted to an optical density at 750 nm of 0.1. After one generation, [³H]phenylalanine was added and the rate of protein synthesis was determined for 60 min. Then clindamycin was added, and its effect was monitored for 2 additional hours.

When a susceptible culture of *B. fragilis* was exposed to clindamycin at a concentration of 4 μg/ml, amino acid incorporation ceased immediately. Even concentrations 10- and 100-fold lower caused amino acid incorporation to stop within 30 min (Fig. 1). After exposure of resistant strain VPI 12256 to as much as 500 μg of clindamycin per ml, amino acid incorporation was 80% of the control after 2 h (Fig. 1).

Confirmation of these in vivo effects of clindamycin on protein synthesis was obtained by examining the effect of the drug on protein synthesis in cell-free extracts of *B. fragilis*. The cell-free extract (S-30) was prepared according to the method of Nirenberg (5), except that the preincubation step was omitted, 10 μg of catalase per ml was present in all buffers except the one

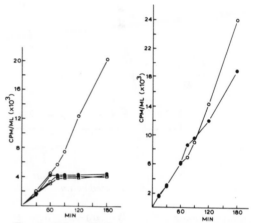

FIG. 1. *Effect of clindamycin on in vivo protein synthesis in susceptible and resistant B. fragilis. [³H]phenylalanine (17 Ci/mol; 0.5 μCi/ml) was added at zero time to all cultures. (Left) At 60 min, clindamycin was added at 4 (●), 0.4 (□), and 0.04 (△) μg/ml to the susceptible strain VPI 2553. (Right) At 60 min, clindamycin was added at 500 μg/ml (○) to the resistant strain VPI 12256.*

for the final dialysis, and 1 mM dithiothreitol was substituted for 6 mM 2-mercaptoethanol at the time of cell breakage. The cell-free extracts were programmed with polyuridylic acid, and protein synthesis was monitored as incorporation of [³H]phenylalanine into acid-insoluble product. The incubation conditions for in vitro protein synthesis were: tris(hydroxymethyl)-aminomethane acetate, pH 8.0, 50 mM; dithiothreitol, 5 mM; magnesium acetate, 20 mM; potassium acetate, 50 mM; adenosine triphosphate, 2 mM; guanosine triphosphate, 0.5 mM; phosphoenolpyruvate, 20 mM; pyruvate kinase, 50 μg/ml; transfer RNA, 300 μg/ml; catalase, 10 μg/ml; [³H]phenylalanine, 2 μCi/ml; and S-30 protein, 7.5 mg/ml. Incubations were for 40 min at 37°C in air.

Amino acid incorporation was stimulated 30-fold by the addition of 40 μg of polyuridylic acid per ml. Incubations containing polyuridylic acid were dependent upon an externally supplied energy-generating system, and all incorporation was abolished by the addition of 30 μg of RNase or 200 μg of puromycin per ml at the start of the incubation.

Amino acid incorporation in the in vitro sys-

TABLE 1. *Effect of clindamycin on cell-free protein synthesis in extracts of susceptible and resistant B. fragilis strains*

Clindamy-cin (μg/ml)	VPI 2553		VPI 12256	
	cpm/mg	% of con-trol	cpm/mg	% of con-trol
0	1,417	100	1,512	100
10	300	21	1,253	83
50	166	12	1,483	98
100	182	12	1,420	94
200	72	5	1,673	111
500			1,743	115

tem derived from a susceptible strain of *B. fragilis* was inhibited by as little as 10 μg of clindamycin per ml. If the S-30 was derived from the resistant strain of *B. fragilis*, even 500 μg of clindamycin per ml did not inhibit protein synthesis (Table 1). The same results were obtained with lincomycin. Neither drug inhibited amino acid incorporation under the direction of polyuridylic acid in a cell-free extract derived from *Escherichia coli*.

Studies aimed at determining whether clindamycin is an irreversible inhibitor of protein synthesis in *B. fragilis* indicated that a portion of the clindamycin bound to a cell-free extract from susceptible cells was released during a prolonged dialysis. After dialysis, amino acid incorporation in a drug-treated, dialyzed extract was 40% of that observed with a dialyzed extract at the same protein concentration. The residual incorporation observed in the drug-treated, di-alyzed extract could be abolished by further addition of clindamycin.

We have developed in vivo and in vitro techniques for studying protein synthesis in the anaerobic bacterium *B. fragilis* and have applied these techniques to studying the point of action of clindamycin, a drug used clinically in the treatment of *Bacteroides* infections. We have shown that the point of action of the drug is at the level of protein synthesis and that protein synthesis in the resistant strain is not affected by the drug. We are currently investigating whether plasmid-coded clindamycin resistance in *B. fragilis* is mediated by methylation of 23S ribosomal RNA as has been shown for induced lincomycin resistance in *Staphylococcus aureus* after exposure to erythromycin (3).

1. **Chang, F. N., and B. Weisblum.** 1967. The specificity of lincomycin binding to ribosomes. Biochemistry **6:**836–843.
2. **Josten, J. J., and P. M. Allen.** 1964. The mode of action of lincomycin. Biochem. Biophys. Res. Commun. **14:** 241–244.
3. **Lai, C. J., and B. Weisblum.** 1971. Altered methylation of ribosomal RNA in an erythromycin resistant strain of *Staphylococcus aureus*. Proc. Natl. Acad. Sci. U.S.A. **68:**856–860.
4. **Munro, R., and D. Vasquez.** 1967. Ribosome catalyzed peptidyl transfer: effects of some inhibitors of protein synthesis. J. Mol. Biol. **28:**161–165.
5. **Nirenberg, M. W.** 1963. Cell-free protein synthesis directed by messenger RNA. Methods Enzymol. **6:**17–23.
6. **Varel, V. H., and M. P. Bryant.** 1974. Nutritional features of *Bacteroides fragilis* subsp. *fragilis*. Appl. Microbiol. **28:**251–257.

Effect of Ribavirin on KB Cell DNA Synthesis

JIMMY W. BARNETT, CHARLES SHIPMAN, JR., AND JOHN C. DRACH*

Dental Research Institute, School of Dentistry, The University of Michigan, Ann Arbor, Michigan 48109, U.S.A.

The synthetic, truncated nucleoside 1-β-D-ribofuranosyl-1,2,4-triazole-3-carboxamide (ribavirin) is an inhibitor of the replication of DNA and RNA viruses (7). The in vitro activity of the compound clearly has carried over to experimental animal models (7), and the drug currently is undergoing clinical evaluation (4, 7). In both in vitro and in vivo evaluations, the drug has shown minimal toxicity in its antiviral dose range (4, 6, 7).

In marked contrast to the low toxicity produced by the drug, ribavirin has been reported to be a potent inhibitor of DNA synthesis in mammalian cell lines (1, 2, 6). In each of these reports (1, 2, 6), DNA synthesis was measured by the incorporation of [³H]thymidine into acid-precipitable material. We have found, however, that ribavirin is a potent inhibitor of thymidine phosphorylation which has led to the misinterpretation that ribavirin is a potent inhibitor of DNA synthesis (J. C. Drach, M. A. Thomas, and C. Shipman, Jr., Annu. Meet. Am. Soc. Microbiol. 1978, A41). We now have confirmed the observation that ribavirin is not a potent inhibitor of mammalian DNA synthesis, and we also report on the biochemical basis by which ribavirin inhibits thymidine phosphorylation.

To extend the initial observations from this

laboratory (Drach et al., Abstr. Annu. Meet. Am. Soc. Microbiol. 1978, A41), we examined DNA synthesis in ribavirin-treated KB cells by means of cytophotometry. Histograms showing the DNA content of ribavirin-treated cells were virtually identical to histograms of untreated cells. In addition, increases in cell number during the duration of these experiments (24 h) were almost the same for treated and untreated cells.

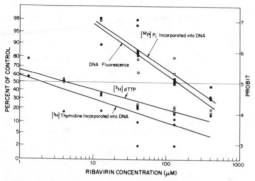

FIG. 1. *Dose-response relationships between riba-virin and parameters related to DNA synthesis. Dose-response relationships were established by linearly regressing probit values of percent inhibition of parameters related to DNA synthesis against log drug concentrations. [^{32}P]orthophosphate and [^{3}H]thy-midine incorporated into DNA were measures of the amount of label in acid-precipitable material after KOH hydrolysis. (Control values were approximately 79,000 and 68,000 cpm, respectively, per 100-µl ali-quot). Amounts of intracellular [^{3}H]dTTP were de-termined by thin-layer chromatography of ethanolic cell extracts. (Control values were approximately 3,200 dpm per 10-µl aliquot). DNA fluorescence was determined by exposing cells to propidium diiodide and passing the nuclei through a flow cytometer.*

Data from two such experiments are summa-rized as dose-response relationships in Fig. 1. Additional data concerning the effect of ribavirin on other measures of DNA synthesis also are presented. These data show that the effect of ribavirin on DNA synthesis as measured by flow cytometry (50% inhibitory concentration [I_{50}] = 150 µM) is virtually identical to its effect on DNA synthesis as measured by [^{32}P]orthophos-phate incorporation (I_{50} = 190 µM). In contrast, both measurements differ greatly from the effect of ribavirin on incorporation of [^{3}H]thymidine into acid-precipitable material (I_{50} = 2 µM). The effects of ribavirin on labeling of DNA and de-oxyribosylthymine triphosphate (dTTP) with [^{3}H]thymidine, however, are closely related (I_{50} = 2 and 4 µM, respectively). We have concluded, therefore, that ribavirin is a potent inhibitor of thymidine phosphorylation, not of DNA synthe-sis.

To elucidate the mechanism by which ribavi-rin inhibits phosphorylation of thymidine, we performed additional studies. Lysates of KB cells were prepared which would phosphorylate [^{3}H]thymidine to the triphosphate level. As can be seen in Table 1, neither ribavirin nor any of its known metabolites (5) inhibited phosphoryl-ation of [^{3}H]thymidine. Therefore, inhibition of phosphorylation in intact cells was most likely not the result of any direct inhibition of thymi-dine or thymidylate kinases by ribavirin or its metabolites.

Since ribavirin and its metabolites had no direct effect on phosphorylation of [^{3}H]thymi-dine, an indirect effect may have caused the observed inhibition. To explore this possibility, we measured the effect of ribavirin treatment on the total dTTP pool size. Lysates from ribavirin-

TABLE 1. *Effect of ribavirin and its known metabolites on in vitro phosphorylation of thymidine*[a]

Compound	Highest concn tested (µM)	Thymi-dine phospho-rylation (% of control)
Ribavirin (1-β-D-ribofuranosyl-1,2,4-triazole-3-carboxamide)	1,000	99
Ribavirin-5'-monophosphate	1,000	93
Ribavirin-5'-diphosphate	200	94
Ribavirin-5'-triphosphate	200	96
Triazole carboxamide moiety (1,2,4-triazole-3-carboxamide)	200	95
Ribavirin carboxylic acid (1-β-D-ribofuranosyl-1,2,4-triazole-3-carboxylic acid)	200	105
Triazole carboxylic acid moiety (1,2,4-triazole-3-carboxylic acid)	100	98
Thymidine triphosphate (positive control)	1	80
	25	4

[a] Phosphorylation of thymidine by KB cell lysates was assayed by incubating the lysate with a reaction mixture consisting of Tris buffer (pH 8.0), [^{3}H]thymidine, MgCl$_2$, ATP, mercaptoethanol, sodium fluoride, and an ATP-regenerating system. Labeled thymidine, dTMP, dTDP, and dTTP were identified by thin-layer chromatography and quantitated by liquid scintillation counting of material eluted from the chromatograms.

treated and untreated KB cells were extracted with 66% ethanol; the extracts were lyophilized to dryness and then reconstituted in water. The dTTP concentrations of the extracts were determined by a DNA polymerase assay with the dTTP to be determined as the limiting substrate. These experiments indicated that the dTTP pool size in cells treated with 131 μM ribavirin (77 nmol/10^9 cells) was seven- to eightfold greater than that in untreated cells (10 nmol/10^9 cells). Lowe et al. (3) also have reported a ribavirin-induced increase in dTTP pool size.

These results suggest that the most probable explanation for inhibition of thymidine phosphorylation in cells treated with ribavirin is that the dTTP pool size increased as a result of ribavirin-induced alterations in de novo dTTP synthesis. Consequently, cellular thymidine kinase activity was reduced as a result of dTTP feedback inhibition. Taken together, the increase in pool size of dTTP and a decrease in the tritium labeling of the pool would result in a significant decline in the specific activity of dTTP and, consequently, a marked drop in the labeling of DNA.

This work was supported by Public Health Service grant DE 02731 from the National Institute of Dental Research.

1. Drach, J. C., and C. Shipman, Jr. 1977. The selective inhibition of viral DNA synthesis by chemotherapeutic agents: an indicator of clinical usefulness? Ann. N.Y. Acad. Sci. 284:396–406.
2. Larsson, A., K. Stenberg, and B. Öberg. 1978. Reversible inhibition of cellular metabolism by ribavirin. Antimicrob. Agents Chemother. 13:154–158.
3. Lowe, J. K., L. Brox, and J. F. Henderson. 1977. Consequences of inhibition of guanine nucleotide synthesis by mycophenolic acid and Virazole. Cancer Res. 37:736–743.
4. Magnussen, C. R., R. G. Douglas, Jr., R. F. Betts, F. K. Roth, and M. P. Meagher. 1977. Double-blind evaluation of oral ribavirin (Virazole) in experimental influenza A virus infection in volunteers. Antimicrob. Agents Chemother. 12:498–502.
5. Miller, J. P., L. J. Kigwana, D. G. Streeter, R. K. Robins, L. N. Simon, and J. Roboz. 1977. The relationship between the metabolism of ribavirin and its proposed mechanism of action. Ann. N.Y. Acad. Sci. 284:211–229.
6. Müller, W. E. G., A. Maidhof, H. Taschner, and R. K. Zahn. 1977. Virazole (1-β-D-ribofuranosyl-1,2,4-triazole-3-carboxamide; a cytostatic agent. Biochem. Pharmacol. 26:1071–1075.
7. Sidwell, R. W., R. K. Robins, and I. W. Hillyard. 1979. Ribavirin: An antiviral agent. Pharmacol. Ther. 6:123–146.

Nature of DNA Damage Induced by Electrolytically Reduced Nitroimidazole Drugs

DAVID I. EDWARDS,* DAVID A. ROWLEY, RICHARD J. KNOX, IRENA M. SKOLIMOWSKI, AND RICHARD C. KNIGHT

Chemotherapy Research Unit, Department of Paramedical Sciences, North East London Polytechnic, London E15 4LZ, England

Much interest is being shown currently in the action of nitroimidazole drugs used clinically both for microbial disease and as radiosensitizers of hypoxic tumors. The basis for the action of such drugs as metronidazole and misonidazole lies in their ability to be reduced via the nitro group to unknown products which then cause the death of susceptible cells. The basis of the selective toxicity of such drugs lies in the redox potential of the nitro group which can only be reduced by anaerobes having redox reactions which are more negative than those found in aerobes (5).

Recently, it has been established, mainly in our laboratory, that reduced nitroimidazole drugs have DNA as their primary target, inhibiting DNA synthesis and causing degradation of DNA in vitro (3, 10). To study the interaction of these drugs with DNA, we have developed an electrolytic method of reduction which occurs at potentials that are biologically relevant and which occurs in the presence of DNA that subsequently can be analyzed for drug-induced damage. The method also lends itself as a most useful model system which can be used to evaluate the potential cytotoxicity of any such drug (6, 8, 9, 11). Briefly, the method involves determining the polarographic half-wave potential of each drug and then reducing it at constant potential in the presence of DNA under N_2, at a voltage which ensures a maximum four- or six-electron reduction but which avoids potentials at which the electrodes and DNA degradatively interact (1).

Drug-induced damage to DNA is measured during the reduction process (which can be monitored spectrophotometrically) by using viscometry, the measurement of DNA melting profiles, its T_m value, and ability to renature under controlled conditions. A decrease in the viscosity of

DNA indicates damage, and alterations in the nature of the melting profile, T_m value, and renaturation indicate stability and changes in the integrity of the helix. Further techniques including hydroxyapatite chromatography and agarose gel electrophoresis indicate strand breakage and reduction of the molecular weight of DNA which can be corroborated further by sucrose gradient sedimentation.

Using the techniques outlined above, we were able to show that a variety of drugs have an increased ability to damage DNA in the order metronidazole, misonidazole, 4-nitroimidazole, 8609 RP, and M&B 4998 (see Fig. 1 for structures). Further, the drug-induced damage was shown to be mediated by a free radical (the one-electron nitro radical anion, $N\dot{O}_2^-$), since damage may be reduced in the presence of aminothiol radical scavengers such as cysteamine or radioprotectors such as cystamine. However, protection against damage by aminothiols was not the same for each drug, but may be correlated with the redox potential or polarographic half-wave potential of the drugs. Thus, the ability of cysteamine to protect against damage depends on the free energies of the drug-aminothiol redox couple. This relationship is valid whether protection against damage to DNA is measured as an increase in DNA viscosity toward normal or as a decrease in the number of single-strand breaks determined by hydroxyapatite chromatography. In all this work it is highly significant that no unreduced drug had any effect on DNA.

More significant was the effect of nitroimida-zole drugs on DNAs of different base composition. Here, it was shown that the ability of a reduced drug to damage DNA depends on the base composition (Fig. 2), those DNAs having a high adenosine plus thymidine (A+T) content being more susceptible to damage than those with low A+T contents.

Examination of the nature of electrolytically reduced metronidazole and misonidazole showed a range of eight products and seven products, respectively. All those from metronidazole have the imidazole ring intact, as do the majority from misonidazole, and chemical tests indicated the presence of both the amine and hydroxylamine derivatives from both drugs. None of the reduction products showed any growth inhibition when tested in liquid and solid culture against *Escherichia coli*, both anaerobically and aerobically, or clostridia. This may indicate a permeability problem because of the increase in the polar nature of the products.

The implications of these results are important insofar as they throw light on the mechanism of action and the selective toxicity of such drugs. Thus, reduction of the nitro group is a vital prerequisite not only for their antimicrobial activity but also for their action as radiosensitizers of hypoxic tumors. Thus, only anaerobes have redox mechanisms of sufficiently low (negative) potential to reduce the nitro group, and this usually occurs via the pyruvate phosphoroclastic reaction (for a review, see 4). It could be postulated that if a susceptible cell had an altered phosphoroclastic or pyruvate dehydrogen-

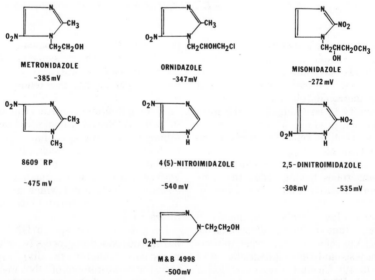

FIG. 1. *Structures of drugs used in this study. The potentials in millivolts indicate the polarographic half-wave potential determined with a mercury cathode and silver/silver chloride anode at pH 7.0.*

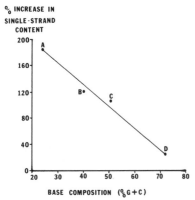

FIG. 2. *Relationship between the extent of DNA damage produced by misonidazole and the base composition of various DNAs (percent guanine plus cytosine). Drug-induced damage was measured as the increase in single-strand content by use of hydroxyapatite chromatography. The reduced misonidazole-nucleotide ratio is 1.0, and the letters A, B, C, and D refer to the DNAs of Clostridium perfringens, calf thymus, Escherichia coli, and Micrococcus lysodeikticus, respectively.*

ase reaction this could lead to drug resistance, and such a mechanism has recently been proposed (2).

The 4-nitroimidazole and the 4-nitropyrazole (8609 RP and M&B 4998, respectively) are inactive as antimicrobial agents because their redox potentials are too negative for reduction of the nitro group to occur. However, when reduction does occur these drugs are far more powerful as DNA strand-breaking agents than metronidazole or misonidazole and may well prove to be useful as potential specific radiosensitizers where radiation alone is able to reduce them.

The selective toxicity of nitroimidazoles to microbes depends not merely upon the redox mechanisms of the anaerobe but also upon the base composition of the DNA. Thus, the protozoans *Trichomonas vaginalis* and *Entamoeba histolytica* have DNA A+T contents of 71%, and clostridia range from 67 to 72% A+T. These, together with *Bacteroides* (59%), are the causative organisms of the majority of diseases for which nitroimidazoles are currently in clinical use. It is highly germane, therefore, that DNAs of high A+T content are more susceptible to damage by nitroimidazoles than those with low A+T contents. *Rhodospirillum and Rhodo-*

pseudomonas acidophila, for example, have low A+T contents (38% and 33%, respectively), and these are 25 times less susceptible to the drugs than the protozoa or the anaerobic bacteria (7).

Equally significant is the fact that the reduced species of the drugs are known to be cytotoxic to both oxic and hypoxic tumor cells so that the DNA damage observed in these in vitro studies could well represent a valuable model of the anticancer effect of nitroimidazole radiosensitizers of hypoxic cells.

We thank the Medical Research Council, Cancer Research Campaign, and Roche Products for financial assistance, and we thank Roche Products Ltd. (Welwyn Garden City, Herts, U.K.) and May and Baker (Dagenham, Essex, U.K.) for misonidazole and metronidazole, M&B 4998 and 8609 RP, respectively. D.A.R. is an S.R.C., C.A.S.E. postgraduate student and R.C.K. is a Cancer Research Campaign Fellow.

1. **Brabec, V., and E. Palecek.** 1976. Interaction of nucleic acids with electrically charged surfaces. III. Surface denaturation of DNA on the mercury electrode in two potential regions. Stud. Biophys. **60:**105–110.
2. **Britz, M. L., and R. G. Wilkinson.** 1979. Isolation and properties of metronidazole resistant mutant of *Bacteroides fragilis*. Antimicrob. Agents Chemother. **16:**19–27.
3. **Edwards, D. I.** 1977. The action of metronidazole on DNA. J. Antimicrob. Chemother. **3:**43–48.
4. **Edwards, D. I.** 1979. Mechanism of antimicrobial action of metronidazole. J. Antimicrob. Chemother. **5:**499–502.
5. **Edwards, D. I., M. Dye, and H. Carne.** 1973. Selective toxicity of antimicrobial nitroheterocyclic drugs. J. Gen. Microbiol. **76:**135–145.
6. **Edwards, D. I., R. C. Knight, and I. Kantor.** 1978. Interaction of nitroimidazole drugs with DNA, p. 714–716. *In* Current chemotherapy, Proceedings of the 10th International Congress of Chemotherapy. American Society for Microbiology, Washington, D.C.
7. **Edwards, D. I., G. E. Mathison, and D. J. Platt.** 1974. Metronidazole—an antimicrobial drug which inhibits photosynthesis. Z. Pflanzenphysiol. **71:**424–427.
8. **Knight, R. C., I. M. Skolimowski, and D. I. Edwards.** 1978. The interaction of reduced metronidazole with DNA. Biochem. Pharmacol. **27:**2089–2093.
9. **Knight, R. C., D. A. Rowley, I. Skolimowski, and D. I. Edwards.** 1979. Mechanism of action of nitroimidazole antimicrobial and antitumour radiosensitivity drugs. Effects of reduced misonidazole on DNA. Int. J. Radiat. Biol. **36:**367–377.
10. **Plant, C. W., and D. I. Edwards.** 1976. The effect of tinidazole, metronidazole and nitrofurazone on nucleic acid synthesis in *Clostridium bifermentans*. J. Antimicrob. Chemother. **2:**203–209.
11. **Rowley, D. A., R. C. Knight, I. M. Skolimowski, and D. I. Edwards.** 1979. The effect of nitroheterocyclic drugs on DNA: an *in vitro* model of cytotoxicity. Biochem. Pharmacol. **28:**3009–3013.

Asymptomatic Eosinophiluria During Penicillin and Cephalosporin Therapy

MARK O. LOVELESS,* CHRIS E. EIDAL, PAUL H. PETEET, AND DAVID N. GILBERT

Providence Medical Center and University of Oregon Health Sciences Center, Portland, Oregon 97213, U.S.A.

The association of eosinophilia with allergic conditions is well known. Some patients administered β-lactam antibiotics develop a syndrome termed allergic interstitial nephritis (AIN) which is characterized by eosinophils, fever, skin rash, and renal failure (1, 2, 6). Kidney biopsy specimens often demonstrate an eosinophilic interstitial inflammatory process. In a recent series of AIN patients, nine were found to have eosinophils in their urine (3). Stimulated by this observation, we prospectively tested urine specimens from patients receiving parenteral penicillin or cephalosporin therapy for the presence of eosinophils (eosinophiluria).

Cellular elements in the urine were collected by centrifugation (5), stained for eosinophils with Pilot's stain, and counted in a hemocytometer. This method will detect a minimum of 100 eosinophils per ml of urine.

Three population groups were studied for the presence of eosinophiluria. One group consisted of patients admitted to the hospital for elective surgery. None of these patients had received antibiotic therapy within the previous 7 days. Their urine was tested only once. The second group was comprised of patients administered a parenteral penicillin or cephalosporin antibiotic, as identified by their pharmacy orders. Urine eosinophils were quantitated pre- or posttherapy and at least once during therapy. None of these patients had any sepsis or symptom suggesting AIN drug allergy. The third group of patients were those seen in consultation for possible AIN or antibiotic-induced hemorrhagic cystitis.

Eosinophils were detected in only 1 of 139 (0.6%) urine specimens from patients admitted to the hospital for elective surgery. There were 27 patients with pyuria (>100 leukocytes/high-power field) and 7 patients with peripheral eosinophil counts above 600 cells/mm^3 of blood.

The results in the patients receiving parenteral penicillins or cephalosporins are shown in Table 1. One patient developed terminal dysuria, urinary frequency, and microscopic hematuria without fever or evidence of renal impairment while receiving methicillin. Eosinophils were detected in his urine. The methicillin was discontinued, and the eosinophiluria was gone when the patient was retested after 28 days. There were no significant differences in duration of antibiotic therapy between those who developed and those who did not develop eosinophiluria. The quantitative urine eosinophil count did not correlate with any specific antibiotic, dosage, or duration of therapy.

During the course of this study, four patients were seen, in consultation, who displayed convincing evidence of either AIN (three patients) or hemorrhagic cystitis (one patient). Eosinophiluria was eliminated within 24 h after corticosteroids were started in two patients and cleared spontaneously in all four patients within 4 weeks after the β-lactam antibiotic was stopped.

The eosinophiluria in patients with AIN is not an unexpected finding and confirms the observations of Galpin et al. (3). The absence of eosinophiluria in the preoperative patients was also expected (4). However, we were surprised to find that over 40% of patients receiving penicillin or cephalosporin had eosinophiluria without any other evidence of an adverse drug reaction.

The significance of this high incidence of asymptomatic eosinophiluria is uncertain. It is conceivable that the appearance of eosinophils in the urine is the only indication of a host allergic response. If so, it would be interesting to know whether these patients develop a positive cutaneous wheal and flare reaction to β-lactum antigens after the urine eosinophils appear.

The anatomic focus of the eosinophiluria is also unknown. Are the cells emanating from the renal interstitium, bladder, some other part of the collecting system, or some combination of these sites? Since none of the patients pro-

TABLE 1. *Eosinophiluria in various patient groups*

Group	No. of patients tested	No. positive for eosino-philuria
Control	139	1 (0.6%)
Antibiotic treated		
Penicillin	21	9 (43%)
Cephalosporin	10	4 (40%)
Both penicillin and cephalosporin	9	4 (44%)
Nephritis/cystitis	4	4 (100%)

gressed to overt AIN and renal failure, we have no evidence that asymptomatic eosinophiluria is causing any serious structural damage to the kidney or other parts of the urinary tract. Future studies should include more sensitive tests of renal function to ascertain whether subtle renal dysfunction is present.

1. **Baldwin, D. S., B. B. Levine, R. T. McCluskey, and G. R. Gallo.** 1973. Renal failure and interstitial nephritis due to penicillin and methicillin. N. Engl. J. Med. **279:** 1245–1252.

2. **Ditlove, J., P. Weidman, M. Bernstein, and S. G. Massry.** 1977. Methicillin nephritis. Medicine (Baltimore) **56:**483–491.

3. **Galpin, J. E., J. H. Shinaberger, T. M. Stanley, et al.** 1978. Acute interstitial nephritis due to methicillin. Am. J. Med. **65:**756–765.

4. **Helgason, S., and B. Lindqvist.** 1972. Eosinophiluria. Scand. J. Urol. Nephrol. **6:**257–259.

5. **Kesson, A. M., J. M. Talbot, and A. Z. Gyory.** 1978. Microscopic examination of the urine. Lancet **2:**809–812.

6. **Nolan, C. M., and R. S. Abernathy.** 1977. Nephropathy associated with methicillin therapy. Arch. Intern. Med. **137:**997–1000.

Renal Function During Cefuroxime Treatment in Patients with Preexisting Renal Impairment

BIRGER TROLLFORS,* MADIS SUURKULA, JOHN D. PRICE, AND RAGNAR NORRBY

Departments of Infectious Diseases and Clinical Physiology, University of Göteborg, S-416 85 Göteborg, Sweden, and Glaxo Group Research Ltd., Greenford, England*

The present study was undertaken to determine the effect of cefuroxime with or without concurrent treatment with furosemide on the renal function of patients with various degrees of preexisting renal impairment. Twenty patients with severe chronic osteitis, caused by *Staphylococcus aureus*, were treated with cefuroxime for 2 weeks. Ten of them received no diuretics (group A) and the other ten were treated with 40 to 60 mg of furosemide per day orally (group B). Five patients with the same types of infections were treated with cephaloridine during 1 week and then received the same dose of cefuroxime during the following week (group C). All had various degrees of renal impairment due to high age and/or diabetes mellitus.

The sodium salt of cefuroxime was used in a dose of 1 g three times per day in most patients. Four patients in group A received 1.5 g three times per day, and one patient in group C was given 1 g twice daily because of elevated serum creatinine.

Glomerular filtration rate (GFR) was measured by plasma clearance of ^{51}Cr-EDTA (1). Urinary β_2-microglobulin was used as a test for proximal tubular function.

Serum concentrations of cefuroxime were assayed in samples drawn before and at 0.5, 1, 2, 3, 4, 6, and 8 h after a 30-min intravenous infusion. Serum half-lives were calculated by use of a two-compartment open model.

The mean daily cefuroxime dose in group A was 63 ± 24 mg/kg of body weight. GFR, serum creatinine, serum β_2-microglobulin, and serum half-life of cefuroxime observed during 2 weeks of treatment are given in Table 1. In all patients these parameters remained within the normal variability of the methods.

In group B the mean daily dose of cefuroxime in 9 of the 10 patients was 43 ± 9 mg/kg of body weight. One patient was given 160 mg of furosemide per day, three patients were given 120 mg/day, three patients were given 80 mg/day, and two patients were given 40 mg/day. The results of the renal function tests and the serum half-lives of cefuroxime (Table 1) showed that all changes in the individual patients were again within the variability of the methods used, except in one patient whose GFR values were 78, 61, and 66 ml/min on treatment days 1, 8, and 15, respectively. This patient had peripheral edema when treatment was started, which is known to give falsely high values of ^{51}Cr-EDTA clearance. One patient in group B, not included in Table 1, was clearly overdosed with cefuroxime in relation to her renal function. She received daily doses of 70 mg of cefuroxime per kg and 80 mg of furosemide per day. After 6 days her GFR had decreased from 23 to 15 ml/min, with corresponding increases of serum creatinine and serum β_2-microglobulin and a prolongation of cefuroxime half-life from 5.7 to 7.2 h. When treatment was stopped, all parameters returned to pretreatment levels during the following 2 to 3 weeks.

The GFR decreased 17 to 19 ml/min in three of the five patients in group C during cephalori-

TABLE 1. ^{51}Cr-EDTA clearance, serum creatinine, serum β_2-microglobulin, and half-life of cefuroxime in two groups of 10 patients during cefuroxime treatment[a]

Group	Day	^{51}Cr-EDTA clearance (ml/min)	Serum creatinine (µmol/liter)	Serum β_2-microglobulin (µg/liter)	Half-life (h)
A	1	68 ± 21	114 ± 22	3,690 ± 1,430	1.8 ± 0.7
	8	72 ± 23	101 ± 28	3,800 ± 1,620	1.6 ± 0.4
	15	74 ± 23	97 ± 31	3,770 ± 1,630	1.5 ± 0.4
B	1	62 ± 23	104 ± 37	5,250 ± 3,420	2.2 ± 1.4
	8	61 ± 20	111 ± 41	5,340 ± 3,510	2.0 ± 1.0
	15	60 ± 20	97 ± 27	4,740 ± 3,130	2.1 ± 1.0

[a] All values are given as the mean ± the SD. Results are for only nine patients in group B because one patient clearly overdosed with cefuroxime in relation to her renal function was not included.

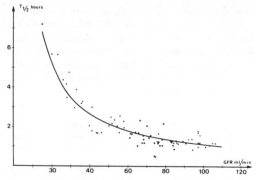

FIG. 1. Correlation between the glomerular filtration rate (GFR) measured by plasma clearance of ^{51}Cr-EDTA and the serum half-life ($T_{1/2}$) of cefuroxime.

dine treatment. In two of them GFR returned to pretreatment levels during cefuroxime treatment while the cefuroxime serum half-life decreased. In the other two patients the GFR was unchanged during both cephaloridine and cefuroxime treatment.

Urine samples on days 1, 8, and 15 with a pH greater than 6 were available from seven patients in group A, seven patients in group B, and five patients in group C. The initial value of urinary β_2-microglobulin (micrograms per micromole of urinary creatinine) varied from 0.004 to 0.95. The values changed little during treatment except in the overdosed patient in group B in whom an increase of the urinary β_2-microglobulin from 0.95 to 24.6 in 6 days was noted.

Figure 1 shows the correlation between the ^{51}Cr-EDTA clearance and the serum half-life of cefuroxime. The correlation coefficient for the logarithmic values of the two parameters was −0.90.

The present study demonstrated that when cefuroxime alone was used in daily doses of up to 116 mg/kg in patients with GFR between 36 and 101 ml/min, neither the GFR nor the proximal tubular function or the serum half-life of the drug itself was affected.

The same parameters were unchanged also when cefuroxime in daily doses up to 56 mg/kg of body weight for 14 days was given to patients with GFR between 29 and 89 ml/min concurrently with moderate doses of furosemide.

However, reduced renal function was observed in one patient with a GFR of only 23 ml/min at the beginning of the treatment receiving 70 mg of cefuroxime/kg of body weight and 80 mg of furosemide per day. The overdosage was due to

a falsely low serum creatinine (108 µmol/liter) reported from a routine laboratory test. When reanalyzed on a saved frozen serum sample, the value was 174 µmol/liter. When the overdosage became obvious, the patient was found to have a decrease of GFR to 15 ml/min, an increase of the cefuroxime half-life, and increased serum and urinary levels of β_2-microglobulin.

The results seen in group C indicate indirectly that cefuroxime is considerably less nephrotoxic than cephaloridine, as the decrease of GFR seen in three patients during cephaloridine treatment did not continue during treatment with the same doses of cefuroxime. Instead, the GFR increased and the serum half-life of cefuroxime decreased during subsequent cefuroxime treatment in two of the patients.

It can be concluded that cefuroxime does not affect the renal function to any measurable extent when used in normal or relatively high doses in patients with markedly, but not severely, reduced renal function irrespective of concurrent administration of furosemide. The logarithmic relation between GFR and serum half-life of cefuroxime (Fig. 1) and the results obtained in the single patient who was overdosed indicate that the cefuroxime dose must be reduced considerably when the GFR is lower than 30 ml/min.

1. Bröchner-Mortensen, J. 1972. A simple method for the determination of glomerulus filtration rate. Scand. J. Clin. Lab. Invest. **30:**271–274.
2. Bröchner-Mortensen, J., and P. Rödbro. 1976. Selection of routine method for determination of glomerular filtration rate in adult patients. Scand. J. Clin. Lab. Invest. **36:**35–43.

E. Pharmacology

Renal Excretion and Reabsorption Processes of Cephapirin, Cephaloridine, Cephalexin, and Cefoxitin

ANNIE ARVIDSSON,* OLOF BORGÅ, AND GUNNAR ALVÁN

Department of Clinical Pharmacology, Karolinska Institute, Huddinge Hospital, S-141 86 Huddinge, Sweden

The mechanism of cephalosporin transport in the mammalian kidney has been extensively studied during the past decade. Cephaloridine, the most nephrotoxic drug in the cephalosporin group, is actively transported into the proximal tubules in rabbits, and a high intracellular drug concentration is obtained (4). In the isolated perfused rat kidney it was demonstrated that cephaloridine is also actively reabsorbed from the luminal side (3). Cephalosporins in humans are mainly excreted via glomerular filtration and tubular secretion. In a series of studies in healthy volunteers we found that besides filtration and secretion cephapirin and cephaloridine are also reabsorbed (1). This was not observed with cefoxitin despite its chemical relation to the cephalosporins.

Plasma and urine specimens were analyzed by high-pressure liquid chromatography. Renal clearance was estimated by dividing the urinary excretion rate during each sampling interval by its midpoint plasma concentration.

Cephapirin and cephaloridine. Cephapirin and cephaloridine were administered by a 10-min infusion in a dose of 1.0 g to five healthy subjects at 1-week intervals. Blood specimens were drawn at 5, 10, 15, 20, and 30 min and once every hour for 8 h after the end of infusion. Urine was collected during 30-min intervals for 2 h and thereafter once every hour for about 12 h after the infusion. Additional 1-h urine collections were obtained between 21 and 30 h after the dose.

Total renal clearance of cephapirin decreased with decreasing plasma concentrations to approximately 5% of initial values (Fig. 1). At plasma concentrations below 2 µg/ml the average total renal clearance was about 10 ml/min. The glomerular filtration rate (GFR) for cephapirin was estimated to be approximately 50 ml/min when corrected for protein binding. The negative value obtained when the GFR is subtracted from total renal clearance thus indicates that reabsorption is greater than active secre-

tion. Considering the high polarity of cephapirin, our data suggest an active or carrier-mediated reabsorption of the drug from the tubular lumen.

As can be seen from Fig. 1, the total renal clearance of cephaloridine also decreased with the plasma concentrations, although this decrease was not so pronounced as in the case of cephapirin. In the subject having the greatest decrease in renal clearance, the reduction was 35% between the first (0 to 0.5 h) and the last (7 to 8 h) urine fractions.

Cephalexin. Cephalexin was administered intravenously in a dose of 0.5 g to five healthy volunteers. Blood and urine samples were collected as described for cephapirin and cephaloridine.

Decreasing renal clearance of cephalexin with decreasing plasma concentrations was noted in two of five subjects. The decrease was about the same as that found for cephaloridine (Fig. 1). Considering that a saturable tubular reabsorption process is an active or carrier-mediated process, it is likely that there will exist interindividual variability.

Cefoxitin. Cefoxitin was administered intravenously in a dose of 2.0 g every 6th h to eight patients undergoing colorectal surgery. Blood samples were drawn prior to the last cefoxitin injection (9th dose, 48 h after surgery) and after that once every hour for 12 h after the last dose.

In this study, which in contrast to the previous ones was performed in patients, there was a great intraindividual variation in renal clearance measured in 12 consecutive 1-h fractions. This was most likely explained by postoperative variations in the condition of the patients. Clearance variations were random and appeared not to be related to plasma concentrations of cefoxitin.

Conclusion. Our studies show that a saturable renal reabsorption process is involved in the elimination of cephapirin and to some extent of cephaloridine and cephalexin. This was observed as a decreasing renal clearance with decreasing

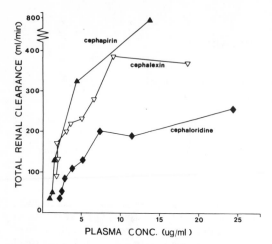

FIG. 1. *Total renal clearance versus plasma concentrations after intravenous administration of 1.0 g of cephapirin, 1.0 g of cephaloridine, and 0.5 g of cephalexin. Each curve represents the results from one subject.*

drug levels. It was not observed with cefoxitin, which, like cefamandole (2), has a renal clearance independent of drug concentrations. For cephalexin the extent of renal reabsorption seemed to vary between individuals. Further studies are needed to establish the clinical significance of these findings with respect to interference with other drugs or endogenous substances.

1. **Arvidsson, A., O. Borgå, and G. Alvan.** 1979. Renal excretion of cephapirin and cephalordine: evidence for saturable tubular reabsorption. Clin. Pharmacol. Ther. **25:**870–876.
2. **Aziz, N. S., J. G. Gambertoglio, E. T. Lin, H. Grausz, and L. S. Benet.** 1978. Pharmacokinetics of cefamandole using a HPLC assay. J. Pharmacokinet. Biopharm. **6:**153–164.
3. **Mitchell, C. J., S. Bullock, and B. D. Ross.** 1977. Renal handling of gentamicin and other antibiotics by the isolated perfused rat kidney. J. Antimicrob. Chemother. **3:**593–600.
4. **Tune, B. M.** 1975. Relationship between the transport and toxicity of cephalosporins in the kidney. J. Infect. Dis. **132:**189–194.

Hydrolysis of Cefamandole Nafate in Patients with Severe Renal Failure

RICHARD NIELSEN, ROBERT WOLEN, FRIEDRICH LUFT,* AND TAKESHI OZAWA

Department of Medicine, Renal Section, Indiana University Medical Center, and Eli Lilly Research Laboratories, Indianapolis, Indiana 46202, U.S.A.

Cefamandole nafate is the *O*-formyl ester of cefamandole (5) and is the pharmaceutical preparation of choice because of its compatibility and stability (4). Cefamandole nafate undergoes hydrolysis to free cefamandole and formate in vitro and in vivo (3, 4, 6). Although no difference is seen between cefamandole and cefamandole nafate in routine assay procedures, specially designed studies have demonstrated a potential difference in potency between cefamandole nafate and cefamandole. Knowledge of the hydrolysis of cefamandole nafate in vivo may be of clinical importance, particularly if cefamandole nafate accumulates in patients with renal failure due to slow hydrolysis. The hydrolysis of cefamandole nafate in patients with diminished renal function has not been described. The present report describes the hydrolysis of the *O*-formyl ester in patients with severe chronic renal failure as compared to subjects with normal renal function.

Ten subjects, five with normal renal function and five chronic hemodialysis patients, were studied. The dialysis patients, who were all studied during the intradialytic period, were all oliguric and had endogenous creatinine clearance rates of less than 2 ml/min. Approval for these studies was obtained from the Indiana University Committee on the Use of Human Subjects in Research.

The cefamandole nafate formulation (Eli Lilly & Co.) contained 1.11 g of cefamandole and 68 mg of sodium carbonate in each vial. The vial contents were diluted with 5% glucose in water and allowed to stand for precisely 15 min prior to infusion. Upon dilution, the initial alkaline pH (ca. 9.0) rapidly falls, with some hydrolysis of the ester to cefamandole and formate (4). Slowing of the hydrolysis occurs as the pH reaches 6 in approximately 5 min, and a very slow hydrolysis takes place thereafter. The 15-min period was chosen to assure that each subject received a uniform drug mixture with 25 to 30% ester hydrolysis in order to minimize variation which could result from random mixing times. A total of 1.5 g of cefamandole nafate per m^2 was infused intravenously into each subject over a 5-min period. Blood samples were collected from 19-gauge butterfly needles into 3-ml disposable syringes containing sufficient heparin to prevent coagulation during the processing period. Preinfusion and postinfusion samples were obtained from a vein in the arm opposite the infusion. Postinfusion samples were obtained at 1, 5, 10, 15, 20, 25, 30, 40, 50, 60, 80, 100, 120, 140, 160, 180, 200, 220, and 240 min after the termination of the infusion.

The primary goal of the sample processing procedure was to reduce to an absolute minimum any potential for hydrolysis of cefamandole nafate in vitro prior to chromatographic analysis. To meet this goal, the plasma was rapidly separated from the cellular components of blood, and a protein denaturant was added to stop any potential enzymatic hydrolysis as well as to change the pH of the sample to a value in the acid range where the ester is stable (4). Each 2-ml sample of blood was centrifuged (Beckman Microfuge, Beckman Instruments, Inc., Palo Alto, Calif.) for 1 min. The plasma was immediately transferred to a tube containing 1 ml of a 10% trichloroacetic acid solution saturated with lithium chloride to precipitate plasma proteins and acidify the sample. A 5-ml portion of ethyl acetate was added, and the mixture was gently extracted by rocking for 10 min. The mixture was then separated by centrifugation at 2,000 rpm for 5 min, and the organic layer was recovered. Water was removed from the organic phase with anhydrous sodium sulfate, after which the extract was taken to dryness in a gentle stream of nitrogen at 30 to 40°C and dissolved in eluting solvent. The chromatography of cefamandole and cefamandole nafate utilized a modification of the method described by Wold et al. (6). The plasma samples were assayed for total drug by the cup plate method (1). The assay does not distinguish between the two forms of the drug, responding equally on a molar basis to either cefamandole or cefamandole nafate.

Calculations for each individual form of the drug utilized the results of the microbiological assay which were proportioned according to the ratio of peak areas for cefamandole and cefamandole nafate as determined by high-pressure liquid chromatography (HPLC). Control samples were run with each set of microbiological and HPLC assays to assure assay consistency. The choice of an assay utilizing a combination of HPLC and microbiology permitted very rapid processing for HPLC since quantitative solvent recovery at each step was not critical to ratio measurement. Rapid processing was essential if the in vitro hydrolysis artifact was to be kept to a minimum.

The pharmacokinetic data were analyzed by means of a two-compartment open model using the IGPHARM program described by Gomeni and Gomeni (2). Comparisons were made by means of Student's t test for unpaired data.

The biological half-life of the terminal phase of the cefamandole nafate ester was significantly longer (18.3 ± 4.5 [SD] min versus 10.35 ± 1.4 min, $P < 0.01$) in the dialysis group as compared to normal subjects. Figure 1 depicts the mean plasma concentrations of cefamandole nafate and cefamandole for the two groups. Since the concentration of cefamandole in the plasma of the dialysis patients changed very little over the study period, pharmacokinetic parameters were not calculated. Data from the subjects most appropriately fit two-compartment open-model kinetics. Using the mean plasma concentrations (C_p) in each group, the equation best describing the initial- and terminal-phase kinetics in normal subjects was given by

$$C_p = 321.73 \exp(-0.4522t)$$
$$+ 156.69 \exp(-0.0754t)$$

whereas the relationship best describing the dialysis patient group was

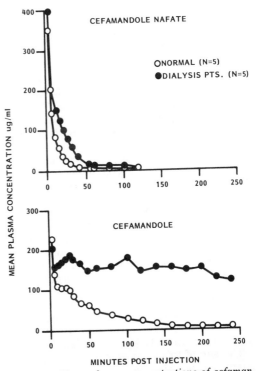

FIG. 1. *Mean plasma concentrations of cefamandole nafate for normal subjects and dialysis patients (upper panel) and the corresponding plasma concentrations of cefamandole (lower panel).*

$C_p = 181.41 \exp(-0.3814t)$

$$+ 290.01 \exp(-0.0529t)$$

The hydrolysis of the cefamandole nafate ester to free cefamandole occurs rapidly in both normal subjects and patients with renal failure. Our data suggest that hydrolysis proceeds sufficiently rapidly in patients with renal failure to allow no accumulation of ester.

In normal subjects, the nafate ester is partially excreted unchanged via the kidneys (6). It is likely that the half-life of cefamandole nafate in normal subjects depends on both hydrolysis in plasma and urinary excretion. Although some cefamandole nafate may be found in bile, the differences in half-life observed in our study groups probably reflect urinary excretion. The disappearance rate of cefamandole nafate observed in the renal failure group may closely approximate the actual rate of hydrolysis in vivo.

1. Brier, G. L., J. Wolny, and J. W. Smith. 1975. Serum bioassay for antimicrobial agents. *In* Technical improvement service no. 21. American Society of Clinical Pathologists, Chicago.
2. Gomeni, C., and R. Gomeni. 1978. IGPHARM: interactive graphic package for pharmacokinetic analysis. Comput. Biomed. Res. 11:345–361.
3. Indelicato, J. M., W. L. Wilham, and B. J. Cerimele. 1976. Conversion of cefamandole nafate to cefamandole sodium. J. Pharm. Sci. 65:1175–1178.
4. Kaiser, G. V., M. Gorman, and J. A. Webber. 1978. Cefamandole—a review of chemistry and microbiology. J. Infect. Dis. 137(Suppl.):510–516.
5. Wick, W. E., and D. Preston. 1972. Biological properties of three 3-heterocyclic-thiomethyl cephalosporin antibiotics. Antimicrob. Agents Chemother. 1:221–234.
6. Wold, J. S., R. R. Joost, H. R. Black, and R. S. Griffith. 1978. Hydrolysis of cefamandole nafate to cefamandole *in vivo*. J. Infect. Dis. 137(Suppl.):S17–S24.

Pharmacokinetics of Cefuroxime and Cefoxitin with Normal, Impaired, and Probenecid Functionally Impaired Kidney Function

CHIEL HEKSTER,* TOM VREE, ROELOF van DALEN, EPPO van der KLEIJN, and JAN HAFKENSCHEID

Departments of Clinical Pharmacy, Intensive Care, and Internal Medicine, St. Radboud Hospital, University of Nijmegen, Nijmegen, The Netherlands*

Cefuroxime and cefoxitin are two newer β-lactamase–resistant cephalosporin derivatives. Cefoxitin is derived from cephamycin C, a naturally occurring substance produced by *Streptomyces lactamdurans*. Cefuroxime is a semisynthetic cephalosporin derivative.

In general, the cephalosporins are eliminated from the body by renal excretion. As nephrotoxicity has been reported for cephalosporin derivatives, their pharmacokinetic behavior in patients with impaired renal function should be known so that the dosage regimen can be adjusted. For the determination of the cephalosporin concentrations in blood and urine, the method of high-performance liquid chromatography (HPLC) was used, being a sensitive, precise, and rapid method, as described by Vree et al. (3). Comparison of the HPLC method and the microbiological assay for cefuroxime resulted in a correlation coefficient of $r = 0.991$, as has been shown by Hekster et al. (2).

The aim of this study was to investigate the pharmacokinetic behavior of cefuroxime and cefoxitin in patients with impaired renal function. For this purpose, the following data were collected: concentrations of cefuroxime and cefoxitin in blood samples, average urine flow and renal excretion rate, biological half-life, apparent volume of distribution, renal clearance of cefuroxime, cefoxitin, and creatinine, and urinary pH in each urine specimen.

Cefuroxime. In patients with normal kidney function about 97% of cefuroxime was excreted unchanged in the urine within 24 h. Its plasma half-life was 1.5 h. Urine flow did not seem to influence the renal excretion rate.

In a patient with an average creatinine clearance of 21 ml/min only 61% of cefuroxime was excreted unchanged within 24 h. The plasma half-life was increased to 11 h.

A linear relationship ($r = 0.93$) between the renal clearance of creatinine and cefuroxime was found in patients with creatinine clearances below 60 ml/min (1). In these patients renal clearance of cefuroxime is related to glomerular filtration as indicated by creatinine clearance, as creatinine clearance can be regarded as a parameter of glomerular filtration.

When in patients with normal renal function probenecid was given as a co-medication to block specifically the tubular excretion, the contribution of the tubular and glomerular pathway to

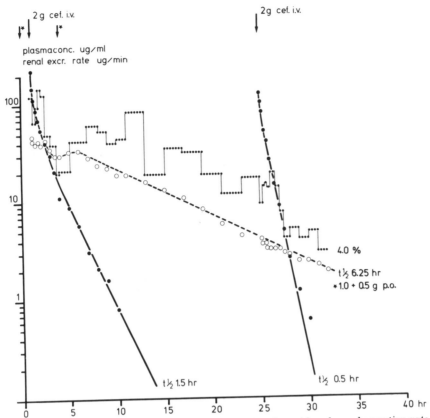

FIG. 1. *Plasma concentration time curves of cefoxitin and probenecid and renal excretion rate of probenecid. Note that cefoxitin was inhibited only in the first dose, at which the plasma concentration of probenecid was above 25 µg/ml.*

the total renal excretion pathway could be determined. Probenecid co-medication influenced cefuroxime kinetics only to a small extent (±25%). This has led to the conclusion that the tubular excretion contribution to the renal elimination is small and that cefuroxime is eliminated from the body mainly by glomerular filtration. Therefore, dosage regimen adjustment in patients with impaired renal function can be carried out on the basis of creatinine clearance.

Cefoxitin. In patients with normal kidney function, 100% of cefoxitin was excreted unchanged in the urine within 24 h. The elimination half-life was 0.5 to 1.0 h. In Fig. 1 the effect of probenecid on cefoxitin kinetics is shown. At 2 h after an oral dose of 1 g of probenecid, cefoxitin was injected intravenously, followed 2 h later by a second dose of 0.5 g of probenecid orally. The elimination half-life of cefoxitin appeared to be 1.5 h. A second dose of cefoxitin (2 g) was given 26 h after the first dose, while probenecid was still present in the plasma at a plasma concentration of about 5 µg/ml.

The elimination half-life of cefoxitin at this low plasma concentration of probenecid was 0.5 h. These studies with different dosages of probenecid, corresponding plasma concentrations, and inhibition of cefoxitin excretion showed that probenecid elicits its inhibitory function at plasma concentrations higher than 25 µg/ml. The renal clearance constant of cefoxitin is composed of glomerular filtration and tubular secretion.

Cefoxitin clearance at low plasma concentrations was found to be mainly by tubular excretion. At higher plasma concentrations the glomerular part of the renal excretion mechanism took part in the elimination of cefoxitin. When probenecid was given as co-medication, only glomerular filtration took place. From the difference in clearance values with and without probenecid co-medication it can be concluded that about 80% by tubular cefoxitin is eliminated about 80% by tubular secretion. Figure 2 shows the relationship between the renal clearance of cefoxitin and creatinine with and without probenecid co-medi-

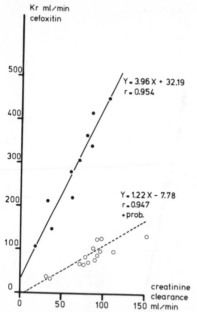

FIG. 2. *Relationship between the renal clearance of cefoxitin and creatinine with (r = 0.974) probenecid co-medication. With probenecid co-medication the ratio between cefoxitin and the creatinine clearance was 1.22, indicating that cefoxitin is cleared by glomerular filtration only.*

cation. It can be seen that without probenecid cefoxitin clearance was about four times the creatinine clearance.

Probenecid blocks tubular secretion but leaves all other renal excretion processes untouched. Thus, probenecid-induced kidney impairment may show the effect of tubular fall out. From Fig. 2 it can be seen that under probenecid co-medication cefoxitin clearance was 1.2 times the creatinine clearance. Thus, in patients with impaired kidney function dosage adjustment of cefoxitin based on creatinine clearance may lead to unpredictable plasma concentrations. Creatinine clearance can serve as a guide for drug dosage adjustment only when the ratio between all renal excretion pathways remains constant. These uncertainties about particular renal excretion mechanisms for a drug in an individual patient require the determination of renal clearance values. Thereafter, drug dosage may be adjusted.

1. **Dalen, R. van, T. B. Vree, J. C. M. Hafkenscheid, and J. S. F. Gimbrère.** 1979. Determination of plasma and renal clearance of cefuroxime and its pharmacokinetics in renal insufficiency. J. Antimicrob. Chemother. **5:**281–292.
2. **Hekster, Y. A., A. M. Baars, T. B. Vree, B. van Klingeren, and A. Rutgers.** 1979. Comparison of the determination of β lactam antibiotic drugs in plasma of rabbits by means of HPLC and of a microbiological assay. Pharm. Weekbl. Sci. Ed. **1:**95–100.
3. **Vree, T. B., Y. A. Hekster, A. M. Baars, and E. van der Kleijn.** 1978. Rapid determination of amoxicillin (Clamoxyl) and ampicillin (Penbritin) in body fluids of man, by means of high performance liquid chromatography. J. Chromatogr. Biomed. Appl. **146:**496–501.

Kinetics of Cefuroxime in Dialysis

PER ÅKE ÖRSTEN,* JOHN D. PRICE, AND KATHRINE DORNBUSCH

St. Erik's Hospital, S-112 82 Stockholm, Sweden

It is important when reviewing the properties of a new cephalosporin to determine its kinetics relative to its antimicrobial capacity in normal healthy volunteers. Fortunately, this gives a good correlation with the levels achieved in most patients, indicating the dose for the control of infection.

In moderate degrees of renal impairment, the fluctuations seen in renal activity make it hard to determine the dose recommendations. It is only, therefore, in severe renal impairment or complete anuric patients that the assessment of the fate of the antibiotic and the dose to be used to achieve satisfactory antimicrobial levels can be determined.

We therefore wished to study the kinetics of cefuroxime in this group of patients and to determine how well the drug is dialyzed from the serum during routine dialysis.

The aim of the study was to examine the kinetics of cefuroxime in patients with known severe renal impairment who are receiving peritoneal dialysis or hemodialysis.

Method. Severely ill patients having infections with concurrent underlying disease and septicemia were treated with cefuroxime for their infection, and serial samples of blood, urine, and dialysate were assayed for cefuroxime levels. The peritoneal dialysis or hemodialysis was carried out on a regular basis. Cefuroxime was given intravenously, 500 or 750 mg every morning (one dose per day). Regular samples of blood and dialysate were then taken when appropriate for assay; urinary output was monitored, and volumes were recorded and sent for cefuroxime assay.

We were able in this way to determine the levels of cefuroxime attained in the serum after a single dose over a 24-h period and to see what effect dialysis had in reducing these levels.

Results. Figure 1 shows the effect of peritoneal dialysis in an 83-year-old male with uremia with myelomatosis, who had been treated with prednisolone and melphalan, aluminium hydroxide and furosemide. He developed a fever and was treated with cloxacillin (4 g/day for 15 days). A urine culture at this time revealed a heavy growth of *Escherichia coli* susceptible to cefuroxime. He was then given cefuroxime, 500 mg/day intravenously, for 8 days. After 24 h he was afebrile. No side effects from cefuroxime were reported.

Figure 2 shows the effect of hemodialysis in a 57-year-old female. On regular hemodialysis (hypertension, renal insufficiency) blood culture grew *Staphylococcus epidermidis* considered to be from an infected fistula. The patient was given cefuroxime, 750 mg/day intravenously, for

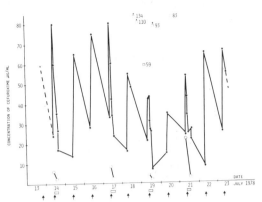

FIG. 2. *Concentration of cefuroxime in (★) serum, (○) dialysis solution, and (□) urine in a 57-year-old female on hemodialysis (□). Dialysis filter: Gambro 13.5 QB/blood, 200 ml/min. Dialysis monitor: Nycotron QB/dialysis solution, 620 ml/min. ↑, 750 mg of cefuroxime intravenously.*

10 days. The symptoms of septicemia disappeared, and no side effects from cefuroxime were seen.

Conclusion. From the limited data it is clear that the levels of cefuroxime in the serum after a single daily administration of cefuroxime in patients with severe renal impairment are well in excess of the MIC for most common pathogens. It is apparent also that the serum levels decrease over a 24-h period from the initial 60 to 80 μg/ml to 20 to 30 μg/ml, with no accumulation in patients on hemodialysis. When the patient is subjected to hemodialysis immediately after the dose of cefuroxime, these lower levels are attained within 4 h.

Cefuroxime is well dialyzed from the serum as unchanged cefuroxime and appears in the urine when this route of excretion is reestablished. In each case the infection was controlled. We feel, therefore, that 750 mg of cefuroxime should be given intravenously on a once-daily basis for these patients. Further studies are in progress.

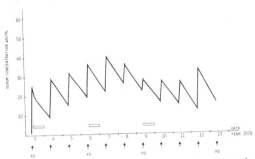

FIG. 1. *Concentration of cefuroxime in serum in an 83-year-old male on peritoneal dialysis (PD; □). ↑, 500 mg of cefuroxime intravenously.*

Pharmacokinetics of Azlocillin in Subjects with Normal and Impaired Renal Function

A. LEROY,* G. HUMBERT, M. GODIN, AND J. P. FILLASTRE

School of Medicine, University of Rouen, Rouen, France

Azlocillin is a semisynthetic broad-spectrum penicillin of the ureidobenzyl-penicillin group. Its antibacterial spectrum includes the β-lactam-ase–nonproducing cocci as well as gram-negative bacilli. It is more effective than carbenicillin against *Pseudomonas aeruginosa*.

The purpose of this study was to investigate the pharmacokinetic properties of azlocillin in subjects with normal renal function and in patients with chronic stable renal insufficiency of various degrees. Five healthy subjects without renal, hepatic, and hematological disease and 16 uremic patients were studied. The five healthy subjects were 22 to 28 years of age, with weights ranging from 59 to 83 kg. Each received a single intravenous (i.v.) dose of 30 mg/kg as a bolus injection (3 min) and 1 week later was given a dose of 80 mg/kg as a 30-min infusion. Thirteen to 16 blood samples were taken regularly after injection during 8 h. Six urine samples were collected during the first 24 h. The 16 patients with renal failure were 18 to 74 years old and were assigned to four groups according to their degree of renal insufficiency, as determined from endogenous creatinine clearance (Ccr): group I, 4 patients with Ccr between 30 and 80 ml/min per 1.73 m^2; group II, 4 patients with Ccr between 10 and 30 ml/min per 1.73 m^2; group III, 4 patients with Ccr below 10 ml/min per 1.73 m^2; and group IV, 4 patients with chronic end-stage renal function undergoing periodic hemodialysis.

A single i.v. dose of 80 mg/kg as a 30-min infusion was given to patients of groups I, II, and III. Patients in group IV received two infusions of 80 mg/kg, one out of dialysis and one prior to a 6-h hemodialysis session. Blood samples were taken at time zero, 30 min (end of infusion) and 45 min, and 1, 1.5, 2, 4, 6, 8, 12, and 24 h (group I), 36 h (group II), and 48 h (groups III and IV). Four to six urine samples were collected. Plated Gambro artificial kidneys were used as dialysis material with constant blood flow of 200 to 250 ml/min and dialysate flow of 800 ml/min. During a 6-h hemodialysis session, blood samples were drawn at time zero, 30 min, and each hour thereafter up to the end of the session. Serum and urine concentrations of azlocillin were determined by the microbiological method of agar diffusion (2, 4). The test strain used was *Bacillus subtilis* ATCC 6633. In healthy subjects, after i.v. injection (3 min) of 30 mg/kg, the pharmacokinetic data were calculated by means of a two-compartment open-body model (5) (Fig. 1).

In the five healthy subjects, after i.v. bolus injection of a single dose of 30 mg/kg, the mean maximal serum concentrations were 263.00 ± 61.67 µg/ml. Serum levels decreased very rapidly and were not detectable at 8 h. The mean elimination serum half-life ($T_{1/2}\beta$) was 0.89 ± 0.08 h, and the rate constant (β) was 0.78 ± 0.06 h^{-1}. Distribution serum half-life ($T_{1/2}\alpha$) was 0.11 ± 0.06 h, and the rate constant (α) was 8.46 ± 5.84 h^{-1}. The volume of the central compartment (V_c) was 7.36 ± 1.76 liters/1.73 m^2 (i.e., 11.4 ±

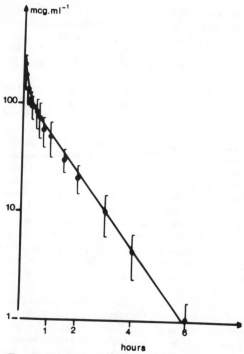

FIG. 1. *Decrease in the serum concentration of azlocillin in healthy subjects after intravenous bolus injection (3 min) of a single dose of 30 mg/kg.*

2.7% of body weight). The apparent volume of distribution (Vd_{ss}) was 14.15 ± 4.18 liters/1.73 m^2 (21.9 ± 5.8% of body weight). The mean serum clearance (C_s) was 215.0 ± 50.5 ml/min per 1.73 m^2; 69.6 ± 12.5% of the injected dose was recovered in urine during 24 h, and the mean renal clearance (C_r) was 145.2 ± 48.5 ml/min per 1.73 m^2. The first-order rate constants k_{12}, k_{21}, and k_e were, respectively, 3.79, 3.71, and 1.75 h^{-1}. After the single dose of 80 mg/kg in the same healthy subjects, serum concentrations obtained at the end of the infusion (30 min) were 409.00 ± 73.94 µg/ml. Elimination serum half-life ($T_{1/2}\beta$) was found to be dose dependent: 1.11 ± 0.17 h ($P < 0.025$). Apparent volume of distribution (V_d area) was 14.56 ± 3.33 liters/1.73 m^2, i.e., 22.8 ± 4.7% of body weight. Serum clearance was 152.9 ± 29.8 and renal clearance was 94.1 ± 18.6 ml/min per 1.73 m^2; 61.8 ± 14.2% of the injected dose was found in urine during the first 24 h.

In uremic patients, after a single dose of 80 mg/kg as a 30-min infusion, $T_{1/2}\beta$ increased in relation to the degree of renal impairment (Table 1): 2.03, 4.01, and 5.66 h in patients with Ccr within 30 to 80, 10 to 30, and <10 ml/min per 1.73 m^2, respectively. In patients on hemodi-

TABLE 1. *Pharmacokinetic data for azlocillin in healthy subjects and in uremic patients after a single intravenous dose of 80 mg/kg as a 30-min infusion*[a]

Renal function[b]	$T_{1/2}\beta$ (h)	β (h^{-1})	AUC (μg/ml per h)	V_d area (liters/kg)	Clearance (mg/min per 1.73 m^2)		Urinary elimination, 0–24 h (%)
					C_s	C_r	
Ccr > 80	1.11 ± 0.17	0.64 ± 0.11	576.4 ± 131.6	0.23 ± 0.05	152.9 ± 29.8	94.1 ± 18.6	61.8 ± 14.2
30 < Ccr < 80	2.03 ± 0.63	0.37 ± 0.10	895.2 ± 176.9	0.26 ± 0.04	101.8 ± 14.0	39.6 ± 9.1	39.4 ± 12.1
10 < Ccr < 30	4.01 ± 0.69	0.18 ± 0.03	1547.6 ± 529.1	0.32 ± 0.10	62.8 ± 25.2	11.0 ± 4.9	20.8 ± 13.7
Ccr < 10	5.66 ± 0.07	0.12 ± 0.001	2251.3 ± 903.0	0.34 ± 0.17	45.8 ± 19.5	5.1 ± 2.6	11.1 ± 7.5
Hemodialyzed patients	6.53 ± 1.67	0.11 ± 0.03	2333.9 ± 569.6	0.32 ± 0.04	37.2 ± 10.0	—	—

[a] All results are given as the mean ± the SD. $T_{1/2}\beta$, elimination serum half-life; β, rate constant; AUC, the area under the serum concentration time curve; V_d area, apparent volume of distribution; C_s, serum clearance; C_r, renal clearance.
[b] Creatinine clearance (Ccr) in milliliters per minute per 1.73 m^2.

alysis, elimination half-life ($T_{1/2}\beta$) was, out of dialysis, 6.53 ± 1.67 h and, on dialysis, 2.81 ± 1.08 h. During a 6-h hemodialysis session, serum concentrations of azlocillin decreased by 85.8 ± 9.6%, and the fraction of drug removed by dialysis was 45.8 ± 14.4%.

In healthy subjects, our results were very similar to those obtained by Fiegel et al. (3) and Lode et al. (6). Results found for the two doses (30 and 80 mg/kg) showed an increase in elimination half-life and a decrease in serum and renal clearances, suggesting that azlocillin pharmacokinetics are dose dependent. The same phenomenon was found by Bergan (1) for mezlocillin. Only 60 to 70% of the dose was recovered in 24-h urine. Azlocillin may be eliminated by extrarenal processes, especially biliary excretion. In uremic patients, the elimination half-life increased with decreases in renal function: 1.11 h in normal subjects to 6.53 h in patients with chronic end-stage renal function. This increase in half-life was important in patients with Ccr below 15 ml/min per 1.73 m^2. Renal insufficiency did not significantly modify apparent volume of distribution. Serum clearance decreased in relation to the degree of renal failure, and the ratio C_s/Ccr was higher in uremic patients than in normal subjects. The decrease in urinary elimination paralleled the degree of renal insufficiency. However, urinary concentrations of azlocillin remained above the MIC for susceptible

organisms for 24 h in patients of groups I, II, and III. The ratio C_r/Ccr was not significantly modified by renal insufficiency. Linear relationships could be established between the pharmacokinetic data and the biological parameters estimating glomerular filtration: half-life ($T_{1/2}\beta$) and serum creatinine (mg/100 ml) ($T_{1/2}\beta$ = 0.285 creatinine + 1.579, n = 17, r = 0.835, P < 0.01), elimination rate constant (β) and Ccr (β = 0.0041 Ccr + 0.1206, n = 21, r = 0.944, P < 0.001). Based upon these pharmacokinetic results, dosage schedules could be proposed according to the degree of renal failure.

1. **Bergan, T.** 1978. Pharmacokinetics of mezlocillin in healthy volunteers. Antimicrob. Agents Chemother. **14:** 801–806.
2. **Chabbert, Y. A., and A. Boulingre.** 1957. Modifications pratiques concernant le dosage des antibiotiques en clinique. Rev. Fr. Etud. Clin. Biol. **2:**636–640.
3. **Fiegel, P., and K. Becker.** 1978. Pharmacokinetics of azlocillin in persons with normal and impaired renal functions. Antimicrob. Agents Chemother. **14:**288–291.
4. **Grove, D. C., and W. A. Randall.** 1955. Assay methods of antibiotics: a laboratory manual, vol. 2, p. 34–36. Medical Encyclopedia, Inc., New York.
5. **Levy, G., and M. Gibaldi.** 1975. Pharmacokinetics, p. 6–18. *In* J. R. Gillette and J. R. Mitchell (ed.), Handbook of experimental pharmacology. New series: concepts in biochemical pharmacology, vol. 28, no. 3. Springer Verlag, Berlin.
6. **Lode, H., U. Niestrath, P. Koeppe, and H. Langmaack.** 1977. Azlocillin and Mezlocillin: zwei neue semisynthetische Acylureidopenicilline. Infection **5:**163–169.

Effect of Hemodialysis and Peritoneal Dialysis on the Pharmacokinetics of Azlocillin and Mezlocillin

RANDOLF SCHURIG,* DIETER KAMPF, KLAUS WEIHERMÜLLER, AND PETER SCHACHT

Department of Nephrology, Klinikum Charlottenburg, Free University of Berlin, Berlin, and Institute of Chemotherapy, Bayer AG, Wuppertal-Elberfeld, Federal Republic of Germany*

The pharmacokinetic behavior of two new semisynthetic acylureido-penicillins, azlocillin and mezlocillin, was studied in patients with end-stage renal failure on maintenance hemodialysis or peritoneal dialysis therapy. The additional purpose of the study was to evaluate the influence of hemodialysis and peritoneal dialysis on the elimination rate in these patients and to define dosage regimens for dialysis patients.

Twenty-four patients with a creatinine clearance of <3 ml/min were investigated (aged 20 to 77 years, mean, 56 years; body weight, 63 ± 12 kg). After intravenous infusion (dosage, 30 to 90 mg/kg) over a period of 30 or 60 min the elimination of the antibiotics was studied without dialysis as well as during a single regular dialysis session. Concentrations in plasma and dialysate were determined microbiologically with the agar plate diffusion method. The decrease in concentrations after the infusion corresponded best with first-order kinetics both with and without dialysis. The following kinetic data were calculated by use of standard equations: rate of elimination, half-life, and total body clearance.

Hemodialysis was performed in a single-pass system (blood flow, 150 to 200 ml/min; dialysate flow, 600 ml/min) with Gambrodialyzers (Lundia optima, 17 and 13.5 μm, respectively; 1 m² of surface area). In peritoneal dialysis a standard dialysate composition with 1.5% glucose was used. Exchange volume was 2 liters, and the dialysate flow was 100 ml/min without intraabdominal dwell time.

As shown in Table 1, in end-stage renal failure the plasma half-life was extended to 6.2 h for azlocillin and to 2.6 h for mezlocillin, suggesting a sixfold and threefold increase of the half-life of azlocillin and mezlocillin, respectively, compared with values in normal renal function (2, 3). However, total body clearance was still 30 ml/min (azlocillin) and 71 ml/min (mezlocillin). This indicates extrarenal, probably hepatic, elimination of both antibiotics. Similar results were described for azlocillin by Fiegel and Becker (1).

With hemodialysis the plasma half-life of azlocillin was decreased by approximately 58% and that of mezlocillin by approximately 46%. The differences in elimination rate and plasma half-life with and without hemodialysis were significant for both antibiotics (t test, P < 0.01).

In 14 patients dialyzer clearance was studied in vivo separately. The mean dialyzer clearance of azlocillin in eight patients was 33 ± 10 ml/min and that of mezlocillin in six patients was 38 ± 8 ml/min. After 4 to 7 h of dialysis, approximately 46 ± 15% of the previously administered dose of azlocillin was recovered in the dialysate. Mean dialysate recovery of mezlocillin was 27 ± 8%.

As demonstrated in Fig. 1, the total body clearance of patients measured during hemodialysis was approximately equal to the sum of dialyzer clearance (A) and total body clearance of patients without dialysis (B). The ratio of dialyzer clearance to total body clearance (without dialysis) was lower for mezlocillin (0.54) than that for azlocillin (1.10). Therefore, the influence of hemodialysis on the reduction of plasma half-life was less pronounced with mezlocillin than with azlocillin (Table 1).

Peritoneal clearance of mezlocillin measured directly was very low: 6.9 ± 3.3 ml/min (six patients). Only 5% of the dose was recovered by the dialysate. Therefore, the elimination of mezlocillin is not influenced by peritoneal dialysis, and plasma half-life remains unchanged during peritoneal dialysis (Table 1).

Despite a significant extrarenal clearance of

TABLE 1. *Pharmacokinetic data (mean ± SD) for patients*

		rate of elimination 1/h	plasma half-life time h	total body clearance ml/min
Azlocillin	without dialysis n = 11	0.14 ± 0.06	6.2 ± 2.8	30 ± 17
	hemodialysis n = 11	0.29 ± 0.08	2.6 ± 0.7	63 ± 22
Mezlocillin	without dialysis n = 8	0.30 ± 0.12	2.6 ± 0.9	71 ± 34
	peritoneal dialysis n = 6	0.35 ± 0.18	2.5 ± 1.3	78 ± 36
	hemodialysis n = 6	0.50 ± 0.16	1.4 ± 0.6	102 ± 28

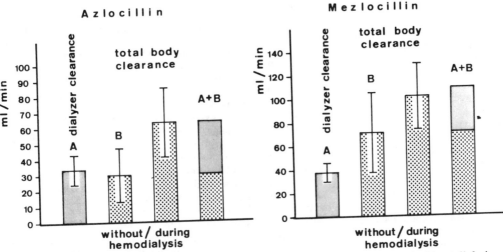

FIG. 1. *Comparison of dialyzer in vivo clearances and total body clearances with and without dialysis.*

both antibiotics, the administered dose must be reduced in patients with oligoanuria. It is recommended that the normal dose (three 5-g doses/day for both antibiotics) be adjusted as follows: azlocillin, first dose 5 g followed by 3.5 g every 12 h; mezlocillin, two 5-g doses/day.

Because of the short duration of hemodialysis, the increased elimination is of no importance for clinical practice. Total daily body clearance after 4 h of hemodialysis was diminished by approximately 16% for azlocillin and 10% for mezlocillin. Consequently, no modification in the reduced

dose of azlocillin or mezlocillin is required for either hemodialysis or peritoneal dialysis.

1. **Fiegel, P., and K. Becker.** 1978. Pharmacokinetics of azlocillin in persons with normal and impaired renal functions. Antimicrob. Agents Chemother. 14:288–291.
2. **Lode, H., U. Niestrath, P. Koeppe, and H. Lang-maack.** 1977. Azlocillin und Mezlocillin: zwei neue semisynthetische Acylureidopenicilline. Infection 5:163–169.
3. **Pancoast, S. J., and H. C. Neu.** 1978. Kinetics of mezlocillin and carbenicillin. Clin. Pharmacol. Ther. 24:108–116.

Pharmacokinetics of Mezlocillin and Azlocillin in Various Degrees of Impaired Renal Function

DIETER KAMPF,* RANDOLF SCHURIG, KLAUS WEIHERMÜLLER, AND DIETER FÖRSTER

Klinikum Charlottenburg, Free University of Berlin, Berlin, Federal Republic of Germany

The new acylureido-penicillins mezlocillin and azlocillin have a wider antibacterial activity than carbenicillin and are drugs of choice in serious infectious diseases. Because of the frequent occurrence of impaired renal function in such situations, we investigated the pharmacokinetic parameters of mezlocillin and azlocillin for various degrees of renal insufficiency.

Sixty-five patients without apparent liver or cardiac disease were studied (36 males, 29 females, aged 18 to 77 years, mean of 47 years). With respect to the degree of renal insufficiency, they were divided into six groups according to the glomerular filtration rate (GFR, milliliters

per minute per 1.73 m²): group I, >80; II, 80 to 40; III, 40 to 20; IV, 20 to 10; V, 10 to 5; and VI, 5 to 0. Patients in group I received mezlocillin only. A single dose (60 mg/kg) of mezlocillin or azlocillin was administered by infusion over a 30-min period. Only part of the patients received 30 or 90 mg of azlocillin per kg. Blood samples were taken regularly over 8 to 12 h. In patients who received mezlocillin, the urine was collected from 0 to 4, 4 to 8, 8 to 12, and 12 to 24 h. Antibiotic activities of mezlocillin and azlocillin were determined by microbiological assay (agar diffusion method; test strain, *Escherichia coli* JBC 4004). The semilogarithmic plot of the serum concentrations was analyzed by the method of least squares. Further calculations were done according to a one-compartment model by use of standard equations.

In the mezlocillin group the mean serum concentration at the end of the infusion was 258.10 μg/ml. The apparent volume of distribution (mean average) amounted to 22.5% of body weight. There were no significant differences in the mean peak serum concentrations or volumes of distribution with respect to the various degrees of renal function. The mean total elimination rate constant of 0.791 h^{-1} in normal renal function showed a modest decline to 0.271 h^{-1} in oligoanuria. The corresponding half-life increased from 0.88 to 2.56 h. In the healthy control the mean urinary recovery rate within 24 h was 65% of the administered dose; 85% of this amount was excreted within the first 4 h. Corresponding to the decline of renal function, the excretion rate decreased as well. However, in patients with a mean GFR of 6.7 ml/min, the excreted portion still amounted to 6.4%. The mean total body clearance of 250.69 ml/min decreased to 60.44 ml/min in oligoanuria, which represents the extrarenal clearance rate. The calculated mean renal clearance rate was 162.95 ml/min in the healthy control.

In the azlocillin group, no patients with normal renal function were studied. Corresponding to the results in the mezlocillin group, there was no significant change in the apparent volume of distribution with increasing renal impairment. The mean value of 20.5% of body weight was quite similar to that for mezlocillin. In addition, the variation of the administered azlocillin dose from 30 to 90 mg/kg was without influence on the volume of distribution. The mean total elimination rate constant of 0.385 h^{-1} in patients with a GFR of 50 ml/min showed a marked decline to 0.142 h^{-1} in oligoanuria. The half-life, which increased from 1.8 to 4.88 h, reached an almost twofold higher value than the corresponding mezlocillin half-life. These differences were due to a lower mean total body clearance of 83.50 ml/min (versus 158.12 ml/min) in patients with a GFR of 50 ml/min and a lower mean extrarenal clearance rate of 30 ml/min (versus 60.44 ml/min for mezlocillin) in oligoanuria. The renal clearance rate was reported to be 111.6 ml/min in the healthy control (1).

The different elimination rate constants, the quite similar volumes of distribution, and the resulting differences in the total body clearance between mezlocillin and azlocillin are finally responsible for the different dosage requirements in renal insufficiency. In the case of mezlocillin no dosage adjustment is required for a GFR of ultimately 10 ml/min. In patients with a GFR lower than 10 ml/min, the dosage interval should be increased from 8 to 12 h. With regard to azlocillin, the same dosage adjustment is indicated in patients with a GFR of 40 to 20 ml/min. A further GFR decline requires an additional dosage reduction. In these cases only 80 or 70% of the usual dose should be administered at 12-h intervals. Therefore, from a pharmacokinetic viewpoint, the use of the acylureido-penicillins, mezlocillin in particular, in various degrees of renal insufficiency is much less complicated and seems to offer advantages, as compared with the cephalosporins or the aminoglycosides.

1. **Lode, H., U. Niestrath, P. Koeppe, and H. Langmaak.** 1977. Azlocillin und Mezlocillin: zwei neue semisynthetische Acylureidopenicilline. Infection **5**:163–169.

Mezlocillin Pharmacokinetics After Single Intravenous Doses to Patients with Various Degrees of Renal Function

NIELS FRIMODT-MOLLER, SVEN MAIGAARD, ROGER D. TOOTHAKER, ROBERT W. BUNDTZEN, MITCHELL V. BRODEY, WILLIAM A. CRAIG,* PETER G. WELLING, AND PAUL O. MADSEN

William S. Middleton Veterans Administration Hospital, Madison, Wisconsin 53705,* and Departments of Surgery and Medicine and School of Pharmacy, University of Wisconsin, Madison, Wisconsin 53706, U.S.A.

Mezlocillin is a recently developed acylureidopenicillin for intravenous administration. In vitro studies have shown this antibiotic to have a spectrum of activity encompassing that of the cephalosporins and penicillins (1, 2). In this study the pharmacokinetics of mezlocillin were examined after single 2- and 4-g intravenous doses to male patients with various degrees of renal impairment.

The subjects were 32 hospitalized male pa-

TABLE 1. *Mezlocillin mean pharmacokinetic parameters*

Group	Dose (g)	$t_{1/2}(\beta)$ (h)	V_1 (liters/kg)	V_{dss} (liters/kg)	AUC (μg·h/ml)	Clearance (ml/min)		Cumulative urinary excretion (%)
						Serum	Renal	
I	2	1.3	0.14	0.28	208	227	148	44.6
	4	1.2	0.10	0.21	326	204	176	55.4
II	2	1.5	0.06	0.15	307	127	70	38.6
	4	1.6	0.09	0.22	919	104	39	46.0
III	2	2.3	0.15	0.36	285	119	4.1	4.0
	4	4.4	0.22	0.33	1,148	68	3.5	1.9

[a] $t_{1/2}(\beta)$, β-phase serum half-life; V_1, apparent volume of the central compartment of the two-compartment open model; V_{dss}, steady-state distribution volume; AUC, area under the mezlocillin concentration in serum curve.

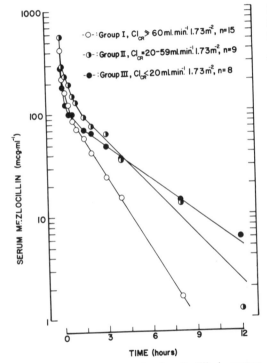

FIG. 1. *Mean serum levels of mezlocillin in groups I, II, and III, with all doses normalized to a value of 40 mg/kg. Cl_cr, creatinine clearance.*

tients suffering from a variety of diseases including renal insufficiency and with no known history of allergy to penicillins. Subjects were divided into three groups on the basis of 24-h creatinine clearance values. Thus, groups I, II, and III had creatinine clearances of ≥60, 20 to 59, and <20 ml/min. Subjects within each group were randomly subdivided to receive either a 2- or a 4-g dose of mezlocillin. Blood samples (5 ml) were taken serially through 12 h after dosing. Urine was collected quantitatively during 0 to 2,

2 to 4, 4 to 6, 6 to 12, and 12 to 24 h postdosing. Serum and urine samples were assayed by a microbiological cup-plate diffusion method.

The mean mezlocillin profiles in serum resulting from the 2- and 4-g doses to the three groups are shown in Fig. 1. Despite the considerable differences in renal function of the three groups, the rates at which mezlocillin was lost from serum did not differ markedly. Mean antibiotic levels in serum were greater than 10 μg/ml for 4 h after the 2- and 4-g doses in group I and for 8 h in group II. In group III, mezlocillin levels >10 μg/ml were maintained for 6 h after the 2-g dose and for 12 h after the 4-g dose.

The results of pharmacokinetic analysis are shown in Table 1. The minor effect of renal function on the rate of mezlocillin clearance from the body is indicated by the small changes in the values of $t_{1/2}(\beta)$ and serum clearance. The mean "β"-phase serum half-life of mezlocillin increased from a value of 1.2 to 1.3 h in group I to 2.3 to 4.4 h in group III, and the plasma clearance decreased from 204 to 227 ml/min to 68 to 119 ml/min. The relatively large values for the apparent volume of the central compartment and the steady-state distribution volume in group III compared to the other groups suggest that tissue take-up of mezlocillin is increased in renal insufficiency.

The cumulative excretion data indicate that, even in cases of relatively good kidney function, only one-half of the mezlocillin dose is cleared unchanged by this route. This proportion was maintained in group II, but dropped to less than 5% of the dose in subjects with severe renal impairment. In all three groups, antibiotic levels were above the MIC for susceptible organisms in subjects who produced urine for a least 12 h postdosing.

This study shows that after intravenous dosage mezlocillin distributes initially into an apparent fluid volume representing approximately

10% of body weight and subsequently into a volume representing approximately 20% of body weight. Distribution equilibrium is achieved within 1 h, and serum levels of antibiotic then decline monoexponentially with a half-life of 1.2 to 1.3 h. The considerable extrarenal elimination of mezlocillin accounts for the only moderate impairment in the clearance of this antibiotic from the serum with declining renal function.

The relatively small effect that renal impairment has on the pharmacokinetics of mezlocillin, and also the adequate urinary levels of antibiotic in patients with variable renal function, make it inappropriate to suggest dose adjustment in patients other than those with severe renal impairment. Even in patients who are functionally anephric, mezlocillin elimination is not markedly inhibited, and the drug is also readily and efficiently cleared during hemodialysis.

1. **Bodey, G. P., and T. Pan.** 1977. Mezlocillin: in vitro studies of a new broad-spectrum penicillin. Antimicrob. Agents Chemother. 11:74–79.
2. **Wise, R., A. P. Gillett, J. M. Andrews, and K. A. Bedford.** 1978. Activity of azlocillin and mezlocillin against gram-negative organisms: comparison with other penicillins. Antimicrob. Agents Chemother. **13:** 559–565.

Chemical Basis of Drug Binding Defects in Uremia

DIANE M. LICHTENWALNER, BYUNGSE SUH,* BENNETT LORBER, AND MICHAEL R. RUDNICK

Section of Infectious Diseases, Temple University Health Sciences Center, Philadelphia, Pennsylvania 19140, U.S.A.

Severe renal failure is associated with protein-binding defects for acidic drugs including penicillins, cephalosporins, sulfonamides, and salicylates. Binding of basic drugs such as trimethoprim, quinidine, and alprenolol tends to be normal or elevated. The uremic binding defect is not corrected by hemodialysis or prolonged exhaustive in vitro dialysis, but is corrected by either successful renal transplantation or activated charcoal treatment of uremic sera at an acidic pH (1). The chemical nature of the compound(s) responsible for defective protein binding and the mechanism(s) involved in the genesis of binding defects in uremia are unknown. Two major hypotheses have been proposed to explain the phenomenon. One possibility is that the binding defect is due to alterations in the serum proteins of uremic patients, more specifically, altered albumin composition (4). Another possibility is that toxic metabolic products which are rapidly removed by the kidneys in normal individuals accumulate in uremia, thus interfering with drug binding (1).

Acidification of serum specimens containing highly bound acidic drugs such as nafcillin and salicylates, followed by extraction with the organic solvent n-butyl chloride (NBC), effectively transfers the drugs into the organic solvent layer (3). Similar treatment of uremic sera at acidic pH (3.0) fully corrected their binding defects for acidic drugs such as nafcillin, salicylate, and sulfamethoxazole. The binding of basic drugs including trimethoprim and quinidine was not affected by the extraction procedure. The results showing the effect of NBC extraction on the binding of various drugs are summarized in Table 1. Binding values were determined by an equilibrium dialysis procedure at 4°C in Krebs-Ringer phosphate buffer, pH 7.4 (2). The values for sulfamethoxazole binding in serum specimens before and after organic solvent treatment in relation to albumin concentration are illustrated in Fig. 1. The corrective procedure by organic solvent extraction was pH dependent, and similar treatment at physiological pH (7.4) did not correct the binding defects.

Further analysis of the organic solvent extract of uremic sera demonstrated that the fraction could induce similar binding defects when it was added to either purified human serum albumin (HSA) or normal sera. The drug binding defect inducer (DBDI) contained in the NBC fraction was shown to be readily transferred to purified HSA when the NBC fraction and HSA were gently mixed at pH 7.4. Thin-layer chromatography of the original NBC extract of uremic sera revealed multiple spots when sprayed with sulfuric acid. Reacidification followed by NBC extraction of the HSA containing DBDI yielded an NBC fraction that was demonstrated to be homogeneous on thin-layer chromatography. This purified fraction induced binding defects for nafcillin, sulfamethoxazole, and salicylate when added to either purified HSA or normal sera.

In acidified uremic sera, the DBDI was readily

TABLE 1. *Effect of n-butyl chloride extraction on serum protein binding of five drugs*

| Drug | Percent protein bound | | | |
| | Normal subjects | | Uremic subjects | |
	Preextraction	Postextraction	Preextraction	Postextraction
Sulfamethoxazole	72.5 ± 1.5^a	73.2 ± 1.2	49.0 ± 13.2	71.2 ± 2.5^b
Nafcillin	87.5 ± 1.4	86.5 ± 2.0	73.3 ± 7.3	85.4 ± 1.1^b
Salicylate	96.3 ± 0.4	96.0 ± 0.6	84.6 ± 9.7	94.8 ± 1.6^b
Trimethoprim	70.8 ± 3.4	69.2 ± 1.3	68.6 ± 2.9	69.1 ± 2.0
Quinidine	80.0 ± 0.5	79.4 ± 0.3	81.4 ± 6.1	81.7 ± 7.3

[a] Values are means ± SD and are derived from six different sera per value.
[b] Values are statistically greater than preextraction values with $P < 0.005$.

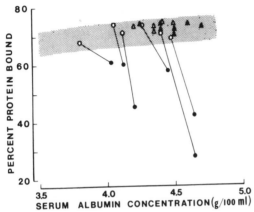

FIG. 1. *Effect of n-butyl chloride extraction on protein binding of sulfamethoxazole. Dotted area represents the 95% confidence limits for protein binding of the drug in normal pooled serum diluted with Krebs-Ringer phosphate buffer to adjust the albumin concentration to appropriate levels. Symbols: ▲ and △, six normal sera, pre- and postextraction, respectively; ● and ○, six uremic sera, pre- and postextraction, respectively.*

filterable through Amicon Diaflo filters with a molecular weight cut-off point of 500. NBC extraction of the ultrafiltrate yielded a fraction which was capable of inducing similar binding defects as described above. Furthermore, DBDI was shown to be dialyzable under appropriate conditions; that is, the binding defect could be partially corrected when uremic sera were dialyzed against HSA solution or normal sera.

In summary, DBDI is a lipid-soluble and apparently acidic compound which has a molecular weight of approximately 500 or less. It is believed that the compound is normally tightly but reversibly bound to human serum albumin at physiological pH but extractable at acidic pH. It is also dialyzable. The above findings strongly support the hypothesis that the protein-binding defects in uremia are due to accumulation of metabolic products that are normally rapidly removed by the kidneys, rather than being an intrinsic defect in albumin molecules.

1. **Craig, W. A., M. A. Evenson, K. P. Sarver, and J. P. Wagnild.** 1976. Correction of protein binding defect in uremic sera by charcoal treatment. J. Lab. Clin. Med. **87**:637–647.
2. **Kunin, C. M.** 1966. Clinical pharmacology of the new penicillins. I. The importance of serum protein binding in determining antimicrobial activity and concentration in serum. Clin. Pharmacol. Ther. **7**:166–188.
3. **Lichtenwalner, D. M., B. Suh, B. Lorber, and A. M. Sugar.** 1979. New rapid assay for nafcillin in serum by spectrofluorometry. Antimicrob. Agents Chemother. **16**:210–213.
4. **Shoeman, D. W., and D. L. Azarnoff.** 1972. The alteration of plasma proteins in uremia as reflected in their ability to bind digitoxin and diphenylhydantoin. Pharmacology **7**:169–177.

Antibiotic Concentrations in Renal Cysts

RICHARD S. MUTHER* AND WILLIAM M. BENNETT

Division of Nephrology, University of Oregon Health Sciences Center, Portland, Oregon 97201, U.S.A.

Genitourinary infection is a major cause of morbidity in patients with renal cystic disease. Despite seemingly adequate antibiotic therapy, these infections usually persist and often progress. One recent report suggests that perinephric abscess may develop in 60% of polycystic patients with urinary tract infections on chronic hemodialysis (3). Indeed, surgical intervention is often necessary to treat infections in both simple renal cysts and polycystic kidney disease (PCKD) (2).

There are several possible explanations for the refractory nature of these infections to antibiotics. Microbes present within cysts may differ from those cultured from urine, fostering ineffective antibiotic therapy. Resistant microorganisms may also exist within these cysts. In addition, poor antibiotic penetration into the renal cysts may contribute to the poor clinical response of these patients.

To examine this latter possibility, we measured the cyst fluid levels of a variety of antibiotics in four patients with simple renal cysts and three patients with PCKD. The mean glomerular filtration rate (GFR) in patients with simple renal cysts was 63 ml/min, and that in patients with PCKD was less than 10 ml/min.

Tobramycin and gentamicin were assayed by the radioenzymatic acetylation method, which has group specificity only; that is, the method cannot distinguish tobramycin from gentamicin, amikacin, or the other aminoglycosides. None of our patients received more than one aminoglycoside, however. Sulfamethoxazole and trimethoprim (given in combination as Bactrim) were detected by chemical assays: sulfamethoxazole by the Bratton-Marshall colorimetric assay and trimethoprim by a spectrofluorometric method. Neither of these drugs interferes with determination of the other. Cephapirin was detected by agar diffusion bioassay. Since this assay measures the ability of the patient's serum or cyst fluid to inhibit the growth of microorganisms, a strain resistant to all other antibiotics must be used.

Antibiotics were started 2 days prior to routine cyst puncture in patients with simple renal cysts. All patients with PCKD had been on therapeutic doses of antibiotics for at least 5 days. Two patients required nephrectomy for progressive renal infection not responsive to antibiotics. Cyst fluid was obtained at the time of surgery. No patient received more than two antibiotics.

In patients with simple renal cysts, gentamicin was detected in only one of three cysts punctured. The mean cyst fluid concentration of gentamicin was only 10% that of serum and 0.3% of urinary levels (Table 1). Bactrim was given to one patient. Despite adequate serum levels, neither sulfamethoxazole nor trimethoprim was detected in the cyst fluid.

In patients with PCKD, several cysts were punctured in each patient. Aminoglycoside antibiotics were found in low concentrations in the cysts of PCKD (Table 1). Tobramycin averaged only 8% of serum levels and 1% of urine levels. The cyst fluid level of gentamicin averaged approximately one-half of serum levels. Sulfamethoxazole apparently had the best performance of all antibiotics tested. Cyst fluid levels averaged 36% of serum and 23% of urinary levels. Despite high serum and urinary levels, cephapirin was poorly concentrated in cysts of polycystic kidneys. Levels averaged 1% of that of urine.

Proximal and distal cysts in PCKD can be distinguished by cyst/serum sodium (1). Aminoglycoside antibiotics were detected only in cysts of proximal nephrons. Neither tobramycin nor gentamicin was detected in distal cysts. Cephapirin, on the other hand, was detected in much greater concentrations in the cysts of distal nephrons.

There are several factors which may influence antibiotic concentrations in renal cysts. These should be considered in light of the fact that the cysts of PCKD are thought to be cysts of single nephrons. The single nephron GFR in humans is at least 10^{-8} liters per min. It would therefore take months for a cyst to reach its usual volume (3 to 5 cm^3) by glomerular filtration alone. This GFR would also seem unlikely to account for any antibiotics detected in renal cysts within 5

TABLE 1. *Antibiotic determinations in patients with simple renal cysts (SC) or polycystic kidney disease (PCKD)*

Patient group	Drug	Concn (µg/ml)[a]			Ratio		
		Serum (S)	Cysts (Cy)	Urine (U)	U/S	Cy/S	Cy/U
SC	Gentamicin	3.7	0.4	135	36.5	0.10	0.003
	Sulfamethoxazole	69	0	—	—	0	0
	Trimethoprim	2.4	0	—	—	0	0
PCKD	Tobramycin	3.7	0.3	28	7.6	0.08	0.01
	Gentamicin	3.1	1.4	—	—	0.45	—
	Sulfamethoxazole	28	10	43	1.5	0.36	0.23
	Trimethoprim	0.6	0	0.6	1	0	0
	Cephapirin	105	15.6	1,300	12.4	0.15	0.01

[a] All values are means.

days. Abnormal tubular function of polycystic nephrons may contribute to the poor antibiotic penetration, particularly of drugs normally transported by the renal tubules, such as the cephalosporins. Dilution of the drug within the cyst is almost sure to occur by the inward movement of water. Drugs may enter the cysts by diffusion across the abnormal cyst epithelium, although this would not seem to account for the discrepancy of drugs detected in proximal versus distal cysts. Diffusion trapping refers to the effect of pH on the diffusibility of drugs. This would not appear to be a significant factor, as distal nephron cysts, with lower pH, would be expected to have a high concentration of organic bases (i.e., aminoglycosides) and a low concentration of organic acids (i.e., cephalosporins). Our results suggest the opposite.

In summary, simultaneous determination of serum, cyst fluid, and urine concentrations of various antibiotics showed low drug levels in both simple renal cysts and PCKD. The reasons for the poor penetration of these drugs remains speculative. These data help explain the poor response of infected renal cysts to antibiotic therapy.

1. **Grantham, J. J.** 1979. Polycystic renal disease, p. 1123–1146. *In* L. E. Early and C. W. Gottschalk (ed.), Strauss and Welt's diseases of the kidney. Little, Brown & Co., Boston.
2. **Patel, N. P., W. R. Pitts, and J. N. Ward.** 1978. Solitary infected renal cyst. Urology **11**:164–167.
3. **Sweet, R., and W. F. Keane.** 1979. Perinephric abscess in patients with polycystic kidney disease undergoing chronic hemodialysis. Nephron **23**:237–240.

Gentamicin Therapy in Children with Renal Failure

SAYOMPORN SIRINAVIN, GEORGE H. McCRACKEN, JR.,* AND JOHN D. NELSON

The University of Texas Health Science Center at Dallas, Southwestern Medical School, Dallas, Texas 75235, U.S.A.

Efficacy and toxicity of aminoglycoside therapy are determined, in part, by the concentrations of drug in serum. Peak concentrations of gentamicin lower than 4 µg/ml may be insufficient for managemennt of infections caused by some coliforms or *Pseudomonas* strains. Additionally, peak concentrations exceeding 12 µg/ml or trough values greater than 2 µg/ml have been associated with increased risk of nephrotoxicity and ototoxicity in adults. The narrow range between therapeutically effective and toxic concentrations of gentamicin in serum must be considered in selecting dosage regimens, particularly in patients with altered renal function. Nomograms and computer programs based on either rates of creatinine clearance or serum creatinine concentration have been developed for adult patients with impaired renal function. To our knowledge, only one study has evaluated gentamicin dosage schedules in pediatric patients with chronic renal insufficiency (4). In that study of older children and young adults (ages, 8 to 17 years), serum half-life ($T_{1/2}$) was estimated from the endogenous creatinine clearance.

From July 1975 to May 1979, infants and children with diminished renal function and infections requiring gentamicin therapy were studied. All patients received the usually recom-

mended amount of 2 or 2.5 mg of gentamicin per kg as the first dose. The dosage schedule of gentamicin in these patients during the first 24 to 48 h was estimated from guidelines established in adults until results of serum assays of gentamicin content were known. Subsequent doses and the intervals of administration were determined on the basis of pharmacokinetic calculations. The clinical course and renal status of every patient were closely monitored.

Serum gentamicin concentrations were measured by a microbioassay method with *Bacillus subtilis* as the test organism. The $T_{1/2}$ of gentamicin was determined by least mean square analysis of the serum concentration-time curve and was calculated by dividing the $\log_{10} 2$ by the slope of the curve. Serum concentrations measured after the first dose of gentamicin or during the terminal washout phase were excluded from analysis.

Twenty-two studies were performed in 18 patients with altered renal function who had constant serum creatinine values (±0.5 mg/100 ml variation) for ≥48 h before sera were obtained for assay. Their ages were from 7 days to 15.5 years (mean, 2.7 years). Ten patients were less than 12 months of age. A statistically significant correlation (Pearson coefficient $R = 0.951$; $P < 0.001$) between gentamicin $T_{1/2}$ and serum creatinine was demonstrated (Fig. 1). The linear regression line was $y = 0.379 + 3.841x$. This equation indicates that $T_{1/2}$ in hours was 3.8 times the serum creatinine value in milligrams per 100 ml. When the ratio of $T_{1/2}$ to serum creatinine was determined for each of the 22 studies, the range was from 1.7 to 9.4 with a mean of 4.4 and a median of 3.9.

In an additional five individuals, studies were performed during a period of unstable serum creatinine values (progressively increasing or decreasing values of ≥ 0.5 mg/100 ml in 24 h). There was no correlation between the $T_{1/2}$ of gentamicin in serum and serum creatinine determined on the same day (Table 1). When renal function stabilized in one patient (number 3) with uric acid nephropathy associated with acute lymphocytic leukemia, repeat measurement of the serum concentration-time curve showed a $T_{1/2}$ value that was 4.2 times the creatinine concentration.

Serum creatinine levels are normally lower in children than in adults because of their smaller muscle mass. This may account for the higher gentamicin $T_{1/2}$ to creatinine ratio observed in infants and children than in adults. Three studies of adults with altered renal function reported

$T_{1/2}$/creatinine values of 2.15, 2.3, and 3.36 (1–3). When serum creatinine concentrations were from 1 to 10 mg/100 ml, the plotted line relating gentamicin $T_{1/2}$ to creatinine in adults was almost parallel to but to the right of that derived in our infants and children. About 60% of our patients were equal to or less than the tenth percentile for weight; however, there was no substantial difference between the ratios for children in this underweight group compared to those with normal percentiles.

Management of pediatric patients with renal failure who require gentamicin therapy is difficult. Serum gentamicin concentrations should be monitored to assure maintenance of therapeutic and nontoxic levels. Determination of half-life from the serum levels must be taken during the steady state, which is usually achieved after three or four half-lives have lapsed. Fitting the serum concentration-time curve to a single exponential (one compartment) term when the curve is actually bioexponential (two compartment) may result in an incorrect estimation of the half-life. This in turn would result in administration of gentamicin at improper intervals with a resultant risk of either subtherapeutic or potentially toxic concentrations of gentamicin in serum.

Although it is desirable to monitor gentamicin concentrations in these patients, many clinical centers do not have facilities to perform the assays. Measurement of endogenous creatinine clearance can be difficult in infants and young children because accurate collection of timed urine specimens is impossible without catheterization. Data from this study indicate that the gentamicin $T_{1/2}$ can be estimated by multiplying the serum creatinine by a factor of four. One-half the usual dose could be given every half-life, three-quarters of the dose every two half-lives, or a full dose every three half-lives. The selection of a regimen depends mainly on the severity of renal functional impairment and avoidance of prolonged periods of subtherapeutic serum concentrations which would occur in patients with

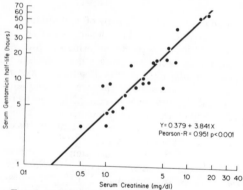

FIG. 1. *Relation between serum gentamicin half-life and serum creatinine concentration in infants and children with altered renal function.*

TABLE 1. *Serum creatinine and gentamicin half-life in five patients with unstable renal function*

Patient	Age	Wt (kg)	Creatinine (mg/100 ml)	Half-life (h)	Ratio[a]	Primary diagnosis
1	1.5 yr	9.5	0.4	4.6	11.5	Congestive heart failure, anuria
2	2 day	2.7	1.2	17.5	14.6	Acute tubular necrosis
3	4.5 yr	16	4.8	5.3	1.1	Acute lymphocytic leukemia, uric acid nephropathy
4	10 mo	10	8	57	7.1	Hemolytic-uremic syndrome (early phase)
5	12 yr	46	7.9	11.1	1.4	Hemolytic-uremic syndrome (diuretic phase)

[a] Half-life/creatinine.

markedly prolonged excretion rates given a full dose every three half-lives. We wish to emphasize that the serum creatinine can only be used to estimate serum half-life when renal function has stabilized. Furthermore, because of the considerable variation in the range of observed ratios, the derived half-life value should be confirmed by pharmacological calculations whenever possible.

1. Barza, M., R. B. Brown, D. Shen, M. Gibaldi, and L. Weinstein. 1975. Predictability of blood level of gentamicin in man. J. Infect. Dis. 132:165–174.

2. Cutler, R. E., A. M. Gyselynck, P. Fleet, and A. W. Forrey. 1972. Correlation of serum creatinine concentration and gentamicin half-life. J. Am. Med. Assoc. 219:1037–1041.

3. McHenry, M. C., T. L. Gavan, R. W. Gifford, et al. 1971. Gentamicin dosages for renal insufficiency: adjustments based on endogenous creatinine clearance and serum creatinine concentration. Ann. Intern. Med. 74:192–197.

4. Yoshioka, H., M. Takimoto, I. Matsuda, and S. Hattori. 1978. Dosage schedule of gentamicin for chronic renal insufficiency in children. Arch. Dis. Child. 53:334–337.

Tobramycin Disposition in Patients on Continuous Ambulatory Peritoneal Dialysis: a Preliminary Study

THOMAS W. PATON* AND M. ARIFIE MANUEL

Sunnybrook Medical Centre and *University of Toronto, Toronto, Ontario, Canada*

The concept of continuous ambulatory peritoneal dialysis (CAPD) is becoming increasingly important as an effective alternative to both hemodialysis and intermittent peritoneal dialysis. Very simply, CAPD uses the continuous presence of peritoneal dialysis solution in the peritoneal cavity except for brief periods of drainage and instillation of fresh solutions four or five times daily. Essentially, CAPD represents a continuous portable dialysis system (2, 3).

Recurring peritonitis is one of the major concerns of CAPD. Treatment consists of intraperitoneal instillation of appropriate antibiotics based on culture and susceptibility data. Systemic infection in these patients requires parenteral administration of antibiotics. Fundamental to the effective management of systemic infection is the dosing frequency of the administered drug. We undertook a study to determine the disposition of tobramycin administered parenterally in these patients on CAPD.

Six uninfected patients stabilized on CAPD were chosen for study. Four of the patients were male. The age (mean ± SEM) was 61.5 ± 3.0 years. The mean serum creatinine before starting CAPD was 12.4 ± 1.98 mg/100 ml, with a mean endogenous creatinine clearance of 6.3 ± 1.38 ml/min. The peritoneal clearance of creatinine was 4.5 ± 0.28 ml/min, and the combined total creatinine clearance was 10.8 ± 1.47 ml/min. The study was approved by the Human Ethics Committee, University of Toronto. Written informed consent was obtained from each patient.

At the beginning of the first of four dwell periods, an intravenous dose of tobramycin was infused over a 1-h period. Four of the patients received 1.5 mg of tobramycin per kg, and the remaining two patients received doses of 1.1 and 1.3 mg/kg. The four dwell periods were scheduled as follows: 0930 to 1400, 1430 to 1900, 1930 to 2400, and 0030 to 0900 h. During the first dwell period blood was drawn for tobramycin determinations at 1 h (end of infusion), midpoint, and the end of the dwell. At the end of each subsequent dwell period plasma and dialysate were assayed for tobramycin. Tobramycin concentrations were determined in duplicate by radioimmunoassay (New England Nuclear Corp.). Tobramycin removal by CAPD was quantitated, and dialysate/plasma ratios were calculated. Half-life ($t_{1/2}$) was determined from the terminal portion of the plasma concentration versus time curve:

$$t_{1/2} = 0.693/K_e$$

where K_e is the elimination rate constant (h^{-1}). The volume of distribution (V_d) was estimated assuming negligible loss of drug during the infusion period by:

$$V_d = dose/C_p$$

where C_p is the concentration at the end of the infusion ($\mu g/ml$). Peritoneal clearance was estimated by dividing the peritoneal excretion rate for each of the four dwell periods by the midpoint plasma concentration for each dwell period. Total tobramycin clearance (Cl) was calculated by the following equation:

$$Cl = dose/AUC$$

where AUC is the area under the curve.

Tobramycin disappearance from plasma was found to be biphasic and independent of dose. Figure 1 represents the plasma and dialysate concentration (mean ± SEM) for the four pa-

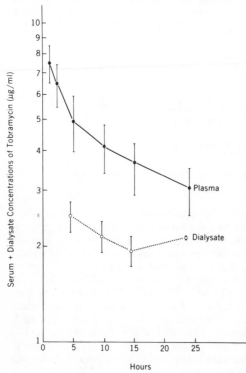

FIG. 1. *Serum and dialysate concentrations of to-bramycin in patients on continuous ambulatory peritoneal dialysis receiving 1.5 mg/kg (mean ± SEM).*

tients receiving 1.5 mg/kg. The mean peak plasma concentration of tobramycin was 7.5 μg/ml. The mean half-life for the entire group was 34.6 h (range, 21 to 70 h), and the mean volume of distribution was 15.2 liters (range, 10.3 to 17.7 liters). Analysis of the tobramycin clearance data revealed a mean dialysate clearance of 4.2 ml/min (range, 2.8 to 5.2 ml/min) and a mean total body clearance of 8.0 ml/min (range, 5.0 to 12.7 ml/min). Table 1 illustrates the concentration of tobramycin in the dialysate after each of the four dwell periods and the amount of the drug removed in the 24-h period.

The amount of tobramycin removed during the 24-h period on CAPD varied with the dose administered. At a dose of 1.5 mg/kg, 20.1 ± 1.6% of the administered dose was removed. At a dose of 1.1 and 1.3 mg/kg, 16.1 and 15.8% were removed, respectively. The mean dialysate/plasma ratio as determined from the four dwell periods was 0.63. The actual concentration of tobramycin in the dialysate decreased with each subsequent dwell period. The highest peritoneal concentration of tobramycin achieved was 3.1 μg/ml.

The results of this investigation suggest that the kinetics of elimination in patients on CAPD are variable. The apparent half-life of elimination of 34.6 h is shorter than the 54 h reported in anephric patients (1). The removal of tobramycin by CAPD was approximately 20% of the given dose in 24 h. If parenteral tobramycin is required, the usual loading dose should be administered, with half the loading dose given every half-life. As a consequence of the variability of tobramycin kinetics in these patients, the dose administered must be verified by plasma tobramycin determinations.

On the basis of this 24-h study, it appears that

TABLE 1. *Tobramycin concentration in the dialysate*

Patient	Dose (mg/kg)	Cpmax[a] (μg/ml)	Dialysate conc. (ug/ml)[b] (Amt removed/dwell (mg))				Total removed (mg) (% of dose)	D/P[c] ratio (mean)
			1	2	3	4		
1	1.5	4.5	3.1(5.95)	2.55(4.55)	2.55(4.70)	2.15(5.16)	20.3(25)	1.04
2	1.5	7.6	1.85(4.18)	1.45(4.32)	1.8(4.32)	2.10(4.56)	16.6(13.8)	0.53
3	1.5	8.9	2.3(6.4)	2.10(6.9)	1.7(5.17)	2.10(4.41)	22.9(15.0)	0.58
4	1.5	8.8	2.8(7.9)	2.5(7.6)	1.7(3.7)	2.15(4.95)	24.3(17.0)	0.365
Mean			2.5(6.1)	2.15(5.8)	1.94(4.5)	2.13(4.8)	20.1(16.5)	0.63
± SEM			0.27(0.77)	0.25(0.83)	0.21(0.31)	0.01(0.17)	1.6(1.46)	0.15
5	1.1	4.25	2.20(5.7)	1.8(3.6)	1.5(3.5)	1.45(3.3)	16.1(26)	0.70
6	1.3	5.8	2.95(5.6)	1.85(4.8)	1.2(2.5)	1.15(2.94)	15.8(26.4)	0.60

[a] Cpmax, maximum serum concentration achieved at the end of a 1-h infusion.
[b] Dialysate concentration at the end of each dwell period.
[c] Dialysate/plasma ratio for tobramycin.

the concentration of tobramycin achieved in the peritoneal cavity would be inadequate for the management of peritonitis. The effect of chronic dosing and infection on the accumulation characteristics of tobramycin cannot be assessed from this study.

1. **Lockwood, W. R., and J. D. Bower.** 1973. Tobramycin and gentamicin concentrations in serum of normal and anephric patients. Antimicrob. Agents Chemother. **3:** 125–129.
2. **Oreopoulos, D. G. M., M. Robson, S. Izatt, S. Clayton, and G. A. deVeber.** 1978. A simple and safe technique for continuous ambulatory peritoneal dialysis (CAPD). Trans. Am. Soc. Artif. Intern. Organs 24:484–489.
3. **Popovich, R. P., J. W. Moncrief, K. D. Nolph, A. J. Ghods, Z. T. Twardowski, and W. K. Pyle.** 1978. Continuous ambulatory peritoneal dialysis. Ann. Intern. Med. **88:**449–456.

Pharmacokinetics of Three Aminoglycosides During Sequential Ultrafiltration-Hemodialysis, a New Dialysis Procedure

J. KOSMIDIS,* K. SOMBOLOS, N. ZEREFOS, AND G. K. DAIKOS

First Department of Propedeutic Medicine, Athens University School of Medicine, Athens, Greece

Many patients undergoing regular hemodialysis often present with fluid retention. Conventional hemodialysis can remove extra fluids, but at a slow rate and with side effects such as hypotension and muscular contractions.

Vacuum ultrafiltration (hemofiltration, diafiltration) is a new dialysis technique especially developed to overcome this problem (1, 3). The usual artificial kidney is used but no dialysis fluid. Instead, a negative pressure is created at the space usually containing the fluid with the help of a vacuum pump. In other words, the filter separates the patient's blood from air in negative pressure. This results in quick removal of large quantities of fluids without side effects. After about 1 h, ultrafiltration is stopped and is followed by conventional hemodialysis (2).

This technique of sequential ultrafiltration-hemodialysis is fairly recent, and information about the kinetics of antibiotics during the procedure is extremely limited. Rumpf and his colleagues (4) gave one 80-mg dose of gentamicin (G) to one patient undergoing vacuum ultrafiltration for 6 h and measured blood levels. They reported that the drug was removed at a rate slower than that expected during conventional hemodialysis.

We decided, therefore, to study the kinetics of G, tobramycin (T), and amikacin (A) prospectively and thoroughly under the above conditions. These drugs are likely to be used in such patients, and since their therapeutic margin is narrow, precise calculation of dosage is necessary.

Twelve patients (seven males and five females) participated in the study. They all had creatinine clearance below 5 ml/min, a fluid overload of at least 2 kg at the time of study, and an arteriovenous fistula. Both vacuum ultrafiltration and hemodialysis were performed with the same dialysis machine (Dasco 505/KL) for all patients. On all occasions, a filter (Gambro Lundia Optima, 13.5 μm [1 m^2]) was used. One hour of vacuum ultrafiltration was followed by 3 h of conventional hemodialysis.

Each patient received one of the following antibiotic doses 2 h before the beginning of a session (four patients for each antibiotic): G, 1.5 mg/kg; T, 1.5 mg/kg; or A, 7.5 mg/kg. All doses were administered as an intravenous injection lasting 5 min. The drug was diluted in 20 ml of 5% dextrose solution.

Blood specimens (arterial and venous) were taken for assay at the beginning and every 20 min during ultrafiltration, every hour during hemodialysis, and at 20 and 44 h after the end of the session. Appropriate ultrafiltrate and dialysate specimens were also taken for calculation of plasma drug clearances. Antibiotic assay was performed with an agar well plate method, using *Bacillus subtilis* as the indicator organism. All standards and specimens were set in triplicate.

Mean values of blood levels and kinetic parameters during ultrafiltration are presented in Table 1, and those for hemodialysis are given in Table 2.

During ultrafiltration, individual arterial and venous blood levels fluctuated so much that the data were unsuitable for calculation of half-life and extraction ratio. These fluctuations were due to changing rates of fluid and drug removal with hemoconcentration, sometimes even resulting in an increase in levels. The arterial blood level at the end of the 1-h ultrafiltration was, however, lowered by an average of 7% for G, 8% for T, and 5% for A. Plasma drug clearances

TABLE 1. *Kinetics during ultrafiltration*[a]

Drug	Levels (µg/ml) at indicated times (min) after starting procedure							% of lowering	Drug clearance (ml/min)
	0	20		40		60			
		A[b]	V	A	V	A	V		
G	6.1	5.7	5.2	5.6	5.3	5.7	5.0	7	14.9
T	5.4	5.8	4.8	5.6	4.5	4.9	4.7	8	16.7
A	28.7	26.1	27.1	27.0	26.9	27.1	24.2	5	28.5

[a] Mean values for four patients for each drug.
[b] A, Arterial blood; V, venous blood.

TABLE 2. *Kinetics during hemodialysis*[a]

Drug	Levels (µg/ml) and ER[b] at indicated times (h) after starting whole procedure							Total % of lowering[c]	$t_{1/2}$ (h)	Drug clearance (ml/min)
	1	2		3		4				
		A[d]	V	A	V	A	V			
G	5.7	4.4	3.6	3.7	2.9	3.3	2.3	47	3.5	76.9
ER		0.18		0.20		0.28				
T	4.9	4.1	3.4	3.5	2.6	2.9	2.2	47	3.9	56.6
ER		0.20		0.27		0.27				
A	27.1	23.1	17.7	20.2	15.2	17.8	13.4	39	3.9	60.0
ER		0.23		0.25		0.24				

[a] Mean values of four patients for each drug.
[b] ER, Extraction ratio.
[c] Due to both ultrafiltration and hemodialysis.
[d] A, Arterial blood; V, venous blood.

averaged 14.9, 16.7, and 28.5 ml/min, respectively, for G, T, and A. These data show that removal of aminoglycosides during vacuum ultrafiltration is small.

Hemodialysis after ultrafiltration was more effective than expected in removing the antibiotics, probably because extra fluids had been already removed and no further hemoconcentration was taking place. Extraction ratios at the end of the 2nd, 3rd, and 4th h were 0.18, 0.20, and 0.28 for G, 0.20, 0.27, and 0.27 for T, and 0.23, 0.25, and 0.24 for A, respectively. Mean serum half-life during this part of the session was 3.5 h for G, 3.9 h for T, and 3.9 h for A. Plasma clearance averaged 76.9, 56.6, and 60.0 ml/min, respectively. The total lowering of blood levels during the whole procedure of sequential ultrafiltration-hemodialysis averaged 47% for G, 47% for T, and 39% for A.

Off dialysis, the blood levels were further lowered, with an average half-life of 23.3 h for G, 31.4 h for T, and 35.0 h for A, data compatible with those of the literature.

For treatment with these aminoglycosides during sequential ultrafiltration-hemodialysis, we recommend loading and presession doses as for conventional hemodialysis. At the end of the session, 50% of a maintenance dose of G and T and 40% of that of A must be added.

1. **Henderson, L. W., A. Besarab, A. S. Michaels, and L. W. Bluemle.** 1967. Blood purification by ultrafiltration and fluid replacement (diafiltration). Trans. Am. Soc. Artif. Intern. Org. **13**:216–222.
2. **Johnson, M. J., S. B. Kurtz, L. A. Brennan, J. H. Ottjes, and A. M. Pierides.** 1977. Longterm trial of separate hemofiltration followed by hemodialysis. Abstr. Kidney Int. **12**:483.
3. **Quellhorst, E., B. Doht, and B. Schuenemann.** 1977. Hemofiltration: treatment of renal failure by ultrafiltration and substitution. J. Dial. **1**:529–542.
4. **Rumpf, K. W., J. Rieger, B. Doht, R. Ansorg, and F. Scheler.** 1977. Drug elimination by hemofiltration. J. Dial. **1**:677–688.

Comparative Nephrotoxicity of SCH 21420 and Amikacin in Rats

LAURA I. RANKIN, FRIEDRICH C. LUFT,* MOO NAHM YUM, REBECCA S. SLOAN, CHARLES B. DINWIDDIE, JR., AND LINDA L. ISAACS

Department of Medicine and Department of Pathology, Indiana University School of Medicine, Indianapolis, Indiana 46223, U.S.A.*

Aminoglycosides are useful antibiotics for treatment of patients with life-threatening bacterial infections; however, their nephrotoxic potential continues to concern clinicians (1). SCH 21420, a new derivative of gentamicin B, has in vitro bactericidal activity which compares favorably with that of currently available aminoglycosides (2, 5). The proposed dose for humans is the same as that of amikacin, 15 mg/kg per day (I. Tabachnick, Schering Corp., personal communication). To compare the relative nephrotoxicities of SCH 21420 and amikacin, we studied the functional and structural effects of both drugs on the kidneys in rats.

Adult male Sprague-Dawley rats weighing 225 to 250 g were randomly assigned to 11 groups of 10 each. Four groups received SCH 21420 at doses of 100, 200, 300, and 600 mg/kg per day. Four groups received the same doses of amikacin. Two groups received saline diluent, and one group received no injections.

On the day before the first injection day (day 0), day 7, and day 14, 24-h urine specimens were collected for volume, osmolality, protein, N-acetylglucosaminidase, and creatinine concentrations. Blood was obtained from the tail for blood urea nitrogen (BUN) determination. On the day of sacrifice (day 15), creatinine was measured in serum and urine for the calculation of creatinine clearance. Kidneys from each animal were weighed and prepared for light microscopy by standard techniques (3). Histological changes were graded as follows by a pathologist unaware of the regimens: grade 0, normal; grade 1, cloudy swelling of proximal tubular epithelium without necrosis; grade 2, necrosis and/or regeneration of 25% of the cortical area; grade 3, necrosis and/or regeneration of 25% but <50% of the cortical area; grade 4, necrosis and/or regeneration of 50% but <75% of the cortical area; and grade 5, necrosis of >75% of the cortical area. Statistical comparisons were performed by one-way analysis of variance. Where differences were shown, Duncan's multiple-range statistic was used for comparisons. Since the saline-injected and non-injected groups were not significantly different, data from these groups were pooled.

The excretion of N-acetylglucosamine was the most sensitive indicator of nephrotoxicity. After 2 weeks of therapy, significant enzymuria compared with controls was observed at all four doses of amikacin and the three higher doses of SCH 21420 ($P < 0.05$). Urinary protein excretion was significantly increased in a dose-related fashion after 7 days of treatment with either drug, but more so with amikacin, at doses of ≥300 mg/kg per day ($P < 0.05$). Amikacin at 600 mg/kg per day increased protein excretion further by day 15 ($P < 0.05$). Amikacin at 300 mg/kg per day increased the BUN by day 15 ($P < 0.05$), whereas amikacin at 600 mg/kg per day increased the BUN by day 7. An additional elevation was observed by day 15 ($P < 0.05$). SCH 21420 caused no BUN elevations until 14 days of treatment with the 600-mg/kg-per-day dose. The changes observed with amikacin at that dose were greater than those with SCH 21420 on both days 7 and 15 ($P < 0.05$). Both drugs decreased urine osmolality at the two higher doses.

The results of creatinine clearance measurements and pathological scores are displayed in Table 1. No change in creatinine clearance was observed until either drug was administered at 600 mg/kg per day. The pathological scores increased in a stepwise fashion as the dose of amikacin was increased. The administration of SCH 21420 at 100 mg/kg per day did not result

TABLE 1. *Creatinine clearance and pathology score at sacrifice[a]*

Drug and dose (mg/kg)	Creatinine clearance (ml/min)[b]	Pathology score[c]
Amikacin		
100	1.3 ± 0.1	1.2 ± 0.2
200	1.4 ± 0.1	3.1 ± 0.2
300	1.2 ± 0.2	3.9 ± 0.3
600	0.7 ± 0.1	4.8 ± 0.1
SCH 21420		
100	1.5 ± 0.1	0.6 ± 0.2[d]
200	1.5 ± 0.1	2.1 ± 0.2[d]
300	1.4 ± 0.2	3.0 ± 0.3[d]
600	0.8 ± 0.1	4.7 ± 0.2

[a] Values are mean ± SEM.
[b] Saline control = 1.5 ± 0.1 ml/min.
[c] Saline control = 0.
[d] Different from corresponding group ($P < 0.05$).

in demonstrable pathological injury; however, above that level, stepwise increases in dose resulted in increased injury. At each dose level except the highest, the histological changes were greater with amikacin ($P < 0.05$).

The data suggest that SCH 21420 compares favorably with amikacin in its nephrotoxic potential at lower doses in rats. SCH 21420 may exhibit a dose-response nephrotoxicity relationship which is initially less steep than that of amikacin. SCH 21420 does, however, cause functional and structural renal injury typical for this class of antimicrobial agents. Since SCH 21420 compares favorably with amikacin in its in vitro activity against many aerobic gram-negative bacilli and *Staphylococcus aureus* (2, 4, 5), and also exhibits documented synergism with penicillin against enterococci (4), it appears that SCH 21420 may be a valuable addition to the aminoglycoside armamentarium.

1. **Appel, B. G., and H. C. Neu.** 1977. The nephrotoxicity of antimicrobial agents. N. Engl. J. Med. **296:**722–728.
2. **Kabins, S. A., and C. Nathan.** 1978. In vitro activity of SCH 21420, derivative of gentamicin B, compared to that of amikacin. Antimicrob. Agents Chemother. **14:** 786–787.
3. **Luft, F. C., R. Bloch, R. S. Sloan, M. N. Yum, R. Costello, and D. R. Maxwell.** 1978. Comparative nephrotoxicity of aminoglycoside antibiotics in rats. J. Infect. Dis. **138:**541–545.
4. **Sanders, S. C., W. E. Sanders, and R. V. Goering.** 1978. *In vitro* studies with SCH 21420 and SCH 22591: activity in comparison with six other aminoglycosides and synergy with penicillin against enterococci. Antimicrob. Agents Chemother. **14:**178–184.
5. **Yu, P. K. W., and J. A. Washington.** 1978. In vitro evaluation of a semisynthetic derivative of gentamicin B (SCH 21420). Antimicrob. Agents Chemother. **13:** 891–892.

Gentamicin-Induced Glomerular Injury

ANDREW P. EVAN, JEFFREY HUSER, P. S. AVASTHI,
LAURA I. RANKIN, AND FRIEDRICH C. LUFT*

Departments of Anatomy and Medicine, University of New Mexico, Albuquerque, New Mexico, and Department of Medicine, Indiana University School of Medicine, Indianapolis, Indiana 46223,* U.S.A.

The renal injury produced by gentamicin is characterized by damage to proximal tubular epithelial cells. Functionally, gentamicin-induced renal injury results in proteinuria, enzymuria, glycosuria, impaired urinary concentrating ability, and a decrease in glomerular filtration rate (2). Recently it was shown that gentamicin administration in rats caused a reduction in glomerular ultrafiltration coefficient (K_f) even at doses which did not substantially impair tubular integrity (1). Although studies of glomerular ultrastructure by transmission electron microscopy failed to reveal any abnormalities, the reduction in K_f was attributed to undetected morphological changes in glomerular filtration area (2). These findings suggested that in addition to its known effect on renal tubular epithelium, gentamicin resulted in glomerular injury as well. The present studies were undertaken to examine the effects of gentamicin on glomerular morphology in an attempt to elucidate the previous observation that even low doses of gentamicin reduce K_f.

Three groups of Sprague-Dawley rats were studied in the first series of experiments. Group I, six normal control rats, was given daily intraperitoneal injections of isotonic saline for 10 days. Group II, eight experimental rats, received intraperitoneal injections of 4 mg of gentamicin per kg (body weight) per day for 10 days. Group III, eight experimental rats, received 40 mg of gentamicin per kg daily for 10 days. On the 12th day, rats were anesthetized and the clearance of inulin (C_I) was determined. Thereafter, the kidneys were perfused with 30 ml of 0.9% NaCl followed by 30 ml of 2.5% glutaraldehyde in 0.075 M sodium cacodylate-HCl buffer, pH 7.4. After in situ fixation, portions of the outer cortex of the kidney were removed, cut into 1-mm cubes, and further fixed in the same fixative for an additional 48 h. Specimens of renal tissue were assigned numbers and read without knowledge of the regimens. Superficial 2-mm sections of renal cortical tissue were obtained from all samples. Small blocks of tissues were routinely prepared for transmission electron microscopy (Philips EM-200 electron microscope). Larger pieces were washed in sodium cacodylate-HCl buffer for 90 min, dehydrated through a series of alcohols to 100% ethanol, fractured in liquid nitrogen, transferred to a Samdri critical-point dryer, and dried with liquid CO_2. Tissues were attached to an aluminum stub and placed in a vacuum evaporator with a rotating stage for gold-palladium coating. Specimens were examined and photographed in an ETEC autoscan

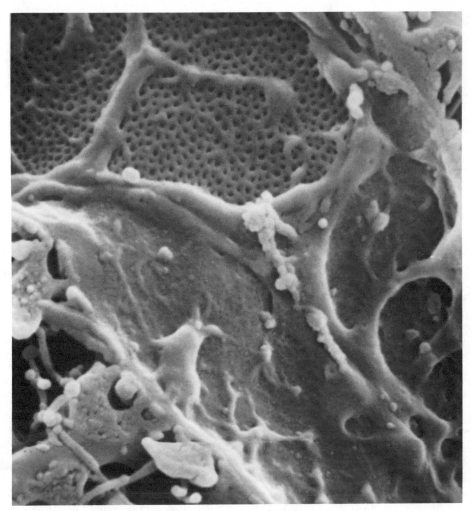

FIG. 1. *Epithelial surface with normal-appearing interdigitating foot processes. Gentamicin administration caused no epithelial changes (×30,000).*

scanning electron microscope operating at an accelerating voltage of 20 kV. Photographs were taken at a minimal tilt (angle of 5°) to render the difference in magnification between foreground and background of the image (perspective error) to minimum.

In the second series of experiments, four groups of eight rats each received the following regimens for 4 weeks: regular diet, sham injection; regular diet, gentamicin at 20 mg/kg per day; 8% salt diet, sham injection; and 8% salt diet, gentamicin at 20 mg/kg per day. At 4 weeks, control and experimental rats were housed in metabolism cages for 48 h, and 24-h urine specimens were collected. The animals were anesthetized with pentobarbital, and blood specimens were obtained for creatinine clearance (C_{Cr}) measurements. Whole-body perfusion with 0.1% procaine in normal saline followed by 2.5% glutaraldehyde in 0.15 M cacodylate-HCl buffer (pH 7.3) was performed. Thereafter the tissue was prepared and studied as described earlier.

C_I was sharply decreased at 10 days by the 40-mg/kg-per-day dose ($P < 0.001$). The 4-mg/kg-per-day dose resulted in changes that approached significance. C_{Cr} was not significantly decreased at 4 weeks of continuous gentamicin treatment at 20 mg/kg per day irrespective of sodium intake.

The architecture of visceral epithelial glomerular cells was normal by scanning and transmission electron microscopy in all experiments. Long primary and secondary processes with slender short interdigitating pedicels of epithelial cells were seen in both control and experimental rats (Fig. 1).

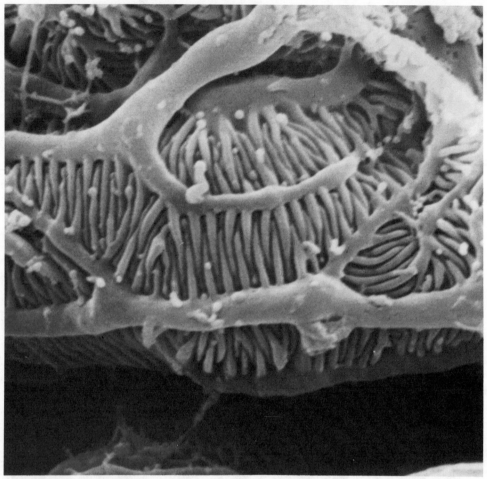

FIG. 2. *Endothelial surface from an animal receiving gentamicin at 20 mg/kg per day and an 8% salt diet for 4 weeks. Although a portion of normal-appearing endothelium with preserved fenestrae is present, a considerable portion shows obliterated fenestrae and bulbous projections (×60,000).*

By scanning electron microscopy, the glomerular changes found in the gentamicin-treated groups were confined to the glomerular endothelial cells. The density and the diameter of the endothelial fenestrae were markedly reduced in the rats treated with gentamicin. The changes were to a degree dose dependent. The reduction in the density and diameter of endothelial cell fenestrae was not uniform in all phases of all capillaries. Marked reduction occurred in fenestral area in groups receiving gentamicin at 40 or 20 mg/kg per day and regular diet as compared with controls. Rats receiving gentamicin at 20 mg/kg per day and 8% salt diet (Fig. 2) and 4 mg/kg per day revealed less prominent, albeit easily detectable, injury.

The present experiments suggest that the previously observed decreases in K_f after gentamicin treatment occur as a consequence of a decrease in the filtration area of glomerular capillaries. The diameter, density, and area of endothelial fenestrae was significantly diminished by all of the regimens used. Previous studies have shown that solute and water traverse the glomerular capillary wall largely through an extracellular pathway consisting of endothelial fenestrae, glomerular basement membrane, rectangular slit diaphragm pores, and filtration slits. The most striking morphological alteration we observed was a reduction in the area of endothelial fenestrae. Since water is predominantly transported through this filtration pathway, a reduction in area would be expected to reduce K_f.

The pathogenesis of the structural alterations we observed remains to be determined. The changes may have resulted from a direct toxic effect of gentamicin on the glomerular capillary endothelial cells. Alternatively, the glomerular endothelial changes may have been produced via a tubular injury. In this context, it should be emphasized that glomerular K_f has been shown to decrease after the infusion of angiotensin II into the renal artery. It is possible that tubular injury initiated the activation of the renin system at the macula densa and that locally released angiotensin II participated in the production of the endothelial alterations.

In conclusion, gentamicin administration results in striking glomerular endothelial injury which is demonstrable by scanning, but not by transmission, electron microscopy. It is likely that the morphological changes explain previously observed changes in K_f after gentamicin treatment.

1. **Baylis, C., H. R. Rennke, and B. M. Brenner.** 1975. Mechanisms of the defect in glomerular ultrafiltration associated with gentamicin administration. Kidney Int. **12:**344–353.
2. **Luft, F. C., R. Bloch, R. S. Sloan, M. N. Yum, R. Costello, and D. R. Maxwell.** 1978. Comparative aminoglycoside nephrotoxicity in rats. J. Infect. Dis. **138:** 541–545.

Renal Subcellular Distribution of Gentamicin During Experimental Nephrotoxicity

SUE J. KOHLHEPP,* SANDY THOMPSON, DON C. HOUGHTON, RODNEY CONNOR, AND DAVID N. GILBERT

Providence Medical Center* and University of Oregon Health Sciences Center, Portland, Oregon 97213, U.S.A.

The potential nephrotoxicity of gentamicin and other aminoglycoside antibiotics is well known. We have used male Fischer rats to characterize many features of aminoglycoside renal injury (2). Histological study has shown cyclical changes in the cells of the proximal tubule during continuous gentamicin administration (1). Lysosome abnormalities appear after 3 days; progressive cellular necrosis is evident after 7 to 10 days; and, finally, cellular regeneration is complete after 17 to 21 days.

It was the purpose of this study to try to correlate the histopathological changes with the intracellular gentamicin distribution over the first 7 days of drug administration.

Male Fischer rats, 200 to 250 g, were given gentamicin, 40 mg/kg per day, in two equally divided doses subcutaneously. The animals were sacrificed after 2 h, 1 day, 3 days, and 7 days of drug exposure. The kidneys were perfused as previously described (2). The cortex of both kidneys was dissected, weighed, minced, and rinsed with tris(hydroxymethyl)aminomethane buffer, pH 7.4. The cortex tissue was homogenized in a glass mortar and pestle. The homogenate was then fractionated by standard differential centrifugation procedures (5). Briefly, the nucleus-whole cell fraction was pelleted by centrifugation for 10 min at 960 × g and verified by microscopic examination. The supernatant was centrifuged at 5,200 × g for 10 min to pellet mitochondria. The resulting supernatant was centrifuged at 25,000 × g for 30 min to pellet lysosomes, and the lysosome supernatant was centrifuged at 48,250 × g for 1 h to pellet ribosomes. The final supernatant was labeled cytosol. All of the pellets and the final supernatant were assayed for acid phosphatase, lactate dehydrogenase (LDH), and protein by standard methods. Gentamicin concentration was determined by radioimmunoassay.

To determine the affinity of gentamicin for subcellular constituents in vitro, gentamicin was added to rat renal homogenates under a variety of conditions. Homogenates from untreated rats were incubated with 650 μg of gentamicin per g of kidney for 2 h at 4 or 37°C and then fractionated as above. In addition, gentamicin, 650 μg per g of kidney, was added in vitro to renal homogenate obtained from rats who had been given 2, 6, or 10 mg of potassium dichromate 48 h previously. Dichromate was chosen because the pathological changes produced were virtually identical to those found after gentamicin administration.

LDH was chosen as a cytosol marker. In subcellular fractions from untreated animals, LDH percentage distribution was as follows: cytosol, 83%; ribosomes, 4%; lysosomes, 4%; mitochondria, 4%; and nucleus-whole cell, 5%. Acid phosphatase did not prove as reliable a marker for lysosomes. The acid phosphatase percentage

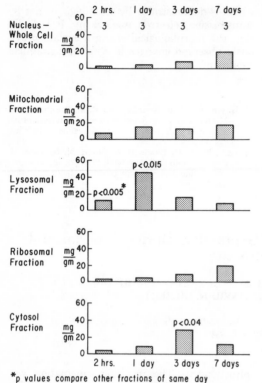

*p values compare other fractions of same day

FIG. 1. *Renal cortical subcellular distribution of gentamicin after various lengths of in vivo administration of gentimicin, 40 mg/kg per day in two divided doses, to male Fischer rats. Each bar represents the mean value of three experimental animals. Results are expressed as milligrams of gentamicin per gram of protein.*

distribution was: cytosol, 24%; ribosomes, 24%; lysosomes, 31%; mitochondria, 13%; and nucleus-whole cell, 8%. Lysosome contamination of other fractions was not evident by electron microscopy.

The distribution of gentamicin in the subcellular fractions over 7 days of in vivo administration is shown in Fig. 1. During the first 24 h, the apparent preferential association with lysosomes was such that the gentamicin concentration in this fraction was statistically greater than that found in any other fraction ($P < 0.02$). By day 3, the lysosome fraction contained little gentamicin and the concentration in the cytosol fraction exceeded that of all other fractions ($P < 0.04$). After 7 days, there was no evidence of preferential association of the drug for any specific fraction.

The in vitro addition of gentamicin produced quite dissimilar results. After incubation at 4°C, gentamicin preferentially associated with the ri-

bosome fraction ($P < 0.01$, compared with all other fractions; Fig. 2). After 37°C, the drug was evenly distributed among all fractions. The difference in gentamicin association with the ribosome fraction may have resulted from loss of ribosome integrity at 37°C.

The results of the in vitro addition of gentamicin to homogenates of potassium dichromate-damaged kidneys is also shown in Fig. 2. Note that these fractionations were all conducted at 4°C. Regardless of the dichromate dose used in vitro, gentamicin was found in greatest concentration in the ribosome fraction ($P < 0.02$).

Previous reports used autoradiography to demonstrate the in vivo association of gentamicin with lysosomes of the renal proximal tubular cells over the first 24 h of drug exposure (3, 4, 6). Our studies extended these observations by following the intracellular gentamicin distribution during 7 days of continuous drug exposure. The results confirmed the early association of gentamicin with lysosomes. This association was

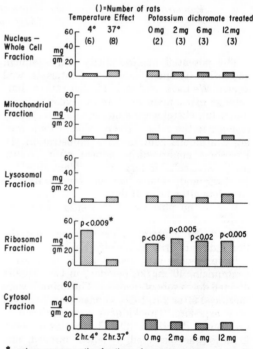

*p values compare other fractions of same treatment

FIG. 2. *Renal cortical subcellular distribution of gentamicin after the in vitro addition of 650 µg of gentamicin per g (wet weight) of kidney cortex. Kidney cortices were obtained from either untreated male Fischer rats or animals given increasing doses of potassium dichromate. Each bar represents the mean value for that group. Results are expressed as milligrams of gentamicin per gram of protein.*

short-lived, and after 3 days the drug was found primarily in the cytosol. After 7 days, the drug was distributed fairly evenly throughout all subcellular fractions. These findings correlate with the histological evidence of lysosomal changes (e.g., cytosegresomes) during the first 1 to 2 days of gentamicin exposure. One could postulate that the shift in gentamicin from the lysosomal cellular fraction to the cytosol is an indication that the histologically damaged lysosomes are unable to continue to sequester the drug. It could be further hypothesized that the generalized subcellular distribution of gentamicin after 7 days of in vivo exposure indicates interaction of the drug with cellular constituents exposed only as progressive necrosis develops.

The results of the in vitro addition of gentamicin to renal homogenates was quite different from the in vivo data. This result argues against the possibility that the in vivo results represent nonspecific binding of gentamicin which might have occurred during the homogenization procedure. To control for the possibility that the in vivo results represented nonspecific binding during homogenization to damaged renal tubules, we produced tubular injury with potassium di-

chromate and then added gentamicin in vitro. The pattern of gentamicin distribution was the same as the pattern of in vitro binding to renal homogenates from untreated control animals.

In summary, these studies demonstrate a cyclical change in the renal subcellular distribution of gentamicin over 7 days of in vivo exposure.

1. **Gilbert, D. N., D. C. Houghton, W. M. Bennett, C. E. Plamp, K. Reger, and G. A. Porter.** 1979. Reversibility of gentamicin nephrotoxicity in rats: recovery during continuous drug administration. Proc. Soc. Exp. Biol. Med. **160**:99–103.
2. **Gilbert, D. N., C. Plamp, P. R. Starr, W. M. Bennett, D. C. Houghton, and G. A. Porter.** 1978. Comparative nephrotoxicity of gentamicin and tobramycin. Antimicrob. Agents Chemother. **13**:34–40.
3. **Just, M., G. Erdmann, and E. Habermann.** 1977. The renal handling of polybasic drugs. I. Gentamicin and aprotinin in intact animals. Naunyn-Schmiedeberg's Arch. Pharmacol. **300**:57–66.
4. **Kuhar, M. J., L. L. Mak, and P. S. Lietman.** 1979. Autoradiographic localization of [^{3}H]gentamicin in the proximal tubules of mice. Antimicrob. Agents Chemother. **15**:131–133.
5. **Lehninger, A. L.** 1975. Biochemistry, p. 380–382. 2nd ed. Worth Publishers, New York.
6. **Silverblatt, F. J., and C. Kuehn.** 1979. Autoradiography of gentamicin uptake by the rat proximal tubule cell. Kidney Int. **15**:335–345.

Gentamicin Binding to Renal Proximal Tubule Brush Border Membranes

RICHARD S. JERAULD* AND FREDRIC J. SILVERBLATT

Wadsworth and Sepulveda Veterans Administration Medical Centers, Los Angeles, California 91343, U.S.A.

Gentamicin injures the epithelium of the renal proximal convoluted tubule. This injury has been associated with the accumulation of high levels of gentamicin in the renal cortex. Autoradiographic studies demonstrate that the major portion of gentamicin that accumulates in the renal cortex enters the proximal tubule cell by pinocytosis from the apical (brush border) side of the cell (3, 6). Filtered gentamicin undergoes pinocytosis when the crypts and invaginations at the base of the brush border membrane pinch off to form apical vesicles. These apical vesicles, with sequestered gentamicin, migrate centripetally and coalesce with preexisting secondary lysosomes. Autoradiographic studies demonstrate that the resulting secondary lysosomes are the site of gentamicin accumulation in the renal cortex.

Several investigators have reported that gentamicin binds in vitro to membrane vesicles de-

rived from the brush border of the proximal tubule cell (4, 5). Brush border membrane vesicles are formed when apical membranes are fragmented and the resulting subunits round up and "reanneal" to form vesicular structures. The present study was undertaken to see whether the in vitro binding of gentamicin to brush border membrane vesicles resulted from gentamicin binding to apical crypts, which might represent the first step in the pinocytosis of gentamicin. This was accomplished by comparing the binding of gentamicin to two different forms of brush border membrane vesicles: one derived from intact sheets of brush border membranes containing apical crypts (whole vesicles), the other derived from sheared microvilli, lacking apical crypts (microvillus vesicles). Although whole brush border vesicles appear to preserve apical crypts capable of binding various substrates, the vesicles are not capable of carrying on pinocytosis in vitro. Whole brush border vesicles were prepared by the method of Aronson and Sacktor (1). Microvillus vesicles were prepared by the method of Beck and Sacktor (2). The quality of membrane preparations was evaluated by the measurement of γ-glutamyltranspeptidase and by electron microscopy.

Binding of gentamicin to brush border membrane vesicles was measured by the membrane filtration technique. Fifty microliters of membrane vesicles, 150 to 300 μg of protein, was incubated for 30 min at 24°C with 50 μl of buffered mannitol (300 mM) containing varying concentrations of tritiated gentamicin (0.1 to 1,000 μM). Preliminary determinations had shown that gentamicin binding occurred in a time-dependent fashion and that binding was 98 to 100% complete within 30 min. Whole membrane vesicles were washed on 5.0-μm membrane filters (Millipore Corp., Bedford, Mass.), and microvillus membrane vesicles were washed on 0.65-μm membrane filters. Standard liquid scintillation counting was used. The concentration of bound gentamicin versus the ratio of bound to free gentamicin was determined for each incubation.

To demonstrate that gentamicin uptake represented binding to the surface of membrane vesicles rather than movement into the interior of the vesicles, gentamicin uptake was measured at different medium osmolarities. (Increasing medium osmolarity reduces intravesicular volume and should reduce the amount of gentamicin within the intravesicular space, but should not affect the amount of gentamicin bound to the vesicle surface.) Medium osmolarity had only a modest effect on gentamicin uptake, suggesting that the majority of gentamicin uptake

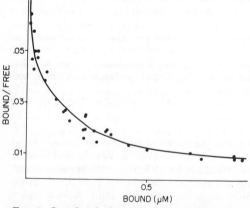

FIG. 1. Scatchard plot of gentamicin binding to whole brush border vesicles (150 μg of protein); tritiated gentamicin concentrations, 0.1 to 100 μM; 30 incubations, 100-μl volume.

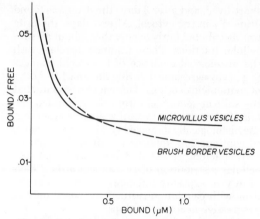

FIG. 2. Representative Scatchard plots of gentamicin binding to microvillus and whole brush border vesicles. Conditions as in Fig. 1.

by whole brush border vesicles represented binding to the vesicle surface rather than movement into the intravesicular space.

Scatchard analysis of gentamicin binding to whole brush border vesicles is depicted in Fig. 1. This type of curvilinear binding plot was observed for both microvillus and whole brush border vesicles. Although there was some variation in the position of individual curves, the gentamicin-binding plots for microvillus and whole brush border vesicles were very similar (Fig. 2).

This consistent pattern of curvilinear Scatchard plots implies that there is not a unique affinity constant for gentamicin binding to brush border membranes. (Calculation of a unique affinity constant requires a linear Scatchard plot.) It should be noted that a straight line drawn tangent to the rightward portion of the Scatchard plots could be used to calculate an affinity constant consistent with the previously reported value of 5 mM^{-1} (5). However, the entirety of each Scatchard plot was clearly curvilinear, consistent with higher orders of gentamicin binding. Interpretation of curvilinear Scatchard plots is not straightforward since they sometimes represent specific binding phenomena (e.g., insulin receptor binding) and sometimes merely result from nonspecific binding. Further investigation will be required to evaluate the specificity of the gentamicin binding demonstrated in this study.

The similar gentamicin binding demonstrated for microvillus and whole brush border vesicles suggests that gentamicin binds exclusively to microvilli, or that it binds equally and perhaps nonspecifically to both microvilli and apical crypts. The present study does not rule out an exclusive, more subtle order of gentamicin binding to apical crypts; however, the gentamicin binding observed under the experimental conditions in this study largely reflects binding to microvilli rather than binding to apical crypts. Since pinocytosis of gentamicin is initiated at the apical crypts, it is unlikely that the gentamicin binding observed in this and similar studies relates to the in vivo phenomena of pinocytosis and intracellular accumulation of gentamicin.

1. **Aronson, P. S., and B. Sacktor.** 1975. The sodium gradient-dependent transport of D-glucose in renal brush border membranes. J. Biol. Chem. **250**:6032–6039.

2. **Beck, J. C., and B. Sacktor.** 1978. The sodium electrochemical potential-mediated uphill transport of D-glucose in renal brush border membrane vesicles. J. Biol. Chem. **253**:5531–5535.

3. **Just, M., G. Erdmann, and E. Habermann.** 1977. The renal handling of polybasic drugs. I. Gentamicin and aprotinin in intact animals. Naunyn-Schmiedeberg's Arch. Pharmacol. **300**:57–66.

4. **Just, M., and E. Habermann.** 1977. The renal handling of polybasic drugs. II. *In vitro* studies with brush border and lysosomal preparations. Naunyn-Schmiedeberg's Arch. Pharmacol. **300**:67–76.

5. **Lipsky, J. J., L. Cheng, B. Sacktor, and P. S. Lietman.** 1979. Gentamicin uptake by renal proximal tubule brush border membranes. Clin. Res. **27**:236A.

6. **Silverblatt, F. J., and C. Kuehn.** 1979. Autoradiography of gentamicin uptake by the rat proximal tubule cell. Kidney Int. **15**:335–345.

Effect of Various Cephalosporins in Combination with Aminoglycosides on the Brush Border Membrane of the Human Kidney

A. W. MONDORF,* J. HUNDT, G. F. SODER, T. STEFANESCU,
G. MACKENRODT, J. E. SCHERBERICH, AND W. SCHOEPPE

Center of Internal Medicine, Department of Nephrology, Johann Wolfgang Goethe-University, Frankfurt, Federal Republic of Germany

The use of aminoglycosides and cephalosporins, alone and in combination, as well as ureidopenicillins to treat serious infections, especially those due to *Pseudomonas aeruginosa* and to certain members of the *Enterobacteriaceae*, is widespread. Clinical experience with these agents has revealed a nephrotoxic potential and the need for more knowledge of all aspects of nephrotoxicity that may occur during clinical use. In particular, there is little knowledge of pathological changes that could reliably be associated with early renal damage. Although standard renal function tests are used extensively to monitor aminoglycoside nephrotoxicity, they indicate functional impairment for which the kidney cannot compensate and hence reflect an amount of damage that is substantially beyond an early stage. Similarly, proteinuria and cylindruria are strong indicators of nephrotoxicity.

Various enzymes that originate in the kidney and other portions of the genitourinary tract are excreted into the urine under normal conditions. In certain disease states, the excretion of some of these enzymes is altered. A known site of aminoglycoside nephrotoxicity is the proximal tubule. We considered the enzymes that originate in this portion of the nephron and began our investigations with alanine aminopeptidase (AAP) (1, 3, 5). On the basis of these observa-tions, we postulated that an abnormal increase in urinary excretion of AAP after drug administration represents pathological alterations in the brush border membrane and that greater enzyme excretion begins at an early stage of developing nephrotoxicity. By using cephalosporins and aminoglycosides in extensive comparative studies in healthy volunteers, we showed that cephalosporins, unlike aminoglycosides, had no nephrotoxic effects (2, 4). We have now completed these studies with investigations on mezlocillin, piperacillin, and combinations of various cephalosporins with aminoglycosides.

By using the applied model, urine was collected 1 or 2 days before application of the drug on 3 consecutive days. Samples were also collected 3 or 6 days after drug application. All examined aminoglycosides in clinically comparable daily dosages (amikacin, 10 mg/kg; gentamicin, 3 mg/kg; netilmicin, 3 mg/kg; ribostamycin, 15 mg/kg; sisomicin, 3 mg/kg; and tobramycin, 3 mg/kg) showed a statistically significant increase after application of the different drugs on the 3rd and 4th days after administration. In all cases, a cumulative increase in AAP elimination was observed. The highest values of AAP activity in urine could, in accordance with the accumulation of the aminoglycosides in tissue of the kidney, be measured 1 day after the last application (2). At the time of greatest AAP

TABLE 1. *AAP activity in 24-h urine samples after treatment with gentamicin alone and in combination[a]*

		AAP activity				
Time	Day	Gentamicin (3 mg/kg per day) with:				Gentamicin, 3 mg/kg per day
		Cephalothin, 8 g/day	Cefuroxime, 6 g/day	Cefazolin, 6 g/day	Cefazedon, 6 g/day	
Before application	−1	2,377	1,514	1,773	2,104	2,149
Application	1	2,098	1,793	2,369	2,516	3,274
	2	3,162	3,027	3,662	3,697	4,575
	3	3,518	4,928	5,980	6,370	5,537
After application	4	6,321	6,803	8,068	8,046	6,154
	5	7,073	5,178	6,318	7,937	4,826
	7	4,687 (6)	2,719	2,796 (6)	4,698	3,042
Mean		4,176	3,708	4,423	5,052	4,422
SE		1,926	1,964	2,372	2,453	1,445

[a] Test groups of 10 healthy subjects given two doses of gentamicin in combination with various cephalosporins were compared with a test group of 15 healthy subjects given gentamicin alone at 3 mg/kg per day (mean values). The cephalosporins were administered intravenously 30 min before gentamicin was injected intramuscularly.

TABLE 2. *AAP activity in 24-h urine samples after treatment with tobramycin alone and in combination*

		AAP activity				
Time	Day	Tobramycin (3 mg/kg per day) with:				Tobramycin, 3 mg/kg per day, n = 15
		Cephalothin, 8 g/day, n = 15	Cefuroxime, 6 g/day, n = 6	Cefoxitin, 6 g/day, n = 10	Cefamandole, 6 g/day, n = 15	
Before application	−1	2,210	1,576	2,652	2,198	2,401
Application	1	2,185	2,018	1,846	2,318	2,440
	2	2,559	2,478	2,559	2,458	3,063
	3	4,241	3,077	2,968	3,657	3,149
After application	4	4,921	4,789	4,822	4,719	4,109
	5	3,498	3,492	3,480	3,402	3,256
	7	2,707	1,941	2,857	2,612	2,407
Mean		3,188	2,767	3,026	3,052	2,975
SE		1,064	1,114	932	920	624

elimination, there were statistically significant differences among the aminoglycosides; tobramycin was statistically significantly different from all the others except netilmicin (3 mg/kg). Doubling the daily dose nearly doubled the AAP activity in the 24-h urine samples. The cephalosporins (cefamandole, cefazedon, cefazolin, cefoxitin, cefotaxime, cefuroxime, cephacetril, cephalothin), piperacillin, and mezlocillin had almost no effect on proximal tubular membranes. With the same model we demonstrated that only cephacetril caused a slight increase in AAP production. During and after application of any of the cephalosporins, piperacillin, or mezlocillin, creatinine in serum and creatinine clearance showed no pathological deviations.

Combinations of gentamicin (3 mg/kg) with cefazedon (6 g), cefazolin (6 g), cefuroxime (6 g), and cephalothin (8 g) and combinations of tobramycin (3 mg/kg) with cefamandole (6 g),

cefoxitin (6 g), cefuroxime (6 g), and cephalothin (8 g) ordered themselves after the potential toxicity of the respective aminoglycoside in the combination (Tables 1, 2). The slight additive effect seen in the combinations with gentamicin on the 1st day after the last application was probably caused by differences in the individual susceptibilities of the test groups, possibly due to different numbers of high responders.

The difference between gentamicin and tobramycin was also evident to a statistically significant degree in their combinations with cephalosporins. A study of the same test group in a 4-month interval made this clear. The combination of cefuroxime and tobramycin produced to a statistically significant degree less enzyme elimination than the combination of cefuroxime with gentamicin. Neither protective nor additive effects of the combination of cephalosporins with aminoglycosides were observable in these studies. At no time, either during or after application of the drug combinations, were kidney function parameters pathologically changed.

This study was supported by grant 207-6 from the Deutsche Forschungsgemeinschaft.

1. Burchardt, U., J. E. Peters, L. Neef, H. Thulin, C. A. Gründig, and R. J. Haschen. 1977. Der diagnostische Wert von Enzymbestimmungen im Harn. Z. Med. Labor.-Diagn. **18**:190–212.

2. Mondorf, A. W., J. Breier, J. Hendus, J. E. Scherberich, G. Mackenrodt, P. M. Shah, W. Stille, and W. Schoeppe. 1978. The effect of aminoglycosides on proximal tubular membranes of the human kidney. Eur. J. Clin. Pharmacol. **13**:133–142.

3. Mondorf, A. W., R. Kinne, J. E. Scherberich, and F. Falkenberg. 1972. Isolierung, enzymatische und immunologische Charakterisierung einer Plasmafraktion vom proximalen Tubulus der menschlichen Niere. Clin. Chim. Acta **37**:25–32.

4. Mondorf, A. W., M. Zegelman, J. Klose, L. Maske, J. E. Scherberich, T. Stefanescu, H. Müller, and W. Schoeppe. 1978. Effect of various cephalosporins on the proximal tubule of the human kidney. Eur. J. Clin. Pharmacol. **13**:357–363.

5. Scherberich, J. E., F. Falkenberg, A. W. Mondorf, H. Müller, and G. Pfleiderer. 1974. Biochemical and immunological studies on isolated brush border membranes of human kidney and their membrane surface proteins. Clin. Chim. Acta **55**:179–197.

Gentamicin Uptake and Nephrotoxicity in Immature Rats

STUART M. MACLEOD* AND WILLIAM A. MAHON

Hospital for Sick Children * *and University of Toronto, Toronto, Canada M5G1X8*

Gentamicin is commonly used to treat newborn babies in spite of its narrow margin of safety and the difficulties inherent in dosage adjustment during a period of rapidly changing renal function. More than 80% of babies weighing less than 1,500 g at birth receive gentamicin during their initial hospitalization in our neonatal intensive care unit. It has been estimated that 5 to 10% of adults receiving gentamicin will experience mild degrees of renal damage (1), but comparable estimates of nephrotoxicity in newborns are not available and the relative sensitivity of the immature kidney tubule to the toxic effects of gentamicin is controversial. We have studied gentamicin uptake and gentamicin-induced biochemical and ultrastructural changes in kidneys of immature Sprague-Dawley rats in a preliminary approach to this question.

Deficiencies in renal function in rats during the first weeks of postnatal life have been well described, and development is analogous to human maturation (2). Changes in both glomerular filtration and tubular transport are relevant to gentamicin toxicity because damage to the proximal tubular cell will be influenced by concentration in glomerular filtrate and by active tubular absorption of the drug. Gentamicin uptake in maturing renal cortical cells may be low, with a corresponding reduction in toxicity.

Rats aged 1 day and 1, 2, 3, and 10 weeks were studied after acute treatment with gentamicin (80 mg/kg) including a tracer dose of tritiated gentamicin (1 μCi/100 g of body weight). Renal uptake of gentamicin was calculated 24 h after dosing by tissue incineration to yield tritiated water. Subcellular distribution was also determined by differential centrifugation. Nephrotoxicity was assessed by measure of enzymuria (3). Concentrations of *N*-acetylglucosaminidase, lactic acid dehydrogenase, and gamma-glutamyl transpeptidase were measured. The disposition of gentamicin at the ages treated is represented in Table 1. Concentrations were lower than those in adult at birth and at 2 and 3 weeks of age and equivalent to adult in animals aged 1 week. Urinary concentrations of *N*-acetylglucosaminidase were increased above control at ages 1 day and 1 week, but enzymuria did not appear to be a reliable marker of renal damage after acute gentamicin dosing. Light microscopy was unremarkable, but electron micrographs showed significant change, with the appearance of cytosegresomes with myeloid bodies in many proximal tubular cells.

Rats aged 1, 2, and 10 weeks at time of sacrifice were treated subchronically with gentamicin (40 mg/kg twice daily) for 7 days (to age 1 week), 14 days (to age 2 weeks), or 5 and 10 days (to age 10 weeks). Treatment for the final 24 h was identical to that used in the acute studies described above, and comparable measurements were made.

Kidney weight relative to control was slightly reduced in subchronically treated 1-week-old rats but increased by 15% in 2-week-old rats and by 32% in adults. Gentamicin uptake as a per-

TABLE 1. *Gentamicin distribution after acute (80 mg/kg) and subchronic (40 mg/kg twice daily) doses*[a]

Dose and age	% Distribution				Total gentamicin concn (μg/g of kidney wt)	Renal concn as % of final dose
	Nuclear	Mitochon-drial	Microsomal	Cytosol		
Acute						
Newborn	25.4 (1.1)	7.3 (0.5)	16.4 (1.0)	50.9 (0.9)	153.1 (5.1)	
1 wk	24.0 (1.1)	7.1 (0.4)	14.2 (1.4)	54.7 (2.1)	253.2 (8.5)	
2 wk	24.3 (1.1)	9.9 (0.9)	16.7 (1.4)	49.1 (2.3)	192.3 (16.0)	
3 wk	29.5 (1.5)	11.7 (0.4)	19.3 (0.7)	39.5 (1.7)	165.0 (6.1)	
Adult	25.4 (0.9)	13.7 (1.2)	16.1 (0.7)	44.1 (1.1)	236.8 (15.2)	
Subchronic						
1 wk	25 (2.1)	8.6 (0.8)	11.8 (1.1)	54.6 (1.1)		2.71 (0.2)
2 wk	43.8 (3.1)	9.3 (3.1)	12.0 (2.6)	34.9 (4.7)		3.46 (0.3)
Adult						
5 days	40.6 (2.5)	13.0 (1.5)	21.7 (0.8)	24.7 (1.0)		2.02 (0.1)
10 days	39.6 (2.7)	10.3 (0.9)	23.1 (1.2)	27.0 (1.2)		1.29 (0.2)

[a] Mean values, with SE given in parentheses.

centage of the final dose is shown in Table 1. Uptake fell in adults treated subchronically relative to that seen after acute dosing, whereas uptake of a subchronic dose in animals aged 1 and 2 weeks remained normal or increased compared with acute dosage controls of the same age or with adults, respectively. This suggests that the uptake pathway for gentamicin in the renal proximal tubular cell is more readily saturable in adults than in rats aged 1 and 2 weeks.

Nephrotoxicity with subchronic treatment for 1 and 2 weeks as reflected in enzymuria was comparable to that seen in adults. Urine lactic acid dehydrogenase (mean ± SE) was 415 ± 25 U of urinary creatinine per mg in 2-week-old animals treated subchronically versus 120 ± 19 U/mg in untreated 2-week-old controls. Urinary N-acetylglucosaminidase was 2,900 ± 400 U of urinary creatinine per mg in 2-week-old rats treated subchronically versus 800 ± 90 U/mg in untreated controls ($P < 0.001$). Urinary gamma-glutamyl transpeptidase fell ($P > 0.05$) in 2-week-old rats receiving subchronic gentamicin treatment, but tripled in adults receiving subchronic treatment for 5 days ($P < 0.01$) and increased by 40% in adults treated for 10 days ($P > 0.05$). With increasing age in subchronically treated rats, the percent binding of gentamicin

in cytosol decreased and urinary concentrations of N-acetylglucosaminidase increased, suggesting that damage may be related to depletion of a cytosol-binding protein.

Light microscopy showed more severe renal tubular damage in subchronically treated immature rats than in adults, although regeneration occurred in both. A unique hydropic degeneration was seen only in some rats aged 1 and 2 weeks. Electron micrographs showed widespread occurrence of cytosegresomes with myeloid bodies in proximal tubular cells, and these were much more prominent than after acute dosing.

Immature rats are not resistant to gentamicin nephrotoxicity and there is, as yet, no clearly identified relationship between toxicity and renal concentration or subcellular distribution.

1. **Barza, M., and M. Lauermann.** 1978. Why monitor serum levels of gentamicin? Clin. Pharmacokin. **3**:202–215.
2. **Hook, J., and W. Hewitt.** 1977. Development of mechanisms for drug excretion. Am. J. Med. **62**:497–506.
3. **Patel, V., F. Luft, M. Yum, B. Patel, W. Zeman, and S. Kleit.** 1975. Enzymuria in gentamicin-induced kidney damage. Antimicrob. Agents Chemother. **7**:364–369.

Resistance of Female Rats to Gentamicin Nephrotoxicity

RICHARD A. PARKER,* WILLIAM M. BENNETT, CHARLES E. PLAMP,
DONALD C. HOUGHTON, DAVID N. GILBERT, AND GEORGE A. PORTER

University of Oregon Health Science Center, Providence Medical Center, Portland, Oregon 97201, U.S.A.

The potential nephrotoxicity of the aminoglycoside antibiotics, particularly gentamicin, has been well established in humans and laboratory animals. The administration of gentamicin twice daily in a total daily dose of 40 mg/kg to male Fischer 344 rats produces progressive but ultimately reversible nonoliguric acute renal failure with a peak impairment in renal function occurring at day 14 of continuous drug administration (1). Numerous factors are known to modify the nephrotoxicity of gentamicin in the laboratory animal. Included in these are age, state of hydration, acid-base status, and the presence of concomitantly administered drugs. The potential role of sex as a determinant of susceptibility to gentamicin-induced nephrotoxicity has not previously been explored. Previous workers have shown, however, that the susceptibility of mice to the nephrotoxic effects of chloroform is dependent on the sex of the animal, females being relatively resistant (2). In addition, Maunsbach has demonstrated ultrastructural differences in the proximal tubules of male and female rat kidneys (3).

In the current study, age-matched adult male and female Fischer 344 rats were treated with 40 mg of gentamicin per kg per day given in two equal doses for time periods ranging from 3 to 21 days. At sacrifice, cardiac blood was obtained for blood urea nitrogen, serum creatinine, and electrolytes. Renal tissue was processed for light microscopy, cortical gentamicin tissue concentration, and cortical slice transport of the organic acid p-aminohippurate. Renal cortical gentamicin content was determined by radioimmunoassay.

The results of gentamicin administration for the various time points are shown in Table 1. At the conclusion of 14 days of drug administration, the male animals developed significantly greater rises in blood urea nitrogen and serum creatinine than those of females ($P < 0.001$). At the same treatment interval, the cortical slice accumulation of p-aminohippurate was significantly lower in the males than in the females ($P < 0.005$), indicating a greater impairment of active transport in the males. At all of the treatment intervals, the females concentrated less gentamicin in the renal cortex than did males. This difference was statistically significant at all times with the exception of 14 days. The comparative histological findings at 14 days were less dramatic than the renal functional differential would have suggested. Females were noted to have generally less severe necrosis of the proximal tubules than did the males. In addition, regenerative activity was less in the female rats at this time point.

In a separate study, female rats were pretreated with testosterone propionate for 10 days before receiving both testosterone and gentamicin for the subsequent 14 days. In spite of achieving circulating levels of testosterone in the females that were comparable to male physiological levels, the response of the females to gentamicin was not altered from that noted previously.

Comparing the female rat response to gentamicin to that of the male reveals that females (i) develop quantitatively less renal dysfunction than do males, (ii) undergo early mild renal injury that is nonprogressive and rapidly healed, and (iii) concentrate significantly less gentami-

TABLE 1. *Nephrotoxicity of gentamicin (40 mg/kg per day) for male (M) and female (F) Fischer 344 rats*

Days of treatment	Blood urea nitrogen (mg/100 ml)		Creatinine (mg/100 ml)		p-Aminohippurate (slice-to-media ratio)		Renal gentamicin concn (µg/g of tissue)	
	M	F	M	F	M	F	M	F
3	20 ± 0.82	20 ± 0.64	1.0 ± 0.34	0.6 ± 0.07	8.6 ± 0.26	7.8 ± 0.52	633 ± 24	454 ± 44[a]
7	21 ± 1.2	26 ± 5.5	0.87 ± 0.02	1.0 ± 0.10	11.5 ± 0.34	7.8 ± 0.76[b]	1,120 ± 60	656 ± 89[a]
10	58 ± 5.1	58 ± 15.0	1.7 ± 0.16	1.9 ± 0.39	4.8 ± 1.2	6.7 ± 1.0[b]	1,168 ± 54	593 ± 31[a]
14	171 ± 28	20 ± 1.2[a]	4.3 ± 0.78	0.93 ± 0.06[a]	1.4 ± 0.14	8.6 ± 0.82	562 ± 25	524 ± 55
21	18 ± 0.29	18 ± 1.0	0.70 ± 0.05	0.93 ± 0.03	6.9 ± 0.99	6.2 ± 0.21	1,484 ± 107	662 ± 28[a]

[a] $P < 0.001$.
[b] $P < 0.005$.

cin in the renal cortex than do males. The basis for these observed differences is unknown. The role of circulating levels of testosterone achieved by its short-term administration to females appears minimal. Other possibilities would include (i) tissue concentrations of testosterone vis-à-vis circulating levels, (ii) a protective effect of estrogen and progesterone, and (iii) genetically determined differences in the renal handling of gentamicin.

Identification of the basis for the sex-related differences may give further insight into the basic mechanism of aminoglycoside nephrotoxicity. In the future, studies evaluating the neph-

rotoxicity of drugs and other toxins should control for the potential modifying role of sex.

1. Gilbert, D. N., D. C. Houghton, W. M. Bennett, C. E. Plamp, K. Reger, and G. A. Porter. 1979. Reversibility of gentamicin nephrotoxicity in rats: recovery during continuous drug administration. Proc. Soc. Exp. Biol. Med. 160:99–103.
2. Krus, S., S. Starzyniski, Z. Zaleska-Rutczynska, and A. Naciazek-Wieniawska. 1974. The role of testosterone in developing chloroform-induced renal tubular necrosis in mice. Nephron 12:275–280.
3. Maunsbach, A. 1966. Observations on the segmentation of the proximal tubule in the rat kidney. J. Ultrastruct. Res. 16:239–258.

Detection of Aminoglycoside Antibiotic-Induced Ototoxicity in Newborns by Brain Stem Response Audiometry

P. A. BERNARD, J. C. PECHÈRE,* R. HÉBERT, P. DÉRY, AND C. CARRIER

Ear, Nose and Throat Department, Department of Microbiology,* and Department of Pediatrics, Laval University, Quebec, Canada

This study compares brain stem response audiometry recordings in neonates treated for 6 to 10 days with either gentamicin or tobramycin at conventional dosages with those of a control group.

Twenty-nine neonates of gestational age between 29 and 42 weeks and weight between 1,000 and 3,500 g were admitted to an intensive care unit and were housed in incubators. Fifteen required aminoglycoside antibiotherapy with either gentamicin (9 cases) or tobramycin (6 cases); 14 other neonates who did not receive aminoglycosides were used as controls. The aminoglycosides were administered intramuscularly at a dose of 5.0 mg/kg per day in two divided doses for neonates under 1 week of age and 7.5 mg/kg per day in three divided doses for neonates 1 to 4 weeks of age. For all neonates, monitoring included brain stem response audiometry recording sessions at days 0, 5, and 10, daily measurements of partial oxygen blood pressure in peripheral capillaries and eventually in arterial blood, and serum creatinine assays and antibiotic serum concentration assays at days 0, 5 ± 2, and 10. In two gentamicin-treated babies, brain stem response audiometry was also performed 40 or 44 days after treatment.

Hypoxemia, a well-known cause of hearing alteration (6), did not occur at any time during the study. In all tested samples, serum creatinine concentrations were less than 1.8 mg/100 ml. In treated neonates, peak antibiotic serum concen-

trations never exceeded 9.4 µg/ml, whereas trough concentrations were below 0.64 µg/ml.

As expected, control neonates showed decreasing latencies of wave V during the period of observation which was attributable to the so-called auditory maturation (4) (Fig. 1). This diminution reached significance after only 5 days when testing at 70-dB sound pressure level (SPL) ($P < 0.01$, Student's t test calculated for paired values, day 0 versus day 5), whereas it took 10 days to obtain a significant difference with a 90-dB SPL stimulus ($P < 0.05$, day 0 versus day 10). In aminoglycoside-treated neonates, unlike the control group, latencies did not decrease with time, latencies being comparable on days 0, 5, and 10 ($P > 0.10$, paired t test; Table 1). Before treatment, all babies shared similar latencies; however, as early as day 5 of observation, latencies were significantly longer in treated babies than in the control babies, the gap becoming even greater at day 10. An analysis of latencies with respect to age, weight, and aminoglycoside serum concentrations failed to detect a significant correlation between either of these factors and the increase in latency ($r^2 < 0.10$). On the other hand, variations between initial and final latency values appeared to be dependent on the total dose of aminoglycoside given per kilogram of body weight (Fig. 2). No statistically significant differences in latency changes could be found between gentamicin- and tobramycin-treated babies even after adjustment for differences in the total dose of aminoglycoside per kilogram of body weight.

The two recordings performed after treatment did not show improvement. In one baby treated with gentamicin for 10 days, latencies were 8.3, 10.7, and 11.2 ms at days 0, 10, and 50, respectively, whereas in another latencies were 10.6, 9.3, and 9.7 ms at days 0, 10 and 54 (70-dB recordings).

For a given age and a given sound intensity, the wave V may be characterized by three parameters: threshold, amplitude, and latency. Due to noise in incubators, the measurement of the threshold may be erroneous below 70-dB SPL. With regard to amplitude, variations between subjects are considerable. In contrast, latency of the wave V is very constant, allowing reliable measurements. It appears from animal studies (1) that sensory hair cell function can be altered without any visible cytological changes. Since aminoglycosides primarily act on calcium of cell membranes (5), a partial blockage of the neurotransmission process (3) may result in an

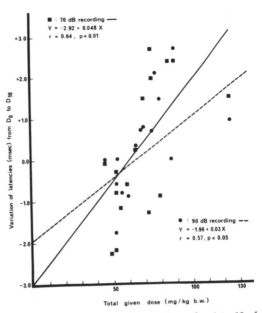

FIG. 2. *Variation of latencies from day 1 to 10 of treatment as a function of the total given dose of aminoglycoside per kilogram of body weight (b.w.).*

impairment of evoked action potentials. Interpretation of the present data should take into account the noise generated by the heat and ventilation systems in the incubators. This noise has been shown to provoke hearing alterations (4) and might have acted synergistically with aminoglycosides, as suggested by some animals studies (2).

In conclusion, short-term aminoglycoside treatments at conventional dosages, given to neonates kept in incubators, appeared to alter the acoustically evoked potentials.

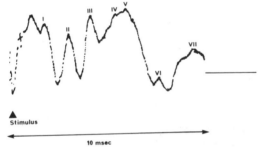

FIG. 1. *Typical recording of brain stem response audiometry in a normal neonate. Stimulus intensity, 70 dB.*

TABLE 1. *Latency results for control and treated neonates*

Parameter	Control	Treated[a]	Significance of difference (t test)
No. of patients	14	15	
Gestational age (wk)	35 ± 4[b]	37 ± 4	NS[c]
Wt (kg)	1.95 ± 0.55	2.55 ± 0.76	$P \le 0.05$
Duration of treatment (days)		8.7 ± 1.3	
Latency at 90-dB SPL			
Day 0	7.98 ± 0.84	8.50 ± 0.99	NS
Day 5	7.75 ± 1.11	9.13 ± 1.90	$P \le 0.05$
Day 10	7.31 ± 1.06	8.87 ± 1.48	$P \le 0.01$
Latency at 70-dB SPL			
Day 0	8.71 ± 1.05	9.42 ± 0.93	NS
Day 5	8.07 ± 1.30	9.91 ± 1.62	$P \le 0.01$
Day 10	7.67 ± 1.12	9.79 ± 1.46	$P \le 0.01$

[a] Total dose of gentamicin or tobramycin, 163 ± 81 mg.
[b] Mean ± SD.
[c] NS, Not significant.

1. **Bernard, P. A., J. C. Pechère, and J. C. Jequier.** 1979. Detection of tobramycin and netilmicin induced ototoxicity in guinea pigs with evoked potentials. J. Infect. Dis. **139**:418–423.
2. **Dayal, V., A. Kokshanian, and D. Mitchell.** 1971. Combined effects of noise and kanamycin. Ann. Otol. **80**:897–902.
3. **Kubinowski, P., and Z. Szreniawski.** 1962. On the mechanisms of the neuromuscular blockade by antibiotics, abstr. 1250. 22nd International Congress of Physiological Sciences, Leiden, The Netherlands. Excerpta Medica, London.
4. **Pujol, R.** 1976. Maturation du systeme auditif. Rev. Laryngol. **97**:551–562.
5. **Schacht, J.** 1974. Interaction of neomycin with phosphoinositide metabolism in guinea pig inner ear and brain tissues. Ann. Otol. **83**:613–618.
6. **Volpe, J.** 1975. Neurological disorders, p. 729–795. *In* G. Avery (ed.), Neonatology, pathophysiology and management of the newborn, vol. 32. Lippincott Co., Toronto.

Gentamicin Inner Ear Susceptibility Is Higher in Newborn than in Adult Cats

PHILIPPE BERNARD,* CLAUDE BOURRET, JEAN-CLAUDE PECHERE, AND JOHN REMINGTON

Otologic Research Laboratory, Laval University, Quebec, Canada

Aminoglycoside antibiotics are widely used in human neonates as soon as a septic state is suspected or demonstrated. Most of these neonates are prematures with an unachieved hearing maturation (1). Since aminoglycosides are commonly considered to be less ototoxic in neonates than in adults, the given daily dosage is usually the same in both groups.

Using an animal model, the aim of this study was to verify this assumption. Cats were chosen because of the similarities in maturation state between kittens during the first month of life and human prematures of 29 to 41 weeks of gestational age. Seven kittens were given 20 mg of gentamicin sulfate per kg daily from birth to day 20 of life. Seven kittens from the same litters did not receive the antibiotic. Two equal groups of seven adult cats underwent similar duration of treatment at two different daily dosages: 20 and 50 mg/kg. Five untreated normal adult cats constituted a control group. All animals were normal before treatment.

Thirty days after the cessation of the treatment (this waiting period allowed a stabilization of eventual cochlear damages), each animal, while under deep anesthesia, was decapitated, and both cochlea were quickly removed for microscopic examination. The anatomical evaluation closely followed the procedure described by Spoendlin and Brun (2): double fixation with glutaraldehyde (0.1 M) and OsO_4 (1%) in phosphate buffer, dehydration, and embedding in Spurr epoxy. After the specimens were trimmed, selected areas of each cochlear turn were examined by electron microscopy after ultrafine sectioning and contrast staining (uranyl acetate and lead citrate) (Fig. 1 and 2).

In the control groups, either adult cats or kittens, no cytological damages could be found in the Corti's organ. Since kittens were sacrificed on day 50, their cochleas had reached the adult stage.

No anatomical damages could be demonstrated in the Corti's organs of 20-mg/kg-treated adult cats. On the other hand, obvious specific aminoglycoside-induced lesions and similar lesions were observed in the Corti's organs of treated kittens (20 mg/kg) and adult cats given a daily dose of 50 mg of gentamicin per kg. These lesions were located in the apex of the three rows of outer hair cells, while the inner hair cells row remained intact. As described by Ylikosky (3), lesions were found in the lower and upper part of the basal coil of the cochlea. There were no hair cell losses and no neural alterations. Cytological changes consisted of a disruption in the regular arrangement of the smooth endoplasmic reticulum along cell walls. Mitochondria were swollen, and crest irregularities formed so-called "myelinic figures" at the apex of the cells. Also at the apex, an increasing number of lysosomes was regularly observed.

The lesions were similar in both 20-mg-treated kittens and 50-mg-treated adult cats. However, they occurred more frequently in kittens (12 abnormal Corti's organs among 14 examined specimens) than in adults (10 abnormal Corti's organs among 14 examined).

These findings lead to the conclusion that gentamicin inner ear susceptibility is higher in newborn than in adult cats.

1. **Stockard, J., J. E. Stockard, and F. W. Sharbrough.** 1979. Brain-stem auditory evoked potentials in neurology, p. 541–567. *In* N. J. Aminoff (ed.), Electrophysiology approaches to neurological diagnosis. Churchill Livingstone, New York.

2. **Spoendlin, H., and J. P. Brun.** 1974. The block-surface technique for evaluation of cochlea pathology. Arch. Otorhinolaryngol. **208:**541–567.

3. **Ylikoski, J.** 1974. Correlative study on cochlear pathology and hearing loss in guinea pigs after intoxication with ototoxic antibiotics. Acta Otolaryngol. Suppl. 326, p. 1–62.

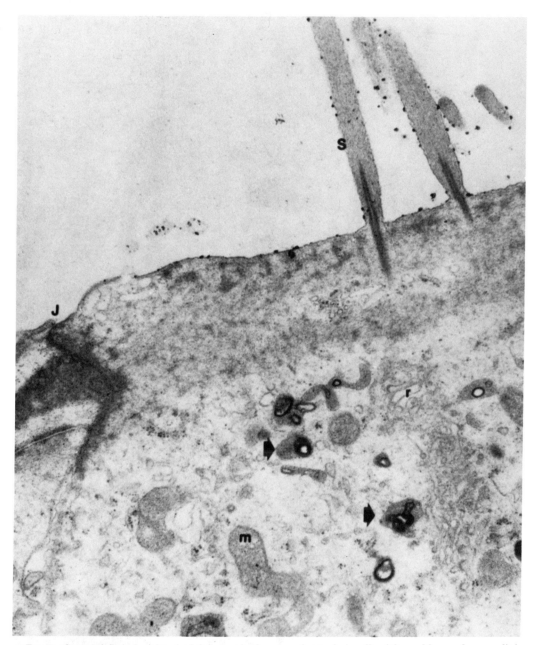

FIG. 1. *Gentamicin-induced typical damages in the apex of outer hair cells of the cochlea, such as myelinic figures (arrow), in mitochondria. Adult cat treated with 50 mg of gentamicin per kg daily over 20 days (×30,000). S, Stereocils; r, endoplasmic reticulum; m, mitochondria; J, cellular junction.*

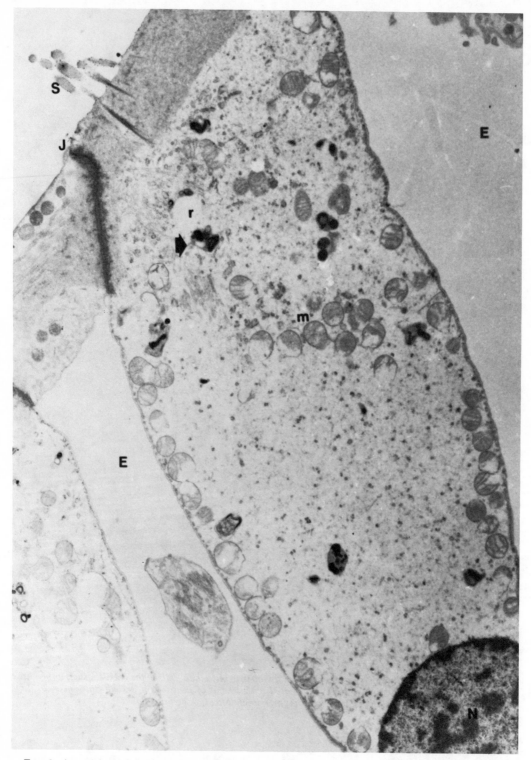

FIG. 2. *Anatomical alterations (arrow) similar to those shown in Fig. 1 when kittens were treated with gentamicin at 20 mg/kg daily for 20 days. Outer hair cell of the basal turn (×12,000). E, Endolymphatic space.*

Influence of Total Dose, Division of Daily Dose, Age, and Pregnancy on Aminoglycoside Ototoxicity

P. J. FEDERSPIL,* W. SCHÄTZLE, M. KAYSER, K. SACK, AND J. SCHENTAG

Department of Oto-Rhino-Laryngology, University of the Saar, Homburg/Saar, and Medizinische Hochschule, Lübeck, Federal Republic of Germany, and State University of New York, Buffalo, New York 14209, U.S.A.

The influence of total dose, division of daily dose, age, and pregnancy on aminoglycoside ototoxicity is of great clinical interest and was studied in an experimental series. These investigations comprised large series of guinea pigs treated simultaneously with tobramycin or one of the other new aminoglycoside antibiotics. Acuity of hearing was determined by the Preyer's pinna reflex and vestibular function was determined by a positional reflex. The topography and extent of hair cell damage was evaluated by phase-contrast microscopic studies of surface preparations of Corti's organ after osmium fixation and a register developed in 1972 (histocochleogram; 1, 3). Electron microscopic studies were performed in the vestibular end organs. The doses were chosen to avoid a high degree of nephrotoxicity or ototoxicity. Functional and histological studies of the kidneys were done in all animals. The tobramycin concentrations were determined in the perilymph, kidney tissues, and sera.

The series with tobramycin, as well as those with gentamicin, sisomicin, amikacin, and netilmicin, showed that the total dose administered is most important for the evaluation of ototoxicity, in addition to uremia and individual sensitivity. In 1972 Waitz (8) had already shown in the cat that the essential parameter for evaluation of the vestibular toxicity of aminoglycoside antibiotics is the total dose administered. Experimental and clinical studies on the ototoxicity of the new aminoglycoside antibiotics demonstrate that there is a threshold for aminoglycoside inner ear damage, and this threshold consists in a certain amount of the total dose of aminoglycoside antibiotic administered. Furthermore, our experimental investigations show that the sensitivity of the ears to the different aminoglycoside antibiotics is the same in all mammalian species studied (2).

The division of the daily dose of tobramycin slightly increases the ototoxicity, as shown in Fig. 1 (4). These results contradict clinical results given by Labovitz et al. (6), who treated two unequal groups of 10 and 11 patients with 1 × 160 and 3 × 60 mg of gentamicin, respectively. On the other hand, our findings confirm the clinical observations of Tompsett (7) concerning the increase in streptomycin ototoxicity after division of the daily dosage and are confirmed by other unpublished experimental data on amikacin (2). Functional and histological studies of the kidneys did not show significant differences among the various groups. The pharmacokinetics of tobramycin in the renal medulla and cortex 24 h after the last injection were not influenced by the division of the daily dosage.

In two groups of seven pregnant guinea pigs, each of which was treated after day 20 of pregnancy (normal duration of pregnancy, 56 days) with 80 mg of tobramycin per kg of body weight for 29 days, no difference in ototoxicity or nephrotoxicity could be found in comparison with the three groups of nonpregnant guinea pigs which simultaneously received treatment with the same dosage of tobramycin. The inner ear hair cell losses of the fetuses were less than those of their mothers (2, 3).

In a group of seven newborn guinea pigs which were treated since day 3 or 4 after birth with 80 mg of tobramycin per kg of body weight for 29 days, an increase in ototoxicity was observed in comparison with the simultaneously treated five

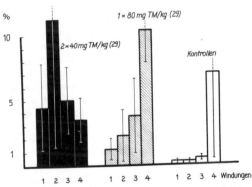

FIG. 1. *Average percentages of degenerated outer hair cells in the different cochlear turns (with SEMs) of three groups of ten guinea pigs each which had each been treated with 40 mg of tobramycin per kg twice a day, 80 mg of tobramycin per kg once a day, and untreated. Kontrollen = controls; Windungen = turns.*

groups of guinea pigs of adolescent or adult age. This increase of cochlear ototoxicity in newborn guinea pigs is statistically significant and important (2, 3). It is probably explained by the different pharmacokinetics of the aminoglycoside antibiotics in the newborn and might be correlated with a higher efficacy of these aminoglycoside antibiotics in the newborn such that a diminution of the administered dosage of 50% could be tolerated. These first data showing a statistically significant increase in tobramycin ototoxicity in newborn guinea pigs may be correlated even to human studies, which have not shown a difference in ototoxicity of the aminoglycoside antibiotics in the neonates because the increase in ototoxicity is not so tremendous that the normal large safety margin of the usual aminoglycoside antibiotics is sufficient to avoid ototoxicity.

Extrapolation of these experimental guinea pig results to humans seems warranted.

1. **Federspil, P.** 1972. Über die Aufzeichnung der Kochleaschäden beim Meerschweinchen. Z. Laryngol. Rhinol. **51**:633–637.
2. **Federspil, P.** 1979. Die klinische Ototoxizität, und ihre Prophylaxe, p. 51–73. *In* K. Hierholzer and N. Rietbrock (ed.), Physiologische und pharmakologische Grundlagen der Therapie, Berliner Seminar 2. Vieweg Verlag, Braunschweig.
3. **Federspil, P.** 1979. Antibiotikaschäden des Ohres. Joh. Ambrosius Barth Verlag, Leipzig.
4. **Federspil, P., W. Schätzle, M. Kayser, and K. Sack.** 1979. Zur Minderung der Ototoxizität und Nephrotoxizität des Tobramycins. Arch. Oto-Rhino-Laryngol. **223**: 238–240.
5. **Hawkins, J. E., Jr.** 1976. Drug ototoxicity. Handbook of sensory physiology, vol. V. Auditory system, part 3: clinical and special topics. Springer-Verlag, Berlin.
6. **Labovitz, E., M. E. Levison, and D. Kaye.** 1974. Single-dose daily gentamicin therapy in urinary tract infection. Antimicrob. Agents Chemother. **6**:465–470.
7. **Tompsett, R.** 1948. Relation of dosage to streptomycin toxicity. Ann. Otol. **57**:181–188.
8. **Waitz, J. A.** 1975. Laboratory evaluation of aminoglycoside antibiotics. Dev. Ind. Microbiol. **16**:161–174.

Evaluation of Ototoxicity of Aminoglycoside Antibiotics in Guinea Pigs by Scanning Electron Microscopy

K. SATO,* M. YOKOTA, AND T. KOEDA

Kanazawa Medical University, Ishikawa Prefecture, and *Central Research Laboratory, Meiji Seika Kaisha, Ltd., Yokohama, Japan*

Auditory hairs on the cuticula of hair cells in Corti's organ are the most important tissue in the auditory conductive system because they first perceive the movement of endolymph induced by the conduction of sound. Accordingly, deformation of the hairs produces impairment of normal auditory conduction which depends solely on the hair's function, resulting in hearing disturbance. On the other hand, sensorineural deafness caused by administration of aminoglycoside antibiotics is well known. Therefore, in the research and development of new substances belonging to the aminoglycoside group of antibiotics, the study of possible ototoxicity in animals is imperative. Experimental evaluation of ototoxicity of the drugs has been conducted physiologically and morphologically, and there have been many reports on the results published. For morphological evaluation, pathohistological, histochemical, and electron microscopic examinations have been employed. Through these studies, it has been shown that aminoglycoside antibiotics primarily affect the outer hair cells in Corti's organ of the cochlea. It has also been clarified that degeneration of hair cells due to aminoglycoside antibiotic adminis-

tration usually starts from the basal end of the basal turn to the upper turns of the cochlea.

In the present study, we examined deformation of the auditory hairs in animals, using a scanning electron microscope, to clarify and compare the ototoxicity of several aminoglycoside antibiotics. Guinea pigs, weighing about 250 g each, were used in our experiment. The animals received intramuscular administration of dibekacin (50 to 75 mg/kg), gentamicin (50 to 75 mg/kg), tobramycin (25 to 75 mg/kg), kanamycin (50 to 200 mg/kg), amikacin (50 to 200 mg/kg), or ribostamycin (200 to 400 mg/kg) daily for 28 days. During the administration, the hearing threshold of all animals was examined by the differential pinna reflex test. Within 5 days after the last injection, the animals were sacrificed, specimens of the cochlea were prepared by the surface preparation technique, and then scanning electron microscopic specimens were obtained by the routine method.

The scanning electron microscopic observations were performed on the surface of the basal turn of the cochlea by using a Hitachi S-430 scanning electron microscope.

Results. The scanning electron microscopic

examination revealed that the deformation of the hairs of the outer hair cells took the form of fanlike spreading, bending, fusion, grapelike formation, and disappearance. When the deformations of hairs by different test drugs were compared, animals receiving dibekacin showed almost normal findings, with slight and scattered fanlike spreading of the first row of outer hair cells (Fig. 1). The ribostamycin group, which received a higher dose than the others, showed findings similar to the dibekacin group. Animals receiving gentamicin in the same dose as dibekacin, however, demonstrated rather highly damaged pictures with grapelike formation or disappearance of the hairs of outer hair cells (Fig. 2). From these findings on the deformation of hairs, it is suggested that under the present experimental conditions, ototoxicity due to aminoglycosides is probably most severe with gentamicin, followed by amikacin, tobramycin, kanamycin, dibekacin, and ribostamycin in that order.

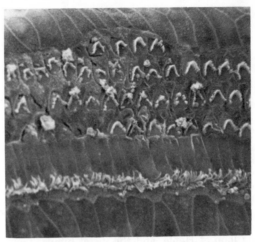

FIG. 2. *Marked deformations of hairs, bending, grapelike formation, and disappearance, on outer hair cells. Guinea pig; hook of the basal turn; gentamicin, 50 mg/kg per day for 28 days (×1,400).*

The present study also revealed that the frequency of deformation of inner hair cells was significantly lower than that of outer hair cells.

We employed a scanning electron microscope as one of the measures for clear, precise, and rapid evaluation of ototoxicity of aminoglycoside antibiotics and found that the severity of ototoxicity due to the drugs can be estimated from the scanning electron microscopic findings on the degree and extent of deformation of the hairs of hair cells in animals.

1. **Akiyoshi, M.** 1977. Advances in clinical pharmacology, vol. 13, p. 374–386. Urban & Schwarzenberg, Baltimore.
2. **Akiyoshi, M., and K. Sato.** 1974. Program Abstr. Intersci. Conf. Antimicrob. Agents Chemother. 14th, 1974, San Francisco, Calif., abstr. no. 16.
3. **Akiyoshi, M., and K. Sato.** 1970. Progress in antimicrobial and anticancer chemotherapy, vol. 1, p. 621–625. University of Tokyo Press, Tokyo.
4. **Hawkins, J. E., and H. Engstrom.** 1963. Acta Otolaryngol. Suppl. **188:**100–107.
5. **Hunter-Duvar, I. M.** 1978. Acta Otolaryngol. Suppl. **351:** 3–23.
6. **Ylikoski, J.** 1974. Acta Otolaryngol. Suppl. **326:**5–22.

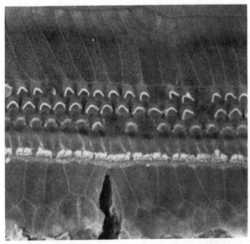

FIG. 1. *Scattered fanlike spreading of hairs on outer hair cells of first row. Hairs of second and third rows show normal appearance. Guinea pig; hook of the basal turn; dibekacin, 75 mg/kg per day intramuscularly for 28 days (×1,100).*

Early Events Related to Gentamicin-Induced Nephrotoxicity

J. P. MORIN,* G. VIOTTE, F. van HOOF, P. TULKENS, and J. P. FILLASTRE

Groupe de Physiopathologie Tissulaire, University of Rouen, Rouen, and Service de Néphrologie, Hôpital de Bois Guillaume, 76230 Bois Guillaume, France, and International Institute of Cellular and Molecular Pathology and the University of Louvain, Brussels, Belgium*

Gentamicin accumulates in the kidney cortex. Using a technique of rabbit kidney nephron microdissection, we have examined the distribution of intrarenal gentamicin along a single nephron from the glomerulus to the collecting duct after injection of G-[^{3}H]gentamicin (100 μCi per animal). No labeled product was found in the glomeruli, the descending and the ascending loop of Henle, and the distal tubule. Low amounts of silver grains were seen in the epithelial cells of the macula densa. Large amounts were found within the proximal tubular cells. The distribution of gentamicin is, however, not homogeneous along the latter structure: we observed an increasing gradient of intracellular gentamicin concentration from the initial to the distal portion of the proximal tubule (Fig. 1). Thus the intracellular concentration of the antibiotic seems to correlate with the concentration gradient of the primary urine solutes along the proximal tubule, which suggests that the uptake of gentamicin in the cells is dependent on its concentration in the tubular fluid.

Fractionation studies of kidney cortices on linear sucrose gradients showed a similar distribution pattern for ^{3}H- or ^{14}C-labeled gentamicin and two lysosomal enzymes, N-acetyl-β-D-glucosaminidase and Cathepsin B. We checked that the amount of radioactivity found in the cortex was exactly that expected from the microbiological assay of the drug in this tissue. If gentamicin was added to a cortex homogenate rather than being injected into the animal, the distributions of the antibiotic and of the lysosomal enzymes were largely dissociated. This indicates that the intrarenal gentamicin is associated with lysosomes, in accordance with the autoradiographic data of Just et al. (2) and Silverblatt and Kuehn (6).

Lysosomes showed prominent alterations after treatment with gentamicin. These alterations consisted mainly in (i) the intralysosomal accumulation of osmiophilic material with a lamellar aspect and a concentric deposition (myeloid bodies); (ii) an enlargement of the lysosomes, which, however, did not appear swollen or overloaded by other material than myeloid bodies. These altered lysosomes, which have been referred earlier as to cytosegrosomes (3),

did not resemble the vacuoles that develop after a nonspecific stimulation of autophagy. Thus we are probably dealing with an impairment of the catabolism (or an increased synthesis and segregation) of a few specific constituents. No alteration of other subcellular structure than lysosomes was observed: the mitochondria maintained their elongated shape, the endoplasmic reticulum remained coated with numerous ribosomes, and its cisternae were as dilated as in the controls. The tubular lumen was occasionally filled with myeloid bodies, although these appeared less tightly packed than those observed in lysosomes.

The biochemical analysis (Table 1) shows that after only 4 mg/kg per day for 8 days, the structural latency of the lysosomal enzyme N-acetyl-β-D-glucosaminidase was significantly decreased, suggesting an alteration of the physical or mechanical properties of the lysosomal membrane. At the same time there was a significant decrease of the activity of the lysosomal sphingomyelinase and of the alanine aminopeptidase (brush border). At larger doses we observed a decrease of the activities of α-D-galactosidase and Cathepsin B (lysosomes) and an increase of the blood urea nitrogen and blood creatinine. Other lysosomal enzymes (α-mannosidase, α-fucosidase, N-acetyl-β-D-glucosaminidase, and Ca-

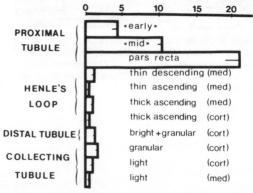

FIG. 1. [^{3}H]gentamicin incorporation in tubular cells (silver grains per 150 μm^2). Distribution of silver grains in autoradiographs of dissected nephrons 6 h after a single injection of tritiated gentamicin to rabbits.

TABLE 1. *Modification of blood urea nitrogen, blood creatinine, lysosomal structural latency, and kidney cortex enzyme levels after gentamicin therapy in rats with increasing doses for 8 days*[a]

Dose (mg/kg)	Structural latency (%)[b] Without incubation	Structural latency (%)[b] Incubation for 60 min, 37°C	Sphingo-myelinase (U/g of protein)	Alanine aminopep-tidase (U/g of protein)	α-D-Galac-tosidase (U/g of protein)	Blood urea nitro-gen (mmol/li-ter)	Creatinine (μmol/li-ter)	Cathepsin B (U/g of protein)
Control	30	100	0.43 ±0.013	81.97 ±6.78	4.39 ±0.28	7.02 ±0.33	48.18 ±1.81	14.35 ±0.57
4	63.76 ±3.17	108.13 ±2.96	0.33 ±0.02	42.92 ±2.22	3.93 ±0.09	7.25 ±0.27	50.0 ±4.08	13.44 ±0.31
10	71.1 ±4.29	129.8 ±4.2	0.27 ±0.02	43.43 ±4.92	3.49 ±0.09	7.12 ±0.56	47.5 ±4.38	12.17 ±1.05
20	77.5 ±0.9	137.7 ±0.21	0.19 ±0.010	50.88 ±4.76	3.88 ±0.27	7.5 ±0.5	56.6 ±6.6	14.50 ±0.86
50	109.7 ±5.66	142.1 ±2.13	0.28 ±0.040	66.37 ±2.21	3.58 ±0.26	8.56 ±1.08	87.5 ±7.5	8.50 ±1.29
100	105.5 ±4.9	141.7 ±2.4	0.12 ±0.03	65.28 ±8.25	2.37 ±0.26	42.5 ±9.5	165.0 ±55.0	3.37 ±0.81

[a] ± Standard deviation.
[b] Of N-acetyl-β-D-glucosaminidase.

thepsin B) or the microsomal enzyme glucose 6-phosphatase were unaffected.

An increase in the cell lipid phosphorus content was observed in Sprague-Dawley rats after a daily dose of 10 mg/kg for 8 days, but was at the limit of the significance in view of the large variation found in the control animals. In Wistar rats, treated with 50 mg/kg, the effect was not significant, although myeloid bodies were prominent. It must be stressed, however, that these assays of lipid phosphorus have been performed on whole kidney cortices, where not all cell types are affected to the same extent. Furthermore, lysosomes may contain only a small proportion of total content of the lipid phosphorus of the tubular cell.

Discussion. Experiments reported in this paper show that intracellular gentamicin is consistently found within the lysosomes of proximal tubule cells (Fig. 1). As discussed earlier (2, 5), endocytosis is the most likely mechanism to account for the intralysosomal storage of gentamicin. Other cell types, including cultured fibroblasts (7), have also been shown to take up aminoglycosides and to store them in their lysosomes. The preferential uptake by tubular cells in vivo is probably related to the concentration of drug in the tubular fluid and to the exceedingly high endocytic activity of these cells.

Gentamicin treatment with dosages inferior to 50 mg/kg for 8 days does not affect other subcellular organelles than lysosomes, on the basis of their ultrastructural appearance. On the other hand, impairment of the lysosomal digestion is strongly suggested by the impairment of the activities of sphingomyelinase, acid α-D-galactosidase, and Cathepsin B, three key enzymes of

phospholipid, glycoside, and protein breakdown, respectively.

The first action of gentamicin seems to be on the sphingomyelinase, and this could explain the deposition of phospholipids in lysosomes (myeloid bodies). This is in accordance with the effects reported for gentamicin on cultured cells where the drug was shown to provoke a lysosomal phospholipidosis associated with a dysfunction of sphingomyelinase (1) and phospholipase A (F. van Hoof, unpublished data). In the kidney, we have not yet assayed the activity of other lysosomal phospholipases. About the impairment of the activities of α-galactosidase and Cathepsin B, for which no accumulation of substrate was detected, it must be stressed that this effect was only observed at large doses and that other glycosidases or proteases were not significantly affected. On the other hand, the lysosomes isolated from gentamicin-treated animals are more labile, suggesting an alteration of their membrane in vivo.

In addition to its effects on lysosomes, gentamicin induces a depression of the activities of the brush-border enzyme alanine aminopeptidase. This result can be explained by an increased urinary excretion of the enzyme as reported by Mondorf et al. (4).

The pathogenesis of the lesions of the lysosomes and of the brush border is not yet understood, nor is their exact relationship with the impairment of the kidney function established. We suggest, however, that they may constitute an early and valuable index of gentamicin toxicity.

We are indebted to F. Andries-Renoird, D. Ghyselen-Grandfils, and D. Falize for excellent technical assistance.

This work was supported by the Belgian Fonds de la Recherche Scientifique Medicale (grant no. 3.4516-79), the U.S. Public Health Service (grant no. 9235), and the French Institut National de la Santé et de la Recherche Médicale (grant no. 76-1176-5). P.T. is chercheur qualifié of the Belgium Fonds National de la Recherche Scientifique.

1. **Aubert-Tulkens, G., F. van Hoof, and P. Tulkens.** 1979. Gentamicin-induced lysosomal phospholipidosis in cultured rat fibroblasts. Lab. Invest. **40:**481–491.

2. **Just, M., G. Erdman, and E. Harbermann.** 1977. The renal handling of polybasic drugs: 1 and 2. Naunyn Schmiedeberg's Arch. Pharmacol. **300:**57–66, 67–76.

3. **Kosek, J. D., R. I. Mazze and M. J. Cousins.** 1974. Nephrotoxicity of gentamicin. Lab. Invest. **30:**48–57.

4. **Mondorf, A. W., M. Zegelman, J. Klose, J. Hendus, and J. Breier.** 1978. Comparative studies on the action of aminoglycosides and cephalosporins on the proximal tubule of the human kidney. J. Antimicrob. Chemother. **4**(Suppl.):53–57.

5. **Morin, J. P., and J. P. Fillastre.** 1979. Aminoglycoside-induced lysosomal dysfunctions in kidney. *In* A. Whelton and H. C. Neu (ed.), The aminoglycosides: microbiology, clinical use, and toxicologic complications. M. Dekker Publisher Inc., New York.

6. **Silverblatt, F. J., and C. Kuehn.** 1979. Autoradiography of gentamicin uptake by the rat proximal tubule cell. Kidney Int. **15:**335–345.

7. **Tulkens, P., and A. Trouet.** 1978. The uptake and intracellular accumulation of aminoglycosides antibiotic in lysosomes of cultured rat fibroblasts. Biochem. Pharmacol. **27:**415–424.

Comparative Nephrotoxicity of Gentamicin and Tobramycin

C. STEWART GOODWIN

University of Western Australia and Department of Microbiology, Royal Perth Hospital, Perth, Western Australia

To compare the toxicity of two antibiotics it is necessary to obtain strictly comparable groups of patients, which may be difficult even in a prospective trial, and so a nonselective analysis was attempted. Between February 1977 and February 1978, every patient in Royal Perth Hospital whose tobramycin treatment was monitored by serum assay of the antibiotic, and who had serum creatinine and urea assays before, during, and after tobramycin treatment, was included in the tobramycin study group. This group comprised 22 adults of whom 8 received both gentamicin and tobramycin, leaving 14 patients unmatched. From the same period of time 14 patients treated with gentamicin were identified who matched the tobramycin group for sex, age, and initial serum creatinine and whose treatment was monitored by antibiotic, creatinine, and urea serum assays.

The clinical diagnoses in the two groups were very similar (Table 1). The initial serum creatinine (normal range, 50 to 120 μmol/liter) in the gentamicin group ranged from 51 to 380 μmol/liter, with a mean of 148.6 μmol/liter, and that in the tobramycin group ranged from 52 to 535 μmol/liter, with a mean of 156.8 μmol/liter. After these two groups had been identified it was found that the mean length of antibiotic treatment was remarkably similar: for the gentamicin group, 15.18 days, and for the tobramycin group, 15.45 days. Also, the mean trough or valley concentration of antibiotic in the gentamicin group was 2.1 mg/liter, and that in the tobramycin group was 2.2 mg/liter.

Frusemide was given to one patient in the tobramycin group and to five patients in the gentamicin group. To eliminate any effect of frusemide, statistical analyses of the gentamicin group were made separately for those who did not receive frusemide, as well as for the whole group.

Cephalosporins, which might have contributed to any nephrotoxic effect, were not given to any patient in the gentamicin group, but four tobramycin patients received cephazolin and one patient received cephalexin. In only one of these patients was there a rise in serum creatinine. The total dose of gentamicin given was, on the average, 2,319 mg, and that of tobramycin was 2,884 mg. This difference was not statistically significant ($t = 0.92$), but there was some relationship between high doses of gentamicin causing a rise in the serum creatinine, whereas the high doses of tobramycin were not associated with a rise in serum creatinine.

Results and discussion. Of the eight patients who received both gentamicin and tobramycin, the serum creatinine rose during treatment with gentamicin in four patients, but in one patient only during treatment with tobramycin. In all these patients, gentamicin was given as the initial drug, and after the creatinine rose, tobramycin was substituted. Of the 22 patients who received tobramycin, the serum creatinine increased in 7 patients by an average of 90%, and at the end of treatment the creatinine level was 49 to 231 μmol/liter, mean 156.9 μmol/liter. Of the 22 patients who received gentamicin, the creatinine increased in 16 patients, and in the 17 who did not receive frusemide it increased in 9 patients by an average of 160%. At the end of treatment in the gentamicin group, the creatinine ranged from 50 to 675 μmol/liter, mean 323.4 μmol/liter. The difference between the two antibiotic groups was statistically significant, both in the whole group ($P < 0.02$; $t = 2.56$, degrees of freedom 42) and comparing those not receiving frusemide ($P < 0.05$; $t = 2.41$, degrees of freedom 36).

The serum urea (normal range, 3 to 8 mmol/liter) increased in 8 patients in the tobramycin group and in 13 patients in the gentamicin group. After gentamicin treatment it ranged from 2.5 to 69.2 mmol/liter, mean 20.41 mmol/liter, whereas in the tobramycin group at the end of treatment it ranged from 1.9 to 13.0 mmol/liter, mean 9.5 mmol/liter.

Comparing the patients who did not receive frusemide, the difference between the two groups is still statistically significant ($P < 0.05$; $t = 2.23$, degrees of freedom 36). After this simple statistical analysis the preliminary conclusion was that gentamicin is more nephrotoxic than tobramycin. More detailed statistical studies were then done using an SPSS computer package. In Table 2 the analysis of variance shows that the only significant variable between the two groups was the antibiotic treatment. Using the technique of Pillai, a nonorthogonal multivariate analysis of variance also showed that the

TABLE 2. *Rises in serum creatinine and urea in patients treated with gentamicin or tobramycin—analysis of variance (log results)*

Determination	Degrees of freedom	Urea		Creatinine	
		Mean squares	F^a	Mean squares	F^a
Sex	1	0.09	<1	1.22	2.99
Antibiotic group	1	2.23	3.24	3.53	8.65^b
Sex × group	1	0.03	<1	0.01	<1
Regression on age	1	1.07	1.55	0.16	<1
Residual error	39	0.69		0.40	

^{a} F 1, 39; 0.05 = 4.10.
^{b} $P < 0.01$.

antibiotic was the only significant variable. Thus gentamicin caused a significantly greater rise in serum creatinine and urea than tobramycin.

In some patients, after the end of antibiotic treatment the raised creatinine or urea may slowly fall. However, in a few of the patients in this study the creatinine rose until the patient died. In this present study the patients were carefully monitored by antibiotic assays, and if the serum trough concentration of antibiotic was >1.5 mg/liter the dose of antibiotic was reduced or the interval between doses was increased. Thus excessive doses of antibiotics were avoided, and very high trough levels were never observed. Any nephrotoxicity would not have been due to excessive doses or accumulation. However, during the common use of these drugs many patients are not monitored by antibiotic assay. Therefore a choice between the two drugs will be based upon the size of the safety margin that remains when they are used thoughtlessly. It would appear that tobramycin has a greater safety margin than gentamicin. The results of this analysis are consistent with all the animal studies reported and with the few human studies which have all shown gentamicin to be more nephrotoxic than tobramycin (1–4).

TABLE 1. *Comparison of diagnoses in two treatment groups*

Diagnosis	Tobramycin	Gentamicin
Urinary calculus	1	1
Septicemia	5	6
Automobile accident	1	2
Pneumonia	3	2
Leukemia and infection	1	0
Osteomyelitis	2	1
Cholecystitis and renal failure	1	1
Post open-heart surgery	1	3
Abdominal wound infection	1	1
Paraplegia, pseudomonas infection	1	1
Post-operative orthopedic infection	2	1
Bronchobiliary fistula	1	0
Umbilical hernia	0	1
Peripheral vascular disease and infection	1	1
Adenocarcinoma	0	1
Epididymitis	1	0

1. Fee, W. E., V. Vierra, and G. R. Lathrop. 1978. Clinical evaluation of aminoglycoside toxicity: tobramycin versus gentamicin, a preliminary report. J. Antimicrob. Chemother. 4(Suppl. A):31–36.
2. Kahlmeter, G. 1979. Nephrotoxicity of gentamicin and tobramycin. Scand. J. Infect. Dis. 18:15–24.
3. Madsen, P. O., T. B. Kjaer, and A. Mosegaard. 1976. Comparison of tobramycin and gentamicin in the treatment of complicated urinary tract infections. J. Infect. Dis. 134(Suppl.):150.
4. Walker, B. D., and L. O. Gentry. 1976. A randomized comparative study of tobramycin and gentamicin in treatments of acute urinary tract infections. J. Infect. Dis. 134(Suppl.):146.

Nephrotoxicity of Gentamicin and Tobramycin in Patients: Pharmacokinetic and Clinical Studies

JEROME J. SCHENTAG,* MARTIN E. PLAUT, AND FRANK B. CERRA

Departments of Pharmaceutics, Medicine, and Surgery, Schools of Pharmacy and Medicine, State University of New York at Buffalo; Buffalo General Hospital; and Clinical Pharmacokinetics Laboratory, Millard Fillmore Hospital, Buffalo, New York 14209, U.S.A.*

Aminoglycoside antibiotics are effective antimicrobial agents, but a narrow margin exists between an effective and a toxic dose. All members of this class are potentially oto- and nephrotoxic, but there are pronounced differences between the available aminoglycosides in animal models (1). Differences in nephrotoxicity in humans have not been clearly shown, perhaps because kidney damage also occurs during diseases and during treatment with agents other than aminoglycoside antibiotics.

Since a better means of discriminating aminoglycoside-induced renal damage from renal damage due to clinical insults might reveal differences between agents, we began a prospective study with three purposes: first, to develop and test a pharmacokinetic method for identifying aminoglycoside-related damage in acutely ill adults; second, to compare this pharmacokinetic methodology with standard clinical assessment in a blind fashion on a group of seriously ill patients given aminoglycosides; and third, to determine whether differences in nephrotoxicity exist between gentamicin (G) and tobramycin (T) when patients are evaluated by both clinical and pharmacokinetic methods.

The pharmacokinetic method was based on quantitation of aminoglycoside tissue accumulation and its effects on renal proximal tubules. We employed a two-compartment pharmacokinetic model to describe aminoglycoside tissue uptake versus time for comparison with indices of renal proximal tubular damage (urinary β_2-microglobulin, urinary cast excretion, and urinary excretion of renal enzymes). These studies established that abnormally high accumulation of aminoglycoside antibiotics in kidney tissue occurs prior to any evidence of tubular damage in patients who later develop aminoglycoside nephrotoxicity (3). We also found that aminoglycoside tissue accumulation remains normal in patients who develop renal failure from other causes. Our proposed explanation for the normal accumulation is that cessation of glomerular filtration due to other clinical insults prevents accumulation of these drugs in renal cortex (4).

We studied 201 patients given 267 courses of G or T. The patients were older adults with serious infections complicating either major medical or surgical disorders. Our responsibilities included dosage selection and adjustments based on measured serum levels. Dosing regimens were selected to maintain therapeutic peak (4.0 to 10.0 $\mu g/ml$) and trough (0.5 to 2.0 $\mu g/ml$) serum concentrations in all study patients.

Of the 267 courses given, clinical assessment could be performed on 258. Nine patients could not be included because of hemodialysis or lack of measurement of serum creatinine after treatment stopped. The clinical criterion for nephrotoxicity was an increase in serum creatinine during therapy or up to 7 days thereafter of 0.5 mg/dl or more. In 13 cases (7 T and 6 G) the creatinine increase was ascribed to another cause, usually septic shock.

Data for pharmacokinetic analysis were available from 240 courses of aminoglycoside therapy. Patients were excluded from pharmacokinetic assessment only if an insufficient number of serum or urine samples prevented the use of a two-compartment pharmacokinetic model or tests of renal tubular damage. This report gives the results in the 240 courses where both clinical and pharmacokinetic analysis could be compared. Results of clinical assessment in 258 courses for nephrotoxicity have been published (2).

The 120 G and 120 T courses were administered to patients of similar age, weight, initial creatinine clearance, and incidence of proven infection (Table 1). One fourth of each group had positive blood cultures. Prior aminoglycosides (usually G) were given twice as frequently to the T group ($P < 0.001$). During treatment, the two groups achieved similar initial trough concentrations, received the same average dosage and duration of treatment, and had on the average 1.1 dosage adjustments made to maintain therapeutic blood levels. Cephalosporins were given concurrently in slightly more T courses, and diuretics (chiefly furosemide) were given in more G courses. Neither difference was significant.

About 75% of infections in each group either were cured or improved with treatment (Table 2). Approximately 25% of patients died, usually as a consequence of underlying disease.

The G group had a greater decrease in creat-

TABLE 1. *Pretherapy and concurrent therapy comparison of 120 G courses and 120 T courses*[a]

Patient group	Age (yrs)	Wt (kg)	Initial creatinine clearance (ml/min)	Proven infection (%)	Positive blood cultures in (%):	Prior[b] aminoglycoside therapy (%)	Initial trough (µg/ml)	Total dosage (g)	Treatment duration (days)	Dose changes in	Concurrent cephalosporins (%)	Concurrent diuretics (%)
G	67 ± 12	66 ± 15	51 ± 27	84	22.5	18	1.6 ± 0.9	1.7 ± 1.2	9.7 ± 5.5	1.1 ± 1.4	30	63
T	66 ± 12	68 ± 13	51 ± 31	91	23	44	1.4 ± 1.0	1.7 ± 1.8	11.3 ± 8.1	1.1 ± 1.5	40	54
Statistical significance (G vs. T)	NS[c]	NS	NS	NS	NS	P < 0.001	NS	NS	NS	NS	NS	NS

[a] Values are given as mean ± 1 standard deviation. (%), Percent of patients. Creatinine clearance values were measured when urine was available, predicted by nomogram in the remainder.
[b] Prior is defined as within 30 days.
[c] NS, Not significant.

TABLE 2. *Nephrotoxicity assessments and response to treatment in 120 G courses and 120 T courses*[a]

Patient group	Infection responded in[b] (%):	Mortality (% died)	Final creatinine clearance (ml/min)	Final serum trough (µg/ml)	Tissue accumulation (mg)[c]	Nephrotoxicity by:		
						Clinical criteria (%)	Pharmacokinetic criteria (%)	Overall agreement (%)
G	73	27	41 ± 27	2.8 ± 2.3	141 ± 133	37	24	76
T	75	23	50 ± 34	2.2 ± 2.2	97 ± 64	22	10	83
Statistical significance (G vs. T)	NS[d]	NS	P < 0.02	P < 0.05	P < 0.01	P < 0.02	P < 0.01	NS

[a] Values are given as mean ± 1 standard deviation, or percent of patients where indicated.
[b] Response is defined as clinical cure or clinical improvement.
[c] Calculated based on a two-compartment pharmacokinetic model confirmed independently by urine or postmortem tissues during 81 courses.
[d] NS, Not significant.

inine clearance ($P < 0.02$), a higher final trough concentration ($P < 0.05$), and greater tissue accumulation ($P < 0.01$) than did the T group. All of these differences were significant and are consistent with the greater incidence of renal damage observed in the G group.

By clinical criteria, 37% of G courses and 22% of T courses were judged nephrotoxic ($P < 0.02$). Pharmacokinetic assessment (based on abnormal tissue accumulation) attributed renal tubular damage to 24% of G and 10% of T courses ($P < 0.01$). Overall agreement between clinical and pharmacokinetic assessments was above 75%, and agreement on nephrotoxic cases alone was 83% on G courses and 67% on T courses.

Our results demonstrate good agreement between pharmacokinetic and clinical criteria when both are applied to acutely ill patients. Use of pharmacokinetic criteria will lower the overall incidence of nephrotoxicity attributed to both G and T. However, we cannot be certain that what is defined here as aminoglycoside damage is solely due to these drugs, since other renal insults are common in patients of this type. Aminoglycoside nephrotoxicity remains a diagnosis of exclusion, even though more specific diagnostic methods are being developed. In the absence of criteria specific enough to distinguish the renal damage due to aminoglycosides from that associated with underlying diseases, even double-blind, randomized studies cannot safely conclude that differences exist between drugs unless the patient groups are first shown to be identical in all other respects.

Since our prospectively studied G and T groups did not differ in base-line risk factors, or in risk factors developing during the treatment period, we propose that differences in renal damage result from differences in the nephrotoxic potential of G and T. Whether our results will be broadly applicable to all categories of aminoglycoside-treated patients remains to be further studied.

1. Luft, F. C., R. Block, R. S. Sloan, M. N. Yum, R. Costello, and D. R. Maxwell. 1978. Comparative nephrotoxicity of aminoglycoside antibiotics in rats. J. Infect. Dis. 138:541–545.
2. Plaut, M. E., J. J. Schentag, and W. J. Jusko. 1979. Nephrotoxicity with gentamicin or tobramycin. Lancet ii:526–527.
3. Schentag, J. J., T. J. Cumbo, W. J. Jusko, and M. E. Plaut. 1978. Gentamicin tissue accumulation and nephrotoxic reactions. J. Am. Med. Assoc. 240:2067–2069.
4. Schentag, J. J., M. E. Plaut, F. B. Cerra, P. B. Wels, P. Walczak, and R. J. Buckley. 1979. Aminoglycoside nephrotoxicity in critically ill surgical patients. J. Surg. Res. 26:270–279.

Tobramycin Is Less Nephrotoxic than Gentamicin: Results of a Double-Blind Clinical Trial

CRAIG R. SMITH,* JAMES J. LIPSKY, OSCAR LASKIN, DAVID HELLMANN, E. DAVID MELLITS, JAMES LONGSTRETH, AND PAUL S. LIETMAN

The Johns Hopkins University, Baltimore, Maryland 21205, U.S.A.

Nephrotoxicity and ototoxicity are major factors limiting the clinical utility of aminoglycoside antibiotics. In experimental animals, tobramycin is less nephrotoxic and ototoxic than gentamicin (3). A few clinical studies have supported these observations (1, 4). However, these trials have included small numbers of patients or have not conformed with methodological standards for comparative drug trials (5). For example, none has been double blind, introducing the possibility that bias may have influenced the results. Because these clinical studies were inconclusive, we conducted a clinical trial to determine whether tobramycin causes less nephrotoxicity or less auditory toxicity than gentamicin. In this prospective, controlled, randomized, double-blind trial we found that tobramycin is less nephrotoxic than gentamicin if patients are treated in the manner to be outlined, and we found that the auditory toxicity of tobramycin and gentamicin does not differ by more than 25%.

Patients with suspected sepsis were candidates for entry into the study. Drug assignments and clinical evaluations were double blind, as previously reported by our group (2). Patients with meningitis, an allergy to penicillin, an infection due to an organism known to be resistant to gentamicin or tobramycin, or antibiotic treatment within the previous 48 h were not entered into the study. The initial aminoglycoside dosage was 2 mg/kg intravenously over 20 to 30 min. Subsequent doses were given every 8 h and adjusted for renal function with the Chan nomogram. Predose and 1-h postdose plasma aminoglycoside concentrations were determined with a radioenzymatic assay within 24 h. Subsequent doses were adjusted to maintain the 1-h postdose plasma level between 5 and 10 µg/ml. Patients also received either methicillin (12 g/day) or nafcillin (9 g/day). Clindamycin (2.4 g/day) was added when a pelvic or gastrointestinal source of infection was suspected and was the only other concurrent antibiotic administered.

Non-antibiotic therapy was not controlled. Predose and 1-h postdose plasma aminoglycoside levels were measured on days 1 and 3, and every alternate day during therapy. Levels were also measured after each dosage change. Serum creatinine was measured before therapy, on days 2, 3, and 4 and on every third day of therapy, and 2 days after therapy. Audiograms were measured at the bedside at 250, 500, 1,000, 2,000, 4,000 and 8,000 Hz on day 1 or 2 and day 7 of therapy and 2 days after therapy. Patients receiving at least nine doses of aminoglycoside and with no other cause of acute renal failure in the previous 72 h were evaluated for nephrotoxicity. Nephrotoxicity was defined as a rise in serum creatinine of over 0.4 mg/100 ml if the initial level was less than 3.0 mg/100 ml, or a rise of over 0.9 mg/100 ml if the initial creatinine was 3.0 mg/100 ml or above. The rise was determined by subtracting the initial creatinine from the highest creatinine during therapy or within 48 h after therapy. Patients who satisfied the definition of nephrotoxicity but who had other causes of acute renal failure were excluded from the comparison because the exact cause of the creatinine increase could not be determined. Patients who received at least nine doses of gentamicin or tobramycin and who were able to cooperate with serial audiograms were evaluated for auditory toxicity. Auditory toxicity was defined as a decrease in auditory threshold of greater than or equal to 15 dB at any frequency in the range of 250 to 8,000 Hz.

The Fisher exact test was used to compare proportions and the Student t test was used to compare means. A one-tailed analysis was decided on before the study was initiated because all available evidence in experimental animals and humans suggested that tobramycin was less nephrotoxic than gentamicin. We selected our sample size to detect a 10% reduction in nephrotoxicity with an estimated control incidence of 15%, $\alpha < 0.05$, and $\beta < 0.2$.

A total of 257 patients were enrolled in the study. Of these, 82 were excluded from the comparison because they received less than nine doses, and 29 had another cause of acute renal failure. Gentamicin and tobramycin were then compared in the remaining 146 patients. Of these, 72 were given gentamicin and 74 received

tobramycin. The two groups did not differ in mean age, initial creatinine, duration of therapy, total dose, and mean predose and 1-h postdose aminoglycoside levels. Neither did the groups differ in the presence of previous renal disease, the presence of urinary tract infection, or the administration of furosemide, nafcillin, methicillin, or clindamycin. The relationship between gentamicin or tobramycin treatment and change in creatinine is shown in Table 1. The mean increase in creatinine was 0.4 mg/100 ml for those given gentamicin and only 0.1 mg/100 ml for those given tobramycin, a difference that is highly statistically significant. The incidence of nephrotoxicity based on our previously mentioned definition and selected at the onset of the study was also greater in the gentamicin group, with 19/72 or 26.4% developing nephrotoxicity compared to 9/74 or 12.2% of those given tobramycin. In the nephrotoxic groups, the severity of the nephrotoxicity was the same with a mean increase in creatinine of 1.3 mg/100 ml.

There were 91 patients compared for auditory toxicity. The other 165 patients were excluded because they received less than nine doses of aminoglycoside or could not cooperate with serial audiograms. Gentamicin was given to 47 patients, and tobramycin was given to 44. These two groups did not differ in mean age, total dose, duration of therapy, initial creatinine, aminoglycoside levels, or number given concurrent furosemide. The relationship between gentamicin or

TABLE 1. *Change in creatinine in patients given gentamicin or tobramycin*

Change in creatinine	No. of patients[a]		Signifi-cance (P)
	Gentamicin (N = 72)	Tobramycin (N = 74)	
No increase	53	65	
Increase	19	9	<0.025
Mean increase (mg/100 ml)	0.4	0.1	<0.005

[a] Number of patients determined by criteria for nephrotoxicity.

TABLE 2. *Change in auditory threshold in patients given gentamicin or tobramycin*

Change in threshold	No. of patients[a]	
	Gentamicin (N = 47)	Tobramycin (N = 44)
No change	42	39
Decrease	5	5
Mean decrease (dB)	21	23

[a] Number of patients determined by criteria for auditory toxicity.

tobramycin treatment and change in auditory threshold is shown in Table 2. Auditory toxicity developed in 5/47 or 10.6% of those given gentamicin and 5/44 or 11.4% of those given tobramycin. These values are not statistically different. With our sample size we would have been able to detect a difference of 25% or greater at the 0.05 level with a beta less than or equal to 0.2. The severity of the auditory toxicity in the two groups was also similar.

In conclusion, we have shown in a prospective, controlled, randomized, double-blind trial that tobramycin is less nephrotoxic than gentamicin if patients are treated in the manner outlined, and we conclude that the auditory toxicity of tobramycin and gentamicin does not differ by more than 25%.

1. Fee, W. E., Jr., V. Vierra, and G. R. Lathrop. 1978. Clinical evaluation of aminoglycoside toxicity: tobramycin versus gentamicin, a preliminary report. J. Antimicrob. Chemother. 4(Suppl. A):31–36.
2. Gifford, R. H., and A. R. Feinstein. 1969. A critique of methodology in studies of anticoagulant therapy for acute myocardial infarction. N. Engl. J. Med. 280:351–357.
3. Gilbert, D. N., C. Plamp, P. Starr, W. M. Bennett, D. C. Houghton, and G. Porter. 1978. Comparative nephrotoxicity of gentamicin and tobramycin in rats. Antimicrob. Agents Chemother. 13:34–40.
4. Schentag, J. J., M. E. Plaut, F. B. Cerra, P. B. Wels, P. Walczak, and R. J. Buckley. 1979. Aminoglycoside nephrotoxicity in critically ill surgical patients. J. Surg. Res. 26:270–279.
5. Smith, C. R., K. L. Baughman, C. Q. Edwards, J. F. Rogers, and P. S. Lietman. 1977. Controlled comparison of amikacin and gentamicin. N. Engl. J. Med. 296:349–353.

Urinary Excretion of β_2-Microglobulin and Other Proteins After Application of Cephalosporins, Aminoglycosides, and Their Combination

M. WEISE, G. JAQUES, M. KELLER, AND A. W. MONDORF

Center of Internal Medicine, Giessen, and Center of Internal Medicine, Frankfurt, Federal Republic of Germany

The increasing clinical application of aminoglycosides and their combination with cephalosporins in the treatment of infections with gram-negative organisms requires accurate knowledge of the possible side effects. Since the kidney is the most important excretory organ for aminoglycosides, it is of principal interest.

For the detection of tubular dysfunction, the renal handling of the low-molecular-weight protein β_2-microglobulin seems to be a very sensitive indicator. This protein is usually freely filtered through the glomerular membrane and nearly completely reabsorbed into the proximal tubular cells, with only about 100 μg excreted in the 24-h final urine. A higher excretion of β_2-microglobulin in the urine is caused by an impaired tubular reabsorption and would indicate a tubular dysfunction.

Another very sensitive marker for tubular damage is the urinary excretion of alanine aminopeptidase. In previous investigations Mondorf and co-workers have shown (1, 2) that alanine aminopeptidase seems to be a principal enzyme of the proximal tubule and an integral constituent of the brush border membrane in the human kidney. This enzyme appears in varying quantities in the urine as a result either of toxic lesions in acute tubular necrosis or of inflammatory processes in the kidney. An increased urinary excretion of alanine aminopeptidase can be used

to assess the degree of membrane alterations possibly produced by cephalosporins and aminoglycosides or their combination.

In a group of 10 informed volunteers we administered cephalothin and tobramycin in recommended dosages of 8 g of cephalothin and 3 mg of tobramycin per kg of body weight twice a day on 3 consecutive days. In the 24-h urine that we collected 1 day before and on the 3 days during administration of the drugs, as well as on days 4, 5, and 7 after the onset of the administration, we determined total protein by using a modification of the Lowry method, β_2-microglobulin with a radioimmunoassay, and alanine aminopeptidase enzymatically. Because β_2-microglobulin is unstable at a pH below 5.7, we excluded those samples with a low pH from determination of this protein.

As can be seen in Fig. 1, there was a significant increase of the elimination of total protein in the urine on days 1, 2, and 3 of the administration of the combination. In contrast to these findings, alanine aminopeptidase as well as β_2-microglobulin showed a cumulative increase in output in the 24-h urine after the onset of the application of the combination: β_2-microglobulin returned to normal on day 3, the last day of application, and alanine aminopeptidase returned to normal on day 4.

This nearly identical behavior of β_2-microglobulin and alanine aminopeptidase indicates an alteration of brush border membranes and tubular function. To our knowledge this behavior corresponds to damage of proximal tubular cells by aminoglycosides, because of their 50-times-higher accumulation in the kidney in comparison to all other organs. Closer observation of these data showed a responder and a nonresponder group. Similar findings could be seen with alanine aminopeptidase. We therefore assume very different individual response to these drugs.

The combination of cefuroxime and tobramycin showed similar results, including the very early elimination of total protein which is obviously not related to the elimination of β_2-microglobulin and alanine aminopeptidase. Here again there was a cumulative increase of β_2-microglobulin and alanine aminopeptidase which lasted 1 day longer for alanine aminopeptidase than for β_2-microglobulin, obviously caused by an induction of the enzyme in the membrane itself. In this group we also could differentiate between responders and non- or low responders.

Cefotaxime application as a single drug showed no effect on the excretion of total protein, alanine aminopeptidase, and β_2-microglobulin. In the case of alanine aminopeptidase, male and female could be clearly separated in their mean values according to the statistically differ-

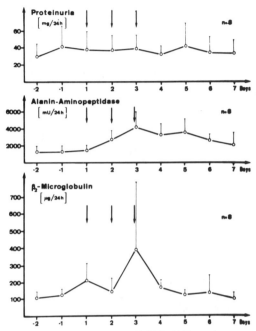

FIG. 2. *Aminoglycoside UK 18892 results.*

ent output of male and female healthy subjects.

In a kinetic study over 3 days, alanine aminopeptidase and total protein showed identical behavior, with a very high output at the beginning of the administration of the drug which was reproducible on days 2 and 3. The standard deviation for alanine aminopeptidase was less than 30%. The profile for β_2-microglobulin in this kinetic study did not show this clear-cut increase at the beginning of the drug administration.

The aminoglycoside UK 18892 showed the cumulative increase of alanine aminopeptidase and β_2-microglobulin as in the combination with cephalosporins, but without any reaction of total protein (Fig. 2).

Obviously the early increase of total protein in the combination was related to cephalosporin in this drug combination. The tubular secretion of cephalosporins is possibly the reason for the increase of total proteinuria.

In summary, the determination of total protein, alanine aminopeptidase, and β_2-microglobulin in the 24-h urine showed various results: (i) the combination of cephalosporins with aminoglycosides had distinct effects on proximal tubular cells related to effects of aminoglycosides alone, reflected by a transient increase of β_2-microglobulin and alanine aminopeptidase; (ii) total proteinuria was only influenced by cephalosporins, which could be clearly demonstrated in kinetic studies with cefotaxime; (iii) the individual response was different in each group in

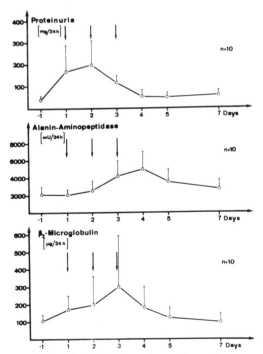

FIG. 1. *Cephalothin + tobramycin results.*

which we could demonstrate responder and non-responder by the output of β_2-microglobulin.

1. Mondorf, A. W., J. Breier, J. Hendus, J. E. Scherberich, G. Mackenrodth, P. M. Shah, W. Stille, and W. Schoeppe. 1978. Effect of aminoglycosides on proximal tubular membranes of the human kidney. Eur. J. Clin. Pharmacol. **13**:133–142.

2. Mondorf, A. W., M. Zegelman, J. Klose, J. Hendus, and J. Breier. 1978. Comparative studies on the action of aminoglycosides and cephalosporins on the proximal tubule of the human kidney. J. Antimicrob. Chemother. **4**(Suppl. A):53–57.

Urinary β_2-Microglobulin and Alanine Aminopeptidase Excretion in Gentamicin-Treated Patients and Untreated Controls

PETER G. DAVEY

East Birmingham Hospital, Birmingham, England

β-Microglobulin (β_2M) is a low-molecular-weight protein that is filtered by the renal glomerulus and reabsorbed by the proximal tubule. With normal tubular function, daily excretion is less than 0.3 mg unless serum levels of β_2M exceed 4.5 mg/liter. Alanine aminopeptidase (AAP) is an enzyme found in the brush border of proximal tubular cells; normal daily excretion is less than 40 IU. Greatly increased excretion of β_2M, up to 20 mg/day, has been reported following surgery or major trauma without increase in serum levels (6), and small increases have been reported with fever (2). Increased excretion of aminopeptidases has been observed following toxic or inflammatory renal damage (4, 5). To study the usefulness of these parameters as markers of aminoglycoside toxicity, a group of 20 control patients and a group of 18 patients who received 19 courses of aminogylcoside treatment have been studied. The control group consisted of seven patients studied after trauma or major surgery, seven patients who had cardiogenic hypotension following myocardial infarction, and a group of six patients with a variety of infections and febrile episodes. The treated group consisted of nine patients treated for complications following surgery, two patients with pyelonephritis who received three treatment courses, and seven patients with a variety of sites of infection. Amikacin was used in one case; all other treatment courses were with gentamicin.

Twenty-four-hour urines were collected from the treated group within 72 h of the start of treatment and then daily until discharge from hospital or for 5 days after the end of treatment. Daily collections were taken from the controls undergoing surgery before and for a week after surgery. Collections were taken from the controls with cardiogenic hypotension during the period of hypotension and from febrile patients while fever persisted. Evidence of renal impair-

ment was defined as a 100% or greater increase in serum creatinine with a 50% or greater decrease in creatinine clearance. Renal impairment developed during the study period in five treated patients but in none of the controls. One of these cases of renal impairment was definitely due to gentamicin; the other four had other possible causes for renal damage.

The peak excretion of β_2M for the controls and treated patients is shown in Fig. 1. One control and one treated patient were eliminated because of serum β_2M levels >4.5 mg/liter. Peak secretion occurred within 4 days of the start of treatment in all cases and preceded the development of renal impairment. Peaks were short-

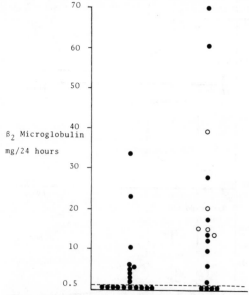

FIG. 1. *Peak excretion of β_2M in controls (n = 19) and aminoglycoside-treated patients (n = 18). Dashed line indicates normal β_2M excretion. (○) Patient with renal impairment developing on treatment.*

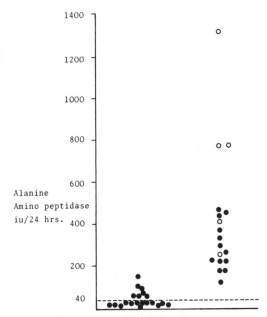

FIG. 2. *Peak excretion of AAP in controls (n = 20) and aminoglycoside-treated patients (n = 19). Dashed line indicates normal AAP excretion. (O) Patient with renal impairment developing on treatment.*

lived, only lasting for 24 h in several cases. Peak excretion of AAP is shown in Fig. 2; peak excretion occurred after 5 to 6 days in most cases, and in contrast to β_2M excretion, the increased level of AAP excretion was sustained for several days.

The overlap between controls and treated patients for β_2M excretion was considerable. Two controls studied after surgery for colonic carcinoma and after multiple injuries excreted 34 and 23 mg/day respectively; both had normal serum β_2M. The two treated patients with the highest urinary β_2M had septicemia with hypotension but did not develop renal impairment. Four of the treated patients showed normal excretion throughout.

Only one of the controls had AAP excretion in the same range as the treated group. Three of the patients with renal damage had excretion well in excess of the rest of the group, and all patients showed abnormal excretion on treatment.

The mechanism for the increased excretion of β_2M following surgery or trauma is unclear; it may be due to tubular damage, increased glomerular filtration, or competition for reabsorption by peptides or amino acids appearing in the urine; amino acids, particularly lysine and arginine, have been shown to compete with β_2M for reabsorption (5). Whatever the mechanism, β_2M excretion is not a suitable test for aminoglycoside toxicity in these patients. The finding of

normal β_2M excretion in some patients prompted further study of its stability in urine. β_2M is known to be unstable in urine with a pH of less than 5.5; significant degradation occurs in 2 h at 37°C but takes 24 h at room temperature (6). Since 24 h urines were used in this study, the effect of longer incubation at body temperature was investigated. Incubation of urine with a pH of 6.0 for 8 h at 37°C produced 50% degradation; no degradation occurred in urine with a pH of 6.5. Finally, the transience of β_2M peaks means that if a single collection is accidentally discarded or if collections are not started from the first day of treatment, peak excretion may be missed.

The AAP results showed that there was almost no overlap between excretion in controls and that in treated patients. This indicates that uncomplicated aminoglycoside treatment has a greater effect on AAP excretion than does the variety of nephrotoxic factors in the control group. However, underlying condition may influence AAP excretion in treated patients, since in the group of treated patients without renal impairment the four with the highest AAP levels were those with underlying conditions likely to cause renal damage, pyelonephritis or septicemia with hypotension. Because of this, patients in comparative studies of aminoglycoside toxicity must be matched for underlying condition.

Three patients with renal impairment had urinary AAP levels well above the rest of the treated group; the patient with definite aminoglycoside nephrotoxicity had the highest excretion of all. Thus AAP excretion may distinguish renal damage caused by aminoglycosides from that due to underlying condition.

In conclusion, AAP excretion is a more promising test than β_2M excretion for the investigation of aminoglycoside toxicity in patients.

1. **Evrin, P. E., and L. Wibell.** 1972. Serum levels and urinary excretion of β_2M in apparently healthy subjects. Scand. J. Clin. Lab. Invest. **29**:59–74.
2. **Hemmingsen, L., and P. Skaarup.** 1977. Urinary excretion of ten plasma proteins in patients with febrile diseases. Acta Med. Scand. **201**:359–364.
3. **Mogensen, C. E., and K. Sølling.** 1977. Studies on renal tubular protein reabsorption: partial and near complete inhibition by certain amino acids. Scand. J. Clin. Lab. Invest. **37**:477–486.
4. **Mondorf, A. W., J. Breier, J. Hendus, J. E. Scherberich, G. Mackenrodt, P. M. Shah, W. Stille, and W. Schoeppe.** 1978. Effect of aminoglycosides on proximal tubular membranes of the human kidney. Eur. J. Clin. Pharmacol. **13**:133–142.
5. **Rabb, W. P.** 1972. Diagnostic value of urinary enzyme determinations. Clin. Chem. **18**:5–25.
6. **Wide, L., and L. Thoren.** 1972. Increased urinary clearance for albumin, B₂-microglobulin, insulin and luteinizing hormone following surgical or accidental trauma. Scand. J. Clin. Lab. Invest. **30**:275–281.

Prospective Comparative Evaluation of Gentamicin Versus Cefuroxime Versus Gentamicin Plus Cefuroxime Renal Toxicity in Humans

H. GIAMARELLOU,* CH. METZIKOFF, G. PETRIKKOS, S. PAPACHRISTOPHOROU, AND G. K. DAIKOS

First Department of Propedeutic Medicine, University of Athens Medical School, King Paul's Hospital, Athens, 609, Greece

It has become a belief that cephalosporins in general augment gentamicin nephrotoxicity in humans. However, most of the data are collected retrospectively from seriously ill patients in whom other predisposing factors coexist. On the other hand, recent studies in rats have demonstrated that cephalothin when given simultaneously with gentamicin protects against gentamicin nephrotoxicity (2). Fanning et al. (3), although retrospectively, provided evidence in humans against the above-mentioned synergistic activity. Giamarellou et al. (5) were the first to show prospectively in humans that gentamicin, whether alone or in combination with various cephalosporins, is consistently nephrotoxic, and that simultaneous administration of the antibiotics is not protective against gentamicin nephrotoxicity.

Cefuroxime, a third-generation β-lactamase-resistant cephalosporin, is claimed to be free from nephrotoxic potential (1). However, cefuroxime is not adequate for treating seriously ill patients; a combination with gentamicin to broaden its spectrum is necessary.

To investigate the possibility of synergism, indifference, or even protection in connection with renal toxicity when both antibiotics are given simultaneously, a prospective randomized trial was designed in 90 patients with normal renal function suffering from a variety of mild to moderate infections, in whom gentamicin plus cefuroxime (group A, 30 patients) was tested, with gentamicin (group B, 30 patients) and cefuroxime (group C, 30 patients) as the control groups. Gentamicin was given at a loading dose of 2 mg intramuscularly every 8 h (three doses), followed by a maintenance dose of 1.5 mg intramuscularly every 8 h; cefuroxime was given at 750 mg intramuscularly every 8 h; and both antibiotics together were given at the same doses intramuscularly and simultaneously at different sites. Patients with predisposing factors influencing renal function, such as cardiorespiratory insufficiency, diabetes mellitus, and nephrolithiasis, were excluded from the study. Renal function was evaluated every other day, and the following were considered as indicators of nephrotoxicity: (i) the persistent presence of cylindruria (> three granular casts per high-power field); (ii) increased β-glycuronidase activity in urine (4); (iii) increased N-α-β-glycosaminidase activity in urine (6); (iv) persistent increase in serum creatinine by more than 400 μg/ml above pretreatment value; and (v) persistent abnormal elevation of blood urea (>50 mg/100 ml). Mean ages in the three groups were 52.4, 52.8, and 48.6 years with mean duration of treatment of 8.8, 8.7, and 8.8 days, respectively.

The incidence of nephrotoxicity in all groups is shown in Table 1 and Fig. 1. It is clear that cefuroxime is not nephrotoxic, although it does not potentiate gentamicin effect on renal function. The results are similar to those of Giamarellou et al. (J. Antimicrob. Chemother., in press) concerning gentamicin versus cephalothin + gentamicin in the production of renal toxicity in humans.

Abnormal N-α-β-glycosaminidase levels in urine have been considered as one of the most sensitive indicators of early nephrotoxicity (6). Although this enzyme, due to technical difficulties, was not measured in all patients, its presence in urine in highly abnormal values in all subjects given gentamicin, but in none treated with cefuroxime, seems to be an obligatory effect of gentamicin on the renal tubular epithelium. On the other hand, detection of abnormal values of N-α-β-glycosaminidase in urine was the earliest indicator of nephrotoxicity, since in almost 70% of the patients it appeared during day 2 of treatment.

The presence of cylindruria and increased β-glycuronidase activity in urine were also considered as quite sensitive indicators of nephrotoxicity. However, elevated urine levels of this enzyme do not appear to be an earlier or more sensitive indicator of nephrotoxicity, since both indices appeared on day 3 of treatment in 63.3% and 73.3% of groups A and B, respectively.

It should be pointed out that whenever trough blood levels of gentamicin were above 2 μg/ml with peak levels exceeding 6 μg/ml, both β-glycuronidase enzymuria and cylindruria were present; their abnormal values indicate therapeutic gentamicin blood levels rather than nephrotoxicity.

TABLE 1. *Incidence of nephrotoxicity in 90 patients administered cefuroxime, gentamicin, and combination[a]*

Parameter	Incidence of nephrotoxicity[b]			χ^{2c}		
	C	G	C + G	C vs. G	C vs. C + G	G vs. C + G
Cylindruria	0/30 (0)	22/30 (73.3)	20/30 (66.6)	31.65*	27.07*	0.07**
β-Glycuronidase urine	2/30 (6.6)	19/30 (63.3)	19/30 (63.3)	14.87*	12.09*	0.03**
NAG[d] urine	0/13 (0)	16/16 (100)	13/13 (100)			
Elevated serum creatinine	0/30 (0)	4/30 (13.3)	5/30 (16.6)	2.41**	3.49**	0
Abnormal blood urea	0/30 (0)	1/30 (3.3)	1/30 (3.3)	0	0	0

[a] C, Cefuroxime; G, gentamicin; C + G, cefuroxime + gentamicin.
[b] Number of patients/total treated (percent).
[c] *, Significant; **, not significant.
[d] NAG, N-α-β-glycosaminidase.

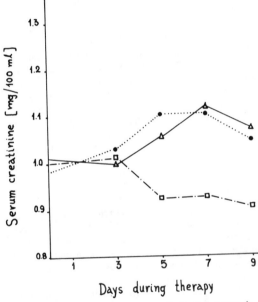

FIG. 1. *Changes in serum creatinine concentration during gentamicin (●), cefuroxime (□), and cefuroxime + gentamicin (△) therapy.*

Among the various predisposing factors in connection with renal toxicity in groups A and B, the following seem to influence the expression of toxicity the most (but at the same extent) in both groups: age > 70 years; male sex; duration of treatment > 10 days; a total daily dose of gentamicin of ≥320 mg as well as a total dose of >3,000 mg; gentamicin trough levels of ≥2 μg/ml; and cholocystographic agents which have a synergistic effect with gentamicin in the production of acute renal failure.

The results were subjected to statistical analysis by the χ^2 test. No statistically significant difference was found in the distribution of age, type of infection, and duration of treatment among the three groups. When the various parameters indicating gentamicin nephrotoxicity were compared with those produced by the combination of gentamicin plus cefuroxime, no statistical difference emerged ($P > 0.1$). However, a highly statistically significant difference was observed between cefuroxime and gentamicin as well as between cefuroxime and gentamicin + cefuroxime ($P < 0.01$).

In conclusion, the results in the study indicate that: (i) gentamicin, whether alone or in combination with cefuroxime, is equally nephrotoxic, and (ii) cefuroxime at the conventional treatment schedule is not nephrotoxic but is also not protective against gentamicin nephrotoxicity.

1. Daikos, G. K., J. C. Kosmidis, Ch. Stathakis, and H. Giamarellou. 1977. Cefuroxime: antimicrobial activity, human pharmacokinetics and therapeutic efficacy. J. Antimicrob. Chemother. 3:555–562.
2. Delinger, P., T. Murphy, V. Pinn, M. Barza, and L. Weinstein. 1976. Protective effect of cephalothin against gentamicin-induced nephrotoxicity in rats. Antimicrob. Agents Chemother. 9:172–178.
3. Fanning, W. L., D. Gump, and H. Jick. 1976. Gentamicin- and cephalothin-associated rises in blood urea nitrogen. Antimicrob. Agents Chemother. 10:80–82.
4. Fishman, W. H., K. Kato, C. L. Anstiss, and S. Green. 1967. Human serum β-glycuronidase; its measurement and some of its properties. Clin. Chim. Acta 15:435–447.
5. Giamarellou, H., G. Petrikkos, P. Doudoulaki, and G. K. Daikos. 1978. Prospective comparative evaluation of gentamicin alone and gentamicin plus various cephalosporins with respect to nephrotoxicity in humans, p. 968–970. In Current chemotherapy, Proceedings of the 10th International Congress of Chemotherapy. American Society for Microbiology, Washington, D.C.
6. Price, R. G., and N. Dance. 1970. The excretion of NAG and β-galactosidase following surgery to the kidneys. Clin. Chim. Acta 27:65–72.

Comparison of Nephrotoxicity of Two Aminoglycosides, Derivatives of Kanamycin A and B, and Amikacin

T. STEFANESCU,* A. W. MONDORF, T. FRANZKE, AND J. E. SCHERBERICH

Center of Internal Medicine, J. W. Goethe University, Frankfurt, Federal Republic of Germany

In our previous studies (2, 3) we demonstrated that a sensitive parameter of damage of the proximal tubules is the enzyme alanine aminopeptidase (AAP), whose increased urinary excretion indicates a lesion of the proximal tubules. The AAP was located in the brush border of the tubular cells as a superficial enzymatic component of the plasma membrane (4, 5).

The urinary increase of the enzyme precedes the modifications of the usual humoral parameter or of the microscopic findings. The normal value of the urinary excretion of AAP was established at 1,000 to 3,500 mU/24 h.

The action on the proximal renal tubules, as demonstrated by urinary excretion of AAP, of two new aminoglycosides, UK 18.892 and UK 31.214, derivatives of kanamycin A and B, respectively, was examined in two groups of healthy, informed volunteers. In a third group of seven volunteers, amikacin in a dosage of 10 mg/kg of body weight daily was studied. For the study of the two new aminoglycosides we selected, from 44 subjectively healthy male candidates, 10 for each aminoglycoside. The criteria of the selection were as follows.

(i) Each patient's medical history should show: no renal diseases, urinary symptoms, or hypertension; no otitis or subjective troubles of the acousticovestibular function (defective hearing, vertigo, or dizziness); no acute hepatitis, other forms of jaundice, or consumptive diseases; no treatment with antibiotics or other potentially nephrotoxic drugs during the last year.

(ii) Clinical examination should present normal findings both of neurological state and in balance tests.

(iii) Laboratory data should demonstrate: normal concentrations in serum of urea, creatinine, uric acid, electrolytes (K^+, Na^+, Ca^{2+}, Cl^-), glutamic oxalacetic transaminase, glutamic pyruvic transaminase, γ-GT, and aminopeptidase; normal values of erythrocytes, leukocytes, and hemoglobin; normal creatinine clearance; no pathological changes in the urine, and normal urine sediment; in the audiogram, no loss of the hearing more than 25 dB; no pathological nystagmus in electronystagmogram.

(iv) Each patient should have normal urinary excretion of AAP.

Of the 44 candidates, we excluded from the study 12 because of modifications in the audiogram, 3 because of vestibular troubles, 1 because of microhematuria, and, 5 because of doubtful medical history.

After a 2-day base-line study period, each of the 10 volunteers in both groups received either UK 18.892 or UK 31.214 intramuscularly at 10 mg/kg of body weight per day, twice a day, over 3 consecutive days. The AAP in 24-h urine was measured daily, 2 days before application, during the 3-day application period, and for 6 days after application. The diagram (Fig. 1) of the daily mean values of the 24-h urinary AAP excretion shows a continuous rise during the application for both aminoglycosides. UK 18.892 AAP excretion peaked at 4,600 mU on the 3rd (last) application day and showed a second peak of 3,950 mU on postapplication day 2. UK 31.214 showed a maximal excretion of AAP of 3,500 mU/24 h on day 1 after application. AAP excretion returned to normal with UK 18.892 on postapplication day 1, and that with UK 31.214 returned to normal on posttreatment day 3. In comparison with amikacin (Fig. 1), administered in the same manner in a dosage of 10 mg/kg of body weight per day, the new aminoglycosides caused a significantly lower AAP excretion. The maximal excretion as mean value was in the amikacin group (6,700 mU/24 h on application day 3), and normal excretion was reached on day 6 after application. Compared with tobramycin (Fig. 2), given to a group of 15 volunteers in the normal therapeutic dosage of 3 mg/kg of body weight per 24 h in the same manner (3 consecutive days) in our former studies, the new aminoglycosides provide similar AAP excretion. The maximal mean value was for tobramycin (4,050 mU of AAP per 24 h) on day 1 after application. On application day 2 and postapplication day 2, the creatinine clearance in the UK 18.892 group was determined. In the UK 31.214 group the creatinine clearance was measured on postapplication day 2. The other humoral and urine examinations were repeated on postapplication day 1, and hearing and balance tests were given on postapplication days 5 and 8 for UK 31.214 and UK 18.892, respectively. All the findings remained normal.

Discussion. The present investigations

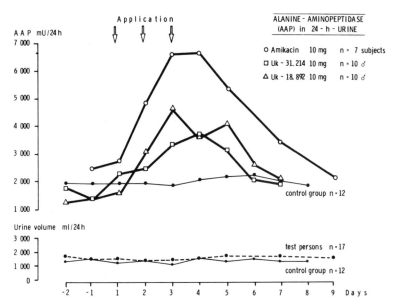

FIG. 1. *Daily mean values of AAP excretion, including the SD, for the two new aminoglycosides compared with those of tobramycin.*

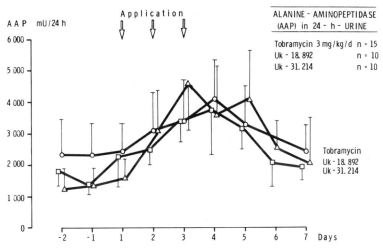

FIG. 2. *Daily mean values of AAP excretion for the two new aminoglycosides compared with those of amikacin and of a control group, including daily diuresis in test persons and the control group.*

showed that the nephrotoxicity of the new derivatives of kanamycin, demonstrated by the urinary excretion of AAP in 24 h, is similar to that of tobramycin and lower than that of amikacin. The new aminoglycosides, like other studied aminoglycosides, have a cumulative effect which increases as the AAP excretion (as maximum of mean values) increases. No other changes of functional renal parameter or of the acousticovestibular function in the audiogram or electronystagmogram after this short administration were found.

1. **Falco, F. G., H. Millard-Smith, and G. M. Arcieri.** 1969. Nephrotoxicity of aminoglycosides and gentamicin. J. Infect. Dis. **119:**406–409.

2. **Mondorf, A. W., J. Breier, J. Hendus, J. E. Scherberich, G. Makenrodt, R. M. Shah, W. Stille, and W. Schoeppe.** 1978. Effects of aminoglycosides on proximal tubular membranes of the human kidney. Eur. J. Clin. Pharmacol. **13:**133–142.

3. **Mondorf, A. W., M. Zegelman, J. Klose, L. Maske, J. E. Scherberich, T. Stefanescu, H. Müller, and W. Schoeppe.** 1978. Effects of various cephalosporins on the proximal tubule of the human kidney. Eur. J. Clin. Pharmacol. **13:**357–363.

4. **Scherberich, J. E., F. Falkenberg, A. W. Mondorf, H. Müller, and G. Pfleiderer.** 1974. Biochemical and

immunological studies on isolated brush border membranes of human kidney and their membrane surface proteins. Clin. Chim. Acta **55**:179–197.

5. **Scherberich, J. E., and W. Mondorf.** 1979. Excretion of kidney brush border antigens as a quantitative indicator of tubular damage. Curr. Probl. Clin. Biochem. **9**:281.

6. **Smith, C. R., K. L. Baughman, C. Q. Edwards, J. F. Rogers, and P. S. Lietman.** 1977. Controlled comparison of amikacin and gentamicin. N. Engl. J. Med. **296:** 349–357.

Clinical Evaluation of Urinary N-Acetyl-β-D-Glucosaminidase Activity in 60 Patients Treated with Aminoglycosides

NAOYUKI HIROKAWA,* ATSUSHI HARUYAMA, SOSUKE OIKE, AND TAKUJI NARUSE

Third Department of Internal Medicine, Gunma University School of Medicine, Maebashi, 371 Japan

Aminoglycoside antibiotics have become very useful in the treatment of severe gram-negative bacterial infections, but their potential nephrotoxicity sometimes poses clinical problems. We recently encountered several patients who had developed renal proximal tubular lesions after gentamicin administration. In this paper, we present the results of comparative studies on nephrotoxicity associated with administration of aminoglycoside antibiotics. The urinary N-acetyl-β-D-glucosaminidase (NAG) activity was used as a sensitive indicator of renal damage induced by the drugs (2–4). The underlying diseases of most of the subjects participating in this study were leukemia or malignant tumors.

The urinary NAG activity was determined by the method of Borooah et al. (1). Urine from each patient was diluted 10 to 40 times, and 0.1 ml was incubated for 1 h with p-nitrophenyl-N-

acetyl-β-D-glucosaminide as the substrate. Then the resulting freed p-nitrophenol was quantitatively determined. The results were expressed in terms of the quantity of free p-nitrophenol. The NAG activity in the urine (collected for 24 h) of 12 control patients with normal renal function was 0.38 ± 0.07 mM per day by this method. No significant changes in NAG activity in the urine were noted, even when the urine was kept for 24 h at room temperature.

Figure 1 shows the changes in urinary NAG activity with time after treatment with gentamicin and dibekacin. As can be seen, the urinary NAG activity tended to be much higher with gentamicin than with dibekacin. Most of the patients given gentamicin showed a peak value within 10 days of administration. Damage to the kidneys was found only in cases where there was a marked rise in this activity. In many patients

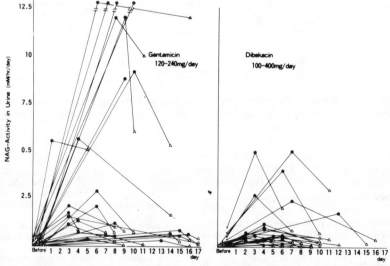

FIG. 1. *Maximal (●) and subsequent minimal (△) values of urinary NAG activities during administration of gentamicin (left) and dibekacin (right).*

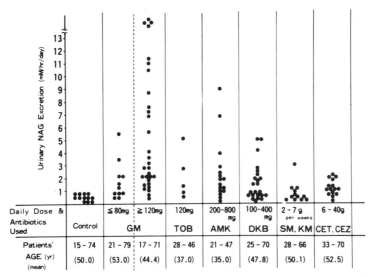

FIG. 2. *Urinary NAG excretion in patients under treatment with antibiotics. Abbreviations: GM, gentamicin; TOB, tobramycin; AMK, amikacin; DKB, dibekacin; SM, streptomycin; KM, kanamycin; CET, cephalothin; CEZ, cefazolin.*

given gentamicin or dibekacin, the urinary NAG activity decreased after reaching the maximum, despite the fact that drug administration was continued.

Figure 2 shows the maximum values of urinary NAG activity during drug administration. Twelve patients free of renal disease served as the control group; their urinary NAG activities were determined without drug administration. Most patients given a daily dose of 120 to 240 mg of gentamicin showed a remarkable increase in NAG activity within 10 days of administration. In some cases, polyuria, proteinuria, a reduction in PSP excretion, and an increase in urinary electrolytes along with reduced serum electrolytes were also observed. But these cases returned to normal within a week after interruption of drug administration. Kidney sections from two autopsied patients who had received gentamicin at 120 to 240 mg/day continuously until death showed distinct necrosis and exfoliation of the proximal tubular epithelial cells. No increase in NAG activity was found in patients given a daily dose of 80 mg of gentamicin. Administration of aminoglycoside drugs other than gentamicin, that is, dibekacin and amikacin, did not produce the marked increase in urinary NAG activity seen with gentamicin. In addition, there was almost no occurrence of polyuria, abnormalities in electrolytes, or reduced

renal function. In addition, administration of antileukemic drugs to patients neither increased the urinary NAG activity nor caused any remarkable renal damage.

In summary, (i) gentamicin was more nephrotoxic than the other aminoglycoside antibiotics tested, histologically showing marked proximal tubular damage in some cases; (ii) polyuria was the first clinical symptom observed, and moderate proteinuria and other disturbances in renal function were also observed in some cases; (iii) renal function impaired by gentamicin returned to normal upon prompt withdrawal of the drug.

We feel that measurement of urinary NAG activity is useful for the early diagnosis and monitoring of nephrotoxic reactions to aminoglycosides.

1. **Borooah, J., D. H. Leaback, and P. G. Walker.** 1961. Studies on glucosaminidase. Biochem. J. **78**:106–110.
2. **Dance, N., and R. G. Price.** 1970. The excretion of N-acetyl-β-D-glucosaminidase and β-galactosidase by patients with renal disease. Clin. Chim. Acta **27**:87–92.
3. **Ellis, B. G., S. M. Tucker, A. E. Thompson, and R. G. Price.** 1975. Presence of serum and tissue forms of N-acetyl-β-D-glucosaminidase in urine from patients with renal disease. Clin. Chim. Acta **64**:195–202.
4. **Wellwood, J. M., B. G. Ellis, R. G. Price, K. Hammond, A. E. Thompson, and N. F. Jones.** 1975. Urinary N-acetyl-β-D-glucosaminidase activity in patients with renal disease. Br. Med. J. **3**:408–411.

Comparison of Amikacin and Gentamicin in Critically Ill Patients

MARGARET A. FRENCH,* FRANK B. CERRA, MARTIN E. PLAUT, AND JEROME J. SCHENTAG

Clinical Pharmacokinetics Laboratory, Millard Fillmore Hospital, and Department of Medicine, State University of New York at Buffalo, Buffalo, New York 14209, U.S.A.*

Amikacin (AMK) and gentamicin (G) are aminoglycoside antibiotics often given to seriously ill patients. These patients commonly have both decreased renal function and concurrent nephrotoxic insults. Both aminoglycosides also cause renal tubular damage, with a frequency cited from 2 to 56%. Correlation was previously sought between increased serum levels and incidence of nephrotoxicity, but elevated serum levels were predictive in only 36% of cases (2).

Both AMK and G are excreted unchanged by glomerular filtration, but total recovery in the urine is not complete at 12 to 24 h (1, 7) because of some tubular reabsorption. G has been detected in urine and serum for prolonged periods after dosing has stopped (4, 6), and both AMK and G concentrate in human kidneys in patients without renal failure given normal doses (3). Although these observations establish that AMK probably has two-compartment characteristics similar to those of G, tobramycin, and netilmicin, the persistence of AMK in patients after multiple-dose regimens has not yet been studied.

The purpose of this study was to describe the two-compartment pharmacokinetics of AMK and then compare these derived parameters with those exhibited by clinically matched patients given G. Finally, we also sought to compare the incidence of nephrotoxicity exhibited by these two drugs in similar patients.

We studied 25 patients receiving multiple-dose treatment with AMK in an intensive care unit. Frequent serum and, when possible, daily 24-h urine samples were collected both during and for a prolonged period after AMK therapy. Postmortem tissue samples were also obtained in six patients. Serum, urine, and tissues were assayed for AMK by radioimmunoassay. Urine was also analyzed for β_2-microglobulin, cast count, and creatinine (5). By using the calculated pharmacokinetic parameters for each patient, the amount of drug in their central and peripheral compartments was predicted and confirmed by tissue samples or urine recovery. One or both of these methods was available on 10 of the 25 patients. The 25 AMK patients were then matched with 25 patients treated with G and studied in an identical manner during the same time period. The matching was performed without knowledge of renal function changes or pharmacokinetic parameters of the G group. Criteria included age, creatinine clearance, concurrent nephrotoxic drugs, and prior aminoglycoside therapy.

Nephrotoxicity attributable to aminoglycoside was defined as an increase in serum creatinine greater than 0.5 mg/100 ml preceded by renal tubular damage (as evidenced by a cast count greater than 500 casts/ml), β_2-microglobulin excretion in excess of 50 mg/24 h, and excessive aminoglycoside tissue accumulation, defined as greater than 200 mg for G and greater than 600 mg for AMK (5).

To analyze variability due to differences in dosing, each patient was also "dosed" by computer simulation for 10 days with a precisely calculated regimen based on body weight and renal function. This regimen, based on individual pharmacokinetic parameters, was also used to compare serum concentrations and tissue accumulation between paired G and AMK patients.

A comparison of the clinical characteristics of G and AMK is presented in Table 1. The two groups were very well matched, as there were no differences in age, sex, base-line renal function, concurrent nephrotoxins, incidence of bacteremia, sites of infections, or duration of therapy. When a 3:1 normalization factor for differences in potency was considered, there were also no differences in total dosage given. The AMK group had a statistically significantly higher prior aminoglycoside exposure ($P < 0.05$).

For both G and AMK, the serum concentrations declined in two phases after the last dose, and the data were fit to the two-compartment open pharmacokinetic model with the aid of a nonlinear least-square regression analysis program (6). Table 2 presents a comparison of mean pharmacokinetic parameters. The patients were similar in their distribution volume and total clearance. The terminal half-life values were in excess of 100 h for both groups, with a trend toward longer values for AMK. The ratio of aminoglycoside clearance to creatinine clearance was 0.8 for both drugs, indicating significant tubular reabsorption. The only significant difference seen between the drugs was the first-order rate constant for drug out of the peripheral compartment (k_{21}). However, the ratio of k_{12}/k_{21} did not differ, suggesting that the slightly longer k_{21} value was due primarily to the longer terminal half-life noted for AMK. There was also no difference between drugs in the predicted amount of drug in the tissue compartment, either when the actual dosing was considered or when the simulated dosing was used (Table 2).

Four patients in the G group and five in the AMK group experienced drug-related renal damage. Only two of the five nephrotoxic AMK patients and none of the four nephrotoxic G patients were given dosing above current recommendations. In absence of major differences in dosing, a possible explanation for slightly greater nephrotoxicity in the AMK group might be their greater exposure to prior aminoglycosides. However, only three of the five (60%) nephrotoxic AMK patients had received prior aminoglycoside therapy, compared with 16 of the 20 (80%) nontoxic AMK patients. Since these results are not statistically different, the greater exposure of AMK-treated patients to prior aminoglycosides does not necessarily emerge as a significant predisposing variable.

AMK, in common with G, tobramycin, and netilmicin, exhibits multicompartment pharma-

TABLE 1. *Comparison of clinical characteristics of AMK and G patients (mean ± SD)*

Parameter	Gentamicin	Amikacin
No. of patients	25	25
Age (yr)	62 ± 15	58 ± 14
Sex (female/male)	15/10	10/15
Surface area (m²)	1.71 ± 0.22	1.73 ± 0.21
Base-line creatinine clearance (ml/min)	46.6 ± 30.3	43.4 ± 40.1
Prior aminoglycoside therapy[a] (no.)	9	19[b]
Concurrent cephalosporins (no.)	9	7
Concurrent other nephrotoxic drugs (no.)	19	18
Both cephalosporins and another concurrent nephrotoxin (no.)	8	6
Site of infection[c]		
Bacteremia	14	18
Soft tissue	9	6
Urinary tract	7	12
Pneumonia	8	11
Dosing		
No. given > recommended	6	7
No. given ≤ recommended	19	18
Days of therapy	9.7 ± 5.5	11.0 ± 6.0
Total dose (mg/kg)	31.73 ± 27.26	40.60 ± 42.67[d]

[a] Less than 1 month prior.

[b] Statistically significant difference (χ^2 = 6.5, $P < 0.05$).

[c] Each patient can have more than one infection site, in addition to bacteremias.

[d] Amikacin divided by three as a normalization factor for potency differences.

TABLE 2. *Comparison of pharmacokinetic values and incidence of nephrotoxicity for amikacin and gentamicin (mean ± SD)*

Parameter	Gentamicin	Amikacin
No. of patients	25	25
Vc, central (liters/kg)	0.257 ± 0.100	0.305 ± 0.088
k_{12}, rate in (h⁻¹)	0.025 + 0.030	0.016 ± 0.015
k_{21}, rate out (h⁻¹)	0.010 ± 0.009	0.005 ± 0.003[a]
k_{12}/k_{21} ratio	2.74 ± 1.80	3.25 ± 2.89
k_{10}, overall elimination rate (h⁻¹)	0.18 ± 0.21	0.10 ± 0.08
TBC[b] (ml/min)	29.53 ± 18.10	33.45 ± 24.60
TBC/creatinine clearance	0.80 ± 0.65	0.78 ± 0.46
Distribution vol, steady state (liters/kg)	0.93 ± 0.49	1.34 ± 0.98
Half-life, terminal (h)	146.5 ± 115.4	187.7 ± 62.5
Amt of drug in tissue at last dose (mg)	117.4 ± 83.1	173.5 ± 186.3[c]
Predicted amt of drug in tissue at last dose with simulated dosing (mg)[d]	149.3 ± 141.7	203.0 ± 166.0[c]
Predicted accumulation/total dose (simulated dosing) %[d]	8.23 ±7.14	9.43 ± 7.17
Aminoglycoside nephrotoxic (no.)	4	5

[a] Statistically significant difference ($P < 0.05$).

[b] TBC, total body clearance.

[c] Amikacin divided by three.

[d] Computer-simulated dosing based on weight, renal function, and individually derived pharmacokinetic parameters in each patient.

cokinetics, with a long terminal half-life. Its pharmacokinetic parameters were similar to those of G in our small groups of clinically matched patients. The incidence of nephrotoxicity attributed to AMK was also similar to that attributed to G.

This study was supported in part by Public Health Service grant 20852 from the National Institutes of Health and by a grant from Bristol Laboratories.

1. **Clarke, J. T., R. D. Libke, C. Regamey, and W. M. M. Kirby.** 1974. Comparative pharmacokinetics of amikacin and kanamycin. Clin. Pharmacol. Ther. 15:610–616.
2. **Dahlgren, J. G., E. T. Anderson, and W. L. Hewitt.** 1975. Gentamicin blood levels: a guide to nephrotoxicity. Antimicrob. Agents Chemother. 8:58–62.
3. **Edwards, C. Q., C. R. S. Smith, K. L. Baughman, J. G. Rogers, and P. S. Lietman.** 1976. Concentrations of gentamicin and amikacin in human kidneys. Antimicrob. Agents Chemother. 9:925–927.
4. **Kahlmeter, G., and C. Kamme.** 1975. Prolonged excretion of gentamicin in a patient with unimpaired renal function. Lancet i:286.
5. **Schentag, J. J., M. E. Plaut, F. B. Cerra, P. B. Wels, P. Walczak, and R. J. Buckley.** 1979. Aminoglycoside nephrotoxicity in critically ill surgical patients. J. Surg. Res. 26:270–279.
6. **Schentag, J. J., W. J. Jusko, M. E. Plaut, T. J. Cumbo, J. W. Vance, and E. Abrutyn.** 1977. Tissue persistence of gentamicin in man. J. Am. Med. Assoc. 238: 327–329.
7. **Wood, M. J., and W. Farrell.** 1976. Comparison of urinary excretion of tobramycin and gentamicin in adults. J. Infect. Dis. 134(Suppl.):S133–S136.

Concentration of Cefoxitin in the Cerebrospinal Fluid in Patients with Meningitis

G. HUMBERT, A. LEROY, J. P. ROGEZ, AND C. CHERUBIN*

Service des Maladies Infectieuses, Hôpital Charles Nicolle, 76038 Rouen, France, and Infectious Disease Service, Brooklyn Jewish Hospital, Brooklyn, New York 11238, U.S.A.

Although the cephalosporin antibiotics are not generally thought to reliably produce adequate therapeutic concentrations in the cerebrospinal fluid (CSF) sufficient for use in central nervous system infections, the nephrotoxic drug cephaloridine and two new cephalosporins, cefamandole and cefoxitin, have been shown to achieve appropriately high CSF levels. Clinical experience in the treatment of meningitis has been disappointing with cefamandole, but much more encouraging with cefoxitin (1, 2). We therefore decided to study the CSF concentrations of cefoxitin achieved in patients with bacterial meningitis who were being treated with the recommended agent for their infection (i.e., ampicillin or penicillin) and who received simultaneous doses of cefoxitin. The use of a penicillinase-producing assay organism has permitted us to determine blood and CSF concentrations of cefoxitin without interference by the presence of ampicillin.

In this study, we used patients on the Service des Maladies Infectieuses at Hôpital Charles Nicolle of the Université de Rouen, Rouen, France, and the Jewish Hospital and Medical Center of Brooklyn, Brooklyn, N.Y. There were three study groups. Group 1 contained 12 patients with nonbacterial meningitis; 11 patients had presumed viral meningitis, and one had a parameningeal focus of infection with signs of moderate inflammation in the CSF but without organisms seen in or grown from the spinal fluid. These patients received 2 g of cefoxitin in a 30-min infusion and had lumbar punctures (LP) 1 or 2 h after the completion of the infusion. Group 2 consisted of 12 patients with bacterial meningitis (mainly meningococcal) who received 12 g of ampicillin intravenously (i.v.) or 20 million U of penicillin i.v. per day along with 2 g of cefoxitin i.v. every 4 h for the first 72 h and then again on the 10th and last day of treatment with an LP 2 h after the infusion. Group 3 contained 14 similar patients (two died within 24 h of the start of therapy) who received, in addition, by the oral route or by i.v. infusion, a 1-g loading dose of probenecid and a 0.5-g continuation dose each 6 to 8 h thereafter.

The assay for cefoxitin was performed with the use of a strain of *Staphylococcus aureus*

(MSD 25935) by the agar diffusion technique. This strain is ampicillin and penicillin resistant.

Results. In group 1, only one of the 17 spinal fluids obtained 1 or 2 h after the infusion in these 12 patients with aseptic meningitis contained detectable levels of cefoxitin. This was a patient who, unlike all the others with presumptive viral meningitis, had a parameningeal focus of infection from an exacerbation of a chronic otitis media, which produced a moderate amount of meningeal inflammation.

Group 2 had considerably more cefoxitin detectable (Table 1); the mean CSF concentrations were 3.2, 4.5, and 2.4 μg/ml. The "simultaneous" serum levels were two to three times the CSF levels, 8.3, 8.8, and 7.6 μg/ml. The group of five patients with LPs at 3 h had mean concentrations of 3.6, 5.3, and 4.0 μg/ml.

Group 3, which received probenecid, had serum levels at the end of the infusion, in general, no higher than those of group 2, but the 2-h serum concentrations were much higher: 57, 35, and 27, μg/ml, respectively. The CSF concentra-

TABLE 1. *Cefoxitin without probenecid*[a]

DAY				DAY 1.	DAY 3	DAY 10-11
DOSE				2 gm	~ 24 gm	6 gm
Pt.	Organism	Age	BUN*			
1.	Meningo.	48	22	12.50	12.50	4.20
2.	Meningo.	48	21	5.20	7.40	6.25
3.	Meningo.	23	20	<1.56	3.12	<1.56
4.	?	65	33	<1.56	4.80	3.20
5.	?	25	24	<1.56	2.20	<1.56
6.	Pneumo.	29	29	4.40	4.80	2.80
7.	Meningo.	16	36	2.00	<1.56	<1.56
8.	Meningo.	19	46	4.60	3.10	2.40
9.	Pneumo.	20	18	4.60	3.50	2.60
10.	Meningo.	41	30	<1.56	3.50	2.50
11.	Meningo.	38	20	2.50	4.50	1.50
12.	Meningo.	25	25	2.75	4.50	3.50
mean				$\bar{x}$ = 3.2	4.50	2.40

[a] CSF concentrations (in micrograms per milliliter) 2 h after a 30-min infusion of 2 g.

* Values in milligrams per decaliter.

TABLE 2. *Cefoxitin with probenecid*[a]

DAY			DAY 1	DAY 2	DAY 3	DAY 4	DAY 5	DAY 6	DAY 10-11
DOSE			2 gm	~12 gm	~24 gm	~36 gm	~48 gm	~60 gm	6 gm
Pt.	Organism	Age BUN							
1.	?	23 27	5.60	—	7.40	—	—	—	3.12
2.	Meningo.	78 41	—	32.40	32.40	16.00	21.00	24.00	7.60
3.	Meningo.	33 40	3.20	—	—	9.60	—	—	3.00
4.	Meningo.	19 36	6.60	—	—	13.00	—	—	3.80
5.	Pneumo.	42 30	2.60	—	—	6.20	—	—	2.50
6.	Pneumo.	20 18	3.00	4.40	—	4.40	—	—	2.80
7.	Pneumo.	50 26	6.00	—	16.00	—	—	—	4.00
8.	Meningo.	20 42	4.60	7.00	—	4.60	—	4.00	<1.56
9.	Meningo.	18 37	6.80	—	15.00	—	—	—	2.80
10.	Pneumo.	20 99	2.40	—	12.50	17.00	12.00	—	6.40
11.	Pneumo.	78 92	15.00	Exitus					
12.	Klebs.	70 65	15.00	Exitus					
13.	Pneumo.	45 20	7.50	—	—	10.00	—	—	7.50
14.	Meningo.	36 28	10.00	—	—	12.00	—	—	8.00
mean			$\bar{x}=8.62$			$\bar{x}=12.30$			$\bar{x}=4.30$

[a] CSF concentrations (micrograms per milliliter).

tions were also higher: 8.6, 12.3, and 4.3 µg/ml (Table 2). The percentage of the serum level in the CSF was between 15 and 35%.

Neither the CSF cell count, protein or glucose value, or renal function showed a clear linear association with spinal fluid concentrations. The age of the patient had the closest relationship to elevated CSF levels: patients 1 and 2 (Table 1) in group 2 were two of the oldest patients (48 years) among the 12 studied; patients 2, 7, 11 and 12 (Table 3) were by far the oldest patients in group 3. All had at least a minor degree of renal insufficiency at the beginning of treatment.

In both groups 2 and 3, the MICs of the common causes of bacterial meningitis (viz., meningococci, pneumococci, *Haemophilus influenzae* group B) were exceeded. What is sought, however, is a better therapy for meningitis due to a gram-negative bacillus other than *Pseudomonas meningitis*. The general recommendations for gram-negative meningitis, chloramphenicol-intrathecal gentamicin, have proved disappointing in practice. The usual explanations given for the frequent treatment failures have been the involvement of the ventricular system, not likely to be reachable by the diffusion of intrathecal aminoglycosides, their pH dependence, and the acid conditions obtained in the CSF in bacterial meningitis, and the considerable discrepancy that exists between the results of disk sensitivity testing for chloramphenicol and the MBC of coliform bacteria (3).

With the administration of 12 g of cefoxitin and 1.5 to 2 g of probenecid per day, CSF levels can regularly be achieved that exceed the MIC and MBC of virtually all clinical *Escherichia coli*, *Klebsiella*, and *Proteus* isolates. Since levels are highest in middle-aged and elderly patients, who are most afflicted by this entity and who probably have a relative degree of renal insufficiency, cefoxitin and probenecid would appear to be a therapy worth consideration in the treatment of gram-negative meningitis.

The future holds even more promise. Two agents, LY127935 (Eli Lilly & Co.) and HR-756 (cefotaxime; Hoechst-Roussel), are presently under investigation; both are 10 to 100 times more active against coliforms and, if they achieve similar CSF concentrations, as has been reported, they could prove to be the agents of choice in the treatment of bacterial meningitis almost regardless of etiology.

1. Massip, P., M. D. Kitzie, V. T. Tran, M. J. Armengaud, and M. Armengaud. 1979. Penetration of cefoxitin into cerebrospinal fluid of dogs with and without exper-

imental meningitis. Rev. Infect. Dis. **1**:132–133.
2. **Nair, S. R., C. E. Cherubin, and M. Weinstein.** 1979. Penetration of cefoxitin into cerebrospinal fluid and treatment of meningitis caused by gram-negative bacteria. Rev. Infect. Dis. **1**:134–142.

3. **Sande, M., R. Sheretz, O. Zak, and L. Strausbaugh.** 1978. Cephalosporin antibiotics in therapy of experimental *Streptococcus pneumoniae* and *Hemophilus influenza* meningitis in rabbits. J. Infect. Dis. **137**:S161–S168.

Cefoxitin Penetration to Cerebrospinal Fluid in Patients with Purulent Meningitis

PAULO A. AYROSA GALVAO, ANDRÉ VILLELA LOMAR, WALDEMAR FRANCISCO,
CID V. FRANCO DE GODOY, AND RAGNAR NORRBY*

*Hospital Emilio Ribas and Department of Microbiology and Immunology, University of Sao Paolo, Sao Paolo, Brazil, and Department of Infectious Diseases, University of Gothenburg, S-416 85 Gothenburg, Sweden**

This study was undertaken in order to evaluate the cerebrospinal fluid (CSF) penetration of cefoxitin in patients with purulent meningitis. Since at that time very limited knowledge was available about the therapeutic efficacy of cefoxitin in cases of meningitis, other antibiotics were given in parallel, and the study concentrated solely on the pharmacokinetics of cefoxitin in CSF.

Twenty-nine patients were entered into the study. The mean age was 34 years (range, 18 to 67 years). Seven of the patients were females, and 22 were males. Four patients were excluded from analysis of CSF concentrations of cefoxitin, either because of insufficient number of samples taken (three patients) or lack of evidence of meningitis (one patient). The remaining 25 patients all had purulent meningitis verified by marked CSF leucocytosis with dominance of polymorphonuclear cells, increased concentrations of protein in CSF, and decreased ratios between CSF and blood glucose. In 18 of the patients, the causative bacterial pathogens were isolated.

None of the patients received systemic antibiotic treatment within 72 h before admission to hospital. Of the patients with verified purulent meningitis, 24 received ampicillin in doses of 12 to 16 g per day intravenously and one received benzylpenicillin, 14.4 g per day intravenously. In addition, all patients received four 2-g doses of cefoxitin (Mefoxin) administered as intravenous bolus injections over 3 to 5 min with 6-h intervals.

Cefoxitin concentrations were studied in serum and CSF samples drawn before the first cefoxitin dose and at 2, 4, or 6 h after the first and third cefoxitin doses. The patients were randomly allocated to the three sampling times. For the cefoxitin assays, a paper disk diffusion technique was used. An ampicillin-resistant strain of *Staphylococcus aureus* was used as test strain.

The serum and CSF concentrations of cefoxitin are given in Fig. 1 and Table 1. All pre-

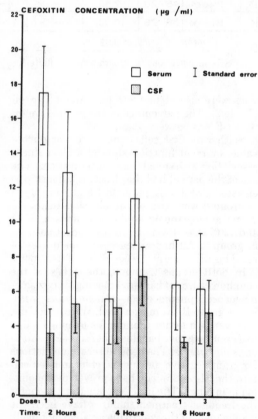

FIG. 1. *Mean cefoxitin concentrations in serum and CSF after intravenous administration of 2 g of cefoxitin to adult patients with purulent meningitis.*

TABLE 1. *Serum and CSF concentrations of cefoxitin*

Patient no.	Serum concn (μg/ml)						CSF concn (μg/ml)					
	Dose 1			Dose 3			Dose 1			Dose 3		
	2 h	4 h	6 h	2 h	4 h	6 h	2 h	4 h	6 h	2 h	4 h	6 h
1			1.8			2.5			2.9 (161)[a]			3.5 (140)
2		13.0			16.0			ND[b]			2.5 (16)	
3	12.5			8.4			2.5 (20)			4.8 (57)		
4	17.0			8.2			1.8 (11)			2.9 (35)		
5	12.0			5.8			1.4 (12)			2.3 (40)		
6	12.5			10.0			1.2 (10)			5.0 (50)		
7		2.0			17.0			1.5 (75)			11.0 (65)	
8	28.0			20.0			2.1 (8)			5.8 (29)		
9			2.3			2.1			2.7 (117)			3.9 (186)
10			2.2			1.8			1.8 (82)			1.2 (67)
11	28.0			35.0			13.2 (47)			17.2 (50)		
12			29.0			35.0			3.2 (11)			22.0 (63)
13			4.0			3.4			2.7 (68)			1.2 (35)
14			8.0			3.4			3.3 (41)			1.5 (44)
15	22.0			7.9			4.8 (22)			2.2 (28)		
16		16.0			22.0			15.0 (84)			15.0 (69)	
17			5.0			2.4			5.8 (116)			4.8 (200)
18			4.0			3.8			3.2 (80)			3.6 (95)
19		3.8			9.6			2.0 (53)			4.0 (42)	
20		7.8			5.0			5.8 (74)			6.0 (120)	
21			3.4			3.3			2.8 (82)			3.1 (94)
22		2.7			8.0			2.2 (81)			6.2 (78)	
23		1.5			2.0			4.0 (267)			3.6 (180)	
24			3.8			4.0			2.3 (61)			3.2 (80)
25	8.0			7.8			1.5 (19)			2.0 (26)		
No.	8	7	10	8	7	10	8	6	10	8	7	10
Mean	17.5	5.6	6.4	12.9	11.4	6.2	3.6 (19)	5.1 (11)	3.1 (82)	5.3 (39)	6.9 (81)	4.8 (100)

[a] Numbers in parentheses are CSF concentrations expressed as percentage of concurrent serum concentrations.

[b] ND, Not done.

cefoxitin samples contained no detectable antibiotic activity. When the patients from whom samples were obtained at the same time after cefoxitin administration were compared, the cefoxitin concentrations in both CSF and serum varied considerably. This was interpreted to be a result of individual variations with respect to weight, renal function, and meningeal inflammation. In all patients, cefoxitin gave detectable CSF concentrations, varying between 1.2 and 22.0 μg/ml.

The cefoxitin CSF concentrations tended to be considerably lower after the first than after the third dose when the results obtained in the individual patients were compared. This was most obvious in the patients sampled 2 h after cefoxitin administration. In these cases, the cefoxitin concentration increased 1.3 to 4.2 times in seven out of eight patients. Higher CSF concentrations in the third than in the first CSF samples were also noted in the patients sampled 4 h after cefoxitin administration, whereas the

concentrations in the samples obtained 6 h after cefoxitin were similar.

Comparing the mean cefoxitin CSF concentrations at various times after administration, higher concentrations were achieved after 4 than after 2 h, both when the absolute cefoxitin concentrations and the concentrations relative to concurrent serum concentrations were compared. At 6 h after cefoxitin administration, the CSF concentrations were lower than at 4 h and similar to those obtained after 2 h.

The patients were followed for adverse reactions to cefoxitin, and the only reported reaction was pain at the infusion site in one patient. No laboratory adverse reactions were observed. Two of the patients with pneumococcal meningitis died of their infection, and the deaths were considered definitely not related to the cefoxitin treatment.

Discussion and conclusions. The most important factor limiting the use of an antibiotic for treatment of bacterial meningitis is difficulty in penetrating the blood-CSF barrier. Most antibiotics have very poor penetration over an intact barrier but penetrate fairly well when the meninges are inflamed. However, even in the presence of marked inflammation, some antibiotics, e.g., the aminoglycosides and the isoxazolylpenicillins, are unable to enter the CSF space in therapeutic concentrations after administration of nontoxic systemic doses. Other limiting factors are inadequate antibacterial spectrum and the increasing frequency of multiple antibiotic resistance in bacterial species causing meningitis, e.g., *Haemophilus influenzae*. Despite the introduction of many new antibiotics during the last decade, chloramphenicol, ampicillin, and benzylpenicillin remain the drugs of choice for use in cases of bacterial meningitis. The cephalosporins, with their wider antibacterial spectrum, have so far given disappointing clinical results.

Cefoxitin has an antibacterial spectrum which is wide and covers most bacterial species causing meningitis, including beta-lactamase-producing strains of *H. influenzae*. Previous studies on its penetration into CSF have demonstrated a low but significant penetration over an intact blood-CSF barrier. High CSF penetration have been reported in a limited number of patients with meningitis. Cefoxitin has also been used successfully for treatment of bacterial meningitis in a few patients. This study demonstrated that cefoxitin penetrated fairly well over inflamed blood-CSF barriers, giving CSF concentrations which were high in relation to concurrent serum concentrations in all patients. The results gave evidence for an accumulation of cefoxitin in CSF when repeated doses were administered. The peak CSF concentration seemed to occur between 2 and 6 h after intravenous administration. This observation indicates that CSF concentrations should be determined not earlier than 2 h after administration of an antibiotic.

If cefoxitin is used for treatment of bacterial meningitis, these results indicate that the drug should be administered in high doses with short intervals, e.g., 4 g four times per day, to adults with normal renal function. This dose is higher than the maximum dose of 12 g presently recommended by the manufacturer, but considering the high degree of safety demonstrated in clinical studies of cefoxitin, a dose of 16 g per day should be well tolerated. With respect to its spectrum, cefoxitin might be an antibiotic suitable for treatment of gram-negative meningitis in compromised patients and in neonates.

Cerebrospinal Fluid Penetration of Cefuroxime

BJORN HOFFSTEDT,* ORJAN JOHANSSON, MATS WALDER, STIG CRONBERG, AND JOHN D. PRICE

General Hospital, S-214 01 Malmo, Sweden, and Glaxo Group Research Ltd., London, England*

Aim of the study. The aim was to investigate the penetrability of cefuroxime into the cerebrospinal fluid (CSF) in cases of meningitis and to follow the penetrability with time to see whether it decreases when the meninges become less inflamed.

Rationale. Rationales for investigating this new beta-lactamase-resistant cephalosporin were (i) the increasing incidence of beta-lactamase-producing *Haemophilus influenzae* resistant to ampicillin and (ii) the need to find an alternative treatment to avoid possible toxic effects seen after chloramphenicol therapy.

Bacteriological methods. Serum and CSF samples were frozen and stored at −20°C until assayed. The cefuroxime concentration was determined microbiologically by the agar well diffusion technique.

The agar used was Oxoid antibiotic agar no. 2, pH adjusted to 7.0. Twenty-five units of penicil-

linase (Leo) per ml was added to the medium after autoclaving. Petri dishes (diameter, 14 cm) with 25 ml of test agar were prepared. The test organism used was a beta-lactamase-producing *Staphylococcus aureus* from Glaxo Research Ltd., London. Standard inoculum was 10^5/ml.

Wells (diameter, 8 mm) were made with a hole punch machine. Each sample and standard antibiotic dilution was tested twice on the same plate. Prediffusion time was 2 h.

Standard antibiotic dilutions, using cefuroxime sodium with pooled human serum and CSF, respectively, as diluents (both previously tested for antimicrobial activity and CSF tested for protein content) were run simultaneously in three control wells. Two standard pools for CSF were used with 0.6 and 1.2 g of CSF protein per liter, respectively, depending on the sample CSF protein.

Method. The patients were given cefuroxime

TABLE 1. *Penetration of cefuroxime into CSF in children*

Patient age	Causative organism	Day of investigation	Protein in CSF (g/liter)	Time after injection (h)	Cefuroxime dose (mg/kg per day)	Cefuroxime concn (μg/ml) in:	
						Serum	CSF
5 mo	Meningococcus	3	1.47	8	100	9.5	2.3
8 mo	Pneumococcus	3	0.90	8	100	10.7	5.2
		9	0.33	8	100	ND[a]	3.3
30 mo	*H. influenzae*	2	0.93	2	100	24.0	6.4
5 yr	Unknown virus	3	0.24	2	100	>50.0	2.6
7 yr	Unknown sterile culture	3	0.62	3	100	7.8	2.7
7 yr	Parotite virus	3	0.87	2	100	2.6	3.2
15 yr	Virus	3	0.40	8	50	5.4	<2

[a] Not done.

TABLE 2. *Penetration of cefuroxime into CSF in adults*

Patient age (yr)	Causative organism	Day of investigation	Protein in CSF (g/liter)	Time after injection (h)	Cefuroxime dose (mg/kg per day)	Cefuroxime concn (μg/ml) in:	
						Serum	CSF
19	Parotite virus	6	0.81	2	75	5.5	2.4
26	Parotite virus	2	1.88	3	60	5.6	3.8
37	Group B streptococcus	3	1.25	3	70	5.5	3.2
		6	1.44	2	70	11.0	2.4
63	Listeria	3	1.25	2	100	ND[a]	7.0
61	Group B streptococcus	3	1.85	2	100	26.2	3.1
		9	0.63	2.5	100	9.5	2.5
68	*H. influenzae*	4	0.37	2	100	28.6	6.0
		9	0.37	2	100	ND	4.0
67	Unknown sterile culture	3	5.4	1/4	60	50.0	24.0
		6	2.5	2	60	38.0	18.0
72	Meningococcus	3	6.25	3	80	55.0	13.0

[a] ND, Not done.

at 50 to 100 mg/kg per day and ampicillin at 100 to 400 mg/kg per day intravenously for 10 days. In five patients (adults), two with viral meningitis and three with bacterial meningitis, ampicillin treatment was stopped after 1 day and cefuroxime treatment was continued alone. All patients had normal renal function.

CSF and serum were obtained on admission by lumbar puncture and venipuncture; the procedure was repeated on the 3rd day of treatment and, in some patients, on days 4, 6, and 9. CSF and serum samples were taken 2, 3, and 8 h after the cefuroxime dose.

Results. Fifteen patients were entered into the study. The age of the patients was 5 months to 72 years (seven were children). Ten patients had bacterial meningitis, and five subsequently developed viral meningitis. Tables 1 and 2 show the etiology, CSF protein, and cefuroxime levels in serum and CSF.

Discussion. Cefuroxime has a penetrability into CSF equal or even superior to that of other beta-lactam antibiotics (1). The levels achieved in the CSF were above 2 μg/ml and exceeded the MICs for the pathogens isolated (listeria excluded). The levels of cefuroxime in CSF during the treatment period decreased only slightly.

We conclude that the pharmacokinetic and antimicrobial properties of cefuroxime are promising for the treatment of bacterial meningitis (neonatal period and immunodeficient hosts excepted). We feel that the data obtained in this study justify using cefuroxime alone for treating bacterial meningitis in a future study.

1. **Thrupp, L. D., J. M. Leedom, D. Ivler, P. F. Wehrle, B. Portnoy, and A. W. Mathies.** 1966. Ampicillin levels in the cerebrospinal fluid during treatment of bacterial meningitis, p. 206–213. Antimicrob. Agents Chemother. 1965.

Penetration of Chloramphenicol into the Cerebrospinal Fluid

IVAN SPIRA, ANDREA NIXDORF, AND HARRY ROSIN*

Institute for Medical Microbiology and Virology, University of Düsseldorf, D-4000 Dusseldorf, Federal Republic of Germany

The penetration of chloramphenicol into the cerebrospinal fluid (CSF) has long been an unresolved problem in chemotherapy. The turbidimetric value obtained from 1950 to 1952 is often cited, according to which chloramphenicol penetrates through healthy meninges with approximately 50% of the serum concentration. Because of (i) the emergence of ampicillin-resistant *Haemophilus influenzae* strains and (ii) a trend to fall back on administration of chloramphenicol in meningitis therapy, it became necessary to investigate the penetration of chloramphenicol by means of modern methods.

We developed a sensitive method to measure the chloramphenicol concentration by means of high-performance liquid chromatography. All serum and CSF samples were extracted three times with ether. For chromatography, we used a reversed-phase column (μ Bondapak C_{18}), a methanol-water mixture (25:75, vol/vol), a flow rate of 3.5 ml/min, and an ultraviolet light de-

tector with a wavelength of 280 nm. The retention time of chloramphenicol was approximately 5 min. Using control runs with pure chloramphenicol and its metabolites assured that the peaks at the 5-min position were exclusively active and not metabolized chloramphenicol. The minimal detectable quantity was on the order of 20 ng of chloramphenicol. Through injection of an internal standard (phenol), the quality of the analysis became independent of technical error. Coefficient of variation of almost 1 for the calibration curve and low coefficients of variation of 0.5 to 1% on replicate analysis indicate the high precision obtained and the good reproducibility of this method.

To systematically investigate the penetration of an antibiotic into the CSF, animal experiments are essential. The pharmacokinetic data obtained from test animals can be related to human beings provided that, among other factors, the serum concentration in the test animal

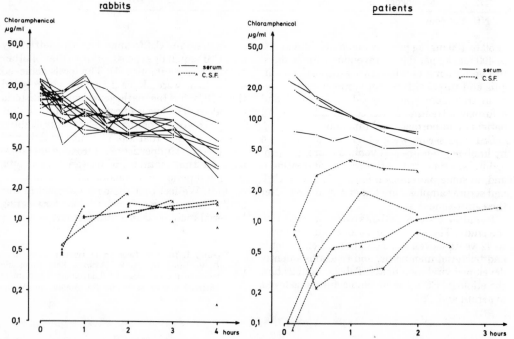

FIG. 1. *Chloramphenicol concentrations in serum and CSF samples of 19 healthy rabbits after an initial i.v. injection of 9 mg of chloramphenicol/kg and subsequent continuous infusion with successively reduced infusion doses and of four patients with tumor of the brain after i.v. injection of 1 g of chloramphenicol.*

is adjusted to the serum concentration used in the therapy of patients. Through an infusion lasting 4 h with a successively reduced dose, which followed a quick intravenous (i.v.) initial injection, a concentration profile of chloramphenicol in the serum of rabbits and a half-life value were simulated as they are used in the therapy of patients (Fig. 1).

The chloramphenicol concentrations in the CSF increased in the patients, as in the rabbits, up to 2 h. Thereafter a statistically significant equilibrium of distribution was reached. The median chloramphenicol concentration in the CSF in the patients amounted to 1.13 μg/ml 2 h after injection; for the rabbits, the concentration was 1.3 μg/ml. This is consistent with a permeation rate from serum of 16.6% for the patients and 14.6% for the rabbits.

In another test series under steady-state conditions, in which a quick initial i.v. injection was followed by continuous chloramphenicol infusion lasting 4 h with a constant serum level in the therapeutical range averaging 16 μg/ml, the mean chloramphenicol concentration in the CSF amounted to only 2.2 μg/ml and the mean percentage permeation rate again was 15%. This is significantly lower than values reported previously in the literature. Nevertheless, this permeation rate of only 15% through healthy meninges is a reasonably good value relative to the conditions found with β-lactam antibiotics and aminoglycosides. According to our results, subsequent treatment of meningitis with chloramphenicol is indicated when, after a decrease of the number of leukocytes in the CSF, adequate penetration of penicillin or ampicillin, for example, is no longer certain. Figure 2 shows chloramphenicol concentrations in serum and CSF of 14 rabbits with experimental meningitis caused by *H. influenzae*. To induce a generalized men-

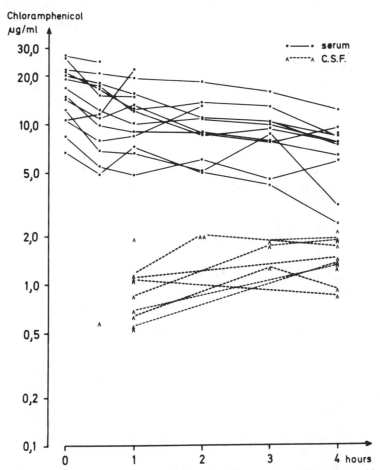

FIG. 2. *Chloramphenicol concentrations in serum and CSF samples of 14 rabbits with H. influenzae meningitis after an initial i.v. injection of 9 mg of chloramphenicol/kg and subsequent continuous infusion with successively reduced infusion doses.*

ingitis, we injected approximately 10^7 live *Haemophilus* organisms into the cisterna magna occipitalis. The CSF specimens taken for chloramphenicol measurements contained between 500 and 13,000 leukocytes/mm^3 (average, 2,700/mm^3). For comparison, most of the children with *Haemophilus* meningitis showed leukocyte levels between 1,000 and 10,000 per mm^3. Also, in the presence of an inflammation the chloramphenicol concentration in the CSF increased up to 2 h, after which an equilibrium of distribution appeared to establish itself. The mean percentage permeation rate for the rabbits infected with meningitis was approximately 25% with reference to the 4-h time point.

We also measured serum and CSF concentrations approximately 4 h after the last chloramphenicol dose in two children, one with meningococcus and one with pneumococcus meningitis, who, after decrease in the number of leukocytes in the CSF, were treated with chloramphenicol. The concentrations in the CSF were 1.48, 1.43, and 4.75 μg of chloramphenicol per ml. These measurements are in good agreement with the results obtained in experimentally induced meningitis. The chloramphenicol concentrations in the CSF do not appear to be always adequate to inhibit all chloramphenicol-susceptible bacteria, i.e., all bacterial strains with an MIC of ≤8 μg of chloramphenicol per ml.

Based on our investigations, we do not regard treatment of *H. influenzae* meningitis with chloramphenicol as an equivalent alternative to high-dose ampicillin therapy. In the very rare case (at least in Germany) that an ampicillin-resistant strain is found, we recommend as initial therapy the combination of ampicillin plus high dosed gentamicin until the results of bacteriological susceptibility testing are obtained. Mostly the treatment can be continued with ampicillin alone. Only against the ampicillin-resistant *Haemophilus* strains chloramphenicol should be preferred for subsequent therapy.

Cerebrospinal Fluid Penetration of Vancomycin in Bacterial Meningitis

DAVID C. REDFIELD,* ARVID UNDERMAN, DEAN NORMAN, AND GARY D. OVERTURF

Communicable Disease Service, Los Angeles County–University of Southern California Medical Center, Los Angeles, California 90033, U.S.A.

The recent occurrence of fatal meningitis caused by multiply antibiotic-resistant, vancomycin-susceptible *Streptococcus pneumoniae* (1) prompted a study of the cerebrospinal fluid (CSF) penetration of vancomycin in patients with bacterial meningitis. Vancomycin has been used successfully to treat meningitis caused by both *Staphylococcus aureus* and *Flavobacterium meningisepticum* (3, 4). Vancomycin has been shown to penetrate rabbit meninges in experimental meningitis (5). Only recently, however, have there been any reports of CSF vancomycin concentrations in patients with central nervous system infection (2).

Sixteen patients with bacterial meningitis were selected for study. Seven children aged 2 months to 16 years and seven adults aged 19 to 56 years, with meningitis caused by *S. pneumoniae* in ten cases, hemolytic streptococci in two cases, and *S. aureus* and *Neisseria meningitidis* in one case each, comprised group I. These patients were treated with ampicillin, 150 to 200 mg/kg per day, and also received an intravenous dose of vancomycin, 10 mg/kg, on days of lumbar puncture. The patient with staphylococcal meningitis received ampicillin and vancomycin for 1 day until culture results were known; the patient then was switched to methicillin therapy and removed from the study. Two adult patients aged 47 and 69 years with meningitis caused by hemolytic streptococci and *S. pneumoniae*, respectively, comprised group II. These patients were treated with vancomycin alone, 40 mg/kg per day in four divided intravenous doses. All patients with bacterial meningitis admitted to this hospital have lumbar puncture on treatment days 1, 2, 3, 7, 10, 14, 18, or 21 in order to monitor response to therapy. The duration of therapy depends on clinical criteria, but all patients receive antibiotics for at least 10 days. Paired serum and CSF samples were collected from all study patients 1 to 3 h after vancomycin infusion on days of lumbar puncture. All specimens were frozen and stored at −20°C until time of vancomycin assay.

Vancomycin concentration was measured by an agar well diffusion microbiological assay using *Bacillus subtilis* as the test organism, with penicillinase added to the medium. Semilog graphs of vancomycin concentration versus the size of the zone of growth inhibition were linear over the range of 3.13 to 50 µg/ml for serum standards and 0.4 to 25 µg/ml for CSF standards. Test samples of CSF containing 0.4 µg or less of vancomycin per ml were enriched by the addition of 0.1 ml of a 4-µg/ml standard vancomycin solution to 0.9 ml of each such CSF sample. This technique allowed measurement of CSF vancomycin concentrations as low as 0.1 µg/ml.

Serum concentration of vancomycin in group I patients ranged from 1.4 to 22 µg/ml, with a median concentration of 12.2 µg/ml. The CSF concentrations in this group ranged from less than 0.1 to 8.5 µg/ml, with a median concentration of 0.4 µg/ml. The percent CSF/serum ratio (CSF/serum concentration × 100) ranged from 1 to 50%, with a median of 4%. The serum concentrations in group II patients ranged from 10.8 to 27.8 µg/ml, with a median of 17.7 µg/ml, and the CSF values ranged from 0.1 to 8.2 µg/ml, with a median of 3.8 µg/ml. The CSF/serum ratio in this group ranged from 1 to 53%, with a median of 22%. Tables 1 and 2 show the relationship of CSF vancomycin concentration and percent CSF/serum ratio to such parameters as early-versus-late days of therapy, CSF protein concentration, and CSF cell counts. For the patients in group I, the CSF vancomycin concentration was higher in association with early days of therapy, high CSF protein concentration, and high cell counts. The CSF/serum ratios were likewise higher in association with high CSF protein concentration and cell counts, and the ratio was observed to decrease in later days of therapy. The patients in group II had higher

CSF concentrations of vancomycin than group I patients. Again there was a direct relationship between both the CSF vancomycin concentration and CSF/serum ratio and the CSF protein concentration and cell count. In contrast to group I, however, patients in group II demonstrated an increase in both CSF vancomycin concentration and CSF/serum ratio over the course of therapy.

A single patient with staphylococcal meningitis, a child in group I, died on treatment day 3. All of the other patients survived. The two patients in group II recovered completely. No patient manifested any unusual signs or symptoms in association with vancomycin administration. Phlebitis was no more or less frequent in these patients than in meningitis patients receiving other antibiotics. There were no cases of fever or rash attributed to vancomycin. All patients had stable renal function during the course of therapy, and no patient manifested any clinically apparent hearing loss or vestibular damage during therapy.

An antibiotic that fails to achieve measurable CSF concentrations in the presence of meningitis is, in general, ineffective in treating central nervous system infections. Efficacy, however, is determined by clinical response to treatment. The appearance of virulent pneumococci resistant not only to penicillin but also to chloramphenicol has signaled the need to investigate alternate drug therapies for pneumococcal meningitis. Vancomycin achieves measurable CSF concentrations in the presence of meningitis. The amount of vancomycin reaching the CSF seems to be proportional to the degree of meningeal inflammation. Although CSF concentrations were low after single-dose infusions, repetitive therapy resulted in CSF accumulation of vancomycin in significant concentration and was associated with an excellent clinical response in a very limited trial. There were no adverse reactions aside from phlebitis associated with the use of vancomycin in this series. Further study of selected cases of meningitis is warranted before vancomycin can be recommended in the treatment of bacterial meningitis.

TABLE 1. *Vancomycin CSF concentration and percent CSF/serum ratio according to day of therapy*[a]

Group	CSF concn (µg/ml) on:		% CSF/serum on:	
	Day ≤3	Day ≥7	Day ≤3	Day ≥7
I	0.7 (0.1–2.6)	0.3 (<0.1–8.5)	6 (1–15)	3 (<1–50)
II	1.1 (0.1–4.5)	5.8 (2.1–8.2)	6 (1–35)	31 (8–53)

[a] For explanation of groups, see text. Values are median, with range in parentheses.

TABLE 2. *Vancomycin CSF concentration and percent CSF/serum ratio according to CSF protein concentration and cell count*[a]

Group	CSF concn (µg/ml)				% CSF/serum			
	CSF protein of:		CSF cells:		CSF protein of:		CSF cells:	
	<100 mg/dl	≥100 mg/dl	<200	≥200	<100 µg/dl	≥100 µg/dl	<200	≥200
I	0.3 (<0.1–1.1)	1.0 (0.3–8.5)	2 (<1–14)	8 (2–50)	0.3 (<0.1–4.1)	0.7 (0.2–2.5)	2 (<1–41)	6 (1–15)
II	1.1 (0.1–2.5)	5.8 (2.5–8.2)	6 (1–9)	37 (22–53)	1.6 (0.1–4.5)	7.0 (2.5–8.2)	7 (1–23)	39 (22–53)

[a] See Table 1.

1. **Appelbaum, P. C., H. J. Koornhof, M. R. Jacobs, et al.** 1977. Multiple-antibiotic resistance of pneumococci-South Africa. Morbid. Mortal. Weekly Rep. **26:**285–286.
2. **Congeni, B. L., J. Tan, S. J. Salstrom, et al.** 1979. Kinetics of vancomycin after intraventricular and intravenous administration. Pediatr. Res. **13:**459.
3. **George, R. M., C. P. Carson, and W. E. Wheeler.** 1961. Epidemic meningitis of the newborn caused by *Flavobacteria*. Am. J. Dis. Child. **101:**296–304.
4. **Hawley, H. B., and D. W. Gump.** 1973. Vancomycin therapy of bacterial meningitis. Am. J. Dis. Child. **126:** 261–264.
5. **Murray, T., L. Strausbaugh, and M. Sande.** 1976. Comparative penetration of antibiotics into the CSF of rabbits with experimental staphylococcal meningitis. Program Abstr. Intersci. Conf. Antimicrob. Agents Chemother. 16th, Chicago, Ill., abstr. no. 246A.

Half-Lives of Penicillins and Cephalosporins in the Cerebrospinal Fluid of Rabbits with Staphylococcal Meningitis

YOSHINO MORIKAWA,* TSUNEKAZU HARUTA, AND YUTAKA KOBAYASHI

Kobe Municipal Central Hospital, Kobe, Japan

We have previously reported the concentrations of antibiotics in serum and cerebrospinal fluid (CSF) at 0.5, 1, and 2 h after administration of eight semisynthetic penicillins to rabbits with experimental staphylococcal meningitis (1). In that experiment, however, it was difficult to evaluate the passage of antibiotics into the CSF, except for apalcillin and cloxacillin, both of which showed an extremely low penetration, because the concentrations in the CSF and simultaneous CSF/serum ratios of concentrations varied widely with sampling time.

This study was designed to analyze the pharmacokinetic properties of antibiotics in the CSF by obtaining half-lives ($T_{1/2}$), maximum concentrations (C_{max}), the time when C_{max} was obtained (T_{max}), and the area under the curve (AUC) in serum and CSF.

Purulent meningitis was induced by intracisternal inoculation of 0.5 ml of *Staphylococcus aureus* FDA 209P suspension containing 10^8

cells per ml into albino rabbits weighing between 2.0 and 2.5 kg. The antibiotics studied in this experiment were penicillins, i.e., methicillin, carbenicillin, penicillin G, and ampicillin, and cephalosporins, i.e., cephalothin, cephacetrile, cefamandole, cefotaxime, cefazolin, cephaloridine, and T-1551. At 24 h after inoculation, rabbits were given each drug intravenously at a dose of 100 mg/kg. Blood from a marginal ear vein and CSF from the cisterna magna were obtained at 15-min intervals for 2 h after administration of each drug. The CSF volume was 50 µl for each sampling. At the time of the experiment, rabbits were anesthetized with 33 mg of amobarbital per kg intravenously. Antibiotic concentrations in serum and CSF were measured by the disk plate method, with *Micrococcus luteus* ATCC 9341 (for T-1551 and cefotaxime) and *Bacillus subtilis* ATCC 6633 (for the nine other drugs) as the indicator organisms. Serum and CSF standards were prepared with phosphate buffer. $T_{1/2}$ in

TABLE 1. *Maximum concentrations (C_{max}), half-lives ($T_{1/2}$), and penetration rates of various antibiotics after intravenous administration of 100 mg of each drug per kg to rabbits with staphylococcal meningitis[a]*

Antibiotic	No. of animals	C_{max} (µg/ml, mean ± SE)			$T_{1/2}$ (min, mean ± SE)			Penetration rate (%)
		CSF	Serum	CSF/ serum (%)	CSF	Serum	CSF/ serum	
Methicillin	9	2.80 ± 0.31 (20 ± 2.5)	152 ± 10.6 (15)	1.8	21.9 ± 2.37	18.0 ± 1.21	1.22	3.0
Carbenicillin	6	9.77 ± 4.28 (23 ± 3.4)	106 ± 8.4 (15)	9.2	42.4 ± 11.9	19.3 ± 1.03	2.20	7.4
Penicillin G	5	2.19 ± 0.09 (18 ± 3.0)	155 ± 22.6 (15)	1.4	37.7 ± 4.58	22.5 ± 1.39	1.68	3.7
Ampicillin	6	5.18 ± 0.75 (38 ± 7.5)	72.3 ± 5.52 (15)	7.2	46.3 ± 2.14	25.7 ± 0.71	1.80	16.4
Cephalothin	6	2.08 ± 0.39 (15 ± 0)	164 ± 7.54 (15)	1.3	26.2 ± 2.58	13.6 ± 0.73	1.93	2.9
Cephacetrile	5	15.9 ± 4.94 (42 ± 14)	135 ± 13.1 (15)	11.8	50.5 ± 7.07	20.5 ± 1.86	2.46	19.9
Cefamandole	6	23.4 ± 6.29 (25 ± 3.2)	184 ± 8.76 (15)	12.7	30.1 ± 2.13	22.6 ± 1.81	1.33	13.7
Cefotaxime	5	5.03 ± 0.55 (21 ± 3.7)	114 ± 17.4 (15)	4.4	55.6 ± 4.98	29.1 ± 2.04	1.91	9.4
Cefazolin	6	9.85 ± 1.35 (43 ± 4.6)	242 ± 15.3 (15)	4.1	72.3 ± 10.3	37.9 ± 5.37	1.91	7.1
Cephaloridine	5	17.4 ± 4.75 (48 ± 7.4)	175 ± 11.6 (15)	9.9	80.3 ± 15.6	42.4 ± 1.24	1.89	12.9
T-1551	5	19.1 ± 7.87 (33 ± 5.6)	109 ± 9.43 (15)	17.5	68.0 ± 14.3	46.3 ± 4.50	1.47	17.4

[a] Numbers in parentheses indicate the time (minutes) when maximum concentrations were obtained.

T1/2 in CSF

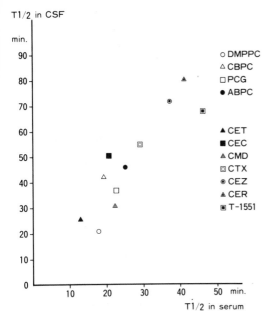

FIG. 1. *Correlation between $T_{1/2}$ in CSF and that in serum after administration of antibiotics to rabbits with staphylococcal meningitis. Abbreviations: DMPPC, methicillin; CBPC, carbenicillin; PCG, penicillin G; ABPC, ampicillin; CET, cephalothin; CEC, cephacetrile; CMD, cefamandole; CTX, cefotaxime; CEZ, cefazolin; CER, cephaloridine.*

CSF and serum were obtained by the method of least squares, assuming that decreasing rates of concentrations were based on the first-order formula. Penetration rates into the CSF were derived as follows: CSF/serum ratios of AUC (percentage).

Table 1 summarizes C_{max}, T_{max}, $T_{1/2}$, and AUC in CSF and serum and their CSF/serum ratios.

Penetration rates into the CSF were as follows: penicillin G, methicillin, cephalothin—under 5%; carbenicillin, cefazolin, cefotaxime—6 to 10%; cephaloridine, cefamandole—11 to 15%; ampicillin, T-1551, cephacetrile—16 to 20%. With reference to the protein binding rate in published data (2, 3), penetration rates were high when protein binding rates were low in penicillins. However, of the cephalosporins, T-1551, with a protein binding rate of over 80%, showed a high penetration rate.

A correlation was found between $T_{1/2}$ in serum and CSF (Fig. 1). CSF/serum ratios of $T_{1/2}$ of each drug showed various values ranging from 1.2 to 2.5, so it appeared obvious that elimination of the drugs from the CSF differed from one drug to another. On the other hand, correlations between CSF/serum ratios of $T_{1/2}$ and other parameters, i.e., CSF/serum ratios of AUC, C_{max} in the CSF, T_{max} in the CSF, and CSF/serum ratios of C_{max}, were not found. Based on these findings, it was speculated that the factors influencing penetration into the CSF were not the same ones influencing elimination from the CSF. Furthermore, there was no correlation between the CSF/serum ratio of $T_{1/2}$ and protein binding rate of a given antibiotic.

1. **Morikawa, Y., T. Haruta, and Y. Kobayashi.** 1978. Passage in semisynthetic penicillins into the cerebrospinal fluid in experimental staphylococcal meningitis in rabbits, p. 582–583. *In* Current chemotherapy, Proceedings of the 10th International Congress of Chemotherapy. American Society for Microbiology, Washington, D.C.
2. **Scholtan, W.** 1968. Die Bindung der Penicilline an die Eiweisskörper des Plasmas und der Gewebsflüssigkeit. Antibiot. Chemother. **14**:53–93.
3. **Vallner, J. J.** 1977. Binding of drugs by albumin and plasma. J. Pharm. Sci. **66**:447–465.

Methicillin Concentration in Human Brain Tissues

PETER T. FRAME,* CHATRCHAI WATANAKUNAKORN, ROBERT L. McLAURIN, AND GHAHREMAN KHODADAD

University of Cincinnati College of Medicine, Cincinnati, Ohio 45267, U.S.A.

Staphylococcus aureus is the most common organism isolated in postoperative craniotomy infections (7) and is an important pathogen in brain abscesses. Since most *S. aureus* isolates are resistant to penicillin G, penicillinase-resistant penicillins are the antibiotics of choice in treating systemic *S. aureus* infections.

Penetration of penicillins into human brain tissue has been studied infrequently. The data

from the literature are summarized in Table 1 (2, 3, 5, 6). Parenterally administered antistaphylococcal penicillins had been examined in only three patients before 1978 (2). In that study, the antibacterial activity of brain abscess pus was determined, but antibiotic concentrations were not reported.

In 1978, we reported the penetration of nafcillin into brain tissue of patients undergoing di-

TABLE 1. *Penetration of penicillins into human brain tissue or brain abscess pus*

Study by reference number	Dose	Tissue studied	No. of levels detected /no. tested	Mean antibiotic concn[a]
Penicillin G				
6	0.375 g of procaine	Normal brain	0/4	<0.019
5	2 g, i.v.[b]	"Relatively normal"	7/9	0.32 (0–1.38)
2	5–12.5 g/24 h	Pus	3/3	32–380 times MIC of infecting organism
3	1–25 g/24 h	Pus	16/26	4.1 (0–11)
Ampicillin				
5	2 g, i.v.	"Relatively normal"	4/8	0.4 (0–20)
2	2–4 g/24 h	Pus	5/6	1.1 (0–3.5)
Cloxacillin				
2	2–6 g/24 h	Pus	5/7	0.79 (0–2)
Nafcillin				
2	18 g/24 h	Pus	0/1	0 times MIC of test organism
Frame, 18th ICAAC, 1978	2 g, i.v.	"Relatively normal"	6/7	1.3 (<0.25–3.2)
		"Abnormal"	5/6	4.3 (<0.36–11)
Methicillin				
2	16–24 g/24 h	Pus	2/2	4–5 times MIC of infecting organism
Frame, 1979	2 g, i.v.	"Relatively normal"	6/10	1.23 (<0.5–3.6)
		"Abnormal"	8/8	2.86 (0.63–5.0)

[a] Concentrations expressed as micrograms per gram of tissue or per milliliter of pus. Numbers in parentheses are range.

[b] i.v., Intravenously.

agnostic craniotomy (P. T. Frame, C. Watanakunakorn, G. Khodadad, and R. McLauren, Program Abstr. Intersci. Conf. Antimicrob. Agents Chemother. 18th, Atlanta, Ga., abstr. no. 28, 1978). In that study, 10 patients received 2-g infusions of nafcillin just after anesthesia induction. Eleven of 13 brain tissue specimens contained nafcillin concentrations, in micrograms per gram of tissue, which equaled or exceeded the MIC of nafcillin for *S. aureus* (0.4 µg/ml).

We recently studied methicillin penetration of brain tissue in an additional 10 patients who were undergoing craniotomy and diagnostic brain biopsy. In this study, patients also received a 2-g infusion of a semisynthetic penicillin, methicillin, just after anesthesia induction. At the time of craniotomy, one or two small samples of the tissue which was removed for therapeutic or diagnostic reasons were separately weighed and frozen at −20°C until assayed. By gross inspection at the operating table, the neurosurgeon designated whether each tissue sample was from the tumor or other pathological area or was "relatively normal" brain tissue from the periphery of the resected lesion.

Methicillin assays were performed by a cupplate bioassay, using *Bacillus subtilis* as the test organism (1, 4). Before the assay, the tissue specimen was washed and then sonicated in a known volume of phosphate-buffered saline at pH 7.4 (PBS). Preliminary studies with human brain tissue obtained at autopsy showed that bioassay standards prepared in PBS only were equivalent to standards prepared with brain tissue and PBS. Thus, the size of the inhibition zone around the brain tissue + PBS cups was compared with zone sizes around cups containing standard methicillin concentrations in PBS. The patient's serum specimen was compared with standards prepared in pooled human serum.

Results are displayed in Fig. 1. Serum concentrations of methicillin were between 19 and 48 µg/ml up to 150 min after the completion of the infusion. Methicillin was detected in 14 of 18 brain tissue specimens. However, a majority of the tissue levels were well below the "susceptible" MIC of methicillin for *S. aureus* (3.0 µg/ml). Only 6 of 18 specimens contained methicillin concentrations which exceeded this level.

In seven of eight patients with two specimens assayed, antibiotic concentrations were higher in "abnormal" tissue than in concurrently obtained "relatively normal" tissue. This finding is in agreement with our previous report in which nafcillin was used.

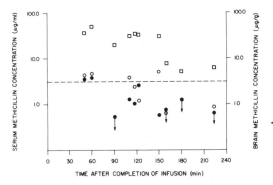

FIG. 1. *Methicillin concentrations in serum* (□) *and brain tissue* (●, *"normal"*; ○, *"abnormal"*) *after a 2-g intravenous infusion. The dotted line at 3 μg/ ml represents the "susceptible" MIC of methicillin for Staphylococcus aureus. The arrows indicate the minimal sensitivity of the assay times the dilution factor for each of the four undetectable concentrations.*

the concentrations detected are similar with the two antibiotics, since nafcillin is more active against *S. aureus*, it may be preferred over methicillin for therapy of intracranial staphylococcal infections and for antibiotic prophylaxis in neurosurgical procedures if prophylaxis is indicated.

In summary, methicillin, like nafcillin, is detected in most brain tissue specimens obtained after a single 2-g intravenous infusion. Although

1. **Bennett, J. V., J. L. Brodie, E. J. Benner, and W. M. M. Kirby.** 1966. Simplified, accurate method for antibiotic assay of clinical specimens. Appl. Microbiol. **14:** 170–177.
2. **Black, P., J. R. Graybill, and P. Charache.** 1973. Penetration of brain abscesses by systemically administered antibiotics. J. Neurosurg. **38:**705–709.
3. **de Louvois, J., P. Gortvai, and R. Hurley.** 1977. Antibiotic treatment of abscesses of the central nervous system. Br. Med. J. **2:**985–987.
4. **Grove, D. C., and W. A. Randall.** 1955. Assay methods of antibiotics. Medical Encyclopedia, New York.
5. **Kramer, P. W., R. S. Griffith, and R. L. Campbell.** 1969. Antibiotic penetration of the brain: a comparative study. J. Neurosurg. **31:**295–302.
6. **Wellman, W. E., H. W. Dodge, Jr., F. R. Heilman, and M. C. Petersen.** 1954. Concentration of antibiotics in the brain. J. Lab. Clin. Med. **43:**275–279.
7. **Wright, R. L.** 1966. A survey of possible etiologic agents in postoperative craniotomy infections. J. Neurosurg. **25:**125–132.

Cefadroxil Levels in Bile in Biliary Infection

A. PALMU,* H. JÄRVINEN, T. HALLYNCK, AND P. J. PIJCK

Second Department of Surgery, University Central Hospital, Helsinki, Finland, and State University, Gent, Belguim*

Disturbances in liver function and biliary obstruction are known to modify biliary concentrations of antibiotics (3, 4). It has also been shown that adequate gallbladder bile concentrations of antibiotics are not attainable in acute cholecystitis because of the obstruction of the cystic duct (2).

In the present investigation biliary levels of cefadroxil, a new semisynthetic oral cephalosporin, were examined from samples obtained during surgery for different biliary diseases and postoperatively from T-tube samples.

Patients and methods. Cefadroxil concentrations were estimated in six patients operated on for acute cholecystitis, in two cases operated on for acalculous cholesterosis, and in four patients with T-tubes. The concentrations of the antibiotic in serum, gallbladder bile, common duct bile, gallbladder wall, and liver tissue were measured during surgery after oral administration of 1,000 mg of cefadroxil at 12-h intervals over the 24 h before the operation. The last dose was given 2 h before surgery. Patients with T-

tubes received 1,000 mg of cefadroxil every 12 h, and serum and bile samples were collected on day 2 after surgery.

Samples. Bile was aspirated from the gallbladder with a fine needle at the beginning of the operation and from the common duct when it was visualized before opening. A venous blood sample was taken simultaneously, and samples of gallbladder wall and liver tissue were taken for antibiotic assay. In patients with T-tubes, common duct bile samples and simultaneous blood samples were taken immediately before drug administration (zero-time sample) and 1, 2, 3, 5, and 7 h after cefadroxil administration.

Microbiological methods. Microbiological assays of cefadroxil in serum and tissue were done with an agar diffusion method, using *Bacillus subtilis* ATCC 6633 for serum and *Sarcina lutea* ATCC 9843 for tissues as test organisms. The determination of the amount of blood in the tissue sample was based upon the comparison of the intensity of the red color of two supernatants: one obtained from the crushing

TABLE 1. *Serum and biliary concentrations of cefadroxil after prophylactic administration[a]*

Patients with:	Concn (mean ± SE)				
	Serum (µg/ml)	Gallbladder bile (µg/ml)	Common duct bile (µg/ml)	Gallbladder wall (µg/g)	Liver tissue (µg/g)
Acute cholecystitis	7.9 ± 3.0	3.7 ± 0.7	3.3 ± 1.3	6.8 ± 3.5	5.1 ± 1.2
Cholesterosis	12.6 ± 0.5	10.3 ± 7.1	7.2 ± 2.0	9.6 ± 0.1	11.0 ± 0

[a] Last dose was administered 2 h before surgery.

TABLE 2. *Serum and common duct bile concentrations of cefadroxil in patients with T-tubes*

Time (h) after administration of drug[a]	Concn (µg/ml, mean ± SE) in:	
	Serum	Common bile duct
0	2.14 ± 1.5	0.7 ± 0.2
1	11.3 ± 4.5	1.7 ± 0.7
2	14.3 ± 4.0	2.7 ± 1.2
3	20.4 ± 6.7	4.5 ± 2.0
5	16.2 ± 4.2	4.5 ± 2.4
7	9.6 ± 2.8	2.5 ± 1.0
12		1.0 ± 0.6

[a] 1,000 mg of cefadroxil administered orally.

and dilution of the tissue samples; the other obtained from the blood samples, crushed and diluted in the same way. Percentage of blood in tissue $(B) = (1/D) \times 100$, where D is dilution of the supernatant of crushed and diluted blood sample to obtain the red color intensity of the supernatant of crushed and diluted tissue samples. Correction of the antibiotic concentration for the blood contamination of the tissue was calculated according to the formula: $C_t = \{[(C_m \times 100) - (C_b \times B)]/(100 - B)\}$, where C_t = calculated antibiotic concentration for blood-free tissue, C_m = measured antibiotic concentration for tissue contaminated with blood, C_b = measured antibiotic concentration for blood, and B = percentage of blood in the tissue samples.

Results. An average serum level of 7.9 ± 3.0 µg/ml, gallbladder bile level of 3.7 ± 0.7 µg/ml, and common duct bile level of 3.3 ± 1.3 µg/ml were attained during acute cholecystitis (Table 1). The corresponding levels in gallbladder wall and liver tissue were 6.8 ± 3.5 and 5.1 ± 1.2 µg/g.

All the cholecystitis patients were found to have cystic duct obstruction. In cholesterosis patients with patent cystic duct, the mean gallbladder and common duct bile levels were 10.3 ± 7.1 and 7.2 ± 2.0 µg/ml, and these patients also had higher tissue concentrations of anti-

biotics than those with acute cholecystitis (9.6 ± 0.1 and 11.0 µg/g).

In T-tube patients a peak serum level of 20.4 ± 6.7 µg/ml and peak common duct bile level of 4.5 ± 2.0 µg/ml were achieved 3 h after oral cefadroxil administration (Table 2).

Discussion. Cefadroxil is a semisynthetic oral cephalosporin which is active against both gram-positive and gram-negative organisms such as various streptococci, *Escherichia coli* and *Klebsiella pneumoniae*, common pathogens in biliary tract infections. The majority of *E. coli* and *K. pneumoniae* species are susceptible to concentrations of 16 µg of cefadroxil or less per ml (1). In the present investigation a peak serum level of 20.4 µg/ml was achieved 3 h after oral administration in patients with T-tubes. The concentrations of cefadroxil in samples obtained during surgery for acute cholecystitis were lower than those in operative samples from cholesterosis patients and postoperative T-tube samples. The principal difference in test groups was that all the cholecystitis patients had a cystic duct obstruction, whereas all the cholesterosis patients had an open cystic duct with functioning gallbladder. Besides the impaired gastrointestinal function in acute phase, which may modify the absorption of the drug, the cystic duct obstruction is the dominating factor which limits the gallbladder bile concentration of cefadroxil as well as other antibiotics in acute cholecystitis.

1. Buck, R. E., and K. E. Price. 1977. Cefadroxil, a new broad-spectrum cephalosporin. Antimicrob. Agents Chemother. 11:324–330.
2. Järvinen, H., O.-V. Renkonen, and A. Palmu. 1978. Antibiotics in acute cholecystitis. Ann. Clin. Res. 10:247–251.
3. Keighley, M. R. B., R. B. Drysdale, A. H. Quaraishi, D. W. Burdon, and J. Alexander-Williams. 1976. Antibiotics in biliary disease: the relative importance of antibiotic concentrations in the bile and serum. Gut 17:495.
4. Mortimer, P. R., D. B. Mackie, and S. Haynes. 1969. Ampicillin levels in human bile in the presence of biliary tract disease. Br. Med. J. 3:88.

Penetration of Cefoxitin into Ascitic Fluid

J. BOURREILLE,* G. LE BIHAN, B. BEAU, A. LEROY, AND G. HUMBERT

Departments of Internal Medicine* and Infectious Diseases, University of Rouen, 76038 Rouen, France

A frequent complication in cirrhotic patients with ascites is spontaneous bacterial peritonitis. Because of the severity of this infection, the development of a new antibiotic agent for treating these patients is always of keen interest. Cefoxitin is a new semisynthetic cephamycin antibiotic, the structure of which confers a high degree of resistance to inactivation by β-lactamase. As a consequence, the antibacterial spectrum of cephoxitin is broader than that of currently available cephalosporins. In vivo and in vitro studies have indicated that cefoxitin is active against many enterobacteriaceae resistant to cephalosporins and also has useful activity against *Bacteroides* species (6, 7). These bacteria are frequently found in ascites of hospitalized cirrhotic patients with spontaneous bacterial peritonitis.

The purpose of this study was to determine concentrations of cefoxitin in ascites after infusion of a single or multiple dose and then to investigate its diffusion into the peritoneal cavity and its therapeutic significance. The 22 patients studied, 19 males and 3 females, had an average age of 65 years and a body weight ranging from 54 to 92 kg. Twenty-one patients suffered from alcoholic cirrhosis of the liver with ascites, and one presented neoplasic ascites secondary to a large-bowel carcinoma. Moderate renal failure was present in two cirrhotic patients (creatininemia, 180 and 130 μmol/liter). Renal function was normal in the other 20 patients. During the course of the study, no other antibiotic or diuretic was administered, and the 21 cirrhotic patients received a 20- to 30-mmol sodium daily diet and water ad libitum.

The 22 patients were classified as follows. Group I included all 22 patients. They received a single continuous 2.0-g intravenous infusion of cefoxitin during 30 min. Serum and ascites specimens were obtained at 0, 0.5 (end of the infusion), 1, 2, 3, 4, and 8 h after antibiotic administration. Moreover, ascites and blood samples were taken from 11 of the 22 patients at 24 h. Group II included 11 of the 22 patients. Cefoxitin was administered every 8 h in a dose of 2.0 g by continuous intravenous infusion over 30 min during 10 days. Serum and ascitic fluid specimens were obtained on day 1 as in the single-dose study and then on days 3 and 10 at zero time (just before the beginning of an infusion),

0.5 h (end of the infusion), and 3 and 8 h after the beginning of the infusion. Total protein, albumin, and creatinine were determined in serum, using the Auto-Analyzer (Technicon SMA 11). Ascitic protein concentration was determined by the same method. Ascitic fluid cell counts and differential cell counts were performed manually.

Cefoxitin was assayed in triplicate in serum and in ascitic fluid, using the agar diffusion microbiological method described by Grove and Randall (5) as modified by Chabert and Boulingre (1). *Staphylococcus aureus* MB 2786 was used as the test organism. The minimal antibiotic concentration detected by this method was ⩽1.56 μg/ml.

Results. (i) Group I. The mean antibiotic concentration in serum at the end of the infusion was 128.2 ± 11.00 μg/ml (mean ± SEM). This value progressively decreased, and the antibiotic concentration was undetectable for 13 of the 22 patients in the 8-h serum specimens. In the 24-h samples, the cefoxitin concentration was detectable in serum in only one sample obtained from a cirrhotic patient with renal failure.

Ascitic fluid levels of cefoxitin increased slowly, reaching a maximal value at 2 h in 16 patients, at 3 h in 4, and at 4 h in 2. The mean maximal antibiotic concentration was 16.16 ± 1.85 μg/ml (mean ± SEM) (Fig. 1). The antibiotic concentration decreased and reached a mean value of 6.73 ± 1.07 μg/ml (mean ± SEM) at 8 h. In 24-h ascitic fluid specimens, the cirrhotic patient with moderate renal failure was the only one in whom the ascitic fluid concentration of cefoxitin was still appreciable (6.10 μg/ml). No correlation was found between the cefoxitin concentration in ascites and ascitic fluid protein ($r = 0.20$), total protein in serum ($r = 0.13$), and number of cells in ascites ($r = 0.16$).

(ii) Group II. No accumulation of the antibiotic was seen in the serum when renal function was normal. In ascitic fluid, the mean cefoxitin concentration was significantly higher on days 3 and 10 than on day 1 in samples obtained at 0.5 h ($P < 0.01$) and 3 h ($P < 0.025$). In 10 patients, no accumulation of the antibiotic was observed in ascitic fluid, as indicated by the trough levels in 8-h samples which were not statistically different on days 1, 3, and 10 (Fig. 2). However, an accumulation of cefoxitin was observed on days

3 and 10 in serum and ascites of a cirrhotic patient with renal failure.

Discussion. In ascitic fluid, the maximal antibiotic concentration was reached at 2 h for

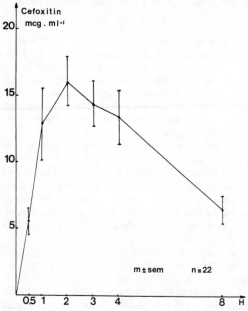

FIG. 1. *Ascitic fluid levels of cefoxitin (mean ± SEM) after a 2.0-g intravenous dose in group I.*

most of the patients. This finding is close to the results of Gerding et al. (2), who administered a 2.0-g intravenous dose of cephalothin. Nevertheless, it is not possible to compare our results and those of previous clinical and experimental studies (2, 4, 8) for at least two reasons: (i) we administered a standard antibiotic dose and not an excessive dose, and (ii) the ascitic fluid volume was not measured in our patients, whereas there seems to be an inverse relation between the antibiotic concentration in ascites and the ascitic fluid volume (8).

Peritoneal inflammation did not seem to alter the ascitic fluid penetration of the antibiotic, as demonstrated by the absence of any relationship between cefoxitin ascitic fluid levels and leukocyte count, neutrophil percentage, or the ascitic fluid protein in these patients.

Gerding et al. (4) have administered different cephalosporins intramuscularly to mongrel dogs with ascites created by inferior vena cava ligation. They observed a slow increase in antibiotic fluid concentration that reached a plateau at 16 to 28 h. In our multiple-dose study, accumulation of cefoxitin was obtained neither in serum nor in ascites when renal function was normal. Nevertheless, ascitic fluid levels were higher in the 0.5- and 3-h specimens on days 3 and 10 than on day 1. This finding may result from a shrinkage of the ascitic volume secondary to low-so-

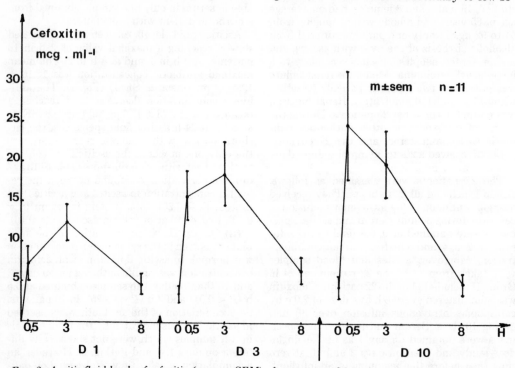

FIG. 2. *Ascitic fluid levels of cefoxitin (mean ± SEM) after a repeated 2.0-g intravenous dose in group II.*

dium diet and to rest prescribed at the beginning of the study; indeed, the mean weight loss reached 4.6 kg in 10 days for 9 of 11 patients. One patient had a stable body weight, and another one gained 4 kg.

The MIC of cefoxitin for most susceptible, infective gram-negative bacteria is 4 to 5 μg/ml. The results of our pharmacokinetic study show that transperitoneal passage of cefoxitin is good and demonstrate the therapeutic efficacy of cefoxitin in infected ascites when administered at a dose of 2.0 g every 8 h regardless the ascitic fluid volume.

1. **Chabert, Y. A., and A. Boulingre.** 1957. Modifications pratiques concernant le dosage des antibiotiques en clinique. Rev. Fr. Etud. Clin. Biol. **2**:636–640.
2. **Gerding, D. N., W. H. Hall, and E. A. Schierl.** 1977. Antibiotic concentrations in ascitic fluid of patients with ascites and bacterial peritonitis. Ann. Intern. Med. **86**: 708–713.
3. **Gerding, D. N., J. P. Kromhout, J. J. Sullivan, and W. H. Hall.** 1976. Antibiotic penetrance of ascitic fluid in dogs. Antimicrob. Agents Chemother. **10**:850–855.
4. **Gerding, D. N., L. R. Peterson, D. C. Legler, W. H. Hall, and E. A. Schierl.** 1978. Ascitic fluid cephalosporin concentrations: influence of protein binding and serum pharmacokinetics. Antimicrob. Agents Chemother. **14**:234–239.
5. **Grove, D. C., and W. A. Randall.** 1955. Assay methods of antibiotics: a laboratory manual. Antibiot. Monogr. **2**:34–36.
6. **Moellering, R. C., M. Dray, and L. J. Kuvz.** 1974. Susceptibility of clinical isolates of bacteria to cefoxitin and cephalotin. Antimicrob. Agents Chemother. **6**:320–323.
7. **Sutter, V. L., and S. M. Finegold.** 1975. Susceptibility of anaerobic bacteria to carbenicillin, cefoxitin and related drugs. J. Infect. Dis. **253**:449–452.
8. **Wilson, D. E., T. C. Chalmers, and M. A. Madoff.** 1967. The passage of cephalothin into and out of ascitic fluid. Am. J. Med. Sci. **253**:449–452.

Tissue Penetration, as Measured by a Blister Technique, and Pharmacokinetics of CGP 7174/E Compared with Carbenicillin

SANDRA BAKER, RICHARD WISE,* ADRIAN P. GILLETT, AND JENNIFER M. ANDREWS

Department of Medical Microbiology, Dudley Road Hospital, Birmingham, England

CGP 7174/E (cefsulodin [SCE 129]) (3) is a novel semisynthetic cephalosporin which, unlike other agents of this class, has a high activity against *Pseudomonas aeruginosa*, being about 16-fold more active than carbenicillin, but it is not active against other pathogenic bacteria.

In this study, the pharmacokinetics of both antibiotics were compared after a rapid intravenous (i.v.) injection of 1 g in healthy volunteers. Since both agents may be used in burn patients to treat pseudomonal infections, the levels of both antibiotics in a chemically induced burn were studied by raising blisters, using a 0.2% cantharides plaster on the forearm.

Eight healthy males aged 21 to 35 years (mean age, 27 years; mean weight, 76.4 kg) volunteered for the study. They had no history of allergy to β-lactams nor evidence of renal disease. Hematological and biomedical profiles were normal. One gram of CGP 7174/E was administered first, and then 2 to 3 months later 1 g of carbenicillin was given (six of the original eight volunteers took part in this phase of the study).

On the night before the study, two 0.2% cantharides plasters (1 by 1 cm) were taped to the forearm in order to induce blister formation. On the morning of the study, the antibiotic was administered by rapid i.v. injection, and blood samples were taken at 15, 30, 45, 60, and 90 min and at 2, 3, 4, 5, 6, 7, and 8 h. Urine samples were collected over 24 h. The two blisters were sampled at 30 and 60 min and then hourly, using a fine needle. The integrity of the blister was maintained by spraying with a fast-drying plastic dressing. The assays were performed as in a previous study (4), using *P. aeruginosa* as indicator organism. The nature of the blister fluid was also studied by routine techniques.

The concentration/time profiles of the two compounds are shown in Fig. 1. The pharmacokinetic parameters are compared in Table 1. The initial fictive concentration of CGP 7174/E was 146 μg/ml and that of carbenicillin was 118 μg/ml, compared with the observed 15-min levels of 71 and 68 μg/ml, respectively, suggesting rapid distribution. The calculated volumes of distribution approximate to the value of the vascular compartment. The serum half-lives of each compound were similar (1.25 to 1.5 h), and both appeared to be eliminated entirely by the renal route, since approximately 90% of the administered dose (i.e., antipseudomonal microbiologically active) was recovered in the urine by 24 h.

Both β-lactams appeared to penetrate rapidly into the blister fluid, reaching maximum levels at 2 to 3 h. Peak blister fluid levels of CGP 7174/E were about twice those of carbenicillin. CGP 7174/E also appeared to penetrate into the fluid

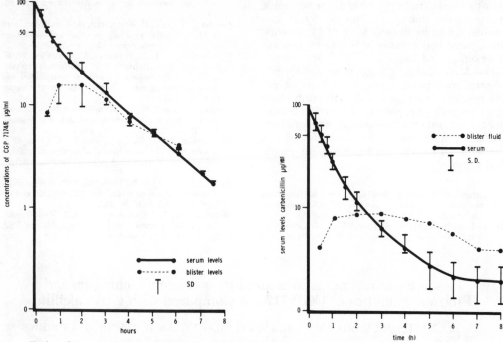

FIG. 1. *Serum and blister fluid levels of CGP 7174/E and carbenicillin after a 1-g i.v. injection.*

TABLE 1. *Comparison of the pharmacokinetics of CGP 7174/E and carbenicillin after 1 g i.v.*

Drug	Serum half-life (h)	Elimination constant (h^{-1})	Initial fictive concn (μg/ml)	Distribution vol (liters)	24-h urine recovery (%)	Peak blister level (μg/ml)	Time of blister level (h)	Terminal blister half-life (h)
CGP 7174/E	1.5	0.46	146	7.0	89.5	15.3	2	2.0
	$(0.21)^a$	(0.07)	(22.2)	(1.03)	(13.0)	(7.1)		
Carbenicillin	1.25	0.55	118	8.5	94.3	8.9	3	2.1
	(0.45)	(0.09)	(24.6)	(1.2)	(12.8)	(1.8)		

^{a} Numbers in parentheses are SD.

somewhat more rapidly. After a 1-g i.v. dose, the levels of CGP 7174/E in the blister fluid exceeded the mode MIC for *P. aeruginosa* (2), but the carbenicillin level in the blister fluid did not.

The blister levels of carbenicillin exceeded those in serum after 2 to 5 h, but the fluid levels of CGP 7174/E approximated to those of serum. The terminal blister fluid half-lives of both agents were similar and approximated to the serum half-life, as would be expected in an open model.

The protein content of the blister fluid was approximately 70% of that of serum, and the total protein albumin ratio was similar to that in serum. The cellular nature of the blister fluid was very variable, 0.6 to 12.3 leukocytes per mm^3, but was made up almost entirely (98%) of polymorphonuclear cells.

It appears that the nature of the blister fluid is similar to that found in burns (2), with a variable cellular and high protein content. It is therefore possible to assume that the kinetics of antibiotics in this fluid will be similar to that in a burn. Both antibiotics penetrate well into this fluid, but the maximal levels of CGP 7174/E were higher than those of carbenicillin. Since CGP 7174/E has higher antipseudomonal activity than carbenicillin, CGP 7174/E may prove to be more efficacious in the treatment of pseudomonal infections in burns. An effective nontoxic antipseudomonal agent would be of considerable use in the management of burns infected with this organism. At infections in other sites, this agent has been shown to be effective (1).

1. **Ahrens, T., W. Vischer, P. Imbhot, J. Fullhaas, O. Zak, and F. Kradolfer.** 1978. Human pharmacology of CGP 7174/E (SCE 129) and initial results of clinical

trials in Europe. *In* Drugs in experimental and clinical research, Proceedings of the 3rd Symposium on Future Trends in Chemotherapy, Tirrena, Italy.

2. **Sevitt, S.** 1957. *In* Burns: pathology and therapeutic applications, p. 37–38. Butterworth, London.

3. **Tosch, W., F. Kradolfer, E. A. Konopka, J. Regos, W. Zimmerman, and O. Zak.** 1978. In vitro characterisation of CGP 7174/E, a cephalosporin active against

Pseudomonas, p. 843–844. *In* Current chemotherapy, Proceedings of the 10th International Congress of Chemotherapy. American Society for Microbiology, Washington, D.C.

4. **Wise, R., B. Cadge, A. P. Gillett, A. Bhamjee, and D. P. Thornhill.** 1979. The pharmacology of cefoxitin and the comparison of two human tissue models. J. Infect. 1(Suppl.):49–56.

Gentamicin Penetration into Abscesses

ZEEV DREZNIK, RENATA SCHWARTZKOPF, ISIDOR T. WOLFSTEIN, AND ETHAN RUBINSTEIN*

Chaim Sheba Medical Center, Sackler School of Medicine, Tel Aviv University, Tel Aviv, Israel

The penetration of gentamicin into abscesses and its therapeutic efficacy in this setting are unknown. We have measured simultaneous blood, interstitial fluid (IF), and abscess fluid concentrations of gentamicin in rats. Interstitial fluid was collected by the dialysis-to-disk method as previously described by Rubinstein et al. (3). Subcutaneous abscesses were induced by contaminating the disk unit with 4.3×10^7 ($\pm 0.7 \times 10^1$) colony-forming units of *Pseudomonas aeruginosa* that was gentamicin susceptible (MIC, 0.8 μg/ml). Seventy-two hours after the implantation, gentamicin (10 mg/kg) was injected intramuscularly. Blood, IF, and abscess fluid specimens were obtained at 0, 30, 90, 150, and 240 min (Fig. 1). To extend the experimental period, some IF and abscess fluid samples were obtained 6, 9, and 24 h after gentamicin administration. At 9 h, whereas blood and IF gentamicin concentrations were undetectable, there was still considerable concentration of gentamicin in the abscess fluid. At 24 h no gentamicin was detected in the abscess fluid. These observations suggest that gentamicin persists in abscesses for extended periods of time. To assess the antibacterial activity of gentamicin in abscesses, the same model was used and gentamicin was administered for 3 days (10 mg/kg per day) twice daily before the actual experiment. Bacterial counts were performed at the time of implantation, after 2 days of gentamicin administration, and 150 min after gentamicin administration on the 3rd day. Bacterial counts were 4.3×10^7 ($\pm 7 \times 10^1$) at implantation, 6×10^7 ($\pm 9 \times 10^1$) after 2 days of therapy and 2.9×10^7 ($\pm 3.2 \times 10^1$) 150 min after administration on the 3rd day, the differences being statistically insignificant.

To assess the failure of gentamicin to eradicate the bacteria from abscesses, pH and pO_2 of the abscess fluid were measured. The pH values

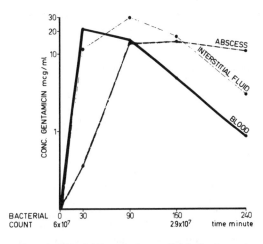

FIG. 1. *Blood, IF, and abscess fluid of rats receiving gentamicin, 10 mg/kg.*

varied between 6.9 and 7.3, and pO_2 in all 12 samples collected was 1 to 3 mm Hg. The low oxygen tension present in abscesses is probably important in the absence of antibacterial activity of the drug. Similar findings were observed by Hays and Mandell (2). These observations suggest that gentamicin penetrates well into abscesses and has a prolonged half-life in this fluid as compared with blood and IF. Despite its adequate penetration, gentamicin fails to cure subcutaneous abscess produced by *P. aeruginosa* or change the bacterial count present in these abscesses. In addition to the inactivation of gentamicin caused by pus as shown by Bryant and Hammond (1), gentamicin, despite adequate penetration into abscesses, is antibacterially inactive. Gentamicin therapy should not be relied upon as a sole agent in the therapy of abscesses even if caused by gentamicin-susceptible bacteria.

1. **Bryant, R. E., and D. Hammond.** 1974. Interaction of purulent material with antibiotics used to treat *Pseudomonas* infections. Antimicrob. Agents Chemother. **6:** 702–706.

2. **Hays, R. C., and G. C. Mandell.** 1974. pO$_2$, pH and redoxy potential of experimental abscesses. Proc. Soc. Exp. Biol. Med. **147:**29–30.

3. **Rubinstein, E., M. Dan, and H. Halkin.** 1978. Interstitial fluid concentrations of antibiotics. Program Abstr. Intersci. Conf. Antimicrob. Agents Chemother. 18th, Atlanta, Ga., abstr. no. 392.

Increased Antibiotic Concentration in Wound Fluid as an Effect of Debrisan Treatment

ANN-CHRISTINE RYDÉN,* CLAES LUNDBERG, DAG CAMPBELL, AND ALVAR SANDKVIST

Department of Biology, Pharmacia AB S-75101 Uppsala, Sweden

The efficacy of parenteral antibiotic treatment of localized infections is closely related to the concentration of the drug that can be obtained at the site of infection. Several recent clinical studies have shown that topical treatment of infected wounds with a dextranomer (Debrisan, Pharmacia AB, Uppsala, Sweden) will enhance healing. As part of our studies of possible underlying mechanisms for the healing-promoting effect, we measured the concentration of two penicillins in wound fluid after parenteral administration in an experimental rat model after topical treatment with dextranomer.

Male Sprague-Dawley rats (weight, 350 to 400 g) were used in the experiments. Two full-thickness skin wounds were produced on the backs of the animals. Metal rings were sewn to the edges of the wounds to inhibit contraction, as described by Campbell (1). One wound was treated with Debrisan, and the other was treated with gauze. The dressings were changed daily. To facilitate these changes and prevent bleeding, Debrisan and gauze were separated from the wound by a porous nylon cloth.

After 1 day, and alternatively after 2 or 4 days, 15 mg of ampicillin, 20% protein bound, or cloxacillin, 92% protein bound, was injected intramuscularly into the rats. The wounds were left occluded but without Debrisan and gauze. Serum samples were drawn from the orbital plexus every half-hour for 2 h and then every hour for 6 h. When blood samples were drawn, weighed filter paper disks were placed on the wound surface for 2 min to absorb wound fluid. The antibiotic concentrations in serum and wound fluid were determined by the plate diffusion method, using filter paper disks with known antibiotic concentrations as standards.

The peak serum concentration was obtained within the first 30 min. The antibiotic was rapidly eliminated from the serum within 3 to 4 h. The maximal concentration in wound fluid was always lower than in serum. The peak concentration was reached after 30 to 60 min. Lower concentrations were maintained in the wound fluid for 5 to 6 h.

The concentration of ampicillin in wound fluid was higher in the Debrisan-treated wounds than in the controls after 4 days of treatment (Fig. 1). At two sampling times, the differences were significant ($P < 0.05$, Student's t-test).

Similar results were obtained after intramuscular injection of cloxacillin (Fig. 2). The concentration of cloxacillin was significantly higher in the Debrisan-treated wounds than in the controls at four sampling times.

Less antibiotic was found in wound fluid after 1 or 2 days of treatment, and no significant differences between Debrisan- and gauze-treated wounds were observed.

The mechanisms behind the differences in wound fluid concentration after 4 days are not fully understood. This wound model does not cause great trauma to the animal. There is only a small inflammatory reaction during the first 2 days, which might explain the low concentration of antibiotic in wound fluid after 1 and 2 days of treatment.

As shown by C. Lundberg and D. Campbell (in press), Debrisan treatment leads to less fluid in wounds than in controls treated with gauze. A Debrisan-treated wound visually has a drier appearance than the gauze-treated control. The absorption effect of Debrisan causing less wound fluid may thus indirectly facilitate the penetration of antibiotics into the fluid.

A more effective removal of bacteria from the wound to the Debrisan layer than to the gauze may be another contributing factor. Penicillinase-producing *Pseudomonas* bacteria have been isolated from both Debrisan- and gauze-treated wounds. Further studies are in progress to monitor the number of bacteria quantitatively on the wound surface and in the tissue to clarify

µg/ml

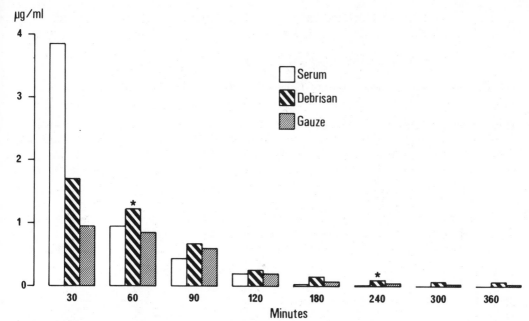

FIG. 1. *Concentration of ampicillin in serum and wound fluid after 4 days of local wound treatment with Debrisan and gauze. Mean of 11 rats. *, P < 0.05, Student's t-test.*

µg/ml

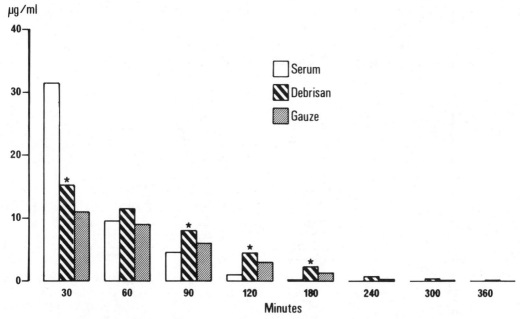

FIG. 2. *Concentration of cloxacillin in serum and wound fluid after 4 days of local wound treatment with Debrisan and gauze. Mean of 12 rats. *, P < 0.05, Student's t-test.*

whether there are significant differences in number of bacteria during the two types of treatment.

Treatment of a wound with Debrisan during antibiotic therapy increases wound fluid concentration of the antibiotic, which may increase the therapeutic effect against infecting organisms.

1. **Campbell, D. E. S.** 1979. Debrisorb-Wirkung. Einige Versuche am Rattenmodell. Extr. Dermatol. **3**(Suppl.):13–20.

Interstitial Fluid Concentrations of Cefoxitin, Cefamandole, and Cefazolin: Comparison Between Protein-Bound and Free-Drug Fraction

ETHAN RUBINSTEIN,* ZVI LANDAU, AND HILLEL HALKIN

Chaim Sheba Medical Center, Tel-Aviv University School of Medicine, Tel-Hashomer, Israel

The concentrations of antimicrobials obtained in the interstitial fluid (IF) are important for curing tissue infections. The protein unbound (=free) fraction of an agent is more meaningful

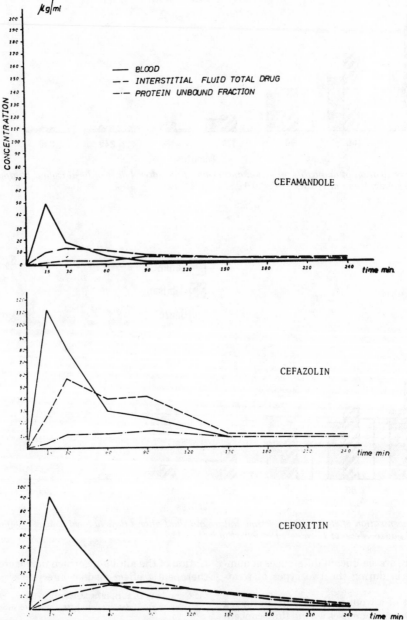

FIG. 1. *Blood, total, and free drug in the IF of rats after a 50-mg intramuscular administration of cefoxitin, cefamandole, and cefazolin.*

TABLE 1. *IF/blood mean 4-h AUC ratio ± SEM*

Fraction	Cefoxitin	Cefa-mandole	Cefazolin
Total	78 ± 0.08	97 ± 0.07	137 ± 0.12[a]
Free	77[b] ± 0.12	53 ± 0.05	54 ± 0.07
Binding to serum protein	37.5%	42%	78%

[a] Different from other two agents at $P < 0.01$.
[b] Different from other two agents at $P < 0.1$.

than the total amount of the drug present, since only the free fraction is active against bacteria (1).

Blood, free, and total IF concentrations of cefoxitin (CFX), cefamandole (CM), and cefazolin (CZ) were measured simultaneously in rats after an intramuscular administration of 50 mg of each agent per kg. Free drug in the IF was obtained by implantation of paper disks enveloped in a dialysis tube; total drug in the IF was obtained by implantation of regular paper disks as previously described (2).

Blood, total, and free-drug concentrations in the IF are shown in Fig. 1. Mean peak blood concentrations for CFX, CM, and CZ were 94, 49, and 112 µg/ml, respectively. Mean peak IF free-drug concentrations were: CFX, 24 µg/ml; CM, 5 µg/ml; and CZ, 19 µg/ml. Peak IF total-drug concentrations were: CFX, 25 µg/ml; CM, 12.5 µg/ml; and CZ, 64 µg/ml. The ratios between mean peak level of the total drug in the IF to mean peak blood levels were 27, 29, and 59% for CFX, CM, and CZ, respectively, whereas the ratios between the mean peak free-drug level in the IF to mean peak blood levels were 27, 11, and 14%, respectively. Mean 4-h area under curve (AUC) values in blood for CFX, CM, and

CZ were 4,343, 1,623, and 5,607 µg/ml, respectively. Mean AUC values of the free-drug fractions in the IF were 3,155, 845, and 2,855 µg/ml per min, respectively, whereas mean AUC values for total drug present in the IF were 3,536, 1,542, and 7,295 µg/ml per min, respectively. The ratios between IF total-drug and free-drug AUC to blood AUC are shown in Table 1.

Protein binding to rat serum was 37.5% for CFX, 42% for CM, and 78% for CZ. Blood half-life values were: CFX, 24.6 min; CM, 22.1 min; and CZ, 30.2 min. The corresponding IF half-life values for the free drug fractions were 74.7, 123, and 133.7 min, respectively.

The results of these studies suggest that CFX and CZ blood and IF concentrations are higher than those of CM. Free IF concentrations of CFX relative to blood concentrations were greater than those of CM and CZ. Binding to rat serum protein in the range of 37.5 to 78% was not a major determinant of IF free-drug concentrations, as has been found previously (3).

CFX and CZ may have an advantage over CM in the treatment of tissue infections caused by susceptible microorganisms. Further studies in infected tissues are needed in order to support these initial observations.

1. **Craig, W. A., and C. M. Kunin.** 1976. Significance of serum protein and tissue binding of antimicrobial agents. Annu. Rev. Med. **27**:287–300.
2. **Rubinstein, E., M. Dan, and H. Halkin.** 1978. Interstitial fluid concentrations of antibiotics. Program Abstr. Intersci. Conf. Antimicrob. Agents Chemother. 18th, Atlanta, Ga., Abstr. no. 392.
3. **Waterman, N. G., M. G. Raff, and L. Scharfenberger.** 1976. Protein binding and concentrations of cephaloridine and cefazolin in serum and interstitial fluid of dogs. J. Infect. Dis. **133**:642–647.

Exudate Levels and Therapeutic Effect of Apalcillin in Inflammatory Tissues of Rats

TAKAO OKUDA,* KENJI IRIE, HIROSHI NOGUCHI, AND TOSHIAKI KOMATSU

Pharmaceuticals Division, Sumitomo Chemical Co., Ltd., Osaka, Japan

Apalcillin (APPC, PC-904) is a broad-spectrum penicillin with potent antibacterial activity against *Pseudomonas aeruginosa, P. cepacia, Escherichia coli,* and *Proteus* species, as reported by Noguchi et al. (2, 3).

Binding rates of APPC with serum protein of humans, bovines, dogs, and rats were high (95 to 98%) and somewhat lower (82%) in mice, but the binding was rather loose and reversible.

The binding rate of APPC to normal liver homogenates (81%) was 76% by the ultracentri-

fugal method, whereas that of cefazolin (CEZ) and dicloxacillin (MDIPC) was 90% and more than 92%, respectively. On the other hand, 92% of APPC was recovered in the supernatant after three washings by centrifugation (CEZ, 96%; MDIPC, <14%). Similar results were obtained with kidney homogenates. The reversibility of APPC to the exudate proteins from granuloma pouches and serum proteins was confirmed by a dilution technique.

These results showed that APPC was highly

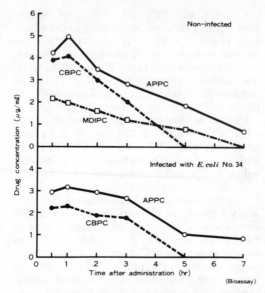

FIG. 1. *Exudate levels of APPC (○), CBPC (●), and MDIPC (□) in rats with granuloma pouches induced by croton oil. Each drug was intravenously given to noninfected rats (upper) and to rats infected with E. coli no. 34 30 min earlier (lower).*

bound to normal tissue components and to the exudate in inflammatory tissues, but the binding was loose and reversible, similar to the findings on a highly protein-bound CEZ.

Kunin et al. (1) reviewed the tissue penetration, other pharmacoparameters, and biological activities of protein-bound antibiotics. Rats may be suitable experimental animals, since binding rates of APPC to rat and human sera were almost identical. The serum level and half-life of APPC were similar to those of carbenicillin (CBPC) after intravenous administration in rats.

Penetration of APPC into inflammatory tissues was studied by using croton oil-induced granuloma pouches in rats. Exudate specimens were subjected to bioassay, with the exudate solution as the standard.

The exudate levels of APPC in the noninfected granuloma pouches were slightly higher than those of CBPC at 0.5, 1, 2, and 3 h after intravenous infection (50 mg/kg), but were more prolonged (Fig. 1). Area under the curve of APPC in the exudate was 1.7 and 2.4 times higher than that of CBPC and MDIPC, respectively. In a separate experiment, the exudate levels of APPC in the pouches, when given 30

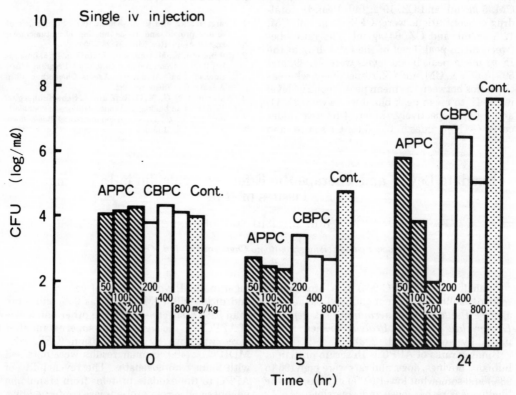

FIG. 2. *Bactericidal activity of APPC and CBPC, intravenously injected at 30 min, against P. aeruginosa KB57 in granuloma pouches in rats.*

min after infection with a clinical isolate of *E. coli* no. 34, were shown to be higher than those of CBPC.

The bactericidal activity of APPC against *E. coli* no. 34 (MIC: APPC, 1.56 µg/ml; CBPC, 3.13 µg/ml) and *P. aeruginosa* KB57 (MIC: APPC, 3.13 µg/ml; CBPC, 50 µg/ml) was examined after the pouches were inoculated with 10^4 cells.

Figure 2 shows the colony-forming units (CFU) per milliliter in the pouches infected with *P. aeruginosa* after administration of APPC with single doses of 50, 100, and 200 mg/kg compared with CBPC at 200, 400, and 800 mg/ kg. At 5 h, the viable count in the control, untreated group increased to 10^5 CFU/ml, whereas that in the treated groups decreased to 10^2 or 10^3 CFU/ml. No significant differences in the counts among the treated groups were observed.

At 24 h, the viable count in the control group increased to greater than 10^8 CFU/ml. That in the APPC group (200 mg/kg) was less than 10^2 CFU/ml, but no bactericidal effects were observed in the group given APPC at 50 mg/kg and CBPC at 200 and 400 mg/kg.

The therapeutic effect of a single 100-mg/kg injection of APPC was found to be greater than that of a 800-mg/kg dose of CBPC.

When the rats were treated twice (0.5 and 5.5 h), the bacterial counts in APPC groups (100 and 50 mg/kg) were 10^2 to 10^3 and 10^5 CFU/ml, respectively, similar to those in the CBPC groups (800 and 400 mg/kg).

Bactericidal effects of APPC were found on the local *E. coli* infection. When the rats were given APPC (200 mg/kg) and CBPC (400 mg/ kg) at 30 min after infection, the viable bacterial count at 24 h decreased to less than 10^2 and $10^{2.6}$ CFU/ml, respectively, whereas that in the control group increased to 10^9 CFU/ml. The decrease in viable cells with 100 mg of APPC per kg was almost the same as with 200 mg of CBPC per ml.

The therapeutic effects of APPC against *E. coli* after two intravenous injections (25 to 100 mg/kg) seemed to correspond with those of CBPC at the two- to fourfold doses of APPC.

1. Kunin, C. M., W. A. Craig, M. Kornguth, and R. Monson. 1973. Influence of binding on the pharmacologic activity of antibiotics. Ann. New York Acad. Sci. 226:214–223.

2. Noguchi, H., Y. Eda, H. Tobiki, T. Nakagome, and T. Komatsu. 1976. PC-904, a novel broad-spectrum semisynthetic penicillin with marked antipseudomonal activity: microbiological evaluation. Antimicrob. Agents Chemother. 9:262–273.

3. Noguchi, H., M. Kubo, S. Kurashige, and S. Mitsuhashi. 1978. Antibacterial activity of apalcillin (PC-904) against gram-negative bacilli, especially ampicillin-, carbenicillin-, and gentamicin-resistant clinical isolates. Antimicrob. Agents Chemother. 13:745–752.

Cefuroxime Levels Attained in Tissues and Wound Exudates from Severely Ischemic Limbs

BARRY R. BULLEN,* COLIN H. RAMSDEN, AND RALPH C. KESTER

University Department of Surgery, St. James's University Hospital, Leeds LS9 7TF, England

The occurrence of sepsis in an arterial graft is a serious disaster which threatens both life and limb. Broad-spectrum antibiotics are commonly used prophylactically during arterial reconstruction of ischemic limbs or specifically to treat established infection where blood flow is reduced. Prophylaxis is aimed at preventing infection from becoming established, particularly in the artificial materials of vascular grafts and sutures. This calls for an antibiotic with a spectrum of activity covering the majority of commonly encountered pathogens. Cephalosporins, as a group, fulfill this requirement quite well, and cefuroxime has a particularly broad spectrum of activity coupled with an enhanced stability to bacterial beta-lactamases. We have measured cefuroxime concentrations in serum, wound exudates, and tissues rendered ischemic by occlusive arterial disease. Twenty patients (mean age, 64 years) underwent either arterial reconstruction (10 patients) or amputation for severe ischemia of the leg. Half of the reconstruction cases received cefuroxime, 1.5 g intravenously (i.v.) with anesthetic induction and 0.75 g intramuscularly (i.m.) every 8 h for 48 h postoperation. The remaining 15 patients received cefuroxime, 0.75 g i.m. with premedication, 1.5 g i.v. with induction of anesthesia, and 0.75 g i.m. every 8 h for 48 h postoperation.

The following specimens were collected: from arterial reconstructions, 2 g of subcutaneous fat from the groin wound and 10 ml of peripheral venous blood before the application of arterial occluding clamps; from amputations, 10 ml of peripheral venous blood and 2-g samples of sub-cutaneous fat and skeletal muscle proximally and distally from the amputated limb. Suction drains were inserted into all wounds, and wound exudate was collected (when available) for two 8-h periods 24 to 48 h postoperation. Specimens were stored as appropriate at −20°C for later batch assay of cefuroxime levels. Tissue levels were corrected for the presence of cefuroxime due to blood contamination.

Results. The time interval between i.m. and i.v. doses of cefuroxime varied from 55 to 160 min (mean, 90 min). The time delay between i.v. dosage and the sampling of blood and tissue ranged from 10 to 70 min (mean, 43 min in reconstruction cases and 20 min in amputation cases).

(i) Serum levels. There was a wide range of serum levels (52 to 287 µg/ml). These serum levels were a reflection of the time interval between i.v. dosage and venous sampling (Tables 1 and 2).

(ii) Tissue levels. Cefuroxime levels (corrected for hemoglobin content) in the subcutaneous fat of arterial reconstruction cases ranged from 0 to 16.5 µg/g (mean, 9.1 µg/g). Corrected cefuroxime levels in the subcutaneous fat of the

amputated limbs varied from 8.8 to 30.3 µg/g (mean, 16.7 µg/g) proximally and from 2.2 to 16.5 µg/g (mean, 9.1 µg/g) distally. The mean corrected cefuroxime level was 17.0 µg/g (5.2 to 53.8 µg/g) in the proximal muscle and 8.9 µg/g (0 to 29.7 µg/g) in the distal muscle.

(iii) Wound exudate levels. Wound exudates from the reconstruction cases had a mean cefuroxime level of 9.2 µg/ml (range, 3.9 to 26.0 µg/ml). This level was lower than that attained in the exudates from amputation stumps, where the cefuroxime concentration ranged from 2.7 to 59.0 µg/ml (mean, 18.9 µg/ml). In 4 cases out of 20, no wound exudate could be collected.

(iv) Wound infection. There were no overtly infected wounds.

Discussion. The efficacy of an antibiotic depends partly on the concentrations attained in the target tissue. It is possible that an effective antibacterial level may be prevented by poor tissue perfusion, as exists in legs affected by occlusive arterial disease.

The serum levels of cefuroxime attained in this study were well above the MICs for the majority of commonly encountered gram-positive and gram-negative pathogens excepting *Pseudomonas*. The wide range of serum levels attained in this study is related to the varying time intervals between administration of the drug and collection of serum samples. It can be seen that the omission of an i.m. dose of cefuroxime with the premedication in the patients of group II made little apparent difference to subsequent serum or tissue levels.

In those patients who underwent arterial reconstruction, the cefuroxime level in subcutaneous fat was unexpectedly higher among those who received a single preoperative dose (Tables 1 and 2). When the corrected tissue levels are considered, low levels were found in 3 of 10 cases, one of these being a sample from the patient with the highest serum level of antibiotic. Uncorrected cefuroxime levels were adequate in every case, and there was no evidence of overt wound sepsis.

In those patients undergoing amputation, corrected cefuroxime concentrations in muscle and subcutaneous fat at the level of section were acceptable in all cases. Low levels of antibiotic were found in 2 of 10 distal fat samples and in 4 of 10 distal muscle samples (in 2 of these, corrected and uncorrected levels were almost identical, indicating almost total ischemia).

Levels of cefuroxime in wound exudates were satisfactory in most patients for prophylaxis against infection. In only one case (an amputation for particularly advanced gangrene) were inadequate concentrations of the drug found.

TABLE 1. *Cefuroxime levels in arterial reconstruction cases*

Time elapsed (min)		Cefuroxime levels		
i.m. to i.v. dose	i.v. dose to sampling	Serum (µg/ml)	Subcutaneous fat (µg/g)	Wound exudate (µg/ml)
82	48	65	15 (7.9)[a]	6.5
55	70	55	8 (7.2)	4.8
				7.2
95	45	87.5	13.3 (1.3)	9.6
				10.6
60	20	90	21.5 (16.5)	7
				5.9
100	35	210	5.3 (0.0)	5.3
				8.3
	45	52	17.5 (13.5)	
	50	72	14 (3.2)	9.8
				14.4
	45	74	14.2 (10.1)	4.5
				4.5
	30	88	19 (15.8)	7.4
				9.2
	45	74	20.8 (15.8)	26
				16
Mean 78.4	43.3	86.8	14.9 (9.1)	9.2
±SD 20.3	13.3	45.3	5.2 (6.2)	5.4

[a] Numbers in parentheses are tissue levels corrected for blood contamination.

TABLE 2. *Cefuroxime levels in amputation cases*

Time elapsed (min)		Cefuroxime levels					Drain Collection ($\mu g/ml$)
i.m. to i.v. dose	i.v. dose to sampling	Serum ($\mu g/ml$)	Muscle ($\mu g/g$)		Subcutaneous fat ($\mu g/g$)		
			Proximal	Distal	Proximal	Distal	
145	15	147.5	22.5	12.9	21.4	13.7	59
			(5.7)[a]	(6.1)	(18.9)	(13.1)	38
60	45	60	19.8	2.8	11.2	2.2	23
			(16)	(2.6)	(10.2)	(2.2)	27
100	20	140	28	22.5	26	39.5	
			(17.1)	(7.4)	(22.6)	(2.4)	
75	20	90	21.1	1.9	22.5	13	33
			(14.8)	(0)	(21.3)	(12.6)	9
60	20	92.5	31	33	14.6	11.2	
			(22.7)	(29.7)	(13.9)	(10.3)	
40	20	92.5	23	19.1	15.4	8	17.5
			(12.9)	(10.3)	(12.7)	(6.6)	15
							12.5
							12.2
95	18	80	20.3	14.4	18.1	17.8	
			(7.5)	(2.8)	(12.8)	(16.5)	
110	20	70	11.5	10.4	9.2	7.3	2.7
			(5.2)	(3.6)	(8.8)	(6.8)	3.2
112	12	215	59	45	31	12	12
			(53.8)	(15)	(30.2)	(11.2)	
160	10	287	22.5	19.5	16	9.4	8.4
			(14.5)	(11.5)	(15.2)	(8.9)	10.5
Mean	95.7	20.0	127.5	25.9	18.2	18.5	13.4	18.9
±SD				±12.7	±13.2	±6.7	±10.1	
	±38.2	±9.5	±7.27	(17.0)	(8.9)	(16.7)	(9.1)	±15.1
				(±14.0)	(±8.6)	(±6.6)	(±4.6)	

[a] Numbers in parentheses are tissue levels corrected for hemoglobin level.

Cefuroxime levels were much higher in the wound exudates from amputation stumps (mean, 18.9 $\mu g/ml$), where muscle had been cut, than in the reconstruction cases (mean 8.2 $\mu g/ml$), where the wound was predominantly in fatty and connective tissue.

We conclude that cefuroxime sodium administered as described provides a useful broad-spectrum antibacterial prophylaxis in vascular surgery even when the tissues are rendered ischemic by occlusive arterial disease. Cefuroxime levels attained in the distal critically ischemic tissues of amputated limbs indicate that the cephalosporin may also be a useful antibiotic for the treatment of soft-tissue infections in ischemic legs.

Anti-*Pseudomonas* Activity in Bronchial Secretions of Patients Receiving Amikacin or Tobramycin as a Continuous Intravenous Infusion

G. MOMBELLI,* L. COPPENS, J. P. THYS, AND J. KLASTERSKY

Department of Medicine, Institut Jules Bordet, Brussels, Belgium

The clinical results of the treatment of *Pseudomonas aeruginosa* pneumonia with systemic aminoglycosides are disappointing (5). Aminoglycoside antibiotics have a low therapeutic-to-toxic ratio, and one of the factors which limit the clinical efficacy of these drugs may be the difficulty to achieve an adequate drug concentration within intrapulmonary sites of infection.

It has been suggested that the antimicrobial drug concentration in bronchial secretions may be a significant determinant of the ultimate outcome in the treatment of tracheobronchial infections (3, 4). Therefore, we measured, in two groups of tracheostomized patients with tracheobronchial infection, the penetration of amikacin and tobramycin, given as continuous infusions, into bronchial secretions, and the bactericidal activities of these drugs in serum and bronchial secretions against 10 strains of *P. aeruginosa*. Continuous infusions of aminoglycosides have been advocated to improve their efficacy (2). Besides, continuous infusions assure a constant blood level and make measurements of the gradient across the blood-bronchus barrier more reliable.

The 13 patients observed had a tracheostomy or an endotracheal tube; all had a tracheobronchial infection and purulent bronchial secretions. The absence of spontaneous antibacterial activity in bronchial secretions was controlled before each experiment. The patients received a loading dose (amikacin, 4 mg/kg; tobramycin, 1 mg/kg) followed by a continuous infusion (ami-

kacin, 7 to 12 mg/kg per 8 h; tobramycin, 2 to 3.5 mg/kg per 8 h). Two samples of serum were obtained at a 2-h interval during the last 4 h of the continuous infusion. Bronchial secretions aspirated through the endotracheal or tracheostomy tube were collected during the same period.

The assay of antibiotics in serum and bronchial secretions was performed as described by Bennett et al. (1). Bronchial secretions were centrifuged, and the bioassay was performed in the supernatant, using a supernatant of pooled bronchial secretions for the standard curve. The percent penetration was defined as: (concentration in bronchial secretions/mean serum concentration) × 100. The inhibitory and bactericidal activities in serum and supernatant of bronchial secretions were measured against 10 strains of *P. aeruginosa* (MIC for amikacin, 1.5 to 6 μg/ml [Table 1]; MIC for tobramycin, 0.03 to 0.7 μg/ml [Table 2]).

The mean serum level ranged between 8.3 and 17.5 μg/ml for amikacin and 2.35 and 5.6 μg/ml

TABLE 1. *Antibiotic concentration and anti-Pseudomonas activity in serum and bronchial secretions under a continuous infusion of amikacin*

Patient no.	Serum (S) single values at 2-h interval	Amikacin levels (μg/ml)		Ratio BS/S (%)	Bactericidal activity against *P. aeruginosa* (median)	
		Mean	Bronchial secretions (BS)		Serum	Bronchial secretions
1	8.2, 8.4	8.3	1.3	15.7	1:4	>1:2
2	14.0, 13.0	13.5	1.3	9.6	1:8	>1:2
3	14.0, 14.0	14.0	1.5	10.7	1:8	1:2
4	10.5, 8.8	9.65	1.4	14.5	1:8	>1:2
5	13, 15	14	2.3	16.4	1:4	1:2
6	18, 15	17.5	4.0	22.8	1:16	1:8
Mean^a		12.8 ± 3.3	2.0 ± 1.0	14.9 ± 4.7		

^{a} ± 1 standard deviation.

TABLE 2. *Antibiotic concentration and anti-Pseudomonas activity in serum and bronchial secretions under a continuous infusion of tobramycin*

Patient no.	Serum (S) single values at 2-h interval	Tobramycin levels (μg/ml)		Ratio BS/S (%)	Bactericidal activity against *P. aeruginosa* (median)	
		Mean	Bronchial secretions (BS)		Serum	Bronchial secretions
1	3.9, 3.4	3.65	0.46	12.6	1:4	>1:2
2	2.5, 4.5	3.5	0.43	12.3	1:8	>1:2
3	3.4, 3.1	3.25	0.56	17.2	1:4	1:2
4	3.4, 3.5	3.45	0.98	28.4	1:8	1:2
5	5.2, 6.0	5.6	2.2	39.3	1:8	1:4
6	2.9, 3.8	3.35	0.1	3	1:4	>1:2
7	2.8, 1.9	2.35	0.23	9.8	1:4	>1:2
Mean^a		3.6 ± 1.0	0.71 ± 0.7	17.5 ± 12.3		

^{a} ± 1 standard deviation.

for tobramycin. The constancy of the serum levels of the drugs is shown by the little variation between samples taken at a 2-h interval. The concentration in bronchial secretions ranged between 1.3 and 4 µg/ml for amikacin and 0.1 and 2.2 µg/ml for tobramycin. There was a rough correlation between levels in serum and in bronchial secretions ($r = 0.772$, $P > 0.05$ for amikacin; $r = 0.894$, $P < 0.01$ for tobramycin). The percent penetration was 14.9 ± 4.7 for amikacin and 17.5 ± 12.3 for tobramycin. This difference is statistically not significant.

Only concentrations superior to 1.5 µg/ml for amikacin and 0.5 µg/ml for tobramycin led to a significant anti-*Pseudomonas* activity in bronchial secretions (median bactericidal activity, ≤1:2). The corresponding serum levels were ≥14 µg/ml for amikacin and ≥3.25 µg/ml for tobramycin. A sustained anti-*Pseudomonas* activity (median bactericidal activity, ≤1:4) was achievable only with very high serum levels (17 µg/ml for amikacin and 5.6 µg/ml for tobramycin). At the given doses there were no significant differences in the bactericidal activity in serum or bronchial secretions achieved with the two drugs.

The rational goal of treatment of a pulmonary infection is to achieve an adequate antimicrobial activity within the intrapulmonary site of infection with minimal toxicity. In bronchopulmonary infections in patients with chronically damaged bronchial tree, antibiotic concentration in bronchial secretions may be a significant determinant of the ultimate outcome of the therapy (3, 4).

There was some correlation between serum and sputum concentration of amikacin and tobramycin, but the percent penetration varied widely from patient to patient. The sputum/ serum ratios of 14.9% for amikacin and 17.5% for tobramycin are somewhat lower than those found by other authors for aminoglycosides (3). However, other studies used intramuscular injections or rapid intravenous administration rather than continuous infusion. Under these conditions, changing serum levels and the accumulation of antibiotic within the bronchial secretions may prevent the measurement of the real percent penetration.

The negative concentration gradient across the blood-bronchus barrier emphasizes the known low therapeutic-to-toxic ratio of aminoglycosides. Several studies have shown how difficult it is to achieve and maintain aminoglycoside concentration in sputum adequate to inhibit *P. aeruginosa*. With a continuous infusion, high serum levels are necessary to maintain a significant activity, and very high levels are required to achieve a sustained anti-*Pseudomonas* activity in bronchial secretions. These results may partly explain the difficulties encountered in the treatment of *P. aeruginosa* bronchopneumonia with classical doses of aminoglycosides.

1. Bennett, J. V., J. L. Brodie, E. J. Brenner, and W. M. M. Kirby. 1966. Simplified, accurate method for antibiotic assay of clinical specimens. Appl. Microbiol. 14: 170–177.
2. Feld, R., M. Valdivieso, G. P. Bodey, and V. Rodriguez. 1977. A comparative trial of sisomicin therapy by intermittent versus continuous infusion. Am. J. Med. Sci. 274:179–188.
3. Lambert, H. P. 1978. Clinical significance of tissue penetration of antibiotics in the respiratory tract. Scand. J. Infect. Dis. Suppl. 14:262–266.
4. May, J. R., and D. M. Devels. 1965. Treatment of chronic bronchitis with ampicillin. Some pharmacological observations. Lancet i:929–933.
5. Stevens, R. M., D. Teres, J. J. Skillman, and D. S. Feingold. 1974. Pneumonia in an intensive care unit: a 30 month experience. Arch. Intern. Med. 134:106–111.

Tropism of Erythromycin for the Respiratory System

F. FRASCHINI,* P. C. BRAGA, V. COPPONI, G. GATTEI, E. GUERRASIO, F. SCAGLIONE, F. VILLA, AND G. SCARPAZZA

Institute of Chemotherapy, University of Milan, Milan, and *INRCA Hospital Casatenovo, Brianza, Italy*

Erythromycin, considered a bacteriostatic antibiotic, performs a bactericidal action in the bronchial lumen (1, 4). This means that erythromycin has a particular tropism for the respiratory apparatus, where it can reach such concentrations as to promote destruction of bacteria rather than bacteriostasis (2, 3, 5, 7).

To verify this hypothesis, we measured the levels of erythromycin in the pulmonary tissue and bronchial secretion in humans. Erythromycin was also measured in the serum and sputum. Our research was carried out by using amoxicillin as a comparison antibiotic. This latter drug was chosen for its being most frequently used in the therapy of respiratory infections and because it is, among semisynthetic penicillins, the one that is most reabsorbed by the gastroenteric mucosa.

This study was carried out on 27 volunteer patients who had to undergo a surgical operation for lung cancer. Two days before the operation, 14 patients were treated with erythromycin and 13 were treated with amoxicillin per os, at a dose of 1.5 g/day, in three administrations at 8-h intervals. The antibiotics were administered at 8:00 a.m., 4:00 p.m., and midnight. A further administration of 0.5 g was given at 8:00 a.m. on the day of surgical operation, which was carried out at 11:00 a.m.

During day 2 of treatment, at 10:00, noon, 4:00 p.m., and midnight, and again at 8:00 a.m. on the day of operation, blood and sputum samples were taken to determine the levels of relevant antibiotic. Before this determination, sputum was carefully homogenized by means of sonication. During surgical operation the removed anatomical piece was washed out via blood vessels with a physiological solution and heparin to get rid of remaining blood. Then, aspiration of secretions present in the lumen of bronchi of second and third order was performed by means of a Pasteur pipette connected with an aspirator. The secretion was first homogenized by sonication, and then the amount of antibiotic present was determined.

Part of the pulmonary tissue not invaded by cancer was removed from the anatomical piece. The pulmonary tissue was carefully homogenized to screen the levels of antibiotic. Microbiological assay for antibiotics was carried out using the agar well diffusion technique with *Sarcina lutea* ATCC 9341 in Mueller-Hinton medium.

Erythromycin reached mean serum levels of 3.08 and 1.30 μg/ml after 2 and 4 h, respectively, of administration (Fig. 1). Amoxicillin reached, at the same times, 6.69 and 2.76 μg/ml, respectively, which is twice as high as erythromycin. At h 8 of administration, amoxicillin barely reached the limits of sensitivity of our dosage method or was completely absent, whereas erythromycin was still present at a mean level little less than 1 μg/ml. Opposite results to those found in the serum at h 2 and 4 were obtained in other organic materials, i.e., pulmonary tissue, bronchial secretion, and sputum. Erythromycin levels in the pulmonary tissue 3 h after administration of 0.5 g of this drug, which followed 2 days of treatment with 1.5 g/day, reached a mean value of 4.71 μg/ml (Fig. 1 and 2). Amoxicillin in the same experimental conditions reached in the lung a mean value equal to 2.40 μg/ml (Fig. 1 and 2). At the same time, in the bronchial secretions, erythromycin reached a mean level of 2.81 μg/ml, whereas amoxicillin barely reached 0.48 μg/ml (Fig. 1 and 2). In the sputum, at various scheduled times, erythromycin exhibited mean values of 0.87 μg/ml after 2 h, 1.67 μg/ml after 4 h, and between 1.18 and 1.58 μg/ml at h 8 (Fig. 1 and 2). At the same times, in the sputum, amoxicillin exhibited values always inferior to those reached by erythromycin and equal to 0.21, 0.51, and 0.04 to 0.05 μg/ml, respectively (Fig. 1 and 2).

The high levels of erythromycin reached in the bronchial secretions and in the pulmonary tissue prove the experimental finding, i.e., that erythromycin performs a bactericidal action in the respiratory tree. In fact, only at the high levels that were found in the pulmonary tissue was erythromycin able to show bactericidal action on bacteria susceptible to it. At lower concentrations, the action of erythromycin is only bacteriostatic (6).

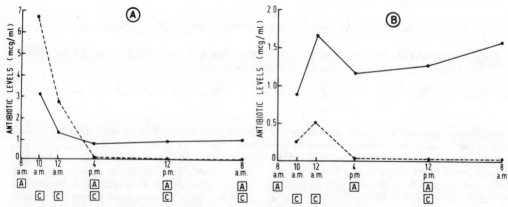

FIG. 1. *Serum (A) and sputum (B) levels of antibiotics in humans. Symbols: (—) erythromycin stearate; (---) amoxicillin; $\boxed{A}$, antibiotic administration (0.5 g/dose); $\boxed{C}$, serum collection.*

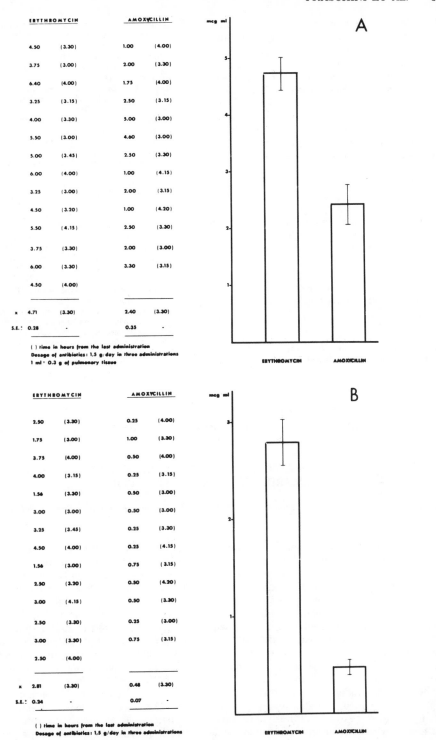

FIG. 2. *Levels of antibiotics (μg/ml) in human pulmonary tissue (A) and in human bronchial secretions (B).*

The study of the kinetic behavior of erythromycin reveals a particular tropism of this antibiotic for the pulmonary apparatus. In fact, the high levels of erythromycin in the lung, bronchial secretions, and sputum do not have correspondingly high levels in the serum. This behavior is completely opposite to that of amoxicillin, which was taken for comparison purposes in this research. In the same experimental conditions, in fact, amoxicillin will reach in the serum levels that are decisively higher than those of erythromycin, whereas in the lung, bronchial secretions, and sputum it will remain at levels much lower than those of erythromycin.

In conclusion, the respiratory apparatus will concentrate erythromycin in an active form, whereas it cannot do anything of the kind with amoxicillin. Last, but not least, the data of this research confirm what was already found concerning the respiratory apparatus, which is that the serum levels of antibiotic do not reflect those present in the pulmonary tissue, bronchial secretions, and sputum.

1. Balbirsingh, M., J. Dorn, A. S. Klainer, R. H. Liss, J. C. Norman, and E. E. Ward. 1978. Clinical, bacteriological and electron microscopic studies of erythromycin bactericidal activity in humans, p. 646–649. *In* W. Siegenthaler and R. Lüthy (ed.), Current chemotherapy, Proceedings of the 10th International Congress of Chemotherapy. American Society for Microbiology, Washington, D.C.
2. Cheng-Chun Lee, R. C. Anderson, and K. Chen. 1953. Tissue distribution of erythromycin in rats. Antibiot. Chemother. 3:920–924.
3. Dubini, F., P. Faraone, C. Guastamacchia, and F. Fraschini. 1976. Ricerca della eritromicina e della spiramicina nella saliva. Dental Cadmos 10:1–6.
4. Fraschini, F., R. Avallon, V. Copponi, G. Fumagalli, F. Mandler, F. Scaglione, and G. Scarpazza. 1979. Bactericidal action of an average dose of erythromycin in the bronchi. Curr. Med. Res. Opin. 6:107–113.
5. Fraschini, F., V. Copponi, F. Dubini, and G. Scarpazza. 1978. Concentration of erythromycin and ampicillin in bronchial secretions of patients with chronic respiratory infections, p. 650–652. *In* W. Siegenthaler and R. Lüthy (ed.), Current chemotherapy, Proceedings of the 10th International Congress of Chemotherapy. American Society for Microbiology, Washington, D.C.
6. Igarashi, K., H. Ishitsuka, and A. Kaji. 1969. Comparative studies on the mechanism of action of lincomycin, streptomycin and erythromycin. Biochem. Biophys. Res. Commun. 37:499–502.
7. Matsumoto, K., and Y. Uzuka. 1976. Concentrations of antibiotics in bronchiolar secretions of the patients with chronic respiratory infections. *In* J. D. Williams and A. M. Geddes (ed.), Chemotherapy, vol. 4. Plenum Press, New York.

Stability of Cephalothin, Cefamandole, Cefuroxime, and Cefoxitin in Acrylic Bone Cement: a Method to Evaluate "In Vivo" Antibiotic Stability

MERCEDES C. GARCÍA-IGLESIAS, CARLOS ITURRATE, JOSÉ M. BORRERO, RICARDO MENA, AND EVELIO J. PEREA*

Departments of Microbiology and Surgery, School of Medicine, University of Seville, Seville-9, Spain*

Our work describes an experimental model which tries to measure the stability of an antibiotic within acrylic bone cement, the diffusion of that antibiotic during the time after implantation, and the antibiotic concentrations in the tissue surrounding the cement cylinder.

We mixed 4 g each of cephalothin, cefamandole, cefuroxime, and cefoxitin with 40 g of acrylic bone cement (Palacos). Before the mixture could solidify, glass cylinders (average interior volume, 294.34 mm^3) were filled in a laminar-flow cabinet under sterile conditions. Once the mixture solidified, the glass cylinders were broken. The average weight of the cylinders was 0.3 g, and 15 cylinders were refrigerated in sterile petri dishes at 4°C; the rest were surgically implanted in the right rear legs of a group of 15 rats, parallel to the previously scraped femur.

Each day antibiotic diffusion was measured in one of the refrigerated cylinders and in one taken from a rat as well as in the surrounding tissue. The antibiotic diffusion from each cylinder placed vertically on an agar surface was determined by a microbiological diffusion method with *Bacillus subtilis* 1904E spore suspension for cefuroxime and *Staphylococcus aureus* ATCC 25923 for all other antibiotics (7).

The tissue was previously twice homogenized in a buffer (pH 6.4) in a Sorvall Omnimixer at rapid speed for 10 min. The homogenized tissue was then centrifuged. Filter paper disks (Schleicher & Schuell, 12.7 mm in diameter) were impregnated with the supernatant (4, 7).

Cephalothin. The diffusion of cephalothin from the refrigerated cylinders remained fairly constant, though a slight decrease occurred in the last 5 days. Figure 1 shows the line of closest fit representing the amounts of antibiotic released by the 15 implanted cylinders, which were extracted daily. The values ranged between 4.5 µg on the first 5 days and 0.6 µg on day 15. Figure 2 shows the tissue concentrations. The concentration was 300 µg/g of tissue on day 1, and a uniform descent was registered as time passed, only 1 µg/g remaining on the last day.

Cefamandole. The refrigerated cylinders registered no lowering of activity for cefamandole. The diffusion rate was much higher than was the case with cephalothin, which had a maximum value of 140 µg on day 1 and 49 µg on day 15, whereas the cefamandole cylinders diffused 620 µg on day 1 and 550 µg on day 15.

Diffusion from implanted cylinders ranged between 70 µg on day 1 and 0.56 on day 15 (Fig. 1). Tissue concentrations (Fig. 2) were 40 µg/g on day 1 and 0.21 µg/g on day 13. On days 14 and 15 no appreciable concentrations could be detected.

Cefoxitin. For cefoxitin the cylinders refrigerated at 4°C maintained constant diffusion values superior to the 1,000-µg maximum value that could be registered on the line. Rat-implanted cylinders registered a diffusion of 510 µg on day 1 and 0.14 µg on day 8, after which no appreciable concentrations were detected (Fig. 1). In the

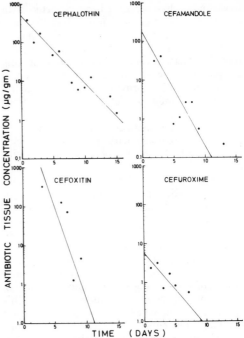

FIG. 2. *Antibiotic concentration in rat tissue surrounding cylinders.*

tissue, concentrations ranged between 332 µg/g on day 3 and 4.71 µg/g on day 9, after which no appreciable concentrations were detected (Fig. 2).

Cefuroxime. Diffusion of cefuroxime from cylinders kept at 4°C was reasonably constant, ranging from 80 µg at the beginning to 22 µg on day 13. Diffusion from implanted cylinders was stable up to day 7 and thereafter showed a decline (Fig. 1). Tissue concentrations were stably maintained during the week 1, after which they could not be detected (Fig. 2).

For an antibiotic to prevent infection after hip replacement, two characteristics are required: that it have a wide antibacterial spectrum and that its activity be maintained afterwards, to prevent colonization by microorganisms brought by the blood to the weakened tissues surrounding the implant area (3).

In practice it is very difficult to judge the role which an antibiotic mixed with cement might play, since infection levels are very low for the majority of the studies published (5). Some authors have tried to develop experimental models, but up now the experiments described have tried to reproduce in vitro the situation of cement in a patient. We have found that they did not achieve this, since the culture medium was changed, at the most, every 24 or 72 h (1–3). A

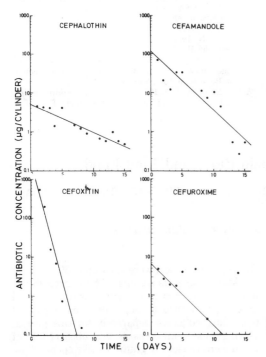

FIG. 1. *Antibiotic diffusion from rat-implanted cylinders.*

mouse model has recently been reported with subcutaneously implanted plugs, but the antibiotic levels were determined only in mouse blood (6). With our model we believe we have created a situation very similar to that occurring in a patient. The amount of cement placed in each rat was 0.3 g, providing a proportion per body weight similar to that ocurring in a patient with an implant.

For as yet unexplained reasons, more antibiotics were released with Palacos than with other cements (1), so we used this cement exclusively.

In experiments in vitro, Hill and colleagues (3) tried fusidic acid, clindamycin, and gentamicin. The first has a short diffusion period, whereas other two were active for 35 and 16 days, respectively. The spectra of the first two were narrow, and the gentamicin, although it had a broad spectrum, was not active against anaerobic bacteria. However, the cephalosporins, of known wide activity, encompassing S. aureus, one of the most frequent agents in this type of infection, have been evaluated either not at all or only superficially (2). Cefamandole, cefoxitin, and cefuroxime have the advantage of acting also upon anaerobic bacteria.

Of the four cephalosporins assayed, cephalothin and cefuroxime registered slight descents in activity in the refrigerated cylinders. In the case of rat-implanted cylinders, cefoxitin showed the greatest antibiotic diffusion and was also the first to disappear, not being detected after the day 10. Cefamandole had persistently high levels. Cefuroxime and cephalothin showed consistently low levels.

Concentrations in tissue surrounding the cement were equally high in cefoxitin and cephalothin, but cefoxitin dissapeared after day 10, whereas cephalothin could be detected as late as day 15. With cefamandole, concentrations were not so high, although they were maintained until day 13. Cefuroxime showed the lowest concentrations and disappeared on day 8.

Although it is essential during an operation to achieve bactericidal levels that can only be obtained through intravenous administration, the risk of periarticular infection carried by the blood could, theoretically, be eliminated by mixing antibiotics with cement, since this would supply prolonged activity, creating a barrier at the infection point. But a final evaluation of the role played by antibiotics in total hip replacement must wait for even more clinical and experimental studies. However, we do believe the method described could facilitate such evaluation.

1. Elson, R. A., A. E. Jephcott, D. B. McGechie, and D. Verettas. 1977. Antibiotic-loaded acrylic cement. J. Bone Joint Surg. 59-B:200-205.
2. Fischer, L. P., G. P. Gonon, J. P. Carret, Y. Vulliez, and G. de Mourgues. 1977. Association métacrylate de méthyle et antibiotiques. Rev. Chir. Orthop. 63:361-372.
3. Hill, J., L. Klenerman, S. Trustey, and R. Blowers. 1977. Diffusion of antibiotics from acrylic bone-cement in vitro. J. Bone Joint Surg. 59-B:197-199.
4. Kaplan, J. M., G. M. McCracken, Jr., and E. Snydeer. 1973. Influence of methodology upon apparent concentrations of antibiotics in tissue. Antimicrob. Agents Chemother. 3:143-146.
5. Moore, N. 1977. Antibiotics in cement. J. Bone Joint Surg. 59-B:129-142.
6. Picknell, B., L. Mizen, and R. Sutherland. 1977. Antibacterial activity of antibiotics in acrylic bone cement. J. Bone Joint Surg. 59-B:302-307.
7. Washington, J. A. 1974. Laboratory procedures in clinical microbiology, p. 309-327. Little, Brown & Co., Boston.

Cefuroxime Concentrations in Blood and Joint Fluid

ASSA LEV-EL,* JACOBO NERUBY, JACOB DUBNER, ALEXANDER KATZNELSON, AND ETHAN RUBINSTEIN

Chaim Sheba Medical Center, Tel-Aviv University, Tel-Hashomer, Israel

Cefuroxime is a new semisynthetic cephalosporin active against both gram-positive and gram-negative bacteria. Its antibacterial spectrum is wider than those of many first-generation cephalosporins (3). Its pharmacokinetics in humans has been previously described (1).

During 1955 through 1975, 104 cases of community-acquired bacterial arthritis were observed at the Chaim Sheba Medical Center.

Gram-positive cocci were isolated in 59 cases (in 46, *Staphylococcus aureus*). The overall distribution of the causative agents has not changed in the years 1975 through 1979, as suggested from data collected separately for this period. During these years 33 cases were observed; 21 of them were caused by gram-positive cocci (16 by *S. aureus*).

Postoperative musculoskeletal infections oc-

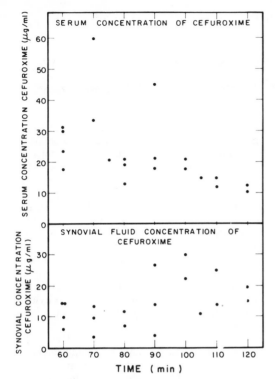

FIG. 1. *Cefuroxime concentration in serum and synovial fluid.*

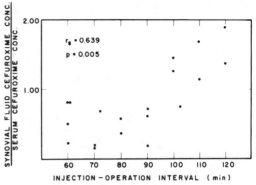

FIG. 2. *Cefuroxime synovial fluid concentration-serum concentration ratio related to the time interval between administration and collection of samples.*

curred in 225 patients (a rate of 7.5% postoperative infections); 37 (16.4%) were caused by *S. aureus. Pseudomonas aeruginosa* was responsible for 23.5% of infections, and 59.9% were due to other gram-negative bacteria. Cefuroxime was active in vitro against most isolates short of *P. aeruginosa.*

To evaluate cefuroxime penetration into joint fluid, 20 patients undergoing knee arthrotomy were given 750 mg of cefuroxime by intramuscular injection. One to two hours later, synovial fluid and serum samples were obtained for cefuroxime assay (during surgery). A tourniquet was applied to the involved limb and inflated ca. 10 min before joint fluid collection. Serum and joint fluid cefuroxime concentrations are shown in Fig. 1. Mean serum cefuroxime concentrations at 60, 90, and 120 min were 32.9, 24.7, and 12.2 μg/ml, respectively. Simultaneous joint fluid concentrations were 8.1, 19.5, and 18.3 μg/ml, respectively.

Joint fluid cefuroxime concentrations ranged from 3.8 to 30 μg/ml. The joint fluid-serum cefuroxime concentration ratio increased from 0.4 at 60 min to 1.51 at 120 min due to increasing joint fluid levels and decreasing serum cefuroxime levels (Fig. 2). This trend was statistically significant ($P \leq 0.005$).

No infections occurred after the operations. No adverse effects were observed. Hematological biochemical and urinary analyses did not disclose any abnormality related to cefuroxime except for slight increases in serum bilirubin concentrations in four patients. These increases could not be directly related to cefuroxime administration.

Cefuroxine penetration into joint fluid compared favorably with those of cephalothin, cefazolin, and cephalexin as previously reported (2, 4).

We conclude that cefuroxime may be a valuable antibiotic agent in the prophylaxis and therapy of joint infections caused by susceptible microorganisms.

1. **Foord, R. D.** 1976. Cefuroxime: human pharmacokinetics. Antimicrob. Agents Chemother. **9**:741–747.
2. **Nelson, J. D., J. B. Howard, and S. Shelton.** 1978. Oral antibiotic therapy for skeletal infections of children. J. Pediatr. **92**:131–134.
3. **O'Callaghan, C. H., R. B. Sykes, A. Griffiths, and J. E. Thornton.** 1976. Cefuroxime, a new cephalosporin antibiotic: activity in vitro. Antimicrob. Agents Chemother. **9**:511–519.
4. **Schurman, D. J., P. Hirshman, G. Kajigama, K. Moser, and D. Burton.** 1978. Cefazolin concentrations in bone and synovial fluid. J. Bone Jt. Surg. **60**:359–362.

Penetration of Two New Cephalosporins, Cefuroxime and Cefotaxime, in Bone

B. PAPATHANASSIOU, J. KOSMIDIS,* C. STATHAKIS, K. MANTOPOULOS, AND G. K. DAIKOS

First Department of Propedeutic Medicine, Athens University School of Medicine, Athens, Greece

Concentration of antibiotics in bone is important both for the successful treatment of osteomyelitis and for prophylaxis from infection after orthopedic operations. Measurement of bone levels, however, presents many problems (5), as a result of which literature data may not be comparable unless the specific set of circumstances is reported. Apart from differences in types of patients and type and site of bone taken, presence of osteomyelitis with or without other bone disease, dosage, time and rapidity of administration of the antibiotic, etc., most important are differences in the technique used. Two approaches for measurement of bone level have been used. One is the extraction of the antibiotic by means of immersion of a fragment in buffer and agitation for several hours. Levels in the eluate are then measured. It is unknown, however, what proportion of the antibiotic is eluted and what remains bound onto the bone. The second approach is to pulverize the bone and suspend it in buffer and then measure the concentration in the suspension. An amount of the drug may, however, be destroyed in this manner. It has been suggested therefore that both techniques must be used and that the results of both must be reported (5).

Cephalosporin antibiotics have been used in prophylaxis against postoperative bone infection. Penetration into bone has been reported satisfactory for cephaloridine, cephalothin, cephradine, and cefazolin (for a review, see reference 5), but Smilack and colleagues (6) could not detect cephalothin in the bone of any of four patients receiving 2 g intravenously every 4 h, and in only one of four receiving cefazolin at 1 g intramuscularly every 8 h were antibiotic levels measurable in bone.

The tendency to increasing resistance rates of bacteria to various antibiotic groups has not left the cephalosporins unaffected. Newer cephalosporins with extended bacterial spectra have been developed, therefore, in order to overcome this phenomenon. Cefuroxime (4) and cefotaxime (3) are two new members of the group, which possess extended antibacterial spectra covering most species resistant to the older cephalosporins. These extended spectra are due to stability of these new compounds to the enzymatic action of β-lactamases from a wide range

of bacteria (2). This enzymatic degradation is most important for the development of bacterial resistance to the older cephalosporins. Both cefuroxime and cefotaxime have been successful in the treatment of infections due to bacteria resistant to the older cephalosporins (1; G. K. Daikos, J. Kosmidis, H. Giamarellou, B. Dranidis, and Ch. Stathakis, Program Abstr. Intersci. Conf. Antimicrob. Agents Chemother. 18th, Atlanta, Ga., abstr. no. 299, 1978).

We decided, therefore, to study the penetration of these two new cephalosporins into human bone in order to see whether they would be good candidates for administration for prophylaxis against postoperative bone infection or in osteomyelitis or both.

Thirteen patients (five males and eight females) were studied. They were aged from 60 to 80 years and were all suffering from hip fractures. No pathology other than degenerative disease was present in their bones. They had not been treated with antibiotics or other substances interfering with cephalosporin kinetics in the recent past, and their renal functions were normal. The antibiotics were administered intramuscularly for 1 or 3 full days before the operation in the following dosages: cefuroxime, 0.75 g or 1.5 g three times daily; cefotaxime, 1 g four times daily or 2 g three times daily. The last injections were planned so that they were administered at various times before operation. Two pieces of cancellous bone were removed, briefly washed with phosphate-buffered saline, pH 7.4, weighed, and then treated in two different ways. One piece was immersed in 1 ml of the above buffer and was agitated for 18 h at 4°C. The following day the concentration of the antibiotic in the buffer was measured and converted into bone concentration as micrograms per gram. The second piece was dried overnight at 4°C, using a vacuum pump, and then crushed with mortar and pestle into a pulp which was subsequently suspended in 1 ml of buffer. Assay of antibiotic was then performed in the suspension, and bone levels were calculated. A simultaneous specimen of blood was obtained with every bone specimen.

Assays were performed by using an agar cup plate technique. A strain of *Bacillus subtilis* was used as the indicator for cefuroxime assays,

TABLE 1. *Concentrations of cefuroxime in bone*

Dose (g)	Duration (days)	Time after last dose (h)	Bone (µg/g)		Serum (µg/ml)
			Eluate	Crushed	
0.75 × 3	1	2	<0.5	<0.5	14
0.75 × 3	3	2	3.9	5.2	18
1.5 × 3	1	2.5	10.5	12.9	19
1.5 × 3	3	2	13.5	12.4	21

TABLE 2. *Concentrations of cefotaxime in bone*

Dose (g)	Duration (days)	Time after last dose (h)	Bone (µg/g)		Serum (µg/ml)
			Eluate	Crushed	
1 × 4	1	2	1.5	1.5	18.2
1 × 4	1	4	<0.5	<0.5	7.2
1 × 4	3	2	1.8	1.6	19.6
1 × 4	3	4	<0.5	<0.5	8.0
1 × 4	3	6	<0.5	<0.5	3.1
2 × 3	1	2	10.7	6.4	34.2
2 × 3	1	2	12.6	15.4	39.0
2 × 3	1	2	7.1	4.5	29.3
2 × 3	1	4	3.3	5.4	15.6

whereas a very susceptible *Escherichia coli* strain was used for cefotaxime measurements. Standards for the bone assays were diluted in buffer.

The results obtained are shown in Tables 1 and 2. Values obtained with the two methods used were generally similar. A dosage of 0.75 g of cefuroxime three times daily did not produce measurable levels after 24 h of treatment, but after 3 days concentrations were 4 to 5 µg/ml. A dosage of 1.5 g three times daily gave very high

bone levels, even within 24 h. Cefotaxime gave lower bone levels. A dosage of 1 g four times daily did not produce levels exceeding 1.8 µg/ml, but 2 g three times daily gave satisfactory levels after 24 h of treatment. Serum levels were always as expected. These results indicate that both antibiotics penetrate well into bone if given in sufficient dosage. The lower levels of cefotaxime may be counterbalanced by a much better in vitro activity against most pathogens. Cefuroxime and cefotaxime may be used for the treatment of osteomyelitis and prophylaxis against postoperative bone infection. A dose of at least 1.5 g three times daily of cefuroxime or 2 g three times daily of cefotaxime must be used. These antibiotics may have to be substituted for the older cephalosporins, especially in localities with high cephalosporin resistance rates.

1. Daikos, G. K., J. Kosmidis, C. Stathakis, and H. Giamarellou. 1977. Cefuroxime: antimicrobial activity, human pharmacokinetics and therapeutic efficacy. J. Antimicrob. Chemother. 3:555–562.
2. Fu, K. P., and H. C. Neu. 1978. Beta-lactamase stability of HR 756, a novel cephalosporin, compared to that of cefuroxime and cefoxitin. Antimicrob. Agents Chemother. 14:322–326.
3. Hamilton-Miller, J. M. T., W. Brumfitt, and A. V. Reynolds. 1978. Cefotaxime (HR 756) a new cephalosporin with exceptional broad-spectrum activity in vitro. J. Antimicrob. Chemother. 4:437–444.
4. O'Callaghan, C. H., R. B. Sykes, D. M. Ryan, R. D. Foord, and P. W. Muggleton. 1976. Cefuroxime—a new cephalosporin antibiotic. J. Antibiot. 29:29–37.
5. Parsons, R. L. 1976. Antibiotics in bone. J. Antimicrob. Chemother. 2:228–231.
6. Smilack, J. D., W. H. Flittie, and T. W. Williams, Jr. 1976. Bone concentrations of antimicrobial agents after parenteral administration. Antimicrob. Agents Chemother. 9:169–171.

Cefadroxil and Cephalexin Concentrations in Prostatic Tissue: Comparison of Tissues Obtained by Transurethral Resection and Transvesical Prostatectomy

TORBEN B. KJAER,* THIERRY HALLYNCK, JANE HESS, AND PETER AGGER

KAS Herlev, University of Copenhagen, and Ringsted Hospital, Denmark, and University of Ghent, Ghent, Belgium*

The prostate is a site of both acute and chronic infections and can be the cause of recurrent urinary infections (3).

It is necessary to achieve sufficiently high concentrations of antibiotic at the site of an infection in order to eliminate its cause. Antibiotic concentrations are different in different

tissues, and the distribution is dependent on the pharmacokinetics of each compound (2, 4). Cefadroxil is a new semisynthetic cefalosporin with a wide antibacterial spectrum. Its activity against gram-positive and gram-negative bacteria is very similar to that of cephalexin (1).

In this study we have tried to see if there is

any difference between the uptakes of these two antibiotics in the prostatic tissue. We have also tried to show that suitable samples for antibiotic analysis can be obtained by transurethral removal of tissue.

Eighteen patients suffering from benign hyperplasia of the prostate gave their written consent to this study. The patients were given 1,000 mg of antibiotics orally at least 2 h before start of anesthesia. Transurethral prostatectomies were carried out in 12 patients, and 6 of these were given cephalexin and the other 6 were given cefadroxil. Transvesical prostatectomies were performed on the remaining six patients, and all six were given cefadroxil. Blood samples were taken immediately before the patients were given the antibiotics and then at roughly hourly intervals up to 1 to 2 h after the removal of the tissue samples. All the samples were stored at 0°C and were then deep frozen to < −20°C as soon as possible after the operation. The samples were kept deep frozen until the analyses were carried out a few weeks later.

Serum was used undiluted. Tissue samples were crushed in a mortar with a pestle and sterile sand and diluted with phosphate buffer at least 20 times.

Microbiological assays of antibiotics in serum and in tissue were done with an agar diffusion method, using *Bacillus subtilis* ATCC 6633 for serum and *Sarcina lutea* ATCC 9843 for tissues as test strains. Serum samples containing high concentrations of cefadroxil were also measured with *Staphylococcus aureus* ATCC 6538 to further validate the assay results.

Tissue samples were obtained during transurethral resection. A part of the mucosa and a little of the prostate tissue was removed by using a cutting electrode while flushing with irrigating fluid continuously. The exposed prostatic tissue had not been in contact with urine, but only with irrigating fluid. Prostatic tissue was removed, taking care that it did not come into contact with either the bladder mucous membrane or urine. In this way we removed roughly 1 g of tissue from each patient for analysis. When we operated transvesically we enucleated the whole gland and cleaned it with a towel. The gland was cut open with a clean knife, and roughly 1 g of tissue was cut out from the middle of the section.

The results of these analyses show that the serum concentrations of cefadroxil (average, 19.84 µg/ml; range, 13.82 to 31.82 µg/ml) were roughly 50% higher than cephalexin concentrations (average, 13.85 µg/ml; range, 7.85 to 18.98 µg/ml) after a dose of 1,000 mg of either antibiotic at roughly the time when the tissue samples were taken. The higher serum concentration

was reflected in higher prostate concentration. Cefadroxil concentrations in the tissue (average, 13.2 µg/ml; range, 5.67 to 15.35 µg/ml) were again 50% higher than cephalexin concentrations (average, 9.03 µg/ml; range, 3.43 to 9.45 µg/ml). The ratio tissue concentration divided by serum concentration was the same for either antibiotic (Table 1). The tissue concentration in either case was roughly half the serum concentration.

Table 1 also shows the relationship between serum and tissue concentrations in the two groups operated either transurethrally or transvesically.

The difference in Table 1 between the ratios in the two cefadroxil-treated groups is around 10%. This observed difference could be real, but is statistically insignificant, given the variations in these small groups. It is possible that small losses of antibiotics can occur when samples are taken transurethrally.

However, the losses from the chips are comparatively small, since even washing the tissue sample for 10 min in irrigating fluid produces only a linear fall in antibiotic concentration, around 30%. In the transurethral procedure the prostatic tissue is only exposed to irrigating fluid for roughly 10 s.

These results show that concentrations in prostatic tissue are approximately half the concentrations in serum for both these antibiotics. This means that since we know the relationship between serum and tissue concentrations, we can, by measuring serum concentrations, adjust

TABLE 1. *Concentrations of cefadroxil and cephalexin in prostatic tissue*

Operation (drug)	Pa-tient	Tissue concn/serum concn (µg/ml)	
		Individual	Mean ± SE
Transurethral resection (cefadroxil)	A	0.46	
	B	0.83	
	C	0.62	0.55 ± 0.07
	D	0.60	
	E	0.30	
	F	0.46	
Transurethral resection (cephalexin)	G	1.08	
	H	0.44	
	I	0.47	0.54 ± 0.11
	J	0.41	
	K	0.43	
	L	0.43	
Prostatectomy (cefadroxil)	M	0.35	
	N	0.43	
	O	0.47	0.59 ± 0.09
	P	0.87	
	Q	0.62	
	R	0.82	

dosages of these antibiotics to ensure that tissue concentrations will be adequate.

Equally important, we have been able to demonstrate that transurethral removal of prostatic tissue is a suitable technique for collecting prostatic tissue samples for antibiotic analysis, when care is taken to ensure that we neither lose antibiotic from the samples nor contaminate them in any way.

1. **Buck, R. E., and K. E. Price.** 1977. Cefadroxil, a new broad-spectrum cephalosporin. Antimicrob. Agents Chemother. **11**:324–330.
2. **Madsen, P. O., T. B. Kjaer, A. Baumueller, and H.-E. Mellin.** 1976. Antimicrobial agents in prostatic fluid and tissue. Infection **4**:(Suppl. 2):154–158.
3. **Meares, E. M., and T. A. Stamey.** 1968. Bacteriologic localisation patterns in bacterial prostatitis and urethritis. Invest. Urol. **5**:492–518.
4. **Stamey, T. A.** 1972. Urinary infection, p. 191–199. The Williams & Wilkins Co., Baltimore.

Alterations in the Protein Binding of Antibiotics During Cardiopulmonary Bypass

FRANK P. POLYAK, BYUNGSE SUH, AND WILLIAM A. CRAIG*

Department of Medicine, William S. Middleton Memorial Veterans Hospital,* and the University of Wisconsin Center for Health Sciences, Madison, Wisconsin 53705, U.S.A.

The binding of antimicrobial agents to serum proteins influences their biological activity and pharmacokinetic behavior (1). In general, high degrees of protein binding restrict drugs to the intravascular space and limit the amount of free, active drug that can reach sites of infection or contamination. Most data on protein binding are obtained from normal subjects. However, these values may not apply in many clinical situations since various drugs and endogenous substances, such as free fatty acids (FFA), can alter the binding of antimicrobials (2).

Patients undergoing cardiopulmonary bypass (CPB) provide an excellent opportunity to study the effects of FFA on the protein binding of antimicrobials. These patients receive short courses of heparin during the bypass procedure, and heparin is well known to increase FFA by activation of lipoprotein lipase (4). This report examines the alterations in serum protein binding of four antibiotics during cardiopulmonary bypass.

After receiving informed consent, sera were obtained from 18 patients undergoing CPB procedures. Samples were obtained on the day before surgery, after induction of anesthesia, 5 min after heparin administration, 15 min and then hourly during CPB, 30 min after the termination of CPB, and the day after surgery. The protein binding of dicloxacillin, penicillin, cefamandole, and cephalothin was measured by equilibrium dialysis. Tracer amounts of the radiolabeled drugs were added to standard solutions of unlabeled antibiotic to facilitate determination of drug concentrations in serum and buffer compartments. Albumin concentrations and FFA levels were also determined for each serum specimen. Molar ratios of FFA to albumin (FFA/ALB) were then calculated for each specimen using a molecular weight of 69,000 for albumin.

The mean values observed for serum albumin, FFA, FFA/ALB, and protein binding of the four antibiotics before, during, and after CPB are shown in Table 1. Mean FFA and FFA/ALB values were higher after induction of anesthesia than on the day prior to surgery. The most marked elevations were observed immediately after the administration of heparin. Pump perfusion resulted in significant hemodilution as reflected by a 30% fall in the serum albumin concentration. FFA levels also fell during CPB. The net effect, however, was that FFA/ALB remained elevated throughout CPB. After termination of CPB, all three parameters returned towards baseline values.

The elevation in FFA/ALB observed during CPB was associated with a significant decrease in the protein binding of dicloxacillin and cefamandole. The reduction in dicloxacillin binding from 96% to the 73 to 84% range represents a four- to sevenfold increase in the fraction of free drug. Similarly, the decrease in binding of cefamandole from 78% to the 48 to 60% range reflects a doubling of the fraction of free drug.

In contrast, elevation in FFA/ALB following anesthesia and heparin administration increased the binding of penicillin. Binding values for this drug fell during CPB but were still higher than baseline values. On the other hand, the protein binding of cephalothin remained relatively constant throughout the period of observation.

In order to better correlate changes in binding with FFA/ALB values, binding ratios per mole of albumin were calculated for each antibiotic in the various patient sera (Table 2). This binding ratio corrects for differences in protein concen-

TABLE 1. *Changes in protein binding, serum albumin concentration, free fatty acid (FFA) level, and the molar ratio of FFA to albumin (FFA/HLB) in 18 patients during cardiopulmonary bypass procedures*

Determination	Day before surgery	Post-anesthesia induction	Post-heparin	During bypass			Post bypass	Day after surgery
				5 min	60 min	120 min		
Albumin (g/100 ml)	3.8[a]	3.5	3.4	2.1	2.3	2.4	2.7	3.0
FFA (mmol/liter)	0.4	1.2	3.1	1.6	1.6	1.7	0.7	0.5
FFA/ALB	0.7	2.4	6.3	5.2	4.8	4.8	1.7	1.1
% Protein bound								
Dicloxacillin	96.3	95.0	83.8	77.6	80.0	73.4	93.1	95.8
Cefamandole	78.3	69.8	51.3	48.1	54.5	60.0	69.0	71.1
Penicillin	53.2	66.7	75.0	61.3	62.4	61.3	57.3	51.0
Cephalothin	66.0	70.1	60.9	60.8	62.7	63.1	60.8	61.4

[a] Mean values.

TABLE 2. *Effect of the molar ratio of FFA to albumin on the binding ratio per mole of albumin for four antibiotics in sera from patients undergoing CPB procedures*

FFA/albumin (molar ratio)	Binding ratio/mole of albumin[a]			
	Dicloxacillin	Cefamandole	Benzylpenicillin	Cephalothin
0:1	57.3 ± 13.4	5.9 ± 0.6	2.0 ± 0.3	3.3 ± 0.8
1:2	48.6 ± 4.9	5.8 ± 1.1	3.2 ± 0.5[c]	4.4 ± 1.1[d]
2:3	35.3 ± 13.6[b]	6.4 ± 1.1	4.4 ± 1.2[c]	4.7 ± 0.8[b]
3:4	16.6 ± 6.1[c]	4.7 ± 0.6[c]	5.1 ± 0.8[c]	5.2 ± 0.9[c]
4:5	8.2 ± 2.3[c]	3.9 ± 1.0[c]	5.8 ± 1.1[c]	5.5 ± 1.0[c]
>5	8.1 ± 2.4[c]	2.6 ± 0.9[c]	6.3 ± 1.5[c]	3.9 ± 0.9

[a] Values are means ± standard deviation for 5 to 17 serum samples.
[b] Statistically different from 0 to 1 FFA/ALB value, $P < 0.01$.
[c] Statistically different from 0 to 1 FFA/ALB value, $P < 0.001$.
[d] Statistically different from 0 to 1 FFA/ALB value, $P < 0.05$.

tration and is defined as the fraction of bound drug divided by the fraction of free drug times the molar concentration of albumin (3). The reduction in the binding ratio seen with dicloxacillin became significant at FFA/ALB values greater than 2 and continued to decrease as the molar ratio increased. Cefamandole behaved similarly except that a significant reduction in binding was not observed until the FFA/ALB value exceeded 3. The binding ratio for penicillin progressively increased as the molar ratio rose. Significant changes occurred as the FFA/ALB exceeded 1. Cephalothin binding behaved simi-

larly until the FFA/ALB value exceeded 5. At these higher molar ratios, binding decreased toward baseline values.

These studies demonstrate that the binding of antimicrobials to serum proteins can be significantly altered during cardiopulmonary bypass procedures. The overall changes in binding are a net result of both the decrease in albumin concentration and the increase in FFA levels. For dicloxacillin and cefamandole, both factors decrease protein binding, resulting in a marked increase in the fraction of free drug. For penicillin and cephalothin the FFA-induced enhancement in protein binding is somewhat negated by the lowered albumin concentration, resulting in little mean change in the fraction of free drug during the bypass procedure. These changes in protein binding may affect the elimination, distribution, and tissue penetrance of prophylactic antibiotics during cardiopulmonary bypass procedures.

1. Craig, W. A., and P. G. Welling. 1977. Protein binding of antimicrobials: clinical pharmacokinetic and therapeutic implications. Clin. Pharmacokinet. 2:252–268.
2. Craig, W. A. 1976. The effect of disease states on serum protein binding of antimicrobials. Infection 4(Suppl.): S137–S141.
3. Nilsen, O. G., D. Fremstad, and S. Jacobsen. 1975. Increased binding of quanidine to serum albumin and lipoproteins in anuric rats. Eur. J. Pharmacol. 33:131–139.
4. Rutstein, D. D., W. P. Castelli, and R. J. Nickerson. 1969. Heparin and human lipid metabolism. Lancet i: 1003–1008.

Binding of Erythromycin Base to Human Plasma Proteins

J. PRANDOTA, J. P. TILLEMENT, P. D'ATHIS, H. CAMPOS, AND J. BARRÉ*

Departements de Pharmacologie et de Pharmacologie Clinique, Faculte de Medecine de Paris XII, Creteil, France

The binding of erythromycin base (EB) to human plasma (HP) proteins was measured by equilibrium dialysis using ^{14}C-labeled EB at approximately 0.68 μM concentration. Pooled HP contained 40 g of human serum albumin/liter and 0.9 g of α_1 acid glycoprotein (α_1AGP)/liter. EB was 64.5 ± 0.4% (mean ± SD) bound to HP. Investigations on isolated plasma proteins dissolved in Sorensen phosphate buffer were carried out using a therapeutic concentration of erythromycin at 0.68 μM. No binding was observed to high- and low-density lipoproteins and gamma globulins, while α_1AGP and human serum albumin bound, respectively, 54.5 ± 0.6% and 8.7 ± 1.6%. The sum of the binding percentages determined on isolated proteins fits with the measurement of EB to HP that is 64.5%.

Erythromycin was also used over a wide range of concentrations (0.68 to 660 μM) on isolated HSA and α_1AGP. For human serum albumin separately, EB binding followed a nonsaturable phenomenon, while for α_1AGP the binding followed a saturable phenomenon characterized by the presence of one single site with an association constant $K = 35,000$ M^{-1}. Those results are not surprising, since other basic drugs such as imipramine and propranolol are known to be bound to α_1AGP as described by Piafsky et al. (2) and Glasson et al. (1). They are also in accordance with Zinneman et al. (3), who reported that EB was bound to α_1 globulin.

Further investigations were carried out to determine the characteristics of EB-HP interactions. The influence of temperature was studied in a plasma pool (containing 0.9 g of α_1AGP/liter). It was observed that the unbound fraction of EB increased linearly with decreasing temperature. The binding percentage varies from 64.5% at 37°C to 25.1% at 4°C. Effect of pH and phosphate buffer molarity significantly affected the affinity of the drug to HP. At pH 6 and 5, the unbound fraction of EB increased about 36 and 48%, respectively, compared with that at pH

7.4. There was no influence of high pH on the drug-HP interaction. A 2.5- and 5-fold increase in phosphate buffer molarity caused an increase of unbound fraction of EB. With distilled water the affinity of the drug to HP increased significantly. So EB-HP interaction appeared to be hydrophobic in nature, which is not surprising since the drug is only 200 mg/100 ml soluble in water.

Some drug interactions between EB and other acidic drugs were also studied. Acetylsalicylic acid, furosemide, phenylbutazone, and warfarin exerted a weak but significant displacing effect on EB binding. Similarly, added concentrations of bilirubin varying from 25 to 75 mg/liter also decreased EB binding to HP. All those compounds are known to be bound to saturable sites of albumin, whereas EB is bound to nonsaturable sites on albumin; so the displacements observed can be assumed to be noncompetitive inhibitions.

In conclusion, there is strong evidence that plasma binding percentage of EB varies according to α_1AGP concentration. It means that, in case of a rise in α_1AGP resulting from an inflammatory syndrome observed in infectious states, EB binding will be greatly increased. It might be of some clinical importance since it is known that only the unbound drug is pharmacologically active.

1. **Glasson, S., R. Zini, P. d'Athis, and J. P. Tillement.** The distribution of bound propranolol between the different human serum proteins. Mol. Pharmacol., in press.

2. **Piafsky, K. M., and A. Borga.** 1977. Plasma protein binding of basic drugs. II. Importance of α_1-acid glycoprotein for interindividual variation. Clin. Pharmacol. Ther. **22**:545–549.

3. **Zinneman, H. H., W. H. Hall, L. Hong, and U. S. Seal.** 1963. Binding of erythromycin, novobiocin, chloramphenicol, chlortetracycline, and nitrofurantoin by serum proteins, p. 637–643. Antimicrob. Agents Chemother. 1962.

Effect of Furosemide on Protein Binding, Extravascular Diffusion, and Urinary Excretion of Cefazolin and Gentamicin in Rabbits

CLAUDE CARBON,* ALAIN CONTREPOIS, ANNE-MARIE VIGNERON, AND SUZANNE LAMOTTE-BARRILLON

Service de Médecine Interne, Hôpital Louis Mourier F 92701 Colombes Cédex, France

Furosemide (F) and antibiotics are commonly used concomitantly. Possible interferences between these drugs deserved further investigation. The purpose of our study was to describe the interactions of F with two antibiotics in common use: cefazolin (CFZ), a highly protein-bound cephalosporin, and gentamicin (G), a poorly protein-bound aminoglycoside. On a previously described animal model (2), we studied the extravascular distribution of these two antibiotics when given alone or in combination with F in rabbits. Single i.m. injections of CFZ (30 mg/kg) and G (1.5 mg/kg) alone or with various doses of F (0.5, 1, and 5 mg/kg) were made. Blood, and extravascular fluid obtained from subcutaneous tissue cages, were measured up to 12 h after the injection. In order to approach the possible mechanisms of interaction between the drugs, we investigated the effect of F on the urinary excretion of the antibiotics in vivo. CFZ or G and inulin were infused at a constant rate for 2 h preceding two control periods of 15-min duration each. Furosemide was then injected i.v. (3 mg/kg). Two experimental periods of 15-min duration each and then two periods of 30 min each followed the diuretic injection. Blood and urine samples for antibiotic, inulin, and sodium assays were collected at the end of each control and experimental clearance period. The fractional excretion of the antibiotic was calculated as the antibiotic/inulin clearance ratio, taking into account the free antibiotic serum concentration. The effect of F on the protein binding of CFZ and G was investigated in vitro by ultracentrifugation according to Peterson (4). Antibiotic concentrations were determined by diffusion in nutrient agar.

In the extravascular diffusion study, the CFZ blood levels were not modified by F i.m. injection. CFZ extravascular levels are reported in Fig. 1. CFZ appeared in tissue cage fluid earlier and at higher levels up to 4 h after F injection, without any dose effect of F. CFZ extravascular peak concentration occurred more rapidly when F was injected. Late tissue cage levels (8 and 12 h) were reduced, these effects depending on the dose of F. Late blood levels of G were reduced by F with a significant dose effect of the diuretic. G extravascular concentrations (Fig. 2) were sig-

nificantly reduced by F without any significant dose effect. G tissue cage peak levels occurred at the same time, whether G was given alone or combined with F.

F did not significantly modify the glomerular filtration rate in either study with CFZ or G. The fractional excretion of CFZ significantly increased during the first two experimental periods (7.68 ± 2.18 and 5.97 ± 0.70) when compared to the control period (4.08 ± 0.73). CFZ blood levels remained identical throughout the study. With G, the fractional excretion significantly increased during the first three experimental periods (1.50 ± 0.36, 1.10 ± 0.30, 1.05 ± 0.50; control period, 0.61 ± 0.05). In vitro, F decreased CFZ protein binding from 80 to 60%, while G protein binding remained minimal (0 to 4%).

Discussion. Our studies outlined two kinds of interactions between F and antibiotics. With CFZ, the major effect of F appeared to be a competitive reduction of serum protein binding.

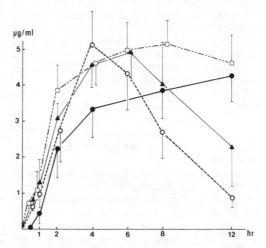

FIG. 1. *Cefazolin extravascular levels obtained after a single i.m. injection of cefazolin (30 mg/kg) alone or combined with three different doses of furosemide (0.5, 1, or 5 mg/kg). Values are means of five experiments and vertical bars represent ± SD. Symbols: ●, antibiotic alone; □, antibiotic + furosemide (0.5 mg/kg); ▲, antibiotic + furosemide (1 mg/kg); ○, antibiotic + furosemide (5 mg/kg).*

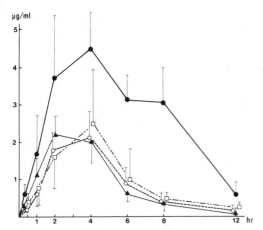

μg/ml

FIG. 2. *Gentamicin extravascular levels obtained after a single i.m. injection of gentamicin (1.5 mg/kg) alone or combined with three different doses of furosemide (0.5, 1, or 5 mg/kg). For symbols, see Fig. 1.*

This was demonstrated in vitro as stated. In vivo, the decrease in the extent of CFZ serum protein binding had two consequences on the kinetics of the antibiotic. The first appeared in the extravascular distribution study. We observed a more rapid diffusion of CFZ at higher levels after furosemide without any dose effect of the diuretic. Extravascular peak concentrations occurred earlier after CFZ + F than after CFZ alone. This F-induced change in the distribution of CFZ was in agreement with the results obtained by Anton and Rodriguez (1) and Kunin (3). The other consequence of the enhanced free CFZ serum level was an increase of the glomerular filtered load. After F i.v. injection, the fractional excretion of CFZ was augmented without any change of the glomerular filtration rate (GFR). Thus, in addition to the augmentation of the glomerular filtered load, a tubular process explained the enhanced urinary excretion of cefazolin. It was difficult to establish precisely the part of reduced reabsorption and the part of increased secretion in this process. F appeared to interfere with G excretion only.

The reduction of G extravascular levels after F, and the absence of modification of early tissue cage levels argued against the competition of F on a potential protein binding of G. Further, G was unbound in vitro. Increased renal excretion of G by F could not be accounted for by a glomerular process. However, we were not able to state precisely which tubular process was involved, i.e., decreased proximal reabsorption by a diuresis effect induced by F, or decreased non-ionic back diffusion in the distal part of the nephron. The tissue cage animal model used in this study allowed a good in vivo approach of antibiotic protein binding through the interference of a displacing agent.

1. **Anton, A. H., and R. E. Rodriguez.** 1973. Drug-induced change in the distribution of sulfonamides in the mother rat and its fetus. Science **180**:974–976.
2. **Carbon, C., A. Contrepois, N. Brion, and S. Lamotte-Barrillon.** 1977. Penetration of cefazolin, cephaloridin, and cefamandole into interstitial fluid in rabbits. Antimicrob. Agents. Chemother. **4**:594–598.
3. **Kunin, C. M.** 1965. Effect of serum binding on the distribution of penicillins in the rabbit. J. Lab. Clin. Med. **65**:406–431.
4. **Peterson, L. R., W. H. Hall, H. H. Zinneman, and D. N. Gerding.** 1977. Standardization of a preparative ultracentrifuge method for quantitative determination of protein binding of seven antibiotics. J. Infect. Dis. **136**:778–783.

Pharmacokinetic Interactions Between Cephalosporins and Furosemide Are Influenced by Administration Time Relationships

J. KOSMIDIS,* A. POLYZOS, AND G. K. DAIKOS

First Department of Propedeutic Medicine, Athens University School of Medicine, King Paul's Hospital, Athens 609, Greece

The recent advent of many new cephalosporins has caused new scientific interest in this group of antibiotics. Nephrotoxicity is the most important adverse reaction, and elucidation of its mechanism would obviously lead to prevention. Several mechanisms have been implicated, such as excessive dosage, especially in preexisting renal failure, shock and other circulatory disturbances, allergic reactions, simultaneous administration of aminoglycosides and other potentially nephrotoxic drugs, and simultaneous treatment with diuretics, especially furosemide (FUR) (1). Several hypotheses have been proposed to explain enhancement of cephalosporin nephrotoxicity by diuretics, among which pharmacokinetic interactions leading to delayed excretion and intracellular trapping of the cephalosporin in the renal tubules seem very plausible.

Potentiation of cephalosporin nephrotoxicity by diuretics seems to depend on administration time relationships, but the few existing reports on pharmacokinetic interactions between cephalosporins and diuretics in humans (2, 3) make no mention of administration time differences. Personal communication with various investigators confirmed the impression that such pharmacokinetic interactions were of unpredictable magnitude. We decided, therefore, to carry out a prospective study of the influence of administration time differences on the pharmacokinetic interactions between cephalosporins and diuretics.

Eighteen healthy volunteers, 13 males and 5 females aged 25 to 40 years and weighing from 65 to 85 kg, all with creatinine clearances >90 ml/min, participated in the study. Nine received cephaloridine (CRD) and nine received cephalothin (CFT). In each of the volunteers three kinetic profiles of the cephalosporin were performed, one without diuretic and two (on later days) after different times of FUR administration. On day 0 one dose of cephalosporin was given without diuretic and a full kinetic profile was conducted. For the next 3 days the volunteer was given a daily morning dose of FUR alone. On day 4 the diuretic was followed by a cephalosporin dose and a second profile was con-

ducted. On day 5 FUR was given alone again and on day 6 the third cephalosporin profile was done, at a different interval of time after the diuretic. The doses given were: CRD, 0.5 g intramuscularly; CFT, 1 g intravenously; and FUR, 40 mg orally. Six volunteers (group A) were studied with FUR given 1 and 3 h before CRD, three (group B) received FUR simultaneously and 2 h before CRD, six (group C) received FUR 2 and 4 h before CFT, and three (group D) were given FUR 1 and 3 h before CFT. In this manner the cephalosporin excretion was expected to occur either at the peak action of FUR or later, extending to periods after completion of diuretic action. Levels of antibiotics in serum and urine were measured using a well plate agar technique and a very susceptible strain of *Bacillus subtilis* as test organism.

A summary of the results is presented in Tables 1 and 2. When the diuretic was given simultaneously or 1 or 2 h before CRD, urinary recovery of the latter during the earlier urinary collections was moderately increased, but the total urinary recovery was not significantly affected and the serum levels showed only slight changes. No significant change in terminal serum half-life was noted. However, when administration of CRD was preceded by FUR by 3 h, a definite effect was noted: excretion of CRD

TABLE 1. *Mean kinetic parameters of CRD given with or without FUR*

Parameter[a]	Without FUR	With FUR given at indicated times (h) before CRD			
		0	1	2	3
Group A					
$T_{1/2}$	94		102 (+9%)[b]		159 (+69%)
8-h UR	84.7		83.4 (−2%)		69.4 (−18%)
Group B					
$T_{1/2}$	104	112 (+8%)		102 (−2%)	
8-h UR	77.3	84.1 (+9%)		82.4 (+7%)	

[a] $T_{1/2}$ = Serum terminal half-life in minutes. 8-h UR = 8-h urinary recovery (percentage of dose).
[b] Percentage of change.

TABLE 2. *Mean kinetic parameters of CFT given with or without FUR*

Parameter[a]	Without FUR	With FUR given at indicated times (h) before CFT:			
		1	2	3	4
Group C					
$T_{1/2\beta}$	43		36 (−16%)[b]		35 (−19%)
$T_{1/2\gamma}$	118		120 (+2%)		162 (+37%)
6-h UR	38.0		74.4 (+96%)		30.7 (−19%)
Group D					
$T_{1/2\beta}$	34	28 (−17%)		27 (−21%)	
$T_{1/2\gamma}$	122	116 (−5%)		128 (+5%)	
6-h UR	34.5	68.7 (+99%)		33.1 (−4%)	

[a] $T_{1/2\beta}$ = Half-life at β-phase (corresponding to CFT elimination) in minutes. $T_{1/2\gamma}$ = Half-life at γ-phase (corresponding to desacetyl-CFT elimination) in minutes. 6-h UR = 6-h urinary recovery of CFT-like activity (percentage of dose).
[b] Percentage of change.

was clearly delayed, with higher serum levels at all times, prolongation of mean terminal serum half-life by 69%, and reduction of mean 8-h urinary recovery by 18%.

The effect on CFT was entirely different. Administration of FUR 1 or 2 h before CFT increased the 6-h urinary recovery of the latter enormously, almost doubling the active amount recovered. On the contrary, when FUR was given 3 or 4 h before CFT it caused a reduction of 6-h urinary recovery by 4 or 19%, respectively. Effects on serum levels were minimal with the exception of the last part of the curve: from 3 to 6 h, where levels were elevated when FUR was given 4 h before CFT. Half-lives in the β-phase (corresponding mainly to CFT elimination) were slightly shortened on all occasions (from 16 to 21%). In the γ-phase, however, which corresponds to elimination of desacetyl-CFT, the effect on half-life was entirely different: whereas administration of FUR 1, 2, or 3 h before CFT had no significant effect, γ-phase half-life was increased by 37% when FUR was given 4 h before CFT.

Our results have clearly shown that pharmacokinetic interactions between cephalosporins and FUR depend on time relationships of drug administration.

These results may be explained as follows: the diuretic at the peak of its action, i.e., 2 h after its administration, increases excretion of CFT by the renal tubules and also slightly increases that of CRD, as a result of increased diuresis. This explains the enormous urinary recovery of CFT under these circumstances, since it was probably excreted before it had time to be metabolized into the less active desacetyl-CFT. The increase of early CRD recovery is also explained. The attempt to excrete a cephalosporin, however, after the diuretic action is completed, which is the case when FUR is administered 3 h before intramuscular CRD or 4 h before intravenous CFT, is met with difficulty. Tubular excretion of CRD and desacetyl-CFT is probably delayed. This may be accompanied by trapping of the cephalosporin inside the renal tubular cells. Since this trapping has been implicated for the nephrotoxicity of the cephalosporins, such a situation should clearly be avoided. Until the mechanism of potentiation of cephalosporin nephrotoxicity by diuretics is completely clarified, we would recommend avoiding administration of a diuretic 3 or 4 h before a cephalosporin.

1. **Foord, R. D.** 1975. Cephaloridine, cephalothin and the kidney. J. Antimicrob. Chemother. 1(Suppl.):119–133.
2. **Norrby, R., K. Stenqvist, and B. Elgefors.** 1976. Interaction between cephaloridine and furosemide in man. Scand. J. Infect. Dis. **8**:209–212.
3. **Trollfors, B., R. Norrby, and K. Kristianson.** 1978. Effects on renal function of treatment with cefoxitin sodium alone or in combination with furosemide. J. Antimicrob. Chemother. 4(Suppl. B):85–89.

Enhancement of Gastrointestinal Absorption of Gentamicin with Nonionic Surfactants

ARDON RUBINSTEIN,* ELKA TOUITOU, AND ETHAN RUBINSTEIN

Department of Medicine, Rokach Hospital, Tel-Aviv; Pharmacy Department, Hebrew University of Jerusalem, Jerusalem; and Infectious Diseases Unit, Chaim Sheba Medical Center, Tel-Hashomer, Israel

The clinical use of aminoglycosides is limited by the inability to administer these agents in a nonparenteral form. The minimal gastrointestinal absorption of aminoglycosides is due to the low lipid solubility of these substances and their existence in a solution in an ionic state. Nonionic surfactants have been previously reported to enhance the intestinal absorption of various substances (1–3). We therefore attempted to increase the intestinal absorption of gentamicin and amikacin in rats.

Rats were starved overnight, and combinations of gentamicin (GM), 12 or 10 mg, and cetomacrogal (CMG), 200 mg/animal, were administered via a gastric tube. Blood GM concentrations were assayed by the disk-diffusion method. Rats given GM or CMG orally, and animals injected with 10 mg of GM i.m. served as controls. Mean peak blood GM concentrations occurred at 30 min and were 25.4 μg/ml in the CMG-GM group; GM administered i.m. resulted in a mean blood peak concentration of 93 μg/ml; and oral GM alone resulted in a peak blood concentration of 1.2 μg/ml. Blood $T\frac{1}{2}$ of the GM-injected group was 43 min and of the group receiving the oral GM-CMG mixture it was 32 min (no significant difference). The area under the curve (AUC) for the GM concentration time curve (over 180 min) was 8,799 μg/ml·min for the i.m. group. For the group that received 12 mg of GM + 200 mg of CMG orally, the AUC was 2,730, for the group that received 10 mg of GM + 200 mg of CMG orally it was 1,965, and for the group that received oral GM it was 90 μg/ml·min. Over a 6-h period animals that received oral GM excreted 2% of the administered dose in the urine, animals that received the CMG-GM mixture excreted 3.7% of the administered dose.

A further experiment evaluating the oral versus rectal absorption of GM was performed. Animals received a semisolid enema containing 10 mg of GM, 1,000 mg of CMG, and 140 mg of polyethylene glycol 400. The oral administration resulted in mean peak blood concentrations of 25.4 μg/ml, whereas the rectal formulation resulted in peak blood levels of 7.2 μg/ml. GM alone administered rectally resulted in nondetectable blood levels. In a further experiment, 10 mg of GM was administered with decreasing dosages of CMG at 200, 100, 50, 25, and 10 mg orally, resulting in peak GM blood levels of 25, 5.8, 4.8, 3, and 1.5 μg/ml, respectively, at later times. Similarly, the gentamicin blood AUC decreased lineary ($r = 0.965$) with decreasing CMG dosages.

In a further experiment, 200 mg of CMG was administered orally 30 min prior to oral administration of 12 mg of GM. Mean blood peak GM levels occurred later (at 60 min) and were lower (mean 8 μg/ml) compared to GM blood levels when both agents were administered simultaneously. In a further experiment, other nonionic surfactants were tested for their ability to increase the intestinal absorption of GM. It was found that Texofore 45, CMG, Brig 35, Brig 30, and Myrj 32 induced high and comparable GM blood levels, while Tween 20 was not efficacious.

Our results suggest that nonionic surfactants may increase the gastrointestinal absorption of otherwise only minimally absorbable agents. The mode of action of the surfactants is unknown, but increased permeability of the intestinal mucosa seems possible. In rats most of the nonionic surfactants are nontoxic, the LD_{50} of CMG is in the range of 5 to 50 g/kg. The enhanced absorption of GM by CMG can be demonstrated in mice, guinea pigs, and rabbits as well.

We conclude: (i) Several nonionic surfactants may increase the gastrointestinal absorption of GM. This is neither specific for GM nor for the species investigated. (ii) The per-oral route of administration results in higher GM blood levels than the per-rectal route. (iii) The gastrointestinal absorption of GM was found to be directly related to the amount of CMG present in the formulation (in the range of 10 to 200 mg of CMG).

1. **Enge, R. H., and S. J. Riggi.** 1969. Intestinal absorption of heparin facilitated by sulfated or unsulfated surfactants. J. Pharm. Sci. **58**:706–710.
2. **Gibadi, M., and S. Feldman.** 1970. Mechanisms of surfactant effects on drug absorption. J. Pharm. Sci. **59**:579–589.
3. **Kreutler, C. J. and W. W. Davis.** 1971. Normal and promoted G.I. absorption of water soluble substances. J. Pharm. Sci. **60**:1835–1838.

Shortcomings in Pharmacokinetic Analysis of Intravenously Administered Amoxicillin

AXEL DALHOFF[1]* AND PETER KOEPPE

Beecham-Wülfing, 4040 Neuss, and Freie Universität Berlin, 1000 Berlin 45, Germany

Pharmacokinetic studies of penicillins are normally conducted by using an open, two-compartment, linear model. Adopting this model, it has been shown that penicillins are eliminated relatively rapidly. As penicillins are normally administered to patients repeatedly for several days or even weeks, it might be of interest and importance for therapy to determine if the penicillins are in fact excreted as rapidly as is normally assumed or if there might be a late, slow phase of disposition which might be essential to an adequate description of the distribution of the drug. Such disposition patterns would indicate a second peripheral compartment, and thus a three-compartment model would describe the distribution of the drug in the body more adequately than does a two-compartment model. The objective of the present study was to compare the pharmacokinetic characteristics of amoxicillin after intravenous administration by means of two- and three-compartment models.

Two-compartment model. For the two-compartment model, identical doses of 250, 500,

[1] Present address: c/o Johann A. Wülfing, Stresemannallee 6, 4040 Neuss, Germany.

and 1,000 mg were administered intravenously to seven healthy volunteers. Because of their different body weights there were discrepancies between the individual doses; therefore, we converted the individual doses to constant relative doses of 4, 8, and 16 mg/kg, respectively. Comparing the coefficients of variation for constant absolute doses and constant relative doses, respectively, it became obvious that the coefficient was lower in the constant-relative-dose group than in the other, and thus the error of the calculations was diminished.

According to the two-compartment model, linearity of concentration versus time curve occurred from 90 min onwards; the distribution constants corresponded to half-times of 8 to 11 min for the first phase of distribution, and for the second phase these values ranged from 59 to 63 min, without exhibiting a significant dose dependency. The second phase of distribution contributed 20 to 25% to the total distribution phase. Also, these values and those for the volumes of distribution were not significantly dose dependent (t test).

The distribution constants, volumes of distribution, and areas under the curves (AUCs) were calculated by using the parameters obtained with the constant relative doses only. There was no significant variation between these parameters and the AUC increases in strict relation to the doses administered (Table 1). Thus, no significant intrasubject or interdose variations occurred, so the individual parameters could be calculated on the basis of a dose of 10 mg/kg by using the constants of the overall average across all doses for total trial observations. The 95% confidence interval was, under these test conditions, ±6% only. The corresponding plot is shown in Fig. 1.

Three-compartment model. The two-compartment model did not represent the best fit of the slopes to the mean values, as the curves declined linearly from 90 min onwards but the mean values deviated from this straight line, indicating a more rapid distribution in the sec-

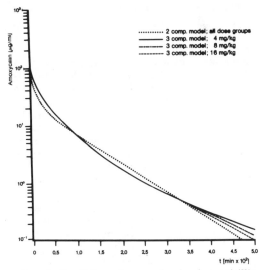

FIG. 1. *Prediction of serum levels of amoxicillin (single intravenous dose of 10 mg/kg).*

ond phase but a slower distribution in the late phase. Therefore, we reanalyzed all the data by means of a three-compartment model.

It became obvious that the third compartment contributed a great deal to the distribution pattern of amoxicillin without affecting the total volume of distribution or total AUC significantly (Table 1). The share of the third phase of distribution as expressed, for example, in the share of the third-phase AUC (AUC_3) values in the total AUC was 20% for the 4-mg/kg-dose group, and for the 8- and 16-mg/kg-dose groups, respectively, the shares were 33 and 43%. These differences between the dose groups were highly significant if the 4-mg/kg-dose group was compared with the 8- and 16-mg/kg-dose group, but the difference was not statistically significant if the 8- and 16-mg/kg-dose groups were compared. Nevertheless, these data indicated a dose-dependent increase of the AUC_3 values insofar as doubling the dosage resulted in AUC_3 values more than twice as high. The introduction of a third compartment was followed by a decrease of the AUC of the central compartment only. As the increase of the AUC_3 values was not proportional to the dose administered, also all the serum values were significantly different from one another if the 4-mg/kg-dose group was compared with the other two dose groups. No significant differences could be observed if the 8-mg/kg-dose group was compared with the 16-mg/kg-dose group. These results, too, indicated a dose dependency of the distribution constants. The partial and total volumes of distribution were significantly different from each other.

TABLE 1. *AUCs calculated by means of two- and three-compartment models*

Dose (mg/kg)	Model (no. of compartments)	μg/h per ml per dose			
		AUC_1	AUC_2	AUC_3	AUC_{total}
4	2	8.69	11.65		20.34
	3	4.34	11.87	4.38	20.59
8	2	16.66	25.42		42.08
	3	5.96	22.33	13.9	42.20
16	2	29.65	52.44		82.10
	3	9.96	36.31	35.73	82.02

The average parameters of each dose group were then used to plot the serum curves which would be expected if 10 mg/kg were administered; in contrast to the calculations made by adopting the two-compartment model, an overall average across all dose groups for total trial observations could not be calculated by means of the three-compartment model, as there occured statistically significant differences between the dose groups. The results are shown in Fig. 1. The slopes clearly point out the differences between the two- and three-compartment models, respectively. Predicting the serum concentrations by means of the two-compartment model, no amoxicillin is present in the serum later than 470 min after dosing, whereas by adopting the three-compartment model, the drug is still available at 500 min and later due to the late phase of disposition.

The prolonged and dose-dependent late phase of distribution of amoxicillin let us assume that the drug might accumulate if administered repeatedly even in relatively low doses. The introduction of a third compartment modified the pharmacokinetic behavior of amoxicillin significantly. The distribution constants and the AUCs were significantly dose dependent. As the K_{13} and K_{31} values indicated, amoxicillin diffused relatively slowly into the second peripheral compartment and back again, and thus the elimination of amoxicillin was prolonged. In contrast, amoxicillin diffused more rapidly from the central compartment to the first peripheral compartment, so the serum concentrations no longer declined linearly and also not in parallel, as the distribution constants were dose dependent. It follows from these facts that more amoxicillin diffused from the central compartment into the peripheral compartments, i.e., "tissue," if the three-compartment model was compared with the two-compartment model.

It has been shown in this study that a two-compartment model does not provide the best fit for serum concentration versus time curves, as the drug seems to persist for prolonged periods in the tissue. A three-compartment model provides for the late phase of distribution of amoxicillin, and an optimal fit of serum concentration versus time curve is obtained. This model substantially revises the pharmacokinetic characterization of amoxicillin disposition, and it is very likely that this assumption is also valid for other penicillins.

Comparative Pharmacokinetics and Microbiological Studies During 8-Day Therapy with Cefadroxil and Cefaclor

H. LODE,* B. HAMPEL, P. KOEPPE, AND J. WAGNER

Medical Department, Klinikum Steglitz, Freie Universität Berlin, 1000 Berlin 45, Germany

For current assessment of new antibiotics, consideration should be given to their pharmacokinetic action throughout the entire duration of therapy and not just after a single application. In addition, the value of new antibiotics is also determined by their possible resistance pressure on intestinal flora.

In a comparative study with eight healthy volunteers, we determined the pharmacokinetic parameters and the influence on fecal flora of two new oral cephalosporins during two 8-day therapy periods. Each of the eight test persons (four males and four females; ages, 21 to 49 years; mean body weight, 63.3 kg) received three 1.0-g doses of cefadroxil (CDX) or cefaclor (CCL) per day with a 4-week interval between the two therapies. The serum concentrations were measured on days 1, 4, and 8 before and 0.25, 0.5, 0.75, 1, 1.5, 2, 3, 4, 6, and 8 h after oral application on an empty stomach. Microbiolog-

ical assay was performed by means of the agar diffusion test (cup plate method [1] in a modification of the method of Reeves and Bywater [8]); test strains were *Sarcina lutea* ATCC 9341 and *Bacillus subtilis* ATCC 6633. The lowest determination levels were 0.3 mg/liter in serum (pH fixed at 7.4) for both antibiotics.

Fecal flora was investigated before, during, and after the antibiotic applications. The parameters were: total count of aerobic fecal bacteria and determinations of enterobacteria, of *Pseudomonas* species, of fungi, and of resistance characteristics. The Wilcoxon signed rank test was used for the analysis of significance of difference (level of significance, $P = 0.05$).

Both cephalosporins showed the typical, previously described characteristics (7) in their serum concentration courses after initial application. CDX evidenced a slow invasion and elimination, with a large area under the serum level curve. The mean maximal concentration was reached between 2 and 3 h and amounted to 27.5 ± 5.1 mg/liter; after 8 h an average value of 2.2 ± 0.5 mg/liter was still measured.

CCL, however, showed a rapid invasion and elimination, with a mean maximal level of 28.7 ± 5.9 mg/liter after 1 h; the 6-h value of CCL was 0.6 ± 0.3 mg/liter. After 8 h, the concentrations were below the threshold of detectability of 0.3 mg/liter.

In the course of the 8-day therapy, there was an accumulation of the CDX serum concentration, with an increase in the maximal levels from 27.5 ± 5.1 mg/liter on day 1 to 33.2 ± 7.7 mg/liter on day 4 and to 35.5 ± 5.9 mg/liter on day 8 (Fig. 1). The trough concentrations (8 h) also showed an increase, from 2.2 ± 0.5 mg/liter on day 1 to 4.3 ± 3.5 mg/liter during day 8. The morning trough concentrations were all clearly higher than the corresponding levels during the day; thus, in the morning, CDX increased to 6.9 ± 3.5 mg/liter. This increase in morning trough concentrations can probably be explained by the retarded invasion during the nocturnal sleep phase.

The mean maximal CCL concentrations did not accumulate during the 8-day treatment, with 28.7 ± 5.8 mg/liter (day 1), 31.5 ± 10.2 mg/liter (day 4), and 29.3 ± 6.4 mg/liter (day 8) (Fig. 2). CCL trough concentrations (8 h) could be detected on day 4 in the morning in two test subjects and on day 8 in three test subjects. During the diurnal periods, on the other hand, CCL concentrations were no longer measurable after 6th h. The serum concentration courses of both cephalosporins on day 8 once again make clear the accumulation of CDX at a dosage of 1.0 g three times daily with a significantly higher mean maximal value and a larger area under the concentration curve than that of CCL.

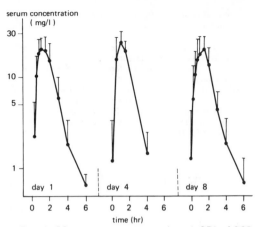

FIG. 2. *Mean serum concentrations (±SD) of CCL in eight volunteers after three applications of 1,000 mg/day on an empty stomach.*

Resistant intestinal flora developed up to day 3 of CDX therapy in seven out of eight volunteers. The bacteria involved were: *Enterobacter hafniae* (3), *Enterobacter cloacae* (4), *Proteus morganii* (3), *Proteus vulgaris* (3), *Citrobacter freundii* (3), *Serratia marcescens* (1), and *Pseudomonas aeruginosa* (1). These bacilli developed parallel resistances to cefazolin, cefaclor, ampicillin, and azlocillin. *Escheria coli* showed no significant fluctuations in number or resistances. The resistant bacilli disappeared 3 weeks after CDX was discontinued.

Resistant strains were detected in all eight test subjects during CCL therapy. The bacteria involved were: *E. hafniae* (6), *E. cloacae* (4), *C. freundii* (5), *P. morganii* (1), *P. vulgaris* (3), *Acinetobacter anitratum* (2), and *E. coli* (2). The parallel resistances resembled those of CDX; the resistant strains disappeared within 1 week after application was discontinued. These microbiological findings on the two cephalosporins correspond to the changes in intestinal flora under tetracyclines (2, 5), ampicillins (6), and cephalexin (3, 4).

The tolerances of both cephalosporin antibiotics were good on the whole; when taken on an empty stomach, CDX resulted in a clearly higher occurrence of epigastric symptoms than did CCL.

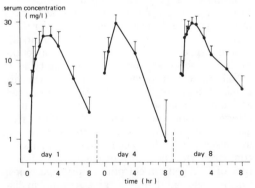

FIG. 1. *Mean serum concentrations (±SD) of CDX in eight volunteers after three applications of 1,000 mg/day on an empty stomach.*

1. **Bennett, J. V., J. L. Brodie, E. J. Benner, and W. M. M. Kirby.** 1966. Simplified, accurate method for antibiotic assay of clinical specimens. Appl. Microbiol. **14:** 170–177.
2. **Datta, N., M. C. Faievs, D. S. Reeves, W. Brumfitt, F. Ørshov, and I. Ørshov.** 1971. R-factors in Escherichia coli in faeces after oral chemotherapy in general practice. Lancet **i:**312–315.

3. **Gaya, H., P. I. Adnitt, and P. Turner.** 1970. Changes in gut flora after cephalexin treatment. Br. Med. J. **3**:624-625.

4. **Hartley, C. L., H. M. Clements, and K. B. Linton.** 1978. Effects of cephalexin, erythromycin and clindamycin on the aerobic gram-negative faecal flora in man. J. Med. Microbiol. **11**:125-135.

5. **Hirsh, D. C., G. C. Burton, and D. C. Blenden.** 1973. Effect of oral tetracycline on the occurrence of tetracycline-resistant strains of *Escherichia coli* in the intestinal tract of humans. Antimicrob. Agents Chemother. **4**:69-71.

6. **Knothe, H.** 1977. Eigenschaften der Chemotherapeutika und deren Einfluß auf die körpereigene Flora. Wochenschr. Kinderheilk. **125**:262-267.

7. **Lode, H., R. Stahlmann, and P. Koeppe.** 1979. Comparative pharmacokinetics of cephalexin, cefaclor, cefadroxil, and CGP 9000. Antimicrob. Agents Chemother. **16**:1-6.

8. **Reeves, D. S., and M. J. Bywater.** 1976. Assay of antimicrobial agents, p. 21-78. *In* J. de Louvois (ed.), Selected topics in clinical bacteriology. Tindall, London.

Preparation and Properties of Liposome-Associated Gentamicin

J. R. MORGAN

Department of Medical Microbiology, Welsh National School of Medicine, Heath Park, Cardiff CF4 4XN, Wales

Liposomes are membrane-limited vesicles which are formed spontaneously when phospholipids are brought into contact with water. During the genesis of a liposome a volume of water will be trapped within the confines of the phospholipid membrane in the intraliposomal space. If any substance is dissolved in the water at the moment of liposome formation, then the solution will be incorporated. A large number of pharmacologically active substances have been trapped inside liposomes, and it has been shown that when such preparations are administered to animals, aspects of the pharmacological activities of the drugs are governed by characteristics attributable to the liposomes. Depending upon the size and surface charge of the liposome will be exhibited such features as prolonged periods of circulation in blood or concentration in certain tissues such as liver and spleen. It has further been shown that liposomes gain entry into cells and thus carry with them the entrapped solutions. This potential as vehicles for drugs and the affinity for the reticuloendothelial system offer interesting possibilities for the use of liposomes as vehicles for antimicrobial agents against infections such as brucellosis and listeriosis that characteristically involve the reticuloendothelial system. This investigation examined the incorporation of gentamicin into liposomes and the behavior of liposome-associated gentamicin when administered to rabbits.

Liposomes carrying no charge (neutral) were prepared from phosphatidylcholine, cationic liposomes were prepared from phosphatidylcholine plus stearylamine, anionic liposomes were prepared from phosphatidylcholine cholesterol and phosphatidylserine, and lipase-resistant liposomes were prepared from dipalmitoylphosphatidylcholine. Liposomes were prepared by drying off the chloroform-methanol solvent containing lipid in a glass vial which then received 2 ml of a 50-mg/ml solution of gentamicin. The resulting liposome suspension was ultrasonicated and separated from free gentamicin by Sephadex G75 gel filtration. Gentamicin assay was performed by radial diffusion from wells cut in agar bearing a lawn of *Klebsiella pneumoniae*. Intraliposomal gentamicin was calculated by subtracting the concentration of free gentamicin in a liposomal suspension from the value obtained after disrupting the liposomes by the addition of Triton X-100.

The entrapment efficiency of anionic, cationic, and neutral liposomes is shown in Table 1, which shows that the percentage of gentamicin entrapped is a function of the lipid concentration and also of the charge carried on the liposomes. Ionic liposomes thus appear to posses a greater intraliposomal space than neutral liposomes. All three types of liposomes were tested at weekly intervals over a 3-week period at +4°C for their capacity to retain gentamicin within the intraliposomal space. No significant leakage of gentamicin was observed from any liposomal type.

Rabbits were intravenously injected with cationic, anionic, or neutral liposome-associated gentamicin, and serum samples were taken at intervals. Estimations were made of both free gentamicin and liposome-associated gentamicin in the serum samples. The results obtained were compared with those of controls receiving injection of free gentamicin plus empty liposomes. Controls showed that detectable gentamicin disappeared from the circulation by 3 h. In contrast, sera taken from rabbits that received a single injection of either cationic or neutral liposome-

TABLE 1. *Entrapment efficiency of cationic, anionic, and neutral liposomes at different lipid concentrations for a gentamicin solution*

liposome charge:	% gentamicin trapped from 100 mg. in 2 ml. using:	
	50 mg lipid.	100 mg lipid.
positive	1·8	3·7
neutral	0·76	1·76
negative	1·77	4·0

TABLE 2. *Rabbit tissue distribution of gentamicin 3 h after intravenous injection of 2 mg of gentamicin per kg associated with cationic, anionic, or neutral liposomes*

Tissue	Gentamicin concn (ug/gm)			
	liposomes			
	cationic	neutral	anionic	control
liver	1·0	0·5	0·9	0
spleen	1·3	0	6·0	0
kidney	1·0	0·5	1·6	9·3
urine	5·6	6·8	0·6	60·0
(free serum	0·9	0·2	0·8	13·3
(liposomal	13·6	13·3	1·6	0

associated gentamicin revealed the presence of high levels of liposome-associated gentamicin up to 24 h after the injection. Free gentamicin was also detectable over this time period. Anionic liposome-associated gentamicin, however, was undetectable, as was concomitant free gentamicin, by 3 h after injection. Liposome-associated gentamicin was prepared from dipalmitoylphosphatidylcholine, which is relatively resistant to pancreatic lipases. This preparation, containing 13 mg of liposomal gentamicin, was administered by intragastric tube to a rabbit. Serum samples taken 1 h later revealed 1.5 μg of free gentamicin per ml, which dropped to 0.8 μg/ml at 2 h and was undetectable at 3 h. The control rabbit received free gentamicin intragastrically and exhibited no detectable gentamicin serum level.

Rabbits were given single intravenous injections of anionic, cationic, or neutral liposome-associated gentamicin and sacrificed 3 h later. Serum, urine, and tissue samples such as liver, spleen, and kidney were obtained. The tissue specimens were homogenized and extracted with distilled water, and the latter was assayed for free gentamicin activity. Table 2 provides data of the gentamicin levels obtained. Controls included animals sacrificed at the time of peak serum gentamicin level and 3 h after an intra-

venous injection of gentamicin, by which time detectable serum gentamicin was not evident. As can be seen, only the liver and spleen of animals receiving liposome-associated gentamicin possessed detectable free gentamicin, with the exception of the spleen of the rabbit receiving neutral liposome-associated gentamicin. Anionic liposome-associated gentamicin appeared in relatively high concentrations in the spleen, which may reflect the rapid disappearance from blood as shown in Table 2 and as described in the previous experiments. Both control and test animals had detectable levels of gentamicin in kidney and urine samples, but the relatively low urine concentrations of the test animals must reflect the low free gentamicin levels present in the serum.

It has been demonstrated that gentamicin can be incorporated within liposomes and once inside retains its location under described conditions. The pharmacology of gentamicin is profoundly altered when enclosed within liposomes. Serum half-life may be greatly prolonged and also tissue distribution may be considerably altered, with a predilection shown for liver and spleen tissue.

Effect of Tinidazole on the Oral, Throat, and Colon Microflora of Humans

CARL E. NORD* AND ANDERS HEIMDAHL

Department of Bacteriology, National Bacteriological Laboratory, and Huddinge University Hospital, Karolinska Institute, Stockholm, Sweden*

The microorganisms in the indigenous flora play an important role both in normal physiological processes and in pathological processes. Disturbances in the distribution of the host mi-

croflora may be associated with different diseases. For example, overgrowth of antibiotic-resistant enterobacteria, staphylococci, and yeasts in the oral cavity may cause stomatitis. Antibiotics have been reported to suppress the normal colon microflora and thereby permit antibiotic-resistant bacteria to increase in number (3). Some of these microorganisms may cause pathological conditions, especially if they are toxin producers.

Tinidazole (1-[-2(ethylsulfonyl)-ethyl]-2-methyl-5-nitroimidazole) is a compound with an antimicrobial spectrum covering protozoa and anaerobic bacteria. It is widely used in the treatment of different protozoal infections, and it is utilized in the treatment of anaerobic infections. However, little information is available concerning the effect of tinidazole on the human microflora. The present study reports on the effects of tinidazole on the human oral, throat, and colon microflora.

Ten volunteers with no history of significant gastrointestinal, hepatic, or renal diseases who had taken no antibiotics during the previous 6 months were studied. They were given 150-mg tinidazole capsules (Fasigyn, Pfizer, Brussels, Belgium) as a loading dose, followed by 150-mg doses at 12-h intervals over a 7-day period.

Collection of specimens. Serum samples were taken prior to the loading dose and 30, 90, 120, 180, 240, and 360 min thereafter. Over the next 7 days, samples were taken every morning 60 min after the intake of the drug. Further samples were taken in the morning 2 days after withdrawal of tinidazole. Saliva samples were collected immediately before the initial dose and then daily 1 h after the drug was swallowed. Further samples were taken 2, 5, and 9 days after the withdrawal of tinidazole. Throat swabs were obtained by pressing dry cotton-tipped sterile swabs against the posterior pharyngeal wall. Stool specimens were collected before drug administration, on the second, fifth, and seventh days during administration, and then 2 and 9 days after withdrawal of the drug.

Processing of specimens. The saliva samples were suspended in prereduced peptone-yeast extract medium, and serial 10-fold dilutions were prepared to 10^{-5}. Each dilution was then inoculated onto two blood agar plates and 10 selective media, as described by Sutter et al. (5). All manipulations were performed in an anaerobic chamber (Coy, Ann Arbor, Mich.) under an atmosphere of 90% (vol/vol) nitrogen and 10% (vol/vol) hydrogen.

The throat swabs were immediately placed in 2 ml of brain heart infusion broth (Difco) and shaken for 2 min. Portions (0.05 ml) of the broth were then inoculated onto different nonselective and selective agar plates. The cultures were examined after incubation aerobically for 24 h and anaerobically for 48 h.

A 1-g sample of feces was homogenized in 9 ml of prereduced peptone-yeast extract medium, and 10-fold serial dilutions were made to 10^{-8}. Duplicate samples (0.1 ml) of the appropriate dilutions were streaked on different nonselective and selective media. All manipulations were performed in the anaerobic chamber mentioned above.

Tinidazole concentrations in serum, saliva, and feces. The serum, saliva, and fecal concentrations were determined by the agar diffusion method. Plates were incubated anaerobically at 37°C for 24 h in GasPak jars (BBL Microbiology Systems, Cockeysville, Md.). The test medium was Penassay seed agar (Difco), and the indicator strain was *Clostridium sporogenes* KE 1.

Serum concentrations varied from 3.5 to 5.4 μg/ml, and saliva concentrations, from 2.9 to 5.9 μg/ml (Table 1). No differences in the concentrations of tinidazole in submandibular, parotid, and mixed saliva were observed. Tinidazole was not detected in the feces.

Effect of tinidazole on the oral, throat, and colon microflora. Bacteria were identified by colonial morphology, Gram stain, and different biochemical and serological tests: enterobacteria by use of the API 20 E (Analytab Products, Inc., Plainview, N.Y.), oxidative-fermentative gram-negative rods by use of an Oxi/Ferm tube (Hoffmann-La Roche, Inc., Nutley, N.J.), staphylococci by the method of Dornbusch et al. (1), and streptococci by the method of Facklam et al. (2). Anaerobic bacteria were identified by biochemical tests and gas-liquid chromatography as described by Holdeman et al. (4).

There were no significant changes in the numbers of aerobic bacteria in the saliva samples collected both during and after the administration of tinidazole. A decrease in the number of fusobacteria was observed (Fig. 1); however, no

TABLE 1. *Mean concentrations of tinidazole in serum, parotid, submandibular, and mixed saliva in 10 volunteers receiving 150-mg tinidazole capsules every 12 h for 7 days*

Day	Mean concn (μg/ml) ± SEM of tinidazole			
	Serum	Mixed saliva	Parotid saliva	Submandibular saliva
1	3.5 ± 0.5	2.9 ± 0.6	3.8 ± 0.6	3.1 ± 0.3
2	4.5 ± 0.5	4.8 ± 0.9	5.8 ± 1.1	5.2 ± 0.7
3	4.7 ± 0.9	5.6 ± 1.3	5.5 ± 0.9	5.5 ± 0.9
4	5.1 ± 1.0	5.5 ± 0.9	5.2 ± 0.8	5.9 ± 0.9
5	5.4 ± 1.1	5.5 ± 0.9	4.1 ± 0.6	5.6 ± 0.7
6	4.1 ± 0.5	5.7 ± 1.2	5.1 ± 0.6	5.8 ± 0.8
7	4.1 ± 0.9	5.6 ± 1.4	4.0 ± 1.1	5.1 ± 0.9

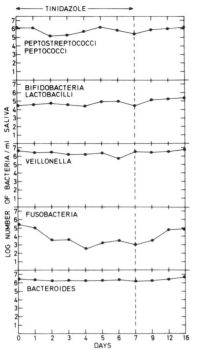

FIG. 1. *Effect of tinidazole on the anaerobic flora in the saliva of 10 volunteers.*

significant changes in the numbers of other obligate anaerobic bacteria occurred. The throat flora was constant during the experimental period and was similar to the saliva flora in all subjects. The fecal flora was also quite stable during the observation period. *Escherichia coli* and *Streptococcus faecalis* were the most common aerobic bacteria, and *Bacteroides fragilis* was the predominant anaerobic species.

Gas chromatographic analysis of volatile fatty acids in saliva and feces. A Varian gas chromatograph 1400 equipped with a glass column (0.9 m by 2 mm [inner diameter]) containing Carbowax 20 M–0.5% H_3PO_4 on 60/80 Carbopack B (Supelco, Bellefonte, Pa.) was used for the analysis of volatile fatty acids. No significant changes in the amounts of acids in the saliva and fecal samples occurred during the observation period.

Conclusions. The normal oral, throat, and colon microflora are relatively stable ecosystems. Some antibacterial agents do not seem to influence the numbers of bacteria or their interrelationships, whereas other antibiotics disturb the balance between different organisms in the normal flora and permit the overgrowth of antibiotic-resistant bacteria. In the present investigation, tinidazole was well tolerated and did not have any effect on the microflora in the mouth, throat, and colon.

1. **Dornbusch, K., C. E. Nord, B. Olsson, and T. Wadström.** 1976. Some properties of coagulase-negative deoxyribonuclease-producing strains of staphylococci from human infections. Med. Microbiol. Immunol. **162:** 143–152.
2. **Facklam, R. R., J. P. Padola, L. G. Tacker, E. L. Wostham, and B. J. Sconyers.** 1974. Presumptive identification of A, B, and D streptococci. Appl. Microbiol. **27:**107–113.
3. **Heimdahl, A., and C. E. Nord.** 1979. Effect of phenoxymethylpenicillin and clindamycin on the oral, throat and faecal microflora of man. Scand. J. Infect. Dis. **11:** 233–242.
4. **Holdeman, L. V., E. C. Cato, and W. E. C. Moore.** 1977. Anaerobe laboratory manual, 4th ed. Virginia Polytechnic Institute and State University, Blacksburg.
5. **Sutter, V. L., V. L. Vargo, and S. M. Finegold.** 1975. Wadsworth anaerobic bacteriology manual. University of California, Los Angeles.

In Vitro Interaction of Hydrocortisone with Antibiotics

I. A. AL-SOWAYGH, A. M. SHIBL, AND Y. HAMMOUDA*

College of Pharmacy, Riyad University, Riyad, Saudi Arabia

Corticosteroids are therapeutically useful in diseases involving inflammatory or neoplastic processes but have the serious side effect of diminishing defenses against infection. Susceptibility to infections of individuals on corticosteroid therapy is therefore expected to be high. The rational use of antibiotics in such cases should be based on thorough calculation of the dosage regimen as well as consideration of any possible drug interaction. The purpose of this investigation was to study the influence of hydrocortisone sodium succinate (HC) on the antibacterial activity of a selection of antibiotics known to have different modes of action.

Strains of *Staphylococcus aureus* (NCTC 6571) and *Pseudomonas aeruginosa* (NCTC 70662) were used. Stock solutions of HC and of the antibiotics were prepared to contain 1 mg/ml and 100 μg/ml, respectively. Twofold serial dilutions of the stock solution were carried out in brain heart infusion broth. Each tube was inoculated with the test organism (10^5 cells per ml), and the MIC was then recorded after incubation at 37°C for 18 h. The interaction between the drug and the antibiotics was recorded as synergistic or antagonistic if at least a two-tube (fourfold) difference in MIC was observed in the presence of HC. In a previous work (1) we reported 300 µg/ml as the MIC of HC against *S. aureus* and *P. aeruginosa*.

The types of interaction between HC and antibiotics are shown in Table 1. Subinhibitory concentrations of HC showed no effect on the antibacterial activity of penicillin or cephaloridine. On the other hand, the same concentrations of HC were found to abolish the antibacterial activity of neomycin, erythromycin, and lincomycin. Since HC has no effect on the antibacterial activity of penicillin or cephaloridine, this eliminates the cell wall as a site of interaction.

Further studies on the mechanism of action of the model combination, HC with neomycin, were carried out. Concentrations of HC below the MIC down to one-half of its value were found necessary to exert its inhibitory effect on the antibiotic. Experiments were conducted to study any possible physical interaction between HC and neomycin. Solutions of HC with the antibiotic in different molecular ratios ranging from 1:1 to 1:6 antibiotic to drug were inspected spectrophotometrically (SP 8-100) in the UV region. Results showed no sign of interaction between HC and the antibiotic in solution. However, HC was found to possess appreciable surface activity (250 µg/ml = 53 dyn/cm). The presence of the antibiotic with HC did not alter its surface activity. The surface activity of HC suggests a possible interaction with bacterial cells. Adsorption experiments were carried out to investigate this assumption. Bacteria were grown overnight at 37°C in brain heart infusion broth, and cells were then washed in phosphate buffer (pH 7.2). To 1 g (net weight) of bacterial cells, 1 mg of HC per ml was added, and the mixture was incubated at 37°C. Samples were taken at intervals and spun at 3,000 × *g* for 10 min. The supernatant was removed, and the presence of HC was determined by using the agar diffusion method. The results (Table 2) show that rapid reduction in HC activity occurred when it was added to the cells, with total abolishment of activity in 5 min. HC activity in the control test during the time of experiment remained unaltered.

TABLE 1. *Interaction between HC and antibiotics as shown by their effect on S. aureus and P. aeruginosa*

Antibiotic	HC[a]	
	S. aureus	P. aeruginosa
Pencillin	N	N
Cephaloridine	N	N
Neomycin	A	A
Lincomycin	A	A
Erythromycin	A	A
Polymyxin	S	S

[a] A, Antagonistic; S, synergistic; N, no effect.

TABLE 2. *Adsorption of HC to bacterial cells at 37°C*

Incubation mixture	Incubation time (min)	HC titer[a]
HC + viable cells	0	8
	1	8
	5	
	15	
HC control	0	8
	15	8

[a] Initial concentration, 1 mg/ml; titers are expressed as reciprocals of the highest dilutions at which HC is active.

Elimination of the cell wall as a site of interaction in addition to the adsorption of HC on the cell membrane led us to investigate the effect of HC on polymyxin B, an antibiotic known to act on the cell membrane. When *S. aureus* or *P. aeruginosa* was incubated with a concentration of polymyxin B too low to affect growth and was then exposed to HC, growth was inhibited.

The data presented in this investigation indicate that adsorption of HC to bacterial cell membrane is possibly a prerequisite for the abolishment of antibiotic activity, as it probably interferes with the free access of neomycin and similar antibiotics into the bacterial cell, where they are supposed to act.

This type of interaction may have clinical implications in patients with diseases such as status asthmaticus who are taking antibiotics while they are on HC therapy. In vivo studies are doubtless essential to explore such interaction.

1. **Hammouda, Y., and A. Shibl.** 1978. *In vitro* activity of certain 11-oxysteroids and progesterone against *S. aureus* and *P. aeruginosa*. Sixth Congress of Arab Pharmacists Union, Tunis, p. 68. Pharm. Soc. Egypt, Cairo.

Pharmacokinetic and Bactericidal Effects of Cephalosporins on a Susceptible Strain of *Klebsiella pneumoniae*

GARY D. RIFKIN* AND GEORGE PACK

Department of Biomedical Sciences, Rockford School of Medicine, Rockford, Illinois 61101, U.S.A.

Traditional methods of assessing the susceptibility of microorganisms to antimicrobial agents subject the organism to constant concentrations of these agents over a set period of time. While easy to perform, these studies do not allow for the normal in vivo changes in concentrations of antibiotics with finite half-lives. To more closely simulate the usual in vivo exposure of microorganisms to antimicrobial agents, we used the dilution analog model of drug pharmacokinetics as adapted by Grasso et al. (1) to compare the antibacterial activity of cephalothin, cefamandole, and cefazolin against a susceptible strain of *Klebsiella pneumoniae*.

In this model, antibiotic-free diluent is pumped into a culture-antibiotic flask at a constant flow rate, and fluid with antibiotic is forced out at an equal rate. The antibiotic depletion rate or half-life is a function of the flow rate, F, and volume of the flask, V, such that $t_{1/2} = (0.693/F)V$. For this series of experiments, the flow rates varied from 0.4 to 1.2 ml/min and volumes varied from 35 to 104 ml.

A 10^{-3} dilution of an overnight growth of *Klebsiella* 630 was placed in the culture-antibiotic flask, yielding an inoculum of 10^5 to 10^6 CFU/ml. The medium and diluent were Mueller-Hinton broth. Volume and flow rate were set to deplete the antibiotic with the desired half-life. After 1 h of incubation at 37°C, a sample was taken for the initial colony count, antibiotic was added to obtain the desired initial concentration, and the pump was started. Samples were collected at intervals dependent on the half-life being tested and assayed for viable bacteria by plating serial dilutions onto the surface of nutrient agar and for antibiotic concentration by the agar diffusion method. Conventional susceptibility tests were performed in Mueller-Hinton broth by the microtiter dilution method. This organism had MICs to cephalothin, cefamandole, and cefazolin of 3.12, 1.56, and 1.56 µg/ml, respectively.

Growth control curves obtained by diluting the cultures at depletion rates equivalent to half-lives of 30, 60, 90, and 120 min gave curves which did not significantly differ from the undiluted or static situation or from each other. This allowed for direct comparison of the antibacterial effects of the antibiotics without correcting for the rate of depletion. The antibacterial activity of cephalothin and cefamandole at starting concentrations of 20 µg/ml and half-lives of 30, 60, and 90 min and cefazolin at a starting concentration of 20 µg/ml and half-lives of 60 and 90 min was determined. All achieved maximum bactericidal activity within 2 to 3 h, and this peak activity level was not dependent on the length of time the antibiotic concentration was above the MIC. At this initial antibiotic concentration, the duration of antibacterial activity was dependent on the depletion rate. When the concentration of antibiotic in the culture-antibiotic flask reached the MIC, regrowth occurred.

A comparison of the antibacterial activity of these three drugs at starting concentrations of 20 µg/ml and depletion rate equivalent to a half-life of 60 min is shown in Fig. 1. While all achieved maximum bactericidal activity by 2 to 3 h, this activity was 10-fold (1 log) greater for cefazolin than for cephalothin or cefamandole. The initial rate of bactericidal action also dif-

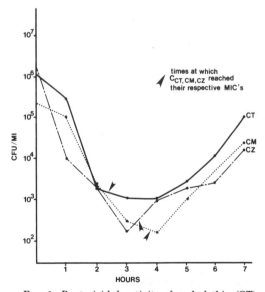

FIG. 1. *Bactericidal activity of cephalothin (CT), cefamandole (CM), and cefazolin (CZ) against Klebsiella pneumoniae 630. $C_{CT,CM,CZ(0)} = 20$ µg/ml; $t_{1/2} = 60$ min.*

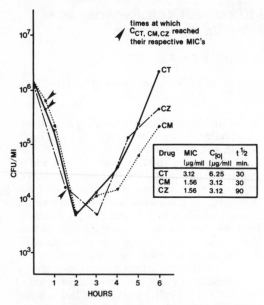

FIG. 2. *Bactericidal activity of cephalothin (CT), cefamandole (CM), and cefazolin (CZ) at twice their MICs for* Klebsiella pneumoniae *630 and at normal serum half-lives.*

Figure 2 depicts the activity of these drugs at twice their MICs and at their normal in vivo half-lives of 30 min for cephalothin and cefamandole and 90 min for cefazolin. Maximum bactericidal activity was again reached at 2 to 3 h. While the rates of killing were the same as with the higher antibiotic concentrations, maximum bactericidal activities were 10- to 100-fold (1 to 2 logs) less. Although the MICs were reached at one half-life (30 min for cephalothin and cefamandole and 90 min for cefazolin), there was continued bactericidal activity for a further 60 to 90 min.

To determine if this continued killing was due to the presence of antibiotic at subinhibitory levels or due to an initial irreversible action of these drugs on the majority of the cell population, we repeated the experiment with the addition of β-lactamase at 30 or 60 min. For cephalothin, regrowth occurred shortly after β-lactamase was added. For cefamandole and cefazolin, however, the addition of β-lactamase did not affect the bactericidal activity, suggesting that these drugs initiated an irreversible killing effect on a larger cell population than occurred with cephalothin.

fered, being 10-fold (1 log) greater for cefazolin in hour 1 than that noted for cephalothin or cefamandole, while in hour 2 the converse occurred.

1. **Grasso, S., G. Meinardi, I. DeCarneri, and V. Tamassia.** 1978. New in vitro model to study the effect of antibiotic concentration and rate of elimination on antibacterial activity. Antimicrob. Agents Chemother. **13:** 570–576.

Response of Bacteria in Infected Fluids to Measured Antibiotic Concentrations

JOHN D. TURNIDGE* AND PETER J. McDONALD

Unit of Clinical Microbiology, Flinders Medical Centre Bedford Park, 5042, Australia

Most antibiotic prescribing is aimed at maintaining greater than the MIC of drug at the site of infection throughout the dosing interval. However, the MIC is a laboratory parameter that does not take into account many of the other factors that may influence the efficacy of antibiotics such as antibody, complement, phagocytosis, local pH, local redox potential, growth rate, and metabolic characteristics of the organism.

We studied the in vivo response of bacteria to measured antibiotic concentrations in (i) the serous exudate of impetigo lesions and (ii) urines infected during catheterization. In six impetigo patients samples of infected fluid were taken at

regular intervals for up to 6 h after the administration of antibiotic. These were divided and the first part was used to determine the viable count of organisms per milliliter by serial 10-fold dilutions. The second part was used to measure the drug level by the agar diffusion technique. Blood taken concurrently was used to measure serum antibiotic level. MIC and MBC were measured by the tube dilution method in Mueller-Hinton broth. All patients were examined on several consecutive days of therapy. Erythromycin and cloxacillin were the antibiotics studied.

One patient was studied as a control over a 6-h period on 3 consecutive days. Without antibiotic therapy a fall of 1 log was noted after 2 to 4 h of hourly sampling, with numbers returning to original levels at 6 h. Thus, a fall of 1 log in other patients was not considered related to antibiotic effect.

Initial lesion fluid demonstrated $10^{9.5}$ colony-forming units or more of mixed *Staphylococcus aureus* and *Streptococcus pyogenes* per ml. Reductions of 10^2 or 10^3 colony-forming units/ml (total numbers) were observed over 4 to 5 h after the first dose in patients receiving "standard" oral erythromycin (250 mg four times a day). *S. pyogenes* diminished more rapidly than *S. aureus* and fell below detectable levels 3 to 6 h after the first dose. Responses observed on the subsequent 2 days after the fifth and ninth doses were less predictable. In general, concentrations were in the range of 10^7 to 10^9 colony-forming units/ml at the time of dosing, followed by falls of 1.5 logs or less over the sampling interval. Organisms were still present in all patients after 4 days of regular therapy.

Erythromycin was not detected in the lesions or blood until day 3 in those patients given regular oral doses. Levels ranging from 0.9 to 5.4 μg/ml were detected in the lesions 1 h after the 9th and 13th doses.

The MICs of all *S. aureus* isolates for erythromycin ranged from 0.15 to 0.3 μg/ml, and all isolates of *S. pyogenes* had an erythromycin MIC of 0.04 μg/ml. No demonstrable change in MIC occurred, even in organisms isolated in the presence of drug levels greater than the MIC.

One patient was given increasing doses of intravenous erythromycin (Fig. 1). In contrast to patients on oral therapy, high erythromycin levels were obtained in both lesions and blood from the first dose. The MIC for both organisms was exceeded by up to 50- to 500-fold for more than 6 h on 3 consecutive days. Falls in viable count of greater than 4 logs were seen on day 1. However, the effect on the bacterial population was much less marked on day 2 despite doubling of the dose, and there was no significant fall in bacterial numbers on day 3 despite a further dose increase.

One patient was given oral cloxacillin. Detectable exudate levels exceeded the MIC by up to 50- to 500-fold for more than 6 h after a dose. With this drug only a modest decrease in bacterial numbers was observed after the initial and fifth cloxacillin doses, despite lesion drug levels above the MIC.

Ten catheter urines were sampled by needle aspiration at regular intervals for up to 7 h after a single dose of antibiotic. The catheter was then removed. Urine viable count and antibiotic levels were determined with the same techniques

as in the impetigo study. The MICs were determined in Mueller-Hinton broth. In addition, in four patients MICs were determined in the patient's own urine collected before antibiotic administration and in control uninfected urine. Antibiotics studied were amoxicillin, cephalexin, and cloxacillin.

After oral antibiotic administration viable counts fell by 2 to 7 logs over 6 to 7 h (Fig. 2). Peak antibiotic levels were detected approximately 2 to 4 h after dosing, with levels of 2,000 to 3,000 μg/ml for amoxicillin, 3,000 to 5,000 μg/ml for cephalexin, and 300 μg/ml for cloxacillin. Antibiotic levels exceeded the MIC and MBC as measured in Mueller-Hinton broth from 30 min after the dose for the duration of the sampling interval in all cases. Peak antibiotic levels exceeded this MIC by 240- to 1,600-fold.

When the MIC and MBC were retested in the patient's own urine in four cases, 4- to 160-fold increases were found. Furthermore, discrepancies appeared between MIC and MBC that were not found when they were performed in Mueller-Hinton broth. Comparable changes in MIC and MBC were found when control urine was used as the broth medium.

To summarize, in most impetigo and urine

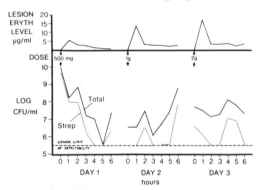

FIG. 1. *Impetigo drug levels and bacterial responses: intravenous erythromycin; S. aureus and group A Streptococcus.*

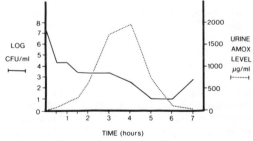

FIG. 2. *Urinary drug level and bacterial response: oral amoxicillin, 1 g; organism, Escherichia coli.*

cases the traditional desired drug effect of greater than MIC concentrations of antibiotic at the site of infection was achieved for several hours after a dose. However, in all impetigo patients organisms persisted in lesions, often despite increasing dosage and in the face of drug levels far in excess of the MIC.

In urinary infections marked variation in the rate of bacterial killing occurred that could not be explained in terms of traditional MIC values. Greatest falls in viable count were observed in some instances before the traditional or urinary MBC was achieved, whereas others had only sluggish killing when the MBC was exceeded for the whole of the sampling period.

The acute effects of antibiotics in urinary infection have been studied previously by Cattell et al. (1) and Waisbren (3), but their results were not compared with in vitro susceptibility testing. From our results, host and local factors appear to play an important role in modifying these acute effects. This has clear implications for antibiotic dosing amounts and intervals. Selwyn (2) has demonstrated an increase in traditional MIC values and discrepancy between MIC and

MBC when measured in the presence of serum. A similar factor is probably operating with the changes in these values that we observed in urine.

Overall there are many factors that need to be considered when predicting antibiotic efficacy. Some of the local factors include pH, redox potential, protein binding, intracellular presence of organisms, growth and metabolic characteristics of the organisms, the phenomenon of tolerance, humoral immunity, and, in the case of urine, the kinetics of urine flow. Our initial observations have suggested that these factors may either contribute to the bactericidal effect or even protect against otherwise predictable bacterial killing.

1. **Cattell, W. R., J. Sardeson, M. B. Sutcliffe, and F. O'Grady.** 1968. Kinetics of urinary bacterial response to antibacterial agents, p. 212–226. *In* F. O'Grady and W. Brumfitt (ed.), Urinary tract infection. Oxford University Press, Oxford.
2. **Selwyn, S.** 1976. Rational choice of penicillins and cephalosporins based on parallel in vitro and in vivo tests. Lancet ii:616–618.
3. **Waisbren, B.** 1965. The proof of efficacy of antibiotics. Am. J. Med. Sci. **250**:406–423.

Human Pharmacokinetics of 5-Episisomicin

RUEDI LÜTHY, REINER MÜNCH, AND JÜRG BLASER*

Department of Medicine, University of Zürich, and Institute for Biomedical Engineering, University of Zürich and Federal Institute of Technology, Zürich, Switzerland

5-Episisomicin (5-ES) is a new semisynthetic stereoisomer of sisomicin (SM), developed by Schering. Compared to gentamicin (GM), tobramycin, and amikacin, it posesses enhanced activity against *Pseudomonas*, *Providencia*, and *Proteus rettgeri*. Its activity against GM-resistant, gram-negative bacteria is comparable to, and for most *Pseudomonas* strains superior to, that of amikacin. Cross-resistance between amikacin and 5-ES is incomplete (5). Animal studies indicated that its nephrotoxicity ranged between those of GM and SM (I. I. A. Tabachnick, personal communication).

The present study was undertaken (i) to determine the pharmacokinetic parameters of 5-ES in humans after a single intramuscular injection of 1 mg/kg of body weight, (ii) to evaluate the local and systemic tolerance, and (iii) to determine the effect of 5-ES on the urinary excretion of alanine-aminopeptidase as a possible indicator of tubular toxicity.

Each of six healthy male volunteers received

an intramuscular injection of 5-ES in a dose of 1 mg/kg of body weight. Thirteen blood samples were drawn at various time intervals over a 24-h period (Fig. 1), and urine was collected quantitatively during eight collection periods beginning 24 h prior to and ending 72 h after injection (Fig. 2). Each serum and urine sample was assayed in quintuplicate with the large-plate agar diffusion method. In addition to a physical examination, a complete laboratory evaluation was performed before and after the study. It included a complete blood count, sedimentation rate, glucose, urea, creatinine, bilirubin, alkaline phosphatase, transaminases, total protein, and complete urinalysis. Twenty-four hour creatinine clearances were measured before, during, and after the study.

The pharmacokinetic parameters (volume of distribution of the central compartment, V_1; rate constants of transfer between the two compartments, k_{12} and k_{21}; and rate constants of absorption and elimination, k_a and k_e) were adapted to

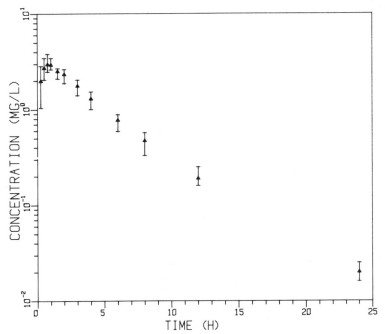

FIG. 1. *Serum concentrations of 5-episisomicin (5-ES), 1 mg/kg intramuscularly (mean and range of six volunteers).*

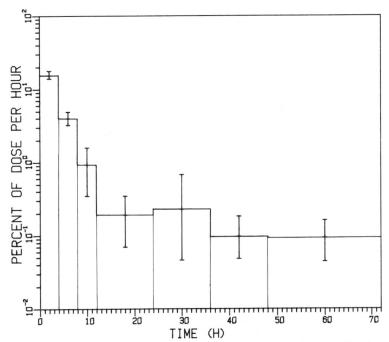

FIG. 2. *Urinary excretion rate of 5-episisomicin (5-ES) (mean and range of six volunteers).*

the experimental serum concentration-time curves with a nonlinear fitting program. The total volume of distribution was defined as V_{Dss} $= V_1 \cdot (1 + k_{12}/k_{21})$ and total body clearance was defined as $Cl_B = V_1 \cdot k_e$.

There is accumulating evidence that after a

bolus injection, the serum concentration-time curves of aminoglycosides follow a triexponential decline. Indeed, graphic and statistical analysis of 5-ES serum concentrations and urinary excretion suggested a similar pharmacokinetic behavior and indicated that the last serum level was already dominated by a γ-phase. However, the last two blood samples were drawn at 12 and 24 h, which did not permit estimation of the two additional parameters describing the terminal elimination phase. Therefore, pharmacokinetic analysis was confined to the time period between 0 and 12 h after injection, using a two-compartment open model.

The observed peak serum concentrations (C_{max}) and the corresponding times (T_{max}) to reach C_{max} were obtained from the individual serum concentration-time data and averaged 3.07 μg/ml (range, 2.68 to 3.33 μg/ml) and 1 h ($r = 0.75$ to 1.50), respectively. The mean serum concentrations were: at 2 h, 2.33 ($r = 1.88$ to 2.64); at 8 h, 0.47 ($r = 0.33$ to 0.57); at 12 h, 0.19 ($r = 0.16$ to 0.25); and at 24 h, 0.02 μg/ml ($r = 0.016$ to 0.025) (Fig. 1). In only one volunteer was the 24-h serum level below our assay limit (<0.016 μg/ml) and was excluded from Fig. 1. Serum levels recorded after 8 h were distinctly higher than expected. Identical intramuscular doses of GM, tobramycin, SM, or netilmicin produce average serum concentrations of 0.3 μg/ml at 8 h compared to 0.47 μg/ml for 5-ES, and serum concentrations of aminoglycosides, which can be attained after a single intramuscular dose of 1 mg/kg at 24 h, are generally below the microbiological assay limits. Urinary excretion, expressed as percentage of the administered dose, averaged 83.1% from 0 to 12 h ($r = 79.6$ to 89.3), 2.2% from 12 to 24 h ($r = 0.8$ to 4.2), 4.0% from 24 to 48 h ($r = 1.1$ to 9.8), 2.2% from 48 to 72 h ($r = 1.1$ to 3.9), and 92.2% from 0 to 72 h ($r = 88.7$ to 99.5). The urinary excretion rate is shown in Fig. 2. In the first 24 h, it decreases exponentially from 15.5%/h in the first 4-h interval to 0.2%/h in the 12-h interval. From 36 to 72 h, the hourly excretion remains constant at a level of approximately 0.01% of the administered dose, which suggests a continuing excretion even beyond the last collection period. A similarly prolonged excretion has been reported for GM, tobramycin, SM, and netilmicin (1-3).

The pharmacokinetic parameters of 5-ES (mean and range) are as follows: β-half-life = 2.99 h (2.38 to 3.23); $V_{Dss} = 0.23$ liter/kg (0.20 to 0.26); $Cl_B = 78.4$ ml/min per 1.73 m^2 (68.0 to 97.4); $k_a = 0.97$ h^{-1} (0.63 to 1.31); and half-life of absorption from the intramuscular depot = 0.76 h (0.53 to 1.10). The β-half-life of 5-ES is distinctly longer than that of other aminoglycosides, which range between 2.0 and 2.4 h. The reported values for the volumes of distribution of GM, tobramycin, SM, and netilmicin, derived from two-compartment analysis, are very similar. In contrast, the total body clearance of 5-ES is slightly lower than that of other aminoglycosides.

Urinary excretion of alanine-aminopeptidase, a possible indicator of tubular toxicity (4), remained within the normal range (1.7 to 13.0 mU/ml) throughout the entire study period. However, a marked increase from base-line excretion (0.5 mU/ml; $r = 0.3$ to 0.9) to the first urine collection period from 0 to 4 h (2.1 mU/ml; $r = 0.6$–4.2) was observed. In the three subsequent urine specimens (4 to 8, 8 to 12, and 12 to 24 h), alanine-aminopeptidase activity nearly returned to pretreatment levels. A considerable rise was again observed in the periods between 24 and 72 h, suggesting a delayed effect of 5-ES on the proximal tubules of the kidney.

The pharmacokinetic profile of 5-ES is characterized by a long β-half-life and a prolonged urinary excretion. No local or systemic side effects attributable to 5-ES were recorded, and all laboratory values remained within the normal range.

1. **Follath, F., P. Spring, M. Wenk, L. Z. Benet, and L. Dettli.** 1978. Comparative pharmacokinetics of sisomicin and netilmicin in healthy volunteers, p. 979–980. *In* Current chemotherapy, Proceedings of the 10th International Congress of Chemotherapy. American Society for Microbiology, Washington, D.C.

2. **Kahlmeter, G., S. Jonsson, and C. Kamme.** 1978. Longstanding post-therapeutic gentamicin serum and urine concentrations in patients with unimpaired renal function. A pharmacokinetic evaluation. J. Antimicrob. Chemother. **4**:143–152.

3. **Kahlmeter, G., S. Jonsson, and C. Kamme.** 1978. Multiple-compartment pharmacokinetics of tobramycin. J. Antimicrob. Chemother. 4 (Suppl. A):5–11.

4. **Mondorf, A. W., J. Breier, J. Hendus, J. E. Scherberich, G. Mackenrodt, P. M. Shah, W. Stille, and W. Schoeppe.** 1978. Effect of aminoglycosides on proximal tubular membranes of the kidney. Eur. J. Clin. Pharmacol. **13**:133–142.

5. **Waitz, J. A., G. H. Miller, E. Moss, Jr., and P. J. S. Chiu.** 1978. Chemotherapeutic evaluation of 5-episisomicin (Sch 22591), a new semisynthetic aminoglycoside. Antimicrob. Agents Chemother. **13**:41–48.

Pharmacology of Intravenous Trimethoprim-Sulfamethoxazole in Children and Adults

GEORGE R. SIBER,* CATHERINE GORHAM, WILLIAM DURBIN, LAWRENCE LESKO, AND MYRON J. LEVIN

Department of Clinical Microbiology, Sidney Farber Cancer Institute, Boston, Massachusetts 02146, U.S.A.

Trimethoprim-sulfamethoxazole (TMP-SMZ; Bactrim [Roche]) has become the drug of choice for the treatment of pneumocystis pneumonia. A major problem has been the unavailability of an intravenous (i.v.) formulation of TMP-SMZ. The oral preparation is frequently difficult to administer and may be unreliably absorbed in severely ill patients (1, 2). We therefore studied the pharmacokinetics of an i.v. preparation of TMP-SMZ (Bactrim) in 22 acutely ill children and adults.

The median age of the patients was 12 years (range, 0.2 to 63 years). Most had serious underlying diseases, including: acute leukemia, 5; lymphoma, 6; solid tumors, 5; and immunodeficiency, 4. Twenty patients were treated for diffuse interstitial pneumonia documented (2 cases) or suspected (18 cases) to be caused by *Pneumocystis carinii*, and two patients had infections with gram-negative organisms resistant to other antibiotics.

Our initial dosage regimen was 150 mg of TMP and 750 mg of SMZ/m^2 given via constant infusion pump (IMED) over 1 h repeated every 8 h. The drug was diluted just before administration in 125 ml of D_5W per ampoule containing 80 mg of TMP and 400 mg of SMZ. The median duration of i.v. therapy was 8.5 days (range, 1 to 32 days).

TMP levels were measured within 48 h of initiation of therapy and every 3 to 5 days thereafter. Blood was sampled before and 65 min, 2 h, 4 h, 6 h, and 8 h after the start of the infusion. TMP levels were also measured after a single oral dose given during i.v. therapy in the 14 patients able to take oral medication. Serum TMP concentrations were measured by high-pressure liquid chromatography.

Based on limited correlations between peak serum TMP levels and therapeutic response of documented pneumocystis pneumonia (1, 2), we chose peak levels between 5 and 10 µg/ml as our goal. In 20 patients who had TMP levels measured on day 2 of i.v. therapy, mean (± SD) concentrations were 2.82 ± 1.44 µg/ml before infusion and 7.02 ± 1.69 µg/ml at 65 min (peak), 5.85 ± 1.62 µg/ml at 2 h, 4.99 ± 1.70 at 4 h, 4.29 ± 1.60 at 6 h, and 3.65 ± 1.6 µg/ml at 8 h after the start of infusion. Only three patients had

peak levels less than 5.0 µg/ml. The mean half-life ($t_{1/2}$; calculated by least-squares regression from serum levels between 2 and 8 h) was 9.6 ± 5.0 h.

Although surface area dosage resulted in higher doses per kilogram in infants and children than in adults, mean peak concentrations and mean peak increments (peak − preinfusion level) were similar in all age groups (Table 1). Trough levels were higher in the older age groups.

Serum TMP levels were directly compared in 12 patients after oral and i.v. administration of the same drug dose on alternate days. Mean peak increments after i.v. dosage (3.81 ± 1.06 µg/ml) were significantly higher than peak increments after oral dosage (1.70 ± 1.17 µg/ml) ($P < 0.001$). Peak increments less than 2 µg/ml occurred after 0 of 12 i.v. doses and 7 of 12 oral doses ($P < 0.01$).

There was a direct correlation between age and the $t_{1/2}$ of TMP ($r = 0.79$, $P < 0.01$) (Table 1). The $t_{1/2}$ of TMP also correlated directly with the serum creatinine ($r = 0.90$, $P < 0.001$) (Fig. 1). This relationship also predicted the age-related change in $t_{1/2}$. The TMP $t_{1/2}$ (in hours) can be estimated by multiplying the serum creatinine (in milligrams per 100 ml) by 12.

In patients with normal renal function, peak levels of TMP increased during the first 48 to 72 h with an every-8-h dosage interval but then reached a steady state in the therapeutic range. In 7 of 22 patients with mild to moderately

TABLE 1. *TMP peak and trough concentrations and half-life in various age groups with a dose of 150 mg of TMP per m^2 every 8 h i.v.*

Age group (yr)	No. of patients	Dose (mg/kg per day)	Mean TMP concn (µg/ml)			Mean TMP $t_{1/2}^b$ (h)
			Peak	Peak increments[a]	Trough	
<1	2	32.2	6.50	4.75	2.95	7.67
1–10	9	20.4	7.18	4.20	3.39	5.49
10–20	5	14.4	7.08	4.29	3.84	8.19
20–63	6	12.4	8.03	3.80	5.27	12.82

[a] Peak increment = peak − preinfusion concentration.

[b] The correlation coefficient between age and $t_{1/2}$ was 0.793, $P < 0.01$.

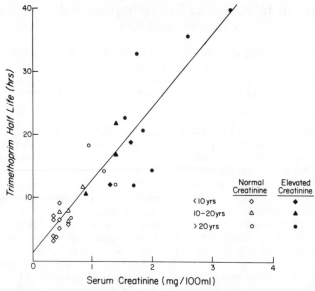

FIG. 1. *Relationship between serum creatinine and the half-life ($t_{1/2}$) of TMP in patients with normal and abnormal renal function.* $t_{1/2} = 1.20 h + 11.4$ *(serum creatinine).* $r = 0.90$; $P < 0.001$.

impaired renal function, accumulation was sufficiently marked (peak levels >10 µg/ml) to require prolongation of the dosage interval.

Adverse effects occurring before or during i.v. TMP-SMZ therapy were renal dysfunction in 7 patients, hepatic dysfunction in 10, fluid overload in 8, and transient facial flushing in 2. In six of seven patients with renal dysfunction, other drugs (aminoglycosides, amphotericin B) were implicated. Hepatic dysfunction was always ascribed to other causes. However, fluid overload was related to the high infusion volume (1,265 ml/1.73 m² per day) in patients with severe underlying cardiopulmonary disease.

We therefore examined the stability of TMP-SMZ in smaller dilution volumes and found that dilution with 50 ml of D$_5$W per ampoule resulted in a stable solution for 2 h at room temperature. TMP levels at dilution volumes of 125 and 50 ml/ampoule were compared in 10 patients on alternate days. Peak levels and $t_{1/2}$'s were similar with both dilutions.

We conclude that a maintenance dose of TMP based on body surface area (150 mg/m²) produces mean peak levels of 6.5 to 8 µg/ml in all age groups. A loading dose of 200 to 250 mg/m² would achieve steady-state levels more rapidly and may be useful in severely ill patients. A dosage interval of 8 h is recommended for children aged 1 to 10 years, and an interval of 12 h is recommended for adults, i.e., dosage every 1 to 1.5 $t_{1/2}$'s. The dosage interval should be prolonged in patients with renal dysfunction. A reasonable guideline for initial treatment based on the data in Fig. 1 is a dosage interval (in hours) equal to the serum creatinine concentration (in milligrams per 100 ml) multiplied by 15. The resulting dosage interval would be 1 to 1.5 times the $t_{1/2}$ of TMP. Serum TMP levels should be monitored in infants, the aged, and patients with renal dysfunction.

1. Hughes, W. T., S. Feldman, S. C. Chaudhary, M. J. Ossi, F. Cox, and S. K. Sanyal. 1978. Comparison of pentamidine isethiocyanate and trimethoprim-sulfamethoxazole in the treatment of *Pneumocystis carinii* pneumonia. J. Pediatr. 92:285–291.
2. Lau, W. K., and L. S. Young. 1976. Trimethoprim-sulfamethoxazole treatment of *Pneumocystis carinii* pneumonia in adults. N. Engl. J. Med. 295:716–718.

Pharmacokinetics of Amikacin and Netilmicin in Cirrhotic Subjects

JONATHAN R. SPICEHANDLER,* LEON BERNHARDT, MICHAEL S. SIMBERKOFF, AND JAMES
J. RAHAL, JR.

Department of Infectious Diseases, New York Veterans Administration Hospital, and New York University
School of Medicine, New York, New York 10010*

Spontaneous peritonitis is a serious sequela of alcoholic cirrhosis, and its incidence may be rising. Although aminoglycosides are the mainstay of therapy, pharmacokinetic data are limited in this area. Our previous experience indicates that in cirrhotic patients, assayed levels of the antibiotic in both serum and ascites have generally been low. This may be the result of overly cautious administration of aminoglycosides in doses that were calculated by estimating the patient's lean body weight (LBW), a method recently proposed by Hull and Sarubbi. In cirrhotic patients with ascites, the difference between whole body weight (WBW) and LBW is due primarily to increased extracellular fluid rather than to body fat. If ascites fluid contributes to the volume of distribution of aminoglycosides, it is likely that in nonobese cirrhotics with ascites (most are nonobese), WBW rather than LBW may be more useful in calculating aminoglycoside dosage. The differences between these weights may be quite large and significantly affect dose and serum levels.

For these reasons, pharmacokinetic evaluation of aminoglycoside usage in cirrhotics is necessary to insure effective serum and ascitic fluid levels for the treatment of bacteremia and peritonitis.

Cirrhotic patients with ascites and nonobese volunteers, who acted as controls, were selected for this study from the Manhattan VA Hospital. After informed consent was obtained, either amikacin at a dose of 7.5 mg/kg of WBW or netilmicin at a dose of 2.0 mg/kg of WBW was administered intravenously over 20 min to both the cirrhotic and control groups. Serum, in the control group, and serum with ascites, in the cirrhotic group, were obtained at 0.5, 1, 2, 4, 6, 8, and 24 h. After the completion of the infusion, amikacin and netilmicin concentrations were determined by bioassay. Plasma volumes were determined on all subjects utilizing a standard isotopic dilution technique.

Mean serum antibiotic concentrations versus time were plotted in controls and cirrhotics, for both amikacin and netilmicin, based on WBW dosage (Fig. 1 and 2). Assuming linear kinetics, projected mean serum antibiotic concentrations versus time were plotted based on LBW dosage.

Mean ascites antibiotic concentrations versus time were plotted in cirrhotics for both amikacin and netilmicin. Serum half-lives ($T_{1/2}$), area under the curves, and experimental volume of distributions were determined using these data.

The amikacin group consisted of five nonobese controls and five cirrhotic patients with ascites. All patients had normal renal function. Calculations for LBW versus WBW revealed a 1.8% mean difference in the controls and a 10.0% difference in the cirrhotics. The mean plasma volumes of controls and cirrhotics were 0.046 and 0.056 liters/kg, respectively.

The netilmicin group consisted of six nonobese controls and six cirrhotic patients with ascites. All patients had normal renal function. Calculations for LBW versus WBW revealed a 2.6% mean difference in the controls and a 11.3% difference in the cirrhotics. The mean plasma volumes of controls and cirrhotics were 0.044 and 0.064 liters/kg, respectively.

Mean amikacin serum concentrations based on WBW dosage were significantly less between controls and cirrhotics only at 0.5 h (31.5 and 22.0 µg/ml). When projected serum concentrations were made utilizing LBW dosage, there was no significant differences in controls but an 11% decrease in serum concentrations in cirrhotics. Plots for both controls and cirrhotics were consistent with a two-compartment open model. Mean amikacin ascites concentrations were greatest at 4 h (7.1 µg/ml) and persisted in the ascitic fluid for up to 24 h (0.7 µg/ml). Terminal elimination rate constants (beta) for controls and cirrhotics were 0.22 and 0.23 h^{-1}, respectively, with corresponding $T_{1/2}$'s of 3.1 and 3.0 h.

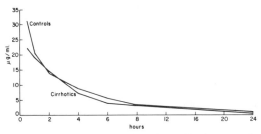

FIG. 1. *Mean serum levels in amikacin controls versus cirrhotics. Dose, 7.5 mg/kg of WBW.*

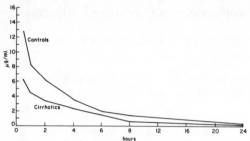

FIG. 2. *Mean serum levels in netilmicin controls versus cirrhotics. Dose, 20 mg/kg of WBW.*

Observed areas under the curve for controls and cirrhotics were 96 and 78 μgh/ml, with experimental volumes of distribution of 0.36 and 0.41 liters/kg, respectively.

Mean netilmicin serum concentrations based on WBW dosage were significantly less between controls and cirrhotics only at 0.5 (12.9 and 6.1 μg/ml) and 1 (8.2 and 4.4 μg/ml) h. When projected serum concentrations were made utilizing LBW dosage, there was no significant differences in controls but a 10% decrease in serum concentrations in cirrhotics. Plots for both controls and cirrhotics were consistent with a two-compartment open model. Mean netilmicin ascites concentrations were greatest at 4 h (1.8 μg/ml) and persisted in the ascitic fluid for up to 24 h (0.1 μg/ml). Beta for controls and cirrhotics were 0.22 and 0.18 h^{-1}, respectively, with corresponding $T_{1/2}$'s of 3.1 and 3.3 h. Observed areas under the curve for controls and cirrhotics were 40 and 28 μg h/ml, with experimental volumes of distribution of 0.23 and 0.40 liters/kg.

The results, utilizing both amikacin and netilmicin, support previous studies of kanamycin, gentamicin, tobramycin, amikacin, and netilmicin showing that the pharmacokinetics of these agents is best described with a two-compartment open model. This model leads to the assumption that the antibiotic is injected into a central compartment which corresponds roughly to the blood volume; an equilibrium is rapidly reached between this central compartment and a larger peripheral compartment corresponding to all the different tissues into which the antibiotic diffuses. A first phase (α) is characterized mainly by the distribution of the antibiotic together with a rapid fall of serum concentrations; it is succeeded by an elimination phase (β) with a slower exponential decline of serum levels.

Our data concerning $T_{1/2}$ and volume of distribution are consistent with previous pharmacokinetic studies of amikacin and netilmicin in a noncirrhotic population. When contrasting these data to a cirrhotic population, clear differences emerge. Serum concentrations are comparable between controls and cirrhotics with both antibiotics, except in the α phase, where cirrhotic concentrations are significantly reduced. If projected serum concentrations based on LBW dosage are used, the differences are even greater. The significantly greater plasma volume in the cirrhotic group, which in turn increases the volume of distribution, could account for these differences.

Antibiotic concentrations in the ascites equilibrates in 4 to 6 h with either agent and detectable concentrations are present for 24 h. Although we have demonstrated reliable systemic antibiotic penetration into the peritoneal fluid, often the levels may be subinhibitory for the common gram-negative pathogens. Utilizing a dosage schedule based on LBW may further decrease these already suboptimal concentrations. Steady-state pharmacokinetics were not performed, but the persistence of antibiotic for 24 h suggests that a cumulative effect may be seen with typical aminoglycoside dosage schedules. Also, the probable additive effect of peritoneal inflammation was not evaluated, although our own previous experience suggests that this occurs.

In conclusion, our data suggest that aminoglycoside dosage in cirrhotics should be based on WBW to reflect the increased volume of distribution in these patients. Our data also support close monitoring of both serum and ascitic fluid for consideration of dosage adjustment in patients who are clinically failing.

Pharmacokinetics of Ampicillin in Liver Impairments, Especially Obstructive Jaundice

TAKASHI KOMATSU,* HAJIME NISHIYA, KOICHIRO IWATA, MICHIO WATANABE, TOMOKO SHIRAISHI, AND OTOHIKO KUNII

The Institute of Medical Science, The University of Tokyo, Tokyo, Japan

The rates of biliary excretion of antibiotics in patients with liver impairments, especially in those with obstructive jaundice, are thought to differ from those under normal liver functional conditions, and, accordingly, the altered pharmacokinetics of antibiotics should have some influence on the antimicrobial effects. We have attempted to make some models of various types of liver impairments and to study the pharmacokinetics of ampicillin (AB-PC).

Acute liver injuries were caused in Wistar male rats by intramuscular injections of 1 ml of carbon tetrachloride (CCl_4) per kg of body weight for 3 days; chronic liver injuries were caused by subcutaneous injections of 1 ml of solutions of equal volumes of CCl_4 and olive oil per kg of body weight twice a week for 5 months.

Obstructive jaundice was caused by inserting a catheter into the common bile duct and stopping the bile excretions by corking the catheter for 24 h. The differences in the pharmacokinetics of AB-PC before and 1 or 2 days after improvement of jaundice were then compared.

Cholangitis was caused by oral administration of 45 mg of α-naphthylisothiocyanate (ANIT) per kg of body weight in the same way as described by Desmet et al. (2). Cholangitic rats were divided into six groups: group 1, rats subjected to a single administration of ANIT; group 2, rats to which ANIT was administered once a day for 4 consecutive days; group 3, rats subjected to ANIT administration for 7 consecutive days; group 4, rats left for 7 days after 7-day administrations of ANIT; and groups 5 and 6, rats left 4 and 7 days, respectively, after a single administration of ANIT.

A dose of 40 mg of AB-PC per kg of body weight was given intramuscularly to each animal in these groups. Serum, bile, and urine were collected, and AB-PC concentrations were determined by microbiological assays with *Bacillus subtilis* ATCC 6633.

Serum liver functional tests (serum glutamic oxalacetic transaminase [SGOT], serum glutamic pyruvic transaminase [SGPT], alkaline phosphatase, bilirubin, lactate dehydrogenase, leucine aminopeptidase [LAP]), zinc turbidity test [ZTT], urea nitrogen, creatinine, etc.) and histological findings were also studied.

The histological findings in the liver in acute injuries caused by CCl_4 showed fatty degenerations, and chronic injuries caused by CCl_4 showed liver cirrhosis. Bile duct obstruction showed clear partial necrosis in the liver but no bile plugs. Bleeding necrosis, the degeneration of cholangial epithelia, and inflammation were found after a single administration of ANIT, and with time regeneration was further increased. The serum liver functional tests were abnormal, except lactate dehydrogenase, LAP, ZTT, urea nitrogen, and creatinine, in almost all of the groups.

Serum levels and biliary and urinary recoveries of AB-PC after administration to rats are shown in Fig. 1 and 2. Serum levels did not differ between the intact group and the group with acute CCl_4 injuries, whereas they were elevated in the group with liver cirrhosis. In the group with obstructive jaundice, the serum levels were the highest and the serum half-life was prolonged.

In the group with acute injuries caused by CCl_4, the biliary excretion rates of AB-PC were decreased to about one-third to one-half of those of the intact group, whereas the rates were increased in the cirrhosis group. In the group with obstructive jaundice, the biliary excretion rates decreased markedly, but they increased after improvements of jaundice.

The urinary excretion rates of AB-PC did not differ distinctly between the intact group and the group with acute injuries, but they increased in the group with liver cirrhosis. In the group with obstructive jaundice, the urinary excretion rates increased, in contrast to the decrease in biliary excretion rates, and decreased after improvements of jaundice, in contrast to the increase in biliary excretion rates.

For the ANIT groups, serum levels and biliary and urinary recoveries of AB-PC are shown in Fig. 2. The biliary excretion rates of AB-PC and biliary excretion volumes showed positive correlations in the cholangitis groups.

It has been known that AB-PC is one of the best antibiotics in biliary excretion, but it has been reported that it shows poor biliary excretion in obstructive jaundice (1, 3).

This study shows the decrease of biliary ex-

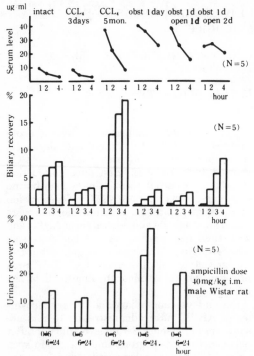

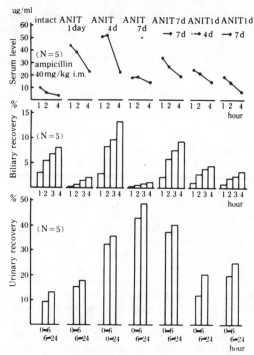

FIG. 1. *Serum levels and biliary and urinary recoveries of ampicillin (AB-PC) in intact rats and rats with acute and chronic liver injuries caused by CCl₄ and obstructive jaundice.*

FIG. 2. *Serum levels and biliary and urinary recoveries of ampicillin (AB-PC) in α-naphthylisothiocyanate (ANIT; 45 mg/kg, per os)-treated rats.*

cretion rates of AB-PC, elevation of serum levels, and increase of urinary excretion rates in cases of obstructive jaundice, whereas after improvement of jaundice, increase in biliary excretion rates, lowering of serum levels, and decrease of urinary excretion rates are shown.

In the case of cholangitis due to ANIT administration, there were no distinct relationships observed among the biliary excretion rates, serum levels, and urinary excretion rates of AB-PC. We think that these results in cholangitis are due to complex factors such as inflammation, degeneration, and regeneration of cholangial epithelia.

As for the increased biliary excretion rates,

elevated serum levels, and increased urinary excretion rates of AB-PC observed in cases of liver cirrhosis, further study is expected to clarify their significance.

In conclusion, it should be considered that the changes of pharmacokinetics of antibiotics in liver impairments, especially in obstructive jaundice, may alter the antimicrobial effects.

1. **Ayliffe, G. A., and A. Davies.** 1965. Ampicillin levels in human bile. Br. J. Pharmacol. **24:**189–193.
2. **Desmet, V. J., B. Krstulovic, and B. Damme.** 1968. Histochemical study of rat liver in alpha-naphthyl isothiocyanate (ANIT) induced cholestasis. Am. J. Pathol. **52:**401–413.
3. **Mortimer, P. R., D. B. Mackie, and S. Haynes.** 1969. Ampicillin levels in human bile in the presence of biliary tract disease. Br. Med. J. **3:**88–89.

Continuous Intravenous Infusion Versus Intermittent Intramuscular Injection of Cefazolin: Effect on Extravascular Penetration

LANCE R. PETERSON,* DALE N. GERDING, AND CLAUDINE E. FASCHING

Infectious Disease Section, Department of Medicine, and Clinical Microbiology Laboratory, Department of Laboratory Medicine and Pathology, Veterans Administration Medical Center, Minneapolis, Minnesota 55417, U.S.A.*

The discovery of antimicrobials initiated investigations into the best method for administering these agents. The purposes of the present report are to (i) demonstrate that for intermittent administration the logarithmic mean of the peak and trough serum concentrations is the important determinant in extravascular penetration, (ii) investigate the influence of the method of administration on extravascular penetration, and (iii) illustrate that both intermittent administration and constant infusion of antibiotics can provide adequate, predictable extravascular antibiotic concentrations.

Animal model. Tissue fluid chambers consist of Visking tubing into which is inserted the tubing from a 21-gauge Butterfly intermittent infusion set. The chambers are placed subcutaneously along the back in rabbits anesthetized with ketamine hydrochloride and subsequently filled with 3 ml of either saline or serum (3).

Antibiotic administration. Cefazolin was administered by either continuous intravenous infusion of 7.5 mg/kg per h or by intermittent intramuscular injection of 30 mg/kg every 4 h for 12 to 26 h.

Specimen collection. Percutaneously, 0.3-ml samples of each serum and saline chamber were obtained at 2-h intervals. Antibiotic serum levels were obtained from the mammary vessels of each rabbit.

Calculations. The log mean serum concentration was used to predict the antibiotic levels within the subcutaneous chambers for the intermittent intramuscular portion of the study. The logarithmic mean of the peak and trough serum concentrations is a mathematical approximation of the drug concentration, which must be maintained by a constant intravenous infusion to give the same extravascular drug concentration as that obtained by intermittent antibiotic administration (1–3). Total (free plus protein bound) chamber fluid drug concentration at equilibrium ($[A_c]$) for both forms of antibiotic administration is determined by: $[A_c] = [A_s] \cdot f_s/f_c$ (equation 1), where $[A_c]$ = total chamber concentration of antibiotic A, $[A_s]$ = log mean total concentration, f_s = free fraction of antibiotic in serum, and f_c = free fraction of antibiotic in chamber fluid.

All results from each animal were normalized to the average peak serum antibiotic concentration obtained during the intermittent study for that animal.

Intermittent intramuscular injection. The normalized log mean total serum concentration was 14.8. Cefazolin concentrations in the serum-filled chambers had reached this level within 10 h. The results based on predictions using the log mean serum calculations are compared to the Visking chamber results interpreted in relation to peak cefazolin serum concentrations in Table 1. Predictions based on the log mean serum calculations were very accurate, whereas comparisons of chamber cefazolin concentrations with peak serum levels made the drug appear to penetrate the high protein-containing fluid (serum) 6.3 times better than into the low protein-containing extravascular fluid (saline).

Constant intravenous infusion. The normalized constant infusion concentration was 30. Cefazolin concentrations in the serum-filled chambers approximated the normalized constant infusion serum concentrations by 26 h. Table 2 presents the data as predicted from equation 1 and as compared with the normalized constant infusion cefazolin concentration. Predictions based on equation 1 again most accurately described the eventual chamber concentration.

TABLE 1. *Results of extravascular cefazolin penetration presented in relation to the log mean serum concentration or in relation to peak cefazolin serum levels*

Visking chamber	Predicted cefazolin concn based on log mean serum level (mean ± range)	Actual mean cefazolin concn found after 8 h (mean ± range)	% Penetration based on comparison with serum peaks
Serum filled	14.8 ± 5.2	17.5 ± 2.5	17.5
Saline filled	0.74 ± 0.26	2.8 ± 0.8[a]	2.8

[a] Higher than predicted levels are due to small amounts of albumin in saline chambers (3).

TABLE 2. *Results of extravascular cefazolin penetration presented as predicted from equation 1 (see text) or in relation to the constant infusion drug concentration*

Visking chamber	Predicted cefazolin concn as derived from equation 1 (mean ± range)	Actual cefazolin concn found at 26 h (mean ± range)	% Penetration based on comparison with constant infusion concn
Serum filled	30 ± 8	27 ± 3	90
Saline filled	1.5 ± 0.4	4 ± 0.2[a]	13.3

[a] Higher than predicted levels are due to small amounts of albumin in saline chambers (3).

Comparison of intermittent versus constant infusion administration. Cefazolin concentrations in the Visking chambers of the constant infusion study were only 59% of those in the intramuscular administration study at 10 h, but equal at 20 h, and the chamber levels in the constant infusion study exceeded those in the intramuscular experiment by 48% at 26 h.

Discussion. At 26 h the constant infusion method was nearly at equilibrium with the extravascular space, and for equal amounts of drug administered, clearly delivered more total drug to the extravascular space. This should be expected if the serum constant infusion antibiotic concentration is measured and found to be greater than the log mean serum level for intermittent administration and if equation 1 correctly describes equilibrium conditions. We feel that it is the logarithmic average of the peak and trough serum concentrations and not the peak serum level that determines equilibrium extravascular conditions, as is demonstrated in this report.

1. Gerding, D. N., L. R. Peterson, D. C. Legler, W. H. Hall, and E. A. Schierl. 1978. Ascitic fluid cephalosporin concentrations: influence of protein binding and serum pharmacokinetics. Antimicrob. Agents Chemother. **14**:234–239.
2. Gerding, D. N., L. R. Peterson, J. K. Salomonson, W. H. Hall, and E. A. Schierl. 1978. Prediction of the concentration of penicillins in ascitic fluid from serum kinetics and protein binding of antibiotics in serum and ascitic fluid of dogs. J. Infect. Dis. **138**:166–173.
3. Peterson, L. R., and D. N. Gerding. 1978. Prediction of cefazolin penetration into high- and low-protein containing extravascular fluid: new method for performing simultaneous studies. Antimicrob. Agents Chemother. **14**:533–538.

Multicompartment Pharmacokinetics of Amikacin

MARKUS WENK,* SAMUEL VOZEH, PIERRE SPRING, AND FERENC FOLLATH

Clinical Pharmacology Unit, Kantonsspital Basel, CH4031 Basel, Switzerland

In previous studies on amikacin, an elimination half-life of 2 h and a volume of distribution of 0.17 liter/kg have been reported (5, 8). Recently, however, a prolonged terminal elimination phase has been described for gentamicin (6) and tobramycin (4) after repetitive administration, and also for netilmicin after a single dose (2). The purpose of the present study was to investigate whether the pharmacokinetics of amikacin follows a similar pattern.

Six patients, aged 22 to 63 years, with various gram-negative infections were treated with amikacin for 7 to 23 days. The antibiotic was administered intravenously at a dose of 250 or 500 mg. Dosage intervals were 8 to 32 h, depending on creatinine clearance, which varied between 13 and 119 ml/min. After the final dose, blood and urine samples were collected at intervals of 1.5 to 24 h over a period of 7 to 10 days. Amikacin concentrations were determined with a radioimmunoassay, the lower limit of measurable concentrations being 0.01 μg/ml.

The individual serum and urine concentrations were simultaneously fitted to a bi-exponential time function: $Cp = A \cdot e^{-\alpha t} + B \cdot e^{-\beta t}$, where A and B are adjusted for multiple dosing (3).

The decay of the amikacin serum concentration after the final dose is shown in Fig. 1. In all six patients the drug concentration shows clearly a biphasic decline. A fast initial phase with a half-life ($t_{1/2\alpha}$) of 1.5 to 8.3 h, which corresponds to the previously assumed "terminal half-life," is followed by a slower terminal phase with a half-life ($t_{1/2\beta}$) between 46 and 122 h. The half-lives and the fractional areas under the serum concentration-time curves (AUC_α and AUC_β) are summarized in Table 1. The presence of a long terminal half-life indicates that, similar to other aminoglycosides, a slowly equilibrating tissue compartment exists also for amikacin. This is in accordance with observations of Edwards et al. (1), who found levels of amikacin up to 1,030 μg/g of renal tissue after repetitive dosing.

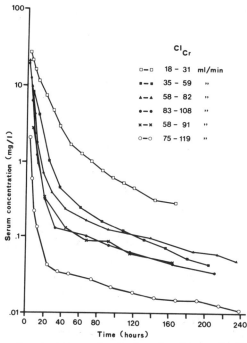

FIG. 1. *Serum concentration of amikacin after the final dose in six patients with different creatinine clearance (Cl$_{cr}$) rates.*

TABLE 1. *Pharmacokinetic data of amikacin in six patients after repetitive dosing*

Patient	Cl$_{cr}$[a] (ml/min)	$t_{1/2\alpha}$ (h)	$t_{1/2\beta}$ (h)	AUC$_\alpha$ (%)	AUC$_\beta$ (%)
1	18–31	8.3	45.7	81.6	18.4
2	58–82	2.6	69.8	95.8	4.2
3	83–108	2.4	69.7	97.3	2.7
4	78–119	1.5	122.0	97.4	2.6
5	35–59	5.6	62.9	95.2	4.8
6	58–91	3.7	98.7	95.4	4.6

[a] Cl$_{cr}$, Creatinine clearance.

Unfortunately, at present, there is no method to prevent accumulation of these antibiotics in deep-tissue compartments on repetitive dosing, even if serum concentrations are carefully monitored. Therefore, during amikacin therapy the clinician should always be aware of this potential danger to toxicity. A better understanding of the pharmacokinetic behavior of aminoglycosides may help in future to overcome these problems.

This work was supported by the Swiss National Research Foundation.

However, the area under the terminal concentration-time curve (AUC$_\beta$) being only about 4% of the total AUC, this terminal phase will not affect serum levels after multiple dosing to any clinically relevant degree. The mean volume of distribution at steady state (Vd$_{ss}$) was found in our study to be 0.69 liter/kg, two to three times higher than previously described (5, 8). Similar values have been given for gentamicin (6), tobramycin (7), and netilmicin (2) when the long terminal elimination phase has not been neglected in pharmacokinetic analysis. As Vd$_{ss}$ is proportional to the average drug amount in the body upon repetitive dosing, amikacin body levels would be considerably underestimated by disregarding the slower elimination phase.

Nephrotoxicity is a major problem also with amikacin therapy. Up to the present time toxic effects of aminoglycosides have usually been related to serum concentrations and not to drug amounts in the body, although this latter parameter may be more relevant to chronic toxicity.

1. **Edwards, C. Q., L. R. Smith, K. L. Baughman, J. F. Rogers, and P. S. Lietman.** 1976. Concentrations of gentamicin and amikacin in human kidneys. Antimicrob. Agents Chemother. **9:**925–927.
2. **Follath, F., P. Spring, M. Wenk, L. Z. Benet, and L. Dettli.** 1978. Comparative pharmacokinetics of sisomicin and netilmicin in healthy volunteers, p. 979–980. *In* Current chemotherapy, Proceedings of the 10th International Congress of Chemotherapy. American Society for Microbiology, Washington, D.C.
3. **Gibaldi, M., and D. Perrier.** 1975. Multiple dosing, p. 119. *In* J. Swarbrick (ed.). Pharmacokinetics. Marcel Dekker, New York.
4. **Kahlmeter, G., S. Jonsson, and C. Kamme.** 1978. Multiple compartment pharmacokinetics of tobramycin, p. 912–915. *In* Current chemotherapy, Proceedings of the 10th International Congress of Chemotherapy. American Society for Microbiology, Washington, D.C.
5. **Lode, H., K. Gruneri, P. Koeppe, and W. Langmaack.** 1976. Pharmacokinetic and clinical studies with amikacin, a new aminoglycoside antibiotic. J. Infect. Dis. **134**(Suppl.):S316–S322.
6. **Schentag, J. J., W. J. Jusko, J. W. Vance, T. J. Cumbo, E. Abrutyn, M. Delattre, and L. M. Gerbracht.** 1977. Gentamicin disposition and tissue accumulation on multiple dosing. J. Pharmacokinet. Biopharm. **5:**559–577.
7. **Schentag, J. J., G. Lasezkay, T. J. Cumbo, M. E. Plaut, and W. J. Jusko.** 1978. Accumulation pharmacokinetics of tobramycin. Antimicrob. Agents Chemother. **13:**649–656.
8. **Walker, J. M., R. Wise, and M. Mitchard.** 1979. The pharmacokinetics of amikacin and gentamicin in volunteers: a comparison of individual differences. J. Antimicrob. Chemother. **5:**95–99.

Predictability of Cure Rate of Aminoglycosides Based on Serum Levels and MIC

S. E. HOLM,* B. HILL, A. LÖWESTAD, AND R. MALLER

Department of Clinical Bacteriology, University of Umeå*; Department of Infectious Diseases, Sundsvall Hospital; Department of Infectious Diseases, Eskilstuna; and Department of Infectious Diseases, University Hospital of Linköping, Linköping, Sweden

A number of clinical studies have been published during recent years aiming at comparative evaluations of aminoglycosides concerning cure rate, frequency of toxic reactions, MICs, and pharmacokinetics (3, 6–11). Usually only one or two of these variables have been the focus of the investigation, which limits the value of the studies since from a clinical point of view, for example, a high cure rate can be accompanied by high toxicity or erratic pharmacokinetics (or both) of the drug. The predictability of the cure rate on the basis of serum levels and susceptibility of the microorganisms to the drug in vitro is another factor of clinical importance (1, 5, 11). The aim of this investigation was to evaluate the adverse reactions during amikacin and gentamicin treatment of patients with severe infections in relation to cure rate, serum levels, and MICs for isolated bacteria.

The study was performed as a multicenter study in Sweden, involving three different departments of infectious diseases and bacteriological laboratories. Fifty patients, mainly with severe infections which were considered suitable for aminoglycoside therapy, were included in the study and given gentamicin or amikacin according to a randomization sheet. Excluded from the study were patients who had earlier received aminoglycoside treatment, pregnant women, and persons younger than 15 years, as well as those with pretreatment cultures revealing high in vitro resistance to the drugs. To several patients included in the study other antibiotics were given simultaneously if necessary, usually penicillin G or ampicillin. Appropriate samples for the bacteriological cultivations were taken from most patients before, during, and 1 to 3 days after treatment. Determination of antibiotic concentration in serum was usually performed on days 2 and 5 as well as on the last day of treatment. The serum samples were drawn immediately before the aminoglycoside injections and 1, 2, and 8 h after gentamicin treatment or 1, 2, and 12 h after amikacin treatment. Triplicates of the serum samples were put in agar wells, which were punched in preseeded plates using antibiotic medium no. 5, pH 7.8. The test strain was Bacillus subtilis. Standard solutions of the two aminoglycosides were analyzed in duplicate simultaneously every day. The MICs of gentamicin and amikacin for isolated strains were determined by the agar plate dilution method. Determination of creatinine clearance and the serum creatinine level and analyses of urine and urine sediments, as well as clinically significant hematological data, were also performed. Nystamograms and audiograms, as well as clinical signs of ototoxicity, were recorded in 27 of the patients, usually before, during, and after the treatment.

Initially, 3 mg of gentamicin per kg of body weight divided in three daily injections or 15 mg of amikacin per kg of body weight divided in two injections were given to the patients. Subsequent dosages and time intervals were individually adjusted so as not to exceed a peak level of 35 μg of amikacin and 10 μg of gentamicin per ml. Critical trough levels chosen for the study were 10 μg/ml for amikacin and 2 μg/ml for gentamicin. The duration of therapy varied between 5 and 14 days.

Twenty-five patients were included in each of the amikacin or gentamicin groups. The average ages were 65 and 64 years, respectively. The types of infections are listed in Table 1. In both groups septicemia and urinary tract infections dominated. No differences were noted in cure rates. The most common microorganism, Escherichia coli, was isolated from 14 of the 50 patients. Other aerobic gram-negative bacteria (Proteus spp., Pseudomonas aeruginosa, Klebsiella pneumoniae) were found in 15 of the patients. It should be noted that from some patients several microorganisms were isolated and that from only 19 of the amikacin-treated patients and 16 of the gentamicin-treated ones could microorganisms of possible etiological significance be isolated. The distribution of the microorganisms was not significantly different between the two groups. Three of the 19 strains had amikacin MICs of >4 μg/ml (two of which were E. coli strains), and 1 of the 16 strains had gentamicin MICs of >2 μg/ml. Although not susceptible to 4 μg of amikacin per ml, all E. coli

TABLE 1. *Types of infection versus clinical response*

	Amikacin		Gentamicin	
Type of infection	Cured or improved	Not cured	Cured or improved	Not cured
Septicemia	14[a]	1	15	
Urinary tract infection	6		4	1
Pneumonia		1	2	
Other	3		2	1

[a] Number of patients.

strains were eradicated in the amikacin group. The clinical cure rate was not noted in two gentamicin-treated patients from whom gentamicin-susceptible strains were isolated (MIC, ≤ 2 μg/ml).

The peak and trough serum concentrations versus given dose are given in Table 2. Two of the patients in the amikacin group and one in the gentamicin group reached peak serum levels >35 and >10 μg, respectively. The trough levels, 10 μg/ml for amikacin and 2 μg/ml for gentamicin, were registered in 2 and 10 patients. Adverse reactions in relation to serum trough levels noted in our study were of the ototoxic and nephrotoxic types. If the number of patients with adverse serum creatinine and creatine clearance findings are combined, the number of patients with signs of nephrotoxicity will be five in the amikacin group and eight in the gentamicin group. One of these amikacin patients also developed a hearing loss. Two of the gentamicin patients showed signs of hearing loss at high frequencies, although the trough levels were <2 μg/ml. Vestibular involvment was registered in two patients; in one of these (the gentamicin patient) it was combined with auditory disturbances.

The differences noted in retrospective versus prospective studies with the same aminoglycoside illustrate the difficulty in clinical evaluation of these drugs. The important relationship among clinical efficiency, laboratory findings, and adverse reactions for amikacin was recently illustrated by Farchione and Chudzik (2). In the present preliminary study the therapeutic ranges of gentamicin and amikacin were compared. It is evident that the clinically reported cure rate was extremely high for both groups of patients, although many patients were old and in severe conditions when antibiotic treatment was initiated. The clinical outcome is, of course, influenced by a number of factors besides the aminoglycoside treatment, as many of them were initially treated in the intensive care ward. The susceptibilities of the isolated microorganisms to the two aminoglycosides were not sig-

TABLE 2. *Serum concentrations versus given dose*

Drug (avg dose/patient)	Serum level (μg/ml)	No. of patients	Mean serum level (μg/ml)
Amikacin (7.9 g)	Peak		
	<35	23	27.0
	>35	2	
	Trough		
	<10	23	6.0
	>10	2	
Gentamicin (2.2 g)	Peak		
	<10	24	5.6
	>10	1	
	Trough		
	>2.0	15	1.7
	<2.0	10	

nificantly different. It is also evident that few of the strains were resistant to these drugs, which is a representative finding for the resistance situation in Sweden. Thus, a comparative study of the efficiency of the two drugs on the basis of differences in MICs for the isolated strains would be hard to do, since a large number of patients must be included. Studies of peak serum and trough levels would, nevertheless, be of value since the predictability of a desired level is of clinical significance in relation to the MIC (although the strains were usually susceptible) and in relation to undesirably high or low serum levels. It is worth noting that trough levels above the desired level were more often found with gentamicin than with amikacin, although the amount of drug given during the treatment period was in the range of the recommended dose regimen. Furthermore, frequent adjustment of the daily doses was made on the basis of determinations of serum drug concentrations. As would be expected from this background, more adverse reactions were found in the gentamicin group. All of these patients had raised serum trough levels of gentamicin.

The results so far indicate that there is no difference between amikacin and gentamicin concerning clinical cure rate and eradication of etiologically significant bacteria. However, critical serum trough levels were more often recorded during gentamicin treatment. This coincided with a greater number of adverse reactions, including nephrotoxicity and ototoxicity. At the present stage of the investigation, serum levels seem to be easier to predict with amikacin, and adjusting the dose is seldom necessary. The MICs of amikacin were two to three times higher than those of gentamicin. However, the ratio of serum peak/MIC was of the same magnitude for the two drugs: 6.5:1 (amikacin) and 5.6:1 (gentamicin). The corresponding ratios for the trough levels were also equivalent, which might be a reflection of the similarity in cure rates.

1. **Barza, M., R. B. Brown, D. Shen, M. Gibaldi, and L. Weinstein.** 1975. Predictability of blood levels of gentamicin in man. J. Infect. Dis. **132:**165–174.
2. **Farchione, L. A., and G. M. Chudzik.** 1978. Serum concentrations and inhibitory ratios during amikacin therapy of gram-negative infections. J. Clin. Pharmacol. **18:**432–438.
3. **Feld, R., M. Valdivieso, G. P. Bodey, and V. Rodriguez.** 1977. Comparison of amikacin and tobramycin in the treatment of infection in patients with cancer. J. Infect. Dis. **135:**61–66.
4. **Hull, J. H., and F. A. Sarubbi.** 1976. Gentamicin serum concentrations: pharmacokinetic predictions. Ann. Intern. Med. **85:**183–189.
5. **Kaye, D., M. E. Levison, and E. D. Labovitz.** 1974. The unpredictability of serum concentrations of gentamicin: pharmacokinetics of gentamicin in patients with normal and abnormal renal function. J. Infect. Dis. **130:**150–154.
6. **Klastersky, J., C. Hensgens, A. Henri, and D. Daneau.** 1974. Comparative clinical study of tobramycin and gentamicin. Antimicrob. Agents Chemother. **5:**133–138.
7. **Lau, W. K., L. S. Young, R. D. Black, D. J. Winston, S. R. Linne, R. J. Weinstein, and W. L. Hewitt.** 1977. Comparative efficacy and toxicity of amikacin/carbenicillin vs gentamicin/carbenicillin in leukopenic patients. A randomized prospective trial. Am. J. Med. **62:**959–966.
8. **Lerner, S. A., R. Seligsdin, and G. J. Matz.** 1977. Comparative clinical studies of ototoxicity and nephrotoxicity of amikacin and gentamicin. Am. J. Med. **62:** 919–923.
9. **Smith, C. R., K. L. Baughman, C. Q. Edwards, J. F. Rogers, and P. S. Lietman.** 1977. Controlled comparison of amikacin and gentamicin. N. Engl. J. Med. **296:** 349.
10. **Wade, J., C. Smith, B. Petty, J. Lipsky, G. Conrad, J. Ellner, and P. Lietman.** 1977. Nephrotoxicity of gentamicin or tobramycin with methicillin or cephalothin, p. 971–972. *In* Current chemotherapy, Proceedings of the 10th International Congress of Chemotherapy. American Society for Microbiology, Washington, D.C.
11. **Walker, J. M., and R. Wise.** 1979. The pharmacokinetics of amikacin and gentamicin in volunteers: a comparison of individual differences. J. Antimicrob. Chemother. **5:** 95–99.

F. Antibiotic Resistance

Penicillin Binding Proteins of Penicillin-Susceptible and -Resistant
Streptococcus pneumoniae

PAUL B. PERCHESON* AND LARRY E. BRYAN

Faculty of Medicine, University of Calgary, Calgary T2N 1N4, Canada

Four strains of *Streptococcus pneumoniae* showing low-level resistance to β-lactam antibiotics were compared with three susceptible *S. pneumoniae* strains. The resistant strains had no change in antibiotic susceptibility to erythromycin, chloramphenicol, tetracycline, or vancomycin. Increased penicillin G, cloxacillin, methicillin, ampicillin, and cephalothin resistance was noted in the resistant strains. There were three similar low-level-resistant strains, D52033, D6848 and D14057, which had MICs for penicillin G of 0.32, 0.16, and 0.32 μg/ml. The three penicillin-susceptible strains, FH25-15, R446, and SPS101, had penicillin G MICs of 0.01, 0.02, and 0.01 μg/ml, respectively. All strains were clinical isolates. Strain SPR110 had a penicillin G MIC of 1.6 μg/ml and was obtained from an immunodeficient child given repeated courses of penicillin G. None of the strains possessed β-lactamase activity when examined with acidometric and bioassay methods on intact and broken cell suspensions. The penicillin resistance of strain SPR110 was not lost after treatment with either acridine orange or ethidium bromide. The penicillin resistance was not explained by a defective murein hydrolase (autolysin) system because all strains still retained their susceptibility to vancomycin, another cell wall inhibitor (MIC = 0.4 to 0.8 μg/ml), and MBCs of penicillin were only twice MICs. A strain with a defective autolytic system causing penicillin resistance should be resistant to all drugs interfering with cell wall synthesis such as D-cycloserine, vancomycin, and cephalexin (3).

PBCs. For penicillin binding component (PBC) assays, cultures of *S. pneumoniae* in late logarithmic growth in Todd-Hewitt broth were collected and washed in 0.05 M tris(hydroxymethyl)aminomethane-hydrochloride buffer at pH 7.4 containing 0.05 M $MgCl_2$ (referred to as "buffer"). The concentrated cell suspension was passed several times through a French pressure cell, and intact cells were removed by low-speed centrifugation (2,000 $\times$ g). A crude membrane fraction was collected by high-speed centrifugation (45,000 $\times$ g for 90 min). This pellet was resuspended in a small volume of buffer, adjusted to 20 mg of protein per ml, frozen, and stored at $-70°C$.

The membrane fraction (20 mg/ml) was incubated with [^{14}C]penicillin G (3.4 μg/ml, final concentration) for 15 min. Uptake of label was terminated by addition of unlabeled penicillin G to a concentration of 2.6 mg/ml. Immediately, a final concentration of 1% sodium dodecyl sulfate was added to denature the PBCs and prevent enzymic loss of labeled penicillin. After 20 min, equal portions were taken from the solubilized incubation mixture and added to the gel sample buffer of Laemmli and Favre (2). Then 2-mercaptoethanol was added (12%, vol:vol), and the mixture was placed in a boiling-water bath for 3 min. After cooling, 30 μl was processed by the discontinuous-buffer, sodium dodecyl sulfate-polyacrylamide slab gel system of Laemmli and Favre (2). A constant current of 20 mA was applied until the sample completely passed out of the 6% acrylamide stacking gel into the 12% separating gel. At this point, the current was increased to 30 mA for the duration of the separation. Detection of the labeled PBCs involved incorporation of 2,5-diphenyloxazole (PPO) into gels according to the fluorographic methods of Bonner and Laskey (1). Gels were exposed to Kodak X-Omat R X-ray film at $-70°C$. Two to four weeks of exposure yielded detectable labeled PBCs. Figure 1 illustrates the PBCs of all seven strains. All penicillin-susceptible strains had four uniformly labeled PBCs. Susceptible strain SPS101 showed an additional faintly labeled PBC associated with PBC 1. The three intermediate penicillin-resistant strains showed comparable levels of penicillin binding by PBCs 1 and 4. However, the uptake of labeled penicillin by PBC 3 was greatly reduced, and its mobility was altered compared with that of the susceptible strains. As well, penicillin uptake by PBC 2 was similarly reduced, and in strain D52033 the PBC had been replaced by two PBCs with altered mobilities. The most penicillin-resistant strain (SPR110) did not have a PBC 3 that bound detectable label at 3.4 μg of

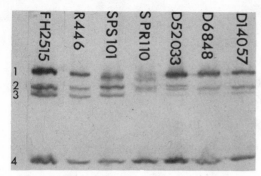

FIG. 1. PBCs of three penicillin-susceptible strains of S. pneumoniae (FH25-15, R446, and SPS101), one penicillin-resistant strain (SPR110), and three strains with intermediate penicillin resistance (D52033, D6848, and D14057). All strains were fractionated on sodium dodecyl sulfate-polyacrylamide gels and exposed to Kodak X-Omat R X-ray film for 32 days (20 mg of protein per ml, 0.5 nmol of [¹⁴C]-penicillin G per mg of cell protein).

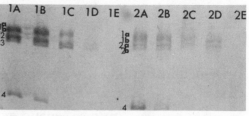

FIG. 2. Affinity of PBCs of strains SPS101 and SPR110 for unlabeled cloxacillin. Cell membrane fractions from SPS101 (columns 1A to 1E) and SPR110 (columns 2A to 2E) at 20 mg of protein per ml were preincubated for 15 min at 30°C with either distilled water (A) or 0.05 (B), 0.5 (C), 5.0 (D) or 50 (E) µg of cloxacillin per ml. These were then incubated with [¹⁴C]penicillin G (0.5 nmol/mg of protein) and treated as described in the text. Exposure of the gel to Kodak X-Omat R X-ray film was for 28 days. Cloxacillin MICs for SPS101 and SPR110 are 0.25 and 32 µg/ml, respectively.

[¹⁴C]penicillin G per ml. PBC 4 in strain SPR110 was similar to that of all other strains. PBC 2 was replaced by two derivatives which had altered mobilities and bound reduced amounts of labeled penicillin. PBC 1b of strain SPR110 bound less labeled penicillin than did the same component of strain SPS101. The affinity of PBCs 1b and 2a of strain SPR110 for cloxacillin, as measured by its ability to compete for [¹⁴C]penicillin G binding, was decreased (see Fig. 2, compare columns 1D and 2D).

Penicillin-resistant strains of S. pneumoniae have reduced binding of [¹⁴C]penicillin G by membrane proteins. The greater the penicillin resistance, the lower the amount of penicillin

bound (see Fig. 1). PBCs 1b and 2a of S. pneumoniae SPR-110 have reduced affinity for cloxacillin. These findings are consistent with the view that penicillin resistance is due to a reduced affinity of these PBCs for penicillin.

1. Bonner, W. M., and R. A. Laskey. 1974. A film detection method for tritium-labelled proteins and nucleic acids in polyacrylamide gels. Eur. J. Biochem. 46:83–88.
2. Laemmli, U. K., and M. Favre. 1973. Maturation of the head of bacteriophage T4. I. DNA packaging events. J. Mol. Biol. 80:575–599.
3. Tomasz, A., and J. V. Holtje. 1977. Murein hydrolases and the lytic and killing action of penicillin, p. 209–215. In D. Schlessinger (ed.), Microbiology—1977. American Society for Microbiology, Washington, D.C.

Mutants of *Pseudomonas aeruginosa* with Altered Susceptibilities to Aminoglycosides and Abnormalities of Terminal Electron Transport

L. E. BRYAN* AND SALLENE KWAN

Microbiology and Infectious Diseases, University of Calgary, Calgary T2N 1N4, Canada

A series of mutants of *Pseudomonas aeruginosa* with increased gentamicin (Gm) resistance was investigated for the basis of their resistance. *P. aeruginosa* PAO503 was treated with ethyl methane sulfonate, and surviving organisms were plated on Gm-selective medium (12.8 µg/ ml). Gm-resistant clones were purified and divided into phenotypes. Three phenotypes were distinguished. All phenotypes had increased resistance by disk and agar dilution methods for

Gm, streptomycin, tobramycin, amikacin, kanamycin, and neomycin, but no changes in susceptibility to carbenicillin, ticarcillin, piperacillin, tetracycline, polymyxin B, chloramphenicol, rifampin, nalidixic acid, and sulfonamides were detected. Each of the phenotypes had several distinguishing properties, but differing patterns of anaerobic growth were the most obvious of these. *P. aeruginosa* PAO2401 did not grow anaerobically in Trypticase soy broth (BBL Microbiology Systems) with 0.4% KNO_3. PAO2403 grew poorly under these conditions, whereas PAO2402 grew equally well anaerobically and aerobically. MICs of Gm were as follows: PAO2401, 150 µg/ml; PAO2403, 100 µg/ml; PAO2402, 25 µg/ml; and PAO503, 4.5 µg/ml by an agar dilution method.

The three mutants and the parent strain were examined for succinate dehydrogenase, NADH dehydrogenase, ubiquinone content, starved whole-cell ATP synthesis, coupling of electron transport to ATP synthesis, and membrane Mg^{2+}–Ca^{2+}-activated ATPase (3, 4). No differences were shown between the mutants and PAO503. PAO2401 was shown to have less than 10% of the cytochrome c_{552} found in the parent PAO503. Nitrate reductase activity (5) examined in cells grown anaerobically (Trypticase soy broth with 0.4% KNO_3, 0.1% KNO_2) was decreased in PAO2401 (0.003 µmol of NO_2 per min per mg of protein) compared with the value found in PAO503 (0.112 µmol of NO_2 per min per mg of protein). A revertant of PAO2401, PAO2404, had parental quantities of cytochrome c_{552} and nitrate reductase. The terminal cytochrome oxidase of PAO2401 utilized oxygen with NADH or succinate as a substrate at a rate 15% that of PAO503. KCN (0.1 mM) inhibited O_2 consumption of PAO503 with NADH or succinate as substrate by 82 and 81%, respectively. For PAO2401, KCN inhibition was 15 and 0%, respectively.

The mutation in PAO2401 was 50% co-transducible with the 8-min $ilvB,C$ marker on the *P. aeruginosa* PAO chromosome. Spontaneous reversion to Gm susceptibility occurred at a frequency of 10^{-5} per viable cell. These findings strongly suggest that the mutation involves a single gene.

Transport of Gm and dihydrostreptomycin (DHS) (1, 2), proline, arginine, glutamine, glucose, and spermidine was compared in PAO503 and PAO2401. PAO2401 showed a marked decrease in transport of Gm (Fig. 1) in both whole cells and spheroplasts compared with PAO503. A similar decrease in transport of DHS (10 µg/ml, nutrient broth) was found for PAO2401. These results also demonstrate that the differential uptake by PAO2401 and PAO503 is retained by spheroplasts and is thus not due to changes in the cell wall. However, no significant differences in transport of proline, arginine, glutamine (Fig. 2), glucose, or spermidine (Fig. 2) were detected. Ribosomal binding of DHS was identical for strains PAO503 and PAO2401. PAO2401 did not inactivate Gm or DHS.

The reduced rate of transport of Gm and DHS

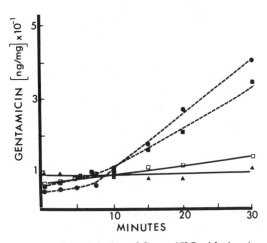

FIG. 1. *Accumulation of Gm at 37°C with time in nutrient broth (BBL Microbiology Systems). Accumulation at 5 µg of Gm per ml by whole cells of P. aeruginosa PAO503 (●-----●) and PAO2401 (▲——▲) and by spheroplasts (2 µg/ml) of PAO503 (■-----■) and PAO2401 (□——□) in nutrient broth with 20% sucrose.*

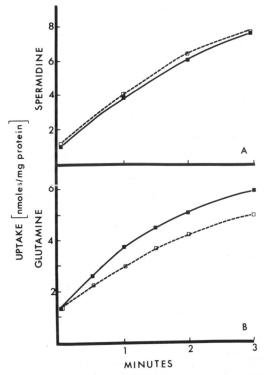

FIG. 2. *Uptake of (A) spermidine and (B) glutamine by whole cells of P. aeruginosa PAO503 (□-----□) and PAO2401 (■——■) in minimal medium containing citrate.*

and normal transport rates for several other compounds in PAO2401 suggest DHS and Gm transport is specifically coupled with terminal electron transport.

PAO2403 was found to accumulate greater than 200 times the amount of nitrite accumulated by PAO503 after overnight growth in Trypticase soy broth with 0.4% KNO_3 and thus has reduced nitrite reductase activity.

Membrane fractions of PAO2402 consume 17% the amount of oxygen used by PAO503 with NADH as substrate and 37% with succinate. KCN (0.1 mM) did not inhibit O_2 consumption by PAO2402 with NADH as substrate but did for PAO503 (79% inhibition). However, KCN inhibition of O_2 consumption with succinate as substrate was the same for PAO503 and PAO2401. Thus, PAO2402 utilizes different terminal oxidase activity than does PAO503.

Mutants PAO2402 and 2403 show reduced rates of Gm and DHS transport. The resistance level for Gm and streptomycin is lower in PAO2402 than for PAO2401 and PAO2403, and the reduction in Gm and DHS transport is also less pronounced. These mutants further illustrate the association between terminal electron transport and aminoglycoside transport.

Another mutant, PAO417-T2, isolated by B. W. Holloway and Carol Crowther at Monash University, Melbourne, Australia, was also examined. This mutant shows at least a fourfold increase in susceptibility to DHS, Gm, and all other aminoglycosides examined. Nitrate reductase activity in 417-T2 is ninefold (0.361 μmol of NO_2 per mg of protein) higher than that of the parent, PAO417 (0.042 μmol of NO_2 per mg of protein) when measured in cells grown anaerobically in Trypticase soy broth with 0.4% KNO_3. It also has about a 50% increase in ubiquinone content (3.2 × 10^{-4} nmol/mg of protein) compared to PAO417 (2.2 × 10^{-4} nmol/mg of pro-

tein). No difference in levels of NADH and succinate dehydrogenases, starved whole-cell ATP, coupling of ATP synthesis to electron transport, and Mg–Ca^{2+}-activated ATPase was found in PAO417 and 417-T2.

All of these mutants show changes in terminal electron transport resulting in a change of aminoglycoside transport and susceptibility. For one of the mutants, these changes have been shown to specifically involve aminoglycosides and not other antibiotics or transport of five other compounds. These findings support a specific association with terminal electron transport and aminoglycoside transport. They are consistent with the view that initial Gm and DHS transport is not a conventional transport system. We believe that DHS and Gm transport involves respiratory quinones or another membrane component coupling electron transport to the development of a cellular proton-motive force (1). However, multiple transport carriers used for cationic substances cannot yet be excluded as transport system for Gm and DHS.

1. **Bryan, L. E., and H. M. Van Den Elzen.** 1977. Effects of membrane-energy mutation and cations on streptomycin and gentamicin accumulation by bacteria: a model for entry of streptomycin and gentamicin in susceptible and resistant bacteria. Antimicrob. Agents Chemother. **12:**163–177.
2. **Bryan, L. E., and H. M. Van Den Elzen.** 1975. Gentamicin accumulation by sensitive strains of *Escherichia coli* and *Pseudomonas aeruginosa.* J. Antibiot. **28:**696–703.
3. **Dills, S. S., and W. J. Dobrogosz.** 1977. Cyclic adenosine 3′,5′-monophosphate regulation of membrane energetics in *Escherichia coli.* J. Bacteriol. **131:**854–856.
4. **van der Beeck, E. G., and A. H. Stouthamer.** 1973. Oxidative phosphorylation in intact bacteria. Arch. Mikrobiol. **89:**327–339.
5. **van Hartinsveldt, J., and A. H. Stouthamer.** 1973. Mapping and characterization of mutants of *Pseudomonas aeruginosa* effective in nitrate respiration and in aerobic or anaerobic growth. J. Gen. Microbiol. **74:**97–106.

Mechanism of Low-Level Aminoglycoside Resistance in *Escherichia coli*

P. DIANNE DAMPER* AND WOLFGANG EPSTEIN

Department of Biochemistry, The University of Chicago, Chicago, Illinois 60637, U.S.A.

Mutants affected in any one of a number of different steps in oxidative metabolism are obtained in selection for low-level resistance to aminoglycoside antibiotics. This type of resistance is due neither to inactivation by enzymes usually encoded on plasmids nor to changes in the ribosomal target. The presumption that up-

take of aminoglycosides is reduced in such mutants has been supported by studies of Bryan and Van Den Elzen (1). They found that uptake of gentamicin and of dihydrostreptomycin was reduced in several mutants defective in aerobic metabolism and moderately resistant to aminoglycosides. The mechanism whereby oxidative defects lead to reduced uptake of these antibiotics has not been established.

We have examined the role of the protonmotive force (PMF), an important energetic intermediate, in resistance to aminoglycosides. The PMF is exerted across the cytoplasmic membrane and is produced by the energy-linked extrusion of protons. It consists of two components, the electrical potential difference across the membrane, $\Delta\Psi$, and the proton concentration difference, ΔpH. The large $\Delta\Psi$, cell interior negative, provides a driving force for the uptake of aminoglycosides, which are polycations at physiological pH. We have compared resistance to the magnitude of $\Delta\Psi$ measured by the uptake of the lipid-soluble cation triphenylmethylphosphonium in EDTA-treated cells (2). Our results suggest that $\Delta\Psi$ is an important factor in determining resistance to aminoglycoside antibiotics.

In wild-type cells, $\Delta\Psi$ can be varied by changing the external pH. Because internal pH and the PMF remain relatively constant, reducing external pH increases the ΔpH component of the PMF, and therefore $\Delta\Psi$ is reduced. The marked increase in resistance at low pH to dihydrostreptomycin and several other aminoglycosides tested was associated with a significant drop in $\Delta\Psi$ (Fig. 1). A *hem* mutant of *Escherichia coli* which is moderately resistant at pH 7.5 had a reduced $\Delta\Psi$ at this pH. At pH 5.5 both $\Delta\Psi$ and

resistance of the mutant were close to those of its wild-type parent (Fig. 1). Proton conductors, such as 2,4-dinitrophenol, will reduce the PMF because they transport protons across the cytoplasmic membrane to short-circuit the PMF. In the presence of 0.6 mM 2,4-dinitrophenol, which moderately inhibits growth, the wild strain became resistant to neomycin at 10 μg/ml (Fig. 2A).

Among the mutants resistant to aminoglyco-

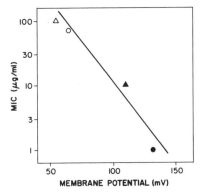

FIG. 1. *Correlation between MIC for dihydrostreptomycin and $\Delta\Psi$. Data are shown for wild-type strain FRAG-5 (O, ●) and its hem-28 derivative (△, ▲). Open symbols are for growth at pH 5.5; closed symbols are for pH 7.5.*

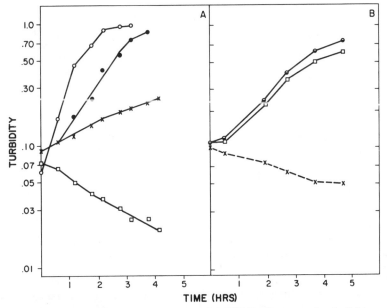

FIG. 2. *(A) Effect of 2,4-dinitrophenol (DNP) on growth inhibition by neomycin of wild-type strain FRAG-5. Symbols: O, control; ●, 0.6 mM DNP; □, 10 μg of neomycin per ml; ×, neomycin plus DNP. (B) Effect of DCCD on proton-leaky uncA strain TK1207. Symbols: O, control; ●, 0.5 mM DCCD; □, 10 μg of neomycin per ml; ×, neomycin plus DCCD.*

sides are ones designated uncA. The uncA mutation abolishes the proton-translocating ATPase, a key component of oxidative phosphorylation, and results in high proton leakage through the proton channel of this ATPase. Treatment with dicyclohexylcarbodiimide (DCCD) abolishes the proton leak by reacting with a protein that forms the proton channel of the ATPase. When a proton-leaky uncA strain was treated with 0.5 mM DCCD, it became susceptible to a concentration of neomycin to which it is resistant in the absence of DCCD (Fig. 2B). This uncA strain had a $\Delta\Psi$ of 78 mV in the absence of DCCD; $\Delta\Psi$ rose to 92 mV after treatment with 0.5 mM DCCD.

In summary, our findings show a correlation between aminoglycoside susceptibility and $\Delta\Psi$. (i) Reducing $\Delta\Psi$ increases resistance: examples include uncA and hem mutants, addition of a proton conductor, and reduction of external pH.

(ii) Increasing $\Delta\Psi$ reduces resistance: the one example studied was addition of DCCD to the proton-leaky uncA mutant. We suggest that the magnitude of $\Delta\Psi$ provides the driving force for aminoglycoside entry, and it is the lower $\Delta\Psi$ in oxidative mutants that accounts for their resistance to aminoglycosides. Our work does not exclude important roles for other factors, such as the permeability barrier of the outer membrane of these gram-negative bacteria.

1. Bryan, L. E., and H. M. Van Den Elzen. 1977. Effects of membrane-energy mutations and cations on streptomycin and gentamicin accumulation by bacteria: a model for entry of streptomycin and gentamicin in susceptible and resistant bacteria. Antimicrob. Agents Chemother. 12:163–177.
2. Damper, P. D., W. Epstein, B. P. Rosen, and E. N. Sorensen. 1979. Thallous ion is accumulated by potassium transport systems in Escherichia coli. Biochemistry 18:4165–4168.

3-N-Aminoglycoside-Acetylating Enzymes Produced by R-Plasmid-Carrying Bacteria Isolated in a General Hospital

R. GOMEZ-LUS,* M. C. RUBIO-CALVO, L. LARRAD, M. NAVARRO, P. LASIERRA, AND M. A. VITORIA

School of Medicine, Saragossa, Spain

Aminoglycoside 3-N-acetyltransferases [AAC(3)s] are widely distributed in clinical isolates of Escherichia coli, Klebsiella pneumoniae, and Pseudomonas aeruginosa. AAC(3)-I was originally isolated from a P. aeruginosa strain by Brzezinska et al. (3); this type of acetylating enzyme confers resistance to gentamicin and sisomicin. AAC(3)-II was isolated from a Klebsiella strain harboring an R plasmid (R176) by Le Goffic et al. (7). This enzyme catalyzes acetylation of the 3-NH_2 group on the deoxystreptamine ring, conferring resistance to gentamicin, sisomicin, tobramycin, and kanamycin A. Biddlecome et al. (2) described a new AAC(3), AAC(3)-III, which inactivates gentamicins, sisomicins, kanamycins, netilmicin, neomycin, and paromomycin. Davies and O'Connor (4) described a plasmid-mediated 3-N-acetylating enzyme, AAC(3)-IV, with a broad substrate range that includes all of the substrates of AAC(3)-III and, in addition, the novel monosubstituted antibiotic apramycin. We have previously isolated several strains of Enterobacteriaceae resistant to gentamicin, sisomicin, tobramycin, netilmicin, and dibekacin but susceptible to kanamycin and amikacin and able to synthetize an acetyltransferase (6). In earlier publications (5, 6) we communicated our primary results concerning the control of plasmids as conducted in the University Hospital of Saragossa; this hospital was inaugurated in 1975 and has an in-patient capacity of approximately 900 beds. From 1 April 1976 to 1 April 1977, a total of 1,360 resistant strains of gram-negative bacilli were isolated; of these, we demonstrated the transference of resistance by conjugation in 428 isolates (31.47%). Among these R-plasmid-harboring strains, 42 (3.08%) conferred resistance to gentamicin and other antibiotics. In our continuing surveillance of resistance patterns, during the period 1 April 1977 to 22 May 1979 we analyzed 2,160 resistant gram-negative bacilli, in which the proportion of gentamicin-resistant isolates increased to 15.50%, a fivefold increase. We report here the AAC(3)s produced by 120 R^+ gentamicin-resistant strains belonging to the genera Escherichia, Klebsiella, Enterobacter, Serratia, Citrobacter, Hafnia, Acinetobacter, and Pseudomonas. Enzymatic activities against 17 aminoglycoside antibiotics were determined as described by Davies and co-workers (1, 3). Two susceptibility profiles were obtained when acetylating activity was determined by the radioactive assay method.

Sixty-nine strains of various species—E. coli

(16), *K. pneumoniae* (15), *Enterobacter cloacae* (4), *Enterobacter aerogenes* (2), *Serratia marcescens* (12), *Hafnia alvei* (1), *Proteus mirabilis* (4), *Proteus morganii* (1), *Proteus vulgaris* (3), *Acinetobacter calcoaceticus* (3), and *P. aeruginosa* (6)—were capable of producing AAC(3)-I and were resistant to gentamicin and sisomicin. Fifty-one strains belonging to the species *E. coli* (15), *K. pneumoniae* (12), *E. cloacae* (9), *Citrobacter freundii* (2) *S. marcescens* (5), *P. mirabilis* (4), *P. morganii* (2), *P. vulgaris* (1), and *Salmonella enteritidis* (1) produced AAC(3)-V and were resistant to gentamicin, sisomicin, tobramycin, dibekacin, and netilmicin. In an attempt to establish a relationship between our provisionally denominated AAC(3)-V and the other classes of AAC(3)s, we decided to compare their substrate ranges and their resistance phenotypes. Thus, we have compared under the same laboratory conditions the following classes of AAC(3) enzymes: I, II, III, IV, and V. First of all we applied the following criteria to assign the AAC(3) group. (i) We confirmed that they did not belong to the AAC(2′) group, since AAC(2′) modifies gentamicin, sisomicin, tobramycin, and netilmicin and also lividomycin A, neomycin B, and butirosin. (ii) We confirmed that the enzymes were not of the AAC(6′) group, since this class, among other distinguishing characteristics, inactivates neomycin B and kanamycins A and B, and is not active on the gentamicin C_1 substrate. (iii) We determined that the substrate profile, was that of an AAC(3), which includes 4,6-deoxystreptamine aminoglycosides.

We may initially classify the five enzymes studied into two groups, the first containing AAC(3)-I, AAC(3)-II, and AAC(3)-V, with activity towards 4,6-deoxystreptamine antibiotics, and the second composed of the AAC(3)-III and AAC(3)-IV, with activity towards 4,6- and 4,5-deoxystreptamine aminoglycosides (Table 1). It should be noted that the first three enzymes possessed the following differential characteristics. (i) AAC(3)-I modified gentamicin and sisomicin, inactivating them, but only moderated tobramycin, kanamycin B, dibekacin, and netilmicin, without inactivation. (ii) AAC(3)-V displayed an elevated activity against gentamicin (100%) and sisomicin (106%) and slightly less against tobramycin, dibekacin, and netilmicin but conferred resistance to all; the activity against kanamycin B was of the order of 37%, and for kanamycin A it is approximately 10%, without inactivation. (iii) For AAC(3)-II there was slightly less activity against sisomicin (89%) than against gentamicin (100%), as compared with the slightly greater activity against sisomicin (106%) than against gentamicin (100%) typical of AAC(3)-V; both enzymes conferred resist-

TABLE 1. *Enzymatic activities* of five AAC(3) classes*

SUBSTRATE	AAC(3)-I E.COLI/ pUZ 1	AAC(3)-II E.COLI/ R 176	AAC(3)-III P.AERUGINOSA PST 1**	AAC(3)-IV E.COLI/ J 225	AAC(3)-V E.COLI/ pUZ 25
GENTAMICIN C₁	100	100	100	100	100
SISOMICIN	147	89	190	118	106
TOBRAMYCIN	32	49	115	120	72
KANAMYCIN A	6	15	71	33	10
KANAMYCIN B	37	50	92	78	37
DIBEKACIN	29	69		126	79
NETILMICIN	38	68		124	63
AMIKACIN	0	0	0	4	0
NEOMYCIN B	0	0	158	94	0
PAROMOMYCIN	0	0	105	53	0
RIBOSTAMYCIN	0	0		89	0
BUTIROSIN	0	0		3	0
LIVIDOMYCIN	0	0			0
APRAMYCIN	0	0		135	0

* Expressed as percentages relative to gentamicin C_1.
** Data taken from reference 2.

TABLE 2. *Effect of 3-N-acetylating enzymes on antibacterial activities of aminoglycosides*

ANTIBIOTIC	AAC(3)-I	AAC(3)-V	AAC(3)-II	AAC(3)-III	AAC(3)-IV
GENTAMICIN C*	+	+	+	+	+
SISOMICIN	+	+	+	+	+
TOBRAMYCIN	-	+	+	+	+
KANAMYCIN A	-	-	+	+	+
NEOMYCIN B	-	-	-	+	+
PAROMOMYCIN	-	-	-	+	+
APRAMYCIN	-	-	-	-	+
5-EPISISOMICIN	-	-	-	+	-

* Gentamicin complex.

ance to gentamicin and sisomicin. The activities against tobramycin (49%), dibekacin (69%), and netilmicin (68%) were expressed as resistance to these antibiotics. In spite of the low degree of substrate activity displayed by the enzyme for kanamycin A (15%), the AAC(3)-II-producing *E. coli* plasmid R176 determined resistance to kanamycin A (16 µg/ml). Paradoxically, AAC(3)-II displayed much greater substrate activity against kanamycin B, but without resistance determination (MIC = 2 µg/ml). The separation of the enzymes of the second group, AAC(3)-III and AAC(3)-IV, is based primarily on the substrate activities for some of the 4,5-deoxystreptamine antibiotics. Basically, AAC(3)-III demonstrated much greater activities against neomycin B (158%) and paromomycin (105%) than did AAC(3)-IV (94 and 53%, respectively), and both enzymes determined resistance to neomycin B and paromomycin. As previously described (4), AAC(3)-IV inactivated apramycin, a valuable distinguishing characteristic. On the other hand, we verified that 5-episisomicin was only inactivated by the AAC(3)-III class. As a practical consequence, the five classes of the AAC(3) enzymes can be easily distinguished by their antibacterial activities (Table 2). We grouped the enzymes from narrow spectrum [AAC(3)-I] to broad [AAC(3)-IV]. The AAC(3)-V activity detected in our strains can be seen to occupy an intermediate position between AAC(3)-I and AAC(3)-II.

1. **Benveniste, R., and J. Davies.** 1971. Enzymatic acetylation of aminoglycoside antibiotics by *Escherichia coli* carrying an R factor. Biochemistry **10**:1787–1796.
2. **Biddlecome, S., M. Haas, J. Davies, G. H. Miller, D. F. Rane, and P. J. L. Daniels.** 1976. Enzymatic modification of aminoglycoside antibiotics: a new 3-N-acetylating enzyme from a *Pseudomonas aeruginosa* isolate. Antimicrob. Agents Chemother. **9**:951–955.
3. **Brzezinska, M., R. Benveniste, J. Davies, D. J. L. Daniels, and J. Weinstein.** 1972. Gentamicin resistance in strains of *Pseudomonas aeruginosa* mediated by enzymatic N-acetylation of the deoxystreptamine moiety. Biochemistry **11**:761–766.
4. **Davies, J., and S. O'Connor.** 1978. Enzymatic modification of aminoglycoside antibiotics: 3-N-acetyltransferase with broad specificity that determines resistance to the novel aminoglycoside apramycin. Antimicrob. Agents Chemother. **14**:69–72.
5. **Gómez-Lus, R.** 1977. Resistencia bacteriana por plásmidos R, p. 275–283. Symposium de infecciones hospitalarias. Monografías Antibióticos S.A., Madrid.
6. **Gómez-Lus, R., M. C. Rubio-Calvo, and L. Larrad Mur.** 1977. Aminoglycoside inactivating enzymes produced by R plasmids of *Escherichia coli, Citrobacter freundii, Klebsiella pneumoniae, Proteus vulgaris, Providencia stuartii,* and *Serratia marcescens.* J. Antimicrob. Chemother **3**(Suppl. C):39–41.
7. **Le Goffic, F., A. Martel, and J. Witchitz.** 1974. 3-N Enzymatic acetylation of gentamicin, tobramycin, and kanamycin by *Escherichia coli* carrying an R factor. Antimicrob. Agents Chemother. **6**:680–684.

Mechanism of Resistance to Penicillin-Aminoglycoside Synergism in *Streptococcus faecium*

CHRISTINE B. WENNERSTEN AND ROBERT C. MOELLERING, JR.*

Infectious Disease Unit, Department of Medicine, Massachusetts General Hospital, and Harvard Medical School, Boston, Massachusetts 02114, U.S.A.*

Streptococcus faecium strains appear to be unique among group D enterococci in that they are consistently resistant to synergism when exposed to penicillin in combination with kanamycin, tobramycin, sisomicin, or netilmicin (2). In addition, some but not all strains are also resistant to penicillin-amikacin and penicillin-streptomycin synergism (2). All strains tested thus far have been killed synergistically by combinations of penicillin with gentamicin (2). Although the mechanism of this resistance to synergism has not been defined, we have demonstrated that these observations have potential clinical significance: only those antimicrobial combinations which produced synergistic killing in vitro were effective in eradicating *S. faecium* from the vegetations of experimentally produced endocarditis in a rabbit model (2). The present study was undertaken to define the mechanism by which resistance to antibiotic synergism occurs among *S. faecium* strains.

Twelve clinical isolates of *S. faecium* from the Bacteriology Laboratory of the Massachusetts General Hospital were utilized in these studies. Antimicrobial susceptibility and synergism determinations, resistance transfer and plasmid curing experiments, identification of plasmid DNA by agarose gel electrophoresis, and assays of aminoglycoside-modifying enzymes were carried out by previously described techniques (1, 2).

Table 1 lists the susceptibilities of 12 strains of *S. faecium* to various aminoglycosidic aminocyclitol antibiotics and details the occurrence or failure of occurrence of synergism when a given strain was exposed to each aminoglycoside in combination with penicillin. The penicillin-gentamicin combination was synergistic against all strains, whereas penicillin-kanamycin, penicillin-tobramycin, and penicillin-netilmicin failed to show synergism against any of the organisms. Penicillin-streptomycin combinations were synergistic only against those strains with MICs of streptomycin of ≤2,000 μg/ml, and penicillin-amikacin was synergistic only against those with MICs of kanamycin of ≤2,000 μg/ml.

Treatment of strain 758 with novobiocin resulted in the loss of high-level resistance to streptomycin and kanamycin but did not significantly alter the MIC of amikacin, tobramycin, or gentamicin (Table 2). In contrast to the parent strains, a novobiocin-treated strain (758A) which had lost high-level resistance to streptomycin and kanamycin was killed synergistically

TABLE 1. *Correlation of MIC of various aminoglycosides with presence or absence of synergism when combined with penicillins against S. faecium*

Strain	Streptomycin		Kanamycin		Amikacin		Tobramycin		Netilmicin		Gentamicin	
	MIC (μg/ml)	Synergism	MIC (μg/ml)	Synergism	MIC (μg/ml)	Synergism	MIC (μg/ml)	Synergism	MIC (μg/ml)	Synergism	MIC (μg/ml)	Synergism
63	>32,000	No	>32,000	No	250	No	1,000	No	125	No	16	Yes
758	>32,000	No	>32,000	No	250	No	500	No	125	No	16	Yes
1140	8,000	No	>32,000	No	1,000	No	2,000	No	250	No	16	Yes
6400	>32,000	No	>32,000	No	1,000	No	1,000	No	250	No	31	Yes
1695	>32,000	No	250	No	62	Yes	250	No	125	No	16	Yes
6216	8,000	No	500	No	62	Yes	500	No	125	No	16	Yes
4379	125	Yes	1,000	No	250	Yes	1,000	No	250	No	31	Yes
4901	125	Yes	2,000	No	125	Yes	8,000	No	500	No	62	Yes
4586	125	Yes	1,000	No	125	Yes	2,000	No	500	No	31	Yes
3482	62	Yes	500	No	125	Yes	1,000	No	125	No	62	Yes
3800	250	Yes	2,000	No	500	Yes	2,000	No	250	No	31	Yes
4900	125	Yes	2,000	No	250	Yes	4,000	No	500	No	62	Yes

TABLE 2. *MIC of aminoglycosides, synergism, and aminoglycoside-modifying activity in S. faecium strain 758 and a novobiocin-treated derivative, strain 758A* [a]

Drug	Strain 758					Strain 758A				
	MIC (μg/ml)	Synergism with penicillin	Aminoglycoside-modifying activity			MIC (μg/ml)	Synergism with penicillin	Aminoglycoside-modifying activity		
			AAC	APH	ANT			AAC	APH	ANT
Streptomycin ..	>32,000	No	0	0	+	125	Yes	0	0	0
Kanamycin	>32,000	No	+	+	0	500	No	+	0	0
Amikacin	250	No	0	+	0	31	Yes	0	0	0
Tobramycin ...	500	No	+	0	0	250	No	+	0	0
Gentamicin	16	Yes	0	0	0	31	Yes	0	0	0

[a] AAC, 6'-Acetyltransferase; APH, 3'-phosphotransferase; ANT, adenylyltransferase; 0, no detectable enzyme activity present; +, enzyme activity present.

by penicillin plus streptomycin and penicillin plus amikacin; however, it retained resistance to penicillin-kanamycin and penicillin-tobramycin synergism. Agarose gel electrophoresis of plasmid DNA from strains 758 and 758A revealed that strain 758A had lost a plasmid band (approximate molecular weight, 15,000 to 20,000) which was present in the parent strain. Transfer experiments revealed the acquisition of high-level resistance to streptomycin and kanamycin in the transconjugants from a mating of strain 758 with *S. faecalis* strain JH2-7. Other strains of *S. faecium* (e.g., 1140) with high-level resistance to streptomycin and kanamycin contained a different plasmid (approximate molecular weight, 40,000) which could also be cured by novobiocin treatment that resulted in loss of high-level resistance. Assays of aminoglycoside-modifying activity revealed the presence of a 3'-phosphotransferase [(APH (3')] with activity against kanamycin and amikacin (Table 2), as well as against butirosin, lividomycin A, neomycin, and ribostamycin, but not against streptomycin, dideoxykanamycin B, tobramycin, gen-

tamicin, sisomicin, and netilmicin in strain 758 but not in 758A. In addition, extracts from strain 758 but not 758A exhibited adenyltransferase activity against streptomycin (Table 2).

Studies of antibiotic synergism utilizing the aminoglycoside analogs gentamicin B and gentamicin B₁ revealed that neither produced synergism against strain 758. However, against novobiocin-cured strain 758A which had lost APH and adenyltransferase activity gentamicin B₁ (but not gentamicin B) was synergistic in combination with penicillin. Gentamicin B and B₁ differ only by the presence of a methyl group on the 6' carbon atom of gentamicin B₁ but not gentamicin B. This suggested that the resistance to synergism when penicillin was combined with gentamicin B (and other aminoglycosidic aminocyclitols, including kanamycin and tobramycin) might be due to enzymatic modification (acetylation) at the 6' position. However, examination of extracts from a number of strains of *S. faecium* revealed only very low-level (two to three times baseline) acetylyltransferase activity against kanamycin and tobramycin, despite testing under a wide range of temperature, pH, and substrate conditions. After serial passage on agar plates with increasing concentrations of kanamycin or tobramycin, strains of *S. faecium* would grow readily on plates containing tobramycin or kanamycin in concentrations of 4,000 to 6,000 µg/ml. Sonic extracts of strains taken from these plates contained definite acetyltransferase activity. The substrate profile of this acetyltransferase confirmed that it was a 6'-acetyltransferase [(AAC (6')] with excellent activity against kanamycins A and B, tobramycin, neomycin, netilmicin, and sisomicin. To date, we have not definitely been able to transfer this enzymatic activity from strains of *S. faecium* to susceptible recipient strains of *S. faecalis* nor have we been able to cure it with novobiocin or other plasmid-curing agents.

These studies thus define several of the mechanisms of the resistance to antimicrobial synergism among *S. faecium* strains. High-level resistance to streptomycin and resistance to penicillin-streptomycin synergism among *S. faecium* strains appears to be determined by a plasmid-mediated adenylyltransferase which modifies streptomycin. Although the genes determining this activity may occur on plasmids of various molecular weights in different strains of *S. faecium*, in all cases tested thus far it appears that the same plasmid also bears the genetic information necessary for the production of a phosphotransferase [APH (3')] which inactivates kanamycin and amikacin and results in resistance to synergism when penicillin is combined with kanamycin or amikacin. This appears similar to the mechanism of resistance to penicillin-streptomycin, penicillin-kanamycin, and penicillin-amikacin synergism which we have recently described in *S. faecalis* (1).

The acetyltransferase [AAC (6')] which we have found in *S. faecium* has not been previously described among streptococci. Although we have not tested all of our strains for enzyme activity, the consistent resistance of *S. faecium* to synergism when exposed to combinations of penicillin with kanamycin, tobramycin, netilmicin, and sisomicin would suggest that AAC [6'] occurs in all of the strains of *S. faecium* which we have seen thus far. Our preliminary studies raise the possibility that the enzyme is inducible. Since we have been unsuccessful in transferring or curing this resistance, it is impossible to be certain whether it is chromosomally mediated or whether the genes that code for its production are found on a plasmid which might also bear the genetic information that defines some or all the species characteristics of *S. faecium*. Irrespective of its genetic basis, the presence of this newly defined enzyme seems to account for the unique resistance of *S. faecium* to synergism by penicillin in combination with kanamycin, tobramycin, netilmicin, or sisomicin. Indeed, among our strains, only penicillin plus gentamicin consistently produced synergistic killing of *S. faecium*.

1. Krogstad, D. J., T. R. Korfhagen, R. C. Moellering, Jr., C. B. Wennersten, M. N. Swartz, S. Perzynski, and J. Davies. 1978. Aminoglycoside-inactivating enzymes in clinical isolates of *Streptococcus faecalis*: an explanation for resistance to antibiotic synergism. J. Clin. Invest. **62**:480–486.
2. Moellering, R. C., Jr., O. M. Korzeniowski, M. A. Sande, and C. B. Wennersten. 1979. Species-specific resistance to antimicrobial synergism among enterococci. J. Infect. Dis. **140**:203–208.

Mechanism of Fusidic Acid Resistance in *Escherichia coli*

ROLF G. WERNER* AND KLAUS H. DANECK

Dr. Karl Thomae GmbH, D-7950, Biberach an der Riss, Federal Republic of Germany

Fusidic acid acts on protein synthesis by stabilizing the ribosome-elongation factor G (EFG)-guanosine diphosphate (GDP) complex and inhibiting the ribosomal binding of aminoacyl-tRNA. Chromosomal fusidic acid-resistant mutants possess a modified EFG with a decreased affinity for the antibiotic. The plasmid-determined resistance in *Staphylococcus aureus* results from an altered cell envelope of the bacteria (1). An *Escherichia coli* DB10 mutant is, in respect to the wild-type strain, with susceptibility to 0.6 µg of erythromycin/ml, 10 µg of fusidic acid/ml, and 5 µg of penicillin G/ml, susceptible to antibiotics which normally fail to penetrate into gram-negative bacteria. Insertion of the R factors R1-1, 222, R28, and R57b results in resistant strains for which MIC values are comparable to those of the wild-type strain *E. coli* K-12 (2). Generally, such an R factor-mediated resistance manifests itself in *Enterobacteriaceae* as an enzymatic inactivation or as a change in the permeability to the antibiotic.

When the biological activity of 10 µg of fusidic acid/ml was determined in the presence of *E. coli* DB10, *E. coli* K-12, and the *E. coli* DB10 strains containing the R factors R1-1, 222, R28, and R57b, no reduction of the activity could be determined, and after extraction from the culture broth no metabolic products could be detected by thin-layer chromatography. These results indicate that there is no enzymatic inactivation of fusidic acid, but that the inactivity of the drug against resistant strains must be due to a decreased permeability. Therefore the protein, lipopolysaccharide, phospholipid, and fatty acid content of all the *E. coli* strains was examined.

Cell envelope protein fractions were prepared by the method of Wu (6) and were separated by disk electrophoresis, which was evaluated by densitometry. For all strains investigated the same protein content could be detected without significant differences in the intensity of the resulting fractions. The lipopolysaccharide sugars were isolated by the method of Galanos et al. (4). After hydrolysis of the lipopolysaccharides and quantitative analysis of the sugar components by gas chromatography, the susceptible, the wild-type, and all R factor-containing strains possessed in the core moiety the same amount of the sugars D-galactose, D-glucose, D-glucosamine, and L-glycero-D-mannoheptose. Bacteria with lipopolysaccharide types Rc, Rd$_1$, Rd$_2$, and Re, displaying a decreased level of galactose and lacking glucosamine, have a higher susceptibility to antibiotics which cannot penetrate into gram-negative bacteria (5). Therefore, if the lipopolysaccharide of the core is identical in susceptible and resistant *E. coli* strains and if galactose and glucosamine are still present, the susceptibility of the *E. coli* DB10 strain could not be explained by the composition of the lipopolysaccharide.

The responsibility of the outer membrane phospholipid composition for the fusidic acid resistance in wild-type and R factor-containing strains, in contrast to the susceptibility of *E. coli* DB10, was determined by investigation of the lysophosphatidylethanolamine, phosphatidylethanolamine, and phosphatidylglycerol. After incubation of the *E. coli* strains for 24 h at 20, 30, and 43°C, the cells were broken and, by use of the method of Folch and Lebaran (3), the phospholipids were extracted and separated by thin-layer chromatography on silica gel; their phosphate content was determined spectrophotometrically. Whereas all strains displayed a temperature-dependent decrease in the overall phospholipid content, the susceptible strain *E. coli* DB10 possessed a smaller amount of phosphatidylethanolamine than the resistant strains (Fig. 1). In all cases the content of cardiolipin

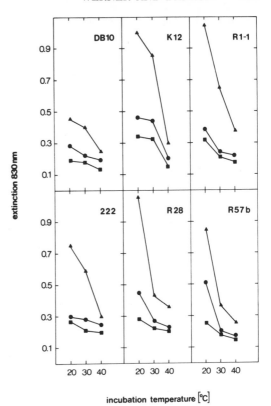

FIG. 1. *Amount of (▲) phosphatidylethanolamine, (●) lysophosphatidylethanolamine, and (■) phosphatidylglycerol after separation by thin-layer chromatography and colorimetric determination at 830 nm in different E. coli strains. E = 0.350 corresponds to 1 µmol of phospholipid.*

was much below that of phosphatidylglycerol and is not shown in Fig. 1.

Because in *E. coli* the fatty acid content remains constant in the stationary phase, the fatty acids of the total phospholipids were analyzed at the end of the logarithmic phase after incubation at 20, 30, and 43°C. After hydrolysis the percentage composition of the fatty acids was calculated after separation by gas chromatography. The results in Table 1 demonstrate that the resistant strains had a larger amount of cyclic fatty acid than the susceptible strain *E. coli* DB10. Otherwise, with an increase in temperature the content of unsaturated fatty acids decreased, whereas the cyclic fatty acid content increased. This implies that at a higher temperature the cyclopropane synthetase is stimulated and the resistance to antibiotic should increase. When the single phospholipids were analyzed for their specific fatty acid content, there was a significant decrease of cyclopropane fatty acids

TABLE 1. *Percentage fatty acid composition of the total phospholipids in relation to growth temperature in the fusidic acid-susceptible and -resistant E. coli strains*

Fatty acid	Temp (°C)	E. coli strain					
		DB10	K-12	R1-1	222	R28	R57b
14:0	20	4.5	1.8	1.4	1.8	1.0	1.5
	30	6.7	5.4	4.2	2.9	2.7	3.1
	43	7.2	6.5	4.9	5.4	3.0	4.7
14:1	20	0.4	0.2	0.1	0.1	0.1	0.2
	30	0.5	0.2	0.1	0.1	0.1	0.2
	43	0.8	0.3	0.1	0.2	0.1	0.1
15 cy[a]	20	—	—	—	—	—	—
	30	—	0.4	0.1	0.1	—	—
	43	0.1	3.1	1.7	0.8	0.4	0.7
16:0	20	43.0	42.9	36.8	40.8	43.3	40.3
	30	41.3	43.8	41.6	40.4	50.5	44.2
	43	44.9	45.5	45.3	49.6	49.2	48.3
16:1	20	34.9	22.8	19.2	18.9	19.9	22.7
	30	34.6	11.4	11.2	17.2	6.7	3.3
	43	27.5	6.2	3.9	5.5	9.7	1.8
17 cy	20	0.7	14.7	11.6	14.6	9.4	12.5
	30	1.2	22.7	21.8	17.5	21.2	30.0
	43	9.9	28.4	30.7	28.4	19.9	32.0
18:0	20	0.3	0.4	0.6	0.5	1.2	0.4
	30	0.3	0.4	0.5	0.4	0.5	0.4
	43	0.5	0.4	0.6	0.5	0.8	0.5
18:1	20	16.2	16.5	29.0	21.2	21.6	21.6
	30	15.4	13.4	17.7	19.6	14.5	10.6
	43	8.9	6.7	6.2	5.5	12.3	3.2
19 cy	20	—	0.7	1.3	2.1	3.5	0.8
	30	—	2.3	2.8	2.9	3.8	8.2
	43	0.2	2.9	6.6	4.1	4.6	8.7

[a] Cyclic.

from lysophosphatidylethanolamine to phosphatidylethanolamine in all strains investigated.

In conclusion, the higher susceptibility of the mutant *E. coli* DB10 to erythromycin, fusidic acid, and penicillin G manifests itself first as a loss of the enzyme cyclopropane fatty acid synthetase and second as a decrease in the phosphatidylethanolamine content. On the other hand, it is obvious from these results that the R factors R1-1, 222, R28, and R57b code for a cyclopropane fatty acid synthetase as well as for enzymes involved in the synthesis of phosphatidylethanolamine.

1. **Copra, I.** 1976. Mechanisms of resistance to fusidic acid in Staphylococcus aureus. J. Gen. Microbiol. **96**:229–238.

2. **Datta, N., R. W. Hedges, D. Becker, and J. Davies.** 1974. Plasmid-determined fusidic acid resistance in the enterobacteriaceae. J. Gen. Microbiol. **83**:191–196.

3. **Folch, J., and F. N. Lebaran.** 1956. The chemistry of the phosphoinositides. Can. J. Biochem. Physiol. **34**:305–319.

4. **Galanos, C., O. Lüderitz, and O. Westphal.** 1969. A new method for extraction of R-lipopolysaccharides. Eur. J. Biochem. **9**:245–249.

5. **Nikaido, H.** 1976. Outer membrane of Salmonella typhimurium transmembrane diffusion of some hydrophobic substances. Biochim. Biophys. Acta **433**:118–132.

6. **Wu, H. C.** 1972. Isolation and characterization of an Escherichia coli mutant with alteration in the outer membrane proteins of the cell envelope. Biochim. Biophys. Acta **290**:274–289.

Mecillinam Resistance and Small Cell Volume: the In Vivo Selection of an *Escherichia coli* Mutant

ALAN G. BARBOUR* AND LEONARD W. MAYER

Division of Infectious Diseases, Department of Medicine, and Department of Pathology, University of Utah College of Medicine, Salt Lake City, Utah 84132, U.S.A.*

We have studied an *Escherichia coli* mutant, isolated from a clinical specimen, with the phenotype of mecillinam resistance, a mucoid character, and a smaller cell mass and volume when compared with the wild type. Mecillinam-susceptible, rod-shaped bacteria become giant spheres during exposure to a wide range of concentrations of mecillinam (2). Although mecillinam had the expected morphological effect of rounding on this mutant (RF292), the mutant's smaller size permitted completion of septation and, thus, division in the presence of mecillinam.

A granulocytopenic patient had a relapse of *E. coli* bacteremia after mecillinam therapy. The pretreatment blood isolate (RF81), the post-treatment isolate (RF292), and a spontaneous revertant of RF292 (RF293) had the same biotype and serotype (O6 H1). RF292 differed from RF81 and RF293 in having mucoid colonies and in being resistant to mecillinam (Table 1). There was slight cross-resistance to thienamycin but not to other β-lactam antibiotics or to non-β-lactam antibiotics, dyes, detergents, azide, and EDTA. RF292 did not possess detectable β-lactamase activity. Neither intact cells nor sonicates inactivated mecillinam. Although RF292 carried a 1.8-megadalton plasmid, both RF81 and RF293 had identically sized plasmids. RF292's plasmid did not express resistance when attempts were made to transform the plasmid into a susceptible recipient. Mucoid, mecillinam-resistant mutants were selected from both RF81 and RF293 plated on mecillinam-containing media.

As one measure of affinity of mecillinam for its target, the minimal concentrations of mecillinam to cause morphological change (MMCC),

i.e., rounding, were determined. In Mueller-Hinton broth the MMCCs for RF81, RF292, and RF293 were 0.015 μg/ml and the MICs were 0.062, 8.0, and 0.062 μg/ml, respectively. The MBC was 8.0 μg/ml for all strains. By the method of Spratt (5), RF292 was found to have penicillin-binding protein 2 (PBP2) in its inner membrane. Binding of [^{14}C]penicillin to PBP2 in isolated membranes was prevented by prior incubation with 0.125 μg of mecillinam/ml.

RF292 has two colony types: radially striated (S) and nonstriated (NS). In distinction to NS colonies, S colonies were nonmucoid at 42°C and did not manifest striations in the presence of mecillinam or on media with high salt concentrations. The frequency of transition of S to NS colonies was 10^{-1} to 10^{-2} per cell per generation. The mechanism of this transition, which resembles phase variation, is unknown.

Growth rates, in minutes per doubling, for RF81, RF292 (S), RF292 (NS), and RF293 were 19.5, 23.6, 26.5, and 19.8 min, respectively. Mean cell masses (optical density at 450 nm/10^9 cells) for these strains were 9.1, 7.6, 3.2, and 9.5, respectively, during early-log-phase growth in Luria broth. When rapidly growing bacteria were exposed to mecillinam, the mean cell masses of both RF81 and RF293 increased exponentially while those of RF292 (S) and RF292 (NS) decreased slightly (Fig. 1). The large mecillinam-treated cells of RF81 and RF293 were sevenfold more susceptible to osmotic lysis in water than the smaller spherical cells of RF292.

In these studies we found the mecillinam resistance to be the result of a chromosomal mutation which occurred and was selected for in vivo. The mechanism of resistance was not in-

TABLE 1. *Susceptibility of E. coli strains to β-lactam antibiotics*[a]

Strain	MIC (μg/ml)					
	Mecillinam	Thienamycin	6-APA[b]	Ampicillin	Cephalothin	Cephalexin
RF81	0.125	0.5	32	4	4	4
RF292	16	4	32	4	4	4
RF293	0.125	0.5	32	2	2	4

[a] Mueller-Hinton agar containing serial twofold dilutions of antibiotic were inoculated with 10^4 colony-forming units of bacteria. Plates were incubated for 18 h at 35°C. The MIC was defined as the lowest concentration of antibiotic which inhibited colony formation.

[b] 6-Aminopenicillanic acid.

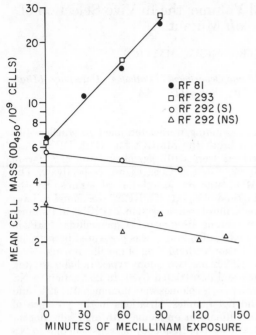

FIG. 1. *Mean cell mass (optical density at 450 nm/10⁹ cells measured by Coulter counter) of growing E. coli strains during exposure to 10 µg of mecillinam per ml in Luria broth. Mecillinam was added to cultures when cell concentration reached 5 × 10⁶ bacteria/ml. Cell counts were continued until the onset of lysis. S, radially striated; NS, nonstriated.*

activation, nonspecific or specific permeability change, or an alteration of binding of mecillinam to the target, PBP2. The resistance of RF292, notably the NS colony type, was associated with a slower growth rate and lesser cell mass and volume when compared with the wild type and

a revertant. A correlation of growth rate and cell volume of bacteria when the nutrient composition of media is altered has been long recognized (4). RF81 and RF293 were resistant to mecillinam but susceptible to ampicillin when grown on minimal media (M9 glucose). A smaller cell volume allowed complete septation of mecillinam-induced spheres. Bacteria unable to finish septation enlarged and became more unstable in a low-osmolality medium. The large number of genes in which a mutation results in the phenotype of slower growth rate may explain the high frequency of mecillinam-resistant "variants" encountered in vitro (1, 3). These mutants, when they occur in vivo, may be less virulent because of slower growth rate. However, they may also allow persistence of infection and relapse of illness.

This work was supported in part by Public Health Service grants AI 107011 and AI 11073 from the National Institute of Allergy and Infectious Diseases and by a grant from Hoffmann-La Roche, Inc.

1. **Greenwood, D., and F. O'Grady.** 1973. FL1060: a new beta lactam antibiotic with novel properties. J. Clin. Pathol. **26**:1–6.
2. **Melchior, N. H., J. Blom, L. Tybring, and A. Birch-Anderson.** 1973. Light and electron microscopy of the early response of *Escherichia coli* to a 6β-amidinopenicillanic acid (FL1060). Acta Pathol. Microbiol. Scand. Sect. B **81**:393–407.
3. **Neu, H. C.** 1976. Mecillinam, a novel penicillanic acid derivative with unusual activity against gram-negative bacteria. Antimicrob. Agents Chemother. **9**:793–799.
4. **Schaechter, M., O. Maaloe, and N. O. Kjeldgaard.** 1958. Dependency on medium and temperature of cell size and chemical composition during balanced growth of *Salmonella typhimurium*. J. Gen. Microbiol. **19**:592–606.
5. **Spratt, B. G.** 1977. Properties of the penicillin-binding proteins of *Escherichia coli* K12. Eur. J. Biochem. **72**:341–352.

Prevalence of Drug Resistance of Bacteria (1975–1978): Results of an International Study

H. LANGMAACK

Paul-Ehrlich-Gesellschaft, "Resistance Group," Klinikhygiene, University Hospital, Freiburg, Federal Republic of Germany

Since 1975 the "Resistance Group" of the Paul-Ehrlich-Gesellschaft für Chemotherapie has studied the prevalence of drug resistance of members of the *Enterobacteriaceae* family, *Pseudomonas aeruginosa*, *Streptococcus faecalis*, and *Staphylococcus aureus* in Central Europe. Twenty-seven departments of medical microbiology in West Germany, Switzerland, and

Austria collaborated in this study. Each laboratory used standardized methods for identification of the bacterial strains and for susceptibility testing. Every year during 1 week in May and November all data on the clinical isolates tested in each laboratory were sent to a computer station for evaluation (4).

As an example I should like to demonstrate

the prevalence of drug resistance of *Escherichia coli*. There has been no significant change in resistance over a 4-year period; however, there may be two exceptions. Firstly, the resistance of *E. coli* to co-trimoxazole seems to have risen from 8 to 16%. This change may have several explanations: it may be due to an increase of R factors coding for trimethoprim resistance markers, to an increase of transposons with the same resistant markers (H. Richards, IV Symposium of Antibiotic Resistance, Abstract 4, Smolinice, Czechoslovakia, June 1979), to a temporary change in resistance, to a local outbreak of resistant bacteria, or to an increase of drug usage.

Secondly, the resistance of *E. coli* to cephalothin varied from 60 to 32%. This change is probably due to the method of evaluation applied (Fig. 1). The breakpoint for sorting out the resistant strains was a zone diameter of 21 mm, as recommended by the German DIN Committee in 1976. Now, in September 1979 (2), the commission has changed the breakpoint to 18 mm. After evaluating, we found a percentage change of 20 to 12% instead of 60 to 30% and not such a drastic change in resistance. To determine which breakpoint is correct, we plotted the

zone diameter against the frequency of *E. coli* strains (Fig. 2).

Alestic et al. (1) recommended that a breakpoint should never divide the wild-type susceptible population but should mark the end of this population, provided that the breakpoint is not inconsistent with clinical experience or the pharmacokinetics of the drug. It is obvious, therefore, that the breakpoint of 21 mm does not represent the real number of *E. coli* strains which are different from the wild-type strains as far as their resistance to cephalothin is concerned, because it divides the bell-shaped curve into two parts.

The 18-mm breakpoint divides the curve roughly at the first quarter, but does not mark the end of the population. We found (W. Mannheim and W. Rehm, Infection, in press) that a breakpoint of 8 to 13 mm separates the strains which developed a mechanism of resistance to cephalothin from the wild-type population. The breakpoint of 8 mm includes ampicillin-resistant strains of *E. coli*, whereas the breakpoint of 13 mm does not. It is worth mentioning that our 13-mm breakpoint is close to that of the NCCLS (3), which is related to MIC values and was

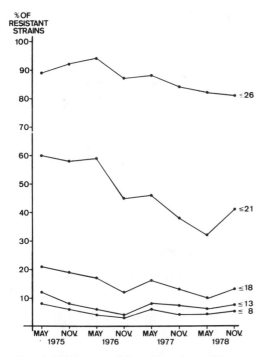

FIG. 1. *Percentage of E. coli strains resistant to cephalothin based on different breakpoints. Zone diameters (millimeters) are shown at the right. (German-DIN-Committee, 1976, 1979, Paul-Ehrlich-Gesellschaft, Resistance Group, 1979.)*

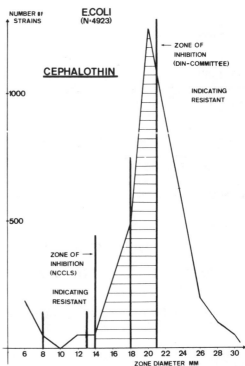

FIG. 2. *Distribution of E. coli strains resistant to cephalothin after plotting the frequency of strains against the zone diameter.*

TABLE 1. *Percentage of resistant bacteria (1975-1978)*[a]

Drug	Escherichia coli		Klebsiella pneumoniae		Proteus mirabilis		Pseudomonas aeruginosa		Streptococcus faecalis	
	Total	Percent	Total	Percent	Total	Percent	Total	Percent	Total	Percent
Ampicillin	4,799	22.1	1,500	92.2	1,442	16.2	1,308	99.2	1,437	1.18
Cephalothin	4,827	46.9	1,536	43.3	1,447	17.0	1,304	99.2	1,419	91.7
Tetracycline	4,810	34.5	1,526	34.7	1,429	95.6	1,323	76.1	1,411	66.9
Chloramphenicol	4,826	19.1	1,536	39.0	1,292	42.3	1,322	88.3	1,437	30.9
Gentamicin	4,839	2.1	1,540	17.6	1,449	3.45	1,337	11.3	1,427	78.3
Tobramycin	1,555	0.64	456	9.43	458	1.96	1,233	5.43	497	81.08
Sisomicin	1,557	0.25	456	3.95	450	1.53	914	6.8	497	43.8
Amikacin	1,554	0.32	456	0.65	457	1.09	965	3.21	497	96.9
Carbenicillin	4,844	18.0	1,525	60.5	1,307	10.5	1,339	18.7	1,213	0.98
Nalidixic acid	4,670	2.3	1,506	10.2	1,273	4.8	1,287	92.5	254	98.4
Nitrofurantoin	4,690	3.1	1,520	8.48	447	60.0	1,294	96.9	1,258	2.5
Co-trimoxazole	4,823	10.3	236	35.6	227	11.09	230	92.6	—	—
Kanamycin	4,772	13.4	1,497	37.2	1,305	11.7	1,308	92.5	255	97.3
Streptomycin	4,611	24.1	1,458	26.2	1,271	13.7	1,275	57.8	1,357	97.4
Erythromycin	—	—	—	—	—	—	—	—	1,393	29.07
Penicillin	—	—	—	—	—	—	—	—	—	—

[a] Resistance standards DIN-58940, part 3, 1976 (2).

determined after considering the pharmacokinetics and the clinical responsiveness of cephalothin.

The percentage of resistant strains based on the 8- to 13-mm breakpoints is shown at the bottom of Fig. 1.

Since we did not find any change in resistance from 1975 through 1978, we can demonstrate the prevalence of resistance of the most frequently isolated bacteria by summarizing all periods (Table 1).

Conclusions. It is impossible to give an overview of all of the work of the multicenter study in this small space. Therefore, I want to emphasize some of the important problems which appeared during our study. (i) Since 1975 there has been no big shift in the prevalence of drug resistance in the most frequently isolated bacteria in Central Europe, a fact which does not exclude changes in local areas. (ii) By sophisticated evaluation of the data it is possible

to find mistakes in the method and in the evaluation of data, especially that concerned with breakpoints, as I have demonstrated with the cephalothin resistance of *E. coli*.

1. **Alestic, K., K. Dornbusch, C. Ericson, L. O. Kallings, C. Kamme, F. Nordbring, R. Norby, and G. Wallmark.** 1978. Resistenzbestamming av bakterier: NY indeling i känslighetsgrupper S., I ode R. Läkartidningen **75**:4346–4348.
2. **Deutsches Institut für Normung e.V.** 1976–1979. Empfindlichkeitsprüfung von bakteriellen Krankheitserregern (außer Mykobakterien) gegen Chemotherapeutica. Entwurf November 1976–September 1979, DIN 58940, Teil 3. Beuthe-Verlag, Berlin.
3. **National Committee for Clinical Laboratory Standards.** 1975. Performance standards for antimicrobial disc susceptibility test. NCCLS, Villanova, Pa.
4. **Paul-Ehrlich-Gesellschaft für Chemotherapie e.V. Arbeitsgemeinschaft "Resistenz."** 1978. Empfindlichkeit klinischer Isolate einiger Enterobacteriacaen, sowie Pseud. aerug., S. aureus und S. faecalis gegenüber verschiedener Chemotherapeutica. Infection **6**:35–44.

Average Percent Antibiotic Resistance in Isolates from Multiple Centers

INTERNATIONAL SURVEY OF ANTIBIOTIC RESISTANCE GROUP; T. F. O'BRIEN,*
COORDINATOR

Peter Bent Brigham Hospital and Harvard Medical School, Boston, Massachusetts 02115, U.S.A.

The International Survey of Antibiotic Resistance Group consists of investigators from 30 centers on five continents who collect and compare susceptibility testing data on clinical isolates from their centers (1). Data on the isolates, including inhibition zone diameter measurements, are computer filed and analyzed by an increasing number of programs for quality con-

TABLE 1. *Species in-day indexes*

Center no.	In-day index[a]					
	Escherichia coli	*Enterobacter cloacae*	*Klebsiella pneumoniae*	*Proteus mirabilis*	*Acinetobacter calcoaceticus*	*Serratia marcescens*
1	1.0	1.8	2.4	1.9	3.2	5.3
25	0.9	2.1	1.4	1.6	2.4	1.5
68	0.8		1.2	1.2	2.3	1.4
80	0.5	0.3	0.8	1.2		1.5
20	0.8	0.9	1.1	0.7	0.9	1.8
19	2.3	4.4	3.3	3.5	2.0	1.7
15	0.7	2.2	1.6	0.8	2.6	1.8
64	0.5	1.1	1.1	1.0	1.4	0.6
88	1.4	2.4	2.9	1.7		4.5
78	0.8	4.0	1.7	1.1	1.0	1.0
60	1.7	3.0	2.7	2.8	2.0	9.4
51	0.8	1.3	1.5		1.5	2.0

[a] In-day index = number of isolates after 8 days of hospitalization/number of isolates during first 8 patient hospital days.

trol, for comparability of sampling, for comparative prevalence of antibiotic resistance, and for presumptive identification of antibiotic resistance mechanisms.

Table 1 illustrates a sampling analysis done on isolates from 12 of these centers. It lists for each of several species of gram-negative bacilli the ratio of number of isolates obtained during the first 8 days of patient hospitalization to the number obtained after 8 days of hospitalization. Values were roughly similar for *Escherichia coli*, suggesting that patterns of culturing over the course of hospitalization in the centers did not differ greatly (2). Other species generally had values one or more times higher than *E. coli*, indicating that they were more often isolated later in patient hospitalization. One center (center 19), which had proportionally higher values for all species, is a rehabilitation hospital with a prolonged average duration of patient hospitalization.

Previous studies have shown substantial differences in prevalence of resistance to individual antibiotics in different parts of the world (3). To compare overall prevalence of antibiotic resistance, we have explored the use of the average percent antibiotic resistance (APAR), defined as the average of the percentages of resistance to each of a set of antibiotics. We computed APAR values for all gram-negative bacilli in samples of isolates recorded from 1976 to 1978 from laboratories of 22 collaborating investigators in Belgium, Brazil, Chile, Colombia, Czechoslovakia, France, Greece, Italy, Israel, Norway, South Africa, Spain, the United States, and Venezuela. The test set of antibiotics, tetracycline, chloramphenicol, kanamycin, ampicillin, cephalothin, and gentamicin, was selected because they are commonly tested and resistance to each is car-

TABLE 2. *P. mirabilis isolates resistant to multiple antibiotics*

Center no.	% Isolates resistant to no. of antibiotics:						
	0	1	2	3	4	5	6
68	1.5	70.7	15.9	7.0	3.5	1.0	0.5
80	2.1	58.4	20.0	12.3	4.9	1.8	0.5
86	0.8	4.8	23.4	16.1	33.8	20.2	0.8
87	0	8.9	28.9	35.6	8.9	15.2	2.2
15	1.3	61.1	9.0	9.7	11.8	6.6	0.6
64	0	69.2	4.8	14.4	8.7	2.9	0
60	0	18.4	50.6	8.1	11.5	2.5	9.2
51	1.4	55.0	22.9	14.0	4.4	2.4	0
1	4.6	85.2	7.8	1.8	0.4	0.1	0
25	1.3	81.9	13.6	2.8	0.3	0.1	0
20	1.7	83.2	12.2	1.7	0.8	0.5	0
3	2.8	85.9	9.9	1.4	0	0	0
21	1.3	94.7	4.0	0	0	0	0

ried mostly by different genes. APAR values for individual centers ranged from 16 to 58, with a median of 40.

The APAR values gave an indication of overall levels of antibiotic resistance and formed the basis of subsequent analyses of multiple variables to determine which were responsible for the differences in these levels. Table 2 is an example of this kind of analysis. It examines for 13 centers the percentages of *Proteus mirabilis* isolates resistant to different numbers of the six antibiotics used in the test set. The five centers listed at the bottom of Table 2 (1, 25, 20, 3, and 21) are located in North America, and the eight above are from other parts of the world. Resistance to multiple antibiotics appears strikingly less prevalent in the lower set.

The relationship shown in Table 2 proved to be a major determinant of the APAR values.

Although less striking in other bacterial species, centers with higher overall APAR values had many more isolates resistant to multiple antibiotics. From center to center there was considerable variation in the species in which multiple resistance predominated. Centers with the higher APAR values tended to have multiple resistance in multiple species. The suggestion, yet unproven, from these observations would be that APAR value correlates with prevalence of plasmids or with prevalence of plasmid-mediated resistance genes. This is supported by the observation of one center in the survey which experienced an appreciable rise in its APAR value after the introduction of a plasmid mediating resistance to multiple antibiotics which

came to circulate in many nosocomial strains in the center.

1. **The International Antibiotic Resistance Survey Group and T. F. O'Brien.** 1978. Multicenter sensitivity studies. International collaborative antibiotic resistance survey, p. 534–536. *In* Current chemotherapy. Proceedings of the 10th International Congress of Chemotherapy. American Society for Microbiology, Washington, D.C.
2. **O'Brien, T. F., J. F. Acar, A. A. Medeiros, R. A. Norton, F. Goldstein, and R. L. Kent.** 1978. International comparison of prevalence of resistance to antibiotics. J. Am. Med. Assoc. **239:**1518–1523.
3. **O'Brien, T. F., R. L. Kent, and A. A. Medeiros.** 1975. A computer surveillance of shifts in the gross patient flora during hospitalization. J. Infect. Dis. **131:**88–96.

Extensive Use of Amikacin in a University Hospital: Observations After 16 Months

WILLIAM M. VALENTI,* ROBERT F. BETTS, STANLEY W. CHAPMAN, PATRICIA H. PINCUS, AND MARJORIE K. MESSNER

Infectious Disease Unit, University of Rochester, Strong Memorial Hospital, Rochester, New York 14642, U.S.A.

Amikacin is frequently used in the treatment of serious gram-negative infections. This drug appears to be particularly useful in the treatment of nosocomial infections due to multiple-drug-resistant gram-negative organisms (1).

Although the overall gram-negative resistance to gentamicin is less than 3% in our hospital, 51% of nosocomial *Pseudomonas aeruginosa* and 75% of *Serratia marcescens* isolates are gentamicin resistant. More than 95% of these two organisms in our hospital are susceptible to amikacin, however. Since nosocomial resistance to amikacin has not been a problem, we substituted amikacin as the aminoglycoside of choice in an attempt to answer certain questions regarding its effects on hospital resistance to aminoglycosides. We also monitored a number of other parameters related to the clinical use of aminoglycosides.

The study was divided into two phases. During the gentamicin period, from September 1977 through April 1978, this drug was used as the aminoglycoside of choice for serious gram-negative infections. The amikacin period began in May 1978 and is continuing at the present time. Gentamicin use was essentially discontinued during this second period, and amikacin was used as the aminoglycoside of choice in adult patients. Amikacin, which accounted for less

than 2% of total aminoglycoside use in the gentamicin period, increased to more than 85% of total aminoglycoside use in the amikacin period. The only control over aminoglycoside use was a restriction program, in effect since 1970, which required approval of the Infectious Disease Unit for use of gentamicin, amikacin, and tobramycin.

During both periods, we studied every fourth patient placed on gentamicin or amikacin for duration and appropriateness of therapy and gram-negative oropharyngeal colonization. Also monitored were the first aminoglycoside serum level submitted and hospital-wide aminoglycoside resistance of all gram-negative isolates.

Twenty-two percent of patients treated with gentamicin or amikacin had gram-negative infections which required gentamicin or amikacin. The remaining infections did not require gentamicin or amikacin, based on culture results, and were later treated with other agents. In the patients requiring gentamicin or amikacin, the mean duration of therapy was 11 days, with 19 of 21 patients treated for >7 days. In patients not requiring gentamicin or amikacin, mean duration of treatment was 5.7 days, and 12 of 74 were treated for >7 days ($P < 0.0001$).

Peak gentamicin levels ranged from 1.8 to 16.8 µg/ml (median, 5.5 µg/ml). Peak amikacin levels ranged from 3 to 50 µg/ml (median, 25 µg/ml).

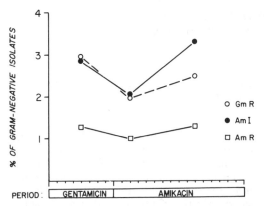

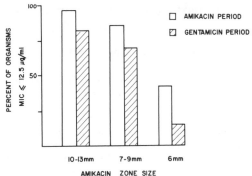

FIG. 1. *Gentamicin and amikacin resistance by period of study. GmR, gentamicin resistance; AmI, intermediate or indeterminate amikacin resistance; AmR, amikacin resistance.*

FIG. 2. *Amikacin zone size versus MIC of amikacin.*

In gentamicin-treated patients, 10 of 71 patients had peak levels less than four times the MIC of gentamicin for *P. aeruginosa* (MIC, 0.8 µg/ml), whereas only 1 of 53 amikacin-treated patients had peak levels less than four times the MIC of amikacin for *P. aeruginosa* (MIC, 1.5 µg/ml; $P < 0.02$).

Oropharyngeal cultures were taken on each patient to monitor gram-negative oropharyngeal colonization 24 h after institution of gentamicin or amikacin treatment. Swabs were placed in enriched broth by the method of Rosenthal (2). Gram-negative oropharyngeal colonization was significantly more frequent after 24 h of gentamicin therapy than after amikacin therapy (52.6% versus 13.3%; $P < 0.0001$).

Gentamicin and amikacin resistance of all clinical isolates submitted to the hospital microbiology laboratory was also monitored (Fig. 1). Using the Kirby-Bauer method, we defined resistance as a gentamicin zone of ≤9 mm or an amikacin zone of ≤12 mm. Intermediate or indeterminate amikacin resistance was defined as a 10- to 13-mm zone of inhibition.

In the first 4 months of the amikacin period, a slight decrease was noted in the percentage of organisms with gentamicin resistance, amikacin resistance, and intermediate amikacin resistance. During the past 8 months, the percentages of organisms showing gentamicin resistance, amikacin resistance, and intermediate amikacin resistance have increased to 2.7%, 1.3%, and 3.4% of all gram-negative isolates, respectively. Neither the decreases nor increases noted in aminoglycoside resistance are statistically significant.

Increased amikacin resistance was not noted when organisms resistant by disk were checked by broth dilution susceptibility tests (Fig. 2). During the gentamicin and amikacin periods, almost all gram-negative organisms with amikacin zone sizes of 10 to 13 mm were susceptible to amikacin, with MICs of ≤12.5 µg/ml.

If the amikacin zone size was 6 mm (no discernible zone size), a disparity was noted between the percentage of organisms susceptible by MIC that were isolated during the gentamicin and amikacin periods of 10% versus 47%, respectively ($P < 0.001$).

In summary, patients who required gentamicin or amikacin were treated with aminoglycosides longer than those who did not require these drugs. Amikacin levels were higher and generally more predictable when compared to the MIC for our *P. aeruginosa* isolates. These higher serum levels may explain the decreased gram-negative oropharyngeal colonization seen in amikacin-treated patients.

Our preliminary data suggest that an increase in absolute amikacin resistance was not seen after 16 months of amikacin use. Amikacin appears to have had an effect on hospital flora, however, by the induction of a diffusion barrier as shown by the apparent disparity between disk diffusion and MICs for organisms with 6-mm zone sizes.

Careful monitoring of patient isolates is necessary to detect changes in amikacin resistance. Disk diffusion susceptibilities may not adequately measure this resistance, however, and broth dilution susceptibility tests may be required to monitor these changes.

1. **Doughty, S. C., R. R. Martin, and S. B. Greenberg.** 1977. Treatment of hospital-acquired infections with amikacin. Am. J. Med. **62:**889–893.
2. **Rosenthal, S., and I. B. Tager.** 1975. Prevalence of gram negative rods in the normal pharyngeal flora. Ann. Intern. Med. **83:**355–357.

Comparison of Trimethoprim-Resistant Strains Isolated from Urinary Tract Infections in Finland and France

J. F. ACAR,* F. W. GOLDSTEIN, M. E. PINTO,[1] R. L. THEN, AND P. TOIVANEN

Hôpital Saint Joseph, Université Pierre et Marie Curie, Paris, France, University of Turku, Turku, Finland, and Hoffmann-La Roche, Basel, Switzerland*

The combination of sulfonamides and trimethoprim has been available in France for clinical use since 1971 (1). In Finland, trimethoprim alone has been used since 1972.

The present study was designed to compare strains resistant to trimethoprim (Tp) isolated from urinary tract infections in France and in Finland. Clinical isolates from urinary tract infections were collected in September and October 1978 in Finland and France. Fifty-five *Enterobacteriaceae* isolates resistant to trimethoprim isolated in Finland were compared to the same number of strains isolated in Paris.

The MIC of trimethoprim was determined by the Steers method on Mueller-Hinton agar with an inoculum of 10^5 bacteria/ml. Resistance to other antibiotics was determined by the disk method (ICS).

Transfer to *Escherichia coli* K-12 j5 Az^r,Ri^r, *E. coli* K-12 C600 Nal^r, and *E. coli* C$_1$ a r-m-Nal^r, incompatibility grouping, mobilization or elimination of the trimethoprim determinant by another plasmid, and curing experiments were performed by methods previously published.

Enzymatic studies were undertaken on 6 trimethoprim-resistant strains isolated in Finland and chosen at random among the 21 strains highly resistant to trimethoprim. Specific activity of the dihydrofolate reductase (DHFR) in the crude extract, estimation of the molecular weight of trimethoprim-sensitive and -resistant DHFR, and separation of the two enzymes were achieved by gel chromatography on Sephadex G-100 and ion-exchange chromatography on DEAE-cellulose.

The MIC of trimethoprim determined for the 55 resistant strains from both countries showed that 48 strains from France (87.3%) had a high level of resistance (MIC > 500 µg/ml) compared to 21 strains (38.2%) from Finland (Table 1).

Resistance to other antibiotics was also more frequent in France than in Finland. The resistance pattern covered a mean range of seven drugs in France compared to three drugs in Finland.

Attempts to transfer the trimethoprim marker

into *E. coli* K-12 failed in the 21 strains from Finland highly resistant to trimethoprim. No mobilization, elimination, or cure of the trimethoprim marker could be obtained in those strains. In contrast, 39 of 48 strains isolated in France could easily transfer the trimethoprim resistance into *E. coli* K-12.

Resistance markers cotransferred with the trimethoprim marker are presented in Table 2. In six cases, sulfonamide was not related to trimethoprim. Incompatibility grouping of the plasmids isolated in 1978 in Paris showed no substantial changes compared to the study in 1972 through 1974. The groups Inc-6 (C) and Inc-FII include 63.7% of the plasmids (2).

Enzymatic studies on six strains from Finland (three *Proteus mirabilis*, two *Citrobacter*, one *E. coli*) demonstrated the presence of a trimethoprim-resistant DHFR very similar to plasmid-mediated DHFR previously described (Table 2) (3, 6, 7). Two strains of *P. mirabilis* showed three different mechanisms of resistance to trimethoprim: production of a trimethoprim-resist-

TABLE 1. *MICs for trimethoprim-resistant strains*

Source and organism	No. of strains susceptible to a concn (µg/ml) of:			Total
	5–50	50–500	>500	
Turku (Finland)				
Escherichia coli	4	5	4	13
Citrobacter	1	2	2	5
Klebsiella	2	7	—	9
Serratia	—	1	—	1
Proteus mirabilis	3	4	13	20
Providencia	—	5	2	7
Total	10	24	21	55
Paris (France)				
E. coli	1	1	22	24
Citrobacter	—	—	7	7
Klebsiella	1	—	9	10
Serratia	—	1	—	1
P. mirabilis	—	1	7	8
Providencia	—	2	3	5
Total	2	5	48	55

[1] Present address: Hospital San Juan de Dios, University of Chile, Santiago, Chile.

TABLE 2. *Inhibition profiles of trimethoprim-sensitive and trimethoprim-resistant dihydrofolate reductases*[a]

Strain	DHFR type[b]	Aminopterin	Trimethoprim	Pyrimetha-mine	Triamterene	2,4-Diamino-6,7-diisopro-pylpteridine
Proteus mirabilis 2623	S	0.0033	0.14[c]	1.0	7.5	0.075
	R	9.0	~100	>100	35	—[d]
Citrobacter 2658	S	0.0024	0.0024	0.69	3.8	0.058
	R	9.1	66	>100	38	20
Citrobacter 3028	S	0.0026	0.0056	3.8	2.4	0.036
	R	10	65	>100	39	25
P. mirabilis 2933	S	0.0084	0.13	1.4	10	0.091
	R	8.0	100	>100	44	—
Escherichia coli 2950 II A	S	0.0033	0.0105	2.0	3.2	0.063
	R	11	62	>100	28	19
P. mirabilis 2950 II B	S	0.0057	0.035	1.31	1.0	0.083
	R	—	100	>100	55	—
E. coli 114 (R 388)	S	0.0028	0.010	1.3	5.0	0.075
	R	—	>100	>100	>100	—
E. coli B	S	0.0022	0.0087	1.37	4.1	0.071
E. coli RT 500	S	0.0018	0.0088	1.4	2.3	0.052
P. mirabilis 1420	S	0.0014	0.0067	1.8	2.0	0.0092

[a] Shown as the IC$_{50}$: 50% inhibitory concentration (micromolar).

[b] DHFR types S and R represent trimethoprim-susceptible and -resistant dihydrofolate reductase, respectively.

[c] Mean of four determinations (IC$_{50}$: 0.15, 0.165, 0.13, and 0.11 μM).

[d] —, Not determined.

ant DHFR, another trimethoprim-resistant DHFR 5 to 20 times more resistant than the normally trimethoprim-sensitive DHFR, and an overproduction of this DHFR.

The comparison between strains isolated in Finland and in France showed that the level of resistance to trimethoprim and the ability to transfer such resistance are different in the two countries. Multiple mechanisms of resistance to trimethoprim were observed in Finnish strains.

1. **Acar, J. F., F. W. Goldstein, and Y. A. Chabbert.** 1973. Synergistic activity of trimethoprim-sulfameth-oxazole combination on Gram negative bacilli: observations in vitro and in vivo. J. Infect. Dis. **128**(Suppl.): 470–477.

2. **Acar, J. F., F. W. Goldstein, Y. A. Chabbert, and G. R. Gerbaud.** 1977. Resistance au trimethoprime, Transférabilité et groupes d'incompatibilité des plasmides. Ann. Inst. Pasteur Paris **128A**:41–47.

3. **Amyes, S. G. B., and J. T. Smith.** 1974. R-factor trimethoprim resistance mechanism: an insusceptible target site. Biochem. Biophys. Res. Commun. **58**:412–418.

4. **Barth, P. T., N. Datta, R. W. Hedges, and N. J. Grinter.** 1976. Transposition of a deoxyribonucleic acid sequence encoding trimethoprim and streptomycin resistances from R 483 to other replicons. J. Bacteriol. **125**:800–810.

5. **Goldstein, F. W.** 1977. Mechanismes de resistance aux sulfamides et au trimethoprime. Bull. Inst. Pasteur Paris **75**:109–139.

6. **Pattishall, K. H., J. F. Acar, J. J. Burchall, F. W. Goldstein, and R. J. Harvey.** 1977. Two distinct types of trimethoprim-resistant dihydrofolate reductases specified by R plasmids of different compatibility groups. J. Biol. Chem. **252**:2319–2323.

7. **Tennhammar, E. B., and O. Skold.** 1979. Trimethoprim resistance plasmids of different origin encode different drug-resistant dihydrofolate reductases. Plasmids **2**: 334–346.

Plasmid-Mediated Trimethoprim Resistance: Detection of the Trimethoprim-Resistance Transposon Tn7, and Cloning and Expression of Plasmid-Encoded Reductase Genes

LYNN P. ELWELL,* MARY FLING, LESLIE WALTON, AND KATHERINE DORNBUSCH

Wellcome Research Laboratories, Research Triangle Park, North Carolina 27709 U.S.A., and Department of Bacteriology, National Bacteriology Laboratory, Stockholm, Sweden*

R plasmid-mediated resistance to trimethoprim has been recognized since 1972 (5). These plasmids specify novel dihydrofolate reductases (DHFRs) which are insensitive to trimethoprim inhibition, yet retain the capacity to bind normal substrates (1). In addition, the trimethoprim resistance determinant has been found to reside within two discrete transposable DNA sequences (transposons), Tn7 (2) and Tn402 (6).

This report concerns itself with two aspects of plasmid-encoded trimethoprim resistance: (i) a method for monitoring the dissemination of Tn7 and (ii) analysis of various plasmid-specified DHFRs by recombinant DNA-*Escherichia coli* minicell techniques.

Detection of Tn7 by use of DNA-DNA hybridization. [³H]thymine-labeled ColE1::Tn7 plasmid DNA and unlabeled whole-cell DNAs were prepared by the method of So et al. (8). DNA-DNA duplex formation between radiolabeled probe DNA and whole-cell DNA was carried out by the S1 endonuclease technique described by Crosa et al. (3). Hybridization results are shown in Table 1.

We draw the following conclusions from these data. (i) Under our experimental conditions, a nucleotide sequence homology value of 52 to 60% indicates the presence of Tn7. (ii) Four trimethoprim-resistant clinical isolates (two from Finland, one from Sweden, and one from Great Britain) harbor plasmids that contain Tn7. (iii) Transposons Tn7 and Tn402 are not closely related based on a homology value of 23% when the Tn7 probe was hybridized against DNA from *E. coli* J53 (R751). This conclusion is supported by restriction endonuclease analysis (M. Fling, unpublished data).

The S1 hybridization procedure is a sensitive and reproducible method for detecting the presence of the Tn7 DNA sequences in R plasmid-containing, trimethoprim-resistant clinical isolates.

Protein expression in *E. coli* minicells by recombinant plasmids specifying trimethoprim-resistant reductases. Using recombinant DNA techniques, we have isolated DNA sequences containing the structural genes for several resistant DHFRs from naturally occurring plasmids and have inserted these sequences into pBR322. Hybrid plasmids were transformed into a minicell-producing *E. coli* strain, and the genetic expression of the cloned genes was analyzed. Isolation and labeling of minicells were done by the method of Dougan and Sherratt (4). Comparison between the polypeptides synthesized in minicells is illustrated in the autoradiograph shown in Fig. 1. Plasmid pFE364, consisting of a 1.6-megadalton *Eco*RI fragment from R67 (type II DHFR) inserted into pBR322, specifies the synthesis of a novel polypeptide with a molecular weight of approximately 9,000 (Fig. 1A and B). Plasmids pFE504 and pFE506, containing the structural gene of the type I reductase harbored by Tn7, specify the synthesis of a novel polypeptide with a molecular mass of approximately 18,000 (Fig. 1D and E). The proteins with molecular weights of 30,000 to 32,000 shown in Fig. 1A through D represent β-lactamase proteins. The protein of 30,000 molecular weight in Fig. 1E is the streptomycin-inactivating enzyme originating in Tn7 (2).

To show that the 9,000-molecular-weight polypeptide was the type II subunit, antibody raised against purified type II DHFR in rabbits was added to the mixture of labeled polypeptides synthesized in minicells harboring pFE364. Protein A-containing *Staphylococcus aureus* cells were added to bind immunoglobulin molecules which were then concentrated by centrifugation through 1 M sucrose. The resultant protein complexes were dissociated with sodium dodecyl sulfate and electrophoresed; the dried gel was autoradiographed. Clearly, the only polypeptide recognized by the anti-DHFR type II antibody was the 9,000-molecular-weight species (data not shown). Smith et al. (7) have recently reported that the R67 reductase has a subunit molecular weight of 8,500. Minicells harboring the trimethoprim-resistance transposon, Tn402, also directed the synthesis of a 9,000-molecular-weight polypeptide that was specifically precipitated by the anti-type II reductase antibody. The 18,000-molecular-weight type I subunit, however, did not antigenically cross-react with this antibody.

TABLE 1. *Hybridization between ³H-labeled ColE1:Tn7 plasmid DNA and unlabeled whole-cell DNAs[a]*

DNA source	Resistances transferred[b]	Origin	Homology[c]
Escherichia coli HB101 (ColE1:Tn7)	Tp, Sm		88
E. coli 185 (F⁻)	—		14
E. coli C600 (pBW1)[d]	Tp, Sm	United Kingdom	57
E. coli C600 (R721)[d]	Tp, Sm	United Kingdom	52
Salmonella typhimurium (pHH1269)[d]	Tp, Sm, Su Km	United Kingdom	60
E. coli J5 (R67)	Tp, Sm, Ap, Cm, Tc, Su, Km	France	22
E. coli J5 (R388)	Tp, Su	United Kingdom	24
E. coli J53 (R751)[e]	Tp	United Kingdom	23
Vibrio cholera (R33)	Tp, Sm, Ap, Su	Africa	24
E. coli (R26)	Tp	Sweden	24
E. coli (R3891)	Tp, Sm, Tc	Finland	56
Citrobacter (R3888)	Tp, Sm, Tc	Finland	57
E. coli (R53)	Tp, Sm	Sweden	58
E. coli (R59)	Tp, Sm, Ap, Tc, Su	United Kingdom	56

[a] Approximately 0.05 µg of ³H-labeled, sheared ColE1:Tn7 DNA (specific activity, 2.4 × 10⁵ cpm/µg) was added to 225 µg of unlabeled, whole-cell DNA in a total volume of 1.5 ml (final NaCl concentration, 0.21 M). DNA mixtures, in tightly sealed glass vials, were heated at 100°C for 10 min. Single strands were allowed to reanneal at 75°C for 3.7 h. At the end of the incubation period, samples were assayed by the S1 endonuclease method described by Crosa (3). Each homology value shown represents the average of three independent experiments. In all cases, the variability between determinations was less than 5%.

[b] Tp, Trimethoprim; Sm, streptomycin; Su, sulfonamide; Km, kanamycin; Ap, ampicillin; Cm, chloramphenicol; Tc, tetracycline;

[c] Percent homology with ³H-labeled ColE1:Tn7.

[d] Strains known to harbor Tn7.

[e] Strain known to harbor Tn402.

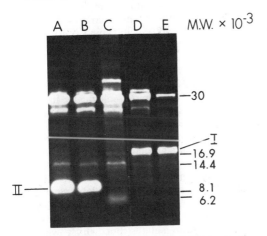

FIG. 1. *Autoradiograph of polypeptides synthesized in minicells carrying plasmids harboring the genes encoding for either the type I or type II reductase. Minicell products were separated by gel electrophoresis in a 15% sodium dodecyl sulfate-polyacrylamide gel. The dried gel was exposed to X-ray film for 11 days. (A and B) Plasmid pFE364, containing the gene for the type II dihydrofolate reductase (DHFR), originally present in the naturally occurring plasmid R67, cloned into pBR322. (C) Plasmid pBR322. (D) Plasmid pFE504, containing the gene for the type I DHFR harbored by the transposon Tn7 cloned into pBR322. (E) Plasmid pFE506, a pared-down derivative of pFE504.*

We conclude the following from these minicell data. (i) The type I reductase encoded by R483 and the type II DHFR specified by R67 are dissimilar enzymes. They differ antigenically and they differ in terms of subunit structure. (ii) The type II reductase determinant can reside within a transposable DNA sequence. This fact may have epidemiological implications in that both the type I and the type II reductases can be expected to disseminate by way of site-specific recombinational mechanisms.

It remains to be seen how universal this apparent diversity among R plasmid-encoded reductases is. The molecular characterization of more of these interesting enzymes, by conventional enzyme purification techniques or by the methods described in this report, should provide the answer.

1. Aymes, S. G. B., and J. T. Smith. 1974. R-factor trimethoprim resistance mechanism: an insusceptible target site. Biochem. Biophys. Res. Commun. **58**:412–418.

2. Barth, P., N. Datta, R. Hedges, and N. Grinter. 1976. Transposition of a DNA sequence encoding trimethoprim and streptomycin resistances from R483 to other replicons. J. Bacteriol. **125**:800–810.

3. Crosa, J., D. Brenner, and S. Falkow. 1973. Use of a single-strand specific nuclease for analysis of bacterial and plasmid deoxyribonucleic acid homo- and heteroduplexes. J. Bacteriol. **115**:904–911.

4. Dougan, G., and D. J. Sherratt. 1977. Changes in protein synthesis on mitomycin C induction of wild-type

and mutant CloDF13 plasmids. J. Bacteriol. **130**:846–851.

5. **Fleming, M. P., N. Datta, and R. N. Gruneberg.** 1972. Trimethoprim resistance determined by R factors. Br. Med. J. **1**:726–728.

6. **Shapiro, J., and P. Sporn.** 1977. Tn*402*: a new transposable element determining trimethoprim resistance that inserts in bacteriophage lambda. J. Bacteriol. **129**:1632–1635.

7. **Smith, S., D. Stone, P. Novak, D. Baccanari, and J. Burchall.** 1979. R plasmid dihydrofolate reductase with subunit structure. J. Biol. Chem. **254**:6222–6225.

8. **So, M., J. Crosa, and S. Falkow.** 1975. Polynucleotide sequence relationship among ENT plasmids and the relationship between ENT and other plasmids. J. Bacteriol. **121**:234–238.

Use of Agarose Gel Electrophoresis of Plasmid DNA as an Epidemiological Marker of Bacterial Strains

L. S. TOMPKINS,* D. R. SCHABERG, AND S. FALKOW

Departments of Microbiology and Immunology, Laboratory Medicine, and Medicine, University of Washington, Seattle, Washington 98195, U.S.A.*

Multiresistant gram-negative organisms have become a common cause of nosocomial epidemics in many hospitals. Epidemiological investigations into the source and mode of spread of these organisms depend on accurate identification of bacterial strains. Methods which have been employed to identify the phenotypes of gram-negative isolates include antibiotic susceptibility patterns, serotyping, bacteriocin typing, phage typing, and biotyping. However, these methods have several limitations: (i) serotyping, phage typing, and bacteriocin typing are not performed by most hospital laboratories and often must be submitted to specialized centers; (ii) antibiograms alone may not be sufficient to differentiate different strains; and (iii) no typing schemes have been developed to identify strains of some species which have caused nosocomial infections.

While investigating the spread of an R factor into various species of *Enterobacteriaceae*, we discovered that the total plasmid complement of nosocomial isolates, as detected by agarose gel electrophoresis (AGE) of plasmid DNA, may be an excellent epidemiological tool for differentiating strains. Our preliminary findings were that all isolates of a given strain, as determined by a single set of phenotypes, showed identical AGE patterns. Conversely, AGE of different strains, even those which had similar antibiograms, produced entirely different patterns.

To prove this association, we examined the plasmid band patterns of isolates collected from nosocomial epidemics due to multiply resistant gram-negative organisms which occurred in seven hospitals in the United States. The majority of isolates were collected during epidemiological investigations carried out by representatives of the Hospital Infections Branch of the Center for Disease Control, which employed prospective culturing of patients, hospital personnel, and environmental sites in order to define reservoirs of infection. Isolates recovered during these studies which had antibiotic resistance patterns similar to the pattern that had become prevalent in the hospital were stocked and subsequently submitted for plasmid analysis and typing of phenotypic markers by use of serotyping (1), bacteriocin typing (2–4), biotyping (1), or a combination of these methods.

In this study, the "epidemic strain" is defined as the organism found most frequently in specimens from infected patients or from colonized patients who were epidemiologically linked to the infected patients. Therefore, all organisms of the same species which had an identical set of phenotypic markers were considered to be isolates of the same epidemic strain. "Co-isolates" are defined as those with different phenotypes than the epidemic strain and thus are different strains. These are organisms isolated during the same period, usually from the same hospital, which had antibiograms similar to those of the epidemic strain isolates but which were recovered from sites or patients who had no apparent epidemiological link to patients infected with the epidemic strain.

DNA for AGE was prepared by lysing 40-ml cultures by the method of Hansen and Olsen (5). In this method, cells are lysed by treatment with lysozyme and sodium dodecyl sulfate. Plasmid DNA is separated from the bulk of chromosomal DNA by heating, alkalinization, and neutralization of the lysate, followed by partial purification of plasmid DNA by precipitation with polyethylene glycol and differential centrifugation. Samples of the partially purified DNA are then applied to 0.7% agarose gels and electrophoresed.

The gel is stained with ethidium bromide and photographed during exposure to long-wave UV light, which permits the DNA to be visualized as discrete bands.

An example of the correlation between phenotypic markers and AGE band patterns is illustrated in Table 1 and Fig. 1. The AGE patterns and phenotypes of isolates from two epidemics due to multiresistant *Serratia marcescens* occurring in Atlanta, Ga., and Seattle, Wash., are compared. In the Atlanta outbreak all isolates of the epidemic strain, serotype ONT:H8, had AGE patterns containing one plasmid (approxi-

mately 15 megadaltons) identical to the isolate shown in column H of Fig. 1. The plasmid patterns of the five co-isolates of five different strains with unique phenotypes, which were recovered from the same hospital, are entirely different both from the epidemic strain isolates and from each other (columns E-G, I, and J, Fig. 1). The antibiograms of two co-isolate strains are identical to the epidemic strain susceptibility pattern (Table 1), showing that an identical antibiogram may be shared by isolates of different strains of multiresistant organisms. The epidemic strain isolates from Seattle all

TABLE 1. *Phenotypic characteristics of isolates from two epidemics due to Serratia marcescens*

Strain	Location	Phenotypic markers[a]	Antibiotic susceptibility[b]
Epidemic	Atlanta	ONT:H8	Ak, Tm
Co-isolate 1	Atlanta	O13:H8	Ak, Tm
Co-isolate 2	Atlanta	ORough:H4	Ak, Tm
Co-isolate 3	Atlanta	O14:H4	Ak, Tm
Co-isolate 4	Atlanta	ONT:HNT	Ak, Tm, Gm, Km, Sm, Tmx
Co-isolate 5	Atlanta	O14:H12	Ak, Tm, Gm, Tmx
Epidemic	Seattle	Bacteriocin type 16	Ak, Tm[I], Gm[I], Km[I]
Co-isolate 1	Seattle	Bacteriocin type 50	Ak

[a] Atlanta strains were serotyped for O + H antigens (1). Seattle strains were bacteriocin typed by the method of Traub (5).

[b] Indicates antibiotics to which the isolates were susceptible by the disk diffusion method. Ak, amikacin; Tm, tobramycin; Gm, gentamicin; Km, kanamycin; Tmx, trimethoprim-sulfamethoxazole. Atlanta and Seattle isolates were resistant to chloramphenicol, tetracycline, sulfonamide, ampicillin, carbenicillin, cephalothin, nitrofurantoin, and polymyxin. Seattle isolates had intermediate (I) susceptibility to Tm, Gm, and Km.

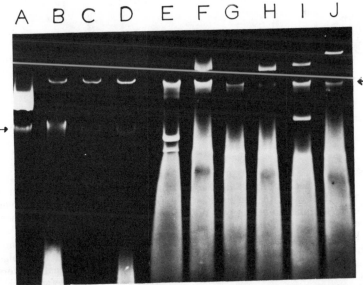

FIG. 1. *Agarose gel electrophoresis of Serratia marcescens isolates from Seattle (columns A–D) and Atlanta (columns E–J). The Seattle epidemic strain isolates are displayed in columns B–D; the co-isolate is shown in column A. An example of the DNA pattern of Atlanta epidemic strain appears in column H; columns E, F, G, I, and J contain DNA from five different co-isolates. Arrows denote the chromosomal DNA bands for the two gels.*

contain a single 45-megadalton plasmid (columns B–D, Fig. 1), whereas the co-isolate contains two plasmids, 12 megadaltons and 50 megadaltons, respectively (column A, Fig. 1).

We examined more than 50 gram-negative multiresistant isolates of four bacterial species isolated from patients in seven different geographical locations. A comparison of other phenotyping systems to AGE band patterns showed that, in every case, organisms which were recovered from a single geographical site and which had identical phenotypes also had identical AGE patterns. Conversely, isolates which were phenotypically different also had different AGE band patterns, so that a common plasmid pattern was not observed in isolates of different strains. In one instance, we observed that a *Providencia stuartii* strain, serotype O42, isolated in Memphis, Tenn., had a plasmid complement which was different from the pattern of a second *P. stuartii* strain of the same serotype isolated in St. Louis, Mo. Therefore, it is likely that the phenotype of an isolate is not co-linked with the organism's ability to carry any particular plasmid complement. However, the plasmid population carried by clinical isolates obtained in a single location appears to be stable enough over fairly long time intervals to allow the laboratory to use AGE in epidemiological investigations.

The function of the majority of extrachromosomal elements in these isolates is unknown. We, and others, have characterized the R factors

obtained from some of these epidemic strains; in two instances, the R factors responsible for the majority of antibiotic resistance markers remained unmodified over the course of several months. The molecular evolution of the other plasmids, however, has not been systematically examined. It seems likely that a particular strain's plasmids might undergo rearrangements, etc., over the course of time, and this would be reflected in the AGE pattern.

AGE of plasmid DNA molecules is a fairly rapid method, requiring approximately 6 h of work spread over 3 days. The test requires no special reagents or biological materials and thus could be applied to many epidemiological studies encountered in large clinical laboratories or in central reference laboratories. AGE of plasmid DNA may be considered as a useful adjunct to (or even replacement for) other methods of differentiating bacterial strains.

1. **Anderson, R. L.** 1978. Typing methods for *Proteus rettgeri.* J. Clin. Microbiol. **8:**715–722.
2. **Edwards, R. P., and W. H. Ewing.** 1972. Identification of Enterobacteriaceae. Burgess Publishing Co., Minneapolis, Minn.
3. **Farmer, J. J., and L. G. Herman.** 1974. Pyocin typing of Pseudomonas aeruginosa. J. Infect. Dis. **130:**534–546.
4. **Hansen, J. B., and R. H. Olsen.** 1978. Isolation of large bacterial plasmids and characterization of the P2 incompatibility group plasmids pMG1 and pMG5. J. Bacteriol. **135:**227–238.
5. **Traub, W. H.** 1972. Bacteriocin typing of *Serratia marcescens* of known serotype-group. Appl. Microbiol. **23:**979–981.

Plasmid Diversity in Multiresistant *Serratia marcescens* Isolates from Affiliated Hospitals

JOSEPH F. JOHN, JR.,* AND WILLIAM F. McNEILL

Veterans Administration Medical Center, Medical University of South Carolina, Charleston, South Carolina 29403, U.S.A.

Multiple-drug resistance is a major problem in *Serratia marcescens* (1). Multiresistant *Serratia marcescens* (MRSM) strains are increasing as a cause of nosocomial infection (4). We previously characterized plasmid types at Medical University Hospital and Charleston County Hospital in Charleston S.C. (Program Abstr. Intersci. Conf. Antimicrob. Agents Chemother. 18th, Atlanta, Ga., abstr. no. 95, 1978), an outbreak dominated by MRSM containing 41-megadalton (conjugative) and 6-megadalton (cryptic) plasmids. Shortly after the appearance of MRSM at Medical University Hospital, an

upsurge of MRSM occurred at the Veterans Administration Medical Center (VAMC), the major affiliate of Medical University Hospital located two blocks away. To discover the possible origin of these plasmids, we studied the relationship among plasmids from newer strains of MRSM at the VAMC and plasmids already characterized at Medical University Hospital.

From July 1977 through April 1979 MRSM were isolated from 78 patients at VAMC. The most common pattern of resistance in the MRSM was ampicillin, carbenicillin, chloramphenicol, tetracycline, trimethoprim, sulfamethoxazole, sulfonamide, streptomycin, gentamicin, tobramycin, kanamycin, and sisomicin. The median MICs in micrograms/milliliter (range given in parentheses) of the aminoglycosides were as follows: gentamicin, 63 (16 to 500); tobramycin, 63 (16 to 250); kanamycin, 250 (125 to >1,000); sisomicin, 31 (16 to 250); amikacin, 4 (1 to 63); and netilmicin, 2 (1 to 16). Agarose gel electrophoresis of cleared lysates disclosed four different large conjugative plasmids (58, 53, 48, and 47 megadaltons), as shown in Fig. 1, and three small cryptic plasmids (4.5, 3.0, and 2.7 megadaltons). One strain containing a 48- and 2.7-megadalton plasmid also contained a 63-megadalton plasmid which cotransferred with the 48-megadalton plasmid. The 48-megadalton plasmid was present in 11 of 17 MRSM screened by agarose gel electrophoresis. These 11 strains came from different parts of the hospital, and most were urinary tract isolates.

Plasmid species of 58, 53, 48, and 47 megadaltons all transferred ampicillin, carbenicillin, sulfonamide, gentamicin, tobramycin, kanamycin, and sisomicin resistance to a susceptible strain of *Escherichia coli*. The 58-, 48-, and 47-megadalton plasmids transferred mercury resistance, and the 48- and 53-megadalton plasmids transferred neomycin resistance. The 47-megadalton species alone encoded for streptomycin and tetracycline resistance. All transcipients were sensitive to chloramphenicol, tetracycline, sulfamethoxazole-trimethoprim, netilmicin, and amikacin. Table 1 shows MICs determined by serial broth dilution for individual plasmid-containing strains. Netilmicin and amikacin were the most active aminoglycosides.

Restriction enzyme analysis of the conjugative plasmids employing enzyme *Hae*II revealed multiple identical cleavage fragments, suggesting relative homology. On the other hand, the

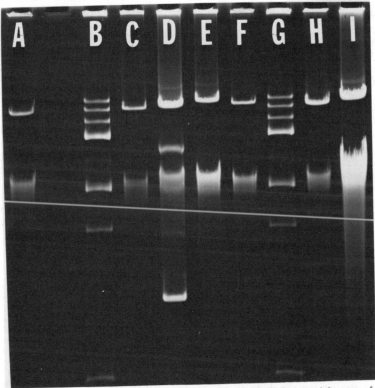

FIG. 1. *Agarose gel electrophoresis of ethanol-precipitated DNA from cleared lysates of multiresistant Serratia marcescens at the Veterans Administration Medical Center. Details of the procedure were outlined by Meyers et al. (2). (B and G) Standard plasmid DNAs ranging in molecular weight from 63×10^6 (uppermost band) to 1.7×10^6 (lowest band). A chromosomal band can be seen in each lysate between 12×10^6 and 14×10^6. (A) Lysate of strain VA9 with one plasmid of molecular weight 47×10^6. (C) Lysate of VA24, one plasmid, 48×10^6. (D) Lysate of VA25, two plasmids, 53×10^6 and 2.7×10^6. (E and I) Lysate of VA109 and VA155, each with one 58×10^6 plasmid. (F and H) Lysate of VA134 and VA142, each with one 53×10^6 plasmid. The lighter bands in lanes D, E, F, H, and I represent open circular DNA.*

TABLE 1. *Plasmid size, aminoglycoside susceptibility, and aminoglycoside-modifying enzymes*

Plasmid size(s) (daltons)	Isolate no.	MIC (μg/ml)[a]						Aminoglyco-side-modifying enzymes[b]
		Gm	Tm	Km	Sis	Net	An	
47×10^6	VA9	125	16	250	125	2	4	AAC(6')-2, ANT(2'')
48×10^6	VA24	31	63	125	63	1	4	AAC(6')-2, ANT(2'')
48×10^6, 61×10^6, 2.7×10^6	VA96	125	125	>1,000	63	2	4	
53×10^6	VA134	125	125	>1,000	31	31	8	AAC(6')-2, ANT(2'')
58×10^6, 2.7×10^6	VA109	63	63	250	31	2	4	AAC(6')-2, ANT(2'')
58×10^6	VA155	500	250	>1,000	250	63	16	

[a] Gm, Gentamicin; Tm, tobramycin; Km, kanamycin; Sis, sisomicin; Net, netilmicin; An, amikacin.
[b] AAC, Aminoglycoside acetyl transferase; ANT, aminoglycoside nucleotidyl transferase.

41-megadalton plasmid from Medical University Hospital had multiple fragments not present in the digestion of the 48-megadalton plasmid from VAMC.

Aminoglycoside-modifying-enzyme determinations performed on sonicates of MRSM by Bristol Laboratories, Syracuse, N.Y., are also shown in Table 1 for four different strains containing four different plasmids. All strains elaborated both a 2''-O-nucleotidyl transferase [ANT(2'')] and a 6-N-acetyl transferase [AAC(6')] which did not modify amikacin. In comparison, the 41-megadalton plasmid from Medical University Hospital elaborated an AAC (3).

Serotyping performed by Walter Traub (3) of strains containing pJFJ9VA, a 47-megadalton plasmid, revealed type O19:H14 and for pJFJ109VA, a 58-megadalton plasmid, type O19:H15. Both strains were nontypable with bacteriocins. In comparison, strains from Medical University Hospital containing different plasmids were also O19 serotype but were bacteriocin type 4 or 63.

As the incidence of MRSM gradually decreased at VAMC, there was a concomitant increase in multiresistant strains of *Providencia rettgeri* and *P. stuartii*. Plasmid analysis of these strains has failed to disclose plasmids of molecular weight similar to those found in MRSM, suggesting that thus far the plasmids of MRSM have been confined to the genus *Serratia*.

From these studies we conclude that some plasmid diversity in MRSM has occurred at VAMC, although there was a predominant, 48-megadalton plasmid. Restriction endonuclease

analysis suggested a large degree of homology among the conjugative plasmids from the VAMC. The finding of elaboration of identical double aminoglycoside-modifying enzymes by these different strains of MRSM also suggests relatedness of these plasmids, although we have not excluded chromosomal loci for either of the enzymes.

An outbreak due to MRSM containing a common plasmid among the affiliated hospitals might have been inferred initially from the antimicrobial susceptibility patterns, the proximity of the hospitals, and exchange of personnel between the hospitals. Using agarose gel for screening of plasmid sizes, restriction endonuclease analysis of purified plasmid DNA, and comparison of aminoglycoside-modifying enzymes, we have excluded the possibility of a common origin of these plasmids. Furthermore, we have not as yet detected plasmids from the MRSM appearing in other enteric bacteria at VAMC.

1. **Cooksey, R. C., G. M. Thorne, and W. E. Farrar, Jr.** 1976. R-factor-mediated antibiotic resistance in *Serratia marcescens* in a general hospital. Antimicrob. Agents Chemother. **10**:123–127.
2. **Meyers, J. A., D. Sanchez, L. P. Elwell, and S. Falkow.** 1976. Simple agarose gel electrophoretic method for the identification and characterization of plasmid deoxyribonucleic acid. J. Bacteriol. **127**:1529–1537.
3. **Traub, W., and I. Kleber.** 1977. Serotyping of *Serratia marcescens*: evaluation of Le Minor's H immobilization test and description of three new flagellar H antigens. J. Clin. Microbiol. **115**:121.
4. **Yu, V. L., C. A. Oakes, K. J. Axnick, et al.** 1979. Patient factors contributing to the emergence of gentamicin-resistant *Serratia marcescens*. Am. J. Med. **66**:468–472.

Identity and Interspecific Transfer of Gentamicin-Resistance Plasmids in *Staphylococcus aureus* and *Staphylococcus epidermidis*

HAROLD W. JAFFE,* HELEN M. SWEENEY, CATHERINE NATHAN, ROBERT A. WEINSTEIN, SHERWIN A. KABINS, AND SIDNEY COHEN

Departments of Microbiology and Medicine, Michael Reese Hospital and Medical Center,* and the Pritzker School of Medicine, University of Chicago, Chicago, Illinois 60616, U.S.A.

In 1977 an outbreak of infections apparently due to single strain of *Staphylococcus aureus* occurred in a Neonatal Special Care Nursery at Michael Reese Hospital. Isolates of this strain were resistant to gentamicin, kanamycin, tobramycin, and sisomicin, as a result of the plasmid-mediated production of inactivating enzymes, but were susceptible to streptomycin, amikacin, and netilmicin (2). From a culture survey of the Nursery during the outbreak, we also obtained two isolates of *S. epidermidis* whose spectrum of aminoglycoside susceptibility and pattern of aminoglycoside enzymatic inactivation were the same as those of the *S. aureus* strain.

To test the hypothesis that resistant strains might have appeared as a result of the interspecific transfer of a single plasmid between these *S. aureus* and *S. epidermidis* isolates, we tried to transfer gentamicin-resistance (Gm^r) plasmids between these bacteria in mixed cultures (Table 1). As donors, we used five isolates of Gm^r *S. aureus* (A1 through A5) obtained from patients during the outbreak and the two isolates of Gm^r *S. epidermidis* (E1 and E2). All five isolates of *S. aureus* had similar phage types and identical antibiograms. The two *S. epidermidis* isolates were indistinguishable with respect to colonial morphology and antibiotic susceptibility. As recipients we used gentamicin-susceptible derivatives of the clinical isolates *S. aureus* A1 (A1s) and *S. epidermidis* E1 (E1s) as well as two natively plasmid-free strains, *S. aureus* PFA and *S. epidermidis* PFE. Donor and recipient strains were suspended in a transfer medium at a concentration of 10^{10} colony-forming units/ml, mixed, incubated at 37°C for 24 h, and then plated on selective media. The seven Gm^r staphylococcal isolates transferred their Gm^r plasmid both intraspecifically and interspecifically, as was shown by the transfer of the aminoglycoside-resistance pattern of the donor and the demonstration by agarose gel electrophoresis of the acquisition of a plasmid by the recipient.

We further tested the possibility of in vivo transfer of the Gm^r plasmid in experiments with mixtures of bacteria on human skin (Table 2). Donor and appropriately marked recipient strains were grown separately; then 10^9 bacteria

of each strain were placed on 4 cm^2 of skin and covered with a plastic dressing. After 6, 18, or 24 h, the test area was uncovered and swabbed, and specimens were plated on selective media. *S. aureus* A1 was shown to transfer its aminoglycoside resistance to its Gm^s derivative, and *S. epidermidis* E1 transferred its resistance both intra- and interspecifically.

If the Gm^r plasmid can be transferred between *S. aureus* and *S. epidermidis*, the physical properties of their Gm^r plasmids should be identical, assuming that no alteration occurs after transfer. As a preliminary test of identity, we determined the molecular weights of the Gm^r plasmids from *S. aureus* A1 and *S. epidermidis* E1 by electron

TABLE 1. *Transfer of the Gm^r plasmid in mixed culture*

Donor strain (Gm^r)	Frequency of transfer^a to recipient strains (Gm^s)			
	S. aureus		*S. epidermidis*	
	A1s	PFA	E1s	PFE
S. aureus				
A1	>2,000	138	78	3
A2	1,200	102	62	2
A3	1,600	89	56	4
A4	>2,000	146	71	1
A5	1,150	92	48	3
S. epidermidis				
E1	110	3	68	16
E2	84	1	52	8

^{a} Colonies per 10^{10} recipient cells.

TABLE 2. *Transfer of the Gm^r plasmid on skin*

Donor strain (Gm^r)	Incubation (h)	Frequency of transfer^a to recipient strains (Gm^s)	
		S. aureus A1s	*S. epidermidis* E1s
S. aureus A1	6	110	Not done
S. epidermidis E1	6	0	0
	18	49	0
	24	0.5	6

^{a} Colonies per 10^9 recipient cells.

microscopy. Based on a comparison of their contour lengths with that of pSH1, a 2.8-megadalton plasmid, the molecular weights of the A1 and E1 Gm^r plasmids were 12.2 megadaltons ± 0.36 (SD) and 12.3 megadaltons ± 0.56, respectively.

As a further test of identity, we used restriction endonuclease digestions to compare the Gm^r plasmids from *S. aureus* and *S. epidermidis*. For these experiments, we transferred Gm^r plasmids from their native hosts to a plasmid-free *S. aureus* strain by transformation or transduction, or in mixed culture. Agarose gel electrophoresis of endonuclease digests of plasmids showed that *Hae*III produced an identical digestion pattern, consisting of eight fragments, from the Gm^r plasmids of all five clinical isolates of *S. aureus* and the two clinical isolates of *S. epidermidis*. Likewise, digestions using the endonucleases *Eco*RI, *Xba*I, and *Hind*III showed no differences among these Gm^r plasmids.

Plasmid transfer between bacterial species is a mechanism for the rapid and widespread dissemination of resistance to multiple antibiotics. Interspecific plasmid transfer is known to occur among members of the *Enterobacteriaceae* family, other gram-negative bacilli, and group B and group D streptococci. Although the hypothesis that interspecific plasmid transfer occurs among the staphylococci has been often proposed, evidence to support this hypothesis has been limited. Witte has reported the transfer of penicillin-resistance and chloramphenicol-resistance plasmids in mixed cultures of *S. aureus* and *S. epidermidis* (3). Novick and associates found that tetracycline-resistance plasmids of *S. aureus* and *S. epidermidis* from diverse sources were structurally identical. They proposed that these plasmids have a common origin (1).

We have shown that gentamicin-resistant *S. aureus* and *S. epidermidis* isolates from infants in a Neonatal Special Care Nursery have Gm^r plasmids which appear to be structurally identical and can be transferred between species in mixed cultures and on human skin. Our findings support the hypothesis that interspecific plasmid transfer occurs among staphylococci in nature.

1. **Iordanescu, S., M. Surdeanu, P. Della Latta, and R. Novick.** 1978. Incompatibility and molecular relationships between small staphylococcal plasmids carrying the same resistance marker. Plasmid 1:468–479.
2. **Vogel, L., C. Nathan, H. M. Sweeney, S. A. Kabins, and S. Cohen.** 1978. Infections due to a gentamicin-resistant *Staphylococcus aureus* strain in a nursery for neonatal infants. Antimicrob. Agents Chemother. 13:466–472.
3. **Witte, W.** 1977. Transfer of drug resistance-plasmids in mixed cultures of staphylococci. Zentralbl. Bakteriol. Parasitenkd. Infektionskr. Hyg. Abt. 1 Orig. Reihe A 237:147–159.

Fecal Carriage of Multiply Resistant Klebsiellae

ELIZABETH T. HOUANG,* P. A. SIMMS, R. A. HORTON, AND M. W. CASEWELL

The London Hospital Medical College, Whitechapel, District Community Physician, Tower Hamlets Health District, Department of Environmental Health, Borough of Tower Hamlets, and St. Thomas's Hospital Medical School, London, SE1, England*

The acquisition of intestinal multiply resistant klebsiellae by hospital patients, who may subsequently acquire infection with the same strain, has been well documented (4), but it is only recently that gentamicin-resistant klebsiellae have caused extensive outbreaks in hospitals in the United Kingdom (1, 2). During one such outbreak, we took the opportunity to investigate the proportion of patients who were unsuspected carriers of the epidemic strain, the duration of fecal carriage, and the contribution of hospital-acquired multiply resistant strains to the non-hospital community by discharged patients. Some details of the outbreak have been reported elsewhere (3).

Gentamicin-resistant isolates of *Klebsiella aerogenes* (*pneumoniae*) were obtained from 61 patients in seven wards. Of 50 isolates that were typed, 48 were capsular (K) type 21, one was K68, and one was nontypable. Of six isolates of K21 tested, five transferred resistance to ampicillin, carbenicillin, chloramphenicol, tetracycline, sulfonamide, streptomycin, kanamycin, neomycin, gentamicin, and tobramycin to *Escherichia coli* K21 J62-1.

An isolation ward was designated for infected or colonized patients, and, except for one patient who required cephalexin, broad-spectrum antibiotic therapy was withheld. Specimens, in addition to those clinically indicated, were obtained as follows. (i) Rectal swabs and urine samples were obtained from 204 apparently un-

TABLE 1. *Carriage of K21 in 28 patients in the isolation ward*

Carriage	No. of patients	Weeks positive
Continuous until discharge	8	1–4
	3	4–6
Continuous until end of survey	4	10
Ended (≥1 negative swab)	9	1–4
	4	4–6

infected patients in the seven wards with known positive patients. Routine clinical specimens had not revealed the epidemic strain in this group. (ii) Weekly rectal swabs and urine were obtained from 28 known positive patients in the isolation ward. (iii) Repeated stools were obtained from five patients known to be excreting gentamicin-resistant klebsiellae at the time of discharge from the hospital and also from three of their spouses. (iv) Single stool specimens were obtained from 100 males attending the venereal disease clinic and from 34 of the nonhospital community who were contacts of patients with diarrhea.

MacConkey agar (containing 10 mg of gentamicin per liter) was used for primary cultures, surface counting of 10-fold dilutions of emulsified stool, and subculture of single-strength MacConkey broth (also containing 10 mg of gentamicin per liter) enrichment cultures. A standard method with paper strips was used for the semiquantitative examination of urine.

Of 204 patients in the seven outbreak wards, 23 (11%) were found to be unsuspected carriers. Fecal or urinary isolates alone were found in 14 (7%) and 5 (3%) patients, respectively, and 4 patients carried the epidemic strain in both feces and urine. Of the 94 patients examined before the wards were closed for cleaning, 17 (18%) had positive fecal swabs. The proportion of unsuspectedly positive patients in individual wards varied from 4 to 50%. Of 110 patients examined after cleaning and reopening of six wards, 6 (6%) were fecal excretors.

The duration of fecal excretion of gentamicin-resistant klebsiellae by the 28 patients admitted to the isolation ward is shown in Table 1. In 10 patients the mean $\log_{10}$ fecal gentamicin-resistant klebsiella count was 4.84 ($\pm$ 1.62). After 6 weeks of isolation, 11 patients had at least two negative stool cultures, but four of the monitored patients (14%) were still positive after 10 weeks. Eight patients were discharged while still excreting multiply resistant klebsiellae. Of the five patients and three spouses who were examined

at regular intervals after discharge, two patients and the spouse of one had negative stool specimens at the time of first stool sampling, 3 and 5 weeks after discharge from hospital. Prolonged excretion was, however, observed in the other three patients (Fig. 1). The highest counts (10^7 to 10^8 klebsiella/g of stool) and most sustained excretion were found in a 59-year-old man (patient A) who had a colostomy and was the only one who received antibiotics at home (repeated courses of co-trimoxazole). One week after the return home of one woman patient (C), her husband also became an intermittent fecal excretor of the same type (K68). Neither was receiving antibiotics.

Gentamicin-resistant klebsiellae, of any serotype, were not found in stools from 100 males attending the venereal disease clinic nor from 34 nonhospitalized contacts of diarrhea.

The results of this study suggest that during hospital outbreaks of gentamicin-resistant klebsiellae there are significant numbers of asymptomatic patients, often unidentified, with multiply resistant fecal klebsiellae who contribute to a "pool" of transferable antibiotic resistance, and who may sustain nosocomial epidemics, continue excreting resistant strains for many weeks, contribute resistant organisms to the nonhospital community, cause intrafamilial spread, and, finally, on readmission, may initiate further hospital outbreaks.

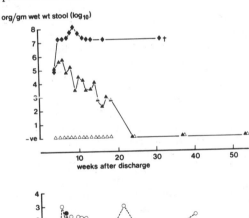

FIG. 1. *Duration of fecal excretion of gentamicin-resistant klebsiellae by three patients and two spouses at home. Patient A (◆) was a 59-year-old male who had a colostomy and received repeated courses of co-trimoxazole. (▲) Patient B and (△) his spouse. (●) Patient C and (○) her spouse.*

1. **Casewell, M. W., M. T. Dalton, M. Webster, and I. Phillips.** 1977. Gentamicin-resistant *Klebsiella aerogenes* in a urological ward. Lancet **2**:444-446.
2. **Curie, K., D. C. E. Speller, R. A. Simpson, M. Stephens, and D. I. Cooke.** 1979. A hospital epidemic caused by gentamicin-resistant *Klebsiella aerogenes.* J. Hyg. **80**:115-123.

3. **Houang, E. T., M. A. L. Evans, and C. N. Simpson.** 1979. Control of hospital epidemic gentamicin-resistant *Klebsiella aerogenes.* Lancet **2**:205.
4. **Selden, R., S. Lee, W. L. L. Wang, J. V. Bennett, and T. C. Eickhoff.** 1971. Nosocomial klebsiella infections: intestinal colonization as a reservoir. Ann. Intern. Med. **74**:657-664.

Genetic Analysis of Multiple-Antibiotic Resistance in *Salmonella dublin*

FRITZ H. KAYSER,* FRANÇOISE HOMBERGER, AND MARLYSE DEVAUD

Institute of Medical Microbiology, University of Zurich, CH-8028 Zurich, Switzerland

Several courses of treatment with immunosuppressive drugs in a patient who had received a cadaver kidney transplant resulted in a septic disease caused by *Salmonella dublin* (1). Strain 1 (HK247), isolated from the blood during the first septic episode, was resistant to chloramphenicol (Cm), streptomycin (Sm), the sulfonamides (Su), and the tetracyclines (Tc) (= R-pattern A). Strain 2 (HK246), isolated several months later, was in addition resistant to ampicillin (Ap), cephalothin (Cp), kanamycin (Km), and gentamicin (Gm). This strain was, however, susceptible to Tc (= R-pattern B). Resistance markers of strain 1 were nontransmissible but could be eliminated, although at low frequencies, by treatment of cultures with regimens known to affect plasmid replication. The complete R-pattern B of strain 2 could be transferred to several enterobacterial receptor strains of different genera, sometimes at high frequencies, as well as to strain 1 and to antibiotic-susceptible variants of this strain. Experiments to eliminate antibiotic resistance from strain 2 easily yielded eliminants, which were susceptible to Ap-Cp-Km-Gm but still resistant to Cm-Sm-Su. The latter resistance markers could be eliminated from the variants at a low frequency, and completely susceptible derivatives of strain HK246 were obtained. Radioactively labeled plasmid DNA was isolated from the *Salmonella* strains by isopycnic centrifugation and was analyzed by sedimentation of DNA in neutral sucrose gradients or by agarose gel electrophoresis (Table 1). Strains HK247 and susceptible variants always contained a cryptic 52-megadalton plasmid. Strain HK246 contained a 52- as well as a 59-megadalton plasmid. Variants of this strain, selected for loss of resistance to β-lactam and/or aminoglycoside antibiotics, contained a 42-together with the 52-megadalton cryptic plasmid. One isolated variant, which was still resistant to Cm-Sm-Su, contained no plasmid DNA at all.

From these results it was concluded that markers of antibiotic resistance in strain HK247 are integrated into the chromosome, whereas multiple-antibiotic resistance in HK246 was due to a 59-megadalton R plasmid. Besides the R markers of this plasmid, strain HK246 also contained copies of the determinants for resistance to Cm-Sm-Su integrated into the chromosome.

The instability of the chromosomal markers in both strains was shown to be due to their location on transposons. Transposition could be demonstrated in an experiment in which the R plasmid R28K, conferring resistance to Ap, was introduced into HK247. In a second mating experiment between HK247(R28K) and *E. coli* K-12, transconjugants were selected for resistance to Ap and for the R-pattern A of HK247. DNA analysis of transconjugants revealed an increase in the molecular weight of R28K from 44×10^6 to 55×10^6. Thus, the transposable sequence was 11 megadaltons in size. An identical experiment showed that the chromosomal R markers of strain HK246 also were transposable.

TABLE 1. *Molecular analysis of plasmid DNA isolated from various Salmonella dublin strains*

Strain	Resistance markers[a]	Mol wt
HK247	Cm-Sm-Su-Tc	52×10^6
HK247 (Tc)[s]	Cm-Sm-Su	52×10^6
HK247 (Cm-Sm-Su-Tc)[s]	—	52×10^6
HK246	Cm-Sm-Su-Ap-Cp-Km-Gm	52×10^6 59×10^6
HK246, type 1 variant	Cm-Sm-Su	52×10^6 42×10^6
HK246, type 2 variant	—	52×10^6 42×10^6
HK246, type 1 variant	Cm-Sm-Su	No plasmid DNA

[a] Cm, Chloramphenicol; Sm, streptomycin; Su, sulfonamides; Tc, tetracycline; Ap, ampicillin; Cp, cephalothin; Km, kanamycin; Gm, gentamicin.

TABLE 2. *Identical characteristics of the Salmonella dublin plasmid pFK17 and the Klebsiella pneumoniae plasmid pFK1*

Property	Result with pFK17 and pFK1
R phenotype	Ap-Cp-Cm-Gm-Km-Sm-Su[a]
Mechanism of resistance	Ap-Cp: TEM-type β-lactamase
	Sm: aminoglycoside 3″-adenylyltransferase [AAD (3″)]
	Km: aminoglycoside 3′-phosphotransferase-1 [APH (3′)-1]
	Gm: aminoglycoside 2″-nucleotidyltransferase [ANT (2″)]
Fertility inhibition	fi+ rep
Host range	Identical
	Incompatibility of pFK1 with the 42-megadalton plasmid of the HK246 type 1 and 2 variants (see Table 1)
Molecular weight	59×10^6
Digestion with restriction endonucleases	Identical fragmentation patterns in *Hind*III and *Sal*I digestion; similar fragmentation patterns in *Sma*I, *Bgl*I, *Bgl*II, and *Eco*RI digestion

[a] Ap, Ampicillin; Cp, cephalothin; Cm, chloramphenicol; Km, kanamycin; Sm, streptomycin; Su, sulfonamides.

From these data it was concluded that *S. dublin* HK246 evolved in vivo from strain HK247 by loss or inactivation of the Tc[r] marker and gain of an R plasmid, probably from the flora endemic in the university hospital. We therefore tried to demonstrate identity between the *Salmonella* plasmid and a plasmid frequently found to be harbored by the hospital flora. From Table 2 it can be seen that the R phenotypes of both plasmids are identical. Both

plasmids were fi+ plasmids and repressed F-pilus formation. Plasmid pFK1 could reside simultaneously in the same host with a variant of plasmid pFK17, which did not contain markers for resistance to β-lactam antibiotics and aminoglycosides. Both plasmids were of the same molecular weight. Digestion of DNA with restriction endonucleases *Hind*III and *Sal*I yielded identical fragmentation patterns. Digestion patterns with *Sma*I, *Bgl*I, *Bgl*II, and *Eco*RI were not totally identical, but were very similar. The differences could be explained by evolutionary changes of the two plasmids, not affecting biological functions but affecting the primary structure of the DNA. Even minor changes of polynucleotide sequences within the cleavage sites for restriction endonucleases will result in a different pattern. Sequence alterations of plasmids were observed and analyzed by Timmis and coworkers in R6-5 (2). From their results, the authors concluded that the primary structure of bacterial plasmids is in a constant flux and that sequence reorganization may be a more widely occurring phenomenon than has been appreciated previously. Evolutionary rearrangement of DNA could also have occurred in the plasmids examined in our study, especially because both plasmids were isolated from different sources at different times and were harbored by different host species.

1. Kayser, F. H., M. Devaud, F. Largiadèr, and U. Binswanger. 1978. Acquisition of multiple antibiotic resistance by *Salmonella dublin* from the gramnegative hospital flora, in a kidney allograft recipient. Zentralbl. Bakteriol. Parasitenkd. Infektionskr. Hyg. Abt. 1 Orig. Reihe A 241:308–318.
2. Timmis, K. N., F. Cabello, J. Andres, A. Nordheim, H. J. Burkhardt, and S. N. Cohen. 1978. Instability of plasmid DNA sequences: macro and micro evolution of the antibiotic resistance plasmids R6-5. Mol. Gen. Genet. 167:11–19.

Characterization of Multiresistant Isolates of *Acinetobacter calcoaceticus* Causing Nosocomial Infections

MARLYSE DEVAUD* AND FRITZ H. KAYSER

Institute of Medical Microbiology, University of Zurich, CH-8028 Zurich, Switzerland

Acinetobacter calcoaceticus is a ubiquitous organism which mainly has been observed in soil, water, food, and lower animals. Only recently has this organism been found to be associated with disease in humans (1, 2). At the Institute of Medical Microbiology in Zurich, we isolate between 250 and 350 strains of *A. cal-*

coaceticus per year from various patient materials. These figures correspond to 1 to 2% of all members of the *Enterobacteriaceae* family and oxidative-fermentative bacteria isolated yearly in our laboratories.

At the end of 1977, we observed a sudden increase in the number of *A. calcoaceticus* strains isolated (Fig. 1). An analysis of our laboratory files revealed that this increase was due to a hospital epidemic, occurring in one of the intensive care units of the university hospital. All cultures isolated from patients in this unit belonged to *A. calcoaceticus* subsp. *anitratus* and were resistant to ampicillin (Ap), gentamicin (Gm), kanamycin (Km), streptomycin (Sm), tetracycline (Tc), chloramphenicol (Cm), and sulfamethoxazole (Su). The isolates were susceptible to tobramycin and amikacin.

An investigation of the mechanism of resistance to aminoglycosides showed that strains produced the aminoglycoside 3-*N*-acetyltransferase, which confers resistance to Gm and sisomicin. In addition, a 3′-*O*-phosphotransferase type 1 enzyme was produced, responsible for high resistance to Km and neomycin, as well as a 3″-*O*-adenylyltransferase, causing resistance to Sm and spectinomycin (Table 1). Resistance to Ap and carbinicillin was due to a TEM-type β-lactamase. All these enzymes are often found in strains of the *Enterobacteriaceae* family and in *Pseudomonas*. The genetic determinants of the enzymes in these organisms mostly are part of plasmids. We suggested, therefore, that an R plasmid was transferred from the nosocomial hospital flora to *Acinetobacter*, which rendered the *Acinetobacter* strain resistant to many antimicrobials.

Various treatments of cultures with agents or procedures known to affect plasmid replication (ethidium bromide, aging of cultures) yielded variants which had become susceptible to Ap and Km alone or to Gm, Ap, Km, Su, and Tc. All variants still were resistant to Cm and Sm.

Transfer of resistance to susceptible strains of the *Acinetobacter* species or to appropriate receptors of the *Enterobacteriaceae* family by mixed cultivation in broth or on agar plates (3, 4) could not be achieved. With the help of the plasmid RP4, however, determinants of resist-

TABLE 1. *Substrate profile of the enzymes produced by Acinetobacter calcoaceticus*[a]

Substrate	AAC (3)	APH (3′)-I	AAD (3″)	MIC (µg/ml)
Gentamicin	+	−	−	>200
Sisomicin	+	−	−	100
Netilmicin	(+)	−	−	12.5
Lividomycin	−	+	−	>200
Butirosin	−	−	−	6.25
Tobramycin	(+)	−	−	3.12
Neomycin	−	+	−	>200
Kanamycin	−	+	−	>200
Amikacin	−	−	−	3.12
Paromomycin	−	+	−	>200
Streptomycin	−	−	+	200
Spectinomycin	−	−	+	200

AAC(3), Aminoglycoside 3-*N*-acetyltransferase; APH(3′)-I, aminoglycoside 3′-*O*-phosphotransferase type I; AAD(3″), aminoglycoside 3″-*O*-adenylyltransferase; +, substrate; −, no substrate; (+), weak substrate.

ance to Gm, Su, Cm, and Sm of an Ap/Km-susceptible variant could be transferred to *Escherichia coli* K-12. Since RP4 carries the markers for resistance to Ap, Km, and Tc, we were not able to prove mobilization of the respective determinants in *Acinetobacter* by the plasmid. Several attempts to mobilize these markers with other plasmids, for instance, with a trimethoprim R plasmid, failed.

Results of elimination and conjugation experiments suggested that antibiotic resistance in *Acinetobacter* might be either due to chromosomal R markers or to R determinants, located on nonconjugative plasmids. In order to differentiate between these two possibilities, plasmid DNA of a representative wild-type strain (no. 67) as well as of two types of susceptible variants (variant 1, susceptible to Ap and Km; variant 2, susceptible, in addition, to Su, Tc, and Gm) was extracted and analyzed by agarose gel electrophoresis. All three strains contained a plasmid with a molecular weight of 6×10^6, which, apparently, has nothing to do with antibiotic resistance in these strains.

From *E. coli* transconjugants, obtained with the helper plasmid RP4, radioactively labeled plasmid DNA was isolated by isopycnic centrifugation in CsCl-ethidium bromide density gradients. The purified DNA was then analyzed by centrifugation in neutral sucrose gradients. Four transconjugants, which had obtained resistance to Cm, Gm, Sm, and Su, and perhaps to Tc, from strain 67, were examined. The molecular weights of the RP4 plasmids of these transconjugants had increased by 15×10^6 or 30×10^6.

The results show that multiple-antibiotic resistance in a strain of *A. calcoaceticus* subsp.

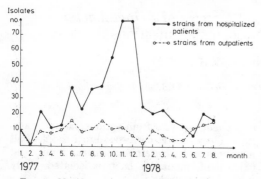

FIG. 1. *Number of Acinetobacter calcoaceticus strains isolated in 1977 and 1978.*

anitratus which caused an epidemic in the intensive care ward of the university hospital is due to chromosomally located markers. It can be suggested that this strain evolved by transfer of an R plasmid from the nosocomial hospital flora to *Acinetobacter* and integration of the R determinants of this plasmid into the *Acinetobacter* chromosome. Such a transfer, however, could not be shown in vitro in mating experiments. The chromosomal DNA sequence carrying the R determinants can be mobilized by the helper plasmid RP4 and transferred with this plasmid to appropriate receptor strains. The molecular weights of the transposed DNA sequences vary between 15×10^6 and 30×10^6. This suggests that the concerned chromosomal

DNA region of *Acinetobacter* is composed of several translocatable DNA pieces.

1. **Buxton, A. E., R. L. Anderson, D. Werdegar, and E. Atlas.** 1978. Nosocomial respiratory tract infection and colonization with *Acinetobacter calcoaceticus.* Am. J. Med. **65:**507–513.
2. **Glew, R. H., R. C. Moellering, and L. J. Kunz.** 1977. Infections with *Acinetobacter calcoaceticus* (Herellea vaginiola): clinical and laboratory studies. Medicine **56:** 79–97.
3. **Olson, R. H., and P. Shipley.** 1973. Host range and properties of the *Pseudomonas aeruginosa* R-factor R1822. J. Bacteriol **113:**772–780.
4. **Towner, K. J., and A. Vivian.** 1976. RP₄-mediated conjugation in *Acinetobacter calcoaceticus.* J. Gen Microbiol. **93:**355–360.

Characterization of a β-Lactamase–Specifying Plasmid from *Haemophilus ducreyi*

J. BRUNTON,* P. BENNETT, J. GRINSTED, M. H. RICHMOND, AND W. ALBRITTON

University of Bristol, Bristol, England, and University of Manitoba, Winnipeg, Manitoba, Canada*

Brunton et al. (2) reported that β-lactamase production in three strains of *Haemophilus ducreyi* was specified by a 6×10^6-dalton plasmid which was designated pJB1. pMR0360 and RSF0885 mediate β-lactamase production in Far Eastern isolates of *Neisseria gonorrhoeae* and *H. parainfluenzae*, respectively. Because these latter plasmids had been shown to be highly related (6), we decided to see whether there was a relationship between them and pJB1. Since restriction endonuclease digestion suggested the presence of at least 2.2×10^6 daltons of TnA sequences in pJB1, we also examined more closely the amount of TnA sequences and their function. We reexamined the molecular weight of pJB1 and found it to be 5.7×10^6.

pJB1 DNA was alkali denatured and renatured in formamide for 30 min. The DNA was spread by use of the formamide technique (3), shadowed with platinum palladium, and examined by electron microscopy. Molecules showed two single-stranded loops whose contour lengths corresponded to 3.2×10^6 and 2.5×10^6 daltons. They were separated by a short double-stranded region. Thus, pJB1 carries an inverted repeat sequence. Heteroduplexes between pJB1 and RSF1010::TnA showed 3.2×10^6 daltons of homologous sequences. The location of the homologous sequences in RSF1010::TnA corresponded to the expected location of the TnA transposon. These results suggested that pJB1 carries the

whole TnA sequence, including both inverted repeats. To demonstrate function of the TnA in pJB1, we transformed the plasmid into *Escherichia coli* JC6310, a *recA* host. pUB307 was mated in, and the two plasmids were grown together for 50 generations. The strain was then mated with a *polA*, nalidixic acid-resistant strain (SF800) (4), and appropriately diluted transconjugants were selected on agar supplemented with (A) tetracycline and nalidixic acid and (B) tetracycline, carbenicillin, and nalidixic acid. Transposition frequency was measured as the number of colonies growing on B divided by the number growing on A and was found to be 10^{-5}. That transposition had occurred was verified by demonstrating 100% cotransfer of tetracycline and carbenicillin resistance in subsequent outcrosses.

Although the minimal copy number of pJB1 was found to be 13, the plasmid was not stably maintained in *E. coli* J53. In the absence of antibiotic selection, 50% of the cells lost the plasmid after 100 generations.

The relationship between pJB1 and pMR0360 was studied by examining heteroduplexes. Figure 1 shows that the two plasmids share 3.3×10^6 daltons of homologous sequences (labeled "a"). Two nonhomologous sequences of 2.4×10^6 and 1.1×10^6 daltons take the form of insertion/deletion loops ("b" and "c," respectively). The nature of the two loops was further examined by

TABLE 1. *Small plasmids responsible for β-lactamase production in Neisseria gonorrhoeae and Haemophilus species*[a]

Plasmid	Original host	Area of origin	Percent TnA	Homology with pMR0360 (%)
RSF0885	*H. parainfluenzae*	San Francisco	30	90[b]
pVE445	*H. influenzae*	West Germany	30–40	95[b]
pJB1	*H. ducreyi*	Winnipeg, Canada	100	58[c]
pMR0360	*N. gonorrhoeae*	Far East	40	100[b]
pMR0200	*N. gonorrhoeae*	West Africa	40	70[b]

[a] pVE445 is described in reference 5; RSF0885, pMR0360, and pMR0200 are described in reference 6. The guanine plus cytosine content of all five plasmids was 0.41.

[b] Assessed by an S1 endonuclease method (5, 6).

[c] Assessed by electron microscope heteroduplex analysis in this study; 58% of pJB1 and 75% of pMR0360 sequences are homologous.

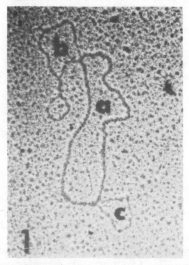

FIG. 1. *Heteroduplex of pMR0360 and pJB1 DNA. The duplex region (a) is 3.3 × 10⁶ daltons. The insertion/deletion loops b and c are 2.4 × 10⁶ and 1.1 × 10⁶ daltons, respectively.*

heteroduplexing DNA cleaved by restriction endonucleases. Loop c was found to be cleaved when HindIII-cut pMR0360 DNA was used, but to be intact when the DNA was cut with PstI. Loop b was not present when a PstI fragment of pJB1 (missing 2.2×10^6 daltons of TnA) was heteroduplexed with PstI-digested pMR0360.

In view of restriction mapping data not presented here, these findings suggested that loop c represents non-TnA sequences of pMR0360 which are not present in pJB1 while loop b represents mostly TnA sequences present in pJB1 but absent in pMR0360.

DNA of RSF0885 and pMR0360, cleaved once within their TnA sequences with BglI was also

heteroduplexed. Here, 3.4×10^6 daltons were homologous while a substitution loop was formed by the short nonhomologous sequences. Restriction mapping suggests that the substitution loop lies outside the TnA sequences.

Table 1 shows the characteristics of the small β-lactamase plasmids studied in *N. gonorrhoeae* and several *Haemophilus* species. All share large portions of their DNA sequences. pJB1 is the first such plasmid to contain a complete and functional TnA sequence. This study shows that three of these plasmids (pJB1, pMR0360, and RSF0885), although highly related, differ from each other in discrete regions. This situation is reminiscent of the streptomycin/sulfonamide resistance plasmids studied by Barth and Grinter (1).

We thank Stanley Falkow for suggesting this study, as well as for providing many bacterial strains.

1. **Barth, P. T., and N. Grinter.** 1974. Comparison of the deoxyribonucleic acid molecular weights and homologies of plasmids conferring linked resistance to streptomycin and sulfonamides. J. Bacteriol. **120:**618–630.

2. **Brunton, J., I. Maclean, A. Ronald, and W. Albritton.** 1979. Plasmid-mediated ampicillin resistance in *Haemophilus ducreyi*. Antimicrob. Agents Chemother. **15:** 294–299.

3. **Davis, R., M. Simon, and N. Davidson.** 1971. Electron microscope heteroduplex methods for mapping regions of base sequence homology in nucleic acids. Methods Enzymol. **21:**413–428.

4. **Gill, R., F. Heffron, G. Dougan, and S. Falkow.** 1978. Analysis sequences transposed by complementation of two classes of transposition-deficient mutants of Tn3. J. Bacteriol. **136:**742–756.

5. **Laufs, R., P. Kaulfers, G. John, and U. Teschner.** 1979. Molecular characterization of a small Haemophilus plasmid specifying β-lactamase. J. Gen. Microbiol. **111:**223–231.

6. **Roberts, M., L. Elwell, and S. Falkow.** 1977. Molecular characterization of two beta-lactamase-specifying plasmids from *Neisseria gonorrhoeae*. J. Bacteriol. **131:** 557–563.

Simple Method of Studying Drug-Induced Loss of Plasmid DNA
(Curing)

JAMES B. JOHNSTON* AND JOHN A. GRUNAU

University of Illinois, Urbana, Illinois 61801, U.S.A.

Drug-induced loss of plasmid was first described by Hirota, who used acridine orange to isolate derivatives of *Escherichia coli* which had lost the F factor (2). The spectrum of agents that have since been used to isolate plasmidless derivatives of plasmid-bearing bacteria includes intercalating dyes, DNA cross-linking agents, an inhibitor of DNA gyrase, surfactants, and high temperatures. Some of these agents are effective against a broad range of plasmids; others apparently are effective against only one or a few plasmids.

In the past a typical experiment involved treatment of the plasmid-bearing strain with drug throughout a growth cycle and assay of the resulting population for the loss of plasmid-specific traits. The design of such experiments assumed that the drug selectively interfered with plasmid replication, giving rise to new, plasmidless cells during growth. However, in our experience the requirement for exposure to drug in the exponential phase of growth is not always absolute. Moreover, the quantitative reproducibility of such experiments is often poor.

To study the phenomenon of drug-induced loss, we have devised a simple assay for the frequency of plasmidless cells in a population. The technique takes advantage of an established method for the isolation of Lac⁻ mutants (4), namely, the inhibition of *lacY*⁺ bacteria by certain β-galactosides. In the presence of *p*-nitrophenyl-β-D-thiogalactoside (PNPTG), derepressed Lac⁺ bacteria cannot form colonies on minimal succinate medium; *lacY* strains grow normally. If the only copies of the *lac* operon reside on plasmid DNA, only plasmidless cells will form colonies on PNPTG agar.

For initial study we chose a derivative of drug resistance factor RP1, plasmid pGC91.14, into which the *lac*-bearing transposon Tn951 has been inserted (1). We chose this plasmid for several reasons. First, RP1 is conjugative and can be transmitted to a very wide range of gram-negative bacteria; therefore, pGC91.14::Tn951 might be used to construct a series of strains with different bacterial hosts. Second, we anticipate that Tn951 can be used to introduce the *lac* genes into other plasmids. Finally, this plasmid carries several other selectable markers (Ap, Kn, Tc, Dps), which can be used to confirm that

Lac⁻ colonies appearing on PNPTG agar are indeed plasmidless. The host chosen for initial study was *Salmonella typhimurium* AA2102 (His⁻ Ser⁻ Arg⁻), a derivative of LT-2 that is plasmidless (R. Olsen, personal communication). The test strain U201 was constructed by the conjugative transfer of pGC91.14::Tn951 into AA2102.

To assay the frequency of plasmidless cells in a population, U201 was plated by the agar overlay technique on Vogel-Bonner E agar containing 0.3% succinate and 25 μg each of L-histidine, L-serine, and L-arginine per ml. The top agar also contained 7 μmol of PNPTG, and 3 μmol of isopropyl-β-D-thiogalactoside as inducer. Appropriate dilutions of the culture were plated on the same medium without the thiogalactosides to obtain the viable count. The ratio of spontaneous Lac⁻ colony-forming units to the total colony-forming units in L-broth culture averaged 6×10^{-4}, ranging from 2×10^{-4} to 1×10^{-3}. There was no difference between the frequencies of Lac⁻ cells measured on PNPTG agar and on lactose-tetrazolium plates. In one experiment, 93% of spontaneous Lac⁻ strains lacked all of the RP1 drug resistance markers; 7% retained these markers and were presumed to have lost the Tn951 transposon rather than the plasmid. During a growth cycle in L-broth, the ratio of plasmidless cells to total colony-forming units did vary perceptibly, but all frequencies fell within the range reported above.

When cells were challenged with acriflavine (Fig. 1), the proportion of plasmidless cells increased. The increase was most dramatic in late stationary phase, apparently due to the preferential death of plasmid-bearing cells. This enrichment of plasmidless cells, therefore, cannot be explained by the model of specific inhibition of plasmid replication by the drug during the growth phase. Rather, this result suggests that the presence of the plasmid, or the expression of one or more plasmid functions, enhances the susceptibility of the strain to the toxic action of acriflavine in stationary phase. It also suggests that the most effective use of acriflavine to obtain plasmidless derivatives may be addition of the drug to stationary-phase cultures.

The action of quinacrine (Fig. 2) contrasted sharply with that of acriflavine. An initial period of cell death was followed by exponential growth of the survivors, during which time the frequency of plasmidless cells in the population was enriched. Independent measurements on U201 and AA2102 in L-broth containing 500 μg of quinacrine per ml showed that the doubling time of the plasmid-bearing strain was longer than that of the plasmidless cells. This could account for most or all of the observed increase in the proportion of plasmidless cells during exponential growth. Quinacrine-induced loss of plasmid DNA could have been occurring in the phase of decelerating growth rate, but we have not yet proved this. Again in contrast to acri-

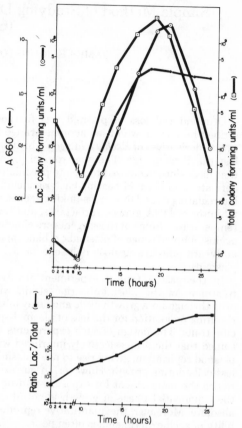

FIG. 2. *Influence of quinacrine on the frequency of plasmidless cells. Experimental details are as for Fig. 1, except that the L-broth contained 500 μg of quinacrine per ml.*

flavine, no differential killing was observed in the death phase.

We have avoided using the term "curing agent" to describe our results. The drugs studied may have induced plasmid loss, but our data suggest that the primary action, certainly of acriflavine and possibly of quinacrine, was to increase the proportion of plasmidless cells in the population by selecting against plasmid-bearing cells.

Novick pointed out 10 years ago that drugs may increase the proportion of plasmidless cells in a population either by strain selection or by inducing plasmid loss. He illustrated his point with novobiocin, which appears to enrich the proportion of plasmidless cells by strain selection (3).

The technique that we have described should permit study of drug-induced plasmid loss in a variety of bacterial hosts and in many plasmid

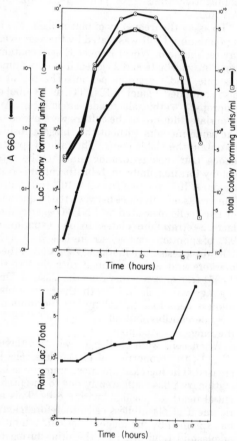

FIG. 1. *Influence of acriflavine on the frequency of plasmidless cells. Stationary phase S. typhimurium U201 was diluted into L-broth containing acriflavine, 40 μg/ml, and incubated at 37°C. The absorbance at 660 nm in an 18-mm tube was determined on appropriate dilutions in a Bausch & Lomb Spectronic 20 colorimeter. Total and Lac⁻ colony-forming units were determined as indicated in the text. The lower panel shows the ratio of Lac⁻ to total colony-forming units.*

incompatibility groups. The assay should permit differentiation between agents that act primarily by strain selection and those that act more directly on plasmid maintenance in the cell.

This work was supported in part by Public Health Service grant 5 T32 ES07001 from the National Institute of Environmental Health Sciences to the University of Illinois.

1. **Cornelis, G., D. Ghosal, and H. Saedler.** 1978. Tn951: a new transposon carrying a lactose operon. Mol. Gen. Genet. **160:**215–224.
2. **Hirota, Y.** 1956. Artificial elimination of the F factor in Bact. coli K12. Nature (London) **178:**92.
3. **Novick, R. P.** 1969. Extrachromosomal inheritance in bacteria. Bacteriol. Rev. **33:**210–263.
4. **Smith, T. F., and J. R. Sadler.** 1971. The nature of lactose operator constitutive mutations. J. Mol. Biol. **59:**273–305.

Cinoxacin, a Synthetic Antibacterial Agent That Inhibits Transfer of R Factors

J. L. OTT* AND R. S. GORDEE

Lilly Research Laboratories, Eli Lilly & Co., Indianapolis, Indiana 46206, U.S.A.

Cinoxacin is an orally active synthetic antimicrobial agent for the treatment of urinary tract infections. Because cinoxacin inhibits DNA replication (2), the effect of this antimicrobial agent on the in vitro transfer of R factors was investigated. Strains of *Escherichia coli* used in these experiments are listed in Table 1. Cultures were incubated for 6 h in brain heart infusion broth and then diluted 1:10 into fresh brain heart infusion broth containing various concentrations of cinoxacin. One-tenth volume of the donor culture was immediately added to the corresponding recipient culture to give the mating mixture. The number of donor, recipient, and transconjugant cells was determined by plate counts on agar containing appropriate antibiotics as the selective agent. The extent of transfer at various time periods was calculated as the percentage of recipients that had received the R factor. In the absence of antibacterial agents, 4.3×10^4 to 1.6×10^7 transconjugants/ml (depending on the R factor transferred and its recipient culture) were detected after 60 min of mating; these numbers corresponded to 0.1 to 8% of the recipients receiving the R factor. The

percentage of inhibition was calculated by determining the extent of transfer in the presence and absence of cinoxacin. The percent inhibition was plotted against the concentration of cinoxacin expressed as log base 2, the slope was cal-

TABLE 1. *Escherichia coli* strains

Strain	Antibiotic markers[a]
DONORS	
15T⁻ R64-11	Tc^r, Sm^r, Su^r
15T⁻ R1-19	Cm^r, Ap^r, Km^r, Sm^r, Su^r
15T⁻ ST	Tc^r, Sm^r, Su^r
15T⁻ JJ-1	Cm^r, Sm^r, Su^r
15T⁻ (Na^r) R64-11	Tc^r, Sm^r, Su^r (Na^r)
15T⁻ (Na^r) JJ-1	Cm^r, Sm^r, Su^r (Na^r)
RECIPIENTS	
15T⁻ (Na^r)	(Na^r)
T3, K-12 substrain	(Rm^r)
T10, K-12 substrain	(Rm^r) (Na^r)

[a] The marker listed first was used for selection. Parentheses indicate resistance on the chromosome, not transferable. TC, tetracycline; Sm, streptomycin; Su, sulfonamide; Cm, chloramphenicol; Ap, ampicillin; Km, kanamycin; Na, nalidixic acid; Rm, rifampin.

TABLE 2. *Concentration of cinoxacin (micrograms per milliliter) to produce 99% inhibition of transfer after 60 min*

Recipient	Donor					
	15T⁻^{a} R64-11	15T⁻^{a} R1-19	15T⁻^{a} ST	15T⁻^{a} JJ1	15T⁻(Na^r)[b] R64-11	15T⁻(Na^r)[b] JJ-1
T3^a	13.0	20.2	11.9	12.4	81.4	57.9
15T⁻(Na^r)[b]	14.5	14.2	9.0	12.4	ND^c	ND^c
T10[b]	12.3	17.9	9.5	17.6	77.8	307

^{a} Susceptible to cinoxacin.
^{b} Resistant to nalidixic acid and cinoxacin.
^{c} Not determinable.

TABLE 3. *Concentration of nalidixic acid (micrograms per milliliter) to produce 99% inhibition of transfer after 60 min*

Recipient	Donor	Nalidixic acid
15T⁻(Naʳ)[a]	15T⁻R64-11[b]	7.2
15T⁻(Naʳ)[a]	15T⁻R1-19[b]	14.1
15T⁻(Naʳ)[a]	15T⁻ST[b]	15.2
15T⁻(Naʳ)[a]	15T⁻JJ[b]	13.7
T3[b]	15T⁻(Naʳ) R64-11[a]	NI[c]
T3[b]	15T⁻(Naʳ)JJ-1[a]	NI[c]

[a] Resistant to nalidixic acid and cinoxacin.
[b] Susceptible to cinoxacin.
[c] No inhibition.

culated by use of linear regression, and the concentration required to produce 99% inhibition was estimated.

The concentration of cinoxacin required to produce 99% inhibition of transfer after 60 min of mating is presented in Table 2. Cinoxacin at concentrations of 11.9 to 20.2 µg/ml inhibited transfer of the R factors when both donors and recipients were susceptible to cinoxacin. At concentrations of cinoxacin comparable to those attained in human urine, ranging from 425 to 750 µg/ml (1), transconjugants were not detected after 60 min of mating, indicating complete inhibition of R-factor transfer in cinoxacin-susceptible strains.

Cinoxacin was also an effective inhibitor of transfer into nalidixic acid-resistant recipients, 15T⁻(Naʳ) and T10. Cinoxacin concentrations of 9.0 to 17.9 µg/ml were required for 99% inhibition (Table 3). When the R factor was present in a nalidixic acid-resistant donor, 57.9 to 307 µg of cinoxacin/ml was required for inhibition.

Cinoxacin and nalidixic acid were equally effective in inhibiting transfer of four R factors into 15T⁻(Naʳ) (Tables 2 and 3). Cinoxacin inhibited transfer of the R64-11 and JJ-1 plasmids from nalidixic acid-resistant donors, whereas nalidixic acid showed no inhibition.

In summary, cinoxacin was found to be an effective inhibitor of the in vitro transfer of a number of R factors. Transfer was inhibited by cinoxacin when the recipient or donor was nalidixic acid resistant. The ability of cinoxacin to inhibit R-factor transfer could be an asset in the treatment of urinary tract infections.

1. Colleen, S., K-E. Andersson, and P.-A Mårdh. 1977. Studies on cinoxacin. 3. Concentrations of cinoxacin in serum, urine and tissues of urological patients. J. Antimicrob. Chemother. 3:579–584.
2. Ott, J. L., and R. S. Gordee. 1978. Inhibition of R-factor transfer by cinoxacin, p. 688–689. *In* Current chemotherapy, Proceedings of the 10th International Congress of Chemotherapy. American Society for Microbiology, Washington, D.C.

Identification of Antibiotic-Inactivating Enzymes by Stepwise Discriminant Analysis of Susceptibility Test Results

R. L. KENT,* T. F. O'BRIEN, A. A. MEDEIROS, J. J. FARRELL, AND M. A. GUZMAN

Peter Bent Brigham Hospital and Harvard Medical School, Boston, Massachusetts 02115, U.S.A.

Stepwise discriminant analysis was used to develop classification functions that provided optimal identification of β-lactamases in one set of bacterial isolates and of aminoglycoside-inactivating enzymes in a second set of isolates solely on the basis of susceptibility test results.

In the first set, isoelectric focusing identified β-lactamases in a selection of 157 clinical isolates of *Escherichia coli*, grouped as TEM (111), OXA-1 (8), OXA-2 and -3 (9), class II (14), and none (15). The feasibility of distinguishing among isolates belonging to these groups on the basis of their inhibition zone diameters for eight β-lactam antibiotics (ampicillin, carbenicillin, cefamandole, cefoxitin, cephaloridine, cephalothin, piperacillin, and ticarcillin) was examined by statistical discriminant analysis.

The rationale for using zone diameters to identify the enzyme present in an isolate is that isolates with the same or very similar resistance mechanisms will tend to have a characteristic antibiogram distinguishing them from other isolates with a different (or no) enzyme. Mean zone diameters around β-lactam disks for *E. coli* isolates in each group provided estimates of characteristic antibiograms resulting from the presence of β-lactamases. Ampicillin zones readily distinguished any enzyme group (mean zone diameters, 6.0 to 6.8 mm) from the no enzyme group (19.4 mm). Mean zones for carbenicillin separated class II isolates (20.4 mm) from isolates with TEM (6.0 mm) or OXA-1 (6.5 mm); low cephalothin zones (averaging 7.1 mm) also characterized class II isolates. Antibiogram profiles for TEM and OXA-1 isolates were differentiated only by small differences in mean zones of inhibition for cephaloridine and cefamandole. Classification will be most successful when zone diameter variation of individual isolates around their characteristic antibiogram are small, relative to the size of mean profile differences between the groups; the opposite would suggest considerable overlap among isolates from different groups.

Discriminant analysis for several groups formalizes this idea in a statistical technique designed, under appropriate assumptions, to provide linear classification functions of the zone diameters that minimizes the probability of incorrectly classified isolates. The method takes into account not only variation of isolate zone diameters for each antibiotic, but also correlations among zone diameters of different antibiotics. Stepwise application of discriminant analysis selects in order those antibiotics which contribute most to distinguishing between resistance enzymes, permitting trade-offs between the accuracy of classifications using a large number of disks and the efficiency of classifications based on a smaller number of disks. At each step, that antibiotic which, on the basis of a variance ratio (F) test, maximized the ratio of between-group differences to within-group variation was entered into the discriminant analysis until all antibiotics significantly differentiating between the enzymes present in isolates had been selected. Antibiotic disks contributing redundant information were identified and not utilized. In developing classification functions and posterior probabilities, equal prior probabilities of 0.20 were assigned to each group.

Ampicillin, carbenicillin, cephaloridine, cefamandole, piperacillin, and cephalothin were selected in successive steps into the discriminant analysis. F-values indicated the level of significance of the disk being added at each step and of the discriminant function for all antibiotics entered up to and including that step. All F-values were highly significant $(P < 0.01)$.

F-values tested the significance of discrimination between all pairs of enzyme groups (Table 1). All pairwise F-values were highly signifi-

TABLE 2. *F-values for pairwise discrimination of aminoglycoside enzyme groups*

Enzyme	F-value		
	ANT-2"	AAC-6'	Both
AAC-6'	92.3		
Both	27.1	99.2	
None	50.4	38.1	81.1

cant $(P < 0.01)$, indicating that meaningful distinctions were achieved between isolates from each pair of groups. Isolates with no β-lactamase (none) were readily distinguished from each enzyme group, as seen in the very large F-values, ranging from 676.0 when paired with TEM to 221.9 with OXA-2,3. The smallest, though still highly significant, F-values occurred for discrimination between TEM and OXA-1 isolates $(F = 7.5)$ and between OXA-1 and OXA-2,3 $(F = 28.0)$.

The linear classification functions, using observed zones around six β-lactam disks, correctly identified the enzyme in 149 of 157 *E. coli* isolates. The similarity of TEM and OXA-1 isolates resulted in 6 of 111 TEM isolates being termed OXA-1 and 2 of 8 OXA-1 isolates being called TEM. All others were correctly identified.

Discriminant analysis was also applied to a second set of 34 clinical isolates of *Serratia marcescens*, previously assayed by the radioactive method for aminoglycoside-inactivating enzymes and susceptibility tested against gentamicin, tobramycin, netilmicin, and amikacin disks. ANT-2" was present in 12 isolates, AAC-6' in 6, both enzymes in 11, and neither enzyme in 5 isolates.

Mean zone diameters for tobramycin were 17.2 mm for isolates with neither enzyme, as compared to 9.1 mm for isolates with ANT-2", 8.5 mm with AAC-6', and 6.0 mm with both enzymes. Average gentamicin zones distinguished ANT-2" (9.5 mm) from AAC-6' (19.5 mm). Isolates with both enzymes had the lowest average zone diameters to all four antibiotics.

Gentamicin, tobramycin, and netilmicin were entered successively into the discriminant analysis. F-values testing the discriminating power of these three antibiotics (Table 2) for each pair of groups were highest (indicating best differentiation) for isolates with AAC-6' and ANT-2" (92.3) and lowest (27.1) for discriminating ANT-2" from the presence of both enzymes. All F-values were highly significant $(P < 0.01)$. Linear classification functions correctly identified all 12 ANT-2" isolates, 5 of 6 isolates with AAC-6', 10 of 11 with both enzymes, and 5 isolates with neither. Only 2 of 24 isolates were incorrectly classified.

TABLE 1. *F-value for pairwise discrimination of β-lactamases*

Enzyme	F-value			
	TEM	OXA-1	OXA-2,3	Class II
OXA-1	7.5			
OXA-2,3	44.7	28.0		
Class II	330.8	149.1	84.2	
None	676.0	269.6	221.9	285.9

The high degree of accuracy achieved in identifying β-lactamases (94.9%) in *E. coli* and aminoglycoside-inactivating enzymes (94.1%) in *S. marcescens* from zone diameters around selected disks strongly suggests the feasibility of procedures for presumptive identification and surveillance of specific resistance mechanisms from routine susceptibility tests.

Easy Method for Evaluating the Structure-Activity Relationship of Penicillinase and Cephalosporinase Inhibition by β-Lactam Antibiotics

L. HUANG, K. JAKUBAS,* AND R. W. BURG

Merck Sharp and Dohme Research Laboratories, Rahway, New Jersey 07065, U.S.A.

The presence of β-lactamases has been detected in the majority of bacteria. The β-lactamases of both gram-positive and gram-negative microorganisms contribute to their resistance to β-lactam antibiotics by catalyzing the hydrolysis of the β-lactam ring. To classify β-lactam antibiotics based on β-lactamase inhibition, an easy and simple spectrophotometric assay has been utilized by modifying the method described by Ullman (6). This method is based on the production of a red pigment under aerobic conditions by the hydrolysis of cephacetrile. As a result of our careful selection of enzyme systems, two completely different types of β-lactamases have been used in the assay. One is a gram-positive inducible exocellular enzyme with penicillinase activity which was obtained from the cultural supernatant of *Bacillus cereus* MB370 after induction with 1 μg of penicillin G per ml.

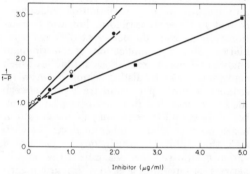

FIG. 2. *Inhibitor concentration versus $1/(1 - P)$. Symbols: ●, thienamycin versus gram-positive β-lactamase; ○, thienamycin versus gram-negative β-lactamase; ■, cefoxitin versus gram-negative β-lactamase.*

The other is a gram-negative inducible intracellular β-lactamase with primarily cephalosporinase activity which was derived from the cell-free extracts of *Pseudomonas aeruginosa* MB979 after induction with 1 g of penicillin G per ml. The enzyme assay was incubated overnight at 37°C with agitation in 0.15 mg of cephacetrile per ml in 0.025 M NaPO$_4$ buffer, pH 7.0. Because of the overnight incubation used in this assay, it is important to establish that there is a linear relationship between the intensity of pigment production and protein concentration. Various enzyme protein concentrations were assayed under constant cephacetrile concentration and incubation time. The linear relationship between optical density at 554 nm and protein concentration for both *Bacillus*- and *Pseudomonas*-inducible β-lactamases is shown in Fig. 1.

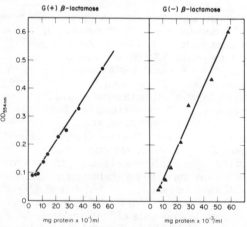

FIG. 1. *Optical density at 554 nm (OD$_{554}$) of pigment production versus enzyme protein concentration after overnight incubation of β-lactamase with 150 μg of cephacetrile per ml. Symbols: ●, gram-positive inducible exocellular β-lactamase; ▲, gram-negative inducible intracellular β-lactamase.*

Inhibition of β-lactamase was evaluated by the decrease in pigment production in the presence of antibiotic. The 50% inhibition (I$_{50}$) of the antibiotic can be calculated based on the linear relationship between inhibitor concentration and a corresponding factor $1/(1 - P)$, where P

TABLE 1. β-Lactamase-inhibiting activity of β-lactam antibiotics

Antibiotic[a]	I_{50} (µg/ml)[b]	
	Gram-positive Bacillus[c]	Gram-negative Pseudomonas[c]
Thienamycin	1.6	1.4
Cefamandole	>50	>50
Cefoxitin	≥50	0.7
Piperacillin	>50	>50
HR-756	>50	2.0
Oxacephamycin	>50	0.1
Cefuroxime	≥50	0.6
Clavulanic acid	1.0	16.0
Azlocillin	>50	22.0
Carbenicillin	>50	2.3
Mezlocillin	>50	32.0
Ticarcillin	>50	4.4
Penicillin G	>50	>50
6-Bromopenicillanic acid	4	3.4
Ampicillin	>50	10.0
Methicillin	>50	0.8

[a] All antibiotics were dissolved in 50% methanol.
[b] I_{50} > 50 µg/ml is considered to be inactive.
[c] β-Lactamase source.

represents the decimal value of percent inhibition, as described by Job et al. (2). This linear relationship is illustrated for thienamycin and cefoxitin as shown in Fig. 2.

The results of systematic analysis of β-lactamase inhibition by various antibiotics are shown in Table 1. Thienamycin is the only β-lactam antibiotic tested that is a potent inhibitor of β-lactamases produced from both gram-positive and gram-negative organisms and is also a potent broad-spectrum antimicrobial agent (3) against many clinically resistant organisms, including P. aeruginosa.

As reported earlier, the semisynthetic anti-staphylococcal penicillins such as methicillin were ineffective against the extracellular β-lactamase of Bacillus (1, 4) but proved to be effective inhibitors of the cephalosporinase produced by Pseudomonas. Of the penicillin derivatives tested, 6-bromopenicillanic acid was the most effective against both β-lactamases. Penicillin G was not active against either enzyme.

The cephalosporin derivatives and the cephamycins are good inhibitors of the gram-negative, chromosomally mediated cephalosporinase but are relatively inactive against the gram-positive penicillinase. Our results confirm previous reports that cefoxitin has been found to be nearly totally resistant to the β-lactamases from gram-negative bacteria (5).

In addition to being a direct and simple assay for β-lactamase inhibition, the overnight incubation of the reaction mixture excludes the detection of inhibitors which are unstable to β-lactamase. This protocol can also be applied to the primary screening of β-lactamase inhibitors of biological origin.

1. Cole, M., S. Elson, and P. D. Fullbrook. 1972. Inhibition of the β-lactamase of Escherichia coli and Klebsiella pneumoniae by semisynthetic penicillins. Biochem. J. 127:295–308.
2. Job, D., C. Cochet, A. Dhien, and E. M. Chambaz. 1978. A rapid method for screening inhibitor effects: determination of I_{50} and its standard deviation. Anal. Biochem. 84:68–77.
3. Kropp, H., J. S. Kahan, F. M. Kahan, J. Sundelof, G. Darland, and J. Birnbaum. 1976. Program Abstr. Intersci. Conf. Antimicrob. Agents Chemother., 6th, Chicago, Ill., abstr. no. 228.
4. Neu, H. C. 1974. The role of beta-lactamases in the resistance of gram negative bacteria to penicillin and cephalosporin derivatives. Infect. Dis. Rev. 11:133–149.
5. Richmond, M. H., and S. Walton. 1976. Comparative study of seven cephalosporins: susceptibility to β-lactamase and ability to penetrate the surface layers of Escherichia coli. Antimicrob. Agents Chemother. 10:219–222.
6. Ullman, U. 1976. A simple screening test for determining the β-lactamase activity of bacteria. Microbios Lett. 3:35–39.

Relationship Between β-Lactamase Activity of Serratia marcescens and Resistance to β-Lactam Antibiotics

J. CHRISTENSON,* E. SQUIRES, W. DeLORENZO, AND R. CLEELAND

Hoffmann-La Roche Inc., Nutley, New Jersey 07110, U.S.A.

Most, if not all, Serratia marcescens strains appear to produce chromosomally determined cephalosporinases (class I β-lactamases). In addition, many strains have been shown to elaborate plasmid-mediated, broad-spectrum β-lactamases (class III). Tsang et al. (4) concluded that β-lactamase production was not solely responsible for resistance to β-lactam antibiotics in the strains studied. They found strains which were resistant to one or more β-lactams but

TABLE 1. *In vivo and in vitro response of S. marcescens strains to ampicillin, carbenicillin, cefazolin, and mecillinam and correlation to β-lactamase specific activities*

Strain[a]	PD$_{50}$ (mg/kg, s.c.)[b]				MIC (μg/ml)[c]			
	Amp	Carb	Cef	Mec	Amp	Carb	Cef	Mec
S217	80	23	127	549	2.7	4.0	576	293
S2	24	369	238	816	131	3.0	853	531
S1	66	16.5	256	856	1.8	1.3	256	258
S147	27	16.8	511	668	1.2	342	320	75
SM	50	34	859	>1,000	37	4.0	384	490
S157	599	611	>1,000	>1,000	8.0	343	576	149
S3	172	167	853	>1,000	12	2.0	768	613
S303	717	107	>1,000	>1,000	92	4.0	1,024	1,024
5805	>1,000	>1,000	>1,000	>1,000	352	1,024	1,024	622
S4	>2,000	>1,000	>1,500	>1,000	1,024	1,024	1,024	441
S247	>2,000	>1,000	>1,000	>1,000	1,024	1,024	1,024	472
S5	>2,000	>1,000	>1,500	~1,000	520	1,024	1,024	117
τ, nitrocefin (*P*)	0.731 (<0.01)	0.636 (<0.01)	0.827 (<0.001)	—[d]	0.595 (<0.01)	0.571 (<0.05)	0.647 (<0.01)	0.061 (NS)
τ, cefazolin (*P*)	0.795 (<0.001)	0.636 (<0.01)	0.810 (<0.001)	—[d]	0.534 (<0.01)	0.636 (<0.01)	0.581 (<0.05)	0 (NS)
τ, cephaloridine (*P*)	0.736 (<0.01)	0.552 (<0.05)	0.731 (<0.01)	—[d]	0.644 (<0.05)	0.454 (NS)[e]	0.580 (<0.05)	0.178 (NS)

[a] The strains are listed in order of increasing specific activity with nitrocefin as the substrate.

[b] Abbreviations: Amp, ampicillin; Carb, carbenicillin; Cef, cefazolin; Mec, mecillinam; PD$_{50}$, 50% protective dose; s.c., subcutaneously. Average of a minimum of three experiments; single treatment immediately after infection.

[c] Average of three to seven determinations by agar dilution assay with a 10^{-5} dilution of an overnight culture and a Steers replicator.

[d] —, All strains exhibited a low response to mecillinam alone; τ values were not calculated.

[e] NS, Not significant (*P* > 0.05).

lacked detectable β-lactamase activity and, conversely, a strain which elaborated considerable β-lactamase but was susceptible to ampicillin, carbenicillin, ticarcillin, and cefoxitin.

Farrar and O'Dell (1) suggested that most *S. marcescens* strains could be divided into two classes: those which were relatively susceptible to ampicillin and carbenicillin and those which were extremely resistant. Both groups tended to be highly resistant to cephalosporins. These authors then showed that the four ampicillin-resistant strains studied all carried plasmids specifying broad-spectrum β-lactamases.

In the present study, we have examined the relationship between the cephalosporinase activities of 12 strains of *S. marcescens* and the response of these strains to ampicillin, carbenicillin, cefazolin, and mecillinam in vitro and in vivo in lethal infections of mice.

All 12 strains produced cell-associated β-lactamase activity which was measurable with nitrocefin, cefazolin, or cephaloridine as the substrate. No β-lactamase activity was detected with ampicillin as the substrate. The enzymes from all 12 strains were markedly inhibited by cloxacillin, but only partially or not at all inhibited by clavulanic acid. These are properties expected of chromosomally mediated cephalosporinases (2, 3).

A strong correlation was found between the cephalosporinase specific activities of the 12 strains and their response, both in vivo and in vitro, to ampicillin, carbenicillin, and cefazolin, but not to mecillinam. Activity in vivo is expressed as the milligram-per-kilogram dose of a given drug required to protect 50% of mice from lethal experimental infections with the respective organism. Activity in vitro is expressed as the MIC in micrograms of a given drug per milliliter for the respective strain by the agar dilution method. Table 1 shows that those strains with higher β-lactamase specific activities for nitrocefin, cefazolin, and cephaloridine also generally had higher 50% protective doses and MIC for ampicillin, carbenicillin, and cefazolin. All strains exhibited a low response to mecillinam in vivo and in vitro. The correlations were quantitated by means of Kendall's rank correlation test (τ). The correlations were found to be significant at the 0.05 level or better in all cases except for mecillinam in vivo and in vitro and carbenicillin MIC with cephaloridine specific activity (Table 1).

The strains were also tested in vivo and in vitro for their response to ampicillin, carbenicillin, and cefazolin in combination with an equal amount of mecillinam. These results are shown in Table 2. Resistance to the combinations was well correlated with β-lactamase specific activity in vivo, but clearly not in vitro.

Pronounced synergy was observed with these combinations in most of the strains. It was observed that those strains with the lower β-lactamase specific activities usually showed synergy, whereas some strains which had relatively high β-lactamase specific activities (S303, 5805,

TABLE 2. *In vivo and in vitro responses of S. marcescens strains to mecillinam in 1:1 combination with ampicillin, carbenicillin, and cefazolin and correlation to β-lactamase specific activities*

Strain[a]	PD$_{50}$ (mg/kg, s.c.)[b]			MIC (μg/ml)[c]		
	1 + 1 Amp + Mec	1 + 1 Carb + Mec	1 + 1 Cef + Mec	1 + 1 Amp + Mec	1 + 1 Carb + Mec	1 + 1 Cef + Mec
S217	15[d]	12.5	17	0.38[d]	1.1	51
S2	7	80	23	17	0.38	8
S1	19	7.5	51	0.6	0.17	4.3
S147	12	4.0	34	0.45	0.06	14.0
SM	17	8.5	46	12	0.27	5.8
S157	179	141	517	0.09	0.13	21
S3	80	113	356	1.3	0.5	24
S303	551	63	637	26	2.3	707
5805	670	>1,000	398	169	129	173
S4	293	>1,000	>1,000	2	48	15
S247	>1,000	>1,000	>1,000	12	4.7	393
S5	591	137	139	0.6	1.2	50
τ, nitrocefin (P)	0.727 (<0.01)	0.588 (<0.05)	0.702 (<0.01)	0.215 (NS)	0.394 (NS)	0.394 (NS)
τ, cefazolin (P)	0.788 (<0.001)	0.588 (<0.05)	0.687 (<0.01)	0.154 (NS)	0.394 (NS)	0.394 (NS)
τ, cephaloridine (P)	0.689 (<0.01)	0.449 (NS)	0.600 (<0.05)	0.270 (NS)	0.467 (NS)	0.378 (NS)

[a] The strains are listed in order of increasing specific activity with nitrocefin as the substrate.

[b] Average of a minimum of three experiments; single treatment immediately after infection. Abbreviations are as in Table 1.

[c] Average of three to seven determinations by agar dilution assay with a 10^{-5} dilution of an overnight culture and a Steers replicator.

[d] PD$_{50}$ and MIC represent the amount of each component in the combination.

S4, and S247) usually did not. However, synergy was consistently observed with strain S5, which had by far the highest β-lactamase specific activity of the strains studied.

The results of the study suggest that the chromosomally determined cephalosporinases of S. marcescens may confer significant resistant to penicillins as well as to cephalosporins. Whether these enzymes are important in mediating resistance to mecillinam is not clear. It should be noted that the designation of these enzymes as cephalosporinases is based on their relatively greater activity toward cephalosporins and not on the absence of activity toward penicillins. In our own experiments, the cephalosporinase assay was considerably more sensitive than the microoiodometric assay used to detect penicillinase activity. Thus, failure to detect activity with ampicillin does not mean that such activity was completely absent.

The poor correlation of β-lactamase specific activity with resistance to mecillinam may be merely a statistical artifact due to the fact that all strains studied were poorly responsive to mecillinam alone. It is also possible that factors other than β-lactamase, such as permeability barriers, are relatively more important in resistance to mecillinam. Further experiments are necessary to test this possibility.

It is interesting to note that β-lactamase specific activity was well correlated with the in vivo response to combinations of mecillinam and ampicillin, carbenicillin, or cefazolin but not with the in vitro response. Thus, in vitro tests may not adequately predict the response of these organisms to such combinations in vivo.

Strain S5 was relatively susceptible to the combinations when compared to other strains with high β-lactamase activity. Whether this is due to a difference in the substrate specificity of the β-lactamase or to a difference in the intrinsic sensitivity of the target enzymes is not clear. In any case, the data show that a high cephalosporinase activity does not preclude a synergistic action of mecillinam with another β-lactam.

1. Farrar, W. E., and N. M. O'Dell. 1976. β-Lactamases and resistance to penicillins and cephalosporins in Serratia marcescens. J. Infect. Dis. 134:245–251.
2. Neu, H. C., and K. P. Fu. 1978. Clavulanic acid, a novel inhibitor of β-lactamases. Antimicrob. Agents Chemother. 14:650–655.
3. Sykes, R. B., and M. Matthew. 1976. The β-lactamases of Gram-negative bacteria and their role in resistance to β-lactam antibiotics. J. Antimicrob. Chemother. 2:115–157.
4. Tsang, J. C., G. A. Sansing, and M. A. Miller. 1975. Relation of beta-lactamase activity to antimicrobial susceptibility in Serratia marcescens. Antimicrob. Agents Chemother. 8:277–281.

Effect of β-Lactamase Production in *Escherichia coli* on Results of Experimental Pyelonephritis Chemotherapy with β-Lactamase-Stable and -Unstable Cephalosporins

H. FREIESLEBEN,* R. MARRE, AND W. HENKEL

Institut für Medizinische Mikrobiologie, Medizinische Hochschule Lübeck, 2400 Lübeck, Federal Republic of Germany

Agar or broth dilution or agar diffusion techniques are used for susceptibility testing. An increasing amount of attention has been focused on β-lactamase production as a further parameter concerning susceptibility to β-lactam antibiotics. It has been shown that there is no correlation between β-lactamase production and susceptibility, determined either by broth dilution or agar diffusion (3). β-Lactamase-positive as well as β-lactamase-negative strains were found among ampicillin-susceptible *Escherichia coli*. An unresolved question is whether β-lactamases influence the outcome of chemotherapy if the infective organism is susceptible to β-lactam antibiotics on the basis of conventional susceptibility tests.

A nalidixic acid-resistant R$^-$ strain of *E. coli* O25:19:12 (*E. coli* R$^-$) and the same strain carrying an R plasmid (*E. coli* R$^+$) were used. The plasmid mediating resistance to ampicillin, gentamicin, kanamycin, neomycin, and paromomycin was transferred from a clinical isolate of *Klebsiella pneumoniae*. The *E. coli* R$^+$ strain produced a β-lactamase of the TEM-I type.

Susceptibility tests were performed according to International Collaborative Study (ICS) recommendations by using the agar diffusion and agar dilution techniques. The inocula were 10^4 and 10^6 colony-forming units per spot. Mueller-Hinton agar (BBL Microbiology Systems) and commercially available disks (Oxoid) containing 30 μg of the cephalosporins were employed.

The rates of hydrolysis of the cephalosporins were determined by spectrophotometry with crude enzyme preparations. Female albino Wistar rats (average weight, 200 g) were used for experimental chemotherapy. The model of estrogen-induced chronic *E. coli* pyelonephritis with its 4-week course and chemotherapy for 1 week has been described previously (1). Acute pyelonephritis was induced without prior estrogen treatment by transurethral infection with the respective strain of *E. coli* (1.3 ml, 10^8 colony-forming units per ml). At 12 h after infection, one dose of the drug (150, 75, and 25 mg/kg) was given intramuscularly. The rats were sacrificed 24 h after infection for determination of the renal viable counts. The mean log number of bacteria per gram of tissue for each group of rats was calculated, and statistical analyses were performed by the U test.

Results of in vitro susceptibility testing are shown in Table 1. The β-lactamase of the R^+ strain was highly active against cefamandole but did not break down cefoxitin or cefuroxime. Increasing the inoculum from 10^4 (ICS recommendations) to 10^6 colony-forming units per spot resulted in distinctly higher cefamandole MICs for the β-lactamase-producing strain.

The results of chemotherapy of acute pyelonephritis are summarized in Table 2. At a dose of 150 mg/kg, both drugs were equally active against the R^- and the R^+ strains. At lower dosages the R^+ strain appeared to be increasingly resistant to cefamandole therapy, whereas the infection with the R^- strain responded fairly well to cefamandole therapy even at a dosage of 25 mg/kg. Chemotherapy with cefuroxime did not result in essential differences between the R^- and R^+ strains.

By using the model of chronic pyelonephritis, cefamandole was compared with cefoxitin. Similar differences in the therapeutic activity between the drugs against the R^+ and R^- strains could be demonstrated.

The results did not show a dose response in the applied dosage range for cefuroxime and cefoxitin against the R^- and R^+ strain and also for cefamandole against the R^- strain. The dose-dependent decrease of therapeutic efficacy of cefamandole against *E. coli* R^+ can be interpreted as a result of β-lactamase production. Because the amount of β-lactamase produced by the bacteria in the kidney is limited, it was probably possible to overcome β-lactamase inactivation by high doses of cefamandole; moderate to low doses, however, increasingly disclosed the influence of β-lactamase production and gave rise to the apparent resistance of the infective organism to therapy. This means that although the presence of a β-lactamase may not

TABLE 1. *In vitro susceptibility and β-lactamase activity of the test strains*

Antibiotic	Agar diffusion zone of inhibition (mm)		Agar dilution MIC (μg/ml)		Hydrolysis rate (μmol/min per ml)	
	E. coli R^-	*E. coli* R^+	*E. coli* R^-	*E. coli* R^+	*E. coli* R^-	*E. coli* R^+
Cefamandole	44	20	0.5^a 1^b	4^a 256^b	0	15.95
Cefoxitin	28	36	2^a 4^b	1^a 4^b	0	0
Cefuroxime	26	28	2^a	1^a	0	0

[a] Standard inoculum (10^4 colony-forming units).
[b] Inoculum of 10^6 colony-forming units.

TABLE 2. *Therapeutic results in acute pyelonephritis of Wistar rats[a]*

Dose (mg/kg)	Mean log no. of bacteria per g of kidney	
	E. coli R^-	*E. coli* R^+
Cefamandole		
150	4.2	4.9
75	4.2	5.3
25	3.8	5.8
Untreated control	6.1	6.2
Cefuroxime		
150	5.3	4.8
75	4.8	5.1
25	5.0	5.0
Untreated control	6.0	6.5

[a] Infection with an R plasmid-carrying, β-lactamase-producing strain (*E. coli* R^+) and its plasmid-free parent strain (*E. coli* R^-).

be evident in MICs determined at the conventional inoculum level, the organism can often produce enough enzyme in vivo to affect the therapeutic outcome significantly. These findings are in keeping with reports by Moxon et al. (2).

It seems that, in the case of cephalosporins, routine susceptibility testing does not always reflect the in vivo activity. Ullmann (3) reported that about 50% of *E. coli* strains were β-lactamase producers, but nevertheless susceptible on the basis of the broth dilution technique. According to the above results, these strains should be considered as intermediate or resistant to compounds unstable to β-lactamase.

We are indebted to C. H. O'Callaghan, Glaxo Research Ltd., Greenford, United Kingdom, for identification of β-lactamase and the determination of the rates of enzymic hydrolysis of the β-lactam compounds.

1. **Commichau, R., H. Freiesleben, K. Sack, C. Krüger, and W. Henkel.** 1976. Model for assessment of activity of antimicrobial agents, p. 317–322. *In* J. D. Williams

750   EPIDEMIOLOGY AND PLASMIDS

and A. M. Geddes (ed.), Chemotherapy, vol. 2. Plenum Press, New York.
2. **Moxon, E. R., A. A. Medeiros, and T. F. O'Brien.** 1977. Beta-lactamase effect on ampicillin treatment of *Haemophilus influenzae* B bacteremia and meningitis in infant rats. Antimicrob. Agents Chemother. **12**:461–464.
3. **Ullmann, U.** 1977. Correlation of minimum inhibitory concentration and β-lactamase activity. Infection **5**: 261–262.

Degradation of Mezlocillin and Other β-Lactam Antibiotics by *Enterobacteriaceae* Compared with Their In Vitro Susceptibilities to the Drugs

C. KRASEMANN AND H. WERNER*

Institute of Medical Microbiology and Immunology, University of Bonn, Bonn, Federal Republic of Germany

Though ample information is available on susceptibility or resistance of newer broad-spectrum penicillins and cephalosporins to certain β-lactamases, the impact of these data on routine susceptibility testing of clinical isolates is little understood.

We, therefore, examined the inactivation ability of 325 randomly selected clinical *Enterobacteriaceae* isolates against mezlocillin and the cephalosporins cefuroxime, cefamandole, and cefoxitin. A comparative susceptibility study, using broth dilution, agar dilution, and agar diffusion tests, was simultaneously performed.

β-Lactamase tests were performed by incubating the *Enterobacteriaceae* strains, in initial concentrations of 5×10^8 cells per ml, with 16 μg of the antibiotic tested per ml in Iso-Sensitest broth for 15 h at 37°C. To evaluate the remaining concentration of the antibiotic, 50 μl of the culture filtrate was applied to nutrient agar plates containing 10^7 *Bacillus subtilis* spores per ml. After 15 h of incubation at 37°C, the inhibition zone was measured, and the remaining concentration of the antibiotic was calculated against a standard curve.

MIC values were determined in Iso-Sensitest broth and on Iso-Sensitest agar plates, using standardized methods. Standardized agar diffusion tests were performed on Iso-Sensitest agar.

The clinical isolates of *Enterobacteriaceae* tested showed remarkable differences in their abilities to degrade mezlocillin, cefuroxime, cefamandole, and cefoxitin. Of 50 *Escherichia coli* strains, 28 did not inactivate mezlocillin, whereas the cephalosporins were less stable (Table 1). Almost 40% of the *Enterobacter* strains did not

TABLE 1. *β-Lactamase activities of Enterobacteriaceae against mezlocillin and three cephalosporins*

	Escherichia coli (n=50)			Citrobacter freundii (n=27)		
	0	+	++	0	+	++
Mezlocillin	28	5	17	6	4	17
Cefamandole	-	33	17	2	4	21
Cefoxitin	11	37	2	9	1	17
Cefuroxime	9	37	4	13	7	7

	Enterobacter spp. (n=52)			Klebsiella spp. (n=50)			Serratia marcescens (n=26)		
	0	+	++	0	+	++	0	+	++
Mezlocillin	21	4	27	2	-	48	3	-	23
Cefamandole	1	5	46	-	1	49	-	-	26
Cefoxitin	13	-	39	48	-	2	1	4	21
Cefuroxime	19	17	16	22	14	14	-	2	24

	P. mirabilis (n=30)			P. vulgaris (n=30)			P. morganii (n=30)			P. rettgeri (n=30)		
	0	+	++	0	+	++	0	+	++	0	+	++
Mezlocillin	25	3	2	13	7	10	5	2	23	12	4	14
Cefamandole	28	-	2	8	-	22	-	1	29	3	4	23
Cefoxitin	23	6	1	18	4	8	4	8	18	15	7	8
Cefuroxime	25	3	2	8	1	21	1	1	28	5	1	24

++ = HIGH ACTIVITY (RESIDUAL ANTIBIOTIC 0 - <4 MCG/ML)
+ = MEDIUM ACTIVITY
0 = NO ACTIVITY

Mezlocillin
Escherichia coli

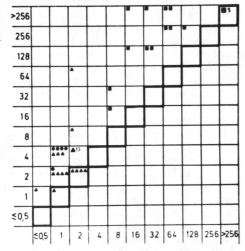

FIG. 1. *Synoptic representation of broth dilution and agar dilution MICs. Symbols:* ■, *strains with high β-lactamase activity;* ●, *strains with medium β-lactamase activity;* ▲, *strains without degradation activity.*

degrade mezlocillin and cefuroxime, whereas cefamandole was resistant to only one strain. With *Klebsiella* spp., the highest stability was found with cefoxitin. None of the antibiotics was resistant to the action of *Serratia marcescens* enzymes (Table 1). However, 30 strains each of *Proteus mirabilis*, *P. vulgaris*, *P. morganii*, and *P. rettgeri* were variably active against the β-lactam antibiotics tested. It seems especially noteworthy that the resistance patterns of the

three cephalosporins to degradation by *Enterobacteriaceae* were far from uniform (Table 1).

With certain species and antibiotics, the results of broth dilution and agar dilution tests were in good agreement. This was true for *E. coli* and cefoxitin as well as cefoxitin and *Klebsiella* spp. With the great majority of *Enterobacteriaceae* and antibiotics, however, the broth dilution tests gave higher MICs than did the agar dilution technique. An example, namely, the mezlocillin MICs obtained with 50 *E. coli* strains, is shown in Fig. 1. These differences in the outcomes of the two quantitative techniques of susceptibility testing did not appear to be dependent on β-lactamase activity (Fig. 1). It has been suggested (1, 2) that the discrepancy between broth and agar dilution MIC measurements of cefamandole against *Enterobacter* could be explained by a high spontaneous mutation rate to resistance.

The generally accepted view that zone sizes tend to be more closely correlated to agar dilution MICs than to the MIC measurements in broth has been confirmed by the present study.

The lack of correlation between β-lactamase production and in vitro susceptibility testing poses the clinically significant problem as to whether certain gram-negative strains have to be regarded as resistant or susceptible.

1. **Findell, C. M., and J. C. Sherris.** 1976. Susceptibility of *Enterobacter* to cefamandole: evidence for a high mutation rate to resistance. Antimicrob. Agents Chemother. 9:970–974.
2. **Ott, J. L., J. R. Turner, and D. F. Mahoney.** 1979. Lack of correlation between β-lactamase production and susceptibility to cefamandole or cefoxitin among spontaneous mutants of *Enterobacteriaceae*. Antimicrob. Agents Chemother. 15:14–19.

Epidemiological Surveillance of Microbial Resistance

M. MANDELLI,* A. GOGLIO, F. MANDLER, G. MARCHIARO, A. MAROCCHI, G. PICERNO, P. POLLINA, L. RADICE ROVEDA, R. RESCALDANI, AND R. VAIANI

Istituto di Ricerche Farmacologiche "Mario Negri," Milan, * *and AMOI Lombardia, Bergamo, Italy*

Antibiotic-resistant bacteria, already a widely recognized cause of worrisome hospital infections, are reported to be spreading in outpatient practice (8). As drugs that were previously effective become less useful, greater morbidity and higher fatality rates can be expected.

In the course of close monitoring of the emergence of resistance patterns, a large degree of variability has been found among hospitals, re-

gions, and countries, emphasizing the importance of continuous surveillance programs based on standardized methods, to permit reliable comparisons of real differences in resistance incidence and profile (1–7). Accurate data are particularly needed in countries where no surveillance policy has ever been enforced, countries which are therefore obliged rather to rely passively on data derived from situations prevailing elsewhere but not necessarily reflecting local needs.

Italy can be considered representative of such countries, for the following main reasons: lack of a serious policy for drug approval and far too much "me too" use of antibiotics (fixed-dose combinations are on the market and are widely used); lack of organized surveillance programs, accompanied by the absence of standardized procedures for hospitals; and total lack of data on the relative weights of ambulatory and hospital antibiotic therapies.

Increased awareness of the drawbacks of this situation suggested the creation in the Lombardy region of a research group whose specific aim was to set up a network of cooperative hospitals where methods could be tested and statistics could be collected on a permanent basis to provide guidelines for therapeutic behavior and a better-controlled drug policy.

Two features of this program merit specific mention: although the group includes research-oriented institutions, most of the parties involved come from general hospitals and are involved full time in routine practice; and close feedback with clinicians has been sought since the very beginning so as to make sure that information obtained is readily understandable and directly useful (specialists in various fields are now full members of the group).

We report the findings after 6 months of intensive and prospective multihospital monitoring on patterns of use of microbiological tests and on differences between microbial resistances in various hospitals assessed by standard microbiological techniques. A total of 35,548 samples have been examined (38.3‰ of daily hospital censuses), and important differences in use of microbiological laboratories in the eight hospitals have been brought to light (requests for bacteriological tests covered from 12.2 to 75.7‰ of daily hospital censuses). The same pattern recurs in the different wards.

Microbiological tests gave positive findings in very few cases or over a large range (from 0.06 to 2.7 for feces and from 6.1 to 49% for blood cultures) or both, probably because the absence of a hospital policy means permissiveness towards physicians' habits. Of the gram-negative bacteria (*Escherichia coli, Proteus* spp., *Pseudomonas aeruginosa, Klebsiella, Enterobacter, Serratia*), which accounted for more than 70% of all bacteria isolated in our hospitals, 8,557 strains were specifically analyzed for their rates of occurrence in outpatients (1/3) and inpatients (2/3). *E. coli* was the species most commonly isolated from all sites and from urine, with different frequencies in in- and outpatients (31.6 and 53.9% for all sites and 36.0 and 55.6% for urines, respectively). *P. aeruginosa* and indole-positive *Proteus* were more common in inpatients.

TABLE 1. *Susceptibilities of gram-negative strains isolated from in- and outpatients*

Antibiotic	Mean % of strains susceptible to antibiotic (interhospital range)				
	E. coli (no. = 3,326)	P. mirabilis (no. = 1,309)	P. aeruginosa (no. = 1,254)	Enterobacter and Serratia (no. = 627)	Klebsiella (no. = 878)
Ampicillin	64.8 (58.8–71.2)	40.9 (23.3–56.3)	8.3 (0–17.8)	24.0 (5.9–38.3)	10.2 (0–22.2)
Carbenicillin	66.5 (41.1–72.9)	44.5 (29.3–63.2)	35.8 (12.2–59.8)	54.1 (20–77.7)	16.7 (0–53.5)
Cephalothin	79.0 (40.5–93.2)	55.4 (26.7–78.9)	6.9 (0–14.9)	16.2 (12.5–25.0)	74.3 (44.4–85.0)
Gentamicin	97.2 (88.6–98.6)	66.1 (47.4–78.9)	61.9 (45.0–85.7)	77.9 (54.8–100.0)	89.1 (75.0–93.7)
Tobramycin	97.1 (87.1–98.5)	83.6 (56.9–95.8)	66.3 (45.0–90.5)	84.3 (70.6–100.0)	93.1 (94.9–100.0)

TABLE 2. *Antibiotic susceptibilities of microbial flora isolated from inpatient (IN) and outpatient (OUT) urines*

Antibiotic	% of strains susceptible to antibiotic									
	E. coli		P. mirabilis		P. aeruginosa		Enterobacter and Serratia		Klebsiella	
	IN (1,418)[a]	OUT (1,124)	IN (724)	OUT (311)	IN (477)	OUT (154)	IN (222)	OUT (72)	IN (289)	OUT (130)
Ampicillin	56.4	71.3	33.7	57.4	7.6	17.7	21.1	32.5	9.6	23.8
Carbenicillin	52.6	66.9	38.1	54.3	26.0	36.5	34.0	55.6	15.6	17.0
Cephalothin	79.6	86.1	54.0	71.0	12.3	24.6	20.2	32.8	69.8	74.5
Gentamicin	92.1	98.8	56.9	86.0	50.0	56.8	69.9	84.7	87.0	90.6
Tobramycin	92.4	96.2	76.3	93.1	51.3	66.4	79.3	84.6	91.6	85.5

[a] Number in parentheses is the number of strains isolated.

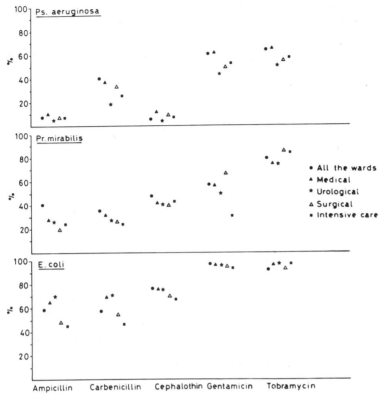

FIG. 1. *Trends of microbial resistance in different wards.*

The patterns of susceptibility to the most widely used antibiotics (ampicillin, carbenicillin, cephalosporins, and aminoglycosides) led to three main observations (Table 1): broad inter-hospital variability for all strains and all drugs except aminoglycosides against *E. coli* and *Klebsiella*, dramatically low susceptibilities of *Proteus mirabilis* and *P. aeruginosa* to specific antibiotics, and major differences from data reported in the international literature (particularly for *P. mirabilis* and *P. aeruginosa*).

Strains isolated from urine differed significantly in out- and inpatients (Table 2). Trends of microbial resistance in the different wards probably reflected different medical habits in antibiotic use (Fig. 1).

Results obtained so far indicate that: antibiotic use and antibiotic policies in hospitals appear to be haphazard, in the sense that personal preferences and uncontrolled and sometimes misinterpreted experience govern practice; the data reported fully justify the need for organized surveillance programs accompanied by standardized procedures for hospitals and problem-oriented studies for ambulatory and hospital antibiotic use; regular review of bacterial susceptibility patterns could help and orient physicians' choices of antimicrobial agents and check the changes in susceptibility patterns of bacterial flora caused by many complex variables, only some of which are known; and the incidence of bacteria in a hospital and their susceptibility to antibiotics are major concerns of the microbiologist, the epidemiologist, and the clinician.

Data reported can be useful for microbiologists in assessing their own clinical laboratories; incidence trends can serve as references for comparing the isolation patterns found in individual laboratories. If they know what the most common species are and where to find them, clinical microbiologists can adjust budgetary, personnel, and technical priorities.

1. **Atkinson, B., and G. More.** 1977. A sample of bacterial isolates in the United States and their susceptibilities to antimicrobial agents, p. 235–256. *In* Significance of medical microbiology in the care of patients. The Williams & Wilkins Co., Baltimore.
2. **Drasar, F. A., W. Farrell, J. Maskell, and J. D. Williams.** 1976. Tobramycin, amikacin, sisomicin, and gentamicin resistant gram-negative rods. Br. Med. J. **2:** 1284–1287.

3. **Driessen, J. H.** 1978. Retrospective studies of resistance patterns of antibiotics in 1975 and 1976, p. 538–540. *In* Current chemotherapy, Proceedings of the 10th International Congress of Chemotherapy. American Society for Microbiology, Washington, D.C.

4. **Grunt, J., V. Kremery, and L. Rosival.** 1978. Monitoring bacterial resistance to restricted antibiotics. Am. J. Hosp. Pharm. **35:**1378–1389.

5. **International Antibiotic Resistance Survey Group and T. F. O'Brien.** 1978. Multicenter sensitivity studies, p. 534–536. *In* Current chemotherapy, Proceedings of the 10th International Congress of Chemotherapy. American Society for Microbiology, Washington, D.C.

6. **Recco, R. A., J. L. Gladstone, S. A. Friedman, and E. H. Gerken.** 1979. Antibiotic control in municipal hospital. J. Am. Med. Assoc. **241:**2283–2286.

7. **Rehm, W. F.** 1978. Prevalence of drug resistance of bacteria: results of an international study, p. 536–538. *In* Current chemotherapy, Proceedings of the 10th International Congress of Chemotherapy. American Society for Microbiology, Washington, D.C.

8. **Schwartz, R., W. Rodriguez, W. Khan, and S. Ross.** 1978. The increasing incidence of ampicillin-resistant *Haemophilus influenzae.* A cause of otitis media. J. Am. Med. Assoc. **239:**320–323.

Characterization of β-Lactamases from *Bacteroides fragilis*

BARBRO OLSSON-LILJEQUIST,* CARL-ERIK NORD, AND KATHRINE DORNBUSCH

Department of Bacteriology, National Bacteriological Laboratory, and Karolinska Institute, S-105 21 Stockholm, Sweden

During the last 10 years the importance of infections caused by anaerobic bacteria has become a well-known fact, much dependent on better cultivation techniques for anaerobic bacteria. Among these, *Bacteroides fragilis* is the anaerobic bacterium most frequently isolated from clinical specimens (2). Unfortunately, it is also one known to be resistant to many antimicrobial agents such as the β-lactam antibiotics (penicillins and cephalosporins), the tetracyclines, and the aminoglycosides, whereas clindamycin, chloramphenicol, and metronidazole in most cases are useful in treatment of such infections.

Most strains of the *B. fragilis* group of organisms produce small amounts of β-lactamase, whereas a limited number of strains have the ability to produce large amounts of the enzyme (4). A correlation can be seen between resistance to β-lactam antibiotics and production of β-lactamase. Weak β-lactamase producers were moderately resistant to most β-lactam antibiotics, whereas strong β-lactamase producers were highly resistant.

Studies of the β-lactamases from *B. fragilis* indicate that they are different from all other β-lactamases found in aerobic gram-negative bacteria (5). Differentiation and characterization of β-lactamases can be done by studying their substrate profile and isoelectric point (pI) (7).

This study reports the characterization of three different β-lactamases from strains of the *B. fragilis* group of organisms.

Strains. Eight strains of the *B. fragilis* group were used in this study. They were identified by the method of Holdeman et al. (3), and their characteristics are listed in Table 1. All strains except *B. distasonis* B98 were strong β-lactamase producers.

Isoelectric focusing. Crude enzyme preparations were submitted to isoelectric focusing in polyacrylamide gel and subsequent staining for β-lactamase activity, as described by Olsson et al. (6).

Determination of kinetic parameters. β-Lactamase assays were performed with the UV method for cephalosporin substrates, and hydrolysis of benzylpenicillin and cephaloridine were compared by using an acidimetric method, as previously described (5). Kinetic parameters K_m and V_{max} were estimated from a least-squares fit to Lineweaver-Burk plots, with substrate concentrations of 0.05 to 0.2 mM.

Transfer experiments. For transfer experiments, filter mating techniques were used, as described by Tally et al. (8). Donor strains were the β-lactamase-producing strains of *B. fragilis*

TABLE 1. *Characterization of strains belonging to the B. fragilis group*

Strain no.	Species	β-Lactamase pI	MIC (μg/ml)[a]			
			Pc	Tc	Rif	Cfx
B34	*B. fragilis*	4.9	>128	<1	<1	4
B105	*B. fragilis*	4.9	>128	>16	<1	4
B122	*B. fragilis*	4.9	>128	>16	<1	2
B147	*B. fragilis*	4.9	>128	>16	<1	8
B70	*B.fragilis*	4.9	128	16	<1	4
B72	*B. uniformis*	5.6	64	16	<1	32
2986	*B. uniformis*	5.3	>128	<1	<1	32
B98	*B. distasonis*		16	<1	>100	32

[a] Pc, Benzylpenicillin; Tc, tetracycline; Rif, rifampin; Cfx, cefoxitin.

TABLE 2. *Kinetic parameters of β-lactamases from B. fragilis and B. uniformis*

Substrate	Strain (pI)							
	B34 (4.9)		B70 (4.9)		B72 (5.6)		2986 (5.3)	
	$V_{max}{}^a$ (rel)	K_m (μM)	V_{max} (rel)	K_m (μM)	V_{max} (rel)	K_m (μM)	V_{max} (rel)	K_m (μM)
Cephaloridine	100	98	100	139	100	108	100	32
Cephalothin	77	67	76	117	134	222	52	43
Cephalexin	6	213	3	96	126	261	28	345
Cefamandole	20	48	17	28	156	214	76	73
Cefuroxime	45	79	36	107	38	64	165	101
Cefazolin	90	247	126	536	139	204	370	48
Cefoxitin	—^{b}		—		—		—	
Benzylpenicillin	3^c	ND^d	3	ND	6	ND	3	ND

^{a} V_{max} relative (rel) to cephaloridine = 100.

^{b} No hydrolysis of substrate detected with the UV or acidimetric method.

^{c} Determined by the acidimetric method with 0.2 mM substrate concentration and related to hydrolysis of cephaloridine measured identically.

^{d} ND, Not determined.

and *B. uniformis*, and *B. distasonis* B98 was used as recipient. Selection of transcipients was done on plates containing benzylpenicillin (50 μg/ml) and rifampin (25 μg/ml).

Determination of pI. β-Lactamases from all strains of *B. fragilis* showed a pI of 4.9. *B. uniformis* strains B72 and 2986 produced β-lactamases with different pI's, 5.6 and 5.3, respectively.

Kinetic parameters. The kinetic parameters K_m and V_{max} for these three β-lactamases were determined with six cephalosporins as substrates (Table 2). For comparison benzylpenicillin was also included, and all three enzymes had very low hydrolyzing activity on this substrate. No hydrolysis of cefoxitin could be detected by any of the three enzymes with either the UV or the acidimetric method. However, it has been shown by a microbiological assay method (1) that *B. uniformis* 2986 is able to inactivate cefoxitin. There was a clear difference between the three enzymes in their affinities for the substrates and their relative rates of hydrolysis. Strains B34 and B70, both producing the pI 4.9 enzyme, showed almost identical patterns, with cephaloridine and cefazolin being the most readily hydrolyzed substrates and cephalexin, cefamandole, and cefuroxime the least well hydrolyzed. However, the affinity of the enzyme is greatest for cefamandole. The β-lactamase produced by strain B72 hydrolyzed all cephalosporins, but cefuroxime more readily than cephaloridine, and the affinity was also highest for cefuroxime. The β-lactamase from strain 2986, on the other hand, was able to hydrolyze both cefuroxime and cefazolin more readily than cephaloridine and, to a lesser extent, cephalothin, cephalexin, and cefamandole.

Transfer of resistance to β-lactam antibiotics. Several transfer experiments were performed with the *B. fragilis* or *B. uniformis* strains as donors and *B. distasonis* strain B98 as recipient. The recipient strain was resistant to rifampin and cefoxitin and had the ability to ferment arabinose and rhamnose. Rifampin was used as selection marker, whereas the other markers were used for control of presumptive transcipients. However, no transcipients were found in any of the mating experiments.

Conclusions. This study shows that at least three different β-lactamases are produced by strains from the *B. fragilis* group of organisms. They are all cephalosporinases, but differ in relative rates of hydrolysis of different cephalosporin substrates and also in their pI's.

There is no evidence so far indicating that the genes coding for resistance to β-lactam antibiotics in *B. fragilis* should be plasmid mediated and transferable. This is in agreement with findings among many aerobic gram-negative bacteria, where species-specific β-lactamases are chromosomally mediated and of the cephalosporinase type.

1. **Dornbusch, K., B. Olsson-Liljequist, and C. E. Nord.** 1980. Antibacterial activity of new beta-lactam antibiotics on cefoxitin-resistant strains of *Bacteroides fragilis*. J. Antimicrob. Chemother. **6:**i–vi.
2. **Finegold, S. M.** 1977. Anaerobic bacteria in human disease. Academic Press Inc., New York.
3. **Holdeman, L. V., E. P. Cato, and W. E. C. Moore.** 1977. Anaerobe laboratory manual, 4th ed. Virginia Polytechnic Institute and State University, Blacksburg.
4. **Olsson, B., K. Dornbusch, and C. E. Nord.** 1977. Susceptibility to beta-lactam antibiotics and production of beta-lactamase in *Bacteroides fragilis*. Med. Microbiol. Immunol. **163:**183–194.
5. **Olsson, B., C. E. Nord, and T. Wadström.** 1976. For-

mation of beta-lactamase in *Bacteroides fragilis*: cell-bound and extracellular activity. Antimicrob. Agents Chemother. **9**:727–735.

6. **Olsson, B., C. E. Nord, T. Wadström, and B. Wretlind.** 1977. Gel electrofocusing combined with zymogram techniques for the characterization of beta-lactamases from gram-negative bacteria. FEMS Microbiol. Lett. **1**: 157–162.

7. **Sykes, R. B., and M. Matthew.** 1976. The beta-lactamases of gram-negative bacteria and their role in resistance to beta-lactam antibiotics. J. Antimicrob. Chemother. **2**:115–157.

8. **Tally, F. P., D. R. Snydman, S. L. Gorbach, and M. H. Malamy.** 1979. Plasmid-mediated, transferable resistance to clindamycin and erythromycin in *Bacteroides fragilis*. J. Infect. Dis. **139**:97–101.

β-Lactamase Activity of Intestinal Saccharolytic *Bacteroides* spp. and Members of the *B. melaninogenicus* and *B. oralis* Groups Determined by Substrate Profiles

RAINER HAMMANN,* HERBERT WERNER, CHRISTINA KRASEMANN, AND HANS J. RUMMEL

Institute of Medical Microbiology and Immunology, University of Bonn, D-5300 Bonn 1, Federal Republic of Germany

In recent years, it has been increasingly recognized (3, 6) that the saccharolytic intestinal *Bacteroides* formerly indiscriminately called *B. fragilis* comprise a variety of species, namely, *B. fragilis, B. thetaiotaomicron, B. vulgatus, B. distasonis, B. eggerthii,* and some other named (7), or so far unnamed, entities (Table 1). *B. fragilis* and *B. thetaiotaomicron* are the species most frequently responsible for severe infections, whereas *B. vulgatus* is predominant in feces and only rarely, if ever, recovered from infectious processes (6). A similar development characterizes the actual taxonomy of the *B. melaninogenicus* and *B. oralis* groups, each of which is at present considered to comprise several species or taxa (1, 2).

The recent findings concerning the diversity of the *Bacteroides* groups mentioned warrant a reassessment of their β-lactamase activities. We therefore tested approximately 100 strains of different species for β-lactamase activity against penicillin G, oxacillin, ampicillin, mezlocillin, cephalothin, cefamandole, and cefoxitin. The strains were selected randomly and comprised clinical as well as normal flora isolates. β-Lactamase tests were performed by incubating the *Bacteroides* strains together with the antibiotic tested at a concentration of 16 µg/ml in a modified brain heart glucose broth anaerobically for 15 h. The remaining concentrations of the antibiotics were evaluated by applying 50-µl samples of the test strain supernatants into wells on nutrient agar plates containing 10^7 *Bacillus subtilis* spores per ml. The plates were incubated aerobically for 8 h. Then the inhibition zones were measured, and the remaining concentrations of the antibiotics were calculated against standard curves.

The substrate profiles of the various strains are shown in Table 1. The 14 *B. fragilis* strains degraded the four penicillin antibiotics as well as cephalothin and cefamandole. With two strains, in addition, inactivation of cefoxitin was observed. *B. thetaiotaomicron* strains degraded all the antibiotics except cefoxitin. Different substrate profiles were observed with *B. vulgatus* strains: some strains did not degrade, or only incompletely degraded, oxacillin and ampicillin, whereas cephalothin was clearly inactivated; most strains, however, were very active against five or more of the substances. Similar substrate profiles were found with *B. uniformis* and *B. variabilis*. The lowest β-lactamase activity was exhibited by *B. distasonis* strains. *B. eggerthii* strains formed two distinct groups, one very active, with most strains degrading up to six antibiotics, and one group completely inactive. The peculiar nature of the *Bacteroides* β-lactamase was best shown by some strains of *B. distasonis*, which acted on cephalothin and/or cefamandole but not on penicillins. A degradation pattern similar to that of *B. uniformis* was found with *Bacteroides* "subspecies a" (3). The one strain of *Bacteroides* "3452 A" (3) was very active too, but the strain of *Bacteroides* "T4-1" (3) remained negative. The strains of unnamed *Bacteroides* species had a substrate profile ranging from completely inactive to strongly active. The majority of the strains degraded fewer than four substances. The two strains of *B. splanchnicus* (7) were also degraders of most of the β-lactam antibiotics, as were the strains of the *B. oralis* group. The *B. melaninogenicus* isolates, however, did not attack any of the antibiotics.

B. fragilis and *B. thetaiotaomicron* strains usually exhibited higher degrading activities

TABLE 1. *β-Lactamase activity of Bacteroides strains*[a]

No. of strains with identical degradation pattern

Antibiotic	B. fragilis			B. thetaiotaomicron					B. vulgatus									B. uniformis					B. eggerthii			B. distasonis			B. variabilis				
	12	1	1	1	1	1	6	1	2	2	1	3	3	1	1	1	6	1	1	1	1	2	3	1	3	3	2	1	1	1	1	1	1
Cephalothin	100	100	100	100	100	100	100	50	100	100	100	100	100	100	100	100	0	100	100	100	100	100	100	100	100	0	50	100	100	100	100	0	100
Cefamandole	100	100	100	100	75	80	100	0	100	100	100	100	100	100	100	50	0	100	0	100	50	100	100	100	100	0	0	0	100	100	100	100	100
Cefoxitin	0	70	100	0	0	0	0	0	0	0	0	0	0	0	0	0	0	0	0	0	0	0	0	0	0	0	0	0	0	0	0	0	0
Penicillin G	100	100	100	100	100	100	100	0	70	100	60	100	100	60	100	100	0	0	100	100	50	100	100	100	100	0	0	0	100	70	70	100	100
Oxacillin	100	100	100	100	100	100	100	0	0	0	50	50	100	50	100	100	0	100	100	0	50	100	100	100	100	0	0	0	100	100	100	100	100
Ampicillin	100	100	100	100	75	100	100	0	0	75	100	100	100	0	0	0	0	50	100	0	0	100	100	100	100	0	0	0	50	100	50	50	100
Mezlocillin	100	100	100	100	100	100	100	0	0	0	0	60	70	0	0	0	0	0	0	0	0	50	100	100	100	0	0	0	0	0	0	50	0

Antibiotic	Bacteroides taxa subsp. a			T4-1,	3452A,	Bacteroides "species"						B. splanchnicus,	B. oralis group		B. melaninogenicus group, 10
	1	1	1	1	1	1	1	1	1	1	6	2	2	4	
Cephalothin	0	100	100	100	100	100	100	100	100	100	0	100	100	100	0
Cefamandole	0	100	100	100	100	100	100	0	100	100	0	100	100	100	0
Cefoxitin	0	0	0	0	0	0	0	0	0	0	0	0	0	0	0
Penicillin G	0	75	50	100	100	100	65	100	100	100	70	100	100	100	0
Oxacillin	0	0	100	100	100	100	0	0	50	0	0	100	100	100	0
Ampicillin	0	60	100	100	100	100	50	50	0	60	0	100	75	100	0
Mezlocillin	0	0	0	100	100	50	0	0	0	0	0	100	70	100	0

[a] Expressed as percentage of antibiotic inactivated.

than members of other species no matter whether they were isolated from clinical or normal flora material. Within the other saccharolytic *Bacteroides* species active normal flora strains as well as clinical isolates with a low β-lactamase activity have been observed.

It remains to be elucidated whether different types of β-lactamases are responsible for the various substrate profiles described in the present paper or other mechanisms are involved (4). It seems noteworthy that no β-lactamase activity was found among 10 members of the *B. melaninogenicus* group, though others have reported positive strains (5).

The finding of two *B. fragilis* strains that inactivated cefoxitin shows that resistance against this substance may be mediated enzymatically and is not necessarily due to lack of a carrier or penetration system.

The technical assistance of I. Werner and J. Ungerechts is gratefully acknowledged.

1. **Finegold, S. M., and E. M. Barnes.** 1977. Report of the ICSB Taxonomic Subcommittee on Gram-Negative Anaerobic Rods: proposal that the saccharolytic and asaccharolytic strains at present classified in the species *Bacteroides melaninogenicus* (Oliver and Wherry) be reclassified in two species as *Bacteroides melaninogenicus* and *Bacteroides asaccharolyticus.* Int. J. Syst. Bacteriol. **27**:388–391.

2. **Holdeman, L. V., and J. L. Johnson.** 1977. *Bacteroides disiens* sp. nov. and *Bacteroides bivius* sp. nov. from human clinical infections. Int. J. Syst. Bacteriol. **27**:337–345.

3. **Johnson, J. L., and D. A. Ault.** 1978. Taxonomy of *Bacteroides.* II. Correlation of phenotypic characteristics with deoxyribonucleic acid homology groupings for *Bacteroides fragilis* and other saccharolytic *Bacteroides* species. Int. J. Syst. Bacteriol. **28**:257–268.

4. **Leung, T., and J. D. Williams.** 1978. β-Lactamases of subspecies of *Bacteroides fragilis.* J. Antimicrob. Chemother. 4:47–54.

5. **Salyers, A. A., J. Wong, and T. D. Wilkins.** 1977. Beta-lactamase activity in strains of *Bacteroides melaninogenicus* and *Bacteroides oralis.* Antimicrob. Agents Chemother. 11:142–246.

6. **Werner, H.** 1974. Differentiation and medical importance of saccharolytic intestinal Bacteroides. Arzneim. Forsch. **24**:340–343.

7. **Werner, H., G. Rintelen, and H. Kunstek-Santos.** 1975. Eine neue buttersäurebildende Bacteroides-Art: B. splanchnicus n. sp. Zentralbl. Bakteriol. Parasitenk. Infektionskr. Hyg. Abt. 1 Orig. Reihe A **231**:133–144.

Cephalosporinase Activity Within the *Bacteroides fragilis* Group and in Strains of *Bacteroides melaninogenicus* and *Bacteroides oralis*

J. M. SHERRILL AND L. R. McCARTHY

Department of Bacteriology and Immunology, University of North Carolina, Chapel Hill, North Carolina 27514, U.S.A.

β-Lactamases are well distributed among most bacteria (6). They are present in both aerobic gram-negative and gram-positive bacteria and are now recognized to occur in anaerobic gram-negative and gram-positive rods (6). The presence of β-lactamases in anaerobic gram-negative rods has only recently been appreciated. It is now recognized that most members of the *Bacteroides fragilis* group and as many as 56% of the *Bacteroides melaninogenicus-Bacteroides oralis* group synthesize a β-lactamase (2). The β-lactamase of *B. fragilis* has been characterized by many as a cephalosporinase, demonstrating greater enzymatic activity with cephalothin than with penicillin (1, 4). More recently, the β-lactamase of the *B. melaninogenicus-B. oralis* group has been characterized by Salyers and co-workers (7). This enzyme is reported to be more active against penicillin than against cephalothin. We elected to more closely examine the β-lactamases of these anaerobic gram-negative rods.

Thirty-four strains of anaerobic gram-negative rods were used for our studies. Included in this collection of organisms were 16 strains representative of the species in the *B. fragilis* group. These were three strains of *B. fragilis*, five of *B. distasonis*, two of *B. vulgatus*, two of *B. ovatus*, and four of *B. thetaiotaomicron*. Eighteen strains of the *B. melaninogenicus-B. oralis* group were also examined. Of these, five were *B. melaninogenicus* subsp. *melaninogenicus*, eight were *B. melaninogenicus* subsp. *intermedius*, three were *B. melaninogenicus* subsp. *asaccharolyticus*, and two were *B. oralis.* Two strains of *B. melaninogenicus* subsp. *asaccharolyticus* and one strain of *B. melaninogenicus* subsp. *intermedius* were provided to us by T. D. Wilkins. These two strains were among those evaluated by Salyers and colleagues (7).

All 34 isolates were tested for their susceptibility to six penicillin and six cephalosporin/cephamycin antibiotics, using the microtiter method described by Thornsberry and Swenson

(10). Table 1 shows the geometric mean MIC obtained with each species of organisms tested with each antibiotic. With the exception of one strain of *B. thetaiotaomicron*, all strains displayed carbenicillin MICs that were ≤ 128 μg/ml. The single *B. thetaiotaomicron* demonstrated a carbenicillin MIC of 256 μg/ml. Of the strains tested, lowest MICs were observed with *B. melaninogenicus* subsp. *asaccharolyticus*. Poor activity with mecillinam was observed with all strains. Of the six cephalosporin/cephamycin antibiotics tested, cefoxitin displayed the greatest activity. With respect to the remaining cephalosporin antibiotics, strains identified as *B. melaninogenicus* and *B. oralis* were significantly more susceptible to cefoxitin than were members of the *B. fragilis* group. Members of the *B. melaninogenicus-B. oralis* group also tended to display lower cephalexin MICs.

We next macrospically examined all organisms for the presence of β-lactamases with the chromogenic cephalosporin nitrocefin. No β-lactamase activity was detected in broth culture supernatants. Examination of both osmotic shockates prepared according to the method of Smith and Wyatt (8) and cellular lysates prepared by sonication revealed that significant β-lactamase activity was present in the cell shockates and lysates.

Shockates and lysates prepared from all strains included in our study were subjected to isoelectric focusing. Isoelectric focusing was carried out with the LKB Multiphor system, using commercially available ampholine gels providing a pH range of 3.5 to 9.5. LKB ampholine plates were prefocused at 1,000 V and 50 mA for 30 min; after sample application, they were run at 1,500 V and 50 mA for 90 min. After focusing, the ampholine gels were stained with nitrocefin (cephalosporin compound 87/312) to locate

bands of β-lactamase activity according to the method of O'Callaghan et al. (3). Without exception, all β-lactamase-producing strains demonstrated a single band of activity at pH 5.4 when shockates were examined. Examination of lysates from all organisms consistently demonstrated two bands of β-lactamase activity. One of these focused at 5.4 and appeared similar to that found in osmotic shockates. The second band of activity present in lysates focused at pH 4.9. When focused gels were stained with Coomassie brilliant blue, shockate specimens revealed the presence of approximately 12 protein bands, whereas lysates revealed the presence of numerous species.

We next examined the strains to determine when the synthesis of the β-lactamase occurred. Growth of a *B. fragilis* strain was monitored by optical density measurements at 620 nm, and the quantity of β-lactamase synthesized was determined by monitoring enzyme activity in broth supernatant and cell lysates using nitrocefin. Similar studies were conducted with a strain of *B. melaninogenicus* subsp. *melaninogenicus*. Greatest β-lactamase synthesis occurred in both organisms examined during logarithmic growth. A dramatic decrease in enzyme activity was observed after each organism established its stationary phase. This decrease in β-lactamase activity could not be attributed to cell lysis since simultaneous agar plate counts failed to demonstrate the same dramatic decrease in viable organisms.

We examined cells and the culture medium for enzyme activity. Total enzymatic activity at each sampling time was defined as the sum of activity present in cell lysates plus culture supernatants. Periplasmic activity was defined as that portion of activity released with osmotic shocking. Cytoplasmic activity was defined as

TABLE 1. *MICs observed with 12 β-lactam antibiotics[a] and 34 strains of Bacteroides*

Organism	No. of strains	MIC (μg/ml, geometric mean)											
		PEN	AMP	MET	OXA	CAR	MEC	CEP	CPL	CLX	CFX	CPS	CFM
B. fragilis	3	11	19	106	27	27	213	96	48	176	4	139	107
B. vulgatus	2	24	24	128	64	48	192	64	32	96	4	24	64
B. ovatus	2	16	32	128	32	96	382	256	64	192	16	192	160
B. distasonis	5	5	20	115	80	43	307	64	34	106	16	45	288
B. thetaiotaomicron	4	32	32	256	104	112	384	160	128	128	20	128	288
B. melaninogenicus subsp. *melaninogenicus*	6	23	7	80	30	3	150	26	31	4	0.3	45	25
B. melaninogenicus subsp. *intermedius*	7	15	14	83	31	23	170	41	31	11	0.6	41	22
B. melaninogenicus subsp. *asaccharolyticus*	3	13	9	11	7	3	37	18	8	11	0.3	8	7
B. oralis	2	32	16	128	96	16	128	32	12	64	0.4	40	64

[a] PEN, Penicillin; AMP, ampicillin; MET, methicillin; OXA, oxacillin; CAR, carbenicillin; MEC, mecillinam; CEP, cephalothin; CPL, cephaloridine; CLX, cephalexin; CFX, cefoxitin; CPS, celospor; CFM, cefamandole.

TABLE 2. *Relative rates of hydolysis observed with the enzymes from nine anaerobes and seven β-lactam antibiotic substrates*

Organism	% Cephaloridine hydrolysis							
	CPL[a]	CEP	CFM	CFX	CPG	CLX	PEN	CAR
B. fragilis	100	88.0	60.1	<1	53.1	30.0	5.8	2.7
B. vulgatus	100	86.0	54.0	<1	53.0	26.2	6.0	2.7
B. distasonis	100	86.6	56.2	<1	46.8	24.7	6.1	2.7
B. ovatus	100	92.3	60.3	<1	55.8	24.6	6.1	2.5
B. thetaiotaomicron	100	94.3	61.2	<1	52.8	31.3	5.8	2.6
B. melaninogenicus subsp. melaninogenicus	100	85.8	60.6	<1	52.5	28.9	5.9	3.1
B. melaninogenicus subsp. intermedius	100	82.0	55.3	<1	47.1	26.8	6.9	3.1
B. melaninogenicus subsp. asaccharolyticus	100	84.8	54.2	<1	47.9	24.5	6.8	2.9
B. oralis	100	86.6	59.7	<1	52.8	29.3	6.4	3.1

[a] CPL, Cephaloridine; CEP, cephalothin; CFM, cefamandole; CFX, cefoxitin; CPG, cephaloglycin; CLX, cephalexin; PEN, penicillin; CAR, carbenicillin.

the activity present in lysates less the activity found in shockates. Similar observations were made with *B. fragilis* and *B. melaninogenicus*. Periplasmic enzyme represented 53 to 56 and 56 to 62% of respective enzyme synthesized in the *B. fragilis* and *B. melaninogenicus* strains examined. Extracellular enzyme is only detectable in low quantities (<1.0%) during logarithmic growth and increases to a maximum of 6 to 7% in late stationary phase. With growth, there is a gradual decrease in the quantity of periplasmic and cytoplasmic enzyme with a corresponding increase in extracellular enzyme.

The same distribution of enzyme, enzyme quantity, and time of enzyme synthesis was noted when these organisms were grown in the presence or absence of penicillin and cephalothin concentrations equivalent to one-fourth of each organism's respective MIC.

We next independently examined the β-lactamases of 20 of the 34 strains studied. Enzyme preparations obtained by osmotic shocking were used. Enzymatic activity against penicillins was assayed by the microiodometric method described by Sykes and Nordstrom (9) and the acidimetric method of Rubin and Smith (5). Activity with cephalosporin substrates was assayed using the spectrophotometric method of O'Callaghan et al. (3). Before testing, all shockates were diluted to yield the same activity (0.02 μmol hydrolyzed/ml per min). All strains demonstrated highest enzymatic activity with cephaloridine (Table 2). The data shown are presented as relative rates of hydrolysis and are relative to the activity observed with cephaloridine. Each enzyme preparation displayed maximal activity against cephalothin and lowest activity with carbenicillin and cefoxitin substrates. In order of decreasing activity all preparations were active against cephaloridine, cephalothin, cefamandole, cephaloglycin, cephalexin, penicillin, carbenicillin, and cefoxitin.

The β-lactamases produced by members of the *B. fragilis* group and the *B. melaninogenicus-B. oralis* group were examined for their susceptibility to known β-lactamase inhibitors. Samples of shockates obtained from each organism were mixed with 0.1 mM concentrations each of four inhibitors and incubated at 35°C for 10 min before measuring enzymatic activity with nitrocefin. An untreated control of each shockate was tested for reference. The enzyme produced by each organism was totally inhibited by *p*-chloromercuribenzoate. Cloxacillin and clavulanic acid inhibited approximately 90% of the enzyme activity present, whereas carbenicillin reduced activity by approximately 50%.

Our results suggest that members of the *B. fragilis* and *B. melaninogenicus-B. oralis* groups produce a β-lactamase that appears to be a cephalosporinase. The similarity of their enzymatic activity with several substrates and the susceptibility of these enzymes to β-lactamase inhibitors suggest that these enzymes are quite similar, if not identical.

1. **Del Bene, V. E., and W. E. Farrar, Jr.** 1973. Cephalosporinase activity *Bacteroides fragilis*. Antimicrob. Agents Chemother. **3**:369–372.
2. **Murray, P. R., and J. E. Rosenblatt.** 1977. Penicillin resistance and penicillinase production in clinical isolates of *Bacteroides melaninogenicus*. Antimicrob. Agents Chemother. **11**:605–608.
3. **O'Callaghan, C. H., P. W. Muggleton, and G. W. Ross.** 1969. Effects of β-lactamase from gram-negative organisms on cephalosporins and penicillins, p. 57–63. Antimicrob. Agents Chemother. 1968.
4. **Olsson, B., C. E. Nord, and T. Wadström.** 1976. Formation of β-lactamase in *Bacteroides fragilis*: cellbound and extracellular activity. Antimicrob. Agents Chemother. **9**:727–735.
5. **Rubin, F. A., and D. H. Smith.** 1973. Characterization of R factor β-lactamases by the acidimetric method. Antimicrob. Agents. Chemother. **3**:68–73.
6. **Richmond, M. H., and R. B. Sykes.** 1973. The β-lactamases of gram-negative bacteria and their possible physiological role. Adv. Microb. Physiol. **9**:31–88.

7. **Salyers, A. A., J. Wong, and T. D. Wilkins.** 1977. Beta-lactamase activity in strains of *Bacteroides melaninogenicus* and *Bacteroides oralis*. Antimicrob. Agents Chemother. **11:**142–146.
8. **Smith, J. T., and J. M. Wyatt.** 1974. Relation of R factor and chromosomal β-lactamase with the periplasmic space. J. Bacteriol. **117:**931–939.

9. **Sykes, R. B., and K. Nordstrom.** 1972. Microiodometric determination of β-lactamase activity. Antimicrob. Agents Chemother. **1:**94–99.
10. **Thornsberry, C., and J. M. Swenson.** 1978. Antimicrobial susceptibility testing of anaerobes. Lab. Med. **9:**43–45.

β-Lactamases of Ampicillin-Resistant *Escherichia coli* from Brazil, France, and the United States

ANTONE A. MEDEIROS,* JOSE XIMENEZ, KAREN BLICKSTEIN-GOLDWORM, THOMAS F. O'BRIEN, AND JACQUES ACAR

The Miriam Hospital and Brown University, Providence, Rhode Island 02906, U.S.A.*; Laborterápica-Bristol, São Paulo, Brazil; Peter Bent Brigham Hospital and the Harvard Medical School, Boston, Massachusetts 02115, U.S.A.; and Hôpital St. Joseph and the Pasteur Institute, Paris, France

Ampicillin-resistant *Escherichia coli* produce β-lactamases which are specified by plasmid or chromosomal genes. These β-lactamases can be characterized according to properties such as substrate range, molecular weight, isoelectric point (pI), inducibility, and sensitivity to inhibition by cloxacillin and *p*-chloromercuribenzoate. Matthew has correlated these properties with the β-lactamase band patterns seen on flatbed analytical isoelectric focusing of crude bacterial extracts (2). By electrofocusing unknown enzymes in parallel with prototypes, it is possible to identify specific β-lactamases in large numbers of bacterial isolates, even when several coexist in the same organism.

Plasmid-mediated β-lactamases (PMB) have been subdivided into 11 types, each of which has a clearly identifiable electrofocusing pattern often made up of a main and satellite bands, with pI's of the main bands generally ranging from 5.2 to 7.7 (4). The TEM-1 type is the most widely distributed and is the most frequent among the bacterial genera except *Pseudomonas*, in which TEM-2 predominates, and possible *Klebsiella*, which frequently possess an SHV-1 type. Among the OXA types which hydrolyze isoxazolyl penicillins, OXA-1 has been found most often in *Klebsiella* and OXA-2 in *Salmonella*. So far OXA-3 has been found only in a few isolates and HMS-1 in a single strain of *Proteus mirabilis*. The remaining four PMBs (PSE-1, PSE-2, PSE-3, and PSE-4) have been found only in *Pseudomonas* and are considered to be *Pseudomonas* specific.

The chromosomally determined β-lactamases (CMB) of *E. coli*, on the other hand, often produce single bands with higher pI's, usually around 8.2. CMBs with low activity can be found in nearly all *E. coli* if highly concentrated cell extracts are electrofocused, but some ampicillin-resistant isolates produce much larger quantites of an identical enzyme (A. A. Medeiros and M. D. Mandel, Abstr. Annu. Meet. Am. Soc. Microbiol. 1979, A32 p. 6). These strains have a characteristic antibiogram, being highly resistant to ampicillin and cephalothin but susceptible to carbenicillin, and may be identified presumptively by using disk antibiotic susceptibility results (5).

Matthew examined by analytical isoelectric focusing 84 separate random strains of PMB-producing *E. coli* from 10 countries excluding China, South America, Eastern Europe, and large parts of Africa and Asia (4). The purpose of this study was to examine by analytical isoelectric focusing all the β-lactamases of a sample of clinical isolates of ampicillin-resistant *E. coli* from a region not previously sampled, Brazil, and from hospitals in the United States and France.

We studied 196 unique clinical isolates from one hospital in France, two in the United States, and several clinical laboratories, both hospital and private, in Brazil. A total of 144 (74%) isolates fell into one of 6 API biotypes, whereas the remainder were distributed among an additional 22 biotypes. A total of 186 (95%) had PMBs: 176 had a single PMB, 6 had two PMBs, 3 had both a CMB and a PMB, and one had a PMB plus an unknown type of β-lactamase. Only 10 isolates, none from Brazil, had a CMB alone. TEM-1 was the most common PMB, occurring in 159 (81.1%) *E. coli* isolates, followed by OXA-1 in 18 (9.2%) (Table 1). SHV-1 was found in six isolates, all from Brazil. The PSE-1 type, not found previously in *Enterobacteriaceae*, occurred in four Brazilian *E. coli* strains of two different biotypes, two of which possessed the TEM-1 enzyme as well. Iodometric assay of β-lactamase activity showed a high hydrolysis rate of carbenicillin by these strains. Four Brazilian *E. coli* isolates had β-lactamases of three unknown types. The β-lactamase of *E. coli* 7259 produced a band between OXA-1 and SHV-1, whereas that of 7181 fell between SHV-1 and OXA-2 (Fig. 1). Both of these enzymes hydrolyze the isoxazolyl penicillins, suggesting that they are new OXA-type β-lactamases, and both are plasmid mediated (G. A. Jacoby and A. A. Medeiros, unpublished data). *E. coli* 7604 had a TEM-1 and a novel β-lactamase with a band between the main bands of TEM-1 and TEM-2.

The TEM-1 β-lactamase was the most common type found in *E. coli* from all regions, consistent with the findings of Matthew (2). However, TEM-2 was not found in any of the isolates in this study and in only 6 of 84 strains studied by Matthew et al. (4). The difference in prevalence between TEM-1 and TEM-2 is puzzling since both are mediated by transposons and confer similar antibiotic resistance levels to their host strains.

Regarding the OXA-type β-lactamases, we found OXA-1 to be the most common, as did Matthew. However, the OXA-3 type found by her in two strains was not present in any of ours.

The PSE-1-type β-lactamase had not been found previously in *Enterobacteriaceae* since it was specified by a plasmid belonging to incompatibility group P2, which transfers only to *Pseudomonas* (2). Preliminary results suggest that the PSE-1 enzyme found in the four Brazilian *E. coli* isolates in this study belongs to a new incompatibility group (R. W. Hedges, personal communication).

All of the *E. coli* isolates specifying PSE-1, those producing SHV-1, a PMB found mainly in *Klebsiella*, and those harboring the three novel β-lactamases were from Brazil, a country not sampled previously by Matthew. Also, five of the six *E. coli* containing more than one PMB were from Brazil. The greater number of different β-lactamase types found in the Brazilian

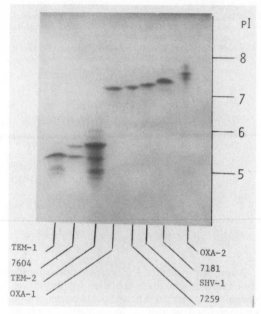

FIG. 1. *Isoelectric focusing patterns of β-lactamases produced by Brazilian isolates 7604, 7259, and 7181 contrasted with prototype β-lactamases of E. coli: R TEM (TEM-1), 1725 RPI (TEM-2), 1527 RGN238 (OXA-1), 1573 R1818 (OXA-2).*

strains suggest that more interchange of resistance genes within and between the bacterial genera has occurred there. The high percentage of resistance of these isolates to other antibiotics (i.e., chloramphenicol, 84%; gentamicin, 11%; tobramycin, 12%) supports this. It is likely that further study of isolates from countries with a high prevalence of antibiotic resistance will detect additional resistance mechanisms not yet recognized.

1. **Hedges, R. W., and M. Matthew.** 1979. Acquisition by *Escherichia coli* of plasmid-borne β-lactamases normally confined to *Pseudomonas* spp. Plasmid **2:**269–278.
2. **Matthew, M.** 1979. Plasmid-mediated β-lactamases of gram-negative bacteria: properties and distribution. J. Antimicrob. Chemother. **5:**349–358.
3. **Matthew, M., A. M. Harris, M. J. Marshall, and G. W. Ross.** 1975. The use of analytical isoelectric focusing for detection and identification of β-lactamases. J. Gen. Microbiol. **88:**169–178.
4. **Matthew, M., R. W. Hedges, and J. T. Smith.** 1979. Types of β-lactamase determined by plasmids in gram-negative bacteria. J. Bacteriol. **138:**657–662.
5. **Medeiros, A. A., R. L. Kent, and T. F. O'Brien.** 1974. Characterization and prevalence of the different mechanisms of resistance to beta-lactam antibiotics in clinical isolates of *Escherichia coli*. Antimicrob. Agents Chemother. **6:**791–801.

TABLE 1. *Distribution by country of different types of plasmid-mediated β-lactamases*

Plasmid-mediated β-lactamases	Brazil		France		U.S.A.		Total	
	No.	%	No.	%	No.	%	No.	%
TEM-1	77	74.0	16	84.2	66	94.3	159	82.4
OXA-1	13	12.5	2	10.5	3	4.3	18	9.3
SHV-1	6	5.8	0	0	0	0	6	3.1
PSE-1	4	3.8	0	0	0	0	4	2.1
OXA-2	0	0	1	5.3	1	1.4	2	1.0
Unknown	4	3.8	0	0	0	0	4	2.1

Biochemical and Immunological Properties of β-Lactamases from *Proteus* Species

CLAUDE MORIN,* ROBERT LETARTE, AND MICHEL COUILLARD

Department of Microbiology, School of Medicine, Laval University, Quebec, Canada G1K 7P4

Although *Proteus* organisms have been recognized as frequent nosocomial pathogens, and although it is known that these organisms, especially those that are indole positive, are often resistant to β-lactam antibiotics (4), very little work has been done on the description and characterization of *Proteus* β-lactamases. Most of the studies have dealt with one or another *Proteus* species, mainly *Proteus morganii* (1, 2, 5). This study was undertaken to identify nine β-lactamases of *Proteus*, representing the four species, in an attempt to compare these enzymes with each other and among species. The nine strains studied included one *P. mirabilis*, two *P. morganii*, three *P. rettgeri*, and three *P. vulgaris*.

The first approach used for the identification of *Proteus* β-lactamases was the detection of the possible presence of TEM-like enzymes among *Proteus* species. This was done based on an immunological neutralization test, using TEM-1 rabbit antiserum (3). Complete neutralization was observed for the *P. mirabilis* strain and two of the three *P. rettgeri* strains. The other *P. rettgeri* strain showed simultaneous production of two different enzymes, including a TEM-like β-lactamase (see Table 1).

Determination of the kinetic constants K_m and V_{max} was done by using a computerized microacidimetric method. Measurements were carried out at pH 7.0 and 37°C. Strains that produce TEM-like β-lactamase were left out of further characterization. The K_m and V_{max} values obtained are listed in Table 2. Summing up the data obtained, especially for V_{max}, it is suggested that a species specificity for the β-lactamases of *P. vulgaris* and *P. morganii* can be hypothesized.

For further characterization, isoelectric focusing of *Proteus* β-lactamases was done on a sucrose-ampholyte density gradient. Isoelectric points (pI), shown in Table 1, were obtained using a specific narrow-range pH gradient after an approximate pI measurement with the conventional pH 3.5 to 10 preparative gradient. The pI's obtained did not confirm species specificity for *Proteus* β-lactamases.

To verify the species specificity hypothesis, two rabbit antisera were prepared with β-lactamases purified by affinity chromatography. The two β-lactamases used for this preparation were those of *P. morganii* Ro9 and *P. vulgaris* Ro104. Results obtained by neutralization with the two antisera are also illustrated in Table 1. No cross-reaction was observed between the species: the antiserum was specific for the β-lactamases of its species.

Summing up the characterization of nine *Proteus* strains highly resistant to β-lactam drugs, it appeared that all the strains exhibited β-lactamase activity. Neutralization assays and isoelectric focusing demonstrated the presence of a TEM-like β-lactamase in *P. mirabilis* and in the three *P. rettgeri* strains. In the latter group, one

TABLE 1. *Results of neutralization assays and isoelectric focusing for the nine Proteus strains*

Strain	Neutralization by:			pI
	Anti-TEM	Anti-Ro9	Anti-Ro104	
P. mirabilis MULB308	+	−	−	ND[a]
P. morganii				
Ro9	−	+	−	8.25
MULB311	−	+	−	6.25
P. rettgeri				
MULB301	+	−	−	9.80 + 5.40
MULB302	+	−	−	ND
MULB313	+	−	−	ND
P. vulgaris				
Ro104	−	−	+	8.45
MULB303	−	−	+	7.30
MULB316	−	−	+	8.20

[a] ND, Not determined.

TABLE 2. *Kinetic constant values obtained by the microacidimetric method at pH 7.0 and 37°C*

Strain	Kinetic con-stant[b]	Antibiotic[a]					
		CTIN	CDIN	CPHR	CZOL	PENI	AMPI
P. vulgaris							
Ro104	K_m	2.8	1.4	0.5	2.7	ND[c]	ND
	V_{max}	100	41	5	144	ND	ND
MULB303	K_m	2.2	3.8	0.8	3.1	0.4	ND
	V_{max}	100	43	6	130	5	ND
MULB316	K_m	6.3	1.9	0.6	2.6	1.7	1.3
	V_{max}	100	46	7	82	13	7
P. morganii							
Ro9	K_m	5.0	5.7	0.3	1.2	2.2	ND
	V_{max}	100	116	3	19	25	ND
MULB311	K_m	4.6	7.3	1.3	1.4	3.2	0.2
	V_{max}	100	133	10	26	28	4
P. rettgeri							
MULB301	K_m	2.6	1.6	0.6	1.1	ND	ND
	V_{max}	100	54	6	46	ND	ND

[a] CTIN, Cephalothin; CDIN, cephaloridine; CPHR, cephradine; CZOL, cefazolin; PENI, penicillin G; AMPI, ampicillin.

[b] K_m is expressed as micromolar concentration. V_{max} is expressed as micromoles of transformed substrate per minute for 100 U of enzyme.

[c] ND, Not determinable.

strain produced simultaneously a TEM-like penicillinase (pI 5.4) and a cephalosporinase (pI 9.8). The β-lactamases found in the three *P. vulgaris* and two *P. morganii* strains exhibited pure cephalosporinase profiles. For these two species, immunological neutralization profiles and kinetic values demonstrated presence of species-specific cephalosporinases. This species specificity hypothesis correlates with the previous observations of Fujii-Kuriyama and collaborators (1), who demonstrated that all of the 11 strains of *P. morganii* in their study were neutralized by a specific antiserum prepared against one of their strains.

1. **Fujii-Kuriyama, Y., M. Yamamoto, and S. Sugawara.** 1977. Purification and properties of β-lactamase from *Proteus morganii.* J. Bacteriol. **131:**726–734.

2. **Hamilton-Miller, J. M. T.** 1963. Inducible cephalosporinase in *Proteus morganii.* Biochem. Biophys. Res. Commun. **13:**43–48.

3. **Le Goffic, F., J. Andrillon-Spiegel, and R. Letarte.** 1974. Immunological study of anti-β-lactamase antibodies by acidimetric methods. Antimicrob. Agents Chemother. **6:**676–680.

4. **Newsom, S. W. B., M. J. Marshall, and A. M. Harris.** 1974. Enterobacteria, β-lactam antibiotics and β-lactamases in clinical practice. J. Med. Microbiol. **7:**473–482.

5. **Yaginuma, S., T. Sawai, S. Yamagishi, and S. Mitsuhashi.** 1974. β-Lactamase formation and resistance of *Proteus morganii* to various penicillins and cephalosporins. Jpn. J. Microbiol. **18:**113–118.

Need of a Combination of Methods for Identifying Beta-Lactamases: the Case of *Enterobacter*

MICHEL COUILLARD,* ROBERT LETARTE, JEAN-CLAUDE PECHERE, AND CLAUDE MORIN

Department of Microbiology, Faculty of Medicine, Laval University, Quebec, G1K 7P4 Canada

β-Lactamases have been studied in many members of *Enterobacteriaceae.* Up to now, three β-lactamases have been characterized in the *Enterobacter* genus: *E. aerogenes* 250 (2) and *E. cloacae* 214 and P99 (1), the latter being the type enzyme of the Richmond class Ia. The value of isoelectric focusing of β-lactamases was pointed out by Matthew et al. (3, 4). Concerning the *Enterobacter* species, they assessed a distribution of four different β-lactamases in 8 strains

of *E. aerogenes* and five β-lactamases in 19 strains of *E. cloacae.* Since then, analytical isoelectric focusing has become a major criterion to differentiate β-lactamases in gram-negative bacteria.

Seventeen strains of *Enterobacter* were studied: P99 and 250 and 15 other strains obtained from M. Matthew. Crude enzymatic extracts were routinely prepared by sonication of organisms collected from an 18-h culture in brain heart infusion broth containing 100 μg of cephaloridine per ml.

Isoelectric focusing on density gradient was performed for all strains. Mean pI values are listed in Table 1, showing that the pI of cephalosporinases ranged from 7.0 to 9.9. *E. aerogenes* 1014E enzymes at pI 6.1 and 5.3 displayed a predominantly penicillinase activity, as well as *E. cloacae* 1683E second enzyme with a pI of 5.2. These will not be included further in this study. These data suggest the presence of several types of β-lactamases inside the genus *Enterobacter*, and a conservative count would give at least 10 different cephalosporinases.

There is a significant difference between some of the values obtained from isoelectric focusing on density gradient and focusing on thin layers of polyacrylamide gel (Table 1). These differences show once again the discrepancy of biochemical values between research teams, as it has been noticed in the past for kinetic values and molecular weights.

The isoelectric focusing technique did not appear sufficient to classify the strains investigated. Therefore, a detailed study was undertaken for each of them.

Specific activity of crude extracts demonstrated various results, even though they were prepared in strictly the same conditions. Extreme values were 1,000-fold apart, ranging from 0.2 to 239.8 U/mg. The β-lactamase of each strain has been purified by affinity chromatography.

Kinetic data were measured by a computerized microacidimetric method. K_m values and substrate profiles were calculated for four β-lactam substrates: benzylpenicillin, cephalosporin C, cephaloridine, and cephalothin. For benzylpenicillin, K_m and V_m values were low and were higher for cephalosporins. Moreover, cloxacillin, carbenicillin, and ampicillin acted as uncompetitive inhibitors for these β-lactamases. However, K_m and V_m results did not allow a significant differentiation of these cephalosporinases.

Molecular weight determinations (Sephadex G-75) were calculated between 28,700 and

TABLE 1. *Isoelectric values of 17 strains of Enterobacter β-lactamases*

Strains	Density gradient	Polyacrylamide gel[a]
E. aerogenes 1014E	7.0 (6.1, 5.3)	6.6
E. cloacae 1686E	7.6	7.4
E. cloacae 346	7.7	
E. cloacae 1671E	7.9	
E. cloacae 366	8.2	
E. cloacae 1672E	8.2	
E. cloacae 204	8.3	
E. cloacae 271	8.3	
E. cloacae P99	8.4	8.0
E. cloacae 1683E	8.6 (5.2)	
E. cloacae 1194E	8.7	
E. aerogenes 1462E	8.8	8.3
E. cloacae 1684E	8.9	
E. aerogenes 250	9.2	
E. cloacae 1673E	9.4	8.0
E. cloacae 284	9.5	
E. aerogenes 1687E	9.9	8.5

[a] See reference 3.

TABLE 2. *Classification of 17 strains of Enterobacter β-lactamases based on four biological parameters*

Type	Sp act	Isoelectric value	Mol wt	Immunological identity			Strains
				P99	250	346	
P99	13.8–239.8	8.2–8.7	28,700–35,700	Yes	No	No	*E. cloacae* 204
							E. cloacae 366
							E. cloacae 1194E
							E. cloacae 1672E
							E. cloacae 1683E
							E. cloacae P99
250	4.4–82.1	8.8–9.9	29,700–31,800	No	Yes	No	*E. aerogenes* 1462E
							E. aerogenes 1687E
							E. aerogenes 250
346	0.3–6.9	7.6–7.9	31,800–32,900	No	No	Yes	*E. cloacae* 346
							E. cloacae 1671E
							E. cloacae 1686E
Unclassified	11.3	7.0	32,200	No	No	No	*E. aerogenes* 1014E
	0.3	8.3	29,900	No	No	ND[a]	*E. cloacae* 271
	0.5	9.5	37,600	No	No	ND	*E. cloacae* 284
	0.2	9.4	30,300	No	No	ND	*E. cloacae* 1673E
	0.2	8.9	38,500	No	No	ND	*E. cloacae* 1684E

[a] ND, Not determined.

38,500. It appears that molecular weight can be used as a criterion of differentiation between cephalosporinases, regarding the extreme values that are present here.

Immunological identification has been performed with β-lactamase antisera prepared in rabbits. The determinations were done by the immunodiffusion technique with three antisera produced against P99, 346, and 250 cephalosporinases. Results are summarized in Table 2. Of the 17 strains, 5 did not show any immunological reaction with the antisera. The others demonstrated a partial or total identity to either of the three cephalosporinases.

Present data allow the classification of *Enterobacter* cephalosporinases into four groups (Table 2), by comparing the most significant biochemical and biological values. These groups are the *E. cloacae* P99-like, the *E. aerogenes* 250-like, the *E. cloacae* 346-like, which is homogeneous, and finally the unclassified ones. Among them, the *E. aerogenes* 1014E seems different, considering its low pI and an absence of immunological relationship with the three former groups. The remaining four unclassified cephalosporinases are characterized by their low specific activity. However, for lack of information concerning their immunological identity, it would be difficult to classify together those β-lactamases, although strains 284 and 1684E look

similar and strains 271 and 1673E could be integrated to the P99 group.

Differentiation between two given strains on the sole basis of their isoelectric values, or their molecular weights, or their specific activities, can lead one to consider as different, enzymes that could be similar if one sums up all the information available concerning their properties. In the case of *Enterobacter*, specific activity, molecular weight, and immunological characterization bring complementary information to the pI value in view of β-lactamase classification. Finally, from the present study, one can count at least five different types in the genus: three for *E. cloacae* and two for *E. aerogenes*.

1. **Jack, G. W., and M. H. Richmond.** 1970. A comparative study of eight distinct β-lactamases synthesized by Gram-negative bacteria. J. Gen. Microbiol. **61:**43–61.
2. **Letarte, R., M. Devaud-Felix, J. C. Pechere, and D. Allard-Leprohon.** 1977. Enzymatic and immunological characterization of a new cephalosporinase from *Enterobacter aerogenes.* Antimicrob. Agents Chemother. **12:**201–205.
3. **Matthew, M., and A. M. Harris.** 1976. Identification of β-lactamases by analytical isoelectric focusing: correlation with bacterial taxonomy. J. Gen. Microbiol. **94:**55–67.
4. **Matthew, M., A. M. Harris, M. J. Marshall, and G. W. Ross.** 1975. The use of analytical isoelectric focusing for detection and identification of β-lactamases. J. Gen. Microbiol. **88:**169–178.

Role of β-Lactamase in the Resistance of *Enterobacteriaceae* to Mecillinam

GER P. A. BONGAERTS,* KRISTIANE M. BRUGGEMAN-OGLE, AND JEANNETTE G. ENGEL

Department of Medical Microbiology, University of Leiden, Leiden, The Netherlands

The 6-β-amidinopenicillanic acid mecillinam {6-β-[(hexahydro-1-H-azepin-1-yl)-methylene amino]-penicillanic acid} belongs to the group of semisynthetic antibiotics derived from penicillanic acid (2). Many studies of this antibiotic have been published, especially on antibacterial activity (4), synergistic effects (8), pharmacokinetics, and mechanism of action (7), but few on mecillinam resistance.

Resistance against mecillinam, as mentioned so far, is concluded to be based on chromosomal mutations (1). These mutations will probably concern a modification of the enzyme, which is the target of mecillinam. This target appears to be different from that of ampicillin, although both enzymes are involved in cell wall synthesis. Only little attention has been paid to destruction

of mecillinam by beta-lactamases. Richmond has studied (5) the relative rate of hydrolysis of the antibiotic by four beta-lactamases in vitro. Only beta-lactamase type III and type IV showed any activity against mecillinam (23 and 7%, respectively) as compared with the activity against penicillin (100%). However, the effect of the presence of this enzyme on the susceptibility of *Escherichia coli* to mecillinam was found to be nil (5).

From a group of ampicillin- and carbenicillin-resistant enterobacterial strains isolated from patients in hospitals in Leiden and Utrecht, strains were selected for mecillinam resistance (MIC $\geq 1\,\mu g/ml$) on McConkey medium without NaCl. The patients concerned had not been treated with mecillinam. In the PAR column of

TABLE 1. *MICs on McConkey medium (without salt) of ampicillin, carbenicillin and mecillinam for 15 selected isolates, 2 reference strains, and E. coli K-12 exconjugates, and the beta-lactamase-mediated hydrolysis rates of benzylpenicillin, ampicillin, carbenicillin, and mecillinam by extracts of the same strains[a]*

| Selected and reference strains | MIC (µg/ml) for | | | | | | % Hydrolysis[b] | | |
| | AMPI | | CARB | | MECI | | | | |
	PAR	EXC	PAR	EXC	PAR	EXC	AMPI	CARB	MECI
K. pneumoniae									
437-2/75	>512	NT	>512	NT	8	NT	62	21	51
E6467	>512	>512	>512	>512	2	1	117	15	190
D8169	>512	NT	>512	NT	2	NT	123	15	125
L111-76	>512	>512	>512	>512	2	2	109	10	178
L117-76	>512	>512	>512	>512	4	1	110	11	196
MM5924	>512	>512	>512	>512	8	4	100	10	200
E. coli									
E7151	>512	>512	>512	>512	2	2	109	10	187
E7125	>512	>512	>512	>512	2	0.5	109	10	187
M5815	>512	>512	>512	>512	8	0.5	97	10	196
K26	>512	>512	>512	>512	2	2	110	10	200
L124-76	>512	>512	>512	>512	2	1	111	10	186
2023-1	>512	>512	>512	>512	4	1	120	10	220
L48367	>512	>512	>512	>512	2	2	104	10	180
Reference strains (see text)									
M739		>512		>512		4	109	10	167
M740		>512		>512		16	120	11	168
Enterobacter cloacae 3579	>512	>512	>512	>512	2	1	107	10	184
Enterobacter liquefaciens L45917	>512	NT	>512	NT	32	NT	110	11	188
E. coli K-12 (Nal[r] Rif[r]) (acceptor)		4		4		0.06			

[a] PAR, Parent strain; EXC, *E. coli* K-12 exconjugate; AMPI, ampicillin; CARB, carbenicillin; MECI, mecillinam; NT, no transfer.

[b] The specific activities are calculated in micromoles of substrate hydrolyzed per minute per milligram of protein at pH 7.0 and 30°C, but presented here in percentages as compared with that against benzylpenicillin (100%).

TABLE 2. *MICs of mecillinam for some bacterial strains on agar medium with low salt concentration (NIH) and on agar media with high salt concentration (NIH + 1% NaCl and Endo agar)*

| Strain | Beta-lactamase[a] | MIC (µg/ml) on: | | |
		NIH	NIH + 1% NaCl	Endo agar
E. coli K-12	−	0.125	2	32
E. coli E7151	+	4	256	>512
E. coli M740	+	16	>512	>512
K. pneumoniae E6467	+	8	>512	>512
E. cloacae 3579	+	1	16	>512
S. aureus IC 146	+	64	>512	—[b]
S. aureus IC 62	−	8	64	—[b]
B. subtilis var. *globigii* NCTC 10073	+	1	4	16

[a] As determined with the nitrocefin test (3).

[b] *S. aureus* does not grow on Endo agar medium.

Table 1, the resistance characteristics of the bacterial strains for ampicillin, carbenicillin, and mecillinam on McConkey medium without NaCl are given. The MICs on NIH medium were the same or somewhat (2×) higher. All these strains were found to be beta-lactamase positive.

Conjugational transfer experiments were performed to investigate the relationship between the presence of beta-lactamase in and the MICs of these strains. The postconjugation mixture was washed with phosphate buffer because of possible interference of beta-lactamase, which was released into the medium due to lysis of cells. At least in two cases, we had observed that the released beta-lactamase hydrolyzed beta-lactam antibiotics in the selection plates.

Three strains did not transfer resistance to ampicillin, carbenicillin, and mecillinam. Mutants of *E. coli* K-12 which were only resistant to mecillinam have been observed on plates inoculated with undiluted and 10-fold-diluted cell suspensions of the conjugation mixtures of these three strains. These mutants did not contain beta-lactamases. The other 12 donor strains as well as the exconjugates were resistant to all the antibiotics mentioned. From this it was concluded that these resistances were due to transferable resistance plasmids. All the parent and exconjugate strains contained beta-lactamases.

Evidence that the mecillinam resistance is caused by beta-lactamase production is given by the following data. Mecillinam is sensitive to beta-lactamase because a pure beta-lactamase preparation derived from *Bacillus cereus* 569/H9 (beta-lactamase Whatman) hydrolyzed mecillinam, although less (6%) than benzylpenicillin (100%), as determined by the iodometric method of Sawai et al (6). All crude extracts of the enterobacterial strains studied and those of the *E. coli* exconjugates possessed hydrolytic activity against mecillinam. A high hydrolysis rate of mecillinam has been found in all cases as compared with the hydrolysis of benzylpenicillin, ampicillin, or carbenicillin (Table 1). Crude extracts of *E. coli* K-12 (strains M739 and M740) containing the TEM-1 and the TEM-2 beta-lactamase, respectively, showed the same pattern. These results together provide strong evidence that the hydrolysis of mecillinam by the crude extracts of the strains studied is caused by beta-lactamases. Additional data (i.e., the hydrolysis rate of cephaloridine and cephalexin, and inhibition by cloxacillin and *p*-chloromercuribenzoic acid) suggest that *Klebsiella pneumoniae* 437-2/75 contains a type IV beta-lactamase, whereas the other strains all contain a TEM-like beta-lactamase (type III). After enzymatic hydrolysis of mecillinam, both by the Whatman beta-lactamase (Whatman Biochemicals Ltd., Maidstone, Kent) and by the crude extract of *E. coli* M740 containing the TEM-2 beta-lactamase, no antibacterial activity towards any of the strains tested was found (MIC > 512 µg/ml). This confirms that these beta-lactamases inactivate mecillinam.

A high salt concentration led to considerable increase of the MIC of mecillinam for *E. coli* K-12 (Table 2). Other authors obtained similar results (4, 8). A great increase of the MIC was shown (Table 2) not only for the beta-lactamase-negative *E. coli* K-12, but also for the beta-lactamase-positive strains of *E. coli* K-12 (the exconjugates) and for the clinical isolates. A less striking effect was observed for the *Staphylococcus aureus* strains and the *Bacillus subtilis* strain. Just like the MICs on NIH (+1% NaCl) medium, the MICs on Endo medium were extremely high.

It is concluded that, by the use of the older beta-lactam antibiotics, a transferable beta-lactamase-mediated mecillinam resistance may arise. Type III beta-lactamases may be responsible for such resistance. This resistance may be underestimated in laboratories due to the use of salt-free media for testing mecillinam susceptibility.

1. Iwaya, M., C. Weldon Jones, J. Khorana, and J. L. Strominger. 1978. Mapping of the mecillinam-resistant, round morphological mutants of *E. coli*. J. Bacteriol. 133:196–202.
2. Lund, F., and L. Tybring. 1972. 6β-Amidinopenicillanic acid—a new group of antibiotics. Nature (London) New Biol. 236:135–137.
3. O'Callaghan, C. H., A. Morris, A. Kirby, and A. H. Shingler. 1972. Novel method for detection of β-lactamases by using a chromogenic cephalosporin substrate. Antimicrob. Agents Chemother. 1:283–288.
4. Reeves, D. S. 1977. Antimicrobial activity of mecillinam. J. Antimicrob. Chemother. 3(Suppl. B):5–11.
5. Richmond, M. H. 1977. *In vitro* studies with mecillinam on *Escherichia coli* and *Pseudomonas aeruginosa*. J. Antimicrob. Chemother. 3(Suppl. B):29–39.
6. Sawai, T., I. Takahashi, and S. Yamagishi. 1978. Iodometric assay method for beta-lactamase with various beta-lactam antibiotics as substrates. Antimicrob. Agents Chemother. 13:910–913.
7. Spratt, B. G. 1977. The mechanism of action of mecillinam. J. Antimicrob. Chemother. 3(Suppl. B):13–19.
8. Tybring, L., and N. H. Melchior. 1975. Mecillinam (FL 1060), a 6β-amidinopenicillanic acid derivative: bactericidal action and synergy in vitro. Antimicrob. Agents Chemother. 8:271–276.

Plasmid-Determined β-Lactamases of *Pseudomonas aeruginosa*

GEORGE A. JACOBY,* LORRAINE SUTTON, AND ANTONE A. MEDEIROS

Massachusetts General Hospital, Boston, Massachusetts 02114,* and the Miriam Hospital, Providence, Rhode Island 02906, U.S.A.

Pseudomonas aeruginosa characteristically produces an inducible β-lactamase active against cephaloridine, penicillin G, and ampicillin but not against carbenicillin (9). One mechanism for enhanced resistance in *P. aeruginosa* is the production of additional constitutive β-lactamases that hydrolyze carbenicillin and that are determined by plasmids. Plasmids found in *P. aeruginosa* can be classified into at least 11 types based on incompatibility. Some have a broad host range, whereas others are transmissible by conjugation only among *Pseudomonas* species or are transfer deficient (Tra⁻). The plasmid-determined β-lactamases of gram-negative bacteria are currently divided into at least 11 types, differing in substrate range, molecular weight, isoelectric point, and other properties (5, 7). Four of these enzymes have been designated *Pseudomonas*-specific (PSE-type) β-lactamases, since they have not been found in other gram-negative bacteria (2). We have previously reported that carbenicillin resistance plasmids of *P. aeruginosa* determine three other β-lactamases in addition to the PSE-types (3), and we have tested the effectiveness of newer β-lactam antibiotics against plasmid-containing, carbenicillin-resistant strains (4). The purpose of this investigation was to extend the characterization of β-lactamase types to a larger group of *Pseudomonas* plasmids and to compare the activities of additional β-lactam antibiotics against plasmid-containing *P. aeruginosa* strains.

Thirty-four plasmids found in *Pseudomonas* determining resistance to carbenicillin have been examined by isoelectric focusing (6) for the type of β-lactamase produced. Nine of the eleven enzyme types have been found. The distribution of β-lactamases on different *Pseudomonas* plasmids, ordered by their incompatibility groups, is given in Table 1. As with plasmids in other gram-negative bacteria (5), TEM-type enzymes were the most common. Eight plasmids produced a TEM-1 enzyme, and 12 plasmids made a TEM-2 β-lactamase. The plasmids involved belonged to five different incompatibility groups, a finding consistent with the determination of TEM-1 and TEM-2 by transposable sequences of DNA. The oxacillin-hydrolyzing enzymes OXA-2 and OXA-3 were the next most common

and were also determined by plasmids belonging to several incompatibility groups. SHV-1 β-lactamase (7) was determined by a single plasmid. PSE-type enzymes were actually uncommon in this collection of plasmids. PSE-1 and PSE-2 were determined by two plasmids each, and PSE-3 and PSE-4 were determined by single plasmids. The confinement of PSE-type enzymes to *Pseudomonas* is reflected by their determination by plasmids that are either Tra⁻ (pMG19, PMG33, and Rms149) or unable to be transferred by conjugation to enterobacteria (RPL11, Rms139, and R151). By genetic manipulations, however, PSE-type β-lactamase genes can be transmitted to *Escherichia coli*, where they function normally (2). Recently, four plasmid-containing *E. coli* isolates from Brazil have been found to make PSE-1 β-lactamase, indicating that this enzyme type must no longer be considered *Pseudomonas* specific (A. A. Medeiros, J. Ximenez, K. Blickstein-Goldworm, T. F. O'Brien, and J. Acar, this volume).

The emergence of carbenicillin-resistant *P. aeruginosa* strains has spurred the development of newer β-lactam antibiotics that are more potent against *Pseudomonas* or more resistant to β-lactamase hydrolysis. To determine their po-

TABLE 1. *Distribution of β-lactamases on Pseudomonas plasmids*

β-Lactamase	Plasmid	Incompatibility group
TEM-1	R527, R1033	P-1
	Rm16a, pMG20, pMG21, Rms165	P-2
	R2, pMG18	P-9
TEM-2	RP1, RP4, Rm16b, R30, R68, RP638	P-1
	pMG23, R40c, R91	P-10
	RP1-1, RP8, RP56Be	P-11
OXA-2	pMG40, pMG44	P-2
	pMG35, pMG48	Unclassified
OXA-3	RIP64	P-3
	pMG25, pMG26	Unclassified
SHV-1	pMG22	P-1
PSE-1	RPL11, Rms139	P-2
PSE-2	pMG33, R151	Unclassified
PSE-3	Rms149	P-6
PSE-4	pMG19	Unclassified

TABLE 2. *Comparative activities of β-lactam antibiotics against plasmid-containing P. aeruginosa strains*

Plasmid	Incompatibility group	β-Lactamase	MIC (µg/ml) of:											
			Carbenicillin	Sulbenicillin	Ticarcillin	Pirbenicillin	Mezlocillin	Nocardicin A	Azlocillin	Piperacillin	Cefsulodin	Cefoperazone	Cefotaxime	LY127935
R⁻			25	20	20	10	100	50	5	5	2	5	20	20
R527	P-1	TEM-1	2,000	2,000	2,000	2,000	400	400	200	200	50	40	20	10
pMG20	P-2	TEM-1	2,000	2,000	2,000	800	200	400	100	100	50	20	20	20
R2	P-9	TEM-1	4,000	4,000	4,000	2,000	800	800	400	400	100	50	20	20
RP1	P-1	TEM-2	8,000	≥4,000	4,000	4,000	800	800	400	400	100	40	20	20
R91	P-10	TEM-2	4,000	4,000	4,000	4,000	800	800	400	400	100	40	20	10
RP1-1	P-11	TEM-2	4,000	4,000	4,000	2,000	400	800	400	200	100	50	20	20
pMG22	P-1	SHV-1	400	400	400	400	200	400	80	40	20	50	20	10
pMG40	P-2	OXA-2	100	100	100	200	100	50	40	20	5	40	20	10
pMG48	?	OXA-2	800	400	800	2,000	400	100	200	100	50	200	20	20
pMG25	?	OXA-3	800	800	800	400	400	50	200	50	20	200	20	20
RIP64	P-3	OXA-3	2,000	2,000	2,000	800	400	50	100	100	20	200	20	20
RPL11	P-2	PSE-1	4,000	≥4,000	4,000	1,000	800	50	200	100	50	50	20	20
R151	?	PSE-2	200	1,000	200	200	200	800	50	50	10	50	20	20
Rms149	P-6	PSE-3	4,000	≥4,000	4,000	800	200	100	100	50	20	20	20	10
pMG19	?	PSE-4	8,000	≥4,000	4,000	1,000	800	50	200	100	50	80	20	10

tential effectiveness against β-lactamase-producing *P. aeruginosa* strains, the MICs for 12 β-lactam antibiotics against 15 otherwise isogenic *P. aeruginosa* strains carrying different β-lactamase-producing plasmids were determined by agar dilution (Table 2). All the R⁺ strains provided resistance to carbenicillin, although the level of resistance varied from an MIC of 100 µg/ml to an MIC of 8,000 µg/ml. MICs for sulbenicillin, ticarcillin, and pirbenicillin were quite similar or only slightly less than those for carbenicillin. MICs for mezlocillin and nocardicin A were 800 µg/ml or less, and for azlocillin and piperacillin they were 400 µg/ml or less; but for each drug at least some plasmids provided enhanced resistance. MICs for cefsulodin (SCE-129) and cefoperazone (T-1551) were 200 µg/ml or less but again were increased by β-lactamase production. The resistance produced by OXA-type enzymes against cefoperazone was particularly striking. Only with cefotaxime (HR-756) and the 1-oxadethiacephalosporin LY127935 (Shionogi no. 6095-S) were the MICs of R⁺ and R⁻ strains equivalent. Both drugs are resistant to hydrolysis by β-lactamases produced by other gram-negative bacteria (1, 8). Evidently, these two new cephalosporin derivatives also resist attack by the nine β-lactamase types studied here and hence are the most likely

of the compounds tested to overcome plasmid-determined resistance in *P. aeruginosa*.

1. **Fu, K. P., and H. C. Neu.** 1978. Beta-lactamase stability of HR 756, a novel cephalosporin, compared to that of cefuroxime and cefoxitin. Antimicrob. Agents Chemother. **14**:322-326.
2. **Hedges, R. W., and M. Matthew.** 1979. Acquisition by *Escherichia coli* of plasmid-borne β-lactamases normally confined to *Pseudomonas* spp. Plasmid **2**:269-278.
3. **Jacoby, G. A., and M. Matthew.** 1979. The distribution of β-lactamase genes on plasmids found in *Pseudomonas*. Plasmid **2**:41-47.
4. **Jacoby, G. A., and L. Sutton.** 1979. Activity of β-lactam antibiotics against *Pseudomonas aeruginosa* carrying R plasmids determining different β-lactamases. Antimicrob. Agents Chemother. **16**:243-245.
5. **Matthew, M.** 1979. Plasmid-mediated β-lactamases of gram-negative bacteria: properties and distribution. J. Antimicrob. Chemother. **5**:349-358.
6. **Matthew, M., A. M. Harris, M. J. Marshall, and G. W. Ross.** 1975. The use of analytical isoelectric focusing for detection and identification of β-lactamases. J. Gen. Microbiol. **88**:169-178.
7. **Matthew, M., R. W. Hedges, and J. T. Smith.** 1979. Types of β-lactamase determined by plasmids in gram-negative bacteria. J. Bacteriol. **138**:657-662.
8. **Neu, H. C., N. Aswapokee, K. P. Fu, and P. Aswapokee.** 1979. Antibacterial activity of a new 1-oxa cephalosporin compared with that of other β-lactam compounds. Antimicrob. Agents Chemother. **16**:141-149.
9. **Sykes, R. B., and M. H. Richmond.** 1971. R factors, beta-lactamase, and carbenicillin-resistant *Pseudomonas aeruginosa*. Lancet **ii**:342-344.

Six Atypical β-Lactamases from *Pseudomonas aeruginosa*

MICHÉLE JOUVENOT* AND YVON MICHEL-BRIAND

Department of Bacteriology, Faculty of Medicine, Besançon, France

Two years ago we reported an increase of the carbenicillin resistance level in *Pseudomonas aeruginosa* related to the greater frequency of constitutive enzymes of the "Dalgleish type" in relation to the substrate profile (1). Since then, we have been particularly interested in the characterization of the isoelectric point (pI) of these penicillinases (PCases), which we report here.

The strains used in this work and their respective β-lactamase activities are shown in Table 1: for the six strains the carbenicillin MICs were higher than 6,000 µg/ml, and the β-lactamase activities were predominantly PCase activities.

Ultrasonically prepared enzymatic extracts were isoelectrically focused on polyacrylamide gel slabs at 400 V for 18 h at 10°C. Then the pH gradient of the gel was recorded at 0.5-cm intervals, and the detection of β-lactamase activity

was obtained by using the chromogenic cephalosporin as a substrate. The focused bands with β-lactamase activity appeared pink on a yellow background.

In our preliminary research, using a pH gradient going from 3.5 to 9.5, we observed that the PCases focused as a main band and satellite bands between pH 5 and pH 6. This led us to use a pH gradient going from 4 to 6.5 to determine the pI of the PCases, and we compared this pI with the pI of well-known β-lactamases focused on the same gel slab.

It appears (Fig. 1) that the PCases from S18, P18, and C18 focused differently from the TEM-2, TEM-1, and Dalgleish enzymes. So, for our PCases, just after the detection of β-lactamase activity, the main band was at pH 5.9, whereas those of the reference enzymes were at pH 5.6, 5.4 and pH 5.3.

TABLE 1. *Origins and substrate profiles of the six β-lactamases studied*

Strain	Origin (hospital unit)	Isolation date	Sero-type	Carbenicillin 99% MIC (μg/ml)	Relative activity of β-lactamase					
					Benzyl-penicillin	Carbeni-cillin	Ampi-cillin	Methi-cillin	Clox-acillin	Cepha-loridine
S27	Pus (urology 1)	8/23/76	10	6,000	100	89	94	2	1	28
S18	Urine (neurosurgery)	7/14/76	11	8,000	100	92	100	1	<1	34
P18	Urine (urology 2)	7/12/76	6	9,000	100	108	102	1	<1	33
C18	Urine (neurosurgery)	7/8/76	6	14,000	100	97	90	1	1	38
T21	Tracheal aspiration (neurosurgery)	7/26/76	6	14,000	100	86	86	1	1	37
G38	Tracheal aspiration (surgery)	11/21/76	6	14,000	100	104	93	1	1	47

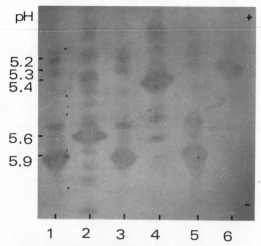

FIG. 1. *Isoelectric focusing patterns on polyacrylamide gel of enzymatic extracts from S18 (1), PAO 2635 (RP1) (2), P18 (3), Escherichia coli (TEM) (4), C18 (5), and Dalgleish strain (6).*

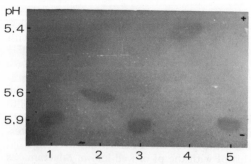

FIG. 2. *Isoelectric focusing patterns on polyacrylamide gel of enzymatic extracts from G38 (1), PAO 2635 (RP1) (2), S27 (3), E. coli (TEM) (4), and T21 (5).*

Ten minutes later there were satellite bands (Fig. 1): the three PCases gave the same satellite bands, but only towards the anode and different from those of the reference enzymes. For the PCases, the satellite bands were at pH 5.6, 5.3 and pH 5.2.

The three other PCases, from G38, S27, and T21, also focused at pH 5.9 (Fig. 2). We must point out that there were also three satellite bands at pH 5.6, 5.3 and pH 5.2, which have not been recorded here.

In conclusion, we can state that there is a striking difference, as regards the pI, between our six PCases and the constitutive β-lactamases commonly found in *P. aeruginosa*, the Dalgleish, TEM-1, and TEM-2 enzymes (Fig. 1 and 2), and also the PSE-1, PSE-2, and PSE-3 enzymes recently described by Matthew (3). So, after 10 determinations, we can assume that the pI is 5.9. Nevertheless, this value was observed by Sawada et al. (4) for a plasmid-determined PCase depending on the R factor Rms 139; but this enzyme was recently described by Matthew as a PSE-1 enzyme with a pI of 5.7. So, we will compare our PCases with a PSE-1 enzyme. Up until now, we have not obtained the transfer of the β-lactamase determinant from our six strains; but before coming to any conclusion, we must try to make this transfer by using helper plasmids as we did for the β-lactamase determinant from the HL strain (2).

It seems that this type of PCase with pI 5.9 could be widespread in the strains isolated in our hospital. So, among the six strains studied, at least three are different as regards the serotypes; moreover, we recently found 10 other strains with this type of PCase, and the number and position of the satellite bands in isoelectric focusing do not vary with the host bacteria.

However, the role of these PCases in carbenicillin resistance cannot be questioned: so, for these enzymes we observed a high hydrolytic activity, and, in the host bacteria, a high carbenicillin MIC, which can be reduced from 14,000 to less than 1 μg/ml by clavulanic acid. This is an important argument which tends to support the striking role played by our PCases in carbenicillin resistance.

1. **Jouvenot, M.** 1978. Carbenicillin resistance and beta-lactamase activity in *Pseudomonas aeruginosa*, p. 484–485. *In* Current chemotherapy, Proceedings of the 10th International Congress of Chemotherapy. American Society for Microbiology, Washington, D.C.

2. **Jouvenot, M., Y. Michel-Briand, and J. M. Laporte.** 1978. Argument en faveur de la localisation plasmidique du gène β-lactamase chez une souche de *Pseudomonas aeruginosa* hautement résistante à la Carbénicilline. C.

R. Acad. Sci. **287**(series D):1067–1070.

3. **Matthew, M.** 1979. Plasmid mediated β-lactamases of gram-negative bacteria: properties and distribution. J. Antimicrob. Chemother. **5**:349–358.

4. **Sawada, Y., S. Yaginuma, M. Tai, S. Iyobe, and S. Mitsuhashi.** 1975. Resistance to β-lactam antibiotics in *Pseudomonas aeruginosa*, p. 391–397. *In* S. Mitsuhashi and H. Hashimoto (ed.), Microbial drug resistance. University of Tokyo Press, Tokyo.

Properties of Some β-Lactamases from Different Strains of *Pseudomonas aeruginosa*

J. REGOES* AND O. ZAK

Research Department, Pharmaceuticals Division, Ciba-Geigy Limited, Basel, Switzerland

In the last few years, some antipseudomonal β-lactams, such as the acylureidopenicillin azlocillin and the cephalosporin compound cefsulodin, have been described (3, 6). In investigations with these substances we have studied the resistance patterns of some isolates of *Pseudomonas aeruginosa* (PA) and some properties of their β-lactamases. Carbenicillin, cefotaxime, and cephaloridine were taken as reference substances.

From a collection of recent clinical isolates of PA, eight strains, some of them resistant to carbenicillin, were selected at random. The MICs of carbenicillin, azlocillin, cefsulodin, and cefotaxime for these strains, as determined by the agar dilution method in brain heart infusion agar (BBL) with an inoculum of 10^6 organisms per ml, are given in Table 1. The susceptibility patterns of the strains were found to differ greatly. This may have been due to individual differences in their β-lactamases, or there may have been only relatively few distinct types of enzyme, but wide variations in cell membrane penetrability or alterations of the sensitivities of target enzymes.

To elucidate this problem, we compared the degrees to which β-lactamases from the selected PA strains were capable of hydrolyzing or were inhibited by various β-lactam molecules. The hydrolysis rates were measured in a spectrophotometer at 200 to 360 nm at the appropriate wavelengths; enzyme inhibition was determined at 515 nm, using 0.1 mM nitrocefin as the substrate in the presence of various inhibitor concentrations.

Table 1 shows the rates, relative to that of benzylpenicillin, at which various β-lactam antibiotics were hydrolyzed by β-lactamases from carbenicillin-susceptible and carbenicillin-resistant PA isolates.

It can be seen that various PA strains produced β-lactamases differing strikingly from one another in their enzymatic properties, such as substrate profile or inhibition. There was no close relationship between the rates of hydrolysis of the β-lactam compounds by the various enzymes and their MICs for the corresponding strains. The most notable example of this was found with PA strain G 15; despite its moderate to good susceptibility to β-lactams, its β-lactamase was the most active of all our PA enzymes against azlocillin, cefsulodin, and cefotaxime. On the other hand, the β-lactamase activity of the most resistant strain, G 54, was found to be significantly lower than that of G 15.

In Table 2 data on the inhibition of the enzymes by cefoxitin and clavulanic acid are included.

On the basis of the available data, we attempted to classify the PA β-lactamases investigated so far. Group 1 β-lactamases, produced by strains 18 S/H, ATCC 12055, 1105, G 77, and G 78, showed similar substrate profiles, were unable to hydrolyze the antipseudomonal β-lactams, and were inhibited by cefoxitin but not by clavulanic acid. These enzymes were considered to be akin to the "Sabath-Abraham" enzymes of PA (5), which belong to the "Id" enzyme class of Richmond and Sykes (4), were mostly inducible and chromosomally mediated, and occurred in all susceptible or resistant PA strains.

Group 2 was represented by β-lactamases isolated from strains G 8, G 15, G 44, and G 54. It was an enzymatically very heterogeneous group which may later prove divisible into subgroups if more strains become available. Strains G 8, G 44, and G 15 were susceptible to carbenicillin, whereas G 54 was resistant to carbenicillin and cefotaxime and moderately susceptible to azlocillin and cefsulodin. These strains formed

TABLE 1. *Substrate profile of some β-lactamases from PA as compared with the corresponding MIC*

Enzyme source (PA strain)	Enzyme group	Relative rate of hydrolysis[a]					MIC (μg/ml)				
		Carbenicillin	Azlocillin	Cefsulodin	Cefotaxime	Cephaloridine	Carbenicillin	Azlocillin	Cefsulodin	Cefotaxime	Cephaloridine
18 S/H[b]		<0.6	66	2	2	3174	>256	>256	64	>256	ND[c]
ATCC 12055[b]		0.06	24	3	0.7	2669	16	2	0.5	8	>128
1105[b]	1	<0.3	95	7	<2	5685	1	0.5	0.5	0.5	ND
G 77[d]		<0.4	17	5	<3	3106	32	2	1	16	ND
G 78[d]		<2	50	12	<9	3200	32	2	2	32	ND
G 8[d]		23	172	69	34	2146	32	4	2	16	ND
G 15[d]	2	139	1237	635	850	2785	64	2	32	1	ND
G 44[d]		17	99	72	20	399	16	2	1	8	ND
G 54[d]		46	28	197	472	835	>256	64	64	>256	ND
PZB 811[d]		1306	469	26	ND	117	>256	256	32	32	ND
PZB 1700[d]	3	1143	484	30	0.3	115	>256	>256	64	32	ND
Dalgleish[b]		1329	475	33	0.4	109	>256	256	8	16	ND

[a] Benzylpenicillin = 1,000; substrate concentrations = 1 mM.
[b] Reference strain.
[c] ND, Not determined.
[d] Recent clinical isolate.

TABLE 2. *Inhibition of some β-lactamases from PA by cefoxitin and clavulanic acid*

Enzyme source (PA strains)	Enzyme group	50% Inhibition (mM) by:	
		Cefoxitin	Clavulanic acid
PA 18 S/H[a]	1	3.8×10^{-4}	7.3×10^{-1}
ATCC 12055[a]		5.4×10^{-4}	$>1.0 \times 10^{-1}$
1105[a]		3.2×10^{-4}	$>1.0 \times 10^{-1}$
G 77[b]		3.6×10^{-4}	$>1.0 \times 10^{-1}$
G 78[b]		3.8×10^{-4}	$>1.0 \times 10^{-1}$
G 8[b]	2	2.2×10^{-4}	$>1.0 \times 10^{-1}$
G 15[b]		4.1×10^{-2}	1.3×10^{-3}
G 44[b]		2.8×10^{-2}	1.0×10^{-1}
G 54[b]		4.0×10^{-3}	2.6×10^{-2}
PZB 811[b]	3	2.7×10^{-1}	7.5×10^{-5}
PZB 1700[b]		4.0×10^{-1}	1.7×10^{-4}
Dalgleish[a]		4.8×10^{-1}	1.3×10^{-4}

[a] Reference strain.
[b] Recent clinical isolate.

widely different β-lactamases which were moderately active against carbenicillin and moderately to highly active against azlocillin, cefsulodin, or cefotaxime. G 15, G 44, and G 54 enzymes were inhibited rather weakly and to various degrees by cefoxitin and clavulanic acid, whereas G 8 was similar in this respect to the enzymes of group 1.

Group 3 consisted of enzymes produced by strains PZB 811 and PZB 1700 which possessed constitutively synthesized β-lactamases of the penicillinase type which were only weakly active against cefsulodin and virtually inactive against cefotaxime. They seemed to be closely related to, or identical with, the "Dalgleish" enzyme (2)

of PA, which is plasmid mediated and belongs to a group of four known plasmid-mediated penicillinases of PA (1).

It may be concluded that different β-lactam-resistant PA strains produce more kinds of β-lactamases than expected. The four strains of group 2 seem to contain four individually different enzymes, but our penicillinase group, group 3, too, may consist of several different enzyme types, according to Matthew (1). No close relationship between MIC and the β-lactamase activity was found. As regards resistance of PA to β-lactam antibiotics, penetrability barriers seem to be at least as important as the hydrolyzing capacity of various β-lactamases.

1. **Matthew, M.** 1979. Plasmid-mediated β-lactamases of gram-negative bacteria: properties and distribution. J. Antimicrob. Chemother. **5**:349–358.
2. **Newsom, S. W. B., R. B. Sykes, and M. H. Richmond.** 1970. Detection of β-lactamase markedly active against carbenicillin in a strain of *Pseudomonas aeruginosa*. J. Bacteriol. **101**:1079–1080.
3. **Nomura, H., T. Fugono, T. Hitaka, I. Minami, T. Azuma, S. Morimoto, and T. Masuda.** 1974. Semisynthetic β-lactam antibiotics. 6. Sulfocephalosporins and their antipseudomonal activities. J. Med. Chem. **17**:1312–1315.
4. **Richmond, M. H., and R. B. Sykes.** 1973. The β-lactamases of gram-negative bacteria and their possible physiological role. Adv. Microb. Physiol. **9**:31–88.
5. **Sabath, L. D., M. Jago, and E. P. Abraham.** 1965. Cephalosporinase and penicillinase activities of a β-lactamase from *Pseudomonas pyocyanea*. Biochem. J. **96**:739–752.
6. **Zak, O., E. A. Konopka, W. Tosch, T. Ahrens, W. Zimmermann, and F. Kradolfer.** 1979. Experimental evaluation of CGP 7174/E (SCE 129), a new injectable cephalosporin antibiotic active against *Pseudomonas aeruginosa*. Drugs Exp. Clin. Res. **5**: 45–59.